ANESTHESIA

Volume 1

Volume 1

ANESTHESIA

Edited by

Ronald D. Miller, M.D.

Professor of Anesthesia and Pharmacology
Department of Anesthesia
University of California, San Francisco
School of Medicine
San Francisco, California

With 31 contributors

Churchill Livingstone
New York, Edinburgh, London, and Melbourne 1981

© Churchill Livingstone Inc. 1981

Distributed in the United Kingdom by Churchill Livingstone,
Robert Stevenson House, 1-3 Baxter's Place, Leith Walk,
Edinburgh EH1 3AF and by associated companies, branches
and representatives throughout the world.

First published 1981
Printed in U.S.A.

ISBN 0-443-08082-8

7 6 5 4 3 2 1

Library of Congress Cataloging in Publication Data

Main entry under title:

Anesthesia.

Bibliography: p.
Includes index.
1. Anesthesia.   I. Miller, Ronald D.,
1939–   [DNLM: 1. Anesthesia. WO 200
A573]
RD81.A54   617'.96   81-6149
ISBN 0-443-08082-8   AACR2

Contributors

David D. Alfery, M.D.
Staff Anesthesiologist, St. Thomas Hospital, Nashville, Tennessee

Jeffrey M. Baden, M.B., B.S., F.F.A.R.C.S.
Assistant Professor of Anesthesia, Department of Anesthesia, Stanford University School of Medicine, Stanford, California; Staff Anesthesiologist, Anesthesiology Service, Veterans Administration Medical Center, Palo Alto, California

R. Dennis Bastron, M.D.
Associate Professor, Department of Anesthesiology, University of Arizona; Chief, Anesthesiology Service, Veterans Administration Medical Center, Tucson, Arizona

Jonathan L. Benumof, M.D.
Associate Professor of Anesthesia, University of California, San Diego, School of Medicine, San Diego, California

Stephen M. Brzica, M.D.
Staff Anesthesiologist, St. Paul Surgical Center, St. Paul, Minnesota

Benjamin G. Covino, Ph.D., M.D.
Professor of Anaesthesia, Harvard Medical School; Chairman, Department of Anesthesia, Brigham and Women's Hospital, Boston, Massachusetts.

Judith H. Donegan, M.D.
Associate Professor, Department of Anesthesiology, The Medical College of Wisconsin, Milwaukee, Wisconsin

John V. Donlon, Jr., M.D.
Assistant Clinical Professor, Anaesthesia, Harvard Medical School; Assistant Clinical Director, Anesthesia, Massachusetts Eye and Ear Infirmary, Boston Massachusetts

Edmond I. Eger II, M.D.
Professor and Vice Chairman for Research, Department of Anesthesia, University of California, San Francisco, School of Medicine, San Francisco, California

Thomas W. Feeley, M.D.

Assistant Professor of Anesthesia, Associate Medical Director, Intensive Care Units, Stanford University School of Medicine, Stanford, California

Adolph H. Giesecke, Jr., M.D.

Jenkins Professor and Chairman, Department of Anesthesiology, University of Texas Southwestern Medical School, Dallas, Texas

George A. Gregory, M.D.

Professor, Departments of Anesthesia and Pediatrics; Director, Pediatric Intensive Care Unit, University of California, San Francisco, School of Medicine, San Francisco, California

Robert F. Hickey, M.D.

Associate Professor, Department of Anesthesia, University of California, San Francisco, School of Medicine; Chief, Anesthesia Services, Veterans Administration Medical Center, San Francisco, California

Carl C. Hug, Jr., M.D., Ph.D.

Professor of Anesthesiology and Pharmacology; Associate Director, Division of Cardiothoracic Anesthesia, Department of Anesthesiology, Emory University School of Medicine, Atlanta, Georgia

Joel A. Kaplan, M.D.

Professor of Anesthesiology; Director, Division of Cardiothoracic Anesthesia, Department of Anesthesiology, Emory University School of Medicine, Atlanta, Georgia

Robert R. Kirby, M.D.

Professor and Chairman, Department of Anesthesiology, Tulane University, School of Medicine, New Orleans, Louisiana

Donald D. Koblin, Ph.D.

Assistant Research Chemist, Department of Anesthesia, University of California, San Francisco, School of Medicine, San Francisco, California

Gershon Levinson, M.D.

Associate Professor of Anesthesia and Obstetrics, Gynecology, and Reproductive Sciences, Department of Anesthesia, University of California, San Francisco, School of Medicine, San Francisco, California

Ronald D. Miller, M.D.

Professor of Anesthesia and Pharmacology, Department of Anesthesia, University of California, San Francisco, School of Medicine, San Francisco, California

Terence M. Murphy, M.B., Ch.B., F.F.A.R.C.S.

Professor of Anesthesia, Director of Clinical Pain Service, University of Washington, School of Medicine, Seattle, Washington

Fredrick K. Orkin, M.D.

Associate Professor of Anesthesiology, Hahnemann Medical College and Hospital; formerly, Assistant Professor of Anesthesia and Research Medicine (Epidemiology), University of Pennsylvania, Philadelphia, Pennsylvania

Edward G. Pavlin, M.D.

Associate Professor of Anesthesiology, University of Washington School of Medicine, Seattle, Washington

Arthur L. Quasha, M.D.

Assistant Clinical Professor, Department of Anesthesia, University of California, San Francisco, School of Medicine, San Francisco, California

Susan A. Rice, Ph.D.

Assistant Professor of Pharmacology and Toxicology in Anesthesia, Department of Anesthesia, Stanford University School of Medicine, Stanford, California; Research Pharmacologist, Anesthesiology Service, Veterans Administration Medical Center, Palo Alto, California

Michael F. Roizen, M.D.

Associate Professor of Anesthesia, Medicine, and Pharmacology, Department of Anesthesia, University of California, San Francisco, School of Medicine, San Francisco, California

Myer H. Rosenthal, M.D.

Associate Professor of Anesthesia, Medicine, and Surgery; Medical Director, Intensive Care Units and Intermediate Intensive Care Unit, Stanford University Medical Center, Stanford, California

John J. Savarese, M.D.

Associate Professor of Anaesthesia, Harvard Medical School; Associate Anesthetist, Massachusetts General Hospital, Boston, Massachusetts

Harvey M. Shapiro, M.D.

Professor of Anesthesiology and Neurosurgery, Department of Neuroanesthesia Research, University of California at San Diego, School of Medicine; Staff Physician, Anesthesia Service, Veteran's Administration Hospital, San Diego, California

Sol M. Shnider, M.D.

Professor and Vice Chairman; Professor of Obstetrics, Gynecology, and Reproductive Sciences; Department of Anesthesia, University of California, San Francisco, School of Medicine, San Francisco, California

Robert A. Smith, B.A., R.R.T.

Clinical Instructor, Department of Anesthesiology, Tulane University School of Medicine, New Orleans, Louisiana; Clinical Specialist, Department of Critical Care Medicine, Memorial Hospital of Jacksonville, Jacksonville, Florida

Theodore H. Stanley, M.D.
Professor of Anesthesiology, Research Professor of Surgery, Department of Anesthesiology, University of Utah, College of Medicine, Salt Lake City, Utah

Robert K. Stoelting, M.D.
Professor and Chairman, Department of Anesthesia, Indiana University School of Medicine, Indianapolis, Indiana

Preface

In recent years an ever-increasing number of monographs on specific aspects of anesthesia have appeared. However, there is still no comprehensive, up-to-date American reference work that covers the entire field of anesthesia. I felt that anesthesiologists would welcome a ready reference to which they could turn for a survey of the current state of the art. And so, when the publisher extended an invitation to organize and edit just such a book, the decision was made—after consultation with friends and colleagues—to accept this major challenge.

The reader will notice that this text, while comprehensive, is not encyclopedic. I assumed that the reader would be familiar with those aspects of elementary anesthesia practice not included in this book. The focus, therefore, is on major areas of new development in anesthesia that have occurred in the last 20 years. While the emphasis of the book is clinical, the physiological and pharmacologic principles on which a sound anesthesia practice can be based are also presented.

The contributors were requested to provide a scholarly analysis of the topic on which they were writing. In some cases, this analysis included challenging the efficacy of rarely challenged dictates in the practice of anesthesia, such as Dr. Roizen's analysis of the traditional preoperative evaluation (Ch. 1) and Dr. Kirby and Mr. Smith's analysis of intensive care units (Ch. 44). The contributors were given no restriction on the number of references that could be cited, and so the reader desiring a more detailed account of a particular subject will find a comprehensive list of references to the literature. Last and perhaps most important, I did not attempt to impose a uniform point of view. For example, the preoperative evaluation and treatment of the patient with hypertension is discussed in several chapters. This allows the reader to evaluate most of the points of view with special reference to the type of surgery being proposed (e.g., hypertension and vascular surgery).

The success of any multiauthored book is in large part dependent on the expertise of the contributors and the degree of their commitment. The contributors to this book were invited because they are acknowledged authorities in their fields. This has truly been a collaborative effort, and for that reason the names of the contributors join mine on the front cover. Without their support and participation, this book would not exist. They have my deepest thanks.

I appreciate the help and flexibility provided by the staff of Churchill Livingstone, especially Donna Balopole, during the entire project. And last—but certainly not least—I am especially grateful to my family and colleagues for their patience during the time *Anesthesia* was in preparation. Their encouragement and understanding were a continuing source of strength.

Ronald D. Miller

Contents

VOLUME 1

Section I. Preparation of the Patient/Use of Anesthetic Agents: Regional Anesthesia

Section II. Physiological Functions During Anesthesia

VOLUME 2

Section III. The Systems and Specific Areas

Section I

Preparation of the Patient/Use of Anesthetic Agents:
Preoperative

1

Routine Preoperative Evaluation

Michael F. Roizen, M.D.

INTRODUCTION

The preoperative meeting of patient and anesthesiologist fulfills three functions: education of the patient about anesthesia in the hope of reducing anxiety (see Ch. 3); acquisition of pertinent information about medical history and physical and mental conditions; and obtaining informed consent. In this chapter, medical history and physical and mental conditions are correlated with the need for preoperative laboratory testing. A major rationale for preoperative medical assessment is reduction in perioperative morbidity by optimizing preoperative status and planning the perioperative management. Other reasons for preoperative assessment include evaluation of risk for anesthesia and surgery and establishment of baseline function with which intraoperative and postoperative abnormalities can be compared. Perioperative mortality and morbidity increase with severity of preexisting disease.[1-5] Therefore preoperative evaluation and treatment should reduce perioperative morbidity and mortality (also see Ch. 2).[3,6,7] Most hospitals and many anesthesia departments have rather arbitrary rules and/or recommendations as to which tests should be performed on a patient prior to elective surgery. In this chapter, I could simply recite these rules and suggest that they be followed. However, in these times of increasingly limited resources, the benefit of these rules and recommendations needs to be examined. Therefore, in this chapter, the effectiveness of the preoperative evaluation is examined and from this analysis specific preoperative assessments are recommended.

PREOPERATIVE SCREENING FOR HEALTHY INDIVIDUALS FOR ROUTINE SURGERY— WHAT SHOULD BE DONE?

The debate concerning what constitutes proper preoperative screening for routine surgery on healthy individuals involves screening for disease before it is apparent, cost/benefit analysis, and medicolegal considerations. The dictum, "there may be minor surgery but there are no minor anesthetics"[6] may be warranted, but complexities of various anesthetics clearly differ. For example, in current practice many anesthetics relieve pain for minor procedures in relatively healthy patients, whereas other anesthetics require manipulation of hemodynamic variables to maintain cardiovascular stability during major vascular procedures. Preoperative assessment for these two diverse types of anesthesia should, of necessity, be different. In this chapter preoperative assessment of patients reputed to be healthy who are undergoing less extensive surgery (i.e. non-cardiac) is considered. The importance of routinely ordering various laboratory examinations is evaluated. In Chapter 2, preoperative examinations for specific diseases, intraoperative procedures, and intraoperative hemodynamic manipulations for complex surgical procedures are discussed. Thus, evaluation of patients with hypertension or on whom a pneumonectomy is planned and those who have certain familial characteristics such as kidney stones or seizures are covered in Chapter 2. Chapter 1 deals solely with routine screening of ambulatory patients, i.e., what preoperative screening should be done on the patient scheduled for an inguinal herniorrhaphy, vein stripping, breast biopsy, tonsillectomy, or hemorrhoidectomy, who has no other known medical problems.

Prior to the introduction of the SMA "6" and "12" panels, tests were ordered singly or in small groups to confirm prior clinical impressions. Thus the results of the history and physical examination dictated what laboratory tests were obtained. Advancing technology and the hope that early presymptomatic diagnosis would lead to longer life and even eventually reduce medical costs led to the widespread use of the screening battery. Even when performed at a cost of about one-twentieth of that in the current hospital laboratory, the multiphasic testing screen (SMA "6" and "12") is difficult to justify for most ambulatory individuals.[8-15] The increasing use of the automated screening battery has magnified two problems that formerly were rare: which tests (if any) should be required preoperatively and what should be done with an unexpectedly "abnormal" laboratory result. It seems axiomatic that the more information known about a patient the better. However, these additional tests have their disadvantages, including the cost of obtaining and processing the blood; additional tests to rule out false positive results; additional referrals to other physicians and consultations; confused and delayed operating room schedules; and, perhaps the most important one being patient

worry (particularly in the case of false positive results). In 1980, about 6 billion laboratory tests will be performed at a cost of 20 billion dollars in the United States.[15] Although the benefits of this additional information preoperatively are not fully known, they are estimated later in this chapter. *However, in most cases, the 15-minute history and physical examination probably is the best screening test preparatory to anesthesia.* Since much of medical school helps the physician learn how to do a history and physical examination, I do not delve into that in any detail here; sample questions I use and physical findings I often seek out are listed near the end of this chapter.

Before answering how preoperative screening may influence the management of anesthesia, I review what percentage of tests are positive in normal healthy patients. Then the influence of these positive results on the management of anesthesia and surgery is examined. From this analysis, specific preoperative screening procedures are recommended from both a medical and cost/benefit point of view.

WHAT IS AN ABNORMAL LABORATORY TEST?

Normal laboratory values are based on the statistical concept of the normal distribution of the Gaussian curve.[15, 16] In large groups of "healthy" individuals, 66 percent of values from the population fall within one standard deviation of the mean value, while 95 percent of values fall within two standard deviations of the mean value. Thus, laboratory values are deemed outside of the normal range if they are more than two standard deviations either above or below the mean. Conversely, in a normal population, 5 percent of healthy individuals will have an abnormal result on any one test.[15-18] For example, if hemoglobin values for healthy men are reported as being between 13.5 and 16.7 g percent, 5 percent of "normal" healthy men will have a test result outside of that range, assuming a Gaussian distribution. Clearly with the use of more extreme normal limits, fewer patients would be labeled as abnormal, but these patients would be more likely to have clinically significant conditions. Of prime importance is knowing what percentage of those abnormal laboratory test values indicate disease.

Data on the incidence of abnormalities in routine preoperative tests are biased by the sample population from which they are derived. This bias will be identified with each screening test. Incidence of abnormalities detected by a preoperative screening test are available from three types of sources. One is health maintenance organization data, such as the Kaiser-Permanente data from Oakland, California.[18] These data are limited, however, because they were derived from a period when the Kaiser-Permanente population was composed mainly of middle-class working people. Thus, these data are biased because they were derived from patients who were healthy enough to work and to walk to an ambulatory clinic. The second source of information is from studies looking at specific questions such as, Are chest roentgenograms worthwhile in individuals under the age of 19 years? or What is the incidence of abnormalities on routine screening chemistry tests? Again, this information is biased by the specific populations studied. The third source of data is epidemiologic studies, such as the Tecumseh and Framingham studies,[19] examining entire populations and the risk of developing certain diseases. Again, this source of data is biased by the community and its environment. For instance, only one black family lived in Tecumseh, Michigan when that study began.[19]

Before evaluating the justification for ordering certain laboratory tests, several caveats are in order. First, as emphasized previously, the history and physical examination will provide some basis for deciding which tests to order. However, because patients frequently enter the hospital the evening before elective surgery, a thorough examination prior to testing is often difficult. That is, if the patient is admitted at 4 p.m. and evaluated by the anesthesiologist at 6 p.m., many hospitals are not organized to perform these diagnostic tests during the night. Then a dilemma arises. Should surgery be delayed until these tests can be performed or should a compromise be made to go ahead with surgery without these tests? This dilemma has led to the arbitrary decision to order routine laboratory roentgenographic and electrocardiographic examinations prior to the history and physical examination. This often justifies acquisitions of some tests routinely in the interest of efficiency (against increased cost from prolonged hospitalization) dependent in part on evening availability of laboratory services.

LABORATORY TEST ABNORMALITIES IN "HEALTHY" POPULATIONS

CHEST ROENTGENOGRAMS

To determine whether preoperative chest roentgenograms are indicated, several questions should be asked. For example, What abnormalities on the chest roentgenogram in a 38-year-old woman scheduled for a vein stripping will influence the anesthetic approach? Then, How likely is it that she has one of those abnormalities? The next question might be, How much does a preoperative chest roentgenogram cost? Then, What is its risk? (radiation effects, false positive test, delaying surgery, patient worry, etc.). Then, Is there a benefit to the patient in obtaining this roentgenogram, and if so what is that benefit worth? The answers to these six questions are what is involved in a physician's decision to order a chest roentgenogram.[20] This cost-benefit analysis will be done for chest roentgenograms as an example of what should ultimately be done for all laboratory tests.

First, what abnormalities on chest roentgenogram would influence the anesthetic approach? By examination of a chest roentgenogram, the degree of chronic lung disease that

Table 1-1. Screening Chest Roentgenograms—Abnormalities Not Previously Known About or Suspected that Might Change Anesthetic Management

Age (years)	Series*	Number of Patients Examined	Percent Abnormalities
< 40	Kaiser[24]	15,978	2.1
< 40	Combined [(21-23,25)]	5,058	1.5
40–50	Sagal[21] & Rees[23]	1,047	8.3
50–60	Sagal[21] & Rees[23]	1,004	22.6
40–59	Kaiser[24]	21,489	7.4
60–70	Sagal[21] & Rees[23]	1,111	31.3
71–80	Rees[23]	76	61.8
> 70	Sagal[21]	832	41.7
≥ 81	Rees[23]	16	68.8
≥ 60	Kaiser[24]	7,196	19.2

* The data presented in these series have been edited to include only abnormalities that might change anesthetic management. Most investigators do not exclude abnormalities known by history or physical examination (see text).

may alter the anesthetic technique probably cannot be detected if it was not detected by the history and physical examination. Certainly tracheal deviation, mediastinal masses, pulmonary nodules, solitary lung masses, aortic aneurysm, pulmonary edema, pneumonia, atelectasis, new fractures of vertebrae, ribs, clavicles, dextrocardia, and cardiomegaly may be important to know about before proceeding to anesthesia and surgery. Table 1-1 indicates that these conditions are first discovered by chest roentgenogram in less than 1.5 percent of the under 40-year-old population.[18,21-25] At the time of this writing, an outpatient anterior-posterior and lateral chest roentgenogram at the University of California, San Francisco costs $30.75 plus $13.75 in professional fees. Thus it costs $44.50 ÷ 0.015 or $2,967 per new positive finding by chest roentgenogram in the unselected 40-year-old and under population.* We do not know the benefit to the surgical patient from knowing of a new positive finding, but let us assume that it reduces anesthetic mortality by 50 percent because of appropriately directed management (I think a reduction this great is unlikely, i.e. it is so difficult to demonstrate that active viral pneu-

monia increases anesthetic risk, that no evidence of that is obtainable in the literature). I selected this high mortality figure to place as much importance on the chest roentgenogram as possible. I also will assume that perioperative "anesthetic" mortality in this under 40-year-old age group is 5 deaths per 1,000 operations. These patients will be assumed to have a mean age of 20 years and an expected survival of 50 to 60 more years of life. Reducing operative mortality increases those years of life; since those years of life are in the future, public health economists discount these years to the present. "The general idea of discounting is a simple one made complicated by the mathematics."[20] Discounting implies that immediate benefit and distant costs are better than vice versa. Although there is no consensus as to what the discount rate should be, the 4 percent discount rate suggested by Neuhauser was chosen using the formula $Pn = \frac{1}{r}(1 - \frac{1}{(1 + r)^n})$ where Pn is the present value, measured in years of life, r is the discount rate (0.04), and n is the number of years saved; using 60 as years of life saved yields a present value of 22.62 years of life per current life saved.

But only patients with abnormal tests who actually have a disease benefit by testing (true

---

* This analysis is patterned after that of Neuhauser[20] with permission of the author.

positive). The predictive false positives (those people with abnormal tests who are healthy) should be subtracted from those people who have abnormal tests and are sick. This subtraction will provide the number of patients who would benefit from testing. If a 10 percent predictive false positive rate is assumed (a low assumption for this analysis as will be discussed below) then the number of patients benefiting per 1,000 roentgenograms is [1.5 percent − 1.5 percent (0.10)] 1,000 = 13.5 patients (true positives). The 50 percent reduction in an operative mortality of 5 per 1,000 is on this basis 13.5 × 0.5 × 0.005 = 0.03375 fewer deaths per 1,000 operations when screening preoperative chest roentgenograms were performed. Translating this into present value as years of life saved per 1,000 roentgenograms gives 0.03375 × 22.62 = 0.7634 total present value years of life saved. In our hospital this 0.7634 years of life saved would cost $44,500 (not including consultative fees, repeat roentgenograms, or other laboratory costs, patient/family worry costs, or extra radiation effect costs); that then means the cost without additional fees would approach $44,500 ÷ 0.7634 or $58,291 per present value year of life saved. But just as there are other costs (repeat laboratory tests, etc.) there are other benefits (treatment of some patients with solitary nodules or mediastinal masses may prolong some lives). We will assume that these costs and benefits are equal or this analysis would go on forever.

The most difficult question to answer is: What evidence is there that *any* change in perioperative anesthetic management because of a chest roentgenogram finding reduces anesthetic morbidity or mortality? The answer is probably that little evidence exists. Then we must ask, How much per year of life saved is too much? Would you as a patient pay $58,291 each in 1980 dollars for each extra year of life you and your family members lived? Although there are philosophical and moral problems in assigning a dollar value to life, this is unfortunately necessary for this kind of analysis. Arbitrarily for the

rest of this chapter in justifying cost benefit analysis I chose $20,000 in 1980 dollars as the cut off for worthwhileness per year of life saved per laboratory test; I also assumed no additional cost from extra tests, time, radiation or other biologic risk incurred by the tests, worry engendered by an incorrect laboratory test, or benefit from the true positive test (for further discussion see Neuhauser[20] or Bunker et al.[26]). In addition, I assumed that each true positive for any test would lead to a 50 percent reduction in perioperative anesthetic morbidity and mortality. I assumed a perioperative anesthetic mortality rate of 5 per 1,000 in the under 40-year-old population, 10 per 1,000 between 40 and 50, 20 per 1,000 between 51 and 60, and 40 per 1,000 above 60 years of age—these rates closely approximate the worst in the literature for elective operations.[1–5] Unless stated, I will assume a 10 percent predictive false positive rate. These assumptions probably give the benefit of doubt to favor the laboratory tests.

Now the issue of false positives, false negatives, the prevalence of disease in the test population, and their meaning to the abnormal (or positive) laboratory test[15,17] will be considered. For example,[16] the *sensitivity* of the test is 95 percent (95 of 100 people with pneumonia will have the radiologist state "pneumonia" or some other significant abnormality on the best roentgenogram report). Second, I assume that the *specificity* of the test is 99 percent (99 of 100 people without pneumonia will have the radiologist read the chest roentgenogram as "without evidence of pneumonia"). Third, I assume that 1.5 percent of the population about to undergo routine elective surgery has pneumonia (1.5 percent is our assumed prevalence of the disease in the population). Given the above assumptions, what is the likelihood that a person with a chest roentgenogram report of "pneumonia" actually has pneumonia. If, for example, 100,000 people have chest roentgenograms, then 1,500 actually have pneumonia and 95/100 or 1,425 who actually have pneumonia will have a chest roentgenogram report of "pneumonia." On the other hand, 98,500 do not have pneumonia. One per hundred of those without pneumonia or 985 who are without pneumonia will actually have the diagnosis "pneumonia" on the chest roentgenogram report. Thus 985 of 2,410 patients or 40.9 percent of patients carrying a roentgenographic reading of pneumonia are actually well. This is what is meant by a *predictive false positive rate* of 40.9 percent. Therefore our 10 percent predictive false positive rate is overestimating the utility of our laboratory test and falsely reducing the cost per positive finding by the same factor. Furthermore, *screening* laboratory tests should produce significant findings not discernible by the history and physical examination. If abnormalities discovered by the history or physical examination are deducted from the true positives and treated as predictive false positives, the cost per unexpected true positive again becomes significantly higher. The cost per positive laboratory test is even greater if more reliable figures are assumed for sensitivity, specificity, and prevalence; sensitivity for chest roentgenograms (positivity in disease) varies between 58 and 75 percent, and specificity (negativity in health) between 97 and 98.7 percent in several studies.[19-33] If a prevalence of pneumonia is assumed to be as much as 0.5 percent in the "healthy" population, and accepting the best sensitivity (75 percent) and specificity (98.3 percent) figures, then 1,691 of 2,066 patients with the chest roentgenographic diagnosis of pneumonia will be predictive false positives (an 82 percent rate). If the same sensitivity and specificity is assumed, but a disease prevalence of 2 percent, then 1,666 of 3,166 patients with the chest roentgenographic diagnosis of pneumonia will be predictive false positives (a 52.6 percent false positive rate). If the prevalence of the disease is 10 percent (and test sensitivity and specificity are as good as the best in the literature) then 1,530 of 8,030 patients labeled by the radiologist as having pneumonia will not have it, so the

predictive false positive rate would be 19 percent.

Data concerning the prevalence of disease in asymptomatic patients are difficult to find. I used assumptions concerning the following to back calculate the prevalence of disease: (1) the incidence of abnormal tests in specific populations; (2) the sensitivity of the test; and (3) the specificity of the test. For example, if 12 percent of chest roentgenograms are abnormal in a population of 10,000 people, we can perform these calculations if, for example, a sensitivity of 60 percent and specificity of 90 percent is assumed. If X represents patients with "roentgenographic discoverable disease" and Y represents healthy individuals, then $0.6X + 0.1Y = (0.12)(10,000)$ and $X + Y = 10,000$. Thus, X really equals 4 percent rather than the 12 percent with abnormal chest roentgenographs.

This detailed analysis shows why knowing the sensitivity, specificity, and especially prevalence of disease in a population group is important to determining the percent of predictive false positives and the cost/benefit analysis of obtaining a laboratory test in a healthy preoperative patient. Also the assumption of only 10 percent predictive false positive data for each laboratory test clearly biases this analysis toward ordering more tests.

Nevertheless, despite these assumptions, which favor ordering laboratory tests, the data in Table 1-1 seem to indicate that preoperative screening chest roentgenography is not cost effective in anyone under the age of 40 years (to reemphasize, by preoperative screening is meant looking for disease not already known about or not evident or not suspected by history or physical examination). Preoperative screening chest roentgenograms probably are not cost effective until the patient is over the age of 60 years, although the data between age 40 and 60 is not explicit enough to allow accurate calculation of the incidence of discovery of new abnormalities on chest roentgenogram. If chest roentgenograms are assumed to be not as good as history and physical examination for diagnosis of significant chronic obstructive pulmonary disease, then no preoperative chest roentgenograms are indicated below the age of 60 on a cost/benefit basis.

This detailed analysis of the efficacy and cost/benefit of chest roentgenograms is undoubtedly tedious to read. However, all laboratory tests must be analyzed in this manner to arrive at logical and valid conclusions. This analysis serves as an example as to how difficult these conclusions are to derive. In all other sections, only the essential data and conclusions are given.

From this type of analysis, chest roentgenograms apparently reveal 1.5 percent new abnormalities in the under 40-year-old population,[18,21-25] approximately 5 percent unsuspected abnormalities in the 40- to 60-year-old population, and 6 to 30 percent new findings in the over 60-year-old population.[21,23,25] Assuming 10 percent false positives and that only tests worth less than $20,000 in 1980 dollars per year of life saved should be done and that each true positive test results in a 50 percent reduction in operative mortality, then preoperative screening chest roentgenograms should be done only in patients 60 years of age or older. The results of this review strongly suggest there is little rationale for chest roentgenograms in preoperative patients under the age of 40 with a pathologic process not associated with chest disease. This review further suggests that screening preoperative chest roentgenograms are cost ineffective in patients between the ages of 40 and 60. This type of analysis coldly ignores the rare patient who may benefit from a screening chest roentgenogram which, in these days of limited resources, many people feel is justified. Although a treatable condition might occasionally be discovered on a screening chest roentgenogram, the socioeconomic benefit is too low to justify the cost. Preoperative screening chest roentgenograms are justifiable for the over 60-year-old population.

ELECTROCARDIOGRAMS

The data on the incidence of electrocardiogram abnormalities were gathered from studies on either working patient populations (Kaiser)[18,24] or epidemiologic surveys of healthy people (Framingham,[34] Tecumseh[19,35]). The abnormalities that may dictate an alteration in anesthetic approach are atrial flutter or fibrillation; atrioventricular block of first, second, or third degree; ST-T changes suggesting ischemia or recent pulmonary embolism; premature ventricular and atrial contractions; left or right ventricular hypertrophy; short PR interval; Wolff-Parkinson-White syndrome; probably recent or old myocardial infarction; prolonged QT segment; and tall peaked T waves. What is the incidence of these findings on preoperative screening tests? What is the incidence of those findings that could not easily be observed on the standard monitor lead I or MCL_5 applied immediately prior to induction of anesthesia in the operating room? Table 1-2 summarizes the available data.[18,34-37] Some caveats are necessary before discussing cost/benefit analysis of preoperative screening electrocardiograms. First, none of these studies excluded patients with histories or physical examinations suggestive of cardiac problems. Second, the studies do not distinguish those findings that are evident on monitor leads versus those only evident on 6- or 12-lead electrocardiograms.

For the purpose of analysis, 50 percent of findings were assumed to be evident on a monitor lead (premature atrial and ventricular beats, atrioventricular blocks of various degrees, short PR intervals, atrial flutter or fibrillation) and further, that 50 percent of the remaining findings (myocardial infarction, left and right ventricular hypertrophy) were evident by history and physical examination. If the assumption that each unexpected finding results in a 50 percent reduction in morbidity is recalled, then certain conclusions can be made. When the cost per electrocardiogram is estimated as $30 and the data in

Table 1-2. Percentage of Patients with Abnormalities as Determined by Screening Electrocardiograms (All Studies are 12 Lead, except for Collen,[18] which is a 6 Lead Study)

Age	Sex	Series	Number of Patients Examined	Total Abnormalities (%)*	Specific Abnormalities (%)			
					"LVH"	Recent or Old MI	ST-T Changes	AV Block
16–19	M	Ostrander[35]	216	20.3	17.8	0	0.9	1.4
16–19	F	Ostrander[35]	242	5.9	1.3	0	4.2	0.4
20–29	M	Ostrander[35]	452	14.0	7.1	0.2	6.0	0.7
20–29	M	Collen[18]	~ 3000	9.6				
20–29	F	Ostrander[35]	577	11.3	0.2	0.2	9.9	1.0
20–29	F	Collen[18]	~ 4000	9.3				
30–39	M	Ostrander[35]	676		3.0	0	6.9	1.3
30–39	M	Collen[18]	~ 4000	12.1				
30–39	F	Ostrander[35]	699		0.4	0.1	11.6	1.6
30–39	F	Collen[18]	~ 5000	11.7				
35–44	M	Kannel[34, 36]			2.9			
35–44	F	Kannel[34, 36]			0.9			
40–49	M	Ostrander[35]	468	~ 24	4.1	1.7	16.1	1.5
40–49	M	Collen[18]	~ 4000	17.6				
40–49	F	Ostrander[35]	474	~ 21	0.6	0.8	17.2	0.6
40–49	F	Collen[18]	~ 5000	15.6				
45–54	M	Kannel[34, 36]			4.8			
45–54	F	Kannel[34, 36]			3.6			
50–59	M	Ostrander[35]	330	~ 30	3.3	5.1	20.8	1.2
50–59	M	Collen[18]	~ 5000	24.9				
50–59	F	Ostrander[35]	327	~ 40	3.4	0.9	32.4	2.1
50–59	F	Collen[18]	~ 6000	20.7				
55–64	M	Kannel[34, 36]			10.1			
55–64	F	Kannel[34, 36]			4.1			
60–69	M	Ostrander[35]	177		8.4	9.0	37.1	4.5
60–69	M	Collen[18]	~ 2000	35.1				
60–69	F	Ostrander[35]	196		10.2	6.1	42.4	4.1
60–69	F	Collen[18]	~ 3000	29.7				
65–74	M	Kannel[34, 36]			7.1			
65–74	F	Kannel[34, 36]			9.6			
> 70	M	Collen[18]	~ 1000	52.2				
> 70	F	Collen[18]	~ 1000	41.2				
70–79	M	Ostrander[35]	100		7.9	9.9	46.5	7.9
70–79	F	Ostrander[35]	119		11.8	2.5	43.8	6.7
> 80	M	Ostrander[35]	26		11.5	7.7	46.2	19.2
> 80	F	Ostrander[35]	43		16.3	4.7	58.2	9.3

* The data portrayed here represent an edited summary of the data given in the several series: edited to select abnormalities that might change anesthetic management. Approximations represent best guess numbers from data not explicitly quantified in the papers.

Table 1-2 are used, then electrocardiograms appear warranted in both men and women over the age of 30 years. However, when the epidemiologically defined sensitivity, specificity, and prevalence of disease pertaining to electrocardiographic diagnosis[35-37] is used (see Table 1-3 for data on left ventricular hypertrophy),[37] then preoperative screening electrocardiograms would be indicated only for men and women over the age of 50 years. But even this screening is unjustified, since reduction in morbidity based on unexpected electrocardiographic findings may not even approximate 50 percent. There are no data that demonstrate a reduction in mortality from routine preoperative electrocardiographic screening. Why did I persist in stating a 50 percent reduction in morbidity for each unexpected finding? Many investigators cite increased morbidity and mortality in patients with recent as opposed to over 6-month-old myocardial infarctions;[38-44] several investigators cite increased morbidity in patients with an electrocardiographic pattern of left ven-

Table 1-3. Effect of Prevalence of Left Ventricular Enlargement Upon Errors in Its Electrocardiographic Recognition

Criteria	Sensitivity (%)	Specificity (%)	Predictive Value of Positives (%) Prevalence			Predictive False Positive Rate (%) Prevalence		
			25%	5%	1%	25%	5%	1%
Romhilt and Estes (5 points)	58	97	87	50	16	13	50	84
Noth, Myers, and Klein	18	98	67	32	8	25	68	92
Schach, Rosenbaum and Katz	18	98	67	24	6	33	76	94
Romhilt et al.	56	89	63	21	5	37	79	95
Allenstein	71	83	58	18	4	42	82	96
Gubner and Underleider	35	87	47	12	3	53	88	97
Goldberger	35	81	38	9	2	62	91	98
Sokolow and Lyon	88	44	34	8	2	66	92	98
Katz	41	73	34	7	2	66	93	98
Goulder and Kissane	12	92	33	7	1	67	93	99
Wilson et al.	94	23	29	6	1	71	94	99

(Galen RS, Gambino SR: The electrocardiogram application of the model to a nonlaboratory test, Beyond Normality: The Predictive Value and Efficiency of Medical Diagnoses. New York, John Wiley & Sons, 1975, pp 99–106.)

tricular hypertrophy.[36,45] One group cites greater than five premature ventricular contractions per minute as an increased risk factor.[3] Since at least two of these three findings can result in the anesthesiologist altering the perioperative course (postponing surgery for 6 months, antiarrhythmic therapy, anesthetic technique), I persisted in the assumption of a 50 percent reduction in morbidity from an unexpected electrocardiographic finding. I, therefore, came to the compromise conclusion that preoperative screening electrocardiograms are indicated for patients over the age of 40 years assuming careful observation of the electrocardiogram before induction of anesthesia.

HEMOGLOBIN, HEMATOCRIT, AND WHITE BLOOD CELL COUNTS

In our hospital, determination of the hemoglobin, hematocrit, and white blood cell count costs $8.00 and any one of these three tests alone costs $7.00. How abnormal must any of these be before different approaches should be taken perioperatively to supposedly healthy individuals undergoing routine ("non-blood-loss") operations?

Wasserman and coworkers[46] found that of 28 patients with uncontrolled polycythemia (hemoglobin greater than 16 g percent) who underwent major surgery, 22 (79 percent) had complications and 10 (36 percent) died. That group was compared to a group of 53 patients with controlled polycythemia (hemoglobin ≤ 16 g percent) who had major surgery, of which 15 (28 percent) had complications and 3 (5 percent) died. Most of the complications in both groups were related to polycythemia (hemorrhage or thrombosis). Although that study has some obvious deficiencies (retrospective, no time frame given, exclusion of "minor" surgery, no statement as to why some patients had their polycythemia controlled and others did not preoperatively), it implies that knowledge and pretreatment of polycythemia decreases perioperative morbidity and mortality. No such evidence exists for normovolemic anemia. Rothstein[47] concluded that theoretically in patients under 3 months of age, hemoglobin should be over 10 g percent, while in children over 3 months of age a hemoglobin of 9 g percent was adequate. Slogoff[48] concluded that theoretically in adults a hematocrit of 20 percent (hemoglobin of about 7 g percent) was adequate. However, no data exist which confirm that treatment of moderate or mild normovolemic anemia prior to non-blood-loss surgery in

Table 1-4. Screening Hemoglobin and White Blood Cell Counts

Age	Sex	Series	Number of Patients Examined	Abnormalities (%)	White Cell Count Abnormalities (%)
< 40	M	Collen[24]	6,941	1.9 ⎫	
< 40	F	Collen[24]	9,037	12.6 ⎭	2.6
40–59	M	Collen[24]	11,832	3.1 ⎫	
40–59	F	Collen[24]	9,657	10.1 ⎭	2.2
≥ 60	M	Collen[24]	4,062	5.6 ⎫	
≥ 60	F	Collen[24]	3,134	5.5 ⎭	1.7
Unspecified Age	Either	Carmalt[50]*	278	30.4	

* Carmalt found 24.5 percent were new abnormalities; 2 patients had hemoglobins < 8 g percent, 17 between 8 and 10 g percent, and 21 between 10 and 12 g percent.

asymptomatic patients decreases perioperative morbidity or mortality. Similarly no data exist with regard to possible harm from abnormal white blood cell counts found preoperatively. I arbitrarily have chosen a hematocrit (or appropriate hemoglobin) value below 29 percent for men and 27 percent for women or above 57 percent for men and 54 percent for women or a white blood cell count below 2,400/m³ or above 16,000/m³ for both men and women as values that deserve pursuance of an alternative diagnosis before anesthesia.[49] How many healthy patients have this degree of abnormality? The limited available data are listed in Table 1-4.[24, 50] If it is assumed that 10 percent of all abnormalities are outside of our "very" abnormal range listed above[50] and if the cost/benefit analysis described in the chest roentgenogram section is used, then preoperative hematocrit or hemoglobin levels (one or the other) should be obtained on all women and on all men over the age of 60 years. White blood cell counts appear to be rarely if ever indicated.

Blood Chemistry

What blood chemistries would have to be abnormal and how abnormal would they have to be before perioperative management should be altered? Abnormal liver or renal function might change the choice and dose of anesthetic or adjuvant drugs—i.e., avoiding or decreasing the dose of pancuronium in renal failure or possibly avoiding halothane in the patient with active liver disease, although the latter conclusion is controversial.[51] Nevertheless about 1 in 700 "healthy" patients is harboring hepatitis and 1 in 3 of those will become jaundiced.[53, 54] The available data on screening blood chemistries is presented in Table 1-5.[24, 52–60] Unexpected abnormalities are reported in from 2 to 10 percent of patients screened,[24, 52–60] and these abnormalities lead to a great deal of additional studies. Approximately 80 percent of the time, these lead to conclusions having no significance for the patient.[24, 52–61] Significant unsolicited abnormal findings arise in 2 to 5 percent of patients studied. Approximately 70 percent of these significant abnormal unexpected chemistry findings are related to blood glucose and blood urea nitrogen (BUN) levels.[24, 52–60] The nine or ten additional tests lead to very few important findings related to anesthesia. In fact the false positive rate is so high (i.e. 96.5 percent for calcium[60]), that the cost/benefit value of most of these tests, even were they free, is negative. If a screening test for hepatitis is desired because its incidence is 0.14 percent and to avoid the legal problems of postanesthetic jaundice, then the three tests (serum glutamic oxaloacetic transaminase) [SGOT], blood glucose, and BUN) seem indicated. These three tests would cost $21 today at our hospital; this is the same cost as the SMA "12," which gives almost all the screening chemistries shown. However, I recommend the specific three, as the cost of pre-

Table 1-5. Screening Blood Chemistries—Percentage of Patients with Abnormalities

Age (Years)	Series	Number of Patients Examined	BUN	Crea-tinine	Glucose	SGOT	Uric Acid	Choles-terol	Albumin	Total Protein	Cal-cium	VDRL	Alkaline PTAse	Billi-rubin	Potas-sium
> 40	Collen et al.[24]	15,978		0.8	4.6	3.6	3.4	1.7	0.4	3.5	1.4	0.8			
40–59	Collen et al.[24]	21,489		1.4	5.6	4.6	4.8	2.7	0.3	4.4	1.3	1.9			
> 60	Collen et al.[24]	7,196		2.7	8.3	4.5	6.0	3.0	0.4	3.9	1.5	2.3			
All	Wataneetawech et al.[53]	6,540				0.234 (9 pts)									
10–54	Schemel et al.[54]	7,620				0.144 (11 pts)									
≥ 18	Schneiderman et al.[55]	547		9.3		1.3							9.7	3.7	
All	Friedman et al.[52]	8,446	3.4	3.3	5.9	2.7	2.7	3.8	1.5	2.5	5.4		3.9	2.4	3.4
> 25	Peery et al.[56]*	1,771	18		21	3.1	36	30	0.5	0.5			1.3		3.6
All	Young et al.[57]*	390	6.4	3.7	7.5						2.0				0
> 18	Thiers VA[58,59]*	623	1.1		5.0		4.5		1.4	2.4	1.0				4.0
15–85	Carmalt et al.[50]*	296	1.4	1.0	2.0	0		0.3	0		0.3		0	0	0.3
All	Boonstra et al.[60]*	12,000									5.0				

* A high percentage of these findings were analyzed in more depth and found to be unimportant clinically.

dictive false positives is so high for the other screening chemistries as to give them a negative cost/benefit ratio even when the first set of screening chemistry results is free. Using my assumptions and method of analysis from the chest roentgenogram section of this chapter and assuming a 2 percent positive rate with a 10 percent predictive false positive rate, all individuals should have SGOT, BUN, and blood glucose values determined. The incidence of significant abnormalities increases with increasing age (e.g. 2.5 percent in those less than 40 years; 5 percent in those 40 to 59 years; and 7.5 percent in those over 60 years), as indicated by the data of Collen et al.[24] Using that incidence progression and a 50 percent predictive false positive rate, then at least from a cost/benefit point of view only the three screening chemistries are indicated and only for individuals over the age of 40 years.

CLOTTING STUDIES

While measurement of the partial thromboplastin time (PTT) and prothrombin time (PT) are useful tests to screen patients with a previous history of bleeding,[62] their value as a routine screening test has been questioned. Robin and Rose[63] examined the PTT values of 1,025 consecutive patients; 143 or 14 percent were prolonged. Twenty-three of these patients did not have a known or suspected clotting disorder by history. Nine of those 23 had a repeat test that yielded normal results. The other 14 all had surgery without further clotting "work up" and without bleeding complications during surgery. Replying to Robin and Rose with a letter to the editor, Baranetsky and Weinstein[64] advocated continued screening PTT determinations. They cited, as evidence, 5 patients with negative bleeding histories, who had abnormal PTT's (out of 2,600 screened with the PTT test). One of these five patients received fresh frozen plasma prior to cholecystostomy; the others underwent operation without bleeding incidents excepting one small hematoma following the traumatic insertion of a pacemaker. The one patient, who did receive fresh frozen plasma prior to cholecystostomy, had previously undergone herniorrhaphy and laminectomy without prior treatment; thus it is not clear that the 2,600 screening PTT determinations benefited any patient. Lorenzi and Cohen[65] found that of 578 patients screened with both the PT and PTT tests, 20 had a PT of $\geq$ 12.5 sec or PTT of $\geq$ 38 sec. Ten of those patients had minor abnormalities defined as a PT between 12.5 and 13 sec or a PTT between 38 and 41 sec. No patient had a note in the chart about this abnormality (perhaps a medicolegal problem if intraoperative bleeding presented a problem); all patients underwent surgery without bleeding problems. Ten patients had a PT of > 13 sec or PTT > 41 sec. Four had known bleeding diathesis (one had hemophilia, one had a bleeding history in admission history, and two were receiving warfarin treatment). Five of the remaining six underwent surgery without any further evaluation of the PT/ PTT abnormalities in the chart and without unusual bleeding during surgery (a medicolegal cost might have resulted from this neglect). The other patient had a normal PT and PTT on a repeated study. Based on these limited data, I believe that little benefit will be obtained from these coagulation tests that are not indicated by history.

PULMONARY FUNCTION TESTS

The suggested tests for patients with a history of lung disease or smoking are described in Chapters 2 and 13. In a patient without history of pulmonary problems, pulmonary function tests are not recommended. The patient's history, especially the maximum tolerated physical activity without shortness of breath, should be used as a guide.

Table 1-6. Indicated Screening Studies on Asymptomatic Healthy Patients Scheduled to Undergo Non-Blood-Loss "Peripheral" Procedures

Age	Males	Females
Under 40	?SGOT/?BUN/?Glucose	Hemoglobin or Hematocrit ?SGOT/?BUN/?Glucose
40–59	Electrocardiogram BUN/Glucose ?SGOT	Hemoglobin or Hematocrit Electrocardiogram BUN/Glucose ?SGOT
Over 60	Hemoglobin or Hematocrit Electrocardiogram Chest x-ray BUN/Glucose ?SGOT	Hemoglobin or Hematocrit Electrocardiogram Chest x-ray BUN/Glucose ?SGOT

? indicates a test that is perhaps indicated on a medicolegal cost benefit basis (see text).

URINALYSIS

In the Kaiser series of 44,663 examinations in 1967 to 1968 (Collen et al.[25]), 8.2 percent of patients had a positive urine glucose concentration and 6.4 percent had a positive urine protein (including menstruating women). Since this is to screen for diabetes or renal disease and since urinalysis at the University of California, San Francisco costs $8.00 and since there appear to be about twice as many false positives with the urine screen as with the blood chemistry screen,[24, 50-60] urinalysis offers no advantage and only duplicates the blood chemistry screen.

SUMMARY OF LABORATORY TESTS (SEE TABLE 1-6)

For the asymptomatic "healthy" patient scheduled to undergo non-blood-loss operations such as breast biopsy, herniorrhaphy, vein stripping, tonsillectomy, and dilatation and curettage, no laboratory tests (or at most SGOT/BUN and blood glucose tests) appear to be indicated below the age of 40 years for males, and only a hemoglobin test below the age of 40 years for females. For patients between 40 and 60 years, an electrocardiogram and determination of BUN and blood glucose levels are indicated for both males and females; females should have a hemoglobin or hematocrit determination as well. After 60 years of age, all patients should have a determination of their hematocrit, BUN and blood glucose levels and an electrocardiogram and chest roentgenogram. An SGOT might also be surveyed for medicolegal reasons in all age groups.

THE MEDICOLEGAL RATIONALE FOR LABORATORY TESTING

If everyone reached the same conclusions from the data as I did, then these conclusions would become the standard of practice. The assumptions used to reach the cost/benefit analysis were skewed to overestimate the predictive value of laboratory testing; thus, for healthy patients one should probably do even less laboratory testing than suggested. We all have a responsibility to provide our patients with optimum care within the bounds of finite resources. If we limit our laboratory use for healthy individuals to that indicated in this chapter, then maybe the government will allow us to practice optimum (and more expensive) medicine for the sick that need more laboratory work (see Ch. 2).

PRACTICAL HISTORY AND PHYSICAL EXAMINATION

As indicated several times, the history and physical examination are usually more important than the various laboratory tests. The following abbreviated approach has been designed especially for preoperative anesthetic evaluation. The questions and physical findings refer to the organ systems that can significantly affect the actions of anesthetics (lungs, liver, kidney), or can be significantly affected by anesthetics (nervous system, cardiovascular system); in addition allergies, drug therapy, and social, family, and personal history relevant to anesthesia are sought. Such a routine (assuming all negative answers and after the introduction) might be as follows:

Have you ever had hepatitis, yellow jaundice, or malaria? Have you recently been exposed to anyone with those conditions?

Have you ever had kidney or renal disease? Do you eat a normal diet? Any bladder infections? Do you get up at night to urinate?

What's the most vigorous thing you've done in the last two weeks?

Do you vacuum, garden, or carry groceries up stairs?

Have you climbed any stairs recently?

How many pillows do you sleep on?

Have you ever had chest pain?

Do you ever wake up short of breath at night?

Have you ever had hypertension (high blood pressure)?

Have you ever had a heart attack or rheumatic fever or been told you had a heart murmur?

Do you smoke? How much?

Do you drink wine or beer or hard liquor? How much?

Do you cough every morning?

Do you cough some mornings?

Have you ever coughed up anything?

Have you had a recent cough or cold?

Have you ever been hospitalized for pneumonia or bronchitis?

Have you ever had a seizure, fit, or convulsion?

Have you ever had an arm or leg go dead on you or be paralyzed or numb?

Do you have pain any place?

Have you ever seen double?

Do you have headaches frequently?

Do you take any medicine or pills or drugs?

Are you pregnant or could you be pregnant?

Do you bleed easily?

Do you bleed when brushing your teeth?

Do you have dentures or false or capped teeth?

Any allergies? Ever have an operation or anesthesia before?

Any family member of yours ever had a problem after anesthesia or surgery?

Then lying and standing blood pressure levels and pulse rates (and a lying blood pressure in the other arm) should be taken. The teeth and jaw should be examined. The patient should be able to follow the examiner's finger in all six eye movement positions. The examiner should then palpate the carotid arteries, examine the jugular venous pulsations, listen to the lungs, palpate and auscultate for heart sounds, apical impulse, and heaves, and ask the patient to walk 10 feet if ambulatory. These are standard procedures in a physical examination to superficially evaluate the cardiorespiratory system, central nervous system, and airway. This type of history and physical examination takes about 15 minutes in the "healthy" adult. I, therefore, feel that this represents the minimum preoperative evaluation for all patients. Clearly, history-taking is one of, if not the best, screens for disease.

OTHER SCREENING LABORATORY TESTS

There are several screening laboratory tests that may increase longevity but which are not needed preoperatively. A case can be made for routine pap smears for detecting cervical and endometrial cancer, for routine testing of stool for occult blood, for urinalysis for bladder cancer (the evidence for microscopic hematuria leading to increased survival over gross hematuria as a screening test is nonexistant), and for urine culture in women over the age of 55 (the evidence that treating asymptomatic bacturia in people over the age of 55 leads to less disease also is nonexistant.) Since these tests will not change what the anesthesiologist does for the patient preoperatively, I do not discuss their yield and cost/benefit analysis in this chapter.

REFERENCES

1. Vacanti CJ, Van Houten RJ, Hill RC: A statistical analysis of the relationship of physical status to postoperative mortality in 68,388 cases. Anesth Analg 49:564, 1970
2. Lewin I, Lerner AG, Green SH, et al: Physical class and physiological status in the prediction of operative mortality in the aged sick. Ann Surg 174:217, 1971
3. Goldman L, Caldera DL, Nussbaum SR, et al: Multifactorial index of cardiac risk in noncardiac surgical procedures. N Engl J Med 297:845, 1977
4. Marx GF, Mateo CV, Orkin LR: Computer analysis of postanesthetic deaths. Anesthesiology 39:54, 1973
5. Ziffren SE, Hartford CE: Comparative mortality for various surgical operations in older versus younger age groups. J Am Geriatr Soc 20:485, 1972
6. Duckett JB: Preoperative assessment of the patient for outpatient anesthesia, Outpatient Anesthesia. Edited by Brown B. Philadelphia, FA Davis, 1978, pp 21-29
7. Okelberry CR: Preadmission testing shortens preoperative length of stay. J Am Hosp Assoc 49:71, 1975
8. Friedman GD: Effects of MHTS on patients, Multiphasic Health Testing Services. Edited by Collen MF. New York, John Wiley & Sons, 1978, Chapter 18
9. Dales LG, Friedman GD, Collen MF: Evaluating periodic multiphasic health checkups: A controlled trial. J Chron Dis 32:385, 1979
10. Grimaldi JV: The worth of occupational health programs. J Occup Med 7:365, 1965
11. Thorner R M, Crumpacker EL: Mortality and periodic examination of executives. Arch Environ Health 3:523, 1961
12. Roberts NJ, Ipsen J, Elpon KO: Mortality among males in periodic-health-examination programs. N Engl J Med 281:20, 1969
13. Kuller L, Tonascia S: Commission on chronic illness follow-up study. Arch Environ Health 21:656, 1970
14. Braren N, Elinson J: Relationship of a clinical examination to mortality rates. Am J Public Health 62:1501, 1972
15. Krieg AF, Gambino R, Galen RS: Why are clinical laboratory tests performed? When are they valid? JAMA 233:76, 1975
16. Gorry GA, Pauker SG, Schwartz WB: The diagnostic importance of the normal finding. N Engl J Med 298:486, 1978
17. Galen RS, Gambino SR: Sensitivity, specificity, prevalence and incidence, Beyond Normality: The Predictive Value and Efficiency of Medical Diagnoses. New York, John Wiley & Sons, 1975, pp 9-14
18. Collen MF (Editor): Multiphasic Health Testing Services. New York, John Wiley & Sons, 1978
19. Napier JA, Johnson BC, Epstein FH: The Tecumseh, Michigan, community health study, Community as an Epidemiologic Laboratory: A Casebook of Community Studies. Edited by Kessler II, Levin ML. Baltimore, Johns Hopkins Press, 1970, pp 25-46
20. Neuhauser D: Cost-effective clinical decision making. Pediatrics 60: 756, 1977
21. Sagal SS, Evens, RG, Forrest JV, et al: Efficacy of routine screening and lateral chest radiographs in a hospital-based population. N Engl J Med 291:1001, 1974
22. Sane SM, Worsing RA, Wiens CW, et al: Value of preoperative chest x-ray examinations in children. Pediatrics 60:669, 1977
23. Rees AM, Roberts CJ, Bligh AS, et al: Routine preoperative chest radiography in non-cardiopulmonary surgery. Br Med J 1:1333, 1976
24. Collen MF, Feldman R, Sieglaub AB, et al: Dollar cost per positive test for automated multiphasic screening. N Engl J Med 283:459, 1970
25. Brill PW, Ewing ML, Donn AA: The value (?) of routine chest radiography in children and adolescents. Pediatrics 52:125, 1973

26. Bunker J, Barnes B, Mosteller F: Costs, Risks, and Benefits of Surgery. New York, Oxford University Press, 1977

27. Cochrane AL, Garland LH: Observer error in the interpretation of chest films. Lancet 2:505, 1952

28. Yerushalmy JT: The statistical assessment of the variability in observer perception and description of roentgenographic pulmonary shadows. Radiol Clin North Am 7:381, 1969

29. Yerushalmy JT: Reliability of chest radiography in the diagnosis of pulmonary lesions. Am J Surg 89:231, 1955

30. Yerushalmy JT, Harkness JT, Cope JH, et al: The role of dual reading in mass radiography. Am Rev Tuberc 61:443, 1950

31. Newell RR, Chamberlain WE, Rigler L: Descriptive classification of pulmonary shadows. Am Rev Tuberc 69:566, 1954

32. Groth-Petersen E, Løvgreen A, Thillemann J: On the reliability of the reading of photofluorograms and the value of dual reading. Acta Tuberc Scand 26:13, 1952

33. Garland LH: On the scientific evaluation of diagnostic procedures. Radiology 52:309, 1949

34. Gordon T, Kannel WB: The Framingham, Massachusetts, study twenty years later, Community as an Epidemiologic Laboratory: A Casebook of Community Studies. Edited by Kessler II, Levin ML. Baltimore, Johns Hopkins Press, 1970, pp 123-146

35. Ostrander LD, Brandt RL, Kjelsberg MO, et al: Electrocardiographic findings among the adult population of a total natural community, Tecumseh, Michigan. Circulation 31:888, 1965

36. Kannel WB, McGee D, Gordon T: A general cardiovascular risk profile: The Framingham study. Am J Cardiol 38:46, 1976

37. Galen RS, Gambino SR: The electrocardiogram application of the model to a nonlaboratory test, Beyond Normality: The Predictive Value and Efficiency of Medical Diagnoses. New York, John Wiley & Sons, 1975, pp 99-106

38. Tarhan S, Moffitt EA, Taylor WF, et al: Myocardial infarction after general anesthesia. JAMA 199:1451, 1972

39. Fraser JG, Ramachandran PR, Davis HS: Anesthesia and recent myocardial infarction. JAMA 199:318, 1967

40. Arkins R, Smessaert AA, Hicks RG: Mortality and morbidity in surgical patients with coronary artery disease. JAMA 190:485, 1964

41. Topkins MJ, Artusio JF: Myocardial infarction and surgery: A five year study. Anesth Analg 43:715, 1964

42. Goldman L et al: Cardiac risk factors and complications in non-cardiac surgery. Medicine 57:357, 1978

43. Steen PA, Tinker JH, Tarhan S: Myocardial reinfarction after anesthesia and surgery. JAMA 239:2566, 1978

44. Mauney FM, Jr., Ebert PA, Sabiston DC: Postoperative myocardial infarction: A study of predisposing factors, diagnosis and mortality in a high risk group of surgical patients. Ann Surg 172:497, 1970

45. Ostrander LO: Serial electrocardiographic findings in a prospective epidemiologic study. Circulation 34:1069, 1966

46. Wasserman LR, Gilbert HS: Surgical bleeding in polycythemia vera. Ann NY Acad Sci 115:122, 1964

47. Rothstein P: What hemoglobin level is adequate in pediatric anesthesia. Anesthesiology Update I:24, 1978

48. Slogoff S: Anesthesia considerations in the anemic patient. Anesthesiology Update II:7, 1979

49. Kowalyshyn TS, Prager D, Young J: Review of the present status of preoperative hemoglobin requirements. Anesth Analg 51:75, 1972

50. Carmalt MHB, Freeman P, Stephens AJH, et al: Value of routine multiple blood tests in patients attending the general practitioner. Br Med J 1:620, 1970

51. Zinn S, Fairley HBF, Eger EI: Personal communication

52. Friedman GD, Goldberg M, Ahuja JN, et al: Biochemical screening tests: Effect of panel size on medical care. Arch Intern Med 129:91, 1972

53. Wataneeyawech M, Kelly KA: Hepatic diseases, unsuspected before surgery. New York State J Med 75:1278, 1975

54. Schemel WH: Unexpected hepatic dysfunction found by multiple laboratory screening. Anesth Analg 55:810, 1976

55. Schneiderman LJ, De Salvo L, Baylor S, et al: The "abnormal" screening laboratory results. Arch Intern Med 129:88, 1972

56. Peery TM: The role of the laboratory in health evaluation, Interim Report No. 77, from the 1964 Technicon International Symposium, New York, NY, as quoted in Schoen I: Clinical chemistry, a retrospective look at routine screening. Calif Med 108:430, 1968

57. Young DM, Drake TGH: Unsolicited laboratory information, presented to the College of American Pathologists, Chicago, 18 Oct 1965, as quoted in Schoen I: Clinical chemistry, a retrospective look at routine screening. Calif Med 108:430, 1968

58. Bryan DJ, Wearne JL, Vian A, et al: Profile of admission chemical data by multichannel automation: An evaluation experiment. Clin Chem 12:137, 1966

59. Schoen I: Clinical chemistry, a retrospective look at routine screening. Calif Med 108:430, 1968

60. Boonstra CE, Jackson CE: The clinical value of routine calcium analyses. Ann Intern Med 57:963, 1962

61. Ahlvin RC: Biochemical screening—A critique. N Engl J Med 283:1084, 1970

62. Nye SW, Graham JB, Brinkhous KM: The partial thromboplastin time as a screening test for the detection of latent bleeders. Am J Med Sci 243:279, 1962

63. Robbins JA, Rose SD: Partial thromboplastin time as a screening test. Ann Intern Med 90:796, 1979

64. Baranetsky NG, Weinstein P: Partial thromboplastin time for screening—Letter to the editor. Ann Intern Med 91:498, 1979

65. Cohen SN: Personal communication

2

Preoperative Evaluation of Patients with Diseases that Require Special Preoperative Evaluation and Intraoperative Management

Michael F. Roizen, M.D.

INTRODUCTION

Patient evaluation in this chapter focuses on those patients who have conditions that require special preoperative evaluation and intraoperative management. Conditions discussed in this chapter are (1) diseases involving the endocrine system, and disorders of nutrition; (2) diseases involving the cardiovascular system; (3) disorders of the respiratory and immune systems; (4) diseases of the central nervous system, neuromuscular diseases, and psychiatric disorders; (5) diseases involving the kidney, infectious diseases, and disorders of electrolytes; (6) diseases involving the gastrointestinal tract or the liver; (7) diseases involving the hematopoetic system, and cancers; and (8) patients receiving drug therapy for chronic and acute medical conditions. (See individual chapters for obstetric and pediatric patients).

Optimizing a patient's preoperative condition is a cooperative venture between the anesthesiologist and the internist, pediatrician, surgeon, or family physician. If the patient's physician cannot state "this patient is in the optimum shape I or anyone I know of can get him in," then the anesthesiologist and the physician should do what is necessary to op-

timize the patient's condition. Not consulting with the primary physician preoperatively is as risky as not checking to see if there is oxygen in the spare tanks. In fact, the statements, "this patient is in optimum shape," and "I feel the mitral stenosis is more severe than the slight degree of mitral insufficiency" are much more useful than one such as "avoid hypoxia and hypotension."[1] The internist, pediatrician, and family practitioner usually have little knowledge of anesthetic problems, physiology, and pharmacology. It is part of the anesthesiologist's job to educate the patient's consultants as to the information needed from the consultation.

DISEASES INVOLVING THE ENDOCRINE SYSTEM AND DISORDERS OF NUTRITION

PANCREATIC MALFUNCTION

PREOPERATIVE DIABETES MELLITUS

The following three aspects of diabetes are discussed:

1. That at least two types of diabetes should be considered;

2. That a current debate exists as to how closely diabetic patients should be controlled vis à vis blood glucose levels (this debate centers on whether normal blood glucose levels are a benefit to diabetic patients but has not progressed to the point of evaluating benefit/risk ratios in awake or anesthetized patients); and

3. That treatment regimens differ depending on how closely the diabetes is controlled. Although close control requires somewhat more effort, either treatment regimen is easy to routinely institute, as is detailed.

The 1978 NIH Classification group[2] segregates diabetic patients into two main types. The insulin-dependent group, which appears to be hereditary with autoimmune association, is composed mainly of juvenile onset diabetics (formerly called juvenile onset or ketosis prone diabetics). The insulin-independent group (presenile senescent islet [β] cells) is composed of drug- and pregnancy-induced and maturity onset diabetics.

The insulin-dependent patient is currently treated with diet and insulin (b.i.d. or t.i.d. by the "tight-control" advocates). The insulin-independent patient previously was treated with diet, weight-control, and oral antidiabetic drugs (acetohexamide [Dymelor], chlorpropramide [Diabinase], tolazamide [Tolinase], tolbutamide [Orinase], or phenformin [DBI]). The University Group Diabetics Program (UGDP) study implied that oral antidiabetic agents might accelerate the atherosclerotic complications of diabetes;[3] therefore the oral antidiabetics have been used less frequently. Oral hypoglycemics may cause hypoglycemia as long as 50 hours after last being taken (chlorpropramide has the longest half-life). Occasionally, a "tight-control advocating" physician will give insulin-independent (maturity onset) diabetic patients insulin, b.i.d.

Diabetes is associated with increased atherosclerosis (e.g., coronary and cerebral), microangiopathy (e.g., retinal and renal), infections, and decreased wound-healing tensile strength. The evidence that hyperglycemia per se accelerates these complications or that tight control of blood sugar decreases the rapidity of disease progression is suggestive, but by no means definite.[4-8]

The perioperative management of the diabetic patient may affect the ultimate surgical outcome. The tight-control advocates adhere to the evidence of increased wound tensile strength and decreased wound infections in diabetic animal models with tight versus poor control of hyperglycemia. Hyperglycemic diabetic patients have an increased incidence of wound infections,[9, 10] a decreased wound tensile strength,[11, 12] and an increased incidence of renal transplant rejections[13] relative to normoglycemic nondiabetics. The debate (and lack of definitive studies to answer the questions) concerns whether control of hyperglycemia per se lessens these complications. Insulin is still primarily used to treat and prevent the severe complications of ketoacidotic and nonketotic hyperosmolar coma. The risk of insulin treatment is hypoglycemia, which is often without symptoms and difficult to diagnose in the anesthetized patient.

The two regimens to control the diabetic patient in the perioperative period are listed below.

Classic (Nontight Control) Regimen

Aim:

Avoid hypoglycemia.

Avoid ketoacidosis and hyperosmolar states.

Protocol:

1. Day before surgery: NPO after midnight with a glass of orange juice at bedside for emergency use.
2. At 6 a.m. on day of surgery, institute IV fluids with plastic cannulae IV using a solution containing 5 percent dextrose at 125 ml/hr/70 kg.
3. After IV is instituted, give ½ of usual a.m. insulin dose subcutaneously.
4. Continue 5 percent dextrose solutions through operative period giving at least 125 ml/hr/70 kg.
5. In recovery room, monitor urine sugars and acetones and blood glucose con-

centrations, and treat with a sliding scale.

Tight Control Regimen 1

Aim:

Keep plasma glucose between 79 and 200 mg/100 ml., which may improve wound healing and prevent wound infections.

Protocol:

1. Evening before operation: obtain preprandial blood glucose level.
2. Through a plastic cannulae, begin IV infusion of 5 percent dextrose in water at 50 ml/hr/70 kg.
3. Piggy back to dextrose infusion, an infusion of regular insulin using an infusion pump—this should be 50 units of regular insulin in 250 ml 0.9 percent sodium chloride; flush the line with 60 ml of infusion mixture and discard before attaching (see Fig. 2-1—this approach is adequate to saturate insulin binding sites on tubing— and see reference 14)
4. Set infusion rate with this equation: insulin (units/hr) = Plasma glucose (mg/100 ml)/150*

   *Note: this denominator should be 100 if patient is taking corticosteroids (≥ 100 mg prednisone per day)
5. Repeat measurements of blood glucose levels every 4 hours as needed with appropriate insulin adjustments to obtain blood glucose levels between 100 and 200 mg/100 ml.
6. Day of surgery: intraoperative fluids and electrolytes managed with nondextrose containing solutions continued as in steps 3 and 4 above.
7. Obtain plasma glucose at start of operation and q 4 hr for the rest of the 24 hour period. Adjust insulin dosage appropriately.

Although our group has not needed to treat hypoglycemia (blood glucose less than 50 mg/100 ml) we have been prepared to do so with 15 ml of 50 percent dextrose in water. Obviously, the insulin infusion should be terminated.

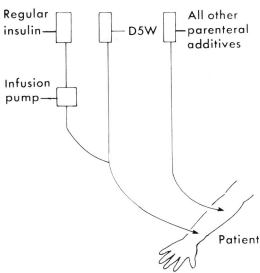

Fig. 2-1 Arrangement of intravenous lines for regular insulin infusion ("tight" control regimen).

Tight Control Regimen 2

Aim:

Same as that of Tight Control Regimen 1.

Protocol:

1. Obtain "feedback mechanical pancreas" and set dials for desired plasma glucose regimen. Institute appropriate two IV lines.

This last regimen may well supersede all others if cost of a mechanical pancreas can be reduced and if control of hyperglycemia is shown to make a meaningful difference.

Other Conditions Associated with Diabetes

In addition to control of diabetes per se, there is an increased incidence of atherosclerosis (and all its complications), microangiopathy (retinal and renal vessels), peripheral neuropathies, autonomic dysfunction, and infection. Abnormalities in those systems should be known about preoperatively, and their treatment (if any is needed, i.e., dialysis) optimized preoperatively.

INSULINOMA AND OTHER CAUSES OF HYPOGLYCEMIA

Hypoglycemia can be caused by such diverse entities as a pancreatic islet cell adenoma or carcinoma, large hepatomas, large sarcomas, alcohol ingestion, hypopituitarism, adrenal insufficiency, after gastric surgery, hereditary fructose intolerance, or galactosemia. The last three entities cause "postprandial reactive hypoglycemia." Since restriction of oral intake prevents severe hypoglycemia, making the patient NPO and infusing small amounts of a solution containing 5 percent dextrose avoids postprandial reactive hypoglycemia.

The other causes of hypoglycemia can cause serious problems in the perioperative period. The symptoms of hypoglycemia fall into two groups: either adrenergic excess (tachycardia, palpitations, tremulousness, or diaphoresis) or neuroglycopenia (headache, confusion, mental sluggishness, seizures, or coma). Since all these symptoms may be masked by anesthesia, the blood glucose levels should be determined to insure that hypoglycemia is not occurring. Since tumor manipulations of insulinomas can result in massive insulin release, this tumor probably should only be operated on in centers where a mechanical pancreas (with its on-line blood glucose analysis and in this case glucose infusion setup) is available. The other causes of hypoglycemia do not release insulin in such vast quantities (or at all), and frequent (every 1 to 2 hour) intraoperative blood glucose determinations and continual dextrose infusion are all that is needed.

DISORDERS OF NUTRITION

HYPERLIPIDEMIAS AND HYPOLIPIDEMIAS

Hyperlipidemia may result from obesity, estrogen or corticoid therapy, uremia, diabetes, hypothyroidism, acromegaly, alcohol ingestion, liver disease, or pregnancy and may cause premature coronary or peripheral vascular disease or pancreatitis.[15] Hypercholesteremia appears to be associated with premature development of atherosclerosis. Most cholesterol is carried in serum by low density lipoproteins (LDL) while about 20 percent of total serum cholesterol is carried by high density lipoproteins (HDL). LDL probably is the atherosclerotic risk factor, while cholesterol carried as HDL is actually protective.[16] HDL is 25 percent higher in women than men; low HDL levels in women are associated with premature atherosclerosis. Cigarette smoking lowers while regular strenuous exercise and small daily intake of alcohol raises HDL levels; octogenarians have a high HDL level.

The drug therapy of hyperlipidemia should concern the anesthesiologist, and diet is the major treatment modality for all types of hyperlipidemia. Clofibrate (Atromid-S)—used to treat hypertriglyceridemia—can cause myopathy, especially in patients with hepatic or renal disease. Cholestyramine binds bile acids, as well as oral anticoagulants, digitalis drugs, and thyroid hormones. Nicotinic acid causes peripheral vasodilation and probably should not be continued through the morning of surgery.

Hypolipidemias are rare diseases often associated with neuropathies, anemia, and renal failure. Anesthetic experience has been so limited, that specific recommendations are not available.

OBESITY

Twenty to 50 percent of adults in the United States weigh more than 20 percent above "normal" body weight. Both obesity itself, its complications, and its treatment have significance for the anesthesiologist. Being 20 percent overweight is associated with a 40 percent increase in the chance of dying of heart disease and a 50 percent increase in the chance of dying of a stroke. Obesity is associated with a higher surgical morbidity and mortality.

While many conditions associated with obesity (diabetes, cholilithiasis, cirrhosis) contribute to morbidity, the main concerns for the anesthesiologist are derangements related to the cardiopulmonary system. Obese patients often have hypertension, which can cause cardiomegaly and left ventricular failure. Care should be taken to use a blood pressure cuff of correct size. The obese, therefore, have limited cardiac reserve and may have a poor tolerance of stress induced by hypotension, hypertension, tachycardia, or fluid overload associated with surgical anesthesia. Airway obstruction frequently occurs because of the abundant soft tissue in the upper airway. Functional residual volume is reduced as the weight of the torso and abdomen make diaphragmatic excursions more difficult. Thus, preoperative assessment, in addition to a history and physical examination accentuating cardiopulmonary problems, should include an electrocardiographic examination (left or right ventricular hypertrophy, ischemia, conduction defects) and if the obesity is severe enough an analysis of arterial blood gases. The latter is needed to quantitate the degree of hypoventilation and to aid in assessment of what numbers to seek when considering extubation of the trachea. Massively obese individuals with carbon dioxide retention have been labelled pickwickian. Other components of the pickwickian syndrome are somnolence, hypoxemia, right heart failure, and secondary polycythemia. These patients often have right ventricular failure (see Ch. 6 for monitoring considerations). More extensive pulmonary function tests and preoperative treatment of any treatable abnormality, such as infectious and bronchospastic components of pulmonary disease, may be indicated in the patient with pulmonary symptoms (smoking, chronic cough, sputum production, wheezing, shortness of breath at rest or on minor exertion). In addition, obese patients have an increased volume of, and acidity of, gastric juice

preoperatively, perhaps indicating the wisdom of premedication with cimetidine or glycopyrrolate.[17] Drastic dieting can cause acidosis, hypokalemia, and hyperuricemia; and protein hydrolyzsate liquid diets are associated with development of intractable ventricular arrhythmias. Metabolic complications of jejunoileal bypass include hypokalemia, hypocalcemia, hypomagnesemia, anemia, renal stones, gout, and liver abnormalities. An attempt to reverse these abnormal conditions should be made prior to anesthesia and may be corrected by infusion of amino acid solutions. Drug treatment of obesity also has implications for the anesthesiologist. For example, amphetamines (and mazindol, probably) given acutely increase anesthetic requirements, while chronically administered amphetamines decrease anesthetic requirements (see Ch. 9). Amphetamines may interfere with the action of vasoactive drugs when the latter are used to treat hypotension or hypertension. Fenfluramine (a drug that inhibits the serotinergic system) may decrease both anesthetic requirement and blood pressure.

ANOREXIA NERVOSA AND STARVATION

Multiple endocrine and metabolic abnormalities occur in the patient beset by anorexia nervosa, a condition of starvation to the point of 40 percent loss of normal weight, hyperactivity, and a psychiatrically distorted body image. Acidosis, hypokalemia, hypocalcemia, hypomagnesemia, hypothermia, diabetes insipidus, and severe endocrine abnormalities mimicking panhypopituitarism need attention prior to anesthesia and surgery. These patients, similar to those with protein deficiency states (kwashiorkor), may have electrocardiographic alterations and cardiomyopathy.[18,19] Total depletion of body potassium makes addition of potassium to glucose solutions useful; however, fluid administration can precipitate pulmonary edema in these patients. Thus, invasive monitoring (radial artery and pulmonary artery catheterization) probably is indicated for those individuals requiring emergency surgery. Elective surgery probably should be delayed until treatment of the identified abnormalities are instituted.

HYPERALIMENTATION (TOTAL PARENTERAL NUTRITION [TPN])

For patients receiving hyperalimentation, hypertonic glucose calories are concentrated in normal daily fluid requirements in solutions containing protein hydrolyzates or synthetic amino acids. To diminish the likelihood of essential fatty acid deficiency, Intralipid, a soybean emulsion, can be added to the solution.[20] The major complications of hyperalimentation are sepsis and metabolic abnormalities. The central lines used for TPN require an absolute aseptic technique and should not be used as an intravenous route for drug administration.

Major metabolic complications of TPN relate to deficiencies and hyperosmolar states that develop. Complications of hypertonic dextrose can develop if the patient has insufficient insulin (diabetes mellitus) to metabolize the sugar or if insulin resistance is present (uremia, burns, sepsis).[20]

Gradual decrease in the infusion rate of TPN prevents the development of hypoglycemia that can occur on abrupt discontinuance. Thus, the infusion rate of TPN should be decreased the night prior to anesthesia and surgery. The main reason for slowing or discontinuing TPN prior to anesthesia is to avoid intraoperative hyperosmolarity secondary to rapid infusion of the solution.[21] Hypophosphatemia is a particularly serious complication that results from administering phosphate-free or phosphate-depleted hyperalimentation solution. The low serum phosphate causes shifts of the oxygen dissociation curve to the left, and thus low 2,3-diphosphoglycerate and ATP require increased

cardiac output for the same oxygen delivery. Hypophosphatemia, when less than 1.0 mg/dl, may cause a hemolytic anemia, cardiac failure, tachypnea, neurologic symptoms, seizures, and death. In addition, trace metal deficiencies associated with long-term TPN include copper (refractory anemia), zinc (impaired wound healing), and magnesium deficiency. Based on the above considerations, I slow TPN beginning the night prior to surgery, substituting 5 or 10 percent dextrose solution preoperatively; measure serum glucose, phosphate, and potassium concentrations preoperatively, and if abnormal, restore them to within normal limits; and maintain strict asepsis.[21]

ADRENAL CORTICAL MALFUNCTION

ADRENAL CORTICAL HORMONE EXCESS

Three major types of hormones—androgen, glucocorticoid, and mineralocorticoid— are secreted by the adrenal cortex; a characteristic clinical syndrome is associated with excess of each. Excess secretion of androgen causes masculinization, pseudopuberty, or female pseudohemaphroditism. With some tumors, this androgen is converted to an estrogenic substance in which case feminization results. No special anesthetic evaluation is needed for patients with that condition.

Excess glucocorticoid secretion produces a moon-faced, plethoric individual, with a centripetal distribution of fat (trunk obesity with skinny extremities), thin skin, easy bruising, and striae; these patients often have osteopenia due to decreased bone matrix formation and impaired calcium absorption, hypertension, protein depletion, a proximal myopathy, fluid retention, and frequently hyperglycemia and even diabetes mellitus (Cushing's syndrome). Special preoperative considerations include regulating diabetes and hypertension and insuring that intravascular fluid volume and electrolyte concentrations are normal. The most common cause of Cushing's syndrome is iatrogenic administration of glucocorticoids for other conditions, such as arthritis, asthma, and allergies. In these cases, the adrenal gland atrophies and cannot respond to stressful situations (i.e., the perioperative period) by secreting more steroid. Thus, additional glucocorticoids are required in the perioperative period. Although the precise amount required has not been established, I give the maximum amount of glucocorticoid equivalent that the body manufactures in response to a maximal stress, about 300 mg/70 kg of hydrocortisone intravenously. The second leading cause of Cushing's syndrome is bilateral adrenal hyperplasia due to increased secretion of ACTH (from either the pituitary or a nonendocrine tumor of lung or pancreas). The third most likely cause of Cushing's syndrome appears to be a primary adrenal tumor. If one of the latter two causes is the etiology of Cushing's syndrome, then no special preoperative preparation above treatment of end-organ results (diabetes, hypertension, fluid and electrolyte abnormalities) probably is required.

Excess mineralocorticoid secretion (common with glucocorticoid excess, as most glucocorticoids have some mineralocorticoid properties) leads to potassium depletion, sodium retention, weakness, hypertension, tetany, polyuria, inability to concentrate urine, and hypokalemic alkalosis; these symptoms constitute hyperaldosteronism, or Conn's syndrome, (a cause of low renin hypertension, as renin secretion is inhibited by the effects of the high aldosterone levels). Intravascular fluid volume, electrolyte concentrations, and renal function should be restored to within normal limits preoperatively by treating the patient with the aldosterone antagonist spironolactone. The effects of spironolactone are slow in onset and continue to increase for 1 to 2 weeks. A patient with a serum potassium level of 2.9 mEq/L may have as little as a 40 mEq or as great as a 400

mEq deficit of body potassium. At least 24 hours are frequently required to restore equilibration. (See Chs. 26 and 27 and section on fluid and electrolyte disorders later in this chapter.) A normal serum potassium level *does not* imply correction of a total body deficit of potassium. Again the efficacy of optimizing the preoperative status of patients with disorders of glucocorticoid or mineralocorticoid secretion has not been clearly established. Our assumption has been that restoring abnormalities to a normal condition is good medicine and therefore will improve mortality and morbidity.

ADRENOCORTICAL INSUFFICIENCY

In addition to withdrawal of, or relative lack of, corticoids given to treat specific diseases, other causes of adrenocortical insufficiency include defects in ACTH secretion and destruction of the adrenal gland by cancer, tuberculosis, or an autoimmune mechanism. Because adrenal insufficiency usually develops slowly, these patients develop a marked pigmentation (from excess ACTH trying to drive an unproductive adrenal) and cardiopenia (apparently secondary to the chronic hypotension). If not stressed, these patients have no problems. Acute adrenal crisis (Addisonian crisis) occurs when even a minor stress (e.g., upper respiratory infection) occurs. To prepare such a patient for surgery and anesthesia, hypovolemia, hyperkalemia, and hyponatremia should be treated preoperatively. Since these patients also cannot respond to stressful situations, we recommend that they be given a maximum stress dose of glucocorticoids (about 300 mg/70 kg/day of hydrocortisone) in the perioperative period.

Hypoaldosteronism or hyporeninemic hypoaldosteronism is a less common condition. This condition can be congenital or appear after unilateral adrenal removal or after prolonged heparin administration and is often associated with diabetes. These patients can have severe hyperkalemia, hyponatremia, and myocardial conduction defects. These defects can be successfully treated by mineralocorticoid supplementation (9-α-fludrocortisone, 0.1 mg/day) preoperatively.

ADRENAL MEDULLARY SYMPATHETIC
HORMONE EXCESS

Less than 0.1 percent of all cases of hypertension are due to pheochromocytoma, catecholamine-producing tumors derived from chromaffin tissue. While usually found in the adrenal medulla, these vascular tumors can occur anywhere, such as in the right atrium, the spleen, the broad ligament of the ovary, or the organ of Zucherkandl at the bifurcation of the aorta. Malignant spread, which occurs in less than 15 percent of cases, usually proceeds to venous and lymphatic channels with a predisposition for the liver. Occasionally this tumor's occurrence is familial and/or can be part of the pluriglandular-neoplastic syndrome known as multiple endocrine adenoma-type II (with medullary carcinoma of the thyroid, and parathyroid adenoma or hyperplasia) or type III (medullary carcinoma of the thyroid, marfanoid appearance, and mucosal neuromas) as an autosomal dominant. Often bilateral tumors are found in the familial form.

Symptoms and signs that may be solicited preoperatively and are suggestive of pheochromocytoma are excessive sweating, headache, orthostatic hypotension, previous hypertensive response to induction of anesthesia or to abdominal examination, paroxysmal attacks of sweating, glucose intolerance, polycythemia, weight loss, and psychological abnormalities.

Although no controlled, randomized, prospective clinical studies have been done on the value of preoperative use of adrenergic blocking drugs, their use is generally recommended in the preoperative period. These drugs probably reduce the perioperative complications of hypertensive crisis, wide blood pressure fluctuations during intraoperative manipulation of the tumor (especially until the venous drainage is obliterated), and perioperative myocardial dysfunction.

Alpha-adrenergic blockade with phentolamine or phenoxybenzamine allows reexpansion of intravascular plasma volume by counteracting the vasoconstrictive effects of high levels of catecholamines; the reexpansion of fluid volume is often followed by a decrease in hematocrit. Because of a longer duration of action, phenoxybenzamine (Dibenzylene) is preferred to phentolamine. This avoids wide fluctuations in drug effect and the need for frequent administration.[22] The long half-life of phenoxybenzamine makes increasing its dose undesirable more often than every 2 or 3 days. Because some patients may be very sensitive to the effects of phenoxybenzamine, it should be given initially in doses of 20 to 30 mg PO per day in once or twice daily doses. Most patients usually require 60 to 250 mg/day. Efficacy of therapy should be judged by reduction in symptoms (especially sweating) and stabilization of blood pressure. In patients who have carbohydrate intolerance because of inhibition of insulin release mediated by α-receptor stimulation, α-adrenergic blockade may produce a reduction in fasting blood sugars.[23, 24] In patients who exhibit ST-T changes on electrocardiogram, long-term preoperative α-adrenergic blockade (2 to 6 months) has been shown to result in electrocardiographic and clinical resolution of catecholamine myocarditis.[25, 26]

Concomitant β-adrenergic blockade with propranolol is suggested for patients who have persistent arrhythmias or tachycardia,[23, 27-31] which may be either precipitated or aggravated by α-adrenergic blockade. These arrhythmias are especially dangerous in patients with cardiac disease. Beta-adrenergic blockade should not be used in the absence of concomitant α-adrenergic blockade because the vasoconstrictive α-adrenergic effects would be left unopposed by blocking the vasodilating β-adrenergic effects; this situation could result in dangerous hypertension.[30]

The optimal duration of therapy with

phenoxybenzamine preoperatively has not been studied. Most patients will require 7 to 14 days of preoperative therapy, as judged by the time required for stabilization of blood pressure and amelioration of symptoms.[23,27] Based on my experience, this is a minimal time. Since the tumor spreads slowly, nothing is lost by waiting until medical therapy has optimized the patient's preoperative condition. Accordingly, the following requirements are recommended:

1. no "in hospital" blood pressure greater than 165/90 torr should be evident for 72 hours prior to surgery,

2. orthostatic hypotension not lower than 90/60 torr for 72 hours should be present,

3. the electrocardiogram should be free of ST-T changes for at least 2 months, and

4. no more than one premature ventricular contraction should be present every 5 minutes.

This management will help insure stability of intraoperative and postoperative blood pressure. Although specific anesthetic drugs have been recommended, I feel that optimal preoperative preparation, a gentle induction of anesthesia, and good communication between surgeon and anesthesiologist is more important. See Tables 2-1 and 2-2 for a comparison of anesthetic drugs. No controlled study exists and virtually all agents including enflurane, fentanyl, and regional anesthesia have been used with success. Because of ease of use, I prefer phenylephrine hydrochloride (Neo-Synephrine) or dopamine for hypotension and nitroprusside for hypertension; phentolamine (Regitine) has too long an onset and duration of action. Once the venous supply is secured and if there is a normal intravascular volume as measured by pulmonary wedge pressure, a normal blood pressure usually results. However some patients become hypotensive, occasionally requiring massive infusions of catecholamines. Rarely patients will remain hypertensive intraoperatively. Postoperatively about 50 percent remain hypertensive for 1 to 3 days—and have markedly elevated but declining plasma catecholamine values—at which time all but 25 percent become normotensive.

HYPOFUNCTION AND ABERRATION IN FUNCTION OF THE SYMPATHETIC NERVOUS SYSTEM

Disorders of this type include Shy Drager syndrome, Riley-Day syndrome, Lesch-Nyhan syndrome, Gill familial dysautonomia, diabetic dysautonomia, and in spinal cord transection patients, autonomic dysfunction.

Although individuals can function well without either of their adrenal medullas,[37] individuals with a deficient peripheral sympathetic nervous system have major problems not only with life but with anesthesia.[38-56] One of the main functions of the sympathetic nervous system appears to be the regulation of blood pressure and intravascular fluid volume when changing position. All of the sympathetic hypofunction syndromes have a common denominator of orthostatic hypotension. This can be caused by deficient intravascular volume, deficient baroreceptor function (as also occurs in carotid disease[57]), abnormalities in central nervous system function (as in Wernicke's or Shy-Drager syndrome[41]), deficient neuronal stores of norepinephrine (idiopathic orthostatic hypotension,[43,45] diabetes[42]), or deficient release of norepinephrine (traumatic spinal cord injury[38,46]).[58] In addition to other abnormalities, such as urinary or fecal retention and deficient heat exchange, individuals with sympathetic hypofunction syndromes often develop renal amyloidosis. Thus, the electrolyte status and especially the intravascular fluid volume status should be evaluated preoperatively. Since many of these patients have cardiac abnormalities, perhaps even for minor procedures preoperative assessment of intravascular fluid volume should be undertaken with the aid of a Swan-Ganz catheter rather than by a central venous pressure

Table 2-1. Results Presented in Studies of Patients Undergoing Surgery for Pheochromocytoma

Study	Number of Patients	Preoperative Treatment	Anesthetic	Complications			
				AR	BP ↑	BP ↓	Mortality
Crout & Brown[32] 1964–1968	1	None	N$_2$O-Meperidine	1	11	(Rx PTA)	0
	3	1 PBZ	Halothane	3			0
	12	11 PBZ	Methoxyflurane	0		8 (Rx pressors)	0
Crandall & Myers[33] 1954–1964	11	—	Ether	NR	8	6 (Rx pressors) (Rx PTA)	0
Gould & Perry[34] 1965–1969	6	None	Ether	1	1	1	0
	20	PBZ	Ether	2	3	0	0
	7	PBZ + PPL	Ether	3	1	0	0
	3	NR	Halothane	3	3	1	0
	2	NR	Methoxyflurane	0	1	0	0
	2	NR	Ether	1	0	1	0
Cooperman et al.[35] 1965–1966	14	14 α-MT 5 PBZ	Halothane	10	NR		0
Desmonts et al.[36]	14 (1964–1965)	None	Thiopental-Narcotic	5 (2 CA)	6	7	4
	50 (1966–1972)	6 α-MT	Halothane	36 (2 CA)	19	7	0
	38 (1973–1976)	None	Innovar	3	15	1	0

Abbreviations used: AR = arrhythmia, BP = blood pressure, PBZ = Phenoxybenzamine, PPL = Propranolol, α-MT = α-Methyltyrosine, PTA = Phentolamine, CA= Cardiac Arrest, NR = Not reported.

Table 2-2. Results of Different Anesthetic Techniques in Pheochromocytoma[32-36]

	Ether	Halothane	Methoxy-flurane	Thiopental-Narcotic	Innovar
Numbers of Patients	46	70	14	14	38
Preoperative Treatment	27	21	11	0	0
Arrhythmia	7	52	0	5	3
Mortality	0	0	0	4	0

measurement (see Ch. 6). Since the sympathetic system function of these patients is not predictable, I usually employ slow gentle induction of anesthesia and treat sympathetic excess or deficiency with careful titration, by infusion, of direct-acting vasoconstrictors (Neo-Synephrine), vasodilators (nitroprusside) or cardiac rate stimulants (isoproterenol), or heart rate depressants (propranolol) rather than of agonists or antagonists that may indirectly release catecholamines. A 20 percent perioperative mortality rate for 2,600 patients with spinal cord transection has been reported,[56] thus indicating that these patients obviously are difficult to manage and deserve particularly close attention.

After reviewing 300 patients with spinal cord injury, Kendrick et al.[59] concluded that autonomic hyperreflexia syndrome does not develop if the lesion is below spinal dermatome T7. If the lesion is above spinal dermatome T7 (the splanchnic outflow), 60 to 70 percent of the patients exhibit extreme vascular instability. The trigger to this instability, or mass reflex involving noradrenergic and motor hypertonus,[46] can be a cutaneous, proprioceptive, or visceral (full bladder is a common initiator) stimulus. The sensation enters the spinal cord and causes a spinal reflex which in normal individuals is inhibited from above. Sudden increases in blood pressure are sensed in the aortic and carotid sinus pressure receptors which results in vagal hyperactivity producing bradycardia, ventricular ectopia, or various degrees of heart block. Reflex vasodilation above the level of the lesion may occur, resulting in flushing of the head and neck. Depending on the time since transection, the anesthesiologist must watch for certain other abnormalities. Acutely (less than 3 weeks from the time of

spinal shock), retention of urine and feces is common and may result in impairment of respiration due to elevated diaphragms; disimpaction is used to cure this respiratory problem. Hyperesthesia is present above the lesion; reflexes and flaccid paralysis are present below the lesion. The intermediate time period (3 days to 6 months) is marked by a hyperkalemic response to depolarizing drugs;[55] the chronic phase is marked by return of muscle tone, a positive Babinski sign, and frequently the occurrence of the hyperreflexia syndromes (mass reflex, see above). Thus, in addition to meticulous attention to perioperative volume and electrolyte status, the anesthesiologist should know—by history and laboratory data—about the status of the patient's myocardial conduction system (ECG), renal function (blood urea nitrogen [BUN]/creatinine), respiratory muscle involvement or lack thereof (FEV_1/FVC, see Ch. 42), chest roentgenogram if history and physical examination leads to a suspicion of atelectasis or pneumonia, temperature control, bone status (pathologic fractures are common as are decubiti), and urine and defecation systems (to prevent postoperative pneumonia or atelectasis from high diaphragm position).

THYROID DYSFUNCTION

HYPERTHYROIDISM

Thyroid Storm

This rare condition results from inadequately treated hyperthyroidism superimposed on another life-threatening condition.[60-62] Although there are several new and different laboratory tests for hyperthyroidism, they have added little additional information to that provided by the older tests.[63]

Thyroxine (T-4) (a product of the thyroid gland) and the more potent 3,5,3, triiodothyronine (T-3, a product of both the thyroid and extrathyroidal enzymatic deiodination of thyroxine) are the major thyroid hormones; this latter peripheral production occurs in many tissues (greatest in liver and kidney) and accounts for 80 percent of the T-3 produced.[64] Thyroid secretion is maintained by pituitary TSH secretion, which in turn is regulated by hypothalamic TRH secretion; it appears that TSH and TRH secretion are negatively regulated by T-4 and T-3. Peripheral T-4 to T-3 conversion is decreased in the normal fetus; in most patients with many illnesses, including acute or chronic starvation; and in patients receiving certain drugs, notably propylthiouracil, propranolol, glucocorticoids, and iopanoic acid (Telepaque). Because of this complexity, diagnosis of hyperthyroidism still rests on a total T-4 level (the majority of which is bound to thyroxine-binding globulin). Because thyroxine-binding globulin is abnormally increased in pregnancy, liver disease, and during estrogen therapy (all of which would elevate total T-4 levels), extra quantity of serum-protein binding sites for T-4 should be determined (by a T-3 resin uptake test). Multiplying total T-4 by T-3 resin uptake will provide a result that helps differentiate euthyroid from hypothyroid or hyperthyroid. The other tests—serum T-3 level, TSH concentration, response to TSH or TRH, thyroid scans with $^{99m}TcO_4$—either help differentiate primary (thyroidal) from pituitary or hypothalamic dysfunction or help decide on medical versus surgical therapeutic options.[65,66]

Hyperthyroidism is usually due to Graves' multinodular diffuse enlargement (also associated with ophthalmopathy, dermopathy) but also can occur during or after pregnancy,[67] accompanying subacute or chronic thyroiditis (with or without neck pain),[68] or because of a thyroid adenoma, choriocarcinoma, or TSH-secreting pituitary adenoma. Regardless of the particular cause of hyperthyroidism, the condition's major manifestations can include weight loss, diarrhea, warm moist skin, weakness of large muscle groups, nervousness, jitteriness, heat intolerance, tachycardia, atrial and ventricular arrhythmias, and heart failure.[69] In the apathetic form of hyperthyroidism, a form found most commonly in those over the age of 60, the cardiac manifestations of thyrotoxicosis —tachycardia, irregular heart beat, heart failure, and occasionally papillary muscle dysfunction—dominate the clinical picture. The proper approach to hyperthyroid patients is to make them pharmacologically euthyroid preoperatively; this effect may take 2 to 6 weeks. Chronically administered antithyroid drugs should be given the morning of surgery. When emergency operations are necessary before the euthyroid state is achieved or in case of hyperthyroidism out of control once surgery has begun, administration of propranolol intravenously, 0.2 to 10 mg, should be titrated to restore a normal heart rate. Also, intravascular fluid volume and electrolyte balance should be restored.[70,71] Propranolol does not invariably prevent thyroid storm, however.[72]

Hypothyroidism

The lack of thyroid hormone results in slow mental function, slow movement, dry skin, intolerance to cold, and bradycardia; in extreme cases cardiomegaly, heart failure, and pericardial and pleural effusions manifest as fatigue, dyspnea, and orthopnea.[69] The condition is often associated with amyloidosis, which may carry with it an enlarged tongue, abnormal cardiac conduction system, and renal disease. Anesthetic requirement is decreased by hypothyroidism.[73] The ideal preoperative management consists of restoring normal thyroid status; I routinely administer the normal T-3 or T-4 dose the morning of surgery even though these drugs have long half-lives (1.4 to 10 days). In patients with myxedema coma requiring emergency surgery, T-3 can be given intravenously (with fear of precipitating myocardial ischemia, however) while supportive therapy to restore normal intravascular fluid, heat, cardiac function, respiratory function, and electrolyte balance is undertaken.

PITUITARY ABNORMALITIES

ANTERIOR PITUITARY HYPERSECRETION

The three most common disorders of pituitary hypersecretion are those related to prolactin excess (amenorrhea, galactorhea, or infertility), ACTH excess (Cushing's disease), or growth hormone excess (acromegaly). In addition to knowing the pathophysiology of the disease involved, the anesthesiologist must know if an air pneumoencephalogram was recently performed. If so, the use of nitrous oxide should be avoided so as to avoid the risk of intracranial hypertension from collection of gas. Otherwise, no special preoperative evaluations are required for patients with the microchromophobe adenomas that most commonly cause prolactin excess[74] or for the transphenoidal surgery now commonly used for their removal.[75] Preoperative preparation of patients with Cushing's disease is included in the discussion of adrenal cortical excess.

Results of growth hormone excess stem both from direct tissue actions of the hormone and stimulation of the production of somatomedins. Excess growth hormone often results in retention of sodium and potassium, inhibition of the peripheral action of insulin (which can result in diabetes mellitus), and the occurrence of premature atherosclerosis (which is often associated with cardiomegaly). Exceptional dyspnea may be related either to heart failure or respiratory insufficiency due to kyphoscoliosis. Cardiac arrhythmias are common.[76] Thus preoperative

evaluation of the patient with acromegaly must begin by determining if the patient has significant cardiac, hypertensive, pulmonary, or diabetic problems. If these conditions are present, then preoperative evaluation should proceed along the lines stressed in those sections.

ANTERIOR PITUITARY HYPOFUNCTION

Anterior pituitary hypofunction results in deficiency of one or more of the following hormones: growth hormone, thyroid-stimulating hormone, adrenocorticotropin, prolactin, or gonadotropins. Preoperative preparation of those individuals deficient in adrenocorticotropin and thyroid-stimulating hormones is discussed above. No special preoperative preparation is required for the patient deficient in prolactin or gonadotropins; deficiency in growth hormone can result in atrophy of cardiac muscle, and this may require a preoperative cardiac evaluation. However, anesthetic problems have not been documented in patients with isolated growth hormone deficiency.

POSTERIOR PITUITARY EXCESS AND DEFICIENCY

Vasopressin (antidiuretic hormone) is the hormone whose secretion is increased with increased serum osmolality, or hypotension. Inappropriate secretion, without relation to serum osmolality, results in hyponatremia and fluid retention. This inappropriate secretion can result from a variety of central nervous system lesions, drugs such as nicotine, narcotics, clofibrate, vincristine, and cyclophosphamide, and ectopic production from tumors. Preoperative treatment includes appropriate treatment of the causative disorders and restriction of water. Occasionally, drugs that inhibit the renal response to ADH (e.g., lithium or demeclocycline) should be administered preoperatively to restore normal intravascular volume and electrolyte status. Lack of ADH results in diabetes insipidus and is caused by pituitary disease, brain tumors, head trauma, or lack of renal response to ADH. Preoperative treatment consists of restoring normal intravascular volume by replacing urine losses plus giving daily fluid requirements intravenously. In severe cases, desmopressin, a vasopressin analogue, is effective for 8 to 24 hours after a single intranasal administration and appears to be warranted preoperatively.[77]

DISORDERS OF CALCIUM METABOLISM

The three substances—parathyroid hormone, calcitonin, and vitamin D—that regulate the serum control of calcium, phosphorus, and magnesium act on bone, kidney, and gut. Parathyroid hormone stimulates bone resorbtion and inhibits renal excretion of calcium, both leading to hypercalcemia. Calcitonin can be considered a parathyroid hormone antagonist. Vitamin D through its metabolites aids in calcium, phosphate, and magnesium absorbtion from the gut and facilitates the bone resorbtive effects of parathyroid hormone.[78]

HYPERCALCEMIA

Hypercalcemia whether due to hyperparathyroidism, malignancy, renal failure, vitamin D intoxication, the milk alkali syndrome, sarcoidosis, or immobilization can present with the same constellation of symptoms: anorexia, vomiting, constipation, polyuria, polydipsia, lethargy, confusion, renal calculi, pancreatitis, bone pain, and psychiatric symptoms. About one third of patients with hypercalcemia are hypertensive; because the latter is a condition that resolves with successful treatment of hypercalcemia,[79] vigorous therapy of mild hypertension in the hypercalcemic patient is not advocated (see

hypertension and cardiovascular disease section). Long-standing hypercalcemia can lead to calcification in the myocardia, blood vessels, brain (which can present as seizures), and kidney (which can present as polyuria unresponsive to vasopressin).

Patients with moderate hypercalcemia who have normal renal and cardiovascular function present no special preoperative management problem. The electrocardiogram should be examined for signs of hypercalcemia (short PR interval, short QT interval) and can be followed intraoperatively for these signs. Severe hypercalcemia can result in a hypovolemic patient. Therefore, normal intravascular volume and electrolyte status should be restored prior to anesthesia and surgery. In emergency situations, vigorous intravascular volume expansion usually can reduce serum calcium to a safe level (less than 14 mg/dl). Administration of furosemide also is often helpful in these emergency situations. Mithramycin will lower calcium levels about 2 mg/dl in 36 to 48 hours, although that amount of time may not be available in an emergency situation. It is especially important to know whether hypercalcemia is chronic, as patients with long-standing hypercalcemia often have serious cardiac, renal, or central nervous system dysfunction.

HYPOCALCEMIA

Hypocalcemia (caused by hypoalbuminemia, one of the hypoparathyroid disorders, hypomagnesemia, or chronic renal disease) usually presents with no cardiovascular disorder. Since in patients with coexisting heart disease, congestive heart failure improves with restoration of calcium and magnesium levels to normal, these ion levels should be normal prior to surgery. QT prolongation is a reliable electrocardiographic sign of hypocalcemia. Sudden decreases in blood calcium concentration (as with chelation therapy) can result in severe hypotension.[80]

DISEASES INVOLVING THE CARDIOVASCULAR SYSTEM

HYPERTENSION

Because of the recent controversy on the appropriateness of preoperative treatment of patients with hypertension, the original articles that stimulated this controversy will be evaluated. Smithwick and Thompson[81] and Brown[82] reported an overall mortality rate in patients with hypertension undergoing sympathectomy between 1935 and 1947 of 2.5 to 3.6 percent respectively, five to six times those of patients with a normal blood pressure undergoing similar operations. Obviously these patients were not randomized to treatment or nontreatment groups, no attempt was made to insure end-organ disease was equivalent in the two groups, etc. In 1929, Sprague analyzed the records of 75 patients with hypertensive cardiac disease and found that 24 (32 percent) died during or shortly after operations employing general anesthesia.[83]

Obviously in the early part of this century severely ill paitents did not do well perioperatively, but whether preoperative treatment would have helped them is not known. The history of drug therapy of hypertension was hampered in the late 1950's and early 1960's by case reports of severe hypotension and bradyarrhythmias in patients receiving antihypertensives prior to surgery; the tailoring of anesthetic dose to patient, and the realization that sympatholytic antihypertensive drugs decreased anesthetic requirement[84] caused these events (or at least reports of them) to cease. A more recent prospective controlled, double-blind VA cooperative study gave a rationale for lifelong treatment of hypertension: such treatment decreased the incidence of stroke, congestive heart failure, and progression to renal insufficiency and to accelerated (malignant) hypertension.[85, 86] Berglund et al.[87] found a decrease in deaths due to myocardial infarction by treatment of patients with mild to moderate hypertension. United States statistics reveal sig-

nificant decreases (greater than 30 percent) in death rate from stroke over the last 12 years. Deaths related to hypertensive cardiovascular disease have decreased dramatically over the last 5 years, accounting for most of the decrease in cardiovascular death in this time period. This strong evidence from the VA studies and epidemiologic data has led to the belief that all patients with a diastolic blood pressure above 90 torr regardless of age should be treated. But should elective surgery be postponed, schedules disrupted, patients and doctors inconvenienced so that treatment can be instituted and stabilized? For the last 9 years anesthesiologists and internists quoted the study of Prys-Roberts et al.[88] Since 1979, Goldman and Caldera's[89] opposing article has been cited. Unfortunately both studies have deficiencies that prevent establishing a definitive answer to this question.

CRITICAL ANALYSIS OF THE DATA OF PRYS-ROBERTS ET AL.[88]

In this study, three groups were compared: 7 elderly controls with normal blood pressure (average mean arterial pressure = 89.5 torr); 7 untreated patients with hypertension, 4 of whom were under treatment (not of blood pressure) for complications of hypertension (average mean arterial pressure was 129.5 torr); 15 patients with hypertension who were being treated (average mean arterial pressure was 129 torr). Thus there was no difference in blood pressure between the treated and untreated patients with hypertension; in addition at least 4 of the 7 untreated patients with hypertension were "sicker" than any of the treated patients with hypertension. It was not described why some patients had their hypertension treated and others did not—it was definitely not done on a random basis. It was not stated whether the patients in different groups had similar surgery. These flaws in the design of the study create serious doubt as to whether the relationship between preoperative treatment of hypertension and peri-

Table 2-3. Treatment Groups in the Study by Goldman and Caldera[89] —
The More Sick Patients Preoperatively are in the Treated Hypertensive Group

Patient Group	Patients with Diastolic Blood Pressure Greater than 100 torr (Number)	Patients with Preoperative BUN Greater than 30 mg (%)	Patients with Preoperative Anginal History or Congestive Heart Failure (%)	Patients with Preoperative History of TIAs (%)	Average Preoperative Systolic Blood Pressure
Treated Hypertensives (n = 79)	0/79	8	47	13	136 ± 2
Unsuccessfully Treated Hypertensives (n = 40)	34/117	13	40	18	154 ± 2
Untreated Hypertensives (n = 77)		1	26	4	161 ± 2

operative morbidity can be objectively evaluated. However, the same dose of thiopental and halothane was given to all groups of patients, and measurements of absolute change in mean arterial blood pressure, cardiac arrhythmias, and electrocardiographic evidence of ischemia were performed. Patients with untreated hypertension had the greatest absolute fall in blood pressure and the highest percentage of arrhythmias and ischemia. The wisdom of administering the same dose of anesthetic to both groups of patients should be questioned. If the anesthetic had been titrated to the anesthetic needs of the patient, would the results be different? This study does indicate that sicker patients preoperatively have more problems perioperatively than healthy patients. This has been shown many times.[90-92] However, from these data the efficacy of preoperative treatment of hypertension cannot be established. This study and others by the same group does provide useful data on hemodynamic consequences of anesthesia with a standard technique on patients who have untreated hypertension.

CRITICAL ANALYSIS OF THE DATA OF GOLDMAN AND CALDERA[89]

In their introduction, Goldman and Caldera state that their study is a prospective one. However, an analysis of their study indicates that the only prospective aspect of their study was that patients were examined preoperatively; hypertensive patients were not randomly allocated into preoperative treatment, undertreatment, and nontreatment groups. They compared the outcomes of three groups: more sick hypertensives, less sick undertreated hypertensives, and less sick untreated moderate hypertensives; the study is thus flawed by lack of preoperative randomization of patients and nonrandom allocation of sicker patients to the treated hypertensive group (Table 2-3), thus biasing the study toward favoring nontreatment.

Only 34 of the 117 patients in the hypertensive groups had diastolic blood pressure of greater than or equal to 100 torr (Table 2-3). If morbid complications were predicted to be 20 percent in the untreated group and treatment predicted to cause a 50 percent reduction in morbidity, then by power analysis[93] Goldman and Caldera[89] would have had to compare about 237 patients to have a confidence level of 0.05 percent and an 80 percent chance of finding such a difference. If a lower complication rate (e.g., 15 percent) and a lesser decrease in the complication rate (e.g., 33 percent) are assumed, then more patients would have to be studied to be 80 percent sure no difference occurred even at the 0.05 level (such as 764 patients for 15 percent complication rate and 33 percent reduction in morbidity by treatment). Thus, three major flaws have been identified: lack of preoperative randomization, allocation of the more sick patients to the treated group, and too few patients from which to conclude that treatment makes no difference. These and other flaws in study design make it impossible to ascertain whether preoperative treatment of hypertension decreases perioperative risk.

RECOMMENDATIONS

Although preoperative systolic blood pressure has been found to be a significant predictor of postoperative morbidity,[94] there are no data that definitively establish whether preoperative treatment of hypertension reduces perioperative risk. Until a good study is performed (unfortunately, these are extremely difficult studies to conduct) I recommend that preoperative treatment of the patient with hypertension be based on the following logic:

1. Education of the patient that lifelong treatment is important.
2. The findings that the absolute perioperative hemodynamic fluctuations are less in treated versus untreated hypertensives (shown by Prys-Roberts et al.[88] and con-

firmed by Goldman and Caldera[89]) and that hemodynamic fluctuations have some relationship with morbidity.

In addition to deciding whether a hypertensive patient needs treatment and ensuring that none of the complications of antihypertensive drugs are present, a search for end-organ damage secondary to hypertension should be conducted: central nervous system changes and coronary artery, myocardial muscle, aortic, carotid, renal, and peripheral vascular changes. For example, the presence of renal disease may alter the choice and dosage of anesthetic drugs; similarly, recent myocardial ischemic changes may lead one to delay elective surgery. Knowing the location of myocardial ischemia may dictate which electrocardiograhic lead should be monitored intraoperatively (see Ch. 7). I also obtain multiple blood pressure readings in both arms in various positions to guide intraoperative blood pressure regulation, as well as to judge the effect and side effects of therapy. Major deviations from preoperative to intraoperative blood pressure levels have been correlated with myocardial ischemia in several studies.[88, 89, 95]

ISCHEMIC HEART DISEASE

The following evidence suggests ischemic heart disease: a history of vice-like chest pain, with or without radiation to the inner arm or neck; dyspnea on exertion, on exposure to cold, with defecation, or after eating; orthopnea; paroxysmal nocturnal dyspnea; nocturnal coughing; nocturia; previous or current peripheral or pulmonary edema; known previous myocardial infarction (MI); a family history of coronary artery disease; diagnosis of MI by electrocardiogram (ECG) or enzymes; and cardiomegaly. Patients with diabetes, hypertension (especially if cigarette smokers or hyperlipidemic[96]), left ventricular hypertrophy on ECG,[97] peripheral vascular disease, or unexplained tachycardia or fa-

tigue should also be suspected of having ischemic heart disease. The more difficult question is how common is ischemic heart disease in asymptomatic patients or in patients with a normal ECG but with other predisposing conditions? Tomatis et al.[98] recorded coronary angiograms on "nearly all patients" who presented for abdominal aortic aneurysm resection or aortoiliac reconstruction; of those with normal ECGs and a history *not* suggestive of coronary artery disease, 38 percent had greater than a 50 percent stenosis of one or more coronary arteries and 14 percent had greater than a 75 percent stenosis of one or more coronary arteries. These percentages of patients with stenosis were the same for asymptomatic patients with an abnormal ECG. However, a normal ECG was not as sensitive in ruling out significant stenosis: 44 percent of patients with a normal ECG and peripheral vascular disease had 50 percent or more stenosis of one or more coronary arteries and 30 percent had a 75 percent or greater stenosis. Benchimol et al.[97] have shown that 15 percent of patients with triple vessel coronary artery disease have a normal resting ECG. The point here is that *the history is the best index of coronary artery disease*, with a sensitivity and specificity of between 80 and 91 percent in most series[97–100] (see Ch. 1 for definition of sensitivity and specificity). The presence of coronary artery disease, its severity, the time that it most recently caused myocardial tissue death, which arteries are affected, its complications, and its treatment are important information because these factors may influence the manner in which anesthesia is given. Numerous epidemiologic studies[95, 101–108] (see Table 2-4) have shown that patients with a documented myocardial infarction within 6 months before an operation have a 5 to 86 percent reinfarction rate postoperatively (1.5 to 10 times as great as patients operated on more than 6 months after a myocardial infarction), with a mortality rate of 23 to 86 percent. After 6 months, the reinfarction rate seems to stabilize at 4 to 6 percent. Rejection for surgery of patients

Table 2-4. Incidence of Perioperative Myocardial Infarction (MI) or Mortality in Patients with Previous MI

Time From MI to Operation (Months)	Arkins et al.[101] 1963 (Mortality)	Topkins & Artusio[102] 1959–1963 (Reinfarction)	(Mortality)	Fraser et al.[103] 1960–1964 (Mortality)	Tarhan et al.[104] 1967–1968 (Reinfarction)	(Mortality)	Sapala et al.[105] 1970 (Reinfarction)	(Mortality)	Steen et al.[106] 1974–1975 (Reinfarction)	(Mortality)	Goldman et al.[107] 1975–1976 (Reinfarction)	(Cardiac Mortality)
0–3	40% 11/27	54.5% 12/22	*	38% 19/38	37% 3/8	*	86% 6/7	86% 6/7	27% 4/15		4.5% 1/22	23% 5/22
4-6	*			*	16% 3/19	*			11% 2/18			
7-12	*	25% 9/36	*	*	5% 2/42	*						
13-18	*	22.4% 11/49	*	*	4% 1/27	*					0% 0/13	8% 1/13
19-24	*			*	4% 1/21	*	5.7% 9/159	1.9% 3/159	5.4% 30/544			
25-36	*	5.9% 3/51	*	*	5% 11/232	*					3.3% 2/66	3.3% 2/66
> 36	*	1.0% 5/493	*	*								
Unknown	*	42.8% 3/7	*	*	9.6% 7/73	*						
Total patients with MI	*	6.5% 43/658	4.7% 31/658	*	6.6% 28/422	3% 15/422	9% 15/166	5.4% 9/166	6.1% 36/587	4.2% 25/587		8.9% 9/109

* Mortality not stated.

less than 6 months from a myocardial infarction should reduce anesthetic mortality. The less severe the coronary artery disease, the closer the patients' anticipated survival curve is to that of patients without coronary artery disease[109] and probably less is the perioperative risk.[110]

Much of the information upon which altered perioperative anesthetic management for ischemic heart disease is based derives from studying patients undergoing aortic to coronary artery bypass grafting procedures (CABG). Although CABG provides relief of angina and improvement in exercise tolerance (much like many "placebo" operations and pills before it[111]), improved survival occurs only for those with significant left main coronary artery disease[112, 113] and for those with mildly to moderately impaired left ventricular function.[114, 115] But recently, a potential new benefit of CABG surgery has been suggested. Several authors suggest that reduced perioperative morbidity during subsequent (noncardiac) operations may be an additional benefit of having survived CABG surgery.[110, 116–118] To provide definitive data for this hypothesis, a randomized, controlled study obviously is necessary: perhaps the intervening CABG surgery consisted of a survival test; that is, the CABG surgery caused reinfarction and/or death in those patients who would have had an MI or died after the noncardiac operation.[110] This appears to be a likely conclusion, since those patients who do poorly during and after CABG surgery are those with poor left ventricular function and increased left ventricular end-diastolic pressure.[119] Patients with these same cardiovascular variables also have an increased perioperative risk after noncardiac surgery.[107] So one proposal to decrease perioperative risk in patients severely disabled with angina (or ischemic heart disease) is to study their coronary arteries and do CABG surgery if the latter is indicated prior to their noncardiac surgery; as stated above, this hypothesis deserves a randomized clinical trial.

To summarize a large number of studies, preoperative findings that correlate with peri-

Table 2-5. New York Heart Association Classification of Angina[120]

I. *Ordinary physical activity does not cause angina,* such as walking or climbing stairs. Angina with strenuous or rapid prolonged exertion at work or recreation or with sexual relations.

II. *Slight limitation of ordinary activity.* Walking or climbing stairs rapidly, walking uphill, walking or stair climbing after meals, or in cold, or in wind, or under emotional stress, or only during a few hours after awakening. Walking more than two blocks on the level or more than one flight of stairs at a normal pace and in normal conditions.

III. *Marked limitation of ordinary physical activity.* Walking one or two blocks on the level and climbing one flight of stairs in normal conditions and at a normal pace. "Comfortable at rest."

IV. *Inability to carry on any physical activity without discomfort—anginal syndrome may be present at rest.*

operative morbidity and that can be corrected prior to operation are (1) recent myocardial infarction (within 6 months),[95, 101–108] (2) severe congestive heart failure (severe enough to produce rales, an S_3 gallop, or jugular venous distention),[105, 107, 119] (3) severity of angina (can be reduced preoperatively—see Table 2-5 for severity scale),[107, 120] (4) rhythm other than sinus,[105, 107] (5) premature atrial contractions,[107] (6) greater than 5 premature ventricular contractions per minute,[105, 107] and (7) BUN greater than 50 mg percent, or potassium less than 3.0 mEq/L.[107] Preoperative factors that correlate with perioperative risk but which cannot be altered include (1) old age (risk increases with increasing age),[90–92, 107, 121–125] (2) significant aortic stenosis,[107] (3) emergency operation,[90, 101, 107, 124] (4) cardiomegaly,[107, 126, 127] (5) history of congestive heart failure,[105, 107] (6) angina, or a history of angina or ischemia by electrocardiogram,[105, 107] (7) abnormal ST segment or inverted or flat T waves on ECG,[107] abnormal QRS on ECG,[107] and (8) significant mitral regurgitant murmur.[107] Significant intraoperative factors that perhaps can be avoided or altered that correlated with perioperative risk are (1) unnecessary use of vasopressors,[128] (2) inadvertent hypotension,[95, 107] (this is debatable, as some authors have found inadvertent hypotension to not be correlated with perioperative morbidity),[121, 125] (3) a high rate-pressure product (heart rate times systolic blood pressure exceeding 11,000),[129] and (4) long operations.[101, 106, 107, 124] Significant intraoperative factors that correlate with perioperative risk and probably cannot be avoided are (1) emergency surgery and (2) thoracic, intraperitoneal, or above the knee amputation operations.[104, 106, 107, 122, 123]

Although the evidence for the factors listed above is fairly substantial, the diligent reader should know that virtually none of the data is from prospective randomized studies that indicate that treatment of the above conditions reduces the perioperative risk to patients with ischemic heart disease. Nevertheless, all logic dictates that such treatment does reduce risk. Thus, the goal in giving anesthesia to patients with ischemic heart disease is to have the patient in optimal shape preoperatively by treating those conditions that correlate with perioperative risk; then one monitors intraoperatively for conditions that correlate with perioperative risk and by that monitoring and attentiveness to detail avoids those circumstances that lead to perioperative risk. Although local anesthesia may reduce the perioperative risk,[92, 105, 130] the epidemiologic studies do not reveal significant differences in perioperative morbidity rates for patients with ischemic heart disease anesthetized with local as opposed to general anesthetics.

The preoperative evaluation should include a review of exercise studies and coronary angiogram to know what ECG lead to monitor for ischemia—the lead on exercise ECG that first reveals ischemia or the surface lead best representative of the stenosed artery should theoretically show ischemia first in the operating room, but no study proving this has been done. If no exercise or coronary angiogram study has been done, precordial lead V_5 is preferred.[129, 131] Since at this time, not much other than maintaining diastolic blood pressure, hemoglobin concentration, and oxygen saturation can be done to increase oxygen supply to the myocardium of patients with coronary artery stenosis, the main thrust of anesthesia practice has been to decrease the determinants of myocardial oxygen demand.[1] The determinants of myocardial oxygen demand are heart rate, ventricular wall tension, and contractile performance.[132] Thus, medical management to accomplish the goal of preserving all viable myocardial tissue possibly includes β-adrenergic blockade (propranolol or metoprolol) to decrease contractility and heart rate, and venodilatation or arteriolar dilatation (nitroglycerin [or its "long acting" analogues], nitroprusside, hydralazine, prazosin) to decrease ventricular wall tension. The goal of anesthesia management should be the same, although no prospective controlled studies document the benefit of preload or afterload reduction or decreased heart rate to perioperative morbidity. The goal of keeping the rate pressure product below anginal threshold appears appropriate, however.[130, 133, 134] The use of Swan-Ganz lines for this type of patient is dealt with in Chapter 6, and the intraoperative management of ischemic heart disease patients is discussed in further detail in Chapter 30. Briefly, I believe drugs given chronically should be continued through the morning of surgery. These patients usually need those drugs (e.g., antihypertensive medications). This subject is covered in more detail in the last section of this chapter. Finally, a patient with a subendocardial myocardial infarction is assumed to be at less perioperative risk than a patient with a transmural myocardial infarction. This is now in question in medical circles.[135] Thus, patients with subendocardial infarctions should be treated no differently than those with transmural infarctions.

VALVULAR HEART DISEASE

Major alterations in the preoperative management of patients with valvular heart disease have been made in anticoagulant usage and etiology. Although preoperative and intraoperative management of patients with valvular heart disease are discussed in Chapter 30, a few important points concerning preoperative care are emphasized here. Of prime importance is realizing that management of stenotic or regurgitant lesions of the same valve is exactly opposite and that the predominant lesion must be established preoperatively. Although the etiology of various forms of valvular heart disease has not changed, the relative frequency has. Rheumatic valvulitis is much less common than it was 10 years ago, and syphilitic aortitis has all but disappeared. Congenital bicuspid aortic stenosis, prolapsed mitral valve, asymmetric septal hypertrophy (subvalvular aortic stenosis), and calcified mitral insufficiency are now common diagnoses. Mitral valve prolapse is perhaps the most frequent valvular abnormality, occurring in about 5 percent of otherwise healthy people and associated with secundum atrial septal defects.[136, 137] This autosomal dominant valvular lesion presents either asymptomatically, or with palpitations, dyspnea, atypical chest pain, dizziness, syncope, or sudden death. Supraventricular arrhythmias (associated with atrioventricular bypass tracts and the preexcitation syndrome) occur in over 50 percent of patients with mitral valve prolapse, ventricular arrhythmias in 45 percent, bradyarrhythmias in 25 percent, and sudden death in 1.4 percent.[137, 138] Transient cerebral ischemic events have lead to the chronic use of anticoagulants in this group, and the potential for endocarditis has led to the recommendation for prophylaxis with antibiotics during predictable bacteremic events.[137, 138] The prognosis and presumably the perioperative risk for patients with valvular heart disease are dependent on the stage of disease. Stenotic lesions progress faster than regurgitant ones, but regurgitant lesions secondary to infective endocarditis or ischemic heart disease can be rapidly fatal. Left ventricular dysfunction is common in the late stage of valvular heart disease.

Preoperative maintenance of drug therapy can be crucial: the patient with aortic stenosis can deteriorate rapidly with the onset of atrial fibrillation or flutter, as the atrial component to left ventricular filling can be critical to maintaining cardiac output. One of the most serious complications of valvular heart surgery and of valvular heart disease prior to surgery are cardiac arrhythmias. Conduction disorders are discussed in the next section of this chapter; chronic antiarrhythmic and ionotropic drug therapy is discussed in the last section of this chapter, but anticoagulant therapy and preoperative antibiotics deserve mention here. Patients with all forms of valvular heart disease as well as with intracardiac (VSD, ASD) or intravascular shunts should have prophylaxis against endocarditis at the time of predictable bacteremic events; endocarditis has occurred in a significant number of patients with subvalvular aortic stenosis (asymmetric septal hypertrophy) and mitral valve prolapse to warrant patients with these lesions to be included in the prophylaxis regimen. Is endotracheal intubation a predictable bacteremic event? Bacteremia follows dental extraction 30 to 80 percent of the time, brushing teeth 20 to 24 percent, use of oral irrigation devices 20 to 24 percent, barium enema 11 percent, transurethral prostate resection 10 to 57 percent, upper gastrointestinal endoscopy 8 percent, nasotracheal intubation 16 percent (4 of 25 patients), and orotracheal intubation 0 percent (0 of 25 patients).[139, 140] Thus, although bacteremia from orotracheal intubation is rare, we believe antimicrobial prophylaxis should be given to valvular heart disease patients before instrumentation of the gall bladder, gastrointestinal tract, oropharynx, and genitourinary tract. Antibiotic choice for prophylaxis should be aimed at the statistically most common pathogen. The guidelines state that all antimicrobial prophylaxis be started 30 minutes to 1 hour prior to predictable bacteremia rather than 24 hours in advance so as to reach therapeutic levels but not to obtain superinfection with unusual pathogens.[141]

Oral anticoagulants can be discontinued safely in patients with prosthetic aortic valves several days in advance to provide a normal prothrombin time preoperatively. Because the risk of thromboembolism is greater with mitral valve prosthesis, rapid reversal of oral anticoagulation with vitamin K should be instituted only the day before surgery, and rapid reanticoagulation with heparin 12 hours postoperatively has proved successful.[142] The patient with a new aortic valve should be reanticoagulated with heparin 2 days postoperatively. Not having the prothrombin time within 20 percent of control does carry an appreciable risk (Tinker JH, Tarhan S, ASA Abstracts 1976, pp 435–436). Regional anesthetic techniques probably should be avoided.[143, 144]

CONDUCTION DISTURBANCES

Bradyarrhythmias, especially if profound or associated with dizziness or syncope, are generally managed with pacemakers. Controversy still exists, however, over the frequency with which chronic bifascicular block (right bundle branch block with left anterior or posterior hemiblock) even with the concomitant presence of first degree heart block progresses to complete heart block and sudden death. Preoperative bifascicular block recently was found not to predispose to intraoperative or postoperative complete heart block; thus, prophylactic preoperative insertion of temporary pacing wires in this condition does not seem warranted.[145] However, a route to pass a temporary pacemaker should be established. The equipment and appropriate personnel should be available.[145]

Premature ventricular contractions (PVCs greater than 5 per minute) on preoperative examination correlate with perioperative cardiac morbidity.[107] Recent studies,[146] however, throw doubt on classic criteria for treating PVCs (R on T, couplets, greater than 3 per minute, multifocality)—see Chapter 7. Chronic antiarrhythmic therapy is discussed in the last section of this Chapter (Ch. 2).

Premature atrial contractions, and rhythm other than sinus, also correlated with perioperative cardiac morbidity in the Massachusetts General Hospital study.[107] Perhaps these arrhythmias are a marker of poor cardiovascular reserve, rather than a specific risk for perioperative cardiac complications.

Preexcitation syndromes[147] is the new name for those supraventricular tachycardias associated with atrioventricular bypass tracts. Successful treatment is predicated upon understanding the clinical and electrophysiological manifestations and uses a preoperative and intraoperative technique tailored to avoid sympathetic and other vasoactive substance release which may lead to tachyarrhythmias.[147, 148]

The types of pacemakers and indications for their use have significantly changed over the past 5 years. Lithium batteries now allow a pacemaker to have a 5- to 10-year life span. Programmable pacemakers allow adjustment of sensitivity and rates. Atrial pacemakers fired by an outside radio frequency source now allow termination of reentrant or preexcitation atrial arrhythmias; similarly, ventricular pacemakers can be used to terminate supraventricular tachycardia and recurrent ventricular tachycardia.[149] Thus, in addition to learning facts about the patient's underlying disease, current condition and drug therapy, the anesthesiologist must preoperatively learn the following:[150, 151]

1. the indication for pacemaker placement, and what rhythm "occurs" if pacemaker does not capture,
2. what type of pacemaker is in place (demand, fixed, or radiofrequency),
3. how to spot deterioration in battery function (increased rate or decreased rate),
4. how to alter modes or how to fire if it is a radiofrequency,
5. the current rate and sensitivity settings,
6. if the pacemaker is currently functioning and how well, and
7. what placement (atrial versus ventricular) has been used.

Demand pacemakers can sense electrocautery which inhibit pacemaker frequency firing and thus can result in asystole for the pacemaker-dependent patient. Most pacemakers can be converted to fixed rate, and the anesthesiologist should have the cardiologist (1) demonstrate how to do this and (2) have the magnet to do it with available in the operating room. In addition, the ground plate should be as far from the pulse generator and lead as possible, a bipolar form of electrocautery should be used, and if possible, some measure of blood flow should be monitored: i.e., Doppler detector or intra-arterial line. The rationale for the latter measure is the electrocautery "hiding" of the electrocardiograms; since asystole could occur during this period, a measure of blood flow is necessary. During the preoperative examination the anesthesiologist must also assess the progression of underlying disease (congestive heart failure, etc.) as well as electrolyte disorders and all systems appropriate to the underlying disease.[150]

DISORDERS OF THE RESPIRATORY AND IMMUNE SYSTEMS

The main purpose of preoperative testing is to identify patients at risk for complications and institute appropriate perioperative therapy. Also preoperative assessment should establish the feasibility of surgical intervention and establish baseline function. Whereas numerous investigators have used pulmonary function tests that define inoperability or high versus low risk groups for pulmonary complications, few have shown reduction of perioperative pulmonary morbidity or motality by any preoperative or intraoperative measures. Since routine preoperative pulmonary testing and care is extensively discussed in Chapters 29 and 42, this discussion is restricted to assessing how effective this care has been shown to be. In fact, only two randomized prospective studies indicate a benefit of preoperative preparation. Stein and Cassara[152] randomly allocated 48 patients into preoperative therapy (cessation of smoking; use of antibiotic treatment of purulent sputum, bronchodilator drugs, postural drainage, chest physical therapy, and ultrasonic nebulizer) or no therapy groups. The no treatment group had a 16 percent mortality and 60 percent morbidity rate, compared to 0 and 20 percent respectively for the treatment group. In addition, the treatment group spent an average of 12 postoperative days in the hospital, compared to 24 days for the 21 survivors in the no treatment group.

Collins et al.[153] also prospectively examined the benefits of preoperative antibiotics, perioperative chest physiotherapy and bronchodilator treatment, and routine postoperative analgesia (morphine) on postoperative respiratory complications in patients with chronic obstructive pulmonary disease. They found a benefit from preoperative antibiotic treatment but no benefit from chest physiotherapy and bronchodilation or from routine analgesia. Several investigators, however, have shown a benefit from prophylactic treatment. These studies usually are nonrandomized or at best poorly controlled, or retrospective and thus probably substantially influenced by the bias of the investigator.[154, 155] Although recent randomized prospective studies show *no* benefit of chest physiotherapy and intermittent positive-pressure breathing on the resolution of pneumonia[156] or postoperative pulmonary complications,[153, 157–162] the two studies cited above[152, 153] and the numerous retrospective studies[154, 155] strongly suggest that preoperative evaluation and treatment of patients with pulmonary disease actually decrease perioperative respiratory complications.

The specific pulmonary function tests that alert one to a high risk group are reviewed in Chapter 42, but as evaluation of dyspnea is especially valuable, this condition is also reviewed here. Boushy et al.[163] found that grades of preoperative dyspnea correlated with postoperative survival. The grades of respiratory dyspnea are listed in Table 2-6. Mittman[164] demonstrated an increased risk of death after thoracic surgery from 8 percent without dyspnea to 56 percent with dyspnea at rest. Similarly, Reichel[165] found that no

Table 2-6. Grade of Dyspnea Caused by Respiratory Problems (Assess in Terms of Walking on the Level at a Normal Pace)[163]

Category	Description
0	No dyspnea while walking on the level at a normal pace
I	"I am able to walk as far as I like provided I take my time"
II	Specific (street) block limitation ("I have to stop for a while after one or two blocks")
III	Dyspnea on mild exertion ("I have to stop and rest while going from the kitchen to the bathroom")
IV	Dyspnea at rest

patients died after pneumonectomy if able to complete a preoperative treadmill test for 4 minutes at 2 miles per hour on level ground. Other than dyspnea, what patient groups or characteristics make respiratory complications more likely? (Also see Chapter 29.) The important findings to search for on the history and physical examination are:

1. Dyspnea.
2. Cough and sputum production. Sputum, if present, should be Gram stained and cultured and appropriate antibiotic treatment should be instituted.
3. Recent respiratory infection. Viral respiratory infections do affect respiratory function, giving rise to increased airflow obstruction that may persist for at least 5 weeks.[166] They also adversely affect respiratory defense mechanisms against bacteria.[167–168]
4. Hemoptysis.
5. Wheezing, and prior use of bronchodilators and corticosteroids. Wheezing often suggests potentially reversible airway obstruction, but is a notoriously bad indicator of the degree of obstruction. Asthmatics have a fourfold increase in perioperative respiratory complications.
6. Pulmonary complications from previous surgery. Prolonged intubation after surgery can be due to many factors, most probably respiratory and neuromuscular disorders.
7. Smoking history. The incidence of respiratory complications is higher among tobacco smokers than nonsmokers.[154, 155, 169]
8. Age, general history, and physical findings. Other disease conditions probably increase respiratory risk, although this has not been adequately documented. Old age definitely increases respiratory risk as it does cardiac risk.[163, 169, 170] Cardiovascular history and examination are obviously important for risk by themselves and especially for signs of pulmonary hypertension, such as right ventricular lift (lift over the lower sternum), fixed and widely split second heart sound, and S_4 gallop at the left sternal border.
9. Breathing frequency and form. Purse lips, cyanosis, and use of accessory muscles should be noted.
10. Body habitus:
    a. Abnormalities of the chest wall—trauma—kyphoscoliosis with restrictive lung disease. Development of a barrel chest is a late manifestation of obstructive lung disease.
    b. Obesity. A weight of 30 percent over ideal weight doubles respiratory complications.[155, 169, 171]
11. Adequacy of upper airway, tracheal deviation, ease of face mask application, ease of endotracheal intubation.
12. Chest examination for rales, rhonchi, wheezing, diaphragmatic excursion, air movement, expiratory to inspiratory time ratio.
13. Site of proposed surgery. Upper abdominal surgery increases perioperative pulmonary risk.[152, 155]

Chapters 29 and 42 review the value of the chest roentgenograms and pulmonary function tests in identifying patients with preoperative pulmonary disease and which tests should be ordered and for whom. If ventilator support will be required postoperatively, I believe preoperative tests should be conducted (this includes anybody with grade II or above dyspnea and anybody with significant abnormalities on the 12 points above).

Despite the lack of definitive data establishing the efficacy of preoperative pulmonary testing and therapy, I recommend the following approach:

1. Eradicate acute and suppress chronic infections by using appropriate diagnostic measures and antibiotic treatment.

2. Relieve bronchospasm by using bronchodilators, and document such relief with FEV_1 measurements (see Chs. 29 and 43).

3. Institute measures to improve sputum clearance to familiarize the patient with respiratory therapy equipment (incentive spirometry) and postural drainage maneuvers. Initiate practice coughing and deep breathing. (See Chs. 29 and 43.)

4. Treat uncompensated right heart failure with digoxin, diuretics, oxygen, and drugs that decrease pulmonary vascular resistance (e.g., hydralazine).

5. Use low dose heparin prophylactically to decrease the incidence of venous thrombosis (and hopefully pulmonary emboli).

6. Encourage reduction or cessation of smoking. Pulmonary function begins to improve in a few weeks after cessation of smoking.[172, 173] Even young people who only smoke ½ to 1 pack of cigarettes per day have abnormalities of respiratory function.[174]

SPECIFIC DISEASES

PULMONARY VASCULAR DISEASES[175]

Pulmonary hypertension secondary to heart disease, parenchymal lung disease, pulmonary embolism, and cor pulmonale from chronic obstructive lung disease are classified as pulmonary vascular diseases. Optimal preoperative treatment of these patients requires treating their underlying disease.[176, 177] If possible, the reactivity of the pulmonary vasculature should be determined, for it may be responsive to pharmacologic vasodilation with agents such as hydralazine, prazosin, tolazoline or phentolamine (Regitine). Monitoring of pulmonary artery pressure is often required; preoperative measures should be

undertaken to insure the patient is not exposed to conditions that elevate pulmonary vascular resistance (hypoxia, hypercarbia, acidosis, lung hyperinflation, cold), decrease systemic vascular resistance, or decrease blood volume (prolonged restriction of fluid intake).

Infectious Diseases of the Lung

Preoperative evaluation and treatment should follow the basic guidelines outlined in the introductory section of this chapter; treatment of the underlying disease should be completed before all but emergency surgery is performed. Viral respiratory infections do affect respiratory function, giving rise to increased airflow obstruction (especially in the small airways) that may persist for at least 5 weeks.[166] They also adversely affect respiratory defense mechanisms against bacteria.[168]

Chronic Obstructive Pulmonary Diseases

Treatment of chronic obstructive diseases (reactive airways) may include use of β-adrenergic drugs, parasympatholytic agents (especially for exercise-induced asthma), and corticosteroids. A trend towards using topical steroids, such as baclomethasone diprorionate, which are inactivated after absorbtion, has begun. However, in large doses these "topical" steroids can cause supression of adrenal function and supplemental systemic corticosteroids may be needed at times of stress. Preoperative assessment must include knowledge of drug regimens and effects, as these drugs can have dangerous interactions with anesthetic agents (see last section of this chapter). An estimated 10 percent of asthmatics have aspirin sensitivity and may react not only to aspirin-containing compounds, but also to tartrazine, yellow dye No. 5, indomethecin, and aminopyrine.[178, 179] Bronchial asthma occurs in 3 to 5 percent of the population and is characterized by reversible airway obstruction. Partially reversible airway obstruction also is often present with chronic bronchitis. A history of chronic cough and sputum production on most days for 3 months per year for at least 2 years usually guarantees the presence of chronic bronchitis. These patients are or almost always have been smokers, although environmental and occupational or genetic predisposition may play a role in the hypertrophy of mucous glands in major airways, hyperplasia of goblet cells, and edema and inflammation of airways. Hyperinflation of airspaces, abnormal dilatation and destruction of acinar units distal to the terminal bronchiole defines emphysema. Cystic fibrosis is characterized by dilatation and hypertrophy of bronchial glands, mucous plugging of peripheral airways, and often bronchitis, bronchiectasis, and bronchiolectasis. For all of these conditions, the measures recommended in the introduction as well as appropriate hydration to allow for mobilization of secretions should be followed.

Interstitial and Immune Lung Diseases

Included in this heterogeneous group of diseases are the hypersensitivity lung diseases, the inorganic dust diseases, radiation-induced lung disease, sarcoidosis, the collagen-vascular disorders (systemic lupis erythematosis, polymyositis, dermatomyositis, Sjogren's syndrome, rheumatoid arthritis, systemic sclerosis), Goodpasture's syndrome, idiopathic pulmonary hemosiderosis, Wegener's granulomatosis, and the autoimmune diseases. Many of these disorders affect blood vessels, the conduction system of the heart, the myocardium, the joints including those of the upper airway and larynx, and the renal, hepatic and/or central nervous systems in addition to the lung; the reader is referred to a textbook of internal medicine to aid in understanding the pathophysiology and full

preoperative assessment of these conditions. The therapy of these conditions includes use of antiinflammatory drugs, corticosteroids, and immunosuppressives.

Neoplasms

Solitary nodules are less than 6 cm in diameter, surrounded by lung parenchyma, and are *not* associated with adenopathy or pleural effusion. The cure rate for bronchogenic carcinoma presenting as a solitary nodule is 40 percent, much better than other presentations.[180] Oat-cell (small cell) carcinoma of the lung and bronchial adenomas are known for their secretion of endocrinologically active substances, such as ACTH-like hormones. Squamous cell cancers in the superior pulmonary sulcus cause characteristic pain in the areas served by the eighth cervical and first and second thoracic nerves and Horner's syndrome. These tumors are now treated with preoperative radiation, and surgical resection leading to an almost 30 percent cure rate.[181]

Allergic Disorders Other Than Lung Diseases and Asthma

Anaphylaxis is the typical immediate hypersensitivity reaction mediated through IgE with vasodilation at the level of the capillary and postcapillary venule leading to erythema, edema, and smooth muscle contraction. The term anaphalactoid reaction denotes an identical or very similar clinical response that is not IgE mediated, and usually not antigen-antibody mediated. Intravenous contrast material is probably the most frequent agent causing anaphalactoid reactions. Since diagnostic (skin and other) tests are helpful only in IgE-mediated reactions, pretesting is not useful in contrast reactions. Pretreatment with diphenhydramine, cimetidine, and corticosteroids have been reported as useful in preventing anaphalactoid reactions due to intravenous contrast material, but use of very large doses of steroids (1 g of methyl predni-solone IV) may be necessary.[182-184] The efficacy of large dose steroid therapy has not been confirmed. The anesthesiologist should be prepared preoperatively to treat a true anaphalactoid response.

The primary immunodeficiency diseases usually present early in life with recurrent infections. Survival due to antibiotic and antibody treatment has led to new prominent features, cancer, and allergic and autoimmune disorders.

Heredity angioedema is an autosomal dominant genetic disease characterized by episodes of angioedema involving the subcutaneous tissues and submucosa of the gastrointestinal tract and the airway and often presenting as abdominal pain. These patients have a deficiency of an inhibitor to the C_1 complement component, or have a functionally impotent inhibitor. Treatment of an acute attack is mainly supportive because epinephrine, antihistamines, and corticosteroids fail to work. Plasma transfusions have been reported to resolve attacks. Attacks can be prevented or decreased in severity by drugs that are either plasmin inhibitors (such as epsilon-aminocaproic acid and tranexamic acid) or androgens (such as Danazol). Because trauma can precipitate acute attacks, prophylactic therapy with Danazol, intravenous epsilon-aminocaproic acid, plasma, or all three is recommended prior to elective surgery.[185]

DISEASES OF THE CENTRAL NERVOUS SYSTEM, NEUROMUSCULAR DISEASES, AND PSYCHIATRIC DISORDERS

Performing the history and physical examination suggested in Chapter 1 should aid in detecting almost all patients with significant neurologic or psychiatric disease. Historical information that might trigger further search includes the previous need for postoperative ventilation in a patient without inordinate lung disease (metabolic neurologic disorders such as porphyria; alcoholic myopathy; other myopathies; neuropathies; and neuromuscular disorders such as myasthenia gravis) and drug therapy (steroids; guanidine; anticonvulsant, anticoagulant, and antiplatelet drugs; lithium; tricyclic antidepressants; phenothiazines; butyrophenones). Although preoperative treatment of the majority of neurologic disorders has not been reported to lessen perioperative morbidity, knowledge of the pathophysiology of these disorders is important in planning intraoperative and postoperative management. Thus preoperative knowledge about these disorders and their associated conditions (such as cardiac arrhythmias with Duchenne muscular dystrophy or respiratory and cardiac muscle weakness in dermatomyositis) may reduce perioperative morbidity. A major thrust of neurologic diagnosis is localization of the lesion in the nervous system. To the outsider this may seem like an intellectual exercise, but to the neurologist localization is essential for the diagnosis and to guide management. The best anesthetic for diagnostic procedures of these conditions may well be the best anesthetic for the surgery of the condition itself. (Disorders with increased intracranial pressure and cerebrovascular disorders are covered in Chs. 25 and 33 respectively.)

COMA

Little is written about anesthesia for the comatose patient, but like all other conditions it is imperative to know *why* the patient is in coma so that drugs can be avoided which will make the coma worse or which will not be metabolized by organs that are not working. First the patient should be observed. Yawning, swallowing, or licking of the lips implies a "light" coma with major brain-stem function intact. If consciousness is depressed but respiration, pupillary response, and eye movements are normal and no focal motor signs are present, metabolic depression is likely (pupillary responses may be abnormal, however, when there is hypoxia, hypothermia, local eye disease, use of eye drops, or drug intoxication with belladonna alkaloids, narcotics, or gluthethemide). Other metabolic causes of coma include uremia, hypoglycemia, hepatic coma, alcohol ingestion, hypophosphatemia, myxedema, and hyperosmolar nonketotic coma. Except in extreme emergencies, such as uncontrolled bleeding or perforated viscus, care should be taken to render the patient as metabolically normal as possible preoperatively to avoid confusion over the etiology of intraoperative problems. However, too rapid correction of uremia or hyperosmolar nonketotic coma can lead to cerebral edema—a shift of water into the brain from a reverse urea effect.

Arms flexed at the elbow implies bilateral hemisphere dysfunction but intact brain stem (decorticate posture), while extension of legs and arms implies bilateral damage to structures at the upper brain stem or deep hemisphere level (bilateral decerebrate posture). Seizures are often seen in uremia and other metabolic encephalopathies. Hyperreflexia and upgoing toes suggests a structural CNS lesion or uremia, hypoglycemia, or hepatic coma; hyporeflexia and downgoing toes with no hemiplegia generally means there is no structural CNS lesion.[186]

EPILEPTIC SEIZURES

Epilesy results from paroxysmal neuronal discharges from abnormally excitable neurons; it can be generalized (arises from deep midline structures in the brain-stem or thalamus, usually without aura or focal features during the seizure) or partial focal motor or sensory (the initial discharge comes from a focal unilateral area of brain, often preceeded by an aura). As with cerebrovascular accidents and coma, knowing the origin may be crucial to understanding the pathophysiology of the patient and guiding his intraoperative and postoperative course. Seizures can arise from alcohol withdrawal, uremia, posttraumatic injury, neoplasm, congenital malformation, birth injury, drug usage (amphetamines), hypercalcemia and hypocalcemia, vascular disease and vascular accidents, or no known cause. The patient with epilepsy requires no special anesthetic management other than for the disease that caused the epilepsy. Anticonvulsant medication levels should be in the therapeutic range[187-190] and continued through the morning of surgery and be given postoperatively. High concentrations of enflurane (especially with hyperventilation) can be associated with electroencephalographic evidence of epileptic activity and tonic clonic movements.[191-193] These seizures do not appear to have any serious sequelae based on lack of reports of sequelae in humans, and some human studies.[191] Enflurane anesthesia does not appear to increase seizure activity in patients with a history of convulsive disorders, and even suppresses seizures induced by electroshock, pentylenetetrazole, strychnine, picrotoxin, or bemegride.[194-196] Thus, other than precautions taken for underlying diseases and current drug therapy, no known perioperative management appears indicated.

INFECTIOUS DISEASES OF THE CNS, DEGENERATIVE CNS DISORDERS, AND HEADACHE

Many of the degenerative central nervous system disorders have been traced to slow virus diseases. We know of no special perioperative anesthetic considerations (other than those for increased intracranial pressure; see Chs. 25 and 33) for the infectious central nervous system disorders.

Parkinson's disease is a degenerative central nervous system disorder that may or may not be due to a virus; clinically, chronic manganese intoxication, phenothiazine or butyrophenone toxicity, Wilson's disease, Huntington's chorea, and carbon monoxide encephalopathy all present with similar features: bradykinesia, rigidity, and tremor. The substantia nigra degenerates, and the clinical signs presumably result from decreased dopamine production in the neurons of the basal ganglia leading to the putamen and caudate. The effects of this dopaminergic deficiency may be compounded by the unopposed cholinergic neurons bordering the basal ganglia. Therapy is thus directed either at increasing neuronal dopaminergic release or receptor response to dopamine or at decreasing cholinergic activity. Anticholinergic agents are first-line drugs and help the tremor more than the rigidity. Since dopamine does not pass the blood-brain barrier, its precursor L-dopa (levodopa) is used. L-dopa, unfortunately, is decarboxylated in the periphery to dopamine, where it can cause nausea, vomiting, and arrhythmias. These side effects are diminished by administration of α-methylhydrazine (Carbidopa), a decarboxylase inhibitor that does not pass through the blood-brain barrier. Refractoriness to L-dopa therapy develops, and its use is now restricted largely to individuals whose symptoms cannot be controlled with anticholinergic medication. Therapy for Parkinson's disease should be continued through the morning of surgery; by this treatment, drooling, the aspiration potential, and ventilatory weakness are apparently diminished.[197-200] Reinstituting therapy promptly after anesthesia is important,[197] as is avoidance of drugs that compete with dopamine at the receptor such as phenothiazines and butyrophenones (droperidol).[201]

Over 90 percent of patients with chronic recurring headaches are diagnosed as having migraine, tension, or cluster headaches. The mechanism of tension or cluster headaches may not be qualitatively different from the mechanism of migraine headaches; all may be manifestations of labile vasomotor regulation.[202] The treatment for cluster and migraine headaches centers around ergotamine and its derivatives. Other therapies that may be effective are propranolol, cyproheptadine, prednisone, antihistamines, tricyclic antidepressants, phenytoin, diuretics, and biofeedback.[203] Giant-cell arteritis and glaucoma are other causes of headache that might benefit from treatment before operation. Other than knowing about the drugs and drug effects that these patients have (see last section of this chapter), no special preoperative workup is indicated for the patient who has a well-delineated cause for his headaches. Acute migraine attacks can sometimes be terminated by ergotamine tartrate aerosol or injection of dihydroergotamine mesylate intravenously, and general anesthesia has been used. I normally continue all prophylactic headache medicines, except aspirin (because of bleeding, see Ch. 28), through the morning of surgery.

BACK, NECK PAIN, AND SPINAL CANAL SYNDROMES

Acute spinal cord injury is covered in the autonomic dysfunction section of this chapter. Little is written about the anesthetic management of syndromes related to herniated disk, spondylosis (usually of advancing age), and congenital narrowing of cervical and lumbar canal giving rise to symptoms of nerve root compression. Other than the common sense approach of seeking neurosurgical consultation or if necessary using awake positioning of these individuals in a comfortable position prior to emergency root-decompressing procedures, no special procedures appear necessary.

DEMYLINATING DISEASES

This is a diffuse group of diseases ranging from those with no as yet known etiology (such as multiple sclerosis) to those that are postinfection or postvaccination (such as Guillain-Barré syndrome) or postantimetabolite treatment of cancer, and patients can present with very diverse symptoms. Apparently, there is a risk of relapse of these diseases immediately postoperatively;[204] thus far no mode of treatment has been shown to alter these disease processes, although ACTH and steroids may ameliorate or abbreviate a relapse, especially of multiple sclerosis.

METABOLIC DISEASES

Included in this category are nervous system dysfunction secondary to porphyrias, alcoholism, uremia, hepatic failure, and vitamin B_{12} deficiency. The periodic paralysis that can accompany thyroid disease is discussed in the neuromuscular disorder section that follows this section.

Alcoholism or heavy alcohol intake is associated with acute alcoholic hepatitis (the activity of which declines as the presumed toxin, alcohol, is withdrawn), a myopathy and cardiomyopathy that can be severe, and withdrawal syndromes. Within 6 to 8 hours of withdrawal the patient may go into a tremulous state that usually subsides within days or weeks. Alcoholic hallucinosis generally occurs within 24 to 36 hours, about the same time as withdrawal seizures. The seizures are generalized grand mal attacks; when focal seizures are manifest, other causes should be sought. Delerium tremens usually appears within 72 hours of withdrawal and is often preceded by tremulousness, hallucinations, or seizures. These three occurrences combined with perceptual distortions, insomnia, psychomotor disturbances, autonomic hyperactivity, and in a large percentage of cases another potentially fatal illness (such as bowel infarction or subdural hematoma) comprise delerium tremens. This syndrome is now treated with benzodiazepines. Nutritional disorders include alcoholic hypoglycemia and hypothermia, alcoholic polyneuropathy, Wernicke-Korsokoff syndrome, and cerebellar degeneration. Alcoholics appear to require a higher dose of anesthesia to prevent movement (R. Barber, personal communication). In alcoholics (2 six-packs of beer or 1 pint of whiskey per day or more), emergency

surgery and anesthesia despite hepatitis (alcoholic) is not associated with increasing abnormalities of liver enzymes (Zinn S, personal communication of a study of 26 patients at San Francisco General Hospital randomly anesthetized with spinal, enflurane, or narcotic-nitrous techniques for emergency orthopedic surgery). In addition, about 20 percent of alcoholics have chronic obstructive pulmonary disease. Thus, the patient who gives a history of heavy use of alcohol necessitates careful examination of many systems to quantify preoperative status.

Hepatic failure can lead to coma with a high output cardiac failure but does not lead to chronic polyneuropathy as does uremia. Uremic polyneuropathy is a distal symmetrical sensorimotor polyneuropathy that may be improved by dialysis. The use of depolarizing muscle relaxants has been questioned in polyneuropathies (see Ch. 17). I believe patients who have a neuropathy associated with uremia should not be given succinylcholine because of a possible exaggerated hyperkalemic response.

Pernicious anemia from vitamin B_{12} deficiency may result in subacute combined degeneration of the spinal cord, with signs similar to that seen with chronic nitrous oxide toxicity. Both pernicious anemia and nitrous oxide toxicity are associated with posterior column (position sense, fine motor skills) and pyramidal tract signs and peripheral neuropathy. Combined system disease can also occur without anemia, as can nitrous oxide poisoning in dentists and N_2O abusers. Patients with B_{12} deficiency and anemia if treated with folate improve hematologically but progress to dementia and severe neuropathy. Thus, administration of 100 μg of vitamin B_{12} intramuscularly before giving folate to the patient who has signs of combined system degeneration may be prudent.

The porphyrias are a metabolic constellation of diseases resulting from an autosomally inherited lack of functional enzymes in the synthesis of hemoglobin. Figure 2-2 depicts the currently accepted abnormalities in

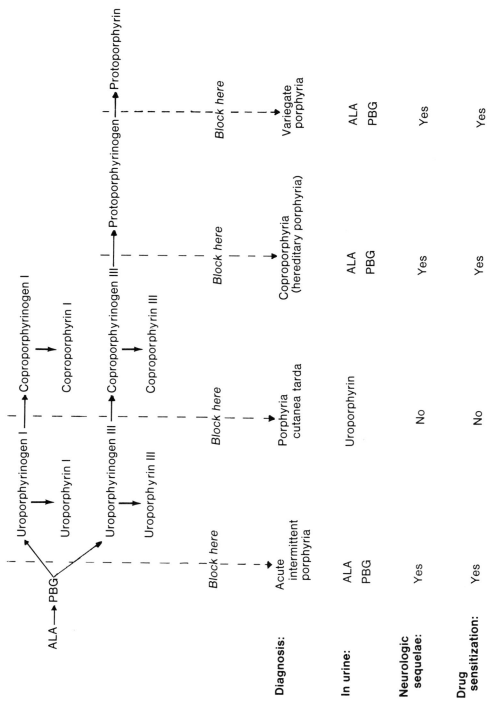

Fig. 2-2 Scheme depicting functional enzyme deficits for some of the "porphyrias." ALA-amino levulinic acid; PBG-porphobilinogen.

this scheme. It is important to note that types 1, 3 and 4 can cause life-threatening neurologic abnormalities; patients with these types of porphyria have either aminolevulinic acid (ALA) or porphobilinogen (PBG) or both in their urine, while those with porphyria cutanea tarda, which is not associated with neurologic sequelae, do not have ALA or PBG in their urine.[205] The typical pattern in acute intermittent porphyria is of acute attacks manifested by colicky pain, nausea, vomiting, severe constipation, psychiatric disorders, and lower motor neuron lesions, which can progress to bulbar paralysis. Certain drugs can induce the enzyme ALA synthetase, exacerbating the disease;[205-209] these sensitizing drugs include barbiturates, meprobamate, chlordiazepoxide, glutethimide, diazepam, hydroxydione, phenytoin, pentazocine, birth control pills, ethyl alcohol, sulfonamides, griseofulvin, and ergot preparations. Patients often have attacks at times of infection, fasting, or menstruation. Glucose administration suppresses ALA synthetase activity and is given to prevent or ablate acute attacks. Drugs used in anesthetic management that are reported as safe[208,209] for patients with porphyria include neostigmine, (Prostigmin), atropine, gallamine, succinylcholine, curare, pancuronium, nitrous oxide, procaine, propanadid, meperidine, fentanyl, morphine, droperidol, promazine, promethazine, and chlorpromazine. Although ketamine has been used,[210] postoperative psychoses might be difficult to differentiate between disease or ketamine effect.

NEUROMUSCULAR DISORDERS

This category includes disorders affecting all major components of the motor unit: motor neuron, peripheral nerve, neuromuscular junction, and muscle. Neuropathies may involve all components of the nerve, producing sensory, motor, and autonomic dysfunction, or may preferentially involve one or the other component. Myopathies may involve proximal or distal muscles or both sets.

Myasthenia gravis (also see Ch. 17) is a deficit caused by partial blockade or destruction of nicotinic acetylcholine receptors by IgG antibodies. It is characterized by fluctuating ophthalmoplegia, ptosis, and bulbar, respiratory, or limb weakness and confirmed by a beneficial response to cholinergic drugs.[211,212] One major problem for the anesthesiologist involves the use of muscle relaxants and their reversal. Since much of the care of myasthenia gravis patients is tailoring the amount of anticholinesterase medication to the maximal muscle strength of the patient compatible with comfort, derangement of the course of the disease intraoperatively could necessitate reassessment of drug dosage. For that reason several researchers recommend withholding all anticholinergic medication for 6 hours preoperatively and reinstituting medicine postoperatively with extreme caution because the sensitivity of these patients may have changed. Small doses of succinylcholine can be used to facilitate endotracheal intubation and tiny doses of nondepolarizing drugs can be used for intraoperative relaxation not obtained by regional anesthesia or volatile agents. Controlled ventilation usually is required for 24 to 48 or more hours postoperatively.[213-217]

The Eaton-Lambert syndrome (myasthenic syndrome) is characterized by proximal limb muscle weakness. Strength or reflexes may increase with repetitive effort. These patients have decreased release of acetylcholine at their neuromuscular junction. Guanidine therapy enhances acetylcholine release from nerve terminals and improves strength. The majority of males with this syndrome have a small-cell carcinoma of the lung or other malignancy, while females often have either malignancy, sarcoidosis, thyroiditis, or collagen vascular disease. These patients also have increased sensitivity to both depolarizing and nondepolarizing muscle relaxants.[214,215]

Dermatomyositis and polymyositis are characterized by proximal limb muscle weakness with dysphagia. These entities are associated with malignancy or collagen vascular disease and often have respiratory muscle and cardiac muscle involvement.

Periodic paralysis is another disease with increased sensitivity to muscle relaxants. Periodic weakness starts in childhood or adolescence and is precipitated by rest after exercise, sleep, stress, cold, surgery, or pregnancy. Hypokalemic and hyperkalemic forms exist and are associated with cardiac arrhythmias but usually spare the respiratory muscles as does thyrotoxic periodic paralysis. Anesthetic management consists of minimizing stress, maintaining normal fluid and electrolyte states, and maintaining normothermia.[218]

Muscular dystrophy patients are surviving into their late twenties. Complicating their diseases are respiratory infections, kyphoscoliosis, contractures, and cardiac abnormalities. Duchenne muscular dystrophy is a sex-linked recessive disease, the most common of the muscular dystrophies. It occurs after age 5; patients experience a rapid progression of muscle disease to incapacity in their teens. Cardiac involvement is common when the disease affects proximal and pelvic muscles, with respiratory failure a common cause of death. Limb-girdle muscular dystrophy is not as severe as Duchenne, occurs later, has heart involvement, and is transmitted as an autosomal recessive. Facioscapulohumoral muscular dystrophy (FSHMD) is a disease of autosomal dominant inheritance and has a mild clinical form in adolescence. Patients with FSHMD live a normal lifespan without an increased risk of cardiac complications, but postoperative respiratory deaths have been recorded. Myotonic dystrophy is a disease in which continued active contraction of muscle persists after cessation of voluntary effort or stimulation. This autosomal-dominant inherited disease has an onset from 20 to 40 years of age and is associated with cardiomyopathy, baldness, testicular atrophy, cataracts, intellectual and emotional abnormalities, and premature death in the 50- to 60-year age range. Weakness and atrophy of

facial, sternocleidomastoid, distal, and pharyngeal muscles occurs. Since the disease involves the muscles themselves and not their innervation, conduction anesthesia cannot produce adequate relaxation of tonic muscles. Gastric dilatation has also been reported to be a problem, as has malignant hyperthermia. But like the other muscular dystrophies, most problems still arise from arrhythmias and respiratory muscle inadequacies. With all of the muscular dystrophies as with all the neuropathies (referred to above) problems related to exaggerated serum potassium release following depolarizing muscle relaxant administration have been reported (see Ch. 17).[219]

Malignant hyperthermia (MH) (also see Ch. 36) in a relative of the patient or in the patient merits careful history and at least a tourniquet test for MH susceptibility and perhaps prophylaxis with dantrolene sodium (Dantrium). In a minority of cases, the MH syndrome has been associated with recognizable musculoskeletal abnormalities such as strabismus, ptosis, myotonic dystrophies, hernias, kyphoscoliosis, muscular dystrophies, central core disease, and marfanoid syndromes; 1 in 14,000 pediatric patients have the syndrome, increasing to 1 in 2,500 in patients requiring squint surgery.[220] Questions to ask the parents include, Does your child get rigid when upset? Does your child sweat profusely when upset? These questions have unproven sensitivity and specificity. More recently Roberts and co-workers[221] have devised a tourniquet test for MH susceptibility. In 7 MH survivors and 20 relatives the test was 100 percent specific and sensitive (however, the number of false positives this test gives is not actually known). With ulnar nerve stimulation and monitoring of thumb contraction tension, a blood pressure cuff should be inflated just above systolic blood pressure for 10 minutes. One minute after release of the blood pressure cuff, normal patients show a decreased thumb tension and MH patients show a tremendous increase. In addition to the anesthesiologist altering his anesthetic technique to a nitrous oxide–narcotic–pancuronium or regional technique, having cooling blankets, fluid, and a purged-with-oxygen anesthetic machine, and using additional temperature and acid-base monitoring techniques, the patient suspected of MH susceptibility should be prophylactically treated with dantrolene sodium 1 to 2 mg/kg orally in 4 divided doses for 2 to 3 days postoperatively.[220, 222] Dantrolene can be given intravenously preoperatively for emergency surgery and can be given intravenously to help stop the MH syndrome once it has begun (see Ch. 36 for treatment of MH once the condition has begun).

AFFECTIVE DISORDERS

Perhaps the most important preoperative consideration for patients with the affective disorders in addition to developing rapport with them is in understanding their drug therapy and its effects and side effects. Lithium, tricyclic antidepressants, phenothiazines, butyrophenones and monamine oxidase inhibitors are used in these patients; these drugs all have potent effects and side effects that are discussed in the last section of this chapter.

RENAL DISEASE, INFECTIOUS DISEASES, AND DISORDERS OF ELECTROLYTES

One may ask why preoperative preparation of the patient with renal disease is discussed in the same section as preoperative preparation of the patient with an infectious disease. Although a common recommendation is that no surgery except emergency or curative (e.g., abscess drainage) be done in patients with infectious disease, it is becoming more evident that renal insufficiency can be caused by antimicrobial agents[223] and that sepsis, not shock, is probably the leading cause of acute postoperative renal failure.[224] The linkage of renal failure with electrolyte disorders is more obvious—the kidney is the end organ for carrying out the regulation of body osmolality and fluid volume and has a major role in excretion of end products of metabolism. In performing these functions, the kidney becomes intimately involved in electrolyte excretion.

Preoperative preparation of the patient with renal insufficiency whose own kidneys are still providing renal function is separated from the patient with end-stage renal disease who has a dialysis machine providing renal function, and from the patient who has a transplanted kidney, because these three groups of patients require quite different preoperative preparation. In addition, acute changes in renal function present quite a different problem from chronic alteration in function. Certain renal diseases require different preoperative preparation than others, but generally renal disease of any etiology presents the same preoperative problems. For more discussion of renal disease also see Chapters 24 and 32.

RENAL DISEASE

Different Causes and Systemic Effects of Different Renal Problems

Patients with glomerular diseases may develop the nephrotic syndrome without any disturbance of tubular function. This is a key differentiation as tubular dysfunction with attendant uremia presents quite a different constellation of problems than simply glomerular diseases with only the nephrotic syndrome. This is not to minimize the effect of the glomerular diseases; the nephrotic syndrome results from massive proteinuria and consequent hypoalbuminemia. The resulting reduction in plasma oncotic pressure diminishes plasma volume, and this calls forth compensatory mechanisms that result in retention of sodium and water. This retained sodium and water lead to another common clinical finding in patients with the nephrotic syndrome: edema. Thus, patients with the nephrotic syndrome may have excess total body water with decreased intravascular volume. In addition, in attempts to decrease edema, diuretics may be used. Thus, the estimation of volume status is an essential preoperative consideration; in patients with diminished tubular renal function who do not yet require a dialysis machine or in those with the nephrotic syndrome with preserved tubular function, hypovolemia appears to be a significant cause of deteriorating tubular renal function.[225–229] Thus, I advocate the same intense preoperative, intraoperative, and postoperative fluid management for patients with the nephrotic syndrome as for patients with diminished tubular function, even though there is not a good randomized study showing that 'tight" control of volume status in these groups of patients preserves renal tubular function or any other measure of perioperative morbidity better than does nontight control of volume status.

Uremia, the end result of renal tubular failure (i.e., concentrating, diluting, acidifying, and filtering function) presents with an array of manifestations. Included in this array are cardiovascular, immunologic, hematologic, neuromuscular, pulmonary, bone, and endocrine alterations. These alterations are ascribed to either the toxic end-products of protein metabolism or to a trade-off of the functions of the kidney. As the number of functioning nephrons diminishes, those nephrons that remain trade off to increase some solute and body composition functions at the expense of other functions, such as phosphate excretion. The accumulation of phosphate causes an increase in parathormone levels, which results in osteodystrophy. This latter alteration can be managed by restriction of dietary phosphate, binding of intestinal phosphate with gels (such as aluminum hydroxide or carbonate), ingestion of supplemental calcium, or parathyroidec-

tomy.[230] Certain alterations of uremia, such as neuropathy, fit better into the toxic metabolite accumulation hypothesis.[231] Peripheral neuropathy is most often sensory and lower extremity but may be motor, is often improved with dialysis, and can be dramatically reversed with a transplantation.[231] As to whether to use a depolarizing muscle relaxant in patients with this neuropathy, see the section on neuropathies in this chapter and Chapter 17.

Autonomic neuropathy may contribute with the altered volume states and cardiac complications of these patients to hypotension during anesthesia. Atherosclerosis is often accelerated in these patients, and hypertension with its attendant consequences is very common. Cardiac failure (especially episodic) is frequently a feature due to the presence of many causes—anemia with increasing myocardial work, hypertension, atherosclerosis, altered volume states. Pericarditis can present only with the sign of a rub or with the symptom of pain (with or without hemorrhage). Tamponade should be ruled out by ultrasound and clinical features if this diagnosis is seriously suspected preoperatively. The degree of anemia generally parallels the degree of uremia, and chronically uremic patients seem to adapt to this well. There are no hard data to substantiate the need to preoperatively transfuse a chronically uremic patient who has existed at even as low a hematocrit as 16 or 18 volume percent preoperatively. One of the major reasons not to transfuse end-stage renal disease patients has recently been disproven: one study showed that the more blood transfusions a transplant recipient has received pretransplant, the greater the chance of successful transplant function.[232] Abnormal coagulation associated with abnormal platelet adhesiveness and decreased factor III activity can occur in uremic patients. Even those uremic patients not receiving corticosteroids or immunosuppressives may demonstrate abnormal immunity, perhaps thus meriting increased attention to the detail of procedures that avoid patient cross-contamination. Patients with uremia exhibit a wide variety of metabolic and endocrinologic disorders[230] including impaired carbohydrate tolerance, insulin resistance, type IV hypertriglyceridemia, hyperparathyroidism, autonomic insufficiency, hyperkalemia, and anion gap acidosis (due to the inability to reabsorb filtered bicarbonate and to excrete sufficient urinary ammonium[233]); they also excrete and pharmacokinetically handle drugs differently. In addition the complications of hemodialysis include hepatitis B (and persistent hepatitis B antigenemia); nutritional deficiencies; electrolyte and fluid excesses, deficiencies, and dysequilibria; and psychological problems. All these symptoms probably must be evaluated prior to surgery because they all can lead to serious perioperative morbidity; there are no data, however, to substantiate that preoperative optimization of these patients reduces perioperative risk.

Patients with kidney stones probably exemplify the value of preoperative optimization. Seventy-five percent of all stones are composed of calcium oxalate. Patients with these stones often take diuretics, avoid calcium rich foods, or restrict their intake of salt. Prevention of dehydration by institution of intravenous fluid therapy at the time the patient is made NPO may be important as it may be for patients with struvate or uric acid stones. Struvate stones often result from urinary infection; uric acid stones can be prevented by treatment with allopurinol, or preoperative hydration, or alkalinazation of the urine. Acidosis may contribute to stone formation. More thorough discussion of renal function and physiology is discussed in Chapter 24, and Chapter 32 deals with the complexities of managing patients for renal and other urologic surgery.

Creatinine clearance appears to be the most accurate means of quantifying the degree of decreased renal function for pharmacokinetic purposes. In the patient with stable renal function this can be approximated with a serum creatinine level—a doubling of creatinine level represents a halving of glomerular filtration rate. Thus, a patient with a stable serum creatinine level of 2 mg/100 ml may have a glomerular filtration rate (GFR) of 60 ml/min, while a stable serum creatinine level of 4 mg/100 ml may be associated with a GFR of 30 ml/min and a stable serum creatinine of 8 mg/100 ml may be associated with a GFR of 15 ml/min or less. Note the accent on the word *stable*. Changing renal function often is associated with a serum creatinine change that lags by several days. The blood urea nitrogen level (BUN) is less useful than serum creatinine, but not altogether meaningless as is seen in the next section.

THE PATIENT WITH INSUFFICIENT BUT FUNCTIONING KIDNEYS

I believe the highest goal of and most skill required for the physician in anesthesia are exemplified by and tested by this group of patients: those in whom insufficient organ (renal) function is to be preserved. The array of uremic symptoms and much perioperative morbidity can probably be avoided by attention to detail in the preoperative and perioperative management of renal insufficiency patients who still use their own kidneys for renal function.[224-229, 234-240] First, studies demonstrate that patients in whom acute renal failure develops after surgery have an extremely high mortality and that acute renal failure perioperatively is most likely to develop in those with preoperative renal insufficiency. Proper preoperative hydration probably decreases mortality following radiocontrast studies.[234-236] To preserve renal function, clues as to the presence of hypovolemia or hypervolemia should be sought from the history and physical examination (e.g., weight loss or gain, thirst, edema, orthostatic hypotension and tachycardia, flat neck veins, dry mucous membranes, decreased skin turgor.) In seriously ill patients, insertion of a pulmonary artery line will allow more precise monitoring of intravascular volume. To preserve normal renal function, infusion of saline, mannitol, or furosemide has been recommended. This should be done cautiously because saline infusions and mannitol can lead to fluid overload and myocardial damage and diuretics given intraoperatively can lead to hypovolemia postoperatively, the latter which can result in the same worsening of renal function that is just postponed. Maintaining normal intravascular fluid volume status can be guided by pulmonary capillary wedge pressure. Despite the above recommendation, I do not routinely give saline, furosemide or mannitol. Other causes of deterioration in function of chronic renal insufficiency are low cardiac output or low renal blood flow (BUN is often increased out of proportion to creatinine increase in prerenal azotemia whether due to fluid depletion from diuretics or cardiac failure), urinary tract infection, nephrotoxic drugs, hypercalcemia, hyperuricemia. Situations that promote these effects should be assiduously avoided and/or treated.

THE DIALYSIS PATIENT

As opposed to the patient using his own kidneys, the patient receiving dialysis no longer has kidneys to lose, so preoperative assessment should be directed towards keeping the function of other organ systems protected and vascular access sites best maintained. Usually this does not require placement of invasive monitoring. Attention must be placed on volume and electrolyte status, which can be ascertained by knowing when the patient was last dialyzed, how much weight he normally gains or loses with dialysis (whether peritoneal or intravascular), and what electrolyte composition he is dialyzed against. Preoperative dialysis may benefit those with hyperkalemia, hypercalcemia, acidosis, neuropathy, and fluid overload, but the resultant disequilibrium or fluid and electrolytes can cause problems.

THE PATIENT WITH A RENAL TRANSPLANT

Over 28,000 patients have received renal transplants (compared to 20,000 currently receiving dialysis in the United States).[241] Approximately 70 percent of those are still alive, although one third are now receiving dialysis.[241] In addition to learning the state of their renal function (which may place the patient in either the normal, insufficient but functioning kidney, or end-stage renal disease using a dialysis machine group) side effects from immunosuppressive drugs should be sought. Because this therapy places these patients at much higher risk of infection, all effort at avoiding invasive monitoring and at preventing patient cross contamination should be taken.

DRUGS IN RENAL FAILURE

Studies have shown that patients with renal azotemia have a threefold or greater risk of an adverse drug reaction than those with normal renal function.[242-244] This increased risk is due to either excessive pharmacologic effects (secondary to high blood levels of a drug or its metabolite [e.g., the metabolite of meperidine]), to physiological alterations in target tissues induced by the uremic state (such as excessive sedation in uremia with standard blood levels of sedative hypnotics), or to excessive administration of electrolytes with drugs (e.g., penicillin standardly has 1.6 mEq of potassium per 1 million units).[242-244] Administration of standard doses of drugs dependent on renal excretion for their elimination can result in drug accumulation and enhanced pharmacologic effect. Information about many drugs anesthesiologists use for-patients with and without renal failure can be found in Bennet et al.[242]

INFECTIOUS DISEASE

Since a common recommendation is that no surgery except emergency or essential (e.g., abscess drainage) be done in patients with infectious disease and also since it is becoming more evident that renal insufficiency can be caused by antimicrobial agents,[223] assessment of renal function and the organ damage present from renal insufficiency should be assessed preoperatively in the patient with infectious disease. Guidelines for prophylactic antibiotics have been summarized elsewhere,[245, 246] and are used to prevent blood stream seeding and sepsis from predictable bacteremic interventions.[245, 246] Sepsis has become a leading cause of postoperative morbidity,[224] probably through a decrease in systemic vascular resistance related to activation of the complement system. Thus attention to antibiotic drug effects must be supplemented by attention to intravascular volume status.[246-248] The degree of impairment of the infected organ and its effect on anesthesia should be assessed. For instance, endocarditis merits examination of volume status, drug therapy and side effects, myocardial function, and renal, lung, neurologic, and hepatic function— those organ systems that endocarditis can effect.

At least two other considerations merit preoperative consideration—patient isolation to avoid contamination and patient infectivity to the physician. These two considerations are the focus of at least two books.[249, 250]

DISORDERS OF ELECTROLYTES

The reader should note that disorders of calcium, magnesium, and phosphate balance were discussed in the section of this chapter on diseases involving the endocrine system and disorders of nutrition.

HYPONATREMIA AND HYPERNATREMIA

Electrolyte disorders are usually detected by measurement of serum electrolyte concentrations. These concentrations reflect water balance relative to electrolyte balance. Thus hyponatremia reflects a relative excess of free water and can occur in the presence of an increase in total body sodium (edematous disorders), with normal total body sodium (excesses of free water as in inappropriate antidiuretic hormone secretion), or with decreases in total body sodium (too aggressive diuretic usage). Definition of the cause defines treatment. The anesthesiologist is faced with the question of what levels of electrolytes require treatment prior to anesthesia. Hyponatremia that develops slowly usually produces few symptoms, but the patient may admit to lethargy and apathy. Chronic hyponatremia is better tolerated than acute hyponatremia because of cell volume regulatory mechanisms that alleviate brain edema; the loss of other solutes from the cell decrease the osmotic movement of water into cells.[251] Despite this, severe chronic hyponatremia (serum sodium $\leq$ 123 mEq/L) can cause brain edema.[251] Acute hyponatremia, however, may be associated with profound cerebral edema with obtundation, coma, convulsions, disordered reflexes, and thermoregulatory control requiring emergency treatment.[251] Depending on the cause and relative total sodium and water content, treatment can range from administration of hypertonic saline or mannitol with or without diuretics to fluid restriction or administration of other drugs.[251-254] In patients with hyponatremia and excess total body water secondary to inappropriate antidiuretic hormone secretion, serum sodium can be corrected by giving 1 mg/kg furosemide and replacement of urinary electrolyte losses with hypertonic saline.[253] In neither acute nor chronic hyponatremia is it necessary to totally restore serum sodium levels to their normal levels; brain swelling symptoms usually disappear at a serum sodium level of 130 mEq/L. This leaves us with the question of what levels of serum sodium make anesthesia more risky. Since no data exist to answer this question, to allow for some error in caring for patients I have arbitrarily chosen a flexible 131 mEq/L concentration as the lower sodium limit for elective surgery. A discussion of intraoperative hyponatremia in transurethral prostatectomy patients can be found in Chapter 32.

Hypernatremia occurs much less commonly than hyponatremia, is often iatrogenic (failure to provide the patient who is unconscious or with a recent stroke deficit of the thirst mechanism with enough free water), and can occur in the presence of a low, normal, or excess content of total body sodium. The primary symptoms of hypernatremia relate to brain cell shrinking; because too rapid correction of hypernatremia can lead to cerebral edema and convulsions, correction should be made gradually. Again, with no data to support this stance, I believe that all elective surgical patients should have serum sodium concentrations of less than 150 mEq/L prior to anesthesia.

HYPOKALEMIA AND HYPERKALEMIA (ALSO SEE CH. 24)

The relationship between the measured serum potassium concentration and the total body potassium stores can best be described by a scattergram.[255-257] Only 2 percent of total body potassium is stored in plasma; 75 percent of the 50 to 60 mEq/L of total body potassium in normal individuals is stored in skeletal muscle, 6 percent in red blood cells, and 5 percent in the liver. Thus a 20 to 25 percent change in serum potassium could represent a 1,000 or more mEq alteration in chronic changes or as little as a 10 to 20 mEq

alteration in acute changes. Acute changes in serum potassium appear (like those for serum sodium[251]) to be tolerated less well than chronic alterations in serum potassium, because of the equilibration between serum and intracellular stores that takes place with chronic changes and returns the resting membrane potential of excitable cells to near normal. Hyperkalemia may result from fictitious elevation (red blood cell hemolysis), exogenous potassium excess (drugs, salt substitutes, excessive banana ingestion), cellular potassium shifts (metabolic acidosis, tissue and muscle damage after burns, depolarizing muscle relaxants, intense catabolism), and decreased renal excretion (renal failure, renal insufficiency with trauma, potassium-sparing diuretics,[252] mineralocorticoid deficiency).

The major danger in anesthetizing patients with disorders of potassium balance appears to be abnormal cardiac function, both electrical[258-260] and muscular pumping.[259,260] Hyperkalemia lowers the cardiac resting membrane potential and decreases the duration of the myocardial action potential and upstroke velocity. This decreased rate of ventricular depolarization and the repolarization beginning in some area of myocardium while others are still being depolarized produces a progressively widening QRS complex that merges with the T wave into a sine wave. There is good correlation between the degree of hyperkalemia and QRS duration above a potassium level of 6.7 mEq/L,[258] which is an even better correlation than that between serum potassium level and T wave changes. However, the earliest manifestations of hyperkalemia are narrowing and peaking of the T wave. While not diagnostic of hyperkalemia, T waves are almost invariably peaked and narrow when serum potassium levels are between 7 and 9 mEq/L. With serum potassium levels over 7 mEq/L, atrial conduction disturbances appear manifest by a decreased P wave amplitude and increased PR duration. Supraventricular tachycardia, atrial fibrillation, ventricular premature beats, ventricular tachycardia, ventricular fibrillation, or sinus arrest may all occur. The electrocardiographic and cardiac alterations of hyperkalemia are potentiated by hypocalcemia and hyponatremia; intravenous administration of saline, bicarbonate, glucose with insulin (1 unit per 2 g glucose), and calcium can reverse the changes by shifting some extracellular potassium intracellularly. Kayexalate enemas can reverse the changes by binding potassium in the gut in exchange for sodium; dialysis against a hypokalemic solution can also be used to decrease serum potassium. Thus, hypoventilation during anesthesia in the hyperkalemic patient can be dangerous,[258–261] as each pH unit change of 0.1 can produce a 0.4 to 1.5 mEq/L change in the opposite direction (i.e., pH change from 7.4 to 7.3 can be associated with a serum potassiuim change of 5.5 to 6.5 mEq/L).[261]

Hypokalemia may be caused by inadequate intake, excessive gastrointestinal losses (diarrhea, vomiting, nasopharyngeal suction, chronic laxative use, exchange resins as in certain wines), excessive renal losses (diuretics, renal tubular acidosis, chronic chloride deficiency, metabolic alkalosis, mineralocorticoid excess, excessive licorice ingestion, antibiotics, ureterosigmoidoscopy, diabetic ketoacidosis), and shifts of potassium from extracellular to intracellular compartments (alkalosis, insulin administration, barium poisoning, periodic paralysis). As with hyperkalemia, knowledge of the cause of the potassium deficiency and its appropriate preoperative evaluation and treatment may be as important as treatment of the potassium deficiency itself. Also like hyperkalemia, hypokalemia may reflect small or vast alterations of total body potassium. Two other similarities to hyperkalemia seem to pertain: acute hypokalemia may be much less well tolerated than chronic hypokalemia and the major worrisome manifestations of hypokalemia affect the circulatory system, both of cardiac and peripheral components. In addition, however, chronic hypokalemia results in weakness, hypoperistalsis, and hypokalemic nephropathy.

The cardiovascular manifestations of hypokalemia include an autonomic neuropathy (which results in orthostatic hypotension and decreased sympathetic reserve), impaired myocardial contractility, and electrical conduction abnormalities that can result in sinus tachycardia, atrial and ventricular arrhythmias, and disturbances of intraventricular conduction that can progress to ventricular fibrillation. That these are real concerns for the hypokalemic patient has been attested to many times.[258–260, 262–264] In addition to arrhythmias, the electrocardiogram reveals some QRS widening, ST segment abnormalities, progressive diminution of the T wave amplitude and progressive U wave amplitude.[258] Surawicz[258] found these changes invariably present below a serum potassium of 2.3 mEq/L. Although U waves are not specific to hypokalemia they are sensitive for it. As mentioned before, repletion of total body potassium deficit for a potassium depletion reflected by a serum deficit of 1 mEq/L (from 4.3 to 3.3 mEq/L) may require 1,000 mEq. Even if this could be given instantaneously (and it should not be repleted at more than 250 mEq/day) it would take 24 to 48 hours to equilibrate in all tissues.[266, 267] The potassium-depleted myocardium is unusually sensitive to digoxin, calcium, and, most importantly, *potassium itself.* Rapid potassium infusion can produce as severe arrhythmias in the hypokalemic patient as does the hypokalemia itself.[268–271]

Thus, making a decision about proceeding with surgery or anesthesia in the face of acute or chronic hyperkalemia, hypokalemia, hyponatremia, or hypernatremia depends on many factors.[272] One must know the etiology and treatment of the underlying condition that caused the electrolyte disturbance and its effect per se on perioperative organ risk and physiology. The urgency of the operation, the degree of electrolyte abnormality, the medications given, the acid-base balance, and the acuteness or chronicity of the electrolyte disturbance all play a role in the decision. As a rule I believe all elective patients should have normal serum potassium, but I will not delay surgery if the serum potassium is above 3.3 and below 5.7 mEq/L, the cause is known, and the patient is otherwise in optimal condition. These are arbitrary numbers. I dialyze all end-stage renal failure patients to the same arbitrary numbers before all surgery except in true emergency cases (e.g., imminent exsanguination). An additional possible intraoperative factor is that in dogs hyponatremia and hypo-osmolality decrease MAC, hypernatremia increases MAC, and hyperkalemia does not affect anesthetic requirements.[273]

GASTROINTESTINAL AND LIVER DISEASE

The reader should see also the discussion of porphyrias in the section on neurologic disease, nutritional deficiencies in the section on disorders of nutrition, and pediatric disorders, such as TE fistula, in Chapter 36.

GASTROINTESTINAL DISEASE

Although preoperative preparation of the gastrointestinal tract per se is often the surgeon's realm and frequently need not be extensively evaluated by the anesthesiologist, gastrointestinal disease can and often does cause derangements in many or all other systems. These disturbances in other systems certainly can affect the safety of anesthesia for the patient. The major advance of correcting not only fluid and electrolyte disorders but also of optimizing nutritional status by either enteral or parenteral routes prior to surgery now allows surgery to be done in patients previously deemed to have too great a risk and perhaps has lessened the risk in others.[20, 21, 274] Still, a thorough evaluation of intravascular fluid volume, electrolyte concentrations, and nutrition is essential, including an evaluation of the supervening side effects of these therapies (e.g., hypophospha-

temia from parenteral nutrition, hyperkalemia or cardiac arrhythmias from too vigorous a treatment of hypokalemia, and congestive failure from too rapid or vigorous a treatment of hypovolemia). In addition to vast alterations of fluid, electrolytes, and nutrition that can occur with such diverse gastrointestinal diseases as neoplasm and pancreatitis, patients with gastrointestinal disorders can have obstruction, vomiting, or hypersecretion of acid and these effects may merit rapid induction of anesthesia with cricoid pressure or awake endotracheal intubation, preoperative nasogastric suction, or preoperative use of histamine-receptor blocking agents (see Ch. 3).[275–277] Clotting abnormalities may need to be corrected, since the fat soluble vitamin K (often malabsorbed) is necessary for synthesis of factors V, VII, IX, and X in the liver (see Ch. 28); liver disease is often associated with gastrointestinal disease and if severe enough can also result in deficiency of clotting factors it synthesizes. Other factors to bear in mind in preoperative evaluation of the patient with gastrointestinal disease is that closed gas spaces expand by absorbing N_2O, which can lead to ischemic injury and/or gastrointestinal viscous rupture,[278] that gastrointestinal surgery predisposes to sepsis, and that sepsis with decreased peripheral vascular resistance can lead to massive fluid requirements, cardiac failure, and renal insufficiency. Recently the wound infection rate has been declining; this may be due to the use of better technique or to more appropriate use of prophylactic antibiotics.[279] The patient with gastrointestinal disease may have anemia from iron, intrinsic factor, folate, or B_{12} deficiency. They may also have neurologic changes of combined system disease; respiratory compromise from peritonitis, abscess,[280] obstruction, previous (and future) incisions, aspiration, or pulmonary embolism from thrombophlebitis from being bedridden or associated with ulcerative colitis; hepatitis, cholangitis, or drug side effects from antibiotics or other medications; massive bleeding with anemia and shock; and psychological derangements. Since gastrointestinal disease can be accompanied by so many diverse associated disorders, a section on proper preoperative assessment would require repetition of the rest of this chapter. The clinician clearly must search for other system involvement in the patient with gastrointestinal disease and preoperatively assess and treat appropriately. Discussion of two specific disease entities—ulcerative colitis and carcinoid tumors—will highlight this point of other system involvement.

Patients with ulcerative colitis often have psychological problems and not uncommonly have phlebitis, iron deficiency, folate deficiency, B_{12} deficiency, anemia, and clotting disorders all from malabsorption. They may be malnourished, dehydrated, have electrolyte abnormalities, have massive bleeding, have closed loops of bowel or bowel perforation or toxic megacolon causing respiratory compromise, and have hepatitis, arthritis, iritis, spondylitis, and diabetes secondary to pancreatitis. Carcinoid tumors usually arise from a primary tumor in the bowel, although lung, liver, and gastric and other sites have been thought to be the location of the primary. Diarrhea with fluid and electrolyte abnormalities is a common presentation. The fascination with these tumors arises because they secrete vasoactive substances such as serotonin, histamine, kinins, and prostaglandins.[281–285] Patients can exhibit hypotension or hypertension with the flush of vasoactive substance release. Vasoactive substances can be released from the tumor by any number of substances including catecholamines. Thus, the anesthesiologist must tread a line between avoiding substances that release histamine (such as curare and morphine) and creating light anesthesia with consequent sympathetic activation by painful stimuli[286–292] and also must be ready and able to treat hypotension, decreased peripheral vascular resistance, bronchospasm and/or hypertension. Alpha-adrenergic

blockade with the phenothiazines, butyrophenones, or phenoxybenzamine and β-adrenergic blockade with propranolol have been advocated to prevent catecholamine-mediated vasoactive substance release, but can lead to hypotension. If severe hypotension develops, the drug of choice is either angiotensin (now commercially unavailable in the United States) or vasopressin. However the vasoactive substances released by carcinoid tumors cause fibrosis of heart valves often resulting in pulmonic stenosis or tricuspid insufficiency. To increase cardiac output in the patient with tricuspid insufficiency, drugs or situations that increase pulmonary vascular resistance (such as angiotensin, vasopressin, acidosis, hypercarbia, and hypothermia should be avoided—see Ch. 30). In addition, if large amounts of serotonin are produced (equal to 200 mg/day of 5-HIAA) then niacin deficiency with pellagra (diarrhea, dermatitis, and dementia) can develop. These patients also often receive antiserotonin drugs (methylsergide) and/or anticholinergic or antihistaminic drugs (Periactin, cyproheptadine, or cimetidine) or antiprostaglandin drugs (aspirin, indomethecin). Many patients also develop bronchospasm with or without the flushing when vasoactive substances are released. Thus, a patient with a carcinoid tumor may be well or may be severely incapacitated by lung, neurologic, nutritional, fluid, electrolyte, and cardiovascular disturbances.[277–281] The point is that the gastrointestinal system by itself may not need extensive preoperative preparation, but gastrointestinal disease can cause disturbances in any or all other systems that require both extensive preoperative preparation to optimize patient condition and preoperative knowledge of disease physiology and effects by anesthesiologists in order to guide patients through the perioperative period smoothly. In addition, the anesthesiologist's understanding of the nature of the surgery probably aids in determining the system involvement caused by gastrointestinal disorder.[293]

LIVER DISEASE

What are the risks of giving anesthesia to patients with acute liver disease who require emergency surgery? What are the risks of giving anesthesia to patients with chronic impairment of liver function? What can be done to minimize these risks? Since hepatic function and physiology is discussed in Chapter 24, I will mention only that the liver serves a synthetic function (proteins, clotting factors, etc.), a detoxifying function for both drugs and products of normal human metabolism, an excretory function, and an energy supply and storage function. Thus, tests of liver function include synthetic tests (cholesterol, protime, albumin levels), cellular integrity tests (SGOT, SGPT, LDH, alkaline phosphatase), detoxifying tests (ammonia level, direct bilirubin level, lidocaine level), and excretory tests (bromosulphalein [BSP] retention, total bilirubin levels). In examining the effect of anesthesia with or without surgery on liver function and in examining ways to reduce risk in patients with preexisting liver disease, investigators have often looked at one or more of these or more commonly at major endpoints of morbidity (jaundice) or mortality. The evidence can be summarized as follows: without anesthesia or surgery approximately one in seven to eight hundred patients who are otherwise healthy and are scheduled for surgery will have abnormal liver function tests, of which one in three will develop jaundice (see Ch. 1 for these studies).[294,295] All anesthetics (general and regional) tested cause transient abnormalities in liver function tests that are magnified by upper intra-abdominal surgery and occur with or without preexisting liver disease.[296-309] Patients with abnormal liver function tests obviously will have more abnormal function tests postoperatively.[296,301-303,305,306] Studies of patients with compromised hepatic function to try to determine how to decrease risk are lacking. In addition to preexisting hepatic disease and the operative site, hypokalemia, hypotension, sepsis, and the need for blood transfusion all contribute to postoperative hepatic dysfunction. Thus, anesthesia and surgery probably exacerbate hepatic disease and this obviously increases morbidity and mortality.[296,298,299,301-303,305,306] The main problem is of worsening hepatic disease (with perhaps its metabolic and central nervous system toxicity), renal failure, and death (in portal hypertension, an albumin less than 3 g/100 ml, serum bilirubin greater than 3 mg/100 ml, and ascites and encephalopathy can result in 50 percent mortality compared to 10 percent when the preoperative serum bilirubin is between 2 and 3 mg/100 ml, serum albumin is between 3 and 3.5 g/100 ml, and encephalopathy is absent).[296-313] The risks of anesthetizing someone with chronic liver disease not requiring portocaval shunt are only sporadically detailed, but appear to be greater than of anesthetizing a healthy patient.[296-313] Should halothane be given to patients with hepatitis or biliary tract disease? The National Halothane Study did not find that halothane caused massive hepatic necrosis or any other hepatic abnormality more frequently than any other anesthetic,[306] and in fact demonstrated its safety in biliary tract surgery. Prospective studies have been contradictory at best as to whether repeat exposures of halothane in a short time-frame cause more elevation of liver enzymes than do alternate anesthetics.[314-316] The incidence of halothane hepatitis is very low, thus very large groups are required to study the problem. The nonhalothane-induced causes of postoperative jaundice and hepatitis is much greater than the incidence of halothane hepatitis, and the absence of differentiating pathologic features make halothane hepatitis difficult to exclude. Thus the strong internist bias makes halothane hepatitis a popular diagnosis, despite the higher incidence of viral and drug hepatitidies.[317-329] The animal models for halothane hepatitis include those with liver hypoxia or PCB pretreatment (all the recent publicity regarding PCB's in the food chain makes me uneasy). Thus, no evidence exists implicating halothane as better or worse than any other anesthetic for the patient with preexisting liver disease (except for halothane hepatitis). But should liver disease worsen postoperatively, the bias is to blame halothane. Anesthesia is certainly less likely than hypoxia, trauma, viral hepatitis, drug hepatitis, or sepsis to cause serious hepatic injury.[294-329] There is no magic timeframe during which repeating exposure to any anesthetic is more dangerous than varying anesthetics or after which repeating anesthesia is as safe as a virgin anesthetic exposure.

What should the physician with hepatitis B do to avoid infecting his patients? That is beyond the scope of this chapter but amply covered already.[330] Liver disease severe enough to induce synthetic injury can impair the detoxification of many drugs[242, 243] including muscle relaxants[331] (see Ch. 17) and disturb coagulation (see Ch. 28). For the latter, fresh frozen plasma may be needed.

HEMATOLOGIC DISORDERS AND ONCOLOGIC DISEASE

HEMATOLOGIC DISORDERS

ANEMIA AND POLYCYTHEMIA IN GENERAL

In Chapter 1, the evidence that normovolemic anemia or polycythemia increases perioperative morbidity was detailed. To review, Wasserman and co-workers[332] found that 22 of 28 patients with uncontrolled polycythemia (hemoglobin greater than 16 g percent) who underwent major surgery had complications and 10 (36 percent) died. Of 53 patients with controlled polycythemia who underwent major surgery, 15 had complications and 3 (5 percent) died. Most of the complications in both groups were related to polycythemia (hemorrhage or thrombosis). Although that study has some obvious deficiencies (retrospective, no time frame given, exclusion of "minor" surgery, no statement as to why some patients had their polycythemia controlled and others did not preoperatively), it implies that knowledge and pretreatment of polycythemia decreases perioperative morbidity and mortality. No such evidence exists for normovolemic anemia. Rothstein[333] concluded that theoretically in patients under 3 months of age, hemoglobin should be over 10 g percent, while in children over 3 months of age a hemoglobin of 9 g percent was adequate. Slogoff[334] concluded that theoretically in adults a hematocrit of 20 percent (hemoglobin of about 7 g percent) was adequate. Perhaps, the duration of anemia is important also, as with time the cardiovascular system adjusts to anemia to increase cardiac output.[334] Thus, whereas there may be no specific preoperative routines for anemia per se, anemia can be a hallmark of many other disease entities that could affect perioperative anesthetic management. For instance, anemia could be a sign of renal insufficiency or a drug reaction, both of which could alter anesthetic management. Thus the cause for the anemia should be known preoperatively. Similarly polycythemia can be secondary to smoking, use of diuretics, or chronic use of androgens, an indicator of hypoxia or other forms of chronic lung/heart disease, or a primary disease (polycythemia vera). Phlebotomies are quite effective for patients whose polycythemia is mild. Recently, it has been shown that cerebral blood flow is improved by keeping the hematocrit below 45 percent.[335, 336] No prospective controlled human trial exists on the decrease in perioperative morbidity or wound healing[334] from treatment of anemia or polycythemia but perhaps the time of most danger to the patient is the early recovery room period when oxygen delivery to the lungs is perhaps at its worst (see Ch. 41). Several forms of anemia present special situations, such as sickle cell anemia, hereditary spherocytosis, and the autoimmune hemolytic anemias.

Sickle Cell Anemia and Related Hemoglobinopathies

The sickle cell syndromes (also see Ch. 28) comprise a family of abnormal hemoglobinopathies due to the genetic transformation of amino acids in the hememoiety.[338–340] A major pathologic feature of sickle cell disease is the aggregation of irreversibly sickled cells in blood vessels. The molecular basis of sickling is aggregation of deoxygenated hemoglobin molecules along their longitudinal axis.[338–344] This distorts the membrane of the cell, resulting in the sickled shape. Irreversible sickled cells become dehydrated and rigid and can cause tissue infarcts by impeding blood flow and oxygen to tissues. Some other abnormal hemoglobins interact with hemoglobin S to various degrees, giving rise to symptomatic disease in patients heterozygous for hemoglobin S and one of the other hemoglobins such as the hemoglobin of thalassemia (hemoglobin C). Two tenths of one percent of the black population in America have sickle thalassemia (hemoglobin SC); these patients also have symptoms suggestive of organ infarction and have end-organ disease. The perioperative considerations of these patients should be similar to those with sickle cell disease (hemoglobin SS) discussed below. Whereas 8 to 10 percent of American blacks have sickle cell trait, 0.2 percent are homozygous for the sickle cell hemoglobin and have the disease. The sickle cell trait should not be considered a disease, because hemoglobin AS cells begin to sickle only when oxygen saturation of hemoglobin is below 20 percent. No difference has been found between normal persons (those with hemoglobin AA) and those with hemoglobin AS in survival rates or occurrence rates of severe disease with the exception of a 50 percent increase in pulmonary infarctions. However, single case reports of a perioperative death and a perioperative brain infarct in two patients with AS disease do exist.[345,346]

The pathologic end-organ damage that occurs in sickle cell states occurs due to three phenomena: sickling of cells in blood vessels, an occurrence that causes infarcts and consequent tissue destruction secondary to tissue ischemia, hemolytic crisis secondary to hemolysis and, aplastic crises that occur with bone marrow exhaustion and can rapidly result in severe anemia. Logic dictates that patients currently in a crisis should not be operated upon except for extreme emergencies, and then only after exchange transfusion.[343–347] Since sickling is increased with lowered oxygen tensions, acidosis, hypothermia, and the presence of more desaturated hemoglobin S, current dictates of therapy include keeping the patient warm, well hydrated, using supplemental oxygen, maintaining a high cardiac output, and avoiding areas of stasis due to pressure. The meticulous attention to these points in those periods when we usually do not pay most careful attention (i.e., waiting in the preinduction area) or when gas exchange may be most unmatched to cardiovascular-metabolic demands (early postoperative period) may be important in lessening morbidity. Following these routine measures with no special emphasis placed on these time periods has led to a 1 percent mortality in several series in patients with sickle cell syndromes.[343,344,346,347] Retrospective review of these patients' charts led those authors to conclude that at most a 0.5 percent mortality rate could be attributed to the sickle cell disease–anesthetic interaction. Can this rate be lessened? Several authors have advocated partial exchange transfusions perioperatively.[348–351] In children with sickle cell disease and acute lung syndromes, partial exchange transfusion resulted in improvement in clinical symptoms and blood oxygenation. Also decreases in serum bilirubin occurred in patients with acute liver injury. Clinical improvement of pneumococcal meningitis and cessation of hematuria in papillary necrosis also accompanied exchange transfusion.[351] The goal of exchange transfusion is to increase the hemoglobin A concentration to 40 percent and hematocrit to 35 percent. The 40 percent figure is an arbitrary one, as no controlled studies have examined ratios of hemoglobin A to S that make blood not able to sickle in vivo. To achieve the 40 percent ratio about 4 units of washed erythrocytes must be exchanged by an efficient but inexpensive system in a 70 kg adult. How great the decrease in perioperative morbidity is after partial exchange transfusion compared to the risks of exchange has not been examined. Until it is, my recommendation is to pay meticulous attention to avoid those factors that increase sickling and to save exchange transfusion for crisis situations. Recently, inducing hyponatremia has been shown to abort acute sickle cell crisis; however, this treatment is still experimental.

In thalassemia, facial deformity has been reported to make endotracheal intubation difficult;[352] this one case report has not been amplified upon, or reported for patients with sickle cell anemia.

Glucose-6-phosphate dehydrogenase (G6-PD) deficiency is also reported to occur in about 8 percent of American black males (it is a sex-linked recessive trait). Red cell hemolysis can occur after administration of drugs that produce substances (such as methemoglobin, glutathione, and hydrogen peroxide) requiring G6PD for detoxification. Drugs to be avoided are sulfa drugs, quinidine, prilocaine, antimalarials, antipyretics, non-narcotic analgesics, vitamin K analogues, and perhaps sodium nitroprusside.

HEREDITARY SPHEROCYTOSIS, ELLIPTOCYTOSIS, AND IMMUNE HEMOLYTIC ANEMIAS

Congenital abnormalities of the erythrocyte membrane are poorly understood. The membrane in hereditary spherocytosis or elliptocytosis is more permeable to cations and more readily undergoes lipid loss when energy of the cell is depleted than does the normal red cell. The role of splenectomy in these diseases is not fully defined, but improves the shortened red cell life span by 100 percent (from 20 to 30 days to 40 to 70 days) in severe disease. Splenectomy does predispose to gram positive septicemia (particularly pneumococcal disease), and perhaps patients should receive pneumococcal vaccine preoperatively prior to when predictable bacteremic events occur. No specific anesthetic problems have been reported for these disorders.

The autoimmune hemolytic anemias include cold antibody, idiopathic (warm), and drug-induced.[353,354] The cold antibody hemolytic anemias are mediated by IgM or IgG antibodies, which cause red cell clumping at or below room temperature. When these patients are transfused, the cells and all fluid infusions must be warm, and as is implied, the patient's temperature must meticulously be maintained at 37°C if hemolysis is to be avoided. Warm antibody or idiopathic hemolytic anemia is a difficult management problem characterized by chronic anemia, antibodies against red cells, positive Coombs' test, and difficulty with cross-matching blood. In elective situations, use of autologous transfusions and blood from rare Rh-negative red cell donors and/or the patient's first degree relatives can be accomplished. In emergency situations, autotransfusions, splenectomy, or corticosteroid treatment possibilities should be explored with a knowledgeable hematologist. Drug-induced hemolytic anemias generally cease with cessation of drug therapy. In emergency situations, the least incompatible cells available should be used for transfusion.

GRANULOCYTOPENIA

In patients with less than 500 granulocytes per ml and established sepsis, granulocyte transfusion has been shown to prolong life.[355,356] Antibiotic prophylaxis logic might dictate giving granulocyte transfusions prophylactically to patients with less than 500 granulocytes per ml and predictable bacteremic events, but this has not been studied.

PLATELET DISORDERS

The inherited platelet disorders are rare, while acquired disorders are quite common. Both present with a history of skin and mucosal bleeding, whereas plasma coagulation defects produce deep tissue or delayed bleeds. Perioperative treatment of the inherited platelet disorders (Glazmann's thrombasthenia, Bernard-Souliep syndrome, Hermansky-Pudlak syndrome) is platelet transfusion. The much commoner acquired disorders may have different therapies. Immune thrombocytopenias, such as lupus erythematosis, idiopathic thrombocytopenic purpura, uremia, and thrombocytosis may respond to steroids, splenectomy, platelet pheresis, or alkylating agents.[357] By far the largest number of platelet defects probably are now drug-related defects in platelet aggregation and release. Aspirin irreversibly acetylates platelet cyclo-oxygenase, the enzyme that converts arachidonic acid to prostaglandin endoperoxidases. Because this enzyme is not regenerated in a platelet's life span in the circulation and is essential for the aggregation of platelets, one aspirin may affect platelet function for a week. All other drugs that inhibit platelet function (vitamin E, indomethecin, sulfinpyrazone, dipyrimidole, tricyclic antidepressants, phenothiazines, furosemide, steroids) do not irreversibly inhibit cyclo-oxygenase function, and thus these drugs disturb platelet function for only 24–48 hours. If emergency surgery is needed prior to aspirin's 8-day period or if the 2-day period for other drugs has expired, 2 to 5 units of platelet concentrates will restore enough platelet function in the 70 kg adult and will restore platelet-induced clotting dysfunction to normal.[358–360] It is apparent that only 30,000 to 50,000 cells/m^3 of normally functioning platelets are needed for normal clotting. One platelet transfusion will increase the platelet count from 4,000 to 20,000 per ml; platelet half-life is about 8 hours.[358–360]

HEMOPHILIA, AND RELATED DISORDERS (ALSO SEE CH. 28)

The disorders of blood coagulation due to plasma coagulation factor defects can be either inherited or acquired. Inherited disorders include X-linked hemophilia A (defect in factor VIII activity), von Willebrand's disease (defect in von Willebrand's component of factor VIII), hemophilia B (a sex-linked deficiency of factor IX activity), and other less common disorders. The sex-linkage of these disorders means that the disease occurs almost exclusively in male offspring of female carriers; males do not transmit the disease to their male offspring. In elective situations, levels of the missing coagulation factor should be assayed 48 hours prior to surgery and a level of 40 percent of normal restored prior to surgery. One unit/kg of body weight normally increases factor concentration by 2 percent. Thus administration of 20 units/kg body weight in the individual essentially devoid of activity is required as an initial dose; since factor VIII has a half-life of 6 to 10 hours and factor IX of 8 to 16 hours, about 1.5 units/hr/kg of factor VIII or 1.5 units/2 hr/kg of factor IX should be given. Additional administration of factors VIII and IX should be guided by the activity of the clotting factors for about 6 to 10 days postoperatively.[361–365] Various preparations are available to give these factors: cryoprecipitate, which contains 20 units/ml, is obtained from regular donors (risk of hepatitis 1/200 5 ml lots) or fresh frozen plasma (which contains 1 unit/ml). Factor IX but not factor VIII is contained in prothrombin complex concentrate, but these may contain activated clotting factors, leading to disseminated intravascular clotting and a high risk of hepatitis. In addition, 0.5 mg/kg of epsilon-aminocaproic acid or tranexamic acid are sometimes administered to these patients as fibrinolytic inhibitors, but they pose a significant risk of disseminated intravascular coagulation. Several additional hazards of modern therapy exist:

acute and chronic hepatitis, psychic trauma, chronic pain with narcotic addiction, and inhibitors to the factors, especially VIII. Approximately 10 percent of patients with either hemophilia A or B develop an antibody that inactivates factors VIII or IX (fresh frozen plasma fails to increase clotting factor activity after incubation with the patient's plasma). These acquired anticoagulants are usually IgG, are poorly removed by plasma pheresis, and are variably responsive to immunosuppressive drugs. Use of prothrombin complex concentrates can be life saving but carries the risk of disseminated intravascular coagulation and hepatitis.

Vitamin K deficiency is reviewed in the section on liver disease. To review, vitamin K dependent clotting factors (II, VII, IX, and X) require vitamin K for the postsynthetic addition of gamma-carboxy groups to glutamate residues; the vitamin K enables the clotting factors to bind calcium and phospholipid. Parenteral vitamin K or fresh frozen plasma can correct these deficiencies.

Patients who come to the operating room having received multiple units of blood (as in massive GI bleeding) may have deficient clotting. This has been demonstrated to be due initially to depletion of platelets (after around 10 to 15 units) and later to coagulation factor depletion (see Ch. 28).[366,367] Treatment of these deficiencies can be corrected with platelet concentrates (each is normally suspended in 50 ml of fresh plasma, thus coagulation factors are also replaced).

The problem of patients on oral anticoagulants is discussed in the cardiac section of this chapter. Regional anesthetic techniques might be avoided in patients who are anticoagulated.[143,144] Reversal of heparin sulfate can be accomplished by using the activated clotting time as a guide and by titrating protamine. Our group usually initially gives approximately 1 mg of protamine per 3 to 4 mg of heparin administered within the last 8 hours.

ONCOLOGIC DISEASE

Patients with malignancy may be essentially healthy (save their yet to be removed malignancy) or desperately ill with nutritional, neurologic, metabolic, endocrinologic, electrolyte, cardiac, pulmonic, renal, hepatic, hematologic, or pharmacologic disability. Thus, knowledge of the other disabilities any patient with malignancy has requires search in all other systems. Common concomitants of malignancy include hypercalcemia either by direct bone invasion, ectopic elaboration of parathyroid hormone or other bone-dissolving substance, uric acid nephropathy, hyponatremia (especially with oat-cell carcinoma of the lung), nausea, vomiting, anorexia, and cachexia, tumor-induced hypoglycemia, intercranial metastases (10 to 20 percent of all cancers), peripheral nerve or spinal cord disorders, meningeal carcinomatosis, toxic neuropathies secondary to anticancer therapy, and paraneoplastic neurologic syndromes (dermatomyositia, Eaton-Lambert, myopathies, and distal neuropathies). Many patients receive large doses of analgesics and should be kept comfortable in the perioperative period; avoidance of drug dependence is of no practical importance in terminally ill patients.[368–370] Marijuana (tetrahydrocannabinol) exerts a central depressive effect on the vomiting center and may be more effective than the phenothiazines in suppressing nausea associated with cancer and its therapy; it decreases anesthetic requirements 15 to 30 percent.[371] The toxicity of cancer chemotherapy relates to the agents used and dose; for radiation therapy, megavoltage sources cause damage above the following doses: lungs 1,500 rads, kidney 2,400 rads, heart 3,000 rads, spinal cord 4,000 rads, intestine 5,500 rads, brain 6,000 rads, and bone 7,500 rads. Alkalating agents cause bone marrow depression, including thrombocytopenia, alopecia, hemorrhagic cystitis, nausea, and vomiting. Nitrosoureas can cause severe hepatic and renal damage, as well as bone marrow toxicity, myalgias, and paresthesia. Folic acid analogues (i.e., methotrexate) result in bone marrow depression, ulcerative stomatitis, pulmonary interstitial infiltrates, gastrointestinal toxicity, and occasionally severe liver dysfunction. Fluorouracil (5-FU) and floxuridine (FUDR), both pyrimidine analogues, cause bone marrow toxicity, megaloblastic anemia and nervous system dysfunction, and hepatic and gastrointestinal alterations. Purine analogues (mercaptopurine, thioquanine) have bone marrow depression as primary toxic effects. Anthracycline antibiotics (doxorubicin, daunorubicin, mithramycin, mitomycin-C, bleomycin) all can cause pulmonary infiltrates, cardiomyopathies (especially doxorubicin and daunorubicin), myelotoxicity, and gastrointestinal, hepatic, and renal disturbances. Vincristine produces peripheral neuropathesia and inappropriate ADH secretion. Vinblastine produces myelotoxocity. The basic rule for dealing with patients receiving cancer chemotherapy is the same as that expressed earlier: when in doubt about side effects, ask two experts.

PATIENTS RECEIVING DRUG THERAPY FOR CHRONIC AND ACUTE MEDICAL CONDITIONS

A steadily increasing number of potent agents of varying degrees of efficacy for the specific and symptomatic treatment of organic and functional diseases are being used. The average hospitalized patient receives eight to ten drugs. Many drugs have side effects that might make the anesthetic period more risky or patient management more arduous. Knowledge of potential side effects can help the anesthesiologist avoid pitfalls that in retrospect and with knowledge of known drug side effects seem careless. Thus, knowledge of common drugs' common side effects and their pharmacology make these pitfalls avoidable. The first step in avoiding these pitfalls is knowing the name and class of every drug, medicine, and over-the-counter preparation the patient is taking and the rationale for his taking that drug. Unnecessary drugs should be discontinued for a period of time of at least 5 half-lives (longer if metabolites of the drug have activity and longer half-lives). Optimal dose to maximize the therapeutic/toxic ratio of needed or beneficial drugs should be arrived at in consultation with the treating physician, and drug side effects should be sought for and either corrected or at least planned for in anesthetic management. For instance, a patient made hypokalemic with diuretics might have that hypokalemia corrected before surgery or at the very minimum not be hyperventilated during surgery. All drug side effects and interactions are not bad and not all must be avoided; knowledge of these effects beforehand allows one to prevent making mistakes that can compound small side effects into life-threatening situations. So many different drugs are being prescribed that virtually no anesthesiologist can be expected to know the class (e.g., "diuretic") let alone the side effects of drugs all patients they anesthetize are receiving without reference to textbooks or other sources of information. Thus, after obtaining a drug history from the patient, the anesthesiologist should learn the drug's class, what diseases it could be prescribed for, and its common side effects. If necessary, the anesthesiologist should return to the patient's bedside to search for signs or symptoms of these conditions or effects. At that point it is useful to review the pharmacology of the drug, decide whether to treat side effects preoperatively, and plan anesthetic management. Obviously, this type of reasoning and planning is best done at least 1 week before anticipated surgery; communication on such topics well in advance between surgeon, internist, and anesthesiologist should be encouraged. Even if not done earlier than the night prior to surgery, such knowledge of and thoughts about other drugs the patient is receiving may be beneficial.

Understanding the side effects of drugs

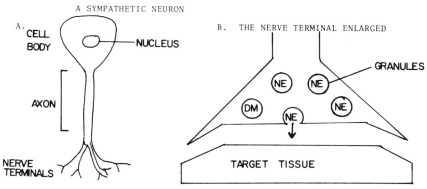

Fig. 2-3 A sympathetic neuron consists of a cell body with its nucleus, a long axon, and multiple nerve terminals. Enzymes responsible for the synthesis of dopamine, norepinephrine, and epinephrine are made in the cell body, transported by a tube system (rapid axoplasmic transport) down the axon to the terminal where the transmitters are made, and stored in granules. (After Axelrod J: Neurotransmitters. Sci Am 230:58, 1974.)

chronically taken that affect the sympathetic nervous system requires some knowledge of basic sympathetic nervous system pharmacology, which will be described below.[372,373]

SYMPATHETIC NERVOUS SYSTEM PHARMACOLOGY
(Also see Ch. 18)

A sympathetic neuron consists of a cell body with its nucleus, a long axon, and multiple nerve terminals. Enzymes responsible for the synthesis of dopamine, norepinephrine, and epinephrine are made in the cell body, transported by a tube system (rapid axoplasmic transport) down the axon to the terminal where the transmitters are made, and then stored in granules (see Fig. 2-3). The sympathetic neuron makes neurotransmitters from either phenylalanine or tyrosine. Tyrosine hydroxylase, the rate-limiting enzyme, aids in converting tyrosine to dopa, which is decarboxylated by *l*-aromatic acid decarboxylase to dopamine. Dopamine is taken up into granules where it remains as itself or is converted by dopamine-β-hydroxylase to norepinephrine. The granules are little packets of neurotransmitters whose

contents are released when an action potential reaches the nerve ending. In some nerve endings (and the adrenal medulla) norepinephrine leaves the granules, is methylated in the cytoplasm to epinephrine, and then reenters a different group of intracellular granules.

Norepinephrine, dopamine, or epinephrine exert their physiological effect by interaction with an appropriate receptor at the target tissue. Three major divisions of catecholamine receptors are α-adrenergic, β-adrenergic, and dopaminergic. These receptors are further subdivided as follows:

Alpha-1—stimulation constricts vascular smooth muscle causing an increase in peripheral vascular resistance.

Alpha-2—stimulation inhibits the release of norepinephrine itself (negative feedback on the sympathetic neuron).

Beta-1—stimulation causes increases in heart rate and strength of contraction.

Beta-2—stimulation causes vascular smooth muscle dilation, airway smooth muscle dilation, uterine smooth muscle relaxation, and a variety of endocrine effects including renin secretion.

Beta-3—stimulation results in a greater re-

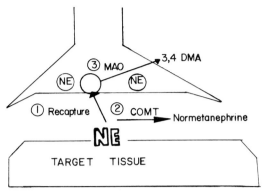

Fig. 2-4 Termination of norepinephrine action. Norepinephrine's (NE) action is terminated mostly through recapture (recycling back into the granules). It may also be terminated by metabolism by (2) catechol-O-methyltransferase (COMT), and/or (3) monamine oxidase (MAO).

lease of norepinephrine from the sympathetic neuron (positive feedback on the sympathetic neuron)

Dopamine—stimulation causes renal vascular dilation and perhaps inhibits acetylcholine release.

The termination of action of sympathomimetic substances is unusual; the nerve ending recaptures most norepinephrine by an active reuptake system (Fig. 2-4). Obviously blockade of this reuptake system permits more norepinephrine to remain free to cause its physiological effects. In addition to this reuptake system, two enzymes metabolically transform catecholamines: monoamine oxidase (MAO) and catechol-O-methyltransferase (COMT) (see Fig. 2-4).

ANTIHYPERTENSIVES

Many antihypertensive agents and almost all mind-altering drugs affect either sympathetic neuronal storage, uptake, metabolism, or release of transmitters. For instance, reserpine and quanethedine (both antihypertensives) deplete the granules of norepineph-

rine, epinephrine, and dopamine both in the brainstem and periphery. The absence of transmitters in sympathetic nerve endings may render drugs such as ephedrine and metaraminol (Aramine) ineffective, since such drugs act by releasing catecholamines (see Fig. 2-5). Guanethedine only affects the peripheral sympathetic system, and depletes granular norepinephrine. Reserpine in amounts clinically used decreases MAC 20 to 30 percent while quanethedine has no effect on anesthetic requirements.[84] In addition to causing a lack of response to indirectly acting vasopressors, reserpine may cause a denervation supersensitivity situation and hyperresponsiveness (with hypertension and/or tachycardia) to usual doses of direct-acting sympathetic amines (such as Neo-Synephrine [phenylephrine], isoproterenol, norepinephrine, epinephrine, and dopamine).[372-374] Thus, in patients who have been treated with drugs that alter sympathetic neurotransmitter release, uptake, metabolism or receptor function, hypotensive, hypertensive or bradycardic problems that need treatment should be treated by titrating doses of direct-acting vasoconstrictors (such as Neo-Synephrine [phenylephrine]), vasodilators (such as nitroprusside), or chronotropes (such as atropine, isoproterenol, or dopamine).

Another group of antihypertensive agents are the false neurotransmitters. False neurotransmitters replace norepinephrine in the granules at the nerve ending. Alpha-methyldopa (Aldomet) becomes α-methyldopamine, which is further metabolized to α-methylnorepinephrine (Fig. 2-6). In some nerve endings and for some receptors, α-methyldopamine or α-methylnorepinephrine (ANE) is more potent than dopamine or norepinephrine as dopaminergic or α stimulants. However, at most nerve endings the false transmitters are less potent stimulants and this is one means by which their antihypertensive action is produced. Alternately, α-methyldopa may act by stimulating the brainstem sympathetic nervous system. When the brainstem sympathetic nervous system antag-

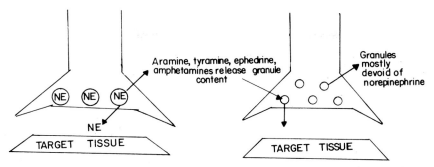

Fig. 2-5 Release of catecholamines. Aramine, tyramine, and ephedrine release the granules' contents. If little norepinephrine is within the granules (as after treatment with Aldomet, reserpine, or guanethedine) then little norepinephrine is released.

onizes the peripheral sympathetic nervous system, the peripheral sympathetic nervous system's activity decreases and the blood pressure is reduced. Alpha-methyldopa through its central effect decreases anesthetic requirements 20 to 40 percent.[84]

Side effects of these neurotransmitter-depleting drugs in addition to altered response to exogenously administered vasopressors are psychic depression, nightmares, drowsiness, nasal stuffiness, diarrhea, bradycardia, and orthostatic hypotension with impotence (reserpine). Guanethedine can cause orthostatic hypotension, bradycardia, asthma, diarrhea,

inhibition of ejaculation; alpha-methyldopa is associated with drowsiness, orthostatic hypotension, bradycardia, diarrhea, acute or chronic hepatitis, cirrhosis, and Coombs' positive hemolytic anemia.[375]

Catecholamine or sympathetic receptor blockers affect the three major divisions of cathecholamine receptors: α-adrenergic, β-adrenergic, and dopaminergic. Subdivisions of these (i.e., beta-1 versus beta-2) imply that drugs are available that can be selective to only one set of receptors: terbutaline is sold over isuprel because terbutaline is said to stimulate beta-2 receptors (to dilate airway

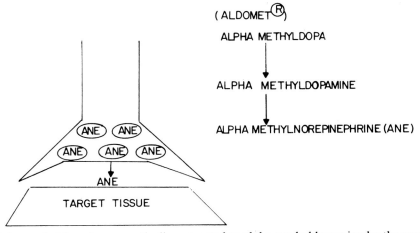

Fig. 2-6 Alpha-methyldopa is enzymatically converted to alpha-methyldopamine by the same enzyme that converts dopa to dopamine. Alpha-methyldopamine is converted to alpha-methylnorepinephrine by the same enzyme that converts dopamine to norepinephrine.

smooth muscle) preferentially, thus avoiding the cardiac stimulant effect of beta-1 stimulants. In fact, selectivity is dose related. A direct beta-2 stimulant will stimulate beta-2 at a specific dose but at a higher dose will stimulate both beta-1 and beta-2 receptors. The effect of a given dose is specific to a given patient. Both beta-1 and beta-2 receptors may be stimulated in one patient by a dose that did not stimulate either beta-1 or beta-2 receptors in another patient. More and more selective blocking drugs are being developed in hopes of widening the margin between beta-1 and beta-2 and α-adrenergic effects.

Propranolol, a β-adrenergic blocker, and metaprolol (Lo-Pressor), a "β-1-adrenergic blocker," are the only widely available β-adrenergic blockers chronically used in the United States. Alpha-adrenergic blockers include regitine, phenoxybenzamine, the phenothiazines, and the butyrophenones (such as droperidol). Dopaminergic receptor antagonists include the antischizophrenic medicines (phenothiazines and butyrophenones). The receptor-blocking drugs block in a dose-related fashion the action of the sympathomimetics at the receptor. Thus, propranolol lowers blood pressure by blocking the effect of norepinephrine and epinephrine in increasing the rate and force of the heart's contractions (and perhaps their effects in increasing renin secretion). To overcome this blockade, one need only to provide more β-stimulant drug. Thus, high doses of vasopressors may be needed to increase blood pressure in a patient receiving large doses of propranolol. When administration of β-adrenergic blocking drugs is terminated, increased levels of sympathetic stimulation often occur, as if the body had responded to their presence by increasing sympathetic neuron activity. Thus, propranolol withdrawal can be accompanied by a hyper-β-adrenergic condition that results in increased myocardial oxygen demands. Administration of propranolol or metoprolol can cause bradycardia, congestive heart failure, tiredness, dizzi-

ness, depression, bronchospasm, and Peyronie's disease.[375] Side effects of the dopaminergic receptor blocking drugs are covered under mood-altering drugs later in this chapter.

Prazocin (Minipress) is an α-1-adrenergic receptor blocker used to treat both hypertension and ischemic cardiomyopathy because it causes both venodilation and arteriodilation. It is associated with dizziness, vertigo, palpitations, depression, dizziness, weakness, and anticholinergic effects.

Brainstem sympathomimetics stimulate α-adrenergic receptors in the brainstem. Clonidine (Catapres), a drug with a 12 to 24 hour half-life, is an α-adrenergic stimulant. Presumably it lowers blood pressure through the central brainstem adrenergic stimulation referred to previously. Its withdrawal can precipitate sudden hypertensive crisis, analogous to withdrawal of propranolol, causing a hyper-β-adrenergic condition referred to above, although the degree of hypertensive crisis following clonidine withdrawal is now being debated. Tricyclic antidepressants, and presumably phenothiazines and the butyrophenones, interfere with its action. Giving a butyrophenone, e.g., droperidol, to a patient chronically receiving clonidine could theoretically precipitate a withdrawal hypertensive crisis, although none have been reported. Clonidine administration can be accompanied by drowsiness, dry mouth, orthostatic hypotension, bradycardia, and impotence.

Two other classes of antihypertensives affect the sympathetic nervous system only indirectly and usually weakly: diuretics and arteriolar dilators. The thiazide diuretics are associated with hypochloremic alkalosis, hypokalemia, hyperglycemia, hyperuricemia, and hypercalcemia; the potassium-sparing diuretic spironolactone is associated with hyperkalemia, hyponatremia, gynecomastia, and impotence. All diuretics can cause dehydration. The thiazide diuretics and furosemide appear to prolong neuromuscular blockade.[376] The arteriolar dilator, hydralazine, can cause a lupus-like condition (usually with renal involvement), nasal congestion, headache, dizziness, congestive heart failure, angina, and GI disturbances.[396]

MOOD-ALTERING DRUGS

Mood-altering drugs are the most frequently prescribed medications in the United States, and include MAO inhibitors (monamine oxidase inhibitors, see Fig. 2-4), phenothiazines, tricyclic antidepressants, and drugs of abuse such as cocaine.

Monamine oxidase inhibitors—isocarboxazide (Marplan), phenelzine (Nardil), pargyline (Eutonyl), and tranylcypromine (Parnate)—irreversibly bind to the enzyme monamine oxidase and thereby increase intraneuronal levels of amine neurotransmitters (serotonin, norepinephrine, dopamine, epinephrine, octopamine). This is associated with both an antidepressive and antihypertensive effect. Interactions may occur as long as 2 weeks after the last dose of this drug and include severe hypertension (especially after taking a food or receiving a medicine that includes indirect sympathetic releasing agents, such as tyramine [in blue cheese] or ephedrine), convulsions, and hyperpyrexia coma (especially after narcotics). Anyone who has witnessed the attempted management of an anesthetic for a patient receiving an MAO inhibitor knows why authors state *"MAO inhibitors should be discontinued at least 2 to 3 weeks before any planned operation."* Emergency surgery of patients receiving MAO inhibitors can be punctuated by hemodynamic instability. Regional block can be attempted to treat postoperative pain; case reports of hyperpyrexic coma following most narcotics exist in man, and animal studies document a 10 to 50 percent incidence of hyperpyrexic coma in animals pretreated with MAO inhibitors who are given any narcotic tested.[191,377-380] These reactions appear to be best treated by supportive therapy.

Alternate drugs for the treatment of severe depression include the tricyclic antidepressants. Tricyclics—amitriptyline (Elavil, Endep), imipramine (Imavate, Tofranil, Presamine), desipramine (Norpramin, Pertofrane), doxepin (Adapin, Sinequan), nortriptyline (Aventyl) and others—block adrenergic reuptake and cause release of transmitters acutely. If chronically given, tricyclics decrease noradrenergic catecholamine stores. They also have atropine-like effects (dry mouth, tachycardia, delerium, urinary retention) and can cause electrocardiographic changes (T wave alterations, QRS prolongation, bundle branch block or other conduction abnormalities, or PVCs). Tricyclic-induced arrhythmias have been successfully treated with physostigmine, but unwanted bradycardia has also been a problem.[375] Drug interactions with tricyclics include those predictable from the drugs' blockade of norepinephrine reuptake (such as interference with the action of guanethedine) and fatal arrhythmias in the presence of halothane and pancuronium.[381]

The effectiveness of phenothiazines and butyrophenones in schizophrenia correlates well with a dopamine receptor blocking action. In addition these drugs possess varying degrees of α-adrenergic blocking potency and parasympathetic stimulation. The phenothiazines—chlorpromazine (Thorazine, Chlor-PZ), promazine (Sparine), triflupromazine (Vesprin), fluphenazine (Prolixin), trifluoperazine (Stelazine), prochlorperizine (Compazine), and numerous others—and the butyrophenones—droperidol and haloperidol (Haldol)—produce sedation, depression, and antihistaminic, antiemetic, and hypothermic responses; in addition they are associated with cholystatic jaundice, impotence, dystonic reactions, and photosensitivity. Other side effects associated with phenothiazines include orthostatic hypotension (partly due to α-adrenergic blockade) and electrocardiographic abnormalities, which include prolongation of the QT or PR intervals, blunting of T waves, ST segment depression, and rarely, PVCs.

There are several important drug interactions with phenothiazine derivatives. Central nervous system depressants are enhanced by concomitant administration of phenothiazines, especially narcotics and barbiturates. Central nervous system seizure threshold is lowered by phenothiazines. They should be avoided in known epileptic patients and in any patient withdrawing from CNS depressant drugs. The antihypertensive effects of guanethidine are blocked by phenothiazines.[375] Lithium carbonate is used to treat manic depression; it is more effective in preventing mania than in relieving depression. Lithium mimics sodium in excitable cells, decreasing the release of neurotransmitters both centrally and peripherally. It prolongs neuromuscular blockade,[382] and may decrease anesthetic requirements because it blocks brainstem noradrenaline, adrenaline, and dopamine release.

Street psychoactive drugs, such as amphetamine and cocaine, both acutely release norepinephrine, epinephrine, and dopamine and block their reuptake. When chronically taken, they deplete the nerve endings of these neurotransmitters.

Drugs that appear to increase central α-adrenergic release increase anesthetic requirement, while drugs that appear to decrease central α-adrenergic release decrease anesthetic requirements (this may not be the mechanism by which they alter anesthetic requirement, but it is a convenient way of remembering the alteration). Drugs that affect only the β-adrenergic system do not alter anesthetic requirements.[84,383–385]

SYMPATHOMIMETICS

Many antiasthmatic drugs (bronchodilators) such as terbutaline, aminophylline, and theophylline are sympathomimetics that can interact with the volatile anesthetics to cause arrhythmias. Halothane (and to some degree most other volatile anesthetics) sensitize the myocardium to exogenous catechol-amines.[386–389] Sensitization means that the dose of exogenous epinephrine administered intravenously needed to produce premature ventricular contractions is lower in halothane anesthetized individuals than in awake individuals. How much epinephrine is it safe to give when halothane is the anesthetic? Katz and Bigger[389] reported that administration of 0.15 ml/kg of a 1/100,000 epinephrine solution per ten minute period not to exceed 0.45 ml/kg of a 1/100,000 solution per hour was safe. Horrigan and others have shown that lidocaine given with epinephrine affords extra protection, and that when enflurane or isoflurane are used they are less sensitizing than halothane.[387,388,390] Since halothane is a potent bronchodilator,[391] it is an acceptable choice, perhaps even the best choice for anesthetizing patients with asthma.[392] However, many asthmatic patients are receiving exogenous catecholamines as chronic bronchodilators. Xanthines are effective bronchodilators because they produce β-adrenergic stimulation in two ways. They cause release of norepinephrine[393,394] and they also inhibit breakdown of cyclic $3'5'$ AMP,[395] the mediator of many of the actions of β-adrenergic agonists.[396] Phosphodiesterase catalyzes the breakdown of cyclic $3'5'$ AMP. Thus, inhibition of phosphodiesterase by theophylline increases the concentration of cyclic $3'5'$ AMP. Marcus et al.[393] and Westfall and Flemming[394] have shown that at least 40 percent of the inotropic effects of aminophylline are due to its ability to directly release norepinephrine. Aminophylline infusion also increases urinary catecholamine excretion.[397] Experimentally, aminophylline decreases the threshold for ventricular fibrillation.[398]

Plasma theophylline levels of 5 mg/L are needed to reduce abnormal elevations of airway resistance. No further beneficial effects are obtained with levels greater than 20 mg/L. Instead, toxic effects start to appear.[399,400] Theophylline (aminophylline is a combination of 85 percent theophylline and 15 percent ethylenediamine) is largely metabolized by the liver, with less than 10 percent excreted unchanged in the urine. The average half-life is 4.4 ± 1.15 hours in adults with a clearance of 1.2 ml/min/kg.[399, 400] Significant liver disease or pulmonary edema can decrease the clearance of the drug, by one half and one third, respectively.[401] Cigarette smokers clear aminophylline more rapidly than nonsmokers.[402]

The interaction between aminophylline and halothane appears to be a predictable, frequent occurrence (12 of 16 dogs anesthetized with 1 percent halothane developed ventricular arrhythmias—8 of 16 ventricular tachycardia or fibrillation—after large dose aminophylline bolus injections).[403-405] Thus, it is advisable to wait three half-lives after the last doses of aminophylline (approximately 13 hours in normal individuals) before using halothane to anesthetize an asthmatic patient. Another anesthetic that is a bronchodilator[391] but is less likely to predispose to catecholamine arrhythmias[387, 388, 390] (such as enflurane) might be an alternative in patients who must receive aminophylline or other exogenous sympathomimetics prior to or during surgery.

OTHER DRUGS

The preoperative management of much drug therapy is discussed in the preceding sections of this chapter dealing with the diseases for which treatment was instituted and thus are not reviewed here. These discussed therapies include anticoagulants (in hematologic section), endocrinologic preparations excluding birth control pills but including corticosteroids (in the section on endocrinologic disease), antihypertensives (earlier in this section and in cardiovascular diseases), anticonvulsants (in the section on neurologic disorders), and cancer chemotherapeutic agents (in the section on oncology).

Antiarrhythmic drugs are local anesthetics (lidocaine, procaine), anticonvulsants (phenytoin) or antihypertensives (propranolol), or primary antiarrhythmics and are covered elsewhere in this chapter or in Chapter 19. Lack of adverse reports does not indicate that all these drugs should be continued through the time of surgery; pharmacokinetic studies have not been completed to tell if anesthesia (or anesthesia with specific agents) alters their volumes of distribution or clearance enough to warrant changing dosage or dosage schedule in the perioperative period. The dearth of reports on this subject may be due to lack of significant drug interaction or lack of awareness that untoward events could be due to this interaction. Disopyramide is similar to quinidine and procainamide in clinical spectrum and is mainly excreted by the kidneys, but hepatic disease increases its half-life.[375] Anticholinergic effects are common, including tachycardia, urinary retention, and psychosis. Cases of hepatitis after its use have been reported.[375] Little is known of the interaction of bretylium and verapamil with anesthetic agents; because bretylium blocks the release of catecholamines, chronic therapy could be and has been associated with hypersensitivity to vasopressors.[375] Quinidine is dependent on renal function for excretion, can have vagolytic effects that can result in decreased atrioventricular block, and is associated with blood dyscrasias and gastrointestinal disturbances.[375] Most of the antiarrhythmic agents enhance the neuromuscular blockade of nondepolarizing neuromuscular blocking agents. Reports in the literature detail this enhancement for quinidine, phenytoin, lidocaine, procainamide, and propranolol;[406-408] no data exist to document this effect with depolarizing muscle relaxants. Many antibiotics are nephrotoxic and/or neurotoxic and many prolong neuromuscular blockade (see Ch. 17).[409-413] The only antibiotics devoid of neuromuscular effects appear to be penicillin G and the cephalosporins.

Digitalis preparations have a limited margin of safety, with increasing toxicity caused by hypokalemia.[414] Since potassium concentrations can fluctuate widely during anesthesia due to fluid shifts and ventilatory acid–base arrangements and since intraoperative arrhythmias caused by digitalis toxicity may be difficult to differentiate from other causes, I have avoided prophylactic digitalization. Digitalis intoxication can present as such diverse arrhythmias as "junctional" escape rhythm, premature ventricular contractions, ventricular bigeminy or trigeminy, junctional tachycardia, paroxysmal atrial tachycardia with or without block, sinus arrest, sinus exit block, Mobitz type I or II blocks, or ventricular tachycardia.[415] However, anesthetic agents appear to protect against digitalis toxicity, at least in animal studies.[416-419] For patients in atrial fibrillation, the ventricular response should guide appropriateness of digitalis dose.

Medications for glaucoma include two organophosphates—echothiophate (Phospholine) and isoflurophate (Floropryl). These drugs inhibit serum cholinesterase, which is responsible for hydrolysis and inactivation of succinylcholine and the "ester" type local anesthetics (such as procaine, chloroprocaine, and tetracaine).[420] These drugs should be avoided in patients treated with organophosphate eye drops.

Magnesium is given to treat eclampsia; it can cause neuromuscular blockade by itself and potentiates neuromuscular blockade by both nondepolarizing and depolarizing muscle relaxants.[421,422]

There is an increased risk of postoperative venous thrombosis in preoperative use of oral contraceptives.[423,424] While some authorities recommend changing from oral contraceptives to topical methods of birth control 2 to 4 weeks before surgery,[425] no controlled study including the incidence of pregnancy has been done to answer the questions of whether or not birth control pills should be stopped prior to surgery.

INTERRUPTION OF A DRUG REGIMEN PRIOR TO SURGERY

As stated earlier, if a drug is needed to treat a patient, it should be continued through the time of surgery. The only exceptions to this are, (1) monamine oxidase inhibitors, (2) anticoagulants if surgical hemostasis is needed, (3) nicotinic acid, and (4) insulin and corticosteroid dosage adjustments. These recommendations mean that the anesthesiologist should be aware of the pharmacology, interactions, and anesthetic implications described above.[191,425-427]

When in doubt about a disease or a drug, my approach is to read about it in *Harrison's Principles of Internal Medicine,* Katz and Kadis' *Anesthesia and Uncommon Diseases,* or Goodman and Gilman's *Pharmacologic Basis of Therapeutics.* Following this, it is wise to learn about the disease from two people who know most about it and then to determine who is best able to care for the patient. Should they be best qualified, one should then watch them care for the patient. Remember, few prospective controlled studies have been done to show that any technique or treatment or preoperative management decreases perioperative risk. Common sense and foreknowledge of potential pitfalls, and diligence in avoiding those pitfalls, however, should reduce avoidable perioperative complications.

REFERENCES

1. Hamilton WK: Do let the blood pressure drop and do use myocardial depressants! Anesthesiology 45:273, 1976
2. Cahill GF Jr: Diabetes mellitus: A brief overview. John Hopkins Med J 143:155, 1978
3. The University Group Diabetes Program: A study of the effects of hypoglycemic agents on vascular complications in patients with adult-onset diabetes. Part I: Design, methods and baseline characteristics. Part II: Mortality Results. Diabetes (suppl) 19:747, 1970
4. Engerman R, Bloodworth JMB, Helson S: Relationship of the microvascular disease in diabetes to metabolic control. Diabetes (suppl) 26:362, 1977
5. Job D, Eschwege E, Guyot-Argenton C, et al: Effect of multiple daily insulin injections on the course of diabetic retinopathy. Diabetes 25:463, 1976
6. Miki E, Idé T, Kuzuya T, et al: Frequency,

degree, and progression with time of proteinuria in diabetic patients. Lancet 1:922, 1972

7. Deckert T, Poulsen JE, Larsen M: Prognosis of diabetics with diabetes onset before the age of thirty-one. II. Factors influencing the prognosis. Diabetologia 14:371, 1978

8. Pirart J: Diabetes mellitus and its degenerative complications: A prospective study of 4,000 patients observed between 1947 and 1973. Diabetes Care 1:168, 1978

9. Cruse PJ, Foord R: A 5-year prospective study of 23,649 surgical wounds. Arch Surg 107:206, 1973

10. Bagdade JD: Phagocytic and microbiological function in diabetes mellitus. Acta Endocrinol 83 (suppl 205):27, 1976

11. Rosen RG, Enquist IF: The healing wound in experimental diabetes. Surgery 50:525, 1961

12. Goodson WH, Hunt TK: Studies of wound healing in experimental diabetes mellitus. J Surg Res 22:221, 1977

13. Anderson RJ, Schafer LA, Olin DB, et al: Infectious risk factors in the immunosuppressed host. Am J Med 54:453, 1973

14. Peterson L, Caldwell J, Hoffman J: Insulin adsorbance to polyvinyl chloride surfaces with implications for constant-infusion therapy. Diabetes 25:72, 1976

15. Brunzell JD, Chait A, Bierman EL: Pathophysiology of lipoprotein transport. Metabolism 27:1109, 1978

16. Glueck CJ, Gartside PS, Steiner PS, et al: Hyperalpha- and hyperbeta-lipoproteinemia in octogenarian kindreds. Atherosclerosis 27:387, 1977

17. Vaughan RW, Bauer S, Wise L: Volume and pH of gastric juice in obese patients. Anesthesiology 43:686, 1975

18. Coke LR: The electrocardiogram in a nutritional deficiency state. Dis Chest 50:314, 1966

19. Wharton BA, Howells GR, McCann RA: Cardiac failure in kwashiorkor. Lancet 2:384, 1967

20. Law DH: Current concepts in nutrition. Total parenteral nutrition. N Engl J Med 297:1104, 1977

21. Sheldon GF, Way L: Total parenteral nutrition: The state of the art. West J Med 127:398, 1977

22. Knapp DR, Holcombe NH, Krueger SA, et al: Qualitative metabolic fate of phenoxybenzamine in rat, dog and man. Drug Metab Dispos 4:164, 1976

23. Melmon KL: Pheochromocytoma, Textbook of Endocrinology, 5th edition. Edited by Williams RH. Philadelphia, WB Saunders, 1974, pp 283–316

24. Vance JE, Buchanan KD, O'Hara D, et al: Insulin and glucogen responses in subjects with pheochromocytoma: Effect of alpha adrenergic blockade. J Clin Endocrin Metab 29:911, 1969

25. Sode J, Getzen LC, Osborne DP: Cardiac arrhythmias and cardiomyopathy associated with pheochromocytomas. Report of three cases. Am J Surg 114:927, 1967

26. Engleman K, Sjoerdsma A: Chronic medical therapy for pheochromocytoma. Ann Intern Med 61:229, 1964

27. Crago RM, Eckholdt JW, Wiswell JG: Pheochromocytoma: Treatment with α- and β-adrenergic blocking drugs. JAMA 202:870, 1967

28. Remine WH, Chong GC, Van Heerden JA, et al: Current management of pheochromocytoma. Ann Surg 179:740, 1974

29. Ross EJ, Prichard BNC, Kaufman L, et al: Preoperative and operative management of patients with pheochromocytoma. Br Med J 1:191, 1967

30. Scott HW, Oates JA, Nies AS, et al: Pheochromocytoma: Present diagnosis and management. Ann Surg 183:587, 1976

31. Sjoerdsma A, Engelman K, Waldmann TA, et al: Pheochromocytoma: Current concepts of diagnosis and treatment. Ann Intern Med 65:1302, 1966

32. Crout JR, Brown BR: Anesthetic management of pheochromocytoma: The value of phenoxybenzamine and methoxyflurane. Anesthesiology 30:29, 1969

33. Crandell DL, Myers RT: Pheochromocytoma: Anesthetic and surgical considerations. JAMA 187:12, 1964

34. Gould AB, Perry LB: The anesthetic management of pheochromocytoma: Cases involving nonexplosive techniques, metastatic tumors, and multiple procedures. Anesth Analg 51:173, 1972

35. Cooperman LH, Engelman K, Mann PEG: Anesthetic management of pheochromocytoma employing halothane and beta adrenergic blockade. Anesthesiology 28:575, 1967

36. Desmonts JM, Houelleur JL, Remond P, et

al: Anesthetic management of patients with pheochromocytoma. Br J Anaesth 49:991, 1977

37. Kopin IJ: Summary remarks, Stress and Catecholamines: Recent Advances. Edited by Usdin E, Kvetnansky RJ, Kopin IJ. New York, Elsevier, 1980

38. Kopin IJ, Lake CR, Ziegler M: Plasma levels of norepinephrine. Ann Intern Med 88:671, 1978

39. Birchfield RI: Postural hypotension in Wernicke's diseases. A manifestation of antonomic nervous system involvement. Am J Med 36:404, 1964

40. Riley CM, Day RL, Greeley DM, et al: Central autonomic dysfunction with defective lacrimation. I. Report of five cases. Pediatrics 3:468, 1949

41. Shy GM, Drager GA: A neurologic syndrome associated with orthostatic hypotension: A clinico-pathologic study. Arch Neurol 2:511, 1960

42. Christensen NJ: Plasma noradrenaline and adrenaline measured by isotope-derivative assay, a review with special reference to diabetes mellitus. Danish Med Bull 26:17, 1979

43. Kontos HA, Richardson DW, Norvell JE: Mechanisms of circulatory dysfunction in orthostatic hypotension. Trans Am Clin Climatol Assoc 87:26, 1975

44. Ziegler MG, Lake CR, Kopin IJ: Deficient sympathetic nervous response in familial dysautonomia. N Engl J Med 294:630, 1976

45. Ziegler MG, Lake CR, Kopin IJ: The sympathetic nervous system defect in primary orthostatic hypotension. N Engl J Med 296:293, 1977

46. Naftchi NE, Wooten GF, Lowman EW, et al: Relationship between serum dopamine-β-hydroxylase activity, catecholamine metabolism, and hemodynamic changes during paroxysmal hypertension in quadraplegia. Circ Res 35:850, 1974

47. Cohen CA: Anesthetic management of a patient with the Shy-Drager syndrome. Anesthesiology 35:95, 1971

48. Kirtchman MM, Schwartz H, Papper EM: Experiences with general anesthesia in patients with familial dysautonomia. JAMA 170:529, 1959

49. McCaughey TJ: Familial dysautonomia as an anesthetic hazard. Can Anaesth Soc J 12:558, 1965

50. Meridy HW, Creighton RE: General anesthesia in eight patients with familial dysautonomia. Can Anaesth Soc J 18:563, 1971

51. Smith RB, Grenvik A: Cardiac arrest following succinylcholine in patients with central nervous system injuries. Anesthesiology 33:558, 1970

52. Ciliberti BJ, Goldfein J, Rovenstine EA: Hypertension during anesthesia in patients with spinal cord injuries. Anesthesiology 15:273, 1954

53. Desmond J: Paraplegia: Problems confronting the anesthesiologist. Can Anaesth Soc J 17:435, 1970

54. Drinker AS, Helrich M: Halothane anesthesia in the paraplegic patient. Anesthesiology 24:399, 1963

55. Gronert GA, Theye RA: Pathophysiology of hyperkalemia induced by succinylcholine. Anesthesiology 43:89, 1975

56. Jousse AT, Wynne-Jones M, Breithaupt DJ: A follow-up study of life expectancy and mortality in traumatic transverse myelitis. Can Med Assoc J 98:770, 1968

57. Wade JG, Larson CP, Hickey RF, et al: Carotid endarterectomy and carotid chemoreceptor and baroreceptor function in man. N Engl J Med 282:823, 1970

58. Thompson PD, Melmon KL: Clinical assessment of autonomic function. Anesthesiology 29:724, 1968

59. Kendrick WW, Scott JW, Jousse AT, et al: Reflex sweating and hypertension in traumatic transverse myelitis. Treatment Serv Bull (Ottawa) 8:437, 1953

60. Mackin JF, Canary JJ, Pittman CS: Thyroid storm and its management. N Engl J Med 291:1396, 1974

61. Roizen MF, Becker CE: Thyroid storm: A review of cases at the University of California, San Francisco. Calif Med 115:5, 1971

62. Das G, Krieger N: Treatment of thyrotoxic storm with intravenous administration of propranolol. Ann Intern Med 70:985, 1969

63. Kaplan MM, Utiger RD: Diagnosis of hyperthyroidism. Clin Endocrinol Metab 7:97, 1978

64. Schimmel M, Utiger RD: Thyroid and peripheral production of thyroid hormones. Review of recent findings and their clinical implications. Ann Intern Med 87:760, 1977

65. Bigos ST, Ridgeway EC, Kourides IA, et al: Spectrum of pituitary alterations with mild

and severe thyroid impairment. J Clin Endocrinol Metab 46:317, 1978

66. Vanderlaan WP: Antithyroid drugs in practice. Mayo Clin Proc 47:962, 1972

67. Burrow GN: Hyperthyroidism during pregnancy. N Engl J Med 298:150, 1978

68. Dorfman SG, Cooperman MT, Nelson RL, et al: Painless thyroiditis and transient hyperthyroidism without goiter. Ann Intern Med 86:24, 1977

69. Bernal J, Refetoff S: The action of thyroid hormone. Clin Endocrinol 6:227, 1977

70. Levey GS: The heart and hyperthyroidism; use of beta-adrenergic blocking drugs. Med Clin North Am 59:1193, 1975

71. Toft ID, Irvine WJ, Sinclair I, et al: Thyroid function after surgical treatment of thyrotoxicosis; A report of 100 cases treated with propranolol before operation. N Engl J Med 298:643, 1978

72. Eriksson M, Rubenfeld S, Garber AJ, et al: Propranolol does not prevent thyroid storm. N Engl J Med 296:263, 1977

73. Babad AA, Eger EI II: The effect of hyperthyroidism and hypothyroidism on halothane and oxygen requirements in dogs. Anesthesiology 29:1087, 1968

74. Frantz AG: Prolactin. N Engl J Med 298:201, 1978

75. Wilson CB, Dempsey LC: Transphenoidal microsurgical removal of 250 pituitary adenomas. J Neurosurg 48:13, 1978

76. McGuffin WL, Sherman BM, Roth J, et al: Acromegaly and cardiovascular disorders: A prospective study. Ann Intern Med 81:11, 1974

77. Cobb WE, Spare S, Reichlin S: Neurogenic diabetes insipidus: Management with 1-DAVP (1-desamino-8-Darginne vasopressin). Ann Intern Med 88:183, 1978

78. Bone HG III, Snyder WH III, Pak CYC: Diagnosis of hyperparathyroidism. Annu Rev Med 28:111, 1977

79. Weidmann P, Massry SG, Coburn JW, et al: Blood pressure effects of acute hypercalcemia. Ann Intern Med 76:741, 1972

80. Shackney S, Hasson J: Precipitous fall in serum calcium, hypotension, and acute renal failure after intravenous phosphate therapy for hypercalcemia. Ann Intern Med 66:906, 1967

81. Smithwick RH, Thompson JE: Splanchni-cectomy for essential hypertension. JAMA 152:1501, 1953

82. Brown BR: Anesthesia and essential hypertension, ASA Refresher Courses in Anesthesiology. Vol 7. Edited by Hershey SG. Philadelphia, JB Lippincott, 1979, pp 41–50

83. Sprague HB: The heart in surgery. An analysis of results of surgery on cardiac patients during the past ten years at the Massachusetts General Hospital. Surg Gynecol Obstet 49:54, 1929

84. Miller RD, Way WL, Eger EI II: The effects of alpha-methyldopa, reserpine, and guanethidine on minimum alveolar anesthetic requirement (MAC). Anesthesiology 29:1153, 1968

85. Veterans Administration Study on Antihypertensive Agents: Effects of treatment on morbidity in hypertension. JAMA 202:1028, 1967

86. Veterans Administration Cooperative Study Group on Antihypertensive Agents: Effects of treatment on morbidity in hypertension: Results in patients with diastolic blood pressure averaging 90 through 114 mm Hg. JAMA 213:1143, 1970

87. Berglund G, Wilhelmen L, Sannerstedt R, et al: Coronary heart-disease after treatment of hypertension. Lancet 1:1, 1978

88. Prys-Roberts C, Meloche R, Foëx P: Studies of anesthesia in relation to hypertension. 1. Cardiovascular responses of treated and untreated patients. Br J Anaesth 43:122, 1971

89. Goldman L, Caldera DL: Risks of general anesthesia and elective operation in the hypertensive patient. Anesthesiology 50:285, 1979

90. Vacanti CJ, Van Houten RJ, Hill RC: A statistical analysis of the relationship of physical status to postoperative morbidity in 68,388 cases. Anesth Analg 49:564, 1970

91. Lewin I, Lerner AG, Green SH, et al: Physical class and physiologic status in the prediction of operative mortality in the aged sick. Ann Surg 174:217, 1971

92. Marx GF, Mateo CV, Orkin LR: Computer analysis of postanesthetic deaths. Anesthesiology 39:54, 1973

93. Fleiss JL: Statistical Methods for Rates and Proportions. New York, John Wiley and Sons, 1973, p 178

94. Schneider AJL, Knoke JD, Zollinger RM Jr,

et al: Morbidity prediction using pre- and intraoperative data. Anesthesiology 51:4, 1979

95. Mauney FM, Ebert PA, Sabiston DC: Postoperative myocardial infarction: A study of predisposing factors, diagnosis and mortality in a high risk group of surgical patients. Ann Surg 172:497, 1970

96. Gordon T, Kannel WB: The Framingham, Massachusetts, study twenty years later, Community as an Epidemiologic Laboratory: A Casebook of Community Studies. Edited by Kessler II, Levin ML: Baltimore, Johns Hopkins Press, 1970, pp 123–146

97. Benchimol A, Harris CL, Desser KB, et al: Resting electrocardiogram in major coronary artery disease. JAMA 224:1489, 1973

98. Tomatis LA, Fierens EE, Verbrugge GP: Evaluation of surgical risk in peripheral vascular disease by coronary angiography: A series of 100 cases. Surgery 71:429, 1972

99. Borer JS, Brensike JF, Redwood DR, et al: Limitations of the electrocardiographic response to exercise in predicting coronary artery disease. N Engl J Med 293:367, 1975

100. Proudfit WL, Shirey EK, Sones FM: Selective CINE coronary angiography: Correlation with clinical finding in 1000 patients. Circulation 33:901, 1966

101. Arkins R, Smessaert AA, Hicks RG: Mortality and morbidity in surgical patients with coronary artery disease. JAMA 190:485, 1964

102. Topkins MJ, Artusio JF: Myocardial infarction and surgery: A five year study. Anesth Analg 43:715, 1964

103. Fraser JG, Ramachandran PR, Davis HS: Anesthesia and recent myocardial infarction. JAMA 199:318, 1967

104. Tarhan S, Moffitt EA, Taylor WF, et al: Myocardial infarction after general anesthesia. JAMA 199:1451, 1972

105. Sapala JA, Ponka JL, Duvernow WFC: Operative and nonoperative risks in the cardiac patient. J Am Geriatr Soc 23:529, 1975

106. Steen PA, Tinker JH, Tarhan S: Myocardial reinfarction after anesthesia and surgery. JAMA 239:2566, 1978

107. Goldman L, Caldera DL, Southwick FS, et al: Cardiac risk factors and complications in non-cardiac surgery. Medicine 57:357, 1978

108. Knapp RB, Topkins MJ, Artusio JF Jr: The cerebrovascular accident and coronary occlusion in anesthesia. JAMA 182:332, 1962

109. Bruschke AVG, Proudfit WL, Sones FM: Progress study of 590 consecutive non surgical cases of coronary disease followed 5–9 years. Circulation 47:1147, 1973

110. Mahar LJ, Steen PA, Tinker JH, et al: Perioperative myocardial infarction in patients with coronary artery disease with and without aorta-coronary bypass grafts. J Thorac Cardiovasc Surg 76:533, 1978

111. Benson H, McCallie DP: Angina pectoris and the placebo effect. N Engl J Med 300:1424, 1979

112. Oberman A, Harrell RR, Russell RO, et al: Surgical versus medical treatment of the left main coronary artery. Lancet 2:591, 1976

113. Takaro T, Hultgren NH, Lipton MJ, et al: The VA cooperative randomized study of surgery for coronary occlusive disease. II. Subgroup with significant left main lesion. Circulation 54 (suppl 3):III-107, 1976

114. Vliestra RE, Assad-Morell JL, Frye RL, et al: Survival predictors in coronary artery disease. Medical and surgical comparisons. Mayo Clin Proc 42:85, 1977

115. Reed RC, Murphy ML, Hultgren HN, Takaro T: Survival of men treated for chronic stable angina pectoris. A cooperative randomized study. J Thorac Cardiovasc Surg 75:1, 1978

116. Scher KS, Tice DA: Operative risk in patients with previous coronary artery bypass. Arch Surg 111:807, 1976

117. McCollum CH, Giarcia-Rinaldi R, Graham JM, et al: Myocardial revascularization prior to subsequent major surgery in patients with coronary artery disease. Surgery 81:302, 1977

118. Crawford ES, Morris GC, Howell JF, et al: Operative risk in patients with previous coronary artery bypass. Ann Thorac Surg 26:215, 1978

119. Hultgren HN, Pfeifer JF, Angell WW, et al: Unstable angina: Comparison of medical and surgical management. Am J Cardiol 39:734, 1977

120. The Criteria Committee of the New York heart Association, Kossman CE (chairman): Diseases of the heart and blood vessels, Nomenclature and Criteria for Diagnosis. 6th edition. Boston, Little Brown, 1964

121. Nachlas MM, Abrams SJ, Goldberg MM: The influence of arteriosclerotic heart disease on surgical risk. Am J Surg 101:447, 1961

122. Santos AL, Gelperin A: Surgical mortality in the elderly. J Am Geriatr Soc 23:42, 1975

123. Ziffren SE, Hartford CE: Comparative mor-

tality for various surgical operations in older versus younger age groups. J Am Geriatr Soc 20:485, 1972

124. Cogbill CL: Operation in the aged. Arch Surg 94:202, 1967

125. Driscoll AC, Hobika JH, Etsten BE, et al: Clinically unrecognized myocardial infarction following surgery. N Engl J Med 264:633, 1961

126. Cohn PF, Gorlin R, Cohn LH, et al: Left ventricular ejection fraction as a prognostic guide in surgical treatment of coronary and valvular heart disease. Am J Cardiol 34:136, 1974

127. Mangano DT, Hedgcock M: Abnormalities of the chest roentgenogram are predictive of ventricular dysfunction in patients with coronary artery disease. Circulation, in press

128. Riles TS, Kopelman I, Imparato AM: Myocardial infarction following carotid endarterectomy: A review of 683 operations. Surgery 85:249, 1979

129. Roy WL, Edelist G, Gilbert B: Myocardial ischemia during non-cardiac surgical procedures in patients with coronary-artery disease. Anesthesiology 51:393, 1979

130. Backer CL, Tinker JH, Robertson DM: Myocardial reinfarction following local anesthesia (abstr). Anesthesiology 51:S61, 1979

131. Kaplan JA, King SB: The precordial electrocardiographic lead (V_5) in patients who have coronary-artery disease. Anesthesiology 45:570, 1976

132. Braunwald E: Thirteenth Bowditch Lecture. The determinants of myocardial oxygen consumption. Physiologist 12:65, 1969

133. Robinson BF: Relation of heart rate and systolic blood pressure to the onset of pain and angina pectoris. Circulation 25:1073, 1967

134. Gobel FL, Nordstrom LA, Nelson RR, et al: The rate pressure product as an index of myocardial oxygen consumption during exercise in patients with angina pectoris. Circulation 57:549, 1978

135. Cannon DS, Levy W, Cohen LS: The short- and long-term prognosis of patients with transmural and nontransmural myocardial infarction. Am J Med 61:452, 1976

136. Devereux RB, Perloff JK, Reichek N, et al: Mitral valve prolapse. Circulation 54:3, 1976

137. Mills P, Rose J, Hillingsworth J, et al: Long-term prognosis of mitral-valve prolapse. N Engl J Med 297:13, 1977

138. Swartz MH, Teicholz LE, Donoso F: Mitral valve prolapse: A review of associated arrhythmias. Am J Med 62:377, 1977

139. Berry FA, Blankenbaker WL, Ball CG: A comparison of bacteremia occurring with nasotracheal and orotracheal intubation. Anesth Analg 52:873, 1973

140. Shull HJ, Greene BM, Allen SD, et al: Bacteremia with upper gastrointestinal endoscopy. Ann Intern Med 83:212, 1975

141. Committee on Prevention of Rheumatic Fever and Bacterial Endocarditis of the American Heart Association: Prevention of bacterial endocarditis. Circulation 56:139A, 1977

142. Katholi RE, Nolan SP, McGuire LB: The management of anticoagulation during noncardiac operations in patients with prosthetic heart valves. A prospective study. Am Heart J 96:163, 1978

143. De Angelis J: Hazards of subdural and epidural anesthesia during anticoagulant therapy: A case report and review. Anesth Analg 51:676, 1972

144. Edelson RN, Chernik NL, Posner JB: Spinal subdural hematomas complicating lumbar puncture. Arch Neurol 31:134, 1974

145. Pastore JO, Yurchak PM, Janis KM, et al: The risk of advanced heart block in surgical patients with right bundle branch block and left axis deviation. Circulation 57:677, 1978

146. Bigger JT Jr, Dresdale RJ, Heissenbuttel RH, et al: Ventricular arrhythmias in ischemic heart disease. Mechanism, prevalence, significance, and management. Prog Cardiovasc Dis 19:255, 1977

147. Gallagher JJ, Pritchett ELC, Sealy WC, et al: The pre-excitation syndromes. Prog Cardiovasc Dis 20:285, 1978

148. Sadowski AR, Moyers JR: Anesthetic management of the Wolff-Parkinson-White syndrome. Anesthesiology 51:553, 1979

149. Josephson ME, Kastor JA: Supraventricular tachycardia: Mechanisms and management. Ann Intern Med 87:346, 1977

150. Simon AB: Perioperative management of the pacemaker patient. Anesthesiology 46:127, 1977

151. Lev M, Kinare SG, Pick A: The pathogenesis of atrioventricular block in coronary disease. Circulation 42:409, 1970

152. Stein M, Cassara EL: Preoperative pulmonary evaluation and therapy for surgery patients. JAMA 211:787, 1970

153. Collins CD, Darke CS, Knowelden J: Chest complications after upper abdominal surgery: Their anticipation and prevention. Br Med J 1:401, 1968

154. Tisi GM: Preoperative evaluation of pulmonary function: Validity, indications, benefits. Am Rev Respir Dis 119:293, 1979

155. Hedley-Whyte J, Burgess GE, Feeley TW, et al: Critical analysis of preventive measures, Applied Physiology of Respiratory Care. Boston, Little, Brown, 1976, pp 119–132

156. Graham WGB, Bradley DA: Efficacy of chest physiotherapy in the resolution of pneumonia. N Engl J Med 299:624, 1978

157. Ziment I: Why are they saying bad things about IPPB? Respir Care 18:677, 1973

158. Baxter WD, Levine RS: An evaluation of intermittent positive pressure breathing in the prevention of postoperative pulmonary complications. Arch Surg 98:795, 1969

159. Cottrell JE, Siker ES: Preoperative intermittent positive pressure breathing therapy in patients with chronic obstructive lung disease: Effect on postoperative pulmonary complications. Anesth Analg 52:258, 1973

160. Noehren TH, Larsry JE, Legters LJ: Intermittent positive pressure breathing for the prevention and management of postoperative pulmonary complications. Surgery 43:658, 1958

161. Noehren TH: Is positive pressure breathing over-rated? Chest 57: 507, 1970

162. Forthman HJ, Shepard A: Postoperative pulmonary complications. South Med J 62:1198, 1969

163. Boushy SF, Billing DM, North LB, et al: Clinical course related to preoperative pulmonary function in patients with bronchogenic carcinoma. Chest 59:383, 1971

164. Mittman C: Assessment of operative risk in thoracic surgery. Am Rev Respir Dis 84:197, 1961

165. Reichel J: Assessment of operative risk of pneumonectomy. Chest 62:570, 1972

166. Hall WJ, Douglas RG, Hyde RW, et al: Pulmonary mechanics after uncomplicated influenza A infection. Am Rev Respir Dis 113: 141, 1976

167. Green GM, Carolin D: The depressant effect of cigarette smoke on the in vitro antibacterial activity of alveolar macrophages. N Engl J Med 276:422, 1967

168. Green GM, Jakab GJ, Low RB, et al: De-
fense mechanisms of the respiratory membrane. Am Rev Respir Dis 115:479, 1977

169. Latimer RG, Dickman M, Day WC, et al: Ventilatory patterns and pulmonary complications after upper abdominal surgery determined by preoperative and postoperative computerized spirometry and blood gas analysis. Am J Surg 122:622, 1971

170. Tarhan S, Moffitt EA, Sessler AD, et al: Risk of anesthesia and surgery in patients with chronic bronchitis and chronic obstructive pulmonary disease. Surgery 74:720, 1973

171. Gould AB: Effect of obesity on respiratory complications following general anesthesia. Anesth Analg 41:448, 1962

172. Buist AS, Sexton GJ, Nagy JM, et al: The effect of smoking cessation and modification on lung function. Am Rev Respir Dis 114:115, 1976

173. McCarthy DS, Craig DB, Cherniack RM: Effect of modification of the smoking habit on lung function. Am Rev Respir Dis 114:103, 1976

174. Neiwoehner DE, Kleinerman J, Rice DB: Pathologic changes in the peripheral airways of young cigarette smokers. N Engl J Med 291:755, 1974

175. Enson Y: Pulmonary heart disease: Relation of pulmonary hypertension to abnormal lung structure and function. Bull NY Acad Med 53:551, 1977

176. Moser KM: Pulmonary embolism. Am Rev Respir Dis 115:829, 1977

177. Edwards WD, Edwards JE: Clinical primary pulmonary hypertension: Three pathologic types. Circulation 56:884, 1977

178. Settipane GA, Dudupakkam RK: Aspirin intolerance. III. Subtypes, familial occurrence and cross reactivity with tartrazine. J Allergy Clin Immunol 56:215, 1975

179. Smith LJ, Slavin RG: Drugs containing tartrazine dye. J Allergy Clin Immunol 58:456, 1976

180. Trunk G, Gracey DR, Byrd RB: The management and evaluation of the solitary pulmonary nodule. Chest 66:236, 1974

181. Paulson DL: Carcinomas in the superior pulmonary sulcus. J Thorac Cardiovasc Surg 70:1095, 1975

182. Millbern SM, Bell SD: Prevention of anaphylaxis to contrast media. Anesthesiology 50:56, 1979

183. Zweiman B, Mishkin MM, Hildreth EA: An

approach to the performance of contrast studies in contrast material-reactive persons. Ann Intern Med 83:159, 1975

184. Miller WL, Doppman JL, Kaplan AP: Renal arteriography following systemic reaction to contrast material. J Allergy Clin Immunol 56:291, 1975

185. Del Pizzo A: Hereditary angioneurotic edema. Anesthesiol Rev 5:41, 1978

186. Plum F, Posner JB: The Diagnosis of Stupor and Coma. 2nd edition. Philadelphia, FA Davis, 1972

187. Kutt H, Louis S: Anticonvulsant drugs. I. Patho-physiological and pharmacological aspects. Drugs 4:227, 1972

188. Kutt H, Louis S: Anticonvulsant drugs. II. Clinical pharmacological and therapeutic aspects. Drugs 4:256, 1972

189. Drugs for epilepsy. Med Lett Drugs Ther 21:25, 1979

190. Hollister LH: Anticonvulsant drugs, Clinical Pharmacology: Basic Principles in Therapeutics. Edited by Melmon KL, Morrelli HF. New York, Macmillan, 1972, pp 499–506

191. Wollman H, Smith AL, Neigh JL, et al: Cerebral blood flow and oxygen consumption in man during electroencephalographic seizure patterns associated with Ethrane anesthesia, Cerebral Blood Flow. Edited by Brock M, Fieschi C, et al. Berlin, Springer Verlag, 1969, pp 246–248

192. Joas TA, Stevens WC, Eger EI II: Electroencephalographic seizure activity in dogs during anesthesia. Br J Anaesth 43:739, 1971

193. Lebowitz MH, Blitt CD, Dillon JB: Enflurane-induced central nervous system excitation and its relation to carbon dioxide tension. Anesth Analg 51:355, 1972

194. Buzello W, Jantzen K, Scholler KL: The influence of Ethrane on the electro- and pentylenetetrazol-convulsions in mice. Anaesthesist 24:118, 1975

195. Kitagawa J, Iwatsubo K, Shigenaga Y, et al: Pharmacologic comparison between enflurane and halothane. Folia Pharmacol Japan 72:211, 1976

196. Opitz A, Brechts B, Stenzel E: Enflurane anaesthesia for epileptic patients. Anaesthesist 26:329, 1977

197. Schwartz AJ, Wollman H: Anesthetic considerations for patients on chronic drug therapy: L-dopa, monamine oxidase inhibitors, tricyclic antidepressants and propranolol,

Refresher Courses in Anesthesiology. Vol 4. Edited by Hershey SG. Philadelphia, JB Lippincott, 1976, pp. 99–111

198. Ngai SH: Parkinsonism, levodopa, and anesthesia. Anesthesiology 37:344, 1972

199. Ngai SH, Wiklund RA: Levodopa and surgical anesthesia. Neurology (suppl) 22:38, 1972

200. Goldberg LI: Levodopa and anesthesia. Anesthesiology 34:1, 1971

201. Wiklund RA, Ngai SH: Rigidity, and pulmonary edema after Innovar in a patient on levodopa therapy: Report of a case. Anesthesiology 35:545, 1971

202. Raskin NH, Appenzeller O: Headache, Major Problems in Internal Medicine. Philadelphia, WB, Saunders, 1980 (in press)

203. Kudrow L: Comparative results of prednisone, methylsergide, and lithium therapy in cluster headache, Current Concepts in Migraine Research. Edited by Greene R. New York, Raven Press, 1978, pp 159–163

204. Baskett PJF, Armstrong R: Anaesthetic problems in multiple sclerosis. Are certain agents contraindicated? Anaesthesia 25:397, 1970

205. Tschudy DP, Valsamis M, Magnussen CR: Acute intermittent porphyria: Clinical and selected research aspects. Ann Intern Med 83:851, 1975

206. Dundee JW, Riding JE: Barbiturate narcosis in porphyria. Anaesthesia 10:55, 1955

207. Eales L: Porphyria and thiopentone. Anesthesiology 27:703, 1966

208. Jackson SH: Hereditary hepatic porphyrias, Anesthesia and Uncommon Diseases. Edited by Katz J, Kadis JB. Philadelphia, WB Saunders, 1973 pp 10–15

209. Mees DE Jr, Frederickson EL: Anesthesia and the porphyrias. South Med J 68:29, 1975

210. Risk SF, Jacobson JH, Silvay G: Ketamine as an induction agent for acute intermittent porphyria. Anesthesiology 46:305, 1977

211. Engle WK, Festoff BW, Patten BM, et al: Myasthenia gravis. Ann Intern Med 81:225, 1974

212. Drachman DB: Myasthenia gravis. N Engl J Med 298:185, 1978

213. Miller RD: Myasthenia gravis, Clinical Anesthesia Edited by Wilkinson PL, Ham J, Miller RD. St. Louis, CV Mosby, 1980, pp 148–150

214. Sokoll MD, Gergis SD: Anesthesia and neu-

romuscular disease. Anesthesiol Rev 2:20, 1975

215. Hedley-Whyte J, Borgess GE, Feeley TW, et al: Respiratory management of peripheral neurologic disease, Applied Physiology of Respiratory Care. Boston, Little, Brown, 1976, pp 245–268

216. Schmidt GB, Patel KP, Grundy EM, et al: The perioperative management of patients with myasthenia gravis: A review. Anesthesiol Rev 4: 29, 1977

217. Rolbin SH, Levinson G, Shnider SM, et al: Anesthetic considerations for myasthenia gravis and pregnancy. Anesth Analg 57:441, 1978

218. Miller J, Katz R: Muscle diseases, Anesthesia and Uncommon Diseases. Edited by Katz J, Kadis L. Philadelphia, WB Saunders, 1973, pp 425–444

219. Rosenberg H, Durbin CG: Anesthesia in the presence of neuromuscular disease. Anesthesiol Update 1:20, 1978

220. Britt BA (Ed): Malignant hyperthermia. Int Anesth Clin 17:1, 1979

221. Roberts J, et al: Tourniquet test for malignant hyperthermia sensitivity. N Engl J Med, 1980 (in press)

222. Pandit SK, Kotary SP, Cohen PJ: Orally administered dantrolene for prophylaxis of maligant hyperthermia. Anesthesiology 50:156, 1979

223. Appel GB, Neu HC: The nephrotoxicity of antimicrobial agents. N Engl J Med 296:663, 722, 784, 1977

224. Fischer RP, Polk HC Jr: Changing etiologic patterns of renal insufficiency in surgical patients (editorial). Surg Gynecol Obstet 140:85, 1975

225. Yamauchi H, Hopper J Jr: Hypovolemic shock and hypotension as a complication in the nephrotic syndrome: A report of ten cases. Ann Intern Med 60:242, 1964

226. Venkatachalam MA, Rennke HG, Sandstrom DJ: The vascular basis for acute renal failure in the rat. Circ Res 38:267, 1976

227. Tasker PRW, MacGregor GA, De Wardener HE: Prophylactic use of intravenous saline in patients with chronic renal failure undergoing major surgery. Lancet 2:911, 1974

228. Brenowitz JB, Williams CD, Edwards WS: Major surgery in patients with chronic renal failure. Am J Surg 134:765, 1977

229. Brown JHJ: Anesthesia for renal transplantation. Anesthesiol Rev 3:22, 1976

230. Feldman HA, Singer I: Endocrinology and metabolism in uremia and dialysis: A clinical review. Medicine 54:345, 1975

231. Raskin NH, Fishman RA: Neurologic disorders in renal failure. N Engl J Med 294:143, 204, 1976

232. Vincenti F, Duca RM, Amend W, et al: Immunologic factors determining survival of cadaver-kidney transplants: The effect of HLA serotyping, cytotoxic antibodies and blood transfusions on graft survival. N Engl J Med 299:793, 1978

233. Oh MS, Carroll HS; The anion gap. N Engl J Med 297:814, 1977

234. Ansari Z, Baldwin DS: Acute renal failure due to radio-contrast agents. Nephron 17:28, 1976

235. Byrd L, Sherman RL: Radiocontrast induced acute renal failure: A clinical and pathophysiological review. Medicine 58:270, 1979

236. Eisenberg RL, Bank WO, Hedgecock MW: Renal failure after major angiography. Am J Med 68:43, 1980

237. Abel RM, Buckley MJ, Austen WL: Etiology, incidence and prognosis of renal failure following cardiac operations. J Thorac Cardiovasc Surg 71:323, 1976

238. Levinsky NG: Pathophysiology of acute renal failure. N Engl J Med 296:1453, 1977

239. Kleinknecht D, Ganeval D, Gonzalez-Duque LA, et al: Furosemide in acute oliguric renal failure: A controlled trial. Nephron 17:51, 1976

240. Anderson RJ, Linas SL, Berns AS, et al: Nonoliguric acute renal failure. N Engl J Med 296:1134, 1977

241. Advisory Committee to the Renal Transplant Registry: The 13th report of the human renal transplant registry. Transplant Proc 9:9, 1977

242. Bennett WM, Singer I, Golper T, et al: Guidelines for drug therapy in renal failure. Ann Intern Med 86:754, 1977

243. Benet L (editor): The effect of disease states on drug pharmacokinetics. Washington D.C., Am Pharmaceutical Assoc/Am Pharmaceutical Sci, 1976

244. Rubin AL, Stenzel KH, Reidenberg MM: Symposium on drug action and metabolism in renal failure. Am J Med 62:459, 1977

245. Keighley MRB: Antibiotics in biliary disease: The relative importance of antibiotic concentrations in the bile and serum. Gut 17:495, 1976

246. Root RK, Hierholzer WJ Jr: Infectious disease, Clinical Pharmacology: Basic Principles in Therapeutics. 2nd edition. Edited by Melmon KL, Morelli HF. New York, Macmillan, 1978, pp 709–801

247. Everett EO, Hirschmann JV: Transient bacteremia and endocarditis prophylaxis: A review. Medicine 56:61, 1977

248. Robinson JA, Klodnycky ML, Loeb HS, et al: Endotoxin, prekallikrein, compliment and systemic vascular resistance: Sequential measurements in man. Am J Med 59:61, 1975

249. Committee on infections Within Hospitals, American Hospital Association: Infection Control in the Hospital. Chicago, American Hosp Assn, 1979

250. Altemeier WA (editor), Committee on Control of Surgical Infections: Manual of Control of Infection in Surgical Patients. Philadelphia, JB Lippincott, 1976

251. Arieff AI, Llacki F, Massry SG: Neurologic manifestations and morbidity of hyponatremia: Correlation with brain water and electrolytes. Medicine 55:121, 1976

252. Seeley JF, Dirks JH: Site of action of diuretic drugs. Kidney Int 11:1, 1977

253. Hantman O, Rossier B, Zohlman R, et al: Rapid correction of hyponatremia in the syndrome of inappropriate antidiuretic hormone. Ann Intern Med 78:870, 1973

254. Forrest JN Jr, Cox M, Hong C, et al: Superiority of demeclocycline over lithium in the treatment of chronic inappropriate secretion of antidiuretic hormone. N Engl J Med 298:173, 1978

255. Birkenfeld LW, Leibman J, O'Meara MP, et al: Total exchangeable sodium, total exchangeable potassium and total body water in edematous patients with cirrhosis of the liver and congestive heart failure. J Clin Invest 37:687, 1958

256. Moore FD, Edelman IS, Olney JM, et al: Body sodium and potassium. III. Interrelated trends in alimentary, renal, and cardiovascular disease; lack of correlation between body stores and plasma concentration. Metabolism 3:334, 1954

257. Muldowney FP, Williams RT: Clinical disturbances in serum sodium and potassium in relation to alteration in total exchangeable sodium, exchangeable potassium and total body water. Am J Med 35:768, 1963

258. Surawicz B: Relationship between electrocardiogram and electrolytes. Am Heart J 73:814, 1967

259. Sack D, Kim ND, Harrison CE Jr: Contractility and subcellular calcium metabolism in chronic potassium deficiency. Am J Physiol 226:756, 1974

260. Wong KC: Electrolyte disturbance and anesthetic considerations, ASA Refresher Courses in Anesthesiology. Vol 6. Edited by Hershey SG. Philadelphia, JB Lippincott, 1978, pp. 187–198

261. Goggin MJ, Joekes AM: Gas exchange in renal failure. I. Dangers of hyperkalaemia during anaesthesia. Br Med J 2:244, 1971

262. Scribner BH, Burnell JM: Interpretation of the serum potassium concentration. Metabolism 5:468, 1959

263. Wright BD, Di Giovanni AJ: Respiratory alkalosis, hypokalemia and repeated ventricular fibrillation associated with mechanical ventilation. Anesth Analg 48:467, 1969

264. Sack D, Kim ND, Harrison CE Jr.: Contractility and subcellular calcium metabolism in chronic potassium deficiency. Am J Physiol 226:756, 1974

265. Lawson NW, Butler GH, Rat CT: Alkalosis and cardiac arrhythmias. Anesth Analg 52:951, 1973

266. Jasani BM, Edmonds CJ: Kinetics of potassium distribution in man using isotope dilution and whole body counting. Metabolism 20:1099, 1971

267. Johnson JE, Hartsuch JM, Zollinger RM, et al: Radiopotassium equilibration in total body potassium: Studies using ^{43}K and ^{42}K. Metabolism 18:663, 1969

268. Surawicz B, Chlebus H, Mazzoleni A: Hemodynamic and electrocardiographic effects of hyperpotassemia. Differences in response to slow and rapid increases in concentration of plasma K. Am Heart J 73:647, 1967

269. Wong KC, Kawamura R, Hodges MR, et al: Acute intravenous administration of potassium chloride to furosemide pretreated dogs. Can Anaesth Soc J 24:203, 1977

270. Kawamura R, Wong KC, Hodges MR: Intravenous potassium chloride in hypokalemic dogs pretreated with digoxin. Anesth Analg 57:108, 1978

271. Aldinger KA, Samaan NA: Hypokalemia with hypercalcemia. Prevalence and significance in treatment. Ann Intern Med 87:571, 1977

272. Wilkinson PL, Ham J, Miller RD: Preoperative hyperkalemia and elective surgery, Clinical Anesthesia: Case Selections from the University of California, San Francisco. St. Louis, CV Mosby, 1980, pp 54–57

273. Tanifuji Y, Eger EI II: Brain sodium, potassium and osmolality: Effect on anesthetic requirement. Anesth Analg 57:404, 1978

274. Heymsfield SB, Bethel RA, Ansley JD: Enteral hyperalimentation: An alternative to central venous hyperalimentation. Ann Intern Med 90:63, 1979

275. Swinton NW, O'Keefe DD: Preoperative evaluation and preparation of the patient with colonic cancer. Surg Clin North Am 50:737, 1970

276. Swinton NW (moderator): Preoperative evaluation of the surgical patient. Dis Colon Rectum 13:175, 1970

277. May RJ, Long BW, Gardner JD: H_2- histamine receptory blocking agents in the Zollinger-Ellison syndrome. Ann Intern Med 87:668, 1977

278. Eger EI II, Saidman LJ: Hazards of nitrous oxide anesthesia in bowel obstruction and pneumothorax. Anesthesiology 26:61, 1965

279. Gregg NB (editor): Trends in surgical wound infection rates. United States Morbidity and Mortality Weekly Report 29:27,33, 1980

280. Skillman JJ, Bushnell LS, Hedley-Whyte J: Peritonitis and respiratory failure after abdominal operations. Ann Surg 170:122, 1961

281. Mengel CE, Kelly MG, Carbone PP: Clinical and biochemical effects of cyclophosphamide in patients with malignant carcinoid. Am J Med 38:396, 1965

282. Tilson MD: Carcinoid syndrome. Surg Clin North Am 54:409, 1974

283. Dory A: Theoretical and clinical considerations in anaesthesia for secreting carcinoid tumors. Can Anaesth Soc J 18:245, 1971

284. Mason RA, Steane PA: Carcinoid syndrome: Its relevance to the anaesthetist. Anaesthetist 31:228, 1976

285. Koppolu SRD, Miller R: Atypical carcinoid syndrome during anesthesia. Anesthesiol Review 4:27, 1977

286. Roizen MF, Moss J, Henry DP, et al: Effect of general anesthetics on handling- and de-capitation-induced increases in sympatho-adrenal discharge. J Pharmacol Exp Ther 204:11, 1978

287. Roizen MF, Wilkinson PL, Chatterjee K, et al: Does anesthesia alter myocardial stress during coronary artery surgery ... A-V myocardial norepinephrine differences, a new index of myocardial stress, Catecholamines and Stress: Recent Advances. Edited by Usdin E, Kvetnansky R, Kopin IJ. New York, Elsevier, 1980, p 211

288. Shnider SM, Wright RG, Levinson G, et al: Uterine blood flow and plasma norepinephrine changes during maternal stress in the pregnant ewe. Anesthesiology 50:524, 1979

289. Reier CE, George JM, Kilman JW: Cortisol and growth hormone response to surgical stress during morphine anesthesia. Anesth Analg 52:1003, 1973

290. Philbin DM, Emerson CW, Coggins CH, et al: Renin, catecholamine and vasopressin response to the "stress" of anesthesia and surgery (abstr). Anesthesiology 51:S121, 1979

291. Philbin DM, Coggins CH: Plasma antidiuretic hormone levels in cardiac surgical patients during morphine and halothane anesthesia. Anesthesiology 49:95, 1978

292. Madsen SN, Brandt MR, Engquist A, et al: Inhibition of plasma cyclic AMP, glucose and cortical response to surgery by epidural analgesia. Br J Surg 64:669, 1977

293. Welch CE, Malt RA: Abdominal surgery. N Engl J Med 300:765, 1979

294. Wataneeyawech M, Kelly KA Jr: Hepatic diseases, unsuspected before surgery. NY State J Med 75:1278, 1975

295. Schemel WH: Unexpected hepatic dysfunction found by multiple laboratory screening. Anesth Analg 55:810, 1976

296. Clark R, Doggart J, Tavery T: Changes in liver function after different types of surgery. Br J Anesth 48:119, 1976

297. Stevens WC, Eger EI II, Joas TA, et al: Comparative toxicity of isoflurane, halothane, fluroxene, and diethyl ether in human volunteers. Can Anaesth Soc J 20:357, 1973

298. Gelman SI: Disturbances in hepatic blood flow during anesthesia and surgery. Arch Surg 111:881, 1976

299. Akdikem S, Flanagan TV, Landmesser CM: A comparative study of serum glutamic pyruvic transaminase changes following an-

esthesia with halothane, methoxyflurane, and other inhalation agents. Anesth Analg 45:819, 1966

300. Strunin L: Preoperative assessment of the patient with liver dysfunction. Br J Anaesth 50:25, 1978

301. Harville DD, Summerskill WH: Surgery in acute hepatitis—Cause and effects. JAMA 184:257, 1963

302. Farman JV: Anaesthesia in the presence of liver disease and for hepatic transplantation. Br J Anaesth 44:946, 1972

303. Viegas O, Stoelting RK: LDH$_5$ changes after cholecystectomy and hysterectomy in patients receiving halothane, enflurane or fentanyl. Anesthesiology 51:556, 1979

304. Smith AA, Volpitto PP, Gramling ZW, et al: Chloroform, halothane and regional anesthesia: A comparative study. Anesth Analg 52:1, 1973

305. Ronk W: Liver function chemistries after enflurane and narcotic-N_2O anesthesia. AANA J 46:507, 1978

306. Bunker JP, Forrest WH, Mosteller F, et al (editors), The National Halothane Study: A study of the possible association between halothane anesthesia and postoperative hepatic necrosis. Washington, U.S. Government Printing Office, 1969

307. McEvan J: Liver function tests following anesthesia. Br J Anaesth 48:1065, 1976

308. Evans C, Evans M, Pollock AV: The incidence and causes of postoperative jaundice. Br J Anaesth 46:520, 1974

309. Whitcomb FF, Trey C, Brausch JW: Preoperative preparation of the jaundiced patient: A review of current practice. Surg Clin North Am 50:663, 1970

310. La Mont JT: Postoperative jaundice. Surg Clin North Am 54:637, 1974

311. Dawson JL: The incidence of postoperative renal failure in obstructive jaundice. Br J Surg 52:663, 1965

312. Child CG, Turcolte JG: The Liver and Portal Hypertension. Philadelphia, WB Saunders, 1964

313. Resnick RH, Iber FL, Ishihara AM, et al: A controlled study of the therapeutic portacaval shunt. Gastroenterology 67:843, 1974

314. Wright R, Eade OE, Chisholm M, et al: Controlled prospective study of the effect on liver function of multiple exposures to halothane. Lancet 6:817, 1975

315. Trowell J, Peto R, Smith AC: Controlled trial of repeated halothane anaesthetics in patients with carcinoma of the uterine cervix treated with radium. Lancet 1:821, 1975

316. Allen PJ, Downing JW: A prospective study of hepatocellular function after repeated exposures to halothane or enflurane in women undergoing radium therapy for cervical cancer. Br J Anaesth 49:1035, 1977

317. Simpson BR, Strunin L, Walton B: Evidence for halothane hepatotoxicity is equivocal, Controversy in Internal Medicine, Vol II. Edited by Ingelfinger FJ, Ebert RV, Finland M, et al. Philadelphia, WB Saunders, 1974, pp. 580–594

318. Carney FMT, Van Dyke RA: Halothane hepatitis: A critical review. Anesth Analg 51:135, 1972

319. Vergani D, Tsantoulas D, Eddleston ALWF, et al: Sensitization to halothane—altered liver components in severe hepatic necrosis after halothane anesthesia. Lancet 2:801, 1978

320. Dykes MHM: Is halothane hepatitis chronic active hepatitis? (editorial). Anesthesiology 46:233, 1977

321. Krugman S, Hoofnagle JH, Gerety RJ, et al: Viral hepatitis, type B. N Engl J Med 290:1331, 1974

322. Thomas FB: Chronic aggressive hepatitis induced by halothane. Ann Intern Med 81:487, 1974

323. Berman M, Alter JH, Ishak KG, et al: The chronic sequelae of Non-A, Non-B hepatitis. Ann Intern Med 91:1, 1979

324. Dykes MHM: Unexplained postoperative fever. JAMA 216:641, 1971

325. Sipes I, Brown B: An animal model of hepatotoxicity associated with halothane anesthesia. Anesthesiology 45:622, 1976

326. Klatskin G, Kimberg DV: Recurrent hepatitis attributable to halothane sensitization in an anesthetist. N Engl J Med 280:515, 1969

327. Douglas HJ, Eger EI II, Biava CG, et al: Hepatic necrosis associated with viral infection after enflurane anesthesia. N Engl J Med 296:553, 1977

328. Gall EA: Report of the pathology panel: National halothane study. Anesthesiology 29:233, 1968

329. Dykes MHM, Gilbert JP, Schur PH, et al: Halothane and the liver: A review of the epidemiologic, immunologic and metabolic as-

pects of the relationship. Can J Surg 15:1, 1972

330. Naulty JS, Reves JG, Tobey RR, et al: Hepatitis and operating room personnel: An approach to diagnosis and management. Anesth Analg 56:360, 1977

331. Duvaldestin P, Agoston S, Henzel D, et al: Pancuronium pharmacokinetics in patients with liver cirrhosis. Br J Anaesth 50:1131, 1978

332. Wasserman LR, Gilbert HS: Surgical bleeding in polycythemia vera. Ann NY Acad Sci 115:122, 1964

333. Rothstein P: What hemoglobin level is adequate in pediatric anesthesia? Anesthesiol Update 1(24):1,1978

334. Slogoff S: Anesthesia considerations in the anemic patient. Anesthesiol Update 2(7):1, 1978

335. Thomas DJ, Du Boulay GH, Marshall J, et al: Cerebral blood flow in polycythaemia. Lancet 2:161, 1977

336. Thomas DJ, Du Boulay GH, Marshall J, et al: Effect of hematocrit on cerebral blood flow in man. Lancet 2:941, 1977

337. Heughan C, Grislis G, Hunt TK: The effect of anemia on wound healing. Ann Surg 179:163, 1974

338. Finch CA: Pathophysiologic aspects of sickle cell anemia (editorial). Am J Med 53:1, 1972

339. Bunn HF, Forget BS, Ranney HM: Sickle cell anemia and related disorders, Human Hemoglobins. Edited by Bunn HF, Forget BS, Ranney HM. Philadelphia, WB Saunders pp 228–281

340. Sheehy TW, Plumb VJ: Treatment of sickle cell disease. Arch Intern Med 137:779, 1977

341. Sears DA: The morbidity of sickle cell trait: A review of the literature. Am J Med 64:1021, 1978

342. Heller P, Best WR, Nelson RB, et al: Clinical implication of sickle cell trait and glucose-6-phosphate dehydrogenase deficiency in hospitalized black male patients. N Engl J Med 300:1001, 1979

343. Price HL: Anesthesia in sickle-cell states. Anesthesiol Update 2(17):1, 1979

344. Searle JF: Anaesthesia in sickle cell states, a review. Anaesthesia 28:48, 1973

345. Dalal FY, Schmidt GB, Bennett EJ, et al: Sickle-cell trait, a report of a postoperative neurological complication. Br J Anaesth 46:387, 1974

346. Oduro KA, Searle JF: Anaesthesia in sickle-cell states: A plea for simplicity. Br Med J 4:596, 1972

347. Homi J, Reynolds J, Skinner A, et al: General anesthesia in sickle-cell disease. Br Med J 1:1599, 1979

348. Trubowitz S: The management of sickle cell anemia. Med Clin North Am 60:933, 1976

349. Morrison JC, Wiser WL: The use of prophylactic partial exchange transfusion in pregnancies associated with sickle cell hemoglobinopathy. Obstet Gynecol 48:516, 1976

350. Morrison JC, Whybrew WD, Bucovaz ET: Use of partial exchange transfusion preoperatively in patients with sickle cell hemoglobinopathies. Am J Obstet Gynecol 132:59, 1978

351. Lanzkowsky P, Shende A, Karayalcin G, et al: Partial exchange tranfusion in sickle cell anemia: Use in children with serious complications. Am J Dis Child 132:1206, 1978

352. Orr D: Difficult intubation: A hazard in thalassemia. A case report. Br J Anaesth 39:585, 1967

353. Frank MM, Schreiber AD, Atkinson JP, et al: Pathophysiology of immune hemolytic anemia. Ann Intern Med 87:210, 1979

354. Loque G, Rosse W: Immunologic mechanisms in autoimmume hemolytic disease. Semin Hematol 13:277, 1976

355. Herzig RH, Herzig GP, Graw RG Jr, et al: Successful granulocyte transfusion therapy for gram negative septisemia. N Engl J Med 296:701, 1977

356. Alavi JB, Root RK, Djerassi I, et al: A randomized clinical trial of granuolocyte transfusion for infection in acute leukemia. N Engl J Med 296:706, 1977

357. Lacey JV, Penner JA: Management of idiopathic thrombocytopenic purpura in the adult. Semin Thromb Hemostas 3:160, 1977

358. Simpson MB: Platelet function and transfusion therapy in the surgical patient, Platelet Physiology and Transfusion. Edited by Schiffer CJ. Washington DC, American Association of Blood Banks, 1978, pp 51–68

359. Davis DW, Steward DT: Unexplained excessive bleeding during operation: Role of acetylsalicylic acid. Can Anaesth Soc J 24:452, 1977

360. Majerus PW, Miletich JP: Relationships between platelets and coagulation factors in hemostasis. Annu Rev Med 29:41, 1978

361. Blatt PM, Brinkhous KM, Culp HR, et al: Anti-hemophilic factor concentrate therapy in von Willebrand's disease. JAMA 236:2770, 1976

362. Evans BE: Dental treatment for hemophiliacs: Evaluation of dental program (1975–1976) at the Mount Sinai Hospital International Hemophilia Training Center. Mt Sinai J Med 44:409, 1977

363. Zauber NP, Levin J: Factor IX levels in patients with hemophilia B (Christmas Disease) following transfusion with concentrates of factor IX or fresh frozen plasma (FFP). Medicine 56:213, 1977

364. Aledort LM: Recent advances in hemophilia. Ann NY Acad Sci 240:1, 1975

365. Gralnick HR, Coller BS, Schulman NR, et al: Factor VIII. Ann Intern Med 86:598, 1977

366. Miller RD: Complications of massive blood transfusions. Anesthesiology 39:82, 1973

367. Sherman LA: Alterations in hemostasis during massive transfusion, Massive Tranfusion. Edited by Nusbacher J. Washington DC, American Association of Blood Banks, 1978, pp 51–68

368. Marks RM, Sachar EJ: Undertreatment of medical inpatients with narcotic analgesics. Ann Intern Med 78:173, 1973

369. Catalano RB: The medical approach to management of pain caused by cancer. Semin Oncol 2:379, 1975

370. Twycross RBG: Choice of strong analgesics in terminal cancer: Diamorphine or morphine. Pain 3:93, 1977

371. Vitez TS, Way WL, Miller RD, et al: Effect of Delta-9-tetrahydrocannabinol on cyclopropane MAC in the rat. Anesthesiology 38:525, 1973

372. Koelle GB: Neurohumoral transmission and the autonomic nervous system, The Pharmacological Basis of Therapeutics. Edited by Goodman LS, Gilman A. New York, Macmillan, 1975, pp 404–444

373. Axelrod J: Neurotransmitters. Sci Am 230:58, 1974

374. Burn JH, Rand MJ: Actions of sympathomimetic amines on animals treated with reserpine. J Physiol 144:314, 1958

375. Drugs of choice. Med Lett Drugs Ther 21:5–64, 1979

376. Miller RD, Sohn YJ, Matteo RS: Enhancement of d-tubocurarine neuromuscular

377. Evans-Prosser CDG: The use of pethidine and morphine in the presence of monamine oxidase inhibitors. Br J Anaesth 40:279, 1968

378. Campbell GD: Dangers of monamine oxidase inhibitors. Br Med J 1:750, 1963

379. Rogers KJ, Thornton JA: The interaction between monamine oxidase inhibitors and narcotic analgesics in mice. Br J Pharmacol 36:470, 1969

380. Sjoqvist F: Psychotropic drugs. 2: Interaction between monamine oxidase (MAO) inhibitors and other substances. Proc R Soc Med 58:967, 1965

381. Edwards RE, Miller RD, Roizen MF, et al: Cardiac effects of imipramine and pancuronium during halothane and enflurane anesthesia. Anesthesiology 50:421, 1979

382. Hill GE, Wong KC: Lithium carbonate and neuromuscular blocking agents. Anesthesiology 46:122, 1977

383. Johnston RR, Way WL, Miller RD: Alteration of anesthetic requirements by amphetamine. Anesthesiology 36:357, 1972

384. Tanifuji Y, Eger EI II: Effect of isoproterenol and propranolol on halothane MAC in dogs. Anesth Analg 55:383, 1976

385. Stoelting RK, Creasser CW, Martz RC: Effect of cocaine adminstration on halothane MAC in dogs. Anesth Analg 54:422, 1975

386. Hall KD, Norris FH: Fluothane sensitization of dog heart to action of epinephrine. Anesthesiology 19:631, 1958

387. Johnston RR, Eger EI II, Wilson C: A comparative interaction of epinephrine with enflurane, isoflurane and halothane in man. Anesth Analg 55:709, 1976

388. Joas TA, Stevens WC: Comparison of the arrhythmic doses of epinephrine during Forane, halothane and enflurane anesthesia in dogs. Anesthesiology 35:48, 1971

389. Katz RL, Bigger JT: Cardiac arrhythmias during anesthesia and operation. Anesthesiology 33:193, 1970

390. Horrigan RW, Eger EI II, Wilson CB: Epinephrine-induced arrhythmias during enflurane anesthesia in man: A nonlinear dose-response relationship and dose-dependent protection from lidocaine. Anesth Analg 57:547, 1978

391. Hirshman CA, Bergman NA: Halothane and enflurane protect against bronchospasm in

an asthma dog model. Anesth Analg 57:629, 1978

392. Shnider SM, Papper EM: Anesthesia for the asthmatic patient. Anesthesiology 22:886, 1961

393. Marcus ML, Skelton CL, Graver LE, et al: Effects of theophylline on myocardial mechanics. Am J Physiol 222:1361, 1972

394. Westfall DP, Flemming WW: Sensitivity changes in the dog heart to norepinephrine, calcium and aminophylline resulting from pretreatment with reserpine. J Pharmacol Exp Ther 159:98, 1968

395. Rall TW, West TC: The potentiation of cardiac inotropic responses to norepinephrine by theophylline. J Pharmacol Exp Ther 139:269, 1963

396. Webb-Johnson DC, Andrews JL: Bronchodilator therapy I. N Engl J Med 297:476, 1977

397. Atuk NO, Blaydes C, Westervelt FB, et al: Effect of aminophylline on urinary excretion of epinephrine and norepinephrine in man. Circulation 35:745, 1967

398. Horwitz LN, Spear JF, Moore EN, et al: Effect of aminophylline on the threshold for initiating ventricular fibrillation during respiratory failure. Am J Cardiol 35:376, 1975

399. Mitenko PA, Ogilvie RI: Pharmacokinetics of intravenous theophylline. Clin Pharmacol Ther 14:509, 1973

400. Patterson JW, Shenfield GM: Bronchodilators. Parts I and II. Br Thorac Tuberc Assoc Rev 4:25, 61, 1974

401. Piafsky KM, Ogilvie RI: Dosage of theophylline in bronchial asthma. N Engl J Med 292:1218, 1975

402. Hunt SN, Jusko WJ, Yurchak AM: Effect of smoking on theophylline disposition. Clin Pharmacol Ther 19:546, 1975

403. Takaori M, Loehning RW: Ventricular arrhythmias induced by aminophylline during halothane anaesthesia in dogs. Can Anaesth Soc J 14:79, 1967

404. Takaori M, Loehning RW: Ventricular arrhythmias during halothane anaesthesia: Effects of isoproterenol, aminophylline, and ephedrine. Can Anaesth Soc J 12:275, 1965

405. Roizen MF, Stevens WC: Multiform ventricular tachycardia due to the interaction of aminophylline and halothane. Anesth Analg 57:738, 1978

406. Harrah MD, Way WL, Katzung BG: The interaction of d-tubocurarine with antiarrhythmic drugs. Anesthesiology 33:406, 1970

407. Telivuo L, Katz RL: The effects of modern intravenous local anesthetics on respiration during partial neuromuscular block in man. Anaesthesia 25:30, 1970

408. Miller RD, Way WL, Katzung BG: The potentiation of neuromuscular blocking agents by quinidine. Anesthesiology 28:1036, 1967

409. Pittinger CB, Eryasa Y, Adamson R: Antibiotic-induced paralysis. Anesth Analg 49:487, 1970

410. Singh YN, Harvey, AL, Marshall IG: Antibiotic induced-paralysis of the mouse phrenic nerve-hemidiaphragm preparation, and reversibility by calcium and by neostigmine. Anesthesiology 48:418, 1978

411. Pittinger CB, Adamson R: Antibiotic blockade of neuromuscular function. Annu Rev Pharmacol 12:169, 1972

412. Becker LD, Miller RD: Clindamycin enhances a non-depolarizing neuromuscular blockade. Anesthesiology 45:84, 1976

413. Sampson IH, Miller, R: Antibiotics: Their relevance to the anesthesiologist, a review. Anesthesiol Rev 5:43, 1978

414. Lown B, Block H, Moore FD: Digitalis, electrolytes, and the surgical patient. Am J Cardiol 6:309, 1960

415. Beller GA, Smith TW, Abelmann WH, et al: Digitalis intoxication. N Engl J Med 284:989, 1971

416. Morrow DH: Anesthesia and digitalis toxicity. VI. Effect of barbiturates and halothane on digoxin toxicity. Anesth Analg 49:305, 1970

417. Pratila MG, Pratilas V: Anesthetic agents and cardiac electromechanical activity. Anesthesiology 49:338, 1978

418. Logic JR, Morrow DH: The effect of halothane on ventricular automaticity. Anesthesiology 36:107, 1972

419. Ivankovich AD, Miletich DJ, Grossman RK, et al: The effect of enflurane, isoflurane, fluroxene, methoxyflurane and diethyl ether on ouabain tolerance in the dog. Anesth Analg 55:360, 1976

420. Pantuck EJ, Pantuck CB: Cholinesterases and anticholinesterases, Muscle Relaxants. Edited by Katz RL. Amsterdam, Excerpta Medica, 1975, pp. 143–162

421. Ghoneim MM, Long JP: The interaction between magnesium and other neuromuscular blocking agents. Anesthesiology 32:23, 1970

422. Del Castillo J, Engback L: The nature of neuromuscular block produced by magnesium. J Physiol (Lond) 124:370, 1954

423. Vessey MD, Doll R, Fairbairn AS, et al: Postoperative thromboembolism and the use of oral contraceptives. Br Med J 3:123, 1970

424. Greene Gr, Sartwell PE: Oral contraceptive use in patients with thromboembolism following surgery, trauma, or infection. Am J Public Health 62:680, 1972

425. Interruption of a drug regimen before anesthesia. Med Lett Drugs Ther 16:19, 1974

426. Cascorbi HF: Perianesthetic problems with nonanesthetic drugs, ASA Refresher Courses in Anesthesiology. Vol 6. Edited by Hershey SG. Philadelphia, JB Lippincott, 1978, pp 15–30

427. Cullen BF, Miller MG: Drug interactions and anesthesia: A review. Anesth Analg 58:413, 1979

3

Psychological Preparation and Preoperative Medication

Robert K. Stoelting, M.D.

Anesthetic management begins with the preoperative psychological preparation of the patient and administration of a drug or drugs selected to produce specific pharmacologic responses prior to the induction of anesthesia. Traditionally, this initial psychological and pharmacologic component of anesthetic management is referred to as preoperative medication.

PREOPERATIVE PSYCHOLOGICAL PREPARATION

The psychological component of preoperative preparation is provided by the anesthesiologist's visit and interview. A thorough description of anesthetic management and events to anticipate in the perioperative period serves to reduce the unknown and establish a personal relationship. The value of this interview is evidenced by its demonstrable calming effect.[1] For example, fewer adult patients are nervous before the induction of anesthesia when a preoperative interview has been conducted as compared with patients receiving pentobarbital but not an interview (Table 3-1). In addition, more patients are judged to be adequately sedated before surgery when an interview has been conducted. In children, careful psychological preparation and well-informed parents to support the child are extremely valuable. Nevertheless, a shortage of time and the fact that some patients' problems do not lend themselves to reassurance may limit the value of the preoperative interview. Therefore, preoperative pharmacologic preparation is often indicated.

Table 3-1. Value of Preoperative Interview Compared with Pentobarbital

	Percentage of Patients			
	Interview	Pentobarbital*	Interview & Pentobarbital*	No Interview No Pentobarbital
Feel nervous	40	61	38	58
Feel drowsy	26	30	38	18
Judged adequately sedated	65	48	71	35

* Two mg/kg intramuscularly 1 hour before surgery.
(Modified from Egbert LD, Battit GE, Turndorf H, et al: The value of the preoperative visit by an anesthetist. JAMA 185:553, 1963 © Copyright 1963, American Medical Association.)

Table 3-2. Drugs and Doses Used for Preoperative Medication

Classification	Drug	Typical Adult Dose (mg)	Route of Administration
Barbiturates	Secobarbital	50–150	Oral, IM
	Pentobarbital	50–150	Oral, IM
Narcotics	Morphine	5–15	IM
	Meperidine	50–100	IM
Tranquilizers and Sedative-Hypnotics	Diazepam	5–10	Oral
	Droperidol	2.5–5	IM
	Hydroxyzine*	50–150	IM
	Promethazine*	25–50	IM
Anticholinergics	Atropine	0.3–0.6	IM
	Scopolamine	0.3–0.5	IM
	Glycopyrrolate	0.2–0.3	IM
Histamine H_2-receptor antagonist	Cimetidine	300	Oral, IM, IV

* May also be classified as antihistamine.

PREOPERATIVE PHARMACOLOGIC PREPARATION

The most important objective of preoperative pharmacologic preparation is anxiety relief. Ideally, patients should enter the preoperative period free from apprehension, sedated but easily arousable, and fully cooperative. Other goals may include analgesia, amnesia, reduction of salivary gland and gastric fluid secretions, elevation of gastric fluid pH, and decreased cardiac vagal activity. No drug or drug combination reliably achieves all these goals. Indeed the number of published articles devoted to preoperative medication emphasizes the ideal drug or drug combination, if such exists, has yet to be discovered.

Pharmacologic preparation should never be routine. The appropriate drug or drugs and doses can be selected only after the psychological and physiological condition of the patient have been evaluated. Drug choice and dose must take into account patient age, weight, physical status, degree of anxiety, tolerance for depressant drugs, prior hospitalizations (especially if the patient is a child), previous adverse experiences with drugs used for preoperative medication (dizziness, nausea, vomiting, "allergy"), duration, and type of surgery. After a thorough evaluation of the patient, it may be appropriate not to include drugs in the preoperative preparation. Examples of patients who should not receive depressant drugs preoperatively might include outpatients, the elderly, the very young, the obtunded patient, the patient in shock, the patient with pulmonary dysfunction, and the patient with intracranial pathology. In contrast, the nervous patient or the patient undergoing life-threatening cancer or cardiac surgery probably deserves pharmacologic attempts to decrease preoperative anxiety and produce sedation.

DRUGS FOR PREOPERATIVE MEDICATION

Drugs used for preoperative medication may be classified as barbiturates, narcotics, tranquilizers and sedative-hypnotics, anticholinergics, and histamine-H_2 receptor antagonists. Examples of drugs and doses used for adult preoperative medication are listed in Table 3-2. Ultimately the specific drug choices are based on a consideration of the goals one wishes to achieve with preoperative pharmacologic preparation balanced against the potential undesirable effects these drugs may produce.

BARBITURATES

Secobarbital and pentobarbital are examples of barbiturates used for preoperative medication. Advantages cited for these drugs include sedation, minimal respiratory depressant effects as evidenced by an unchanged ventilatory response to carbon dioxide,[2] minimal circulatory depression, rarity of nausea and vomiting, and effectiveness when administered orally. Disadvantages include lack of analgesia, disorientation, especially if administered to patients in pain, and absence of a specific pharmacologic antagonist. Enzyme induction is not a consideration with the doses used for preoperative medication. The rare patient with acute intermittent porphyria should not receive barbiturates, as these drugs may precipitate an acute exacerbation of this disease.

NARCOTICS

Morphine and meperidine are the narcotics most frequently used. Fentanyl has an inappropriate onset and too short a duration of action to justify recommending its use as preoperative medication. Advantages cited for narcotics include facilitation of anesthetic induction, reduction in anesthetic requirements, production of preoperative and postoperative analgesia, ease of controlled ventilation intraoperatively, and reversibility with naloxone. Many of these advantages are no longer valid. For example, potent and rapidly acting intravenous drugs insure a rapid and pleasant induction of anesthesia regardless of preoperative medication. The decrease in inhalation anesthetic requirements produced by morphine is probably clinically insignificant.[3] Pain is rare preoperatively while postoperative analgesia is best achieved with intravenous drugs administered near the end of surgery. When a nitrous oxide–narcotic anesthetic technique is planned, initial narcotic administration is more logically given intravenously before induction of anesthesia rather than intramuscularly as part of the preoperative medication.

Adverse side effects of narcotics when used for preoperative medication are several. Although narcotics exert no significant depressant effects on the myocardium, they do produce relaxation of peripheral vascular smooth muscle manifested as orthostatic hypotension. In contrast to barbiturates, narcotics used for preoperative medication depress the medullary respiratory center as evidenced by decreased responsiveness to carbon dioxide.[2] The euphoric effect of narcotics in patients with pain may be dysphoria in the absence of pain. Nausea and vomiting have been attributed to a specific narcotic effect on the vestibular apparatus or stimulation of the chemoreceptor trigger zone. Narcotic induced smooth muscle constriction may be manifest as choledochoduodenal sphincter spasm[4] causing some to question the use of narcotics in patients with biliary tract disease. Antidiuretic hormone release, although attributed to morphine, has not been documented to occur in man.[5]

TRANQUILIZERS AND SEDATIVE-HYPNOTICS

Examples of this class of drugs used for preoperative medication include diazepam, droperidol, hydroxyzine, and promethazine. Hydroxyzine and promethazine may also be classified as antihistamines.

Diazepam is considered to be specific for relief of anxiety. In addition, vomiting and significant cardiorespiratory depression do not occur. Disadvantages include discomfort at the injection site following intramuscular or intravenous administration, prolonged duration of action, and unreliable systemic absorption after intramuscular injection. Indeed, diazepam blood levels are greater following oral administration than after intramuscular injection.[6] In animals diazepam increases the seizure threshold for lidocaine but there is no evidence in man that diazepam used as preoperative medication reduces the likelihood of local anesthetic toxicity.[7] Elderly patients or those with severe liver dysfunction may be sensitive to the depressant effects of diazepam.[8] Therefore, it would seem prudent to reduce the diazepam dose in such patients.

Droperidol is used for anxiety relief and is a potent antiemetic. A major disadvantage is the occasional patient who develops acute anxiety following droperidol.[9] These patients express a fear of death and may refuse a previously agreed upon elective operative procedure. In addition, this drug is a dopaminergic receptor blocker and may produce extrapyrimidal symptoms.[10] Therefore, patients with known paralysis agitans should not receive this drug. Finally, droperidol is a mild alpha-adrenergic blocker, which may detract from its use in patients with a reduced blood volume.

Hydroxyzine and promethazine manifest antihistaminic, antiemetic, and sedative properties. These drugs may add to the sedative effects of narcotics. For example, promethazine combined with meperidine does not increase respiratory depression from meperidine or alter the incidence of nausea and vomiting but does produce an additive sedative effect.[11]

ANTICHOLINERGICS

Atropine, scopolamine, and glycopyrrolate are examples of anticholinergics used in preoperative medication. These drugs are competitive inhibitors of the muscarinic actions of acetylcholine. Atropine and scopolamine are tertiary amines and can cross lipid barriers such as the blood brain barrier, placenta, and gastrointestinal tract. In contrast, glycopyrrolate acts only on peripheral cholinergic receptors, as its quaternary ammonium structure prevents it from crossing lipid barriers in significant amounts.[12]

The sensitivity of peripheral cholinergic receptors differs such that low doses of an an-

ticholinergic may be sufficient to inhibit salivation but large doses are necessary for cardiac or gastrointestinal effects.[12] Furthermore, reponses to various anticholinergics are dependent on the dose used for preoperative medication.[12] For example, scopolamine has significant effects on the central nervous system and is a potent antisialagogue. In contrast, atropine has minimal effects on the central nervous system and is a more effective cardiac vagolytic than scopolamine. Glycopyrrolate has no central nervous system effects and produces minimal cardiovascular and visual effects. As an antisialagogue glycopyrrolate is more potent and longer lasting than atropine.

Routine inclusion of an anticholinergic in the preoperative medication is not necessary. However, an anticholinergic may be combined with other drugs for the purposes of producing an antisialagogue effect, providing sedative and amnesic effects, decreasing gastric hydrogen ion secretion, and preventing reflex bradycardia. In addition, intramuscular atropine or glycopyrrolate may serve as a placebo in patients who expect an injection preoperatively.

ANTISIALAGOGUE EFFECT

The need for including an anticholinergic in the preoperative medication to produce an antisialagogue effect has been questioned, since currently used inhalation anesthetics do not stimulate excessive upper airway secretions. Nevertheless, more satisfactory conditions during general anesthesia due to decreased secretions are likely when an anticholinergic is administered preoperatively.[13] An antisialagogue effect is particularly important for intraoral operations or when topical anesthesia is necessary, as excessive secretions may interfere with the surgery or impair production of topical anesthesia by diluting the local anesthetic.

The potential discomfort of a dry mouth in an awake patient is an important consideration. Certainly, preoperative anticholinergic administration for an antisialagogue effect is not necessary when regional anesthesia is planned. Nevertheless, anxiety, fluid deprivation, and other drugs used in preoperative medication[14] may produce a dry mouth even in the absence of an anticholinergic.

PRODUCTION OF SEDATIVE AND AMNESIC EFFECTS

Scopolamine produces useful sedative effects particularly in combination with other drugs used for preoperative medication. Scopolamine is 8 to 9 times more potent than atropine in this respect.[12] Patient acceptance of morphine as preoperative medication is better when this drug is combined with scopolamine rather than atropine.[15] Sedative effects following glycopyrrolate would be unlikely, since the quaternary ammonium structure of this drug prevents easy passage into the central nervous system.

Despite the clinical impression that scopolamine is a potent amnesic, at least one study does not support this view when the drug is used alone.[16] In this report, all patients receiving scopolamine 0.5 mg intravenously remembered their arrival in the operating room when questioned 24 hours later. In contrast, the incidence of amnesia for entering the operating room was 32 percent with 5 to 10 mg of diazepam given intravenously and 50 percent with diazepam plus scopolamine confirming that scopolamine contributed significantly to the amnesic effects of diazepam.

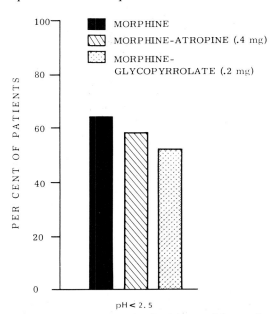

Fig. 3-1 The percentage of patients with gastric fluid pH below 2.5 at the time of anesthetic induction was not different ($P > 0.05$) with or without the inclusion of an anticholinergic in the preoperative medication. All drugs were administered intramuscularly 1 to 1.5 hours before induction of anesthesia.[17]

cantly raising gastric fluid pH or reducing gastric fluid volume as compared with patients not receiving an anticholinergic.[17] For example, about 60 percent of patients have a gastric fluid pH below 2.5 immediately following induction of anesthesia with or without inclusion of atropine (0.4 mg) or glycopyrrolate (0.2 mg) in the preoperative medication[17] (Fig. 3-1). Increasing the glycopyrrolate dose to 0.3 mg is not more effective in increasing gastric fluid pH above 2.5.[18]

DECREASED GASTRIC HYDROGEN ION SECRETION

The value of an anticholinergic in elevating gastric fluid pH is questionable. Atropine or glycopyrrolate administered intramuscularly 1 to 1.5 hours before induction of anesthesia in adult patients is not effective in signifi-

PREVENTION OF REFLEX BRADYCARDIA

Prevention of reflex bradycardia seems unlikely with the timing and dose of intramuscular anticholinergic typically administered for preoperative medication. If an anticholinergic is selected to prevent reflex bradycardia, the most logical approach is to administer atropine or glycopyrrolate intravenously shortly before the anticipated need.[19] Vagal responses may be more active in children; therefore, intravenous atropine is often administered immediately before induction of anesthesia.

SIDE EFFECTS

Undesirable side effects of anticholinergics may include (1) central nervous system toxicity, (2) relaxation of the lower esophageal sphincter, (3) heart rate changes, (4) mydriasis and cycloplegia, (5) elevation of body temperature, (6) drying of airway secretions, and (7) increased physiological dead space.

Central Nervous System Toxicity

The central anticholinergic syndrome represents toxic central nervous system effects of anticholinergics. Symptoms include restlessness, agitation, prolonged somnolence after anesthesia, and in extreme cases convulsions and coma. Toxicity is most likely to follow scopolamine but the incidence should be low with the doses used for preoperative medication. Central nervous system toxicity is even less likely with atropine. Nevertheless, elderly patients may be particularly susceptible to central toxic effects from both scopolamine and atropine.[20] A central anticholinergic syndrome after glycopyrrolate is unlikely, since this drug is unable to easily cross the blood brain barrier.

Physostigmine (1 to 2 mg intravenously) is effective in reversing the central anticholinergic syndrome produced by atropine or scopolamine.[21] Simultaneous administration of glycopyrrolate intravenously should be an effective method for preventing undesirable peripheral muscarinic effects (bradycardia, salivation) produced by physostigmine. Toxicity attributed to scopolamine or atropine may also be the response to pain in the presence of incomplete recovery from the mental-inhibiting effects of the anesthetic.

Relaxation of the Lower Esophageal Sphincter

Atropine, scopolamine, and glycopyrrolate in doses used for preoperative medication decrease the resting tone of the lower esophageal sphincter.[22] This sphincter is a 2 to 5 cm zone of increased intraluminal pressure at the gastroesophageal junction and is assumed to be an important determinant in the prevention of gastric reflux. Conceivably, reduction in sphincter tone produced by inclusion of an anticholinergic in the preoperative medication could increase the risk of gastroesophageal reflux. Lower esophageal sphincter tone is also decreased by morphine, meperidine, droperidol, and promethazine.[23]

Heart Rate Changes

Theoretically, heart rate may increase after intramuscular anticholinergic administration. When a tachycardia would be undesirable, scopolamine or glycopyrrolate are better choices than atropine because these drugs manifest less cardioaccelerator effects.[12] Nevertheless, the most likely cardiac response after intramuscular atropine as used in preoperative medication is heart-rate slowing. This is believed to be secondary to central vagal stimulation before a sufficient atropine blood concentration is established in the periphery to offset this central effect.[12]

Atropine administered to a pregnant patient may result in loss of fetal beat to beat variability removing an early sign of fetal hypoxia. Glycopyrrolate would seem less likely to produce this effect, since it is unable to easily cross the placenta.

Mydriasis and Cycloplegia

Atropine and scopolamine may produce mydriasis and cycloplegia such that patients may experience visual impairment postoperatively. Scopolamine has a greater mydriatic effect than atropine.[24] Conceivably, mydriasis could interfere with drainage of aqueous humor from the anterior chamber of the eye. Despite this response, an anticholinergic may be safely included in the preoperative medication of a patient with glaucoma.[24] However, miotic eye drops should be continued and atropine or glycopyrrolate would seem a more prudent choice than scopolamine.

Elevation of Body Temperature

An anticholinergic may result in elevation of body temperature by suppressing sweat glands which are innervated by cholinergic nerves via the sympathetic nervous system.[12] Prevention of sweating by this mechanism in children may further increase body temperature especially if there is preexisting fever.

Drying of Airway Secretions

In addition to the discomfort of a dry mouth, the drying and thickening of mucus makes it difficult for cilia to clear secretions. Therefore, perhaps anticholinergics should be avoided in patients who benefit from thin secretions.

Increased Physiological Dead Space

Atropine or scopolamine increase physiological dead space 20 to 25 percent.[2] This is compensated for by increased minute ventilation such that arterial PCO_2 does not increase. This increased minute ventilation should not be interpreted as antagonism of

Table 3-3. Percentage of Patients with Gastric Fluid pH Samples

Preoperative Medication	Below 2.5	2.5 to 5.0	Above 5
Morphine Atropine	60	34	6
Morphine Atropine Cimetidine*	16**	24	60**

* 300 mg orally 1 to 1.5 hours before induction of anesthesia.
** $P < 0.05$ compared with morphine-atropine.
(Modified from Stoelting RK: Gastric fluid pH in patients receiving cimetidine. Anesth Analg 57:675, 1978.)

ventilatory depression produced by concomitantly administered drugs such as narcotics. Alone, anticholinergics do not alter the ventilatory responses to carbon dioxide.[2]

HISTAMINE H_2-RECEPTOR ANTAGONIST

Cimetidine is a histamine H_2-receptor antagonist that counters the ability of histamine to induce secretion of gastric fluid with a high hydrogen ion concentration. Therefore, this drug offers a pharmacologic approach for increasing gastric fluid pH preoperatively. Indeed, oral cimetidine (300 mg) administered to adult patients 1 to 1.5 hours before induction of anesthesia increases the gastric fluid pH above 2.5 in over 80 percent of patients[25] (Table 3-3). In this study gastric fluid volume was not detectably altered by cimetidine. In another report intravenous cimetidine (300 mg) 2 hours before induction of anesthesia reduced gastric fluid volume and increased gastric fluid pH above 2.5 in 11 of 11 patients.[18] Preoperative antacids also increase gastric fluid pH at the time of anesthetic induction but in contrast to cimetidine increase gastric fluid volume.[17] Furthermore, antacids may have adverse effects on the tracheobronchial tree if they are aspirated.[26, 27]

Routine inclusion of cimetidine in the preoperative medication has been suggested.[25]

Cimetidine would be particularly appropriate before emergency surgery in unprepared patients, in patients with symptoms of gastroesophageal reflux and when anesthesia administered via a mask is planned or when a prolonged induction of anesthesia is anticipated. Obese patients have a lower gastric fluid pH and higher gastric fluid volume than their non-obese counterparts[28] and therefore cimetidine administration would seem logical in this group. Likewise, outpatients may have large acidic gastric volumes which may reflect the lack of a preoperative interview and medication to decrease anxiety.[29] Use of cimetidine in pregnant patients is attractive but should be weighed against an unknown effect of this drug on the fetus. Despite clear evidence that cimetidine increases gastric fluid pH, there are no data to confirm increased patient safety should aspiration of gastric contents occur in those receiving cimetidine for premedication. Furthermore, cimetidine probably will not alter the incidence of vomiting or regurgitation in the preoperative period.

EVALUATION OF DRUGS USED FOR PREOPERATIVE MEDICATION

Precise methods to quantify the value of drugs used for preoperative medication are not available.[30] Although anxiety relief is an important goal of preoperative medication, there is no reliable method to measure this subjective response. Sedation is a more objective measurement but it must be remembered that drowsiness does not insure relief of anxiety.[14] Comparison of studies on preoperative medication is hampered by different drug doses, sites, and methods of injection and by varying times for measuring responses. Differences in emotional states of patients and what the patient expects from the preoperative medication may also play a role in the evaluation of a drug or drug combination.

Despite these complexities, Forrest et al.[14] provided useful information on preoperative medication administered to adult patients prior to elective operations. These investigators evaluated responses following intramuscular pentobarbital, secobarbital, diazepam, hydroxyzine, morphine, and meperidine. With the exception of diazepam, all drugs produced dose-related sedation 0.5 to 1 hour after injection. According to patient evaluation, no drug at any dose had a significant effect on apprehension relative to the placebo, thus emphasizing that sedation does not equal anxiety relief. However, those who received a placebo were more apprehensive in the operating room than when interviewed earlier in their rooms. Interestingly, anesthesiologists, who did not know which drug had been given, rated preoperative medication satisfactory in 37 to 63 percent of patients receiving placebo and 43 to 67 percent of drug-treated patients. This finding certainly creates doubt as to the value of drugs given preoperatively. The two most frequent side effects described by patients were dry mouth and slurred speech (Table 3-4). Nausea was an infrequent complaint and vomiting did not occur in any patient. Severe pain at the intramuscular injection site was infrequent (2 percent) and the incidence was not increased for any specific drug.

RECOMMENDED APPROACH TO PREOPERATIVE MEDICATION

An outline of the recommended approach to preoperative medication is shown in Table 3-5. Preoperative medication begins with the anesthesiologist's interview, explanation of the planned anesthetic management, and discussion of any questions or concerns the patient or other interested parties may pose. The importance of this personal contact, ideally the day before elective surgery, is well documented.[1] After the interview is concluded, the decision as to the need for pharmacologic preparation is made and the specific drug or

Table 3-4. Percentage of Patients Reporting Side Effects After Intramuscular Preoperative Medication

Medication	Dry Mouth	Slurred Speech	Dizzy	Nauseated	Vomiting
Pentobarbital 50 mg	30	20	10	7	0
Pentobarbital 150 mg	28	38	10	7	0
Secobarbital 50 mg	34	21	3	7	0
Secobarbital 150 mg	47	43	13	10	0
Placebo	26	23	6	10	0
Diazepam 5 mg	30	10	3	3	0
Diazepam 10 mg	37	30	13	0	0
Hydroxyzine 50 mg	50	27	3	3	0
Hydroxyzine 100 mg	37	30	3	0	0
Placebo	27	23	3	10	0
Morphine 5 mg	77	33	13	3	0
Morphine 10 mg	88*	33	17	10	0
Meperidine 50 mg	83*	33	17	20	0
Meperidine 100 mg	87*	57*	23	3	0
Placebo	50	17	13	17	0

* Significantly different from placebo control ($P<0.05$).
(Modified from Forrest WH, Brown CR, Brown BW: Subjective responses to six common preoperative medications. Anesthesiology 47:241, 1977.)

Table 3-5. Recommended Approach to Preoperative Medication

1. Patient interview by anesthesiologist the day before elective surgery
2. Flurazepam orally the evening before surgery to prevent insomnia
3. Diazepam orally 1 to 2 hours before induction of anesthesia
   Substitute morphine intramuscularly if analgesia is desired
   Scopolamine intramuscularly at the same time as diazepam or morphine if reliable sedation and amnesia are desired—otherwise recommendation number 5
4. Cimetidine orally 1 to 2 hours before induction of anesthesia
5. Glycopyrrolate intramuscularly when patient is sent to the operating room

drugs and doses to be administered are determined. Insomnia is common the night before surgery; flurazepam (15 to 30 mg orally) most closely mimics natural sleep and would seem a better choice than a barbiturate for the prevention of insomnia.

Medication designed to decrease anxiety and produce sedation in the immediate preoperative period is most appropriately administered 1 to 2 hours before induction of anesthesia. Intramuscular injections are unpleasant whereas oral administration is ideal.

Oral cimetidine is also conveniently administered at this time. The small amount of water (30 to 45 ml) needed for oral administration of drugs is negligible with respect to gastric fluid volume. If pain is present preoperatively or preparation for anesthesia is likely to be uncomfortable (invasive monitoring, nerve blocks) an intramuscular narcotic is indicated.

Intramuscular administration of scopolamine at the same time as an oral drug or intramuscular narcotic is administered is indicated when one wishes to exploit the amnesic and sedative effects of this anticholinergic. It seems to be a valid clinical impression that scopolamine contributes significantly to the sedative effect of narcotics or tranquilizers. The combination of intramuscular morphine and scopolamine is ideal for producing tranquility and sedation in patients most deserving of aggressive pharmacologic preoperative medication.

Routine antiemetic therapy is not necessary, since most patients do not need this type of prophylaxis. It is best to identify those at risk (ocular surgery, past history of vomiting) and administer an intravenous antiemetic such as benzquinamide or droperidol

15 to 20 minutes before the end of the operation.

An anticholinergic selected to produce an antisialagogue effect is most appropriately administered intramuscularly immediately before the patient is sent to the operating room. If the anticholinergic is given 1 to 2 hours before induction of anesthesia, the patient is more likely to be uncomfortable from a dry mouth. Glycopyrrolate is the most logical drug if an antisialagogue response without central nervous system effects is desired. The sequence of an oral barbiturate or diazepam and cimetidine followed later by intramuscular glycopyrrolate allows all drugs to be given at the time most appropriate for achieving an optimal desirable effect.

REFERENCES

1. Egbert LD, Battit GE, Turndorf H, et al: The value of the preoperative visit by an anesthetist. JAMA 185:553, 1963
2. Smith TC, Stephen GW, Zeiger L, et al: Effects of premedicant drugs on respiration and gas exchange in man. Anesthesiology 28:883, 1967
3. Saidman LJ, Eger EI II: Effect of nitrous oxide and of narcotic premedication on the alveolar concentration of halothane required for anesthesia. Anesthesiology 25:302, 1964
4. Greenstein AJ, Kayman A, Singer A, et al: A comparative study of pentazocine and meperidine on the biliary passage pressure. Am J Gastroenterol 58:417, 1972
5. Philbin DM, Coggins CH: Plasma antidiuretic hormone levels in cardiac surgical patients during morphine and halothane anesthesia. Anesthesiology 49:95, 1978
6. Hillestad L, Hansen T, Melsom H, et al: Diazepam metabolism in normal man. 1. Serum concentrations and clinical effects after intravenous, intramuscular and oral administration. Clin Pharm Ther 16:479, 1974
7. Moore DC, Balfour RI, Fitzgibbons D: Convulsive arterial plasma levels of bupivacaine and the response to diazepam therapy. Anesthesiology 50:454, 1979
8. Koltz U, Avant GR, Hoyumpa A, et al: The effects of age and liver disease on the disposition and elimination of diazepam in adult man. J Clin Invest 55:347, 1975
9. Lee CM, Yeakel AE: Patient refusal of surgery following Innovar premedication, Anesth Analg 54:225, 1975
10. Patton CM: Rapid induction of acute dyskinesia by droperidol. Anesthesiology 43:126, 1975
11. Keats AS, Telford J, Jurosu Y: "Protentiation" of meperidine by promethazine. Anesthesiology 22:34, 1961
12. Mirakhur RK: Anticholinergic drugs. Br J Anaesth 51:671, 1979
13. Falick YS, Smiler BG: Is anticholinergic premedication necessary? Anesthesiology 43:472, 1975
14. Forrest WH, Brown CR, Brown BW: Subjective responses to six common preoperative medications. Anesthesiology 47:241, 1977
15. Conner JT, Bellville JW, Wender R, et al: Morphine, scopolamine, and atropine as intravenous surgical premedicants. Anesth Analg 56:606, 1977
16. Frumin MJ, Herekar VR, Jarvik ME: Amnesic actions of diazepam and scopolamine in man. Anesthesiology 45:406, 1976
17. Stoelting RK: Responses to atropine, glycopyrrolate, and Riopan of gastric fluid pH and volume in adult patients. Anesthesiology 48:367, 1978
18. Maliniak K, Vakil AH: Pre-anesthetic cimetidine and gastric pH. Anesth Analg 58:309, 1979
19. Meyers EF, Tomeldan SA: Glycopyrrolate compared with atropine in prevention of the oculocardiac reflex during eye-muscle surgery. Anesthesiology 51:350, 1979
20. Smith DS, Orkin FK, Gardner SM, et al: Prolonged sedation in the elderly after intraoperative atropin administration. Anesthesiology 51:348, 1979
21. Holzgrafe RE, Vondrell JJ, Mintz SM: Reversal of postoperative reactions to scopolamine with physostigmine. Anesth Analg 52:921, 1973
22. Brock-Utne JG, Rubin J, Welman S, et al: The effect of glycopyrrolate (Robinul) on the lower oesophageal sphincter. Canad Anaesth Soc J 25:144, 1978
23. Sehhati GH: The effect of premedicant drugs on the lower esophageal sphincter (LES). Anaesthetist 26:489, 1977
24. Garde JF, Aston R, Endler GC, et al: Racial

mydriatic responses to belladonna premedication. Anesth Analg 57:572, 1978

25. Stoelting RK: Gastric fluild pH in patients receiving cimetidine. Anesth Analg 57:675, 1978
26. Gibbs CP, Schwartz DJ, Wynne JW, et al: Antacid pulmonary aspiration in the dog. Anesthesiology 51:380, 1979
27. Bond VK, Stoelting RK, Gupta CD: Pulmonary aspiration syndrome after inhalation of gastric fluid containing antacids. Anesthesiology 51:452, 1979
28. Vaughn RW, Bauer S, Wise L: Volume and pH of gastric juice in obese patients. Anesthesiology 43:686, 1975
29. Ong BY, Palahniuk RJ, Cumming M: Gastric volume and pH in out-patients. Canad Anaesth Soc J 25:36, 1978
30. Norris W: The quantitative assessment of premedication. Br J Anaesth 41:778, 1969

4

The Immediate Preinduction Period

Ronald D. Miller, M.D.

INTRODUCTION

One of the main obligations of the anesthesiologist is to prepare the patient and operating room for a safe anesthetic. In this chapter, the tasks that should be completed from the time the patient enters the operating room until induction of anesthesia are described. The considerations presented in this chapter apply to all patients undergoing all types of anesthesia and surgery, even the most simple and routine type. More specific preparation and monitoring for specialized types of anesthesia and surgery will be covered in the appropriate chapters (e.g., Swan Ganz catheters in Ch. 6).

The anesthesiologist should develop a routine which assures that the operating room, its equipment, and the patient are prepared for safe anesthesia. Apparently, some anesthesiologists are not using an adequate routine. Cooper et al.,[1] using a modified critical-incident analysis technique, evaluated preventable mishaps resulting from human error that could have or actually did contribute to anesthetic risk. Of 277 incidents, 47 percent of them occurred during the time from entry of the patient into the operating room until the surgical incision. Eighty-two percent of these incidents were secondary to human error and

14 percent were due to overt equipment error. The most common errors, with the most common listed first, are breathing circuit disconnection, inadvertent gas flow change, syringe swap, gas supply problem, intravenous apparatus disconnection, and laryngoscope malfunction.

Cooper et al.[1] concluded that associated factors also contributed to errors, some of which listed in order of occurrence are inadequate total experience, inadequate familiarity with equipment, poor communication with other members of the surgical team, haste, inattention or carelessness, fatigue, excessive dependence on other personnel, and failure to perform a normal check.

Although several factors obviously contribute to these preventable mishaps in the preinduction of anesthesia period, knowing how the anesthetic equipment works and ensuring that this equipment is functioning properly will eliminate many of the errors. Obviously, the anesthesiologist must develop a checklist and acquire the discipline to utilize it every time an anesthetic is administered. Airline pilots run through a mandatory checklist before starting a flight; this same principle applies to starting an anesthetic. The following questions are the most important ones for the anesthesiologist to ask.

QUESTIONS THE ANESTHESIOLOGIST SHOULD ASK

Is the Central and Cylinder Source of Oxygen and Nitrous Oxide Functioning?

Most hospitals pipe oxygen and often nitrous oxide from large cylinders in central locations in the hospital. Coupling systems at wall outlets and machines are designed to prevent accidental interchange of nitrous oxide and oxygen. Despite this system, nitrous oxide and oxygen lines have been occasionally accidentally switched resulting in severe morbidity and even death.

Feeley and Hedley-Whyte[2] surveyed hospitals with anesthesia residency training programs to ascertain the frequency and types of complications encountered with the use of bulk supplies of oxygen and nitrous oxide. A total of 76 incidents were reported, 3 of which led to death. In one hospital, tanks used for central oxygen were marked to contain oxygen but in fact contained nitrogen. Use of these tanks was felt to contribute to the deaths of two infants. Another patient died while being anesthetized in a new operating room where the oxygen and nitrous oxide pipes were crossed. I am aware of three deaths caused by this same mistake; fortunately these problems are usually, but not always, detected before serious damage to a patient occurs. The most frequent malfunction was insufficient oxygen pressure (Table 4-1). Feeley and Hedley-Whyte[2] concluded that the major problem was that most hospitals have no formal system of inspection to assure that hospitals and gas suppliers comply with the National Fire Protection Association regulations. Although compliance is required by the Joint Commission on Accreditation of Hospitals, their inspection apparently is often inadequate. Obviously, all physicians should be aware of designs and hazards of medical gas delivery systems and whether their own

Table 4-1. Reported Malfunctions of Gas Delivery Systems

Malfunction	Number of Reports
Insufficient oxygen pressure	37
Excessive oxygen and nitrous oxide pressure	7
Crossed pipelines	6
Depletion of Nitrous oxide	5
Failure of low-pressure alarm	4
Leaks in nitrous oxide pipeline	3
Leaks in wall connectors	2
Freezing of nitrous oxide regulators	2
Low oxygen flow	2
Others	8
Total	76

(Modified from Feeley TW, Hedley-Whyte J: Bulk oxygen and nitrous oxide delivery systems. Anesthesiology 44:301, 1976.)

hospital complies with regulations. On a day by day basis, routine use of an oxygen analyzer in the anesthetic system should allow the anesthesiologist to immediately detect when defects in central gas delivery systems have occurred.

Smaller cylinders attached to the anesthetic machine should be available as a backup in case the central source of gases fails. These smaller cylinders should be checked before each administration of anesthetic. The anesthetic machines have pressure gauges to determine the gas pressure in these smaller cylinders. In the case of oxygen, the pressure on the gauge is proportional to the volume of gas in the cylinder. This is because temperature in the operating rooms is above the critical temperature of oxygen (the critical temperature is that at which a gas cannot be liquified by pressure). Therefore when the pressure gauge reads 1200 psi, the tank is 66 percent full of oxygen, as compared to a pressure of 1800 psi.

In the case of nitrous oxide, the cylinder pressure does not reflect the volume of gas available. This is because nitrous oxide is stored as a liquid. As gas is withdrawn from the cylinder it is replaced by an equal volume vaporized from the liquid without change in pressure until all the liquid is exhausted. In

Table 4-2. Checklist for Evaluation of an Anesthetic Machine *Prior* to Its Use

1. Date of last inspection and servicing. (Ideally, maintenance should be performed every 3 to 6 months.)
2. Oxygen tank pressure (with flow meters off) indicates an oxygen supply sufficient for the expected duration of the case.
3. Oxygen flow meter ball or float rotates freely without sticking to side or top of flow meter tube.
4. Nitrous oxide flow meter ball or float rotates freely and is not jammed at top of flow meter tube; nitrous oxide is turned off before starting anesthesia.
5. Oxygen flush valve fills reservoir bag rapidly when it is opened and the breathing circuit is closed (i.e., by the anesthesiologist placing a thumb over the mask of endotracheal tube connector and with the pop-off valve closed).
6. Breathing circuit holds a steady positive pressure when circuit is closed and flow of fresh oxygen is turned off to ascertain the absence of leaks.
7. Pop-off valve releases positive pressure when it is opened.
8. The anesthesiologist breathes into the anesthetic system to detect any unexpected resistance in the circuit (e.g., malfunctioning valve).
9. Carbon dioxide absorbent is not depleted (i.e., see color indicator).
10. Volatile anesthetic vaporizers are filled adequately.
11. Sniff test—no smell of anesthetic when vaporizer is off: intensity of odor is appropriate when vaporizer is turned on to a low or medium concentration.
12. Suction bottle is empty and suction apparatus develops greater than 25 torr of negative pressure.
13. Oxygen analyzer is turned on and is calibrated appropriately.

this manner, greater volumes can be stored in cylinders if they liquify at room temperature. For example, 420 gallons of nitrous oxide can be stored in an E cylinder at 750 psi and only 165 gallons of oxygen in an E cylinder at 1800 psi.

Has the Anesthetic Machine Been Checked Thoroughly?

As outlined by Cooper et al.,[1] the failure to perform a proper check is associated with a large fraction of errors designated as preventable mishaps. Although the check will vary somewhat depending on the anesthetic system being used (see Ch. 5 for a detailed description of various anesthetic systems), several checks apply to all anesthetic systems (see Table 4-2). In essence, the anesthesiologist should confirm that the gas sources from the central source and cylinders are adequate. Is the vaporizer full of anesthetic? Does the circuit have any leaks or unexpected resistance? Is the absorbent satisfactory? I strongly recommend that the anesthesiologist apply the mask to his own face and breath through the circuit; this will confirm that the circuit does not offer a high resistance to breathing such as from a malfunctioning valve. Also, an excessive concentration of anesthetic that could occur from an undetected open flow meter may be detected. Lastly, by smelling the outflow from the anesthetic machine, the anesthesiologist can even check to see whether the vaporizer is functioning. The "calibrated nose" is a very useful clinical tool. As stated in Cullen and Larson,[3] the advantages of preventing inadvertent exposure to the patient of dangerously high concentrations of anesthetic outweigh the highly unlikely toxic effects to the anesthesiologist from an occasional sniff of the machine outflow.

Is the Anesthetic Work Area Organized Properly?

A carefully organized work space should lessen the chance of overt error and increase the chance of being effective in a crisis situation. As indicated earlier, an inadvertent syringe swap is a common cause of preventable anesthetic mishaps. These errors probably could be prevented by simply labelling the syringes. The anesthesiologist must develop a checklist that is meticulously followed. Although several such checklists have been recommended,[4] the anesthesiologist probably should develop one that suits his needs. Obviously, surgery can be delayed by the anesthesiologist who has an unrealistic checklist that takes too much time to follow. However, if the operating room and, specifically, anesthetic work area are adequately prepared before the first case, an adequate check in between cases should take less than 5 minutes.

Is the Intravenous Functioning Properly?

A well-functioning intravenous line is an obvious necessity for most anesthetics and surgery. Although the techniques of establishing an intravenous line have been adequately described in most introductory texts of anesthesia,[3] I have a few preferences.

Often patients are subjected to unnecessary discomfort in an effort to establish a large bore intravenous line prior to induction of anesthesia. Patients enter the operating room with veins that are often collapsed because of fear or cold. In this situation, I prefer to use an inhalational induction of anesthesia or to find a small vein with a fine needle through which drugs such as thiopental can be infused. After anesthesia has been induced, these veins probably will be dilated and a larger, more suitable line can then be established.

Basically, three kinds of needles are used: the "butterfly needle," intracath, and extracath. The butterfly is very good for small veins, such as the scalp vein of an infant. However, movement will cause the solid needle to puncture the vein and "infiltrate." The intracath has a plastic catheter introduced through the needle, while an extracath has the plastic catheter introduced over the needle. The latter is preferred because it causes less bleeding at the puncture site of the vein.

A vein that is easily seen and reasonably straight should be selected. The dorsum of the hand frequently has such veins. If the vein is collapsed because of cold or the patient's fear, measures can be taken to dilate the vein. These measures are dependent on drainage, application of moist heat, or gentle rubbing or tapping of the puncture site. Too often the novice will firmly pound the patient's hand or arm instead of using gentle rubbing. The former is nonproductive and uncomfortable for the patient.

Details of venipuncture have been described in various introductory texts of anesthesia.[3,5] Whether the bevel of the needle should be up or down when puncturing the vein is one aspect of the technique on which there is disagreement. Cullen and Larson[3] advocate having the bevel down. They argue that there is less possibility of puncturing the vein wall furthermost from the skin and less likelihood of leak from part of the bevel being out of the vein. Also, the bevel-down technique allows one to see the dimple produced in the vein ahead of the needle just before the needle enters the vein. Lastly, the bevel-down technique facilitates securing the needle flat against the skin, a procedure that Cullen and Larson[3] feel is advantageous. Despite these convincing reasons, Dripps, Eckenhoff, and Vandam[5] recommend keeping the bevel up until the vein has been punctured; this is my preference because it facilitates entry into the vein. If the bevel-up technique is selected, the needle should be rotated 180 degrees after the vein has been entered to lessen the chance of puncturing the vein wall that is furthermost from the skin. A common error of the novice is attempting to slide the catheter off the introducing needle prematurely. Too often, although the needle has penetrated the vein, the plastic catheter is still outside the vein. Therefore, if an extracath is used, the entire unit should be advanced into the vein a few millimeters before sliding the catheter off the introducing needle.

Probably the most common complication in using a plastic catheter is thrombophlebitis. My practice is to use 1 percent iodine or Betadine as an antiseptic. I then apply an antibiotic ointment to the insertion site and cover it with a small sterile dressing. Admittedly, the efficacy of each one of these maneuvers has not been established.

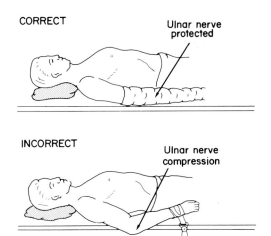

CORRECT — Ulnar nerve protected

INCORRECT — Ulnar nerve compression

Fig. 4-1 In the supine position, the ulnar nerve can be protected from injury; but by permitting the elbow to hang over the edge of the table, pressure may induce injury to the ulnar nerve.

Is the Patient in a Position that Will Not Cause Complications?

After he is anesthetized, the patient obviously does not know whether he is in a position that may lead to a peripheral neuropathy or pressure necrosis. Placing the patient in the position of surgery before anesthesia is induced will help identify areas of undue pressure. Frequently, however, the patient can be positioned only after anesthesia has been induced. Thus, the anesthesiologist must be aware of areas of the body that are especially vulnerable to injury. This usually occurs where nerves are in their long anatomic course and often superficially distributed.

Supine Position. Of 72 postoperative peripheral nerve complications, 33 occurred in the supine position. Of these, 14 involved the brachial plexus,[5] with the ulnar nerve being the most common[6] probably because of its superficial path along the median elbow. This injury can be prevented by proper padding and positioning (Fig. 4-1). If the arm is extended, then risk of brachial plexus injury develops; stretch to the brachial plexus should be avoided. A guide to follow is to palpate the tension of the pectoralis major muscle (Fig. 4-2). If it is relaxed, then tension on the brachial plexus is unlikely.

Prone Position. This position can result in several complications from pressure. The eye may be contused or penetrated from pressure with the face down. To assure that pressure is not being applied to the eye, the bony orbit should be palpated. If the entire orbit can be easily palpated with no obstruction, then no undue pressure probably is being applied to the eye. The brachial plexus can be injured if it is stretched or by pressure from improperly placed support. The ulnar nerve is especially vulnerable when the elbow is placed against sharp edges of the table;

CORRECT   INCORRECT

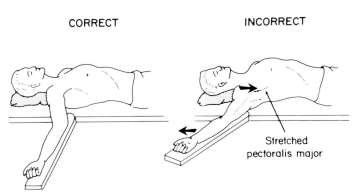

Stretched pectoralis major

Fig. 4-2 If the arm is extended at an angle of more than 90 degrees, an injury to the brachial plexus may result. An additional guide is to feel whether the pectoralis major muscle is tense. If so, then tension on the brachial plexus may also be present.

CORRECT

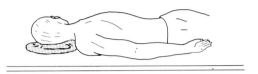

INCORRECT

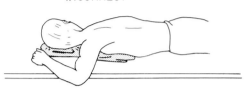

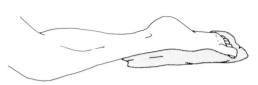

Fig. 4-3 In the prone position, injury to the lower brachial plexus, or ulnar nerve, or both can be avoided.

Fig. 4-4 In the prone position, proper placement can prevent injury to the foot from pressure.

flexion of the table makes the danger more likely (Fig. 4-3). Injury to the nerves and tendons of the dorsum of the foot may occur if the foot rests against the metal edge of the table; proper padding can prevent this complication (Fig. 4-4). The femoral cutaneous nerve of the thigh can be compressed against the supporting devices under the plexus causing a syndrome called meralgia paresthetica. These are only a few of the many problems that can result from the prone position. The reader is referred to an excellent chapter by Smith that deals with the problems associated with the prone position.[7]

Lateral Decubitus Position. In this position, padding or pillows should be placed under the head (Fig. 4-5) and between the

knees and elbows (Fig. 4-6). If the head is improperly supported (Fig. 4-5), compression to the dependent arm may occur and may impair neurovascular function to that extremity. The pillow between the knees and elbows will help distribute the weight of the upper extremity to the dependent extremity more evenly. Lastly, the brachial plexus can be compressed if the body is pressing on the dependent axilla. A small roll under the upper chest and not the axilla will take the weight off the arm (Fig. 4-6). (See Thomas[8] for more details.)

Lithotomy Position. Four nerves are most likely to be damaged in the lithotomy position.[9] The obturator nerve can be compressed by undue flexion of the thigh to the

CORRECT

INCORRECT

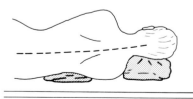

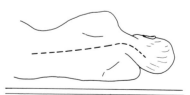

Fig. 4-5 Proper position of the head reduces pressure on the dependent arm in the lateral decubitus position.

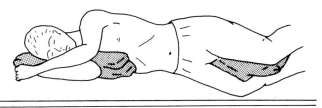

Fig. 4-6 In the lateral decubitus position, pillows between legs and elbows help distribute the weight of the upper extremity to that of the lower extremity.

groin. The saphenous nerve may be compressed against the medial aspect of the knee brace. The femoral nerve can be damaged by excessive angulation of the thigh with consequent compression to the nerve trunk. Lastly, the common peroneal nerve courses around the head of the fibula at the tibial condyles after penetrating various fascial planes; prolonged pressure at this point, by compression on the lateral aspect of the knee, can damage this nerve. These neuropathies can be prevented by cushioning the ankle and the knee against pressure from the metal stirrup. Wrapping a towel around the knee and ankle is effective in attenuating pressure. When positioning the patient, the legs should be elevated and flexed together. The thighs should be flexed no more than 90 degrees before rotating the stirrups laterally. (See Goldstein[9] for details.)

In summary, there obviously are many other less commonly used positions. The reader is referred to an excellent book edited by Martin[7-9] in which the various positions are discussed in detail. Most complications can be prevented by using good sense by which excessive pressure or angulation of the body is avoided.

SUMMARY

To prepare the patient and operating room for a safe anesthetic, the following preanesthetic checklist is recommended (E. I. Eger, II, personal communication).

Recommended Preanesthetic Checklist

A. Before first case of day
  1. Machine checkout (Table 4-2)
  2. Check and calibrate monitors
     a. Electrocardiogram
     b. Strain gauge
     c. Thermometers
     d. Other transducers
  3. Check emergency drug supply
     a. Lidocaine
     b. Bicarbonate
     c. Cardiotonics (isoproterenal, epinephrine, ephedrine, and other pressors)
     d. Propranolol
     e. Atropine
B. Before each case of day
  1. Recheck machine for leaks
  2. Set up intravenous and infusion devices
  3. Check airways (oropharyngeal, nasopharyngeal, endotracheal, bite blocks)
  4. Check laryngoscope (extra blade available)
  5. Minimum drugs drawn up and labeled—thiopental, succinylcholine (vasopressor if regional technique)
  6. Patient arrives: check
     a. Identification, consent
     b. NPO
     c. Permits
     d. Premedications and effect
     e. Special orders (steroids, diabetes, etc.)
     f. Laboratory work not available previous evening
     g. Status of ordered blood
     h. Dentures
     i. Intravenous (contains additives?)
  7. Attach to the patient:
     a. Blood pressure cuff and stethoscope
     b. Precordial stethoscope
     c. Other monitors
     d. Intravenous line
     e. Electrocardiogram
  8. Check all monitors—record initial values
  9. Position patient for induction of anesthesia
     a. Prevent nerve injury
     b. Use comfortable restraints as indicated

REFERENCES

1. Cooper JB, Newbower RS, Long CD, et al: Preventable anesthesia mishaps: A study of human factors. Anesthesiology 49:339, 1978
2. Feeley TW, Hedley-Whyte J: Bulk oxygen and nitrous oxide delivery systems: Design and dangers. Anesthesiology 44:301, 1976
3. Cullen SC, Larson CP Jr: Essentials of Anesthetic Practice. Chicago, Yearbook Medical Publishers, 1974, pp 112–118
4. Friedman G, Cunningham MA: Preanesthetic checklists of equipment and drugs. Anesth Rev 10:44, 1979
5. Parks BJ: Postoperative peripheral neuropathies. Surgery 74:348, 1973
6. Miller RG, Camp PE: Postoperative ulnar neuropathy. JAMA 242:1636, 1979
7. Smith RH: The prone position, Positioning in Anesthesia and Surgery, Edited by Martin JT. Philadelphia, WB Saunders, 1978, pp 32–43
8. Thomas AN: The lateral decubitus position, Positioning in Anesthesia and Surgery. Edited by Martin JT. Philadelphia, WB Saunders, 1978, pp 116–124
9. Goldstein PJ: The lithotomy position, Positioning in Anesthesia and Surgery. Edited by Martin JT. Philadelphia, WB Saunders, 1978, pp 142–151

Section I

Preparation of the Patient/Use of Anesthetic Agents: Intraoperative

5

Anesthetic Systems

Fredrick K. Orkin, M.D.

INTRODUCTION

The anesthetic system is the assembly of components that delivers anesthetic gases from the flowmeters of the anesthetic machine to the mask or tracheal tube. Functionally, the system comprises those pieces of anesthetic equipment through which the patient breathes. Properly chosen and used, the anesthetic system is a convenient and efficient way to deliver anesthetic gases (and oxygen) and remove exhaled carbon dioxide. In contrast, a poorly designed or improperly used system prolongs the induction of (and recovery from) anesthesia and risks more serious problems and complications, largely of a respiratory nature.

This chapter presents the principles underlying the safe use of anesthetic systems—sometimes loosely termed anesthetic or breathing circuits—and their components, such as carbon dioxide absorbers, volatile anesthetic vaporizers, and excess gas scavenging equipment. Because of limited space and the rapidity with which equipment is modified and replaced, the reader is referred to other sources for discussion of the historic development of this equipment[1] and manufacturer-specific details.[2–6]

EQUIPMENT AND ADVERSE ANESTHETIC OUTCOMES

Depending upon the definition and other details of the study, approximately six anesthetic-related deaths occur for every ten thousand operations;[7] less studied, anesthetic-related morbidity undoubtedly occurs considerably more frequently. More importantly, however, are two very sobering facts: first, since anesthesia is rarely therapeutic apart from the surgical procedure, significant risk is assumed without any hope of improving the patient's condition; second, 50 to 87 percent of adverse anesthetic outcomes have been deemed *preventable*[8–13] (see Ch. 4). The more prominent problems identified are breathing system disconnections and connection errors;[14, 15] associated factors include the anesthesiologist having inadequate total experience, inadequate familiarity with the equipment, and failure to check equipment properly prior to use (Fig. 5-1). As anesthesiology continues to evolve into a more exact science, fewer adverse outcomes related to inadequate medical knowledge should occur. Instead, an increasing portion of the risk of anesthesia will be attributable to preventable factors such as misuse of breathing systems.

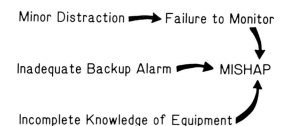

Minor Distraction ➡ Failure to Monitor

Inadequate Backup Alarm ➡ MISHAP

Incomplete Knowledge of Equipment

Fig. 5-1 Incomplete knowledge of equipment, coupled with minor distraction in the operating room and inadequate backup alarms, is viewed as an important predisposing factor leading to anesthetic mishaps. (Courtesy of Jeffrey B. Cooper, Ph.D., Massachusetts General Hospital.)

Herein lies the necessity of becoming knowledgeable about anesthesia systems.

PHYSICAL PRINCIPLES

GAS FLOW AND RESISTANCE

Anesthetic gases flow from the anesthesia machine to the patient in response to a pressure gradient that exists between the gas pressure regulators or reducing valves at the machine (usually about 345 kPa or 50 lb/in^2) and the patient (atmospheric pressure). The gas flow rate through a straight tube of uniform bore is proportional to the pressure gradient and the *fourth* power of the radius, and is related inversely to the viscosity of the gas and the length of the tube. These relationships are summarized in the Hagen-Poiseuille equation:

$$\dot{Q} = \frac{\pi p r^4}{8\eta l} \qquad (1)$$

where $\dot{Q}$ is the flow rate in cubic meters per second, p is the pressure gradient in Newtons per square meter, r is the radius in meters, l is the length of the tube in meters, and η is the viscosity of the gas in Newton-seconds per square meter. Thus, for a given pressure gradient and tube length, the critical determinant of flow rate is the radius of the tube,

since this term is present in the Hagen-Poiseuille equation raised to the fourth power. Alternatively, since the pressure gradient required to effect flow is a measure of the resistance to flow, resistance is also directly proportional to the flow rate, but inversely related to the *fourth* power of the radius.

LAMINAR FLOW

The molecules comprising the gas typically move in paths parallel to the sides of the tube, and, hence, the flow is termed laminar. Laminar flow is characterized by adherence to the Hagen-Poiseuille equation and a parabolic flow pattern in which the highest velocity is at the center of the lumen and least (zero) at the wall of the tube. This pattern of different velocities reflects the underlying differences in shear forces between apposed particle layers that retard particle movement. The shear force is greatest at the periphery because the tubing wall is immobile, and the force is progressively smaller toward the center of the tube (Fig. 5-2a).

TURBULENT FLOW

When the flow rate exceeds a critical velocity, the flow loses its parabolic velocity profile, becomes disorderly, and is termed turbulent (Fig. 5-2b). The critical velocity is itself proportional to the viscosity of the gas and is related inversely to the density of the gas and the radius of the tube (Fig 5-3). These relationships are summarized as follows:

$$v_c = \frac{k\eta}{\rho r} \qquad (2)$$

where v_c is the critical velocity in centimeters per second, k is a constant known as the Reynold's number (approximately 2,000), η is the viscosity in Newtons per square meter, ρ is the density of the gas in grams per cubic centimeter, and r is the radius of the tube in centimeters. Laminar flow can also

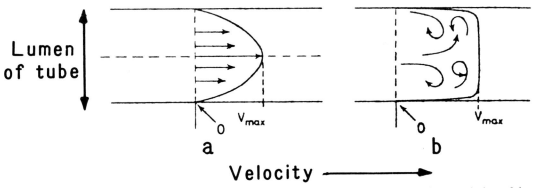

Fig. 5-2 Flow profiles characterizing (a) laminar and (b) turbulent flow. (Reprinted by permission of the publisher from (with modification) Hill DW: Physics Applied to Anaesthesia. 4th edition. London: Butterworths (Publishers) Ltd. 1980.)

become turbulent as a result of irregularities in the tube lumen, such as abrupt narrowing, turns, or branching. When turbulent flow exists, the relationship between pressure gradient (or resistance) and flow rate is no longer governed by the Hagen-Poiseuille equation. Instead, the pressure gradient required (or the resistance encountered)

during turbulent flow varies as the *square* of the flow rate. Hence, given the high flow rates present during turbulent flow, this is an inefficient way to move gas, since a much greater pressure gradient must be generated—or, alternatively, a much greater resistance must be overcome—than during laminar flow.

Fig. 5-3 Approximate critical flow rates of helium, air, oxygen, nitrogen, nitrous oxide, and cyclopropane at room temperature through smooth, straight tubes of various internal diameters. For a given diameter, there is a critical flow rate, which is dependent upon gas viscosity and density, above which laminar flow becomes turbulent. (Values for air taken from reference 2; values for other gases calculated.)

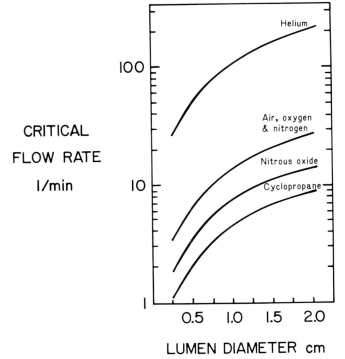

A special case of turbulence exists when a gas flows through an orifice that may be considered a very unusual tube whose diameter is considerably larger than its length. Although flow through an orifice can be laminar at low flow rates, the flow through such an aperture is generally at least partially turbulent. Empirical evidence indicates that the flow rate across an orifice is given by the following expression:

$$\dot{Q} \propto r^2 \sqrt{\frac{p}{\rho}} \qquad (3)$$

where $\dot{Q}$ is the flow rate, r is the radius of the orifice, p is the pressure gradient, and ρ is the density of the gas. Thus, as in the more general case of turbulence, the pressure gradient (or resistance) varies as the square of the flow rate; however, in this special case, the flow rate is dependent upon the density rather than the viscosity of the gas.

CLINICAL IMPORTANCE

Much of the equipment to be discussed in this chapter constitutes a tubular extension to the patient's upper airway. Because peak inspiratory flows as high as 60 L/min are reached during *resting* spontaneous ventilation in man, anesthetic systems can add considerable resistance to respiration.[16-21] The resistance imparted by any system is determined most by those portions having the smallest bore, typically the tracheal tube and connector (Fig. 5-4). For example, the resistance of a Mapleson A (Magill) breathing system is 0.25 cm H_2O (25 N/m^2) at a constant flow rate of 50 L/min; adding a tracheal tube having an internal diameter of 10 mm with a curved connector increases the resistance to 2.5 cm H_2O (250 N/m^2); and, finally, changing the curved connector to a right-angle one increases the pressure drop across the system to 5.0 cm H_2O (500 N/m^2).[22]

To counter increased respiratory resistance, the spontaneously breathing patient

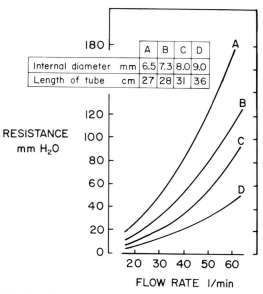

	A	B	C	D
Internal diameter mm	6.5	7.3	8.0	9.0
Length of tube cm	27	28	31	36

Fig. 5-4 Resistance as a function of trachael tube internal diameter (ID) and flow rate. The relationship between flow rate and resistance is not linear—that is, the flow is not laminar—particularly as the lumen becomes smaller, because most of the flow rates depicted are above the critical velocities. Note also that flow rate must always be specified with values of resistance. (Modified from Macintosh R, Mushin WW, Epstein HG: Physics for the Anaesthetist. 3rd edition. Oxford, Blackwell Scientific Publications, 1963.)

must generate a greater pressure gradient, which constitutes an increase in the work of breathing, to effect the same exchange of gas, or suffer hypoventilation.[23, 24] In response to a mean increase of 241 percent in inspiratory resistance, infants in one study tolerated a mean increase of 205 percent in the work of breathing without carbon dioxide retention and acidosis.[25] However, these infants lacked cardiorespiratory disease, and, it should be emphasized, hypercarbia and acidosis are *late* signs of respiratory decompensation. Increasing the inspiratory resistance further resulted in extremely variable responses. In a study of unselected surgical patients, some of whom had cardiorespiratory disease, the imposition of increased respiratory resistance resulted in an immediate, presumably reflex increase in inspiratory pressure generated to partially counter the added resistance; an increase in minute ventilation occurred during the next few minutes. Breathing through resistors that simulated the resistance of pediatric endotracheal tubes having an external diameter of 24 French and 16 French (approximately 5.5 mm and 3.5 mm internal diameter, respectively), these adults experienced mean reductions of 7 and 21 percent in minute ventilation, respectively. There was marked scatter in their responses, with some patients maintaining a near-normal minute ventilation inspiring against 17 cm H_2O, whereas one patient became apneic at 12 cm H_2O.[26]

The added respiratory resistance due to anesthesia equipment is somewhat less clinically relevant now that assisted and controlled ventilation have supplanted spontaneous respiration during anesthesia. However, respiratory resistance remains an important consideration in the intensive care unit, where a patient may breathe spontaneously for a considerable period (e.g., T-piece trial, intermittent mandatory ventilation) through a tracheal tube whose lumen can be encroached upon progressively by inspissated secretions.

Minimizing respiratory resistance requires that components of the anesthetic system have the shortest length and greatest diameter practicable; hence, the corrugated breathing system tubing has a very large bore, and the tracheal tube should be the largest that can be accommodated. Sharp bends and other sudden changes in lumen size should be avoided; similarly, curved tracheal tube connectors (e.g., Magill) are preferable to right-angled ones (e.g., Cobb, Rowbotham). In clinical circumstances that simulate a narrow orifice, such as croup and tracheal stenosis, the use of a gas having a lower density than air, such as helium, as the carrier for oxygen results in improved gas flow (Fig. 5-3). A mixture of 80 percent helium in oxygen in place of air or oxygen augments gas flow rate by approximately 75 percent, thereby decreasing the work of breathing.[27]

CARBON DIOXIDE ELIMINATION

REBREATHING

Carbon dioxide is continuously produced in the body as a result of cellular metabolism and transported to the lungs for elimination via pulmonary ventilation. An anesthetic breathing system can impair carbon dioxide elimination because the breathing system—effectively a tubular extension of the patient's upper airway—adds apparatus dead space to the patient's physiological dead space; the latter includes the anatomic dead space (volume in nonventilating conducting airways) and alveolar dead space (volume in ventilated, nonperfused alveoli). Upon the imposition of the additional dead space, the patient breathes again, or rebreathes, a volume of his expired gases that approximates that of the added dead space.

Physiological Effects

Although the effects of rebreathing depend upon the volume and composition of the gas that is rebreathed, one cannot predict the physiological responses precisely in the clinical setting.[28] The volume of rebreathing can differ from that determined volumetrically because of turbulence and other peculiarities of gas flow; moreover, the patient's anatomic dead space can vary, affecting the volume of total dead space. The composition of the rebreathed gas depends upon which portion of the dead space is rebreathed. The composition of the gas in the apparatus dead space varies with the arrangement of components comprising the given breathing system. Gas in the anatomic dead space has a composition resembling that of the inspired concentration but is saturated with water vapor within a few degrees of body temperature. Alveolar gas is also saturated and contains 5 to 6 percent carbon dioxide.

Altered Inspired Concentrations. Rebreathing alveolar gas whose carbon dioxide has not been removed necessarily results in an increased $PaCO_2$. Although an awake, healthy person can tolerate even large increases in dead space by increasing minute ventilation, the anesthetized patient generally cannot compensate for even small amounts of rebreathing (see Chs. 13 and 22). The increase in the carbon dioxide concentration in alveolar air, coupled with the uptake of oxygen and nitrogen washout early during anesthesia, results in a decreased inspired concentration of oxygen. Rebreathing also causes a discrepancy between delivered and inspired concentrations of inhaled agents, because the rebreathed gas is a mixture of fresh gas and expired gas. Hence, during induction of anesthesia, when the alveolar concentration of anesthetic is lower than the inspired, rebreathing dilutes the inspired concentration, reducing the alveolar concentration and prolonging induction of anesthesia. In contrast, rebreathing slows the elimination of anesthetic during emergence by maintaining a higher alveolar concentration of anesthetic.

Heat and Water Retention. Since anesthetic gases are dry and at ambient temperature and expired gas is saturated with water vapor at body temperature, rebreathing conserves heat and water.

CARBON DIOXIDE ABSORPTION

Gas warfare during World War I provided the impetus for finding a way to remove expired carbon dioxide from the totally closed breathing system of the gas mask.[29] A general approach resulted that involves a chemical neutralization of an acid by a base.[30] The carbon dioxide combines with water to form carbonic acid, which ionizes readily, releasing hydrogen ion, the acid. The base is the hydroxyl ion resulting from the ionization of the hydroxide salt of the alkali metals (e.g., potassium, sodium) and of the alkaline earth metals (e.g., barium, calcium). The carbon dioxide absorbent is actually a mixture of the hydroxide salts, which are fused and then crushed into granular fragments having a large surface area for absorption of the carbon dioxide.

Granule Size

The size of the granules represents a compromise between absorptive activity and resistance to air flow: absorptive activity increases as granule size decreases because total surface area increases; but, the smaller the granules, the smaller the interstices through which gas must flow and, hence, the greater the resistance. Empirically, the optimal granule size has been found to be 4 to 8 mesh.[31] (A granule size of 4 mesh will pass through a screen having four or fewer wires per inch.)

Water Content

Although a small amount of water may be present in the hydrated salt, water is added to the granules by the manufacturer prior to sealing in an air-tight package. Additional water is needed to raise the total water content to a level at which the particular absorbent mixture absorbs optimally: too much water reduces the surface area available for absorption, whereas too little water effectively retards the formation of carbonic acid.[32] (Inadequate moisture is also associated with adsorption of sufficient halothane to prolong the induction of anesthesia.[33]) The water also dissipates some of the heat generated in the exothermic neutralization reaction.

Indicator

An indicator is a dye whose color depends upon hydrogen ion concentration, which is mixed throughout the absorbent.[34] When the hydrogen ion concentration rises above a level specific for the given dye, a color change becomes apparent through a transparent canister, indicating that the absorptive capacity has been reached and the absorbent should be changed. If the absorbent is not changed, the color often reverts during disuse; however, minimal regeneration will have occurred, and, upon reuse, the dye quickly changes color again.[35] Commonly used indicators and their colors are listed in Table 5-1.

Channeling

Loose packing of the granules in a carbon dioxide canister, or poor design of the canister, results in the gas passing preferentially through the canister by way of paths of very low resistance. Such "channeling" is particularly likely to occur along the sides of the canister[30] and results, in turn, in exhaustion of the granules constituting the low resistance paths, with passage of carbon dioxide through the canister if the absorbent is not changed. Shaking the canister gently prior to use can reduce the likelihood of channeling without substantially increasing resistance to air flow.

Absorptive Capacity

The maximum volume of carbon dioxide that can be absorbed is approximately 26 L of carbon dioxide per 100 g of the commonly used absorbents.[36] Usually considerably less carbon dioxide is actually absorbed due to diverse factors such as canister design, moisture content, degree of channeling, and the particular end-point used to detect exhaustion. For example, only 10 to 15 L of carbon

Table 5-1. Indicators used in Carbon Dioxide Absorbents

Indicator	Color when Absorbent Fresh	Color when Absorbent Exhausted
Phenolphthalein	Colorless	Pink
Ethyl violet	Colorless	Purple
Clayton yellow	Red	Yellow
Ethyl orange	Orange	Yellow
Mimosa Z	Red	Colorless

(Modified from Dorsch JA, Dorsch SE: Understanding Anesthesia Equipment: Construction, Care and Complications. Baltimore. © (1975) The Williams & Wilkins Co., Baltimore.)

dioxide per 100 g is absorbed in a single-chambered canister, whereas 18–20 L is absorbed in a dual-chambered design. In the latter, the chamber through which the expired gas flows first is discarded when the indicator changes color, the second chamber is moved to the position formerly occupied by the first, and a new chamber containing fresh absorbent is added to the canister.

Incompatibility with Trichloroethylene

During 1943 and 1944 some two dozen case reports of cranial nerve injuries following trichloroethylene anesthesia appeared.[37] The patients emerged from anesthesia with an unusual amount of nausea and vomiting, often with concomitant headache. During the next few days, bilateral facial numbness (cranial nerve V) and weakness (VII), loss of corneal reflexes (V), oculomotor palsy (III), hoarseness (X), weakness of the tongue (XII), diminished hearing (VIII), and constriction of visual fields (II) occurred. Although these signs and symptoms vanished in some patients within a few months, most had permanent facial numbness and weakness and several died with encephalitis. No effective therapy was found. Analysis of the case reports indicated that all affected patients had received trichloroethylene anesthesia administered via breathing systems containing a carbon dioxide absorber or had followed patients who had received the agent through the same breathing system. At the same time, trichloroethylene was found to decompose to neurotoxic agents (e.g., dichloroacetylene, phosgene) in the presence of alkali and heat—circumstances characterizing conditions in the carbon dioxide absorber.

Although the intentional use of this anesthetic in breathing systems with carbon dioxide absorbers ended with the publicity that the syndrome attracted, and although this agent has been abandoned in the United States, trichloroethylene is still used in other countries on occasion, and this complication may occur. For example, a patient who self-administered trichloroethylene by hand-held inhaler during obstetric labor may receive general anesthesia soon thereafter for removal of retained placental fragments and exhale residual amounts of the agent into the absorber. Or, this agent may be inadvertently substituted for another volatile agent when filling a vaporizer.[38]

Soda Lime

The most commonly used absorbent today, soda lime, is a mixture whose composition has evolved over six decades (Table 5-2). Although the principal component is calcium hydroxide, smaller amounts of the more active sodium and potassium hydroxides are present as activators. Silica is added to give hardness to the mixture, minimizing the formation of alkaline dust. Such dust can be forced out of the canister into the breathing system and even into the patient's lungs, where it can cause respiratory irritation that can present as bronchospasm.[39,40]

The following reactions describe the absorption of carbon dioxide by soda lime:

$$CO_2 + H_2O \rightarrow H_2CO_3$$
$$H_2CO_3 + 2\ NaOH\ (and\ KOH)$$
$$\rightarrow Na_2CO_3\ (and\ K_2CO_3) + 2\ H_2O + heat$$
$$Na_2CO_3\ (and\ K_2CO_3) + Ca(OH)_2$$
$$\rightarrow CaCO_3 + 2\ NaOH\ (and\ KOH)$$

Table 5-2. Approximate Composition of "Wet" Soda Lime

Ingredient	Percentage of Wet Weight
Sodium hydroxide	4.0
Potassium hydroxide	1.0
Water	14–19
Silica	0.2
Calcium hydroxide	Balance

Some carbon dioxide reacts directly, but more slowly, with the calcium hydroxide:

$$CO_2 + Ca(OH)_2 \rightarrow H_2O + CaCO_3 + heat$$

The heat generated is termed the heat of neutralization and amounts to about 13.7 kcal/mole of carbon dioxide (22.4 L) absorbed.

Baralyme

Baralyme is a newer, but less commonly used, absorbent that is composed of 80 percent calcium hydroxide and 20 percent barium hydroxide; the latter serves as an activator. Unlike soda lime, baralyme contains moisture as the bound *water of crystallization* in the octahydrate salt of barium hydroxide. This water binds the absorbent sufficiently so that no silica is necessary. The bound water also accounts for baralyme's greater stability in water content and, thus, its greater reliability of performance in dry environments, as compared with soda lime.[41] Because optimal activity requires a water content of 11 to 14 percent, additional water is added.

Carbon dioxide absorption proceeds as follows:

$$Ba(OH)_2 \cdot 8H_2O + CO_2$$
$$\rightarrow BaCO_3 + 9\ H_2O + heat$$
$$9\ H_2O + 9\ CO_2 \rightarrow 9\ H_2CO_3$$
$$9\ H_2CO_3 + 9\ Ca(OH)_2$$
$$\rightarrow CaCO_3 + 18\ H_2O + heat$$

Heat production is similar to that occurring with soda lime.[42]

VAPORIZATION

All of the commonly used, potent general anesthetics are volatile liquids at room temperature and atmospheric pressure. These agents must be transformed into the vapor phase for clinical use. The safe use of vaporizers for these agents requires an understanding of vaporization. The concepts reviewed here also explain and suggest preventive measures for the cold stress resulting from the evaporation of water from the airway when the patient breathes dry gas through the anesthetic system.

THE PHENOMENON OF VAPORIZATION

According to the kinetic theory of matter, the molecules comprising matter are in constant, random motion. Motion requires energy, and the velocity with which the molecules move and the number of collisions per unit time reflect the amount of energy imparted to the matter. As a form of energy, heat is both a source of energy and a representation of the average kinetic energy of the molecules in the given matter. Thus, a higher temperature connotes a greater number of collisions per unit time and a higher velocity; and upon losing energy, the matter has a lower temperature and the constituent molecules are less active.

Consider a closed container in which there is both liquid and air. Within the densely packed array of molecules comprising the liquid are two types of motion: the bulk of the molecules move about randomly because intermolecular attractive forces are rather symmetrically applied about each molecule and, thus, negate each other. An asymmetrical arrangement of intermolecular forces, however, is applied to the small number of molecules at the liquid-air interface. This is because surrounding a given molecule at the surface there are many more molecules within the liquid than in the air above. As a result, there is a net attractive force pulling the surface molecules into the liquid—a force that must be overcome if the surface molecules are to enter the air, where their relatively sparse density constitutes a vapor. Hence, the transition from the liquid to the vapor phase requires energy. The *heat of vaporization* of a liquid is the number of calories required at a specified temperature to convert 1 g of the liquid into a vapor (Table 5-3). The heat of vaporization is temperature-dependent; the colder the liquid, the greater the amount of energy needed to vaporize a given amount of liquid. As a result of the energy expenditure incurred in vaporization, the aggregate energy of the remaining liquid decreases and, thus, the temperature of the liquid falls.

Vaporization does not continue indefinitely in this hypothetical closed container, but rather ceases when an equilibrium is reached between the liquid and vapor phases such that the number of molecules in the vapor phase is constant. That is, as many molecules leave the liquid as reenter it per unit time. The molecules in the vapor phase collide with each other and the walls of the container, creating a pressure that is termed the vapor pressure, or saturated vapor pressure to emphasize that at equilibrium the vapor phase contains a maximal number of molecules of anesthetic agent per unit space. Like the heat of vaporization, vapor pressure is also temperature-dependent; a higher temperature is associated with a greater number of molecules in the vapor phase and, thus, a higher vapor pressure. The relationship between vapor pressure and temperature is given by the Antoine equation:[43]

$$\log P = A - \frac{B}{t + c} \qquad (4)$$

where P is the pressure, t is the temperature in °C, and A, B, and C are constants derived experimentally. Constants for the volatile anesthetics are listed in Table 5-3, which also includes room temperature values for the

Table 5-3. Physical Properties of Volatile Anesthetic Agents and Water

	Molecular Weight	Boiling Point (°C,760 torr)	Vapor Pressure (20°C,760 torr)	Liquid Density (g/ml,20°C)	Vapor Density (g/L,20°C)	Heat of Vaporization (cal/g,20°C)	Antoine A ($\frac{kPa}{torr}$)	Equation B	Constants C
Chloroform	119.0	61.2	160	1.50	4.12	64	5.978 / 6.854	1125.05	222.0
Diethyl ether	74.1	34.6	440	0.71	2.55	87	6.151 / 7.027	1109.58	233.2
Divinyl ether	70.0	28.3	550	0.77	2.42	90	6.094 / 6.970	1044.14	227.0
Ethyl chloride	65	12.3	1003	0.90	2.22	92	6.514 / 7.390	1269.62	269.2
Halothane	197	50.2	243	1.86	8.90	35	5.892 / 6.768	1043.70	218.3
Methoxyflurane	165	104.7	23	1.42	6.68	58.6	6.206 / 7.082	1336.58	213.5
Trichloroethylene	131	87.1	60	1.47	4.53	58	5.961 / 6.837	1198.48	216.4
Enflurane	184.5	56.5	175	1.5125*	7.54*	42*	6.112 / 6.988	1107.84	213.1
Isoflurane	184.5	48.5	239	1.5125*	7.54*	41*	4.822 / 5.698	536.46	141.0
Water	18	100	17.5	1.00		540	7.167 / 8.043	1716.98	232.5

* Values at 25°C.

(Modified from Dorsch JA, Dorsch SE: Understanding Anesthetic Equipment: Construction, Care and Complications. © (1975) The Williams & Wilkins Co., Baltimore, except for Antoine constants, which are taken from Rogers RC, Hill GE: Equations for vapour pressure versus temperature. Br J Anaesth 50:415, 1978.)

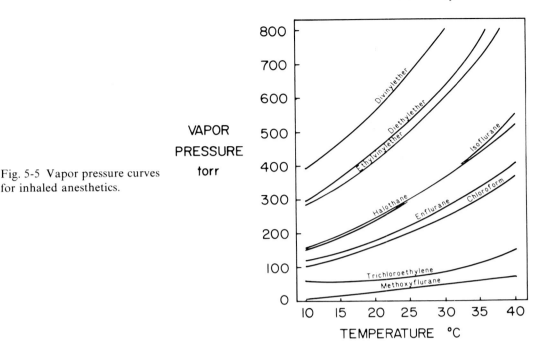

VAPOR
PRESSURE
torr

Fig. 5-5 Vapor pressure curves
for inhaled anesthetics.

vapor pressure. Such an equation facilitates the generation of vapor pressure curves for each agent (Fig. 5-5).

If a hole is made in the container, molecules in the vapor phase can escape and the equilibrium is upset. More molecules leave the liquid than reenter it, resulting in a progressive decrease in the tempeature of the remaining liquid.

THE IDEAL ANESTHETIC VAPORIZER

From the foregoing it would seem that a simple vaporizer might consist of an otherwise closed container with oxygen (or a mixture of oxygen and nitrous oxide) flowing through the space above the liquid anesthetic. However, such a laudably simple design would present several problems in actual use. As vaporization proceeds, as in the case of the closed container with the hole, the temperature of the remaining liquid would decrease; with time, progressively less vaporization would occur. The maximum concentration

delivered by this device is given by the quotient of the vapor pressure of the given anesthetic at a specified temperature and atmospheric pressure. For example, if the anesthetic is halothane, the vapor pressure at room temperature is 243 torr (Table 5-3), or about one third of atmospheric pressure (243/760); hence, the gas existing from this vaporizer under optimal circumstances would be 32 percent halothane, a most certainly lethal concentration. It is very unlikely, though, that the carrier gas would have sufficient contact with the halothane vapor to equilibrate completely, so the effluent gas would contain a lower concentration of halothane. Similarly, the higher the flow rate of the carrier gas, the less time afforded for equilibration, and the lower the concentration of halothane in the effluent gas. Hence, the performance of this vaporizer is not only unknown—the output can vary between lethal concentrations of anesthetic and, perhaps, no anesthetic—but also uncontrollable.

An "ideal anesthetic vaporizer" would satisfy these deficiencies, as well as the attributes measure of the amount of heat required to change the temperature of a substance—and a very high thermal conductivity—a measure of the speed with which heat flows through a substance. Hence, copper serves as a reservoir for heat and readily gives it up to the anesthetic liquid, whose temperature is thereby maintained. Some designs also include a bi-metallic strip that functions as a thermostat to counter a decrease in vaporizer temperature by allowing more carrier gas to pass through the vaporizing chamber; an ambient temperature water bath, which serves as a heat reservoir, and an electric heater are present in other designs. Safety is enhanced by designing the vaporizer with the anesthetic liquid-filling port in a relatively low position to prevent overfilling of the vaporizer. This diminishes the possibility that anesthetic *liquid* may be carried into the breathing system and even into the patient's lungs, usually resulting in death.[44-46]

listed in Table 5-4. That there are more than a dozen different vaporizer designs should suggest, however, that the "ideal" has not been achieved.

VAPORIZER DESIGN

There are three general approaches to vaporizer design: flow-over, bubble-through, and a combination of both. Because the designs are so numerous, technical, and ever-changing, only a few representative approaches are mentioned here, following some general comments. There are several excellent sources of further information.[3-5]

Common Features

Since the vapor pressure of commonly-used volatile anesthetics ensures a saturation concentration well above clinical concentrations (recall the saturation vapor pressure of 32 percent for halothane), vaporizer design includes some provision for diluting the vapor generated. Vaporization-induced lowering of the liquid temperature is largely prevented in many designs through the use of copper in the construction of the vaporizer. Copper has a relatively high specific heat—a

Flow-Over Vaporizers

As the name suggests, in flow-over vaporizers the carrier gas flows over the anesthetic liquid, carrying vapor out of the vaporizer. Vaporization is enhanced by increasing the area of contact between carrier gas and anesthetic liquid by means of baffles and/or wicks, as well as by directing the carrier gas as close to the liquid as possible. The saturation concentration is diluted to clinical concentrations through the use of a variable bypass that diverts the major portion of the carrier gas away from the vaporizing chamber (Fig. 5-6).

Assuming equilibration of the carrier gas with the anesthetic vapor, the carrier gas becomes saturated with vapor and the concentration of anesthetic leaving the vaporizing chamber is expressed in the same fashion as in the case of the closed container:

$$\frac{\%\text{ anesthetic}}{\text{leaving chamber}} = \frac{P_a}{P_b} \times 100\% \quad (5)$$

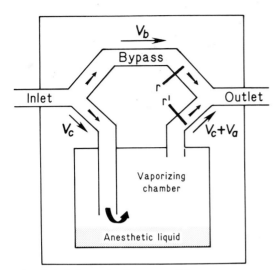

Fig. 5-6 Schematic diagram of flow-over vaporizer design. The incoming gas flow is divided between a bypass route and a vaporizing chamber inlet according to the ratio of the resistances (r, r'). The resistance on the outlet is usually calibrated in volume percent. A vaporization-induced decrease in liquid temperature and, hence, vaporization results in an increasing flow through the chamber, maintaining the ratio of flow through the two resistance points.

where P_a is the vapor pressure of the anesthetic and P_b is the barometric pressure. Since the pressure exerted by a mixture of gases is the sum of the partial pressures of the individual gases (Dalton's law of partial pressures), equation 5 may be rewritten:

$$\% \text{ anesthetic leaving chamber} = \frac{V_a}{V_a + V_c} \times 100\% \quad (6)$$

where V_a is the volume of anesthetic vapor and V_c is the volume of carrier gas. Similarly, the concentration of the anesthetic in the gas at the vaporizer's outlet may be expressed as follows:

$$\% \text{ anesthetic leaving chamber} = \frac{V_a}{V_a + V_b + V_c} \times 100\% \quad (7)$$

where V_b is the bypass gas flow and the denominator represents the total gas flow. Since V_a is not measured, equations 5 and 6 can be

solved for V_a and the result substituted into equation 7 to obtain a more useful expression for the concentration of anesthetic at the outlet:

$$\% \text{ anesthetic leaving vaporizer} = \frac{V_a \cdot P_a}{V_b(P_b - P_a) + V_b \cdot P_b} \times 100\% \quad (8)$$

The Agent-Specific, Calibrated Vaporizer. In the commonly-used modern vaporizer, the desired concentration is obtained by turning a knob that alters the ratio of gas flowing through the bypass to that flowing through the vaporizing chamber (Fig. 5-7). Settings of the knob are calibrated directly in volume percent, obviating the need for computation. Temperature- and flow-compensating mechanisms ensure constant output at a given setting—except in low-flow and closed systems, where the gas flows are below those for which the vaporizer is calibrated. Yet, the penalty for this technologic progress is the possibility that the wrong anesthetic agent will be put into the vaporizer, resulting in the delivery of a high and usually unknown concentration. This error is particularly hazardous when a highly volatile agent is used in a vaporizer designed for one of lower volatility.[47,49] The likelihood of causing this error is minimized with a pin-indexing system at the filling port, similar to that used for compressed gas tanks at the anesthesia machine; yet, this safety feature is present in few vaporizers. In the end, as in other aspects of clinical practice, there is no substitute for increased vigilance (see Ch. 4).

Open-Drop Administration. In 1847, Simpson administered chloroform by pouring small quantities of the volatile liquid on a handkerchief held over his patient's nose and mouth. Open-drop administration survives in primitive circumstances with a Schimmelbusch mask, a wire frame that supports several layers of gauze (Fig. 5-8). This "vaporizer" is satisfactory only for the more volatile agents—most of which are flammable and,

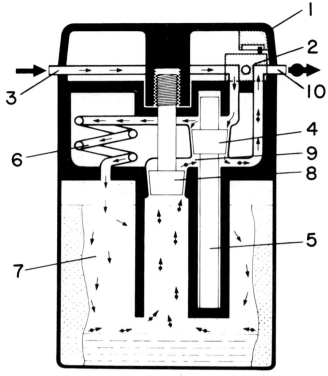

Fig. 5-7 Schematic diagram of Dräger "Vapor 19." This is a modern flow-over, temperature- and flow-compensated, agent-specific vaporizer, with models available for use with enflurane and with halothane. Turning a knob (1) to desired concentration (volume percent) opens a shunt (2) that permits carrier gas (oxygen or an oxygen–nitrous oxide mixture) entering the inlet (3) to reach a cone (4) with a temperature-compensating expansion rod (5), which diverts a small portion of the flow into a long spiral tube (6) that permits compensation for pressure changes in the breathing system (e.g., consequent to different modes of respiration) before reaching the vaporizing chamber (7). Saturated carrier gas leaves the vaporizing chamber at a control cone (8) that regulates the concentration delivered according to the position of the knob (1), mixes with the bypass carrier gas (9), and exits the vaporizer through the outlet (10). (Modified from North American Dräger Company brochure.)

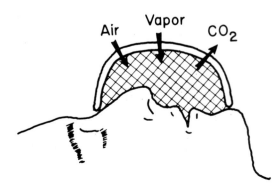

Fig. 5-8 Schematic diagram of open-drop administration using the Schimmelbusch mask with gauze moistened with a highly volatile anesthetic agent. Rebreathing can be diminished by insufflating oxygen under the mask.

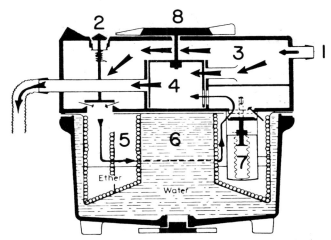

Fig. 5-9 Schematic diagram of the EMO (Epstein-Macintosh-Oxford) inhaler. This is a flow-over, temperature-compensated, agent-specific vaporizer, with models available for use with halothane, diethyl ether, and less commonly used agents. Air enters the inlet (1) and, upon turning the vaporizer "on" (2), the flow divides at a bypass (3). One stream flows into a mixing chamber (4); the other stream flows above the mixing chamber before entering the donut-shaped vaporizing chamber (5), surrounded by water (6), which is lined by wicks and contains a temperature-compensating mechanism (7) that regulates gas flow above at the vaporizing outlet en route to the mixing chamber. The ratio between the bypass and vaporizing chamber flows is determined by changing the diameter of apertures in the mixing chamber, according to control lever (8) settings. (Reproduced by courtesy of Penlon Ltd. Reprinted, with relabelling, by permission of the publisher from Hill DW: Physics Applied to Anaesthesia. 4th edition. London: Butterworths (Publishers) Ltd. 1980.)

hence, rarely used—and, even then, only with small children. Delivered concentration is unknown and difficult to control, and the mask often becomes so cold (and thereby diminishes subsequent vaporization) that it must be changed frequently to avoid prolonging the induction. This "vaporizer" is discussed further as an example of an open-breathing system.

The EMO Inhaler. As equally portable as open-drop administration but much more controllable is the EMO (Epstein Macintosh Oxford) inhaler, which was developed for use in field conditions and other circumstances where nitrous oxide, and even oxygen, may not be available.[49] As with the open-drop mask, the patient's own inspiratory effort is the motive force; air is drawn through a low-resistance, temperature-compensated device whose delivered concentration is set with a calibrated lever (Fig. 5-9). Vaporization-in-duced changes in the anesthetic liquid temperature are minimized by a temperature-compensating mechanism and a water bath. A foot-operated bellows is available for assisted and controlled respiration.

The Ohio No. 8 Bottle. Much less commonly used now, this example of a flow-over vaporizer deserves a passing mention because, unlike the other vaporizers described here, it is used as part of the semiclosed or closed breathing system and is often found on older anesthetic machines. It consists of a glass jar, a wick with a large surface area, and a valve that permits the diversion of any or all of the breathing system flow through the vaporizing chamber. Designed for diethyl ether and used more recently with methoxyflurane, this vaporizer can be used with any volatile agent. Although a simple device and less wasteful of anesthetic than the open-drop mask, it is not calibrated and there is no provision for maintaining the temperature of the liquid anesthetic. Hence, the delivered concentration is unknown and, as vaporization proceeds, progressively decreases at any given setting.

Bubble-Through Vaporizers

In the bubble-through design, efficient vaporization is achieved by increasing the surface area available for vaporization through the use of very small bubbles. The smaller the bubble, the greater the surface/volume ratio of the bubble and, thus, the more likely that the gas within the bubble will become saturated with anesthetic vapor when in contact with anesthetic liquid. Fine bubbles are formed by passing oxygen through a porous plate or sintered bronze disk at the bottom of the liquid-filled vaporizing chamber. Because these vaporizers lack a temperature-compensation mechanism and a dilution bypass, the effluent gas contains a very high concentration of the anesthetic vapor in oxygen, as determined by the vapor pressure of the given anesthetic at the ambient temperature. To make this device clinically useful, the oxygen carrier gas is regulated with a flow meter and the effluent gas is diluted in the manifold of the anesthesia machine with the other gases (e.g., oxygen, nitrous oxide) that are being administered. The concentration of anesthetic delivered to the breathing system can be calculated by using equation 8, with the oxygen flow to the kettle substituted for V_c and the other gas flows substituted for V_b. Although bubble-through vaporizers are less convenient to use because they are not calibrated, clinical "rules of thumb" are quickly learned (e.g., with enflurane, 100 ml oxygen through the kettle at 20°C with other flows totalling 3 L produces a 1 percent concentration). Moreover, these vaporizers can be used with all volatile agents and with all flows, including those used for low-flow and closed-system techniques.

The Copper Kettle. This prototype bubble-through vaporizer is constructed entirely of copper because of this element's high heat capacity and thermal conductivity (Fig. 5-10).[50] Thermal stability is enhanced by its attachment to the copper work surface of the anesthesia machine.

Vernitrol. Constructed of bronze, this vaporizer is an integral part of one brand of anesthesia machine. The bronze serves as a ready heat reservoir to stabilize the vaporizer temperature.

Flow-Over, Bubble-Through Vaporizers

This combination design is not used in the United States, although it is used in England in the Boyle's Bottle.

VAPORIZER LOCATION

The vaporizer may be located proximal to the anesthetic breathing system (out-of-system) or within the breathing system (in-system). In the former, more common location, the vaporizer receives its inflow directly from the flow meters of the anesthesia machine or more distally somewhere between the common gas delivery of the machine and the breathing system. In this out-of-system location, the vaporizer receives only fresh gas; thus, the concentration of volatile anesthetic in the vaporizer effluent is dependent only upon considerations such as vaporizer characteristics, vaporizer setting, and ambient temperature. In contrast, the in-system vaporizer (e.g., Ohio No. 8) is located within a circle breathing system and, hence, its inflow contains a varying and unknown mixture of fresh gas and expired anesthetic. The concentration of volatile anesthetic leaving the in-circle vaporizer depends upon the same considerations as in the case of the out-of-system vaporizer but is modified by the com-

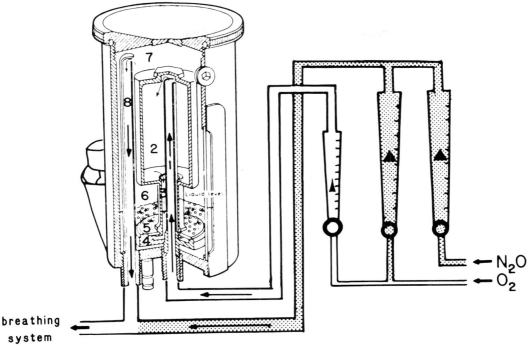

Fig. 5-10 Schematic diagram of the Copper Kettle vaporizer. A metered oxygen flow enters the inlet at the base of the vaporizer, travels up a center tube (1) to the loving cup (2) (which dissipates the effect of sudden surges of gas), turns downward (3), and passes through a sintered bronze disk (5). The resultant bubbles rise through the anesthetic liquid (6) in the vaporizing chamber (7), and the saturated vapor exists through an outlet tube (8) where it is diluted by joining other gases in the manifold of the anesthesia machine en route to the machine gas delivery. (Reproduced by courtesy of Foregger Co. Reprinted, with modification, by permission of the publisher from Hill DW: Physics Applied to Anaesthesia. 4th edition. London: Butterworths (Publishers) Ltd. 1980.)

position of the gas entering the vaporizer. The latter is particularly sensitive to fresh gas flow and the patient's minute ventilation, as will be discussed when the circle breathing system is described. Thus, the gas exiting from the in-system vaporizer has a very unpredictable and potentially very high concentration of volatile anesthetic.

HUMIDIFICATION

Humidification—the process of adding moisture (water vapor) to a gas—is merely a subset of vaporization. Although the underlying physical principles are the same, humidification assumes special importance be-cause it occurs within the patient who then incurs the deleterious side effects of vaporization such as heat loss.

Air passing through the nose en route to the lungs is subjected to the air conditioning function of the upper airway, which consists of warming, humidification, and filtering. Before reaching the carina, the air rises to within a few percent of body temperature and of saturation with water vapor. Inhalational anesthesia prevents such air conditioning when administration is via a tracheal tube that bypasses the upper airway. A more consistent problem, however, is that anesthetic gases are water-free because water would otherwise condense and freeze in the pressure-reducing valves of the anesthesia machine's high pressure system. Anesthetic gases also are generally at room temperature, although the temperature can be somewhat lower if the gas sources are machine-mounted gas cylinders.

Bypassing the upper airway and using such dry gases leads to cytologic damage to the respiratory ciliated epithelium in as short a period as 1 hour.[51,52] Continued inhalation of dry gas has been associated in dogs with increased pulmonary shunting and reduced compliance.[53] Whether these changes produce an increased incidence of postoperative pulmonary complications is not known.[54] Breathing dry gas for several hours can result in drying of secretions, crusting, and, when an endotracheal tube is used, even airway obstruction from inspissated secretions. However, the more frequently cited problems of "dry gas" breathing are the water and heat losses that occur because the respiratory mucosa adds water and warmth so that air is at body temperature and fully saturated with water in the lungs. Discussion of these losses requires an understanding of the ways in which the water content of a gas is quantitated.

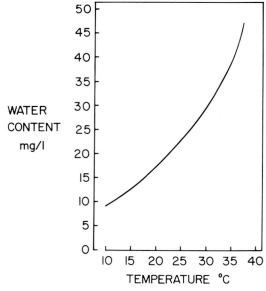

Fig. 5-11 Absolute water content of saturated gas as a function of temperature.

HUMIDITY

Two terms are used to express the water content of a gas: the weight of water vapor in a given volume of gas (in mg/L) at a specified temperature is the absolute humidity; the ratio of absolute humidity of a gas sample to the absolute humidity of that sample if it were saturated with water at that temperature is termed the relative humidity. Because the absolute water content of saturated gas is an exponential function of temperature (Fig. 5-11), the relative humidity of a given sample of gas changes markedly upon entering the body. For example, the relative humidity of gas saturated at room temperature is only 38 percent at body temperature. Generally, however, absolute humidity, expressed in terms of mg/L,

is more useful when considering the water and heat loss consequent to humidification.

WATER LOSS

The respiratory moisture loss can be quantitated simply as the product of the minute ventilation and the gradient existing between the water content of the inspired and expired air. The minute ventilation may be measured or estimated from a nomogram,[55-57] and the water content of expired air (i.e., fully saturated air at 37° C) may be taken as 45 mg/L. Hence, the hourly respiratory water loss can be estimated as follows:

Respiratory water loss per hour =
$$60 \, \dot{V}_E \, (45 - A_t)$$

where A is the water content at temperature t° C. For the 70-kg adult breathing air with a relative humidity of 50 percent at room temperature (i.e., a water content of 9 mg/L) the respiratory water loss is approximately 13 g/hr, which agrees reasonably well with empirical observations of 250 to 300 g/day.[58] Even using a non–rebreathing system with dry gases, the respiratory water loss would rise only to about 16 g/hr. Such a loss is small compared to daily fluid requirements and is easily replaced by intravenous fluids, without any special effort. Values proportional to their smaller minute ventilation are obtained in children. Clearly, the magnitude of the respiratory water loss is too small to argue cogently for instituting humidification of anesthetic gases solely to counter water loss.

RESPIRATORY HEAT LOSS

There are two ways in which heat loss via the respiratory tract occurs. The first and quantitatively less important way is the warming of inspired gases to body temperature. The heat expended is dependent upon the minute ventilation, the temperature gradient, and the specific heat of the gases and may be estimated as follows:

Heat loss due to warming =
$$\dot{V}_E\ (37 - t)\ (\text{specific heat})$$

where t is the temperature ($^{\circ}$C) of the inspired gas. Under particularly adverse circumstances, such as the open-drop administration of ether, the temperature of the inspired gas can drop to 0°C, and the rate of heat expenditure to warm this gas to body temperature approximates 90 cal/min in the adult. However, with currently-used breathing systems the inspired gas is at room temperature, so the heat loss due to warming is less than half as much.

The more important way in which heat is lost via the respiratory tract is vaporization. In addition to having a lower temperature, the inspired air also has a lower water content than the expired air. Heat is expended to vaporize a sufficient amount of water to saturate the inspired air at body temperature. For each gram of water vaporized, 580 cal must be supplied by the patient. The resultant heat

loss constitutes a clinically significant threat to the temperature homeostasis of infants and children during general anesthesia, which renders the body poikilothermic. Herein lies the principal rationale for the use of a humidifier. Humidification can also reduce heat loss sufficiently to reduce, in turn, the incidence of postoperative shivering.[59, 60]

HUMIDIFIERS

The simplest method of raising the water content of anesthetic gases, merely wetting the lumen of the breathing system tubing, results in a water content of about 22 mg/L.[61] With either the adult circle breathing system[62] or a pediatric semiopen system,[63] a water content as high as 29 mg/L may be obtained by passing inspired gas through the soda lime canister, which is heated by the exothermic reaction that occurs with carbon dioxide absorption; heating enables the gas to hold more water (Fig. 5-11). Respiratory moisture can also be conserved by placing a fine-mesh gauze condenser, the so-called artificial nose, just proximal to the tracheal tube.[64] Moisture from the warm, moist expired gas condenses on the cooler gauze, which is warmed by the gas; cool, otherwise dry inspired gas is warmed and humidified as it passes through the warm, moist gauze. Unfortunately, the condenser effect requires such a fine mesh that considerable respiratory resistance and dead space result, undesirable characteristics for a device that would find greatest use in infants and small children. Obtaining a higher water content requires a considerably more complex design that involves heating water in contact with inspired gas and/or nebulizing water to effect supersaturation of the inspired gas. With improved efficiency of humidification comes a variety of potentially serious complications, including nosocomial infection secondary to bacterial contamination,[65-69] particularly in conjunction with the use of mechanical

Table 5-5. Attributes Desired in an Anesthetic Breathing System

Accuracy and precision in delivery of anesthetics and oxygen
Small dead space and efficient elimination of expired carbon dioxide
Low respiratory resistance
Conservation of respiratory moisture
Convenience and safety in clinical use

ventilators; water intoxication[70] and increased respiratory resistance[71] from nebulizers, especially in infants; hyperthermia[72] and tracheal "burns" from excessively heated inspired gas; and electrocution, explosion, and other problems related to malfunction of electrical equipment. These hazards, as well as the bulkiness of the devices, explain why humidifiers are used infrequently.

BREATHING SYSTEMS

The design of anesthetic breathing systems has been an evolutionary process, albeit a haphazard one. The systems available today possess in varying degrees desirable characteristics (Table 5-5). New knowledge has prompted modifications in available systems, as well as a return to breathing systems abandoned decades ago; an example of the latter is the renewed interest in the closed system at a time when there is concern about anesthetic pollution of the operating room. Although the ideal breathing system is not at hand, the variety of systems available satisfy diverse clinical requirements reasonably well. Hence, the anesthesiologist must be sufficiently familiar with the available systems to be able to choose the most appropriate one, as well as to be aware of potential problems with each.

The systems are described here according to a classification scheme (Table 5-6) based solely upon the presence of a gas reservoir and rebreathing of expired gases.[73] This scheme represents the simplest yet most functionally adequate one among the many

proposed.[74] Nonetheless, because distinctions between systems are blurred (e.g., a semiclosed system functions as a closed system when all expired gases except carbon dioxide are rebreathed), the plea has been made that the components and fresh gas flow be stated when describing a given system.[75]

OPEN SYSTEMS

Lacking a reservoir and rebreathing, open systems are the simplest and least expensive systems, if not the most primitive systems. Because they have no physical connection to the patient's airway, open systems do not impose respiratory resistance. Yet, many disadvantages limit their use. The lack of physical connection to the airway results necessarily in the spillage of large quantities of anesthetics into the operating room, loss of respiratory moisture, inability to control ventilation, and, when flammable agents are used, an increased risk of explosion. The major disadvantage is the unstable anesthetic level: when the anesthetic level is light, for example, during induction and emergence, the patient has a relatively large tidal volume whose peak flow rate—instantaneously as high as 50 L/min in the adult and child and 10 L/min in the infant[76]—exceeds that delivered. Hence, there is increased dilution of the anesthetic agents with room air, and the anesthetic concentration decreases. In contrast, as the anesthetic level deepens, the patient's tidal volume decreases and less dilution with room air occurs, resulting in an increasing anesthetic concentration. Light anesthesia begets lighter anesthesia, and deep anesthesia, deeper.

Insufflation

In insufflation, the anesthetic is administered directly from the anesthesia machine's delivery hose or from a mask held above the face. This technique is useful for inducing an-

Table 5-6. Classification of Anesthetic Breathing Systems

Breathing System	Reservoir	Rebreathing
Open	No	No
Semiopen	Yes	No
Semiclosed	Yes	Partial
Closed	Yes	Complete

(Moyers J: A nomenclature for methods of inhalation anesthesia. Anesthesiology 14:609, 1953.)

esthesia in the child ("steal induction") and in bronchoscopy and laryngoscopy.

OPEN-DROP ADMINISTRATION

An inhaled agent with a high vapor pressure and moderate potency (e.g., diethyl ether, halothane) is administered dropwise onto layers of gauze held in a Schimmelbusch mask (Fig. 5-7). Once the mask is lowered onto the face, this technique is no longer strictly nonrebreathing. Elimination of expired carbon dioxide is impeded when water condenses and freezes in the gauze mesh as the mask temperature drops consequent to vaporization. The carbon dioxide trapped under the mask also dilutes the room air, resulting in hypoxemia. Oxygen insufflation under the mask with an "ether hook" treats both problems but increases the hazard of explosion. However, the condensation of respiratory moisture on the mask results in the inhalation of very dry (and cold) gas. For these reasons this technique is rarely used, although its portability favors use in disaster and other field circumstances.

SEMIOPEN SYSTEMS WITH NONREBREATHING VALVES

As in the open system, the semiopen system allows no rebreathing; however, the latter does include a reservoir bag. The addition of a nonrebreathing valve[77]—a device that directs fresh gas into the patient and expired gas out of the system—permits a lower fresh gas flow to be used, often as low as that equal to the patient's minute ventilation (Fig. 5-12). The principal advantage of the semiopen system is that the composition of the inspired gas approximates that delivered to the system and, thus, the concentrations of inspired gases can be changed rapidly. Also, the presence of the reservoir bag enables assisted and controlled ventilation, including tactile assessment of pulmonary compliance.

Numerous disadvantages, however, mostly relating to the nonrebreathing valve, have relegated this system to use in resuscitative equipment: the bulky valve must be located immediately proximal to the patient, a location that may be inconvenient in many circumstances; and the valve adds considerable respiratory resistance so that its use in infants and, given the high flow rates needed which further increase the resistance, in adults is unwise.[78] In addition, condensation of respiratory moisture makes the valve stick. With the more commonly used valves (e.g., Fink, Stephen-Slater, Ruben), respiratory obstruction occurs when minute ventilation exceeds fresh gas flow. The Steen valve prevents this by permitting ambient gas to enter; this pre-

Fig. 5-12 Semiclosed breathing system with a Ruben nonbreathing valve and a reservoir bag.

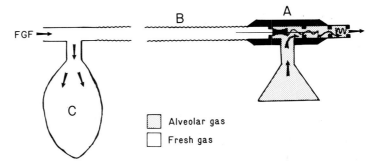

FGF ➡

B   A

C

☐ Alveolar gas
☐ Fresh gas

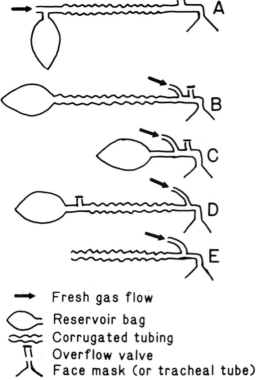

→ Fresh gas flow
Reservoir bag
Corrugated tubing
Overflow valve
Face mask (or tracheal tube)

Fig. 5-13 Semiopen breathing circuits, as classified by Mapleson. (Redrawn from Mapleson WW: The elimination of rebreathing in various semiclosed anaesthetic systems. Br J Anaesth 26:323, 1954.)

vents a cardiorespiratory catastrophe such as a pneumothorax but dilutes the anesthetic concentration. All nonrebreathing valves are subject to occlusion of the exit port—for example, when excessive fresh gas flow jams the valve in the inspiratory position—unless a pressure-relief device is placed elsewhere in the system. Like the open system, there is no conservation of respiratory moisture.

SEMIOPEN SYSTEMS WITHOUT VALVES

These semiopen systems grossly resemble those with nonrebreathing valves except that an overflow (relief, or "popoff") valve is substituted. Because the overflow is not interposed between the fresh gas flow and the patient, these semiopen systems are regarded as not having valves. These systems generally share the same components, arrangements (Fig. 5-13) of which affect their performance with respect to the efficiency of expired carbon dioxide elimination (Fig. 5-14). The classification scheme is the one proposed by Mapleson.[79]

THE MAPLESON A SYSTEM

Often referred to as the Magill attachment, or system, the Mapleson A system is particularly efficient in eliminating carbon dioxide during spontaneous ventilation. In fact, rebreathing does not occur with this system until fresh gas flow decreases to a value equal to the patient's *alveolar* ventilation.[80,81] In clinical usage, however, fresh gas flow should equal or exceed the patient's minute ventilation.[79] This efficiency results from the fact that during expiration the fresh gas flow flushes expired carbon dioxide out the overflow valve. During inspiration, the patient inhales fresh gas from both the fresh gas inflow and the reservoir bag, which then collapses. Upon expiration, dead space gas and then alveolar gas enter the expiratory limb. The reservoir bag fills as the expired gases meet the fresh gas flow, and the pressure within the system increases. Later in expiration, the pressure rises sufficiently to force the overflow valve to open, and alveolar gas exits. If fresh gas flow is high enough, dead space gas also exits, although whether this occurs is of little physiological consequence.

During assisted or controlled ventilation, this system is much less efficient.[82] This is because, with tightening of the overflow valve and squeezing of the bag, gas exits from the system during *inspiration* rather than expiration. Thus, expired gas and some fresh gas collect in the expiratory limb during expiration and enter the patient during inspiration before the pressure within the system rises

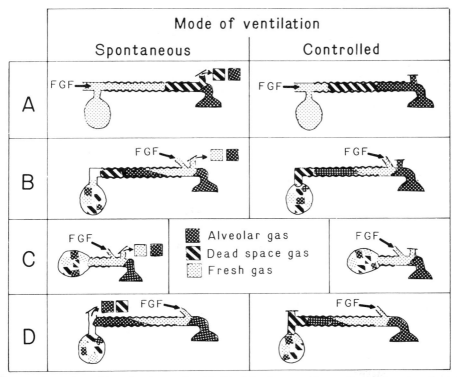

Fig. 5-14 Semiopen breathing circuits, as classified by Mapleson, with gas disposition at end-expiration, during spontaneous and controlled ventilation. FGF=fresh gas flow. (Redrawn from Sykes MK: Rebreathing circuits: A review. Br J Anaesth 40:666, 1968.)

sufficiently to force the overflow valve open. The fresh gas flow required to prevent rebreathing during assisted or controlled ventilation with this system is dependent upon not only the fresh gas flow but also the tidal volume, respiratory rate, and rate of pressure rise within the system during inspiration. Since this system is so inefficient under these circumstances and the fresh gas flow requirement cannot be estimated easily, this system is generally used only with spontaneous ventilation.

THE MAPLESON B SYSTEM

Moving the fresh gas inflow to the end of the expiratory limb near the patient, just distal to the overflow valve, results in a breathing system that, although not as efficient as the A

system during spontaneous ventilation, is clinically useful and behaves in a similar way for any mode of ventilation. The location of fresh gas inflow allows expired gas (and some fresh gas) to collect in the reservoir bag and expiratory limb during exhalation. The bag fills with a mixture of dead space, alveolar, and fresh gas, whereas the corrugated tubing receives alveolar and fresh gas. Once the bag has filled and the pressure in the system has risen sufficiently, the overflow valve opens, allowing mostly fresh gas to exit. Upon inspiration, with lowering of pressure within the system, the overflow valve closes, and the patient receives fresh gas, as well as gas from the expiratory limb. The fresh gas flow rate determines the composition of the inspired mixture: with high flows, the mixture consists of fresh gas and some alveolar gas; whereas, with lower flows, a greater proportion of alveolar gas will be inhaled. A fresh gas flow of at least twice the minute ventilation is needed to minimize rebreathing.[28, 82]

THE MAPLESON C SYSTEM

The Mapleson C system is a Mapleson B system whose expiratory limb has been shortened (i.e., the corrugated tubing has been removed). As a result, the inspired gas contains more alveolar gas than is the case with the B system, and a fresh gas flow of at least twice the minute ventilation is needed to prevent rebreathing.[28] This system may also be used for spontaneous, assisted, or controlled ventilation.

THE MAPLESON D SYSTEM

In the Mapleson D system, a commonly used system, the arrangement of components most closely resembles that in the B system except that the overflow valve is located at the reservoir bag. Not insignificantly, however, exchanging the locations of the fresh gas inflow and overflow valve converts a D system to an A system. As a result of this altered configuration and the flushing effect of the fresh gas flow, with the Mapleson D system there is greater efficiency of carbon dioxide elimination during assisted or controlled ventilation than during spontaneous ventilation.[28] In fact, during assisted or controlled ventilation with the D system, the flushing effect forces alveolar and dead space gas out the overflow valve, resulting in an inspired mixture of almost solely fresh gas, when using a fresh gas flow as low as twice minute ventilation.[28]

During spontaneous ventilation, the D system is as complicated as the A system is during controlled ventilation: fresh gas and alveolar gas flow down the expiratory limb during expiration. Once the bag has filled and pressure has risen within the system, the overflow valve opens, thus allowing some of

this mixture to exit. Upon inspiration, the patient inhales fresh gas and gas from the expiratory limb. The latter may be fresh gas or a mixture of fresh gas and alveolar gas, depending upon the duration of the expiratory pause and patient's tidal volume, as well as on the fresh gas flow. A short expiratory pause does not permit much flushing by the fresh gas, regardless of its flow rate; similarly, a tidal volume greater than can be satisfied by the fresh gas flow results in the inhalation of gas containing expired carbon dioxide from further down the expiratory limb.

The Bain System

In the Bain system, a recent modification of the Mapleson D system, fresh gas flows through a narrow tube within the corrugated expiratory limb (Fig. 5-15).[83] Among the claimed advantages of this configuration are the warming of the fresh gas by the surrounding expired gases in the expiratory limb, improved humidification as a result of partial rebreathing at the patient end of the expiratory limb,[84] reduced weight (because they are supplied as disposable, plastic items), sterility (again, because they are single-use items), ease of scavenging waste anesthetic gases from an overflow valve), and the convenience and safety of having the overflow valve further from the patient (especially in the case of head and neck surgery). Since the configuration is that of the Mapleson D system, the same flow considerations apply. However, during controlled ventilation, a fresh gas flow rate as low as 70 ml/kg body weight will maintain normocarbia, with 100 ml/kg producing mild hyperventilation.[85, 86] Although similar flow rates *may* prove satisfactory during spontaneous ventilation in some patients, a fresh gas flow of 200 to 300 ml/kg is recommended.[87, 88] This more conservative recommendation recognizes that the patient may not be able to increase his

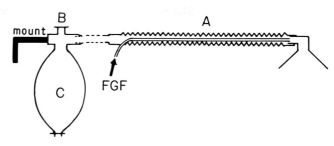

Fig. 5-15 Schematic diagram of a Bain breathing system showing fresh gas flow (FGF) into modified Mapleson D system (A), overflow valve (B), and reservoir bag (C). (Relabelled from Bain JA, Spoerel WE: A streamlined anaesthetic system. Can Anaesth Soc J 19:426, 1972.)

minute ventilation, or at least increase it sufficiently, due to impaired respiratory drive secondary to anesthetics and other drugs, increased carbon dioxide production secondary to hyperthermia, or increased apparatus or physiological dead space. The price paid for the simplicity of this potentially "universal" breathing system[89] is a group of new complications and concerns that include increased respiratory resistance due to a relatively high flow rate through the narrow bore of the inner tube, unrecognized disconnection[90] or misconnection[91] of the inner tube with severe hypercarbia, absence of flow due to unrecognized kinking of the inner tube,[92] and, as might be expected, hypercarbia from an inadequate fresh gas flow during spontaneous ventilation.[93]

THE MAPLESON E SYSTEM

The Mapleson E system involves the use of the T-piece introduced in 1937 by Ayre as a means of supplying, without cumbersome equipment near the surgical field, endotracheal anesthesia for children undergoing cra-

nial surgery and cleft palate repair.[94-96] In its original design, this device consists of a tube, whose internal diameter is 1 cm, that receives fresh gas from a smaller side arm (Fig. 5-16). During expiration, both expired gas and fresh gas flow down the open expiratory limb. During inspiration, varying ratios of fresh gas and expired gas can be inhaled, depending upon the fresh gas flow rate and the volume of the expiratory limb. With an expiratory limb whose volume is one third the patient's tidal volume, a fresh gas flow of about three times minute ventilation avoids rebreathing during spontaneous ventilation. Flow rates as low as twice minute ventilation can prevent rebreathing if the expiratory pause increases and/or the inspiratory flow rate decreases. Although there is no reservoir bag, respiration can be controlled by intermittent occlusion of the expiratory limb, which forces fresh gas into the trachea. Assisted and controlled ventilation is facilitated by the Jackson-Rees modification of the Ayre's T-piece—the addition of a reservoir bag at the end of the expiratory limb, with an adjustable aperture at the open end of the bag.[97] The T-piece system has minimal dead space and respiratory re-

Fig. 5-16 Ayre's T-piece breathing system, with gas disposition at end-expiration shown. FGF=fresh gas flow. (Redrawn from Sykes MK: Rebreathing circuits: A review. Br J Anaesth 40:666, 1968.)

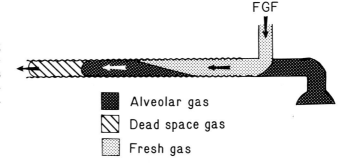

■ Alveolar gas

◩ Dead space gas

▦ Fresh gas

sistance and can be used with a mask or tracheal tube, but this system still wastes large volumes of anesthetics.

OVERVIEW

Comparing the various Mapleson systems, it is apparent that during spontaneous ventilation the most efficient in eliminating carbon dioxide is the A system, followed by the D, C, and B. During controlled ventilation, the most efficient is the D system, followed by the B, C, and A.[98] Although these systems are simple, lightweight, sturdy, easy to clean, and offer low resistance to respiration, the high flow rates needed incur loss of respiratory moisture and pollute the operating room. The Bain system addresses many of these problems but, as noted, introduces some new ones. The high flow, however, does result in the inspired mixture having a composition very similar to that being delivered from the anesthesia machine' and, thus, enables rapid changes in the concentrations of gases inspired.

SEMICLOSED BREATHING SYSTEMS

Currently the most commonly used breathing system for adults is the semiclosed system, which has a reservoir bag and provides partial rebreathing of expired gases. Rebreathing is permissible in this system because a carbon dioxide absorber is used. As a result, there is some conservation of respiratory moisture and the magnitude of the fresh gas inflow is not a paramount concern.

THE CIRCLE SYSTEM

The circle system, the most widely used example of the semiclosed system, is named for the overall arrangement of components and, thus, is a true breathing *circuit*.

Components

To prevent excessive rebreathing, unidirectional valves are placed in the system so that the gases flow in only one direction, generally making a pass through the carbon dioxide absorber each time around. The principal conduit for the circle gases is a wide-bore, corrugated ("elephant") hose that offers little resistance; even the properly-filled carbon dioxide canister adds little respiratory resistance, due to its large cross-sectional area. Other components include an overflow valve to permit the escape of excess gases, a reservoir bag, and a Y connector to attach the mask or tracheal tube to the breathing system. Optional components include bacterial filters, a circulator, and an in-system (e.g., Ohio No. 8) vaporizer. As with the Mapleson systems, the arrangement of these components determines the behavior of the system.

Prevention of CO_2 Rebreathing

To prevent the rebreathing of expired carbon dioxide in the circle system, the arrangement of components must obey three rules: (1) a one-way valve must be located between the patient and rebreathing bag on both the inspiratory and expiratory limbs of the circuit; (2) fresh gas inflow must not enter the circuit between the overflow valve and the patient; and (3) the overflow valve must not be located between the patient and the inspiratory valve.[99]

Conservation of Fresh Gases

Avoiding rebreathing of carbon dioxide, however, does not ensure the most efficient use of the fresh gas inflow. In the more efficient arrangements, the overflow valve is located on the expiratory limb, often near the patient, to preferentially vent alveolar gas: this arrangement results in a higher inspired concentration of anesthetic and oxygen, as

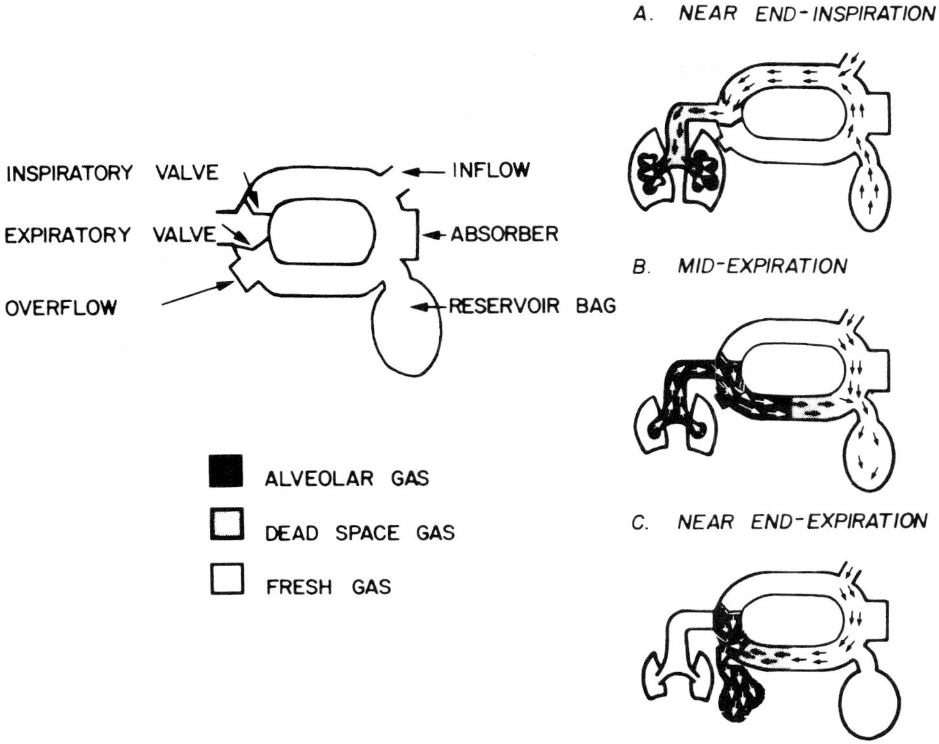

A. NEAR END-INSPIRATION

INSPIRATORY VALVE

EXPIRATORY VALVE

OVERFLOW

INFLOW

ABSORBER

RESERVOIR BAG

B. MID-EXPIRATION

■ ALVEOLAR GAS

□ DEAD SPACE GAS

□ FRESH GAS

C. NEAR END-EXPIRATION

Fig. 5-17 Circle breathing system with optimal arrangement of components. (Redrawn from Eger EI II: Anesthetic Uptake and Action. Baltimore, Williams & Wilkins, 1974. © (1974) EI Eger II, M.D.)

well as prolongs the life of the absorber.[101] In the most efficient system for both spontaneous and controlled ventilation (Fig. 5-17), the overflow valve is close to the patient on the expiratory limb but just distal to the expiratory valve, fresh gas enters the circuit between the absorber and inspiratory valve, and the reservoir bag is located between the absorber and expiratory valve.[101] As in the Mapleson A (Magill) system, fresh gas flushes alveolar gas preferentially before any dead space gas leaves the circuit. At end-inspiration, fresh gas fills the inspiratory limb. With the beginning of expiration, dead space gas and then alveolar gas flows down the expiratory limb, forcing the fresh gas ahead into the reservoir bag, which simultaneously receives fresh gas in a retrograde fashion. Once the bag has filled and the pressure within the circuit has risen sufficiently, the overflow valve opens,

allowing the escape of alveolar gas; this escape is hastened by retrograde flow of fresh gas in the expiratory limb. The presence and location of the one-way valves enables the same high efficiency regardless of whether ventilation is spontaneous or controlled. With this arrangement, the inspired concentration is equal to the inflow concentration when the fresh gas inflow is equal to or exceeds the alveolar minute ventilation.[101] Unfortunately, this optimal arrangement is impractical in the clinical setting because the relatively bulky valves and overflow are located near the patient.

A more practical, although somewhat less efficient, arrangement is shown in Figure 5-18. This arrangement is less efficient because moving the overflow down the expiratory limb further from the patient permits mixing of alveolar and dead space gas. Hence, when

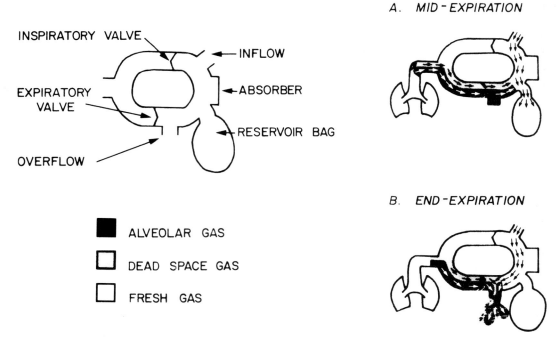

INSPIRATORY VALVE

INFLOW

EXPIRATORY VALVE

ABSORBER

RESERVOIR BAG

OVERFLOW

A. MID-EXPIRATION

B. END-EXPIRATION

■ ALVEOLAR GAS

□ DEAD SPACE GAS

□ FRESH GAS

Fig. 5-18 Circle breathing system whose components are arranged in a less efficient way than the arrangement shown in Figure 5-17. The pairing of dead space gas with alveolar gas indicates complete mixing. (Redrawn from Eger EI II: Anesthetic Uptake and Action. Baltimore, Williams & Wilkins, 1974. © (1974) EI Eger II, M.D.)

the overflow opens, dead space gas is lost with alveolar gas.

Vaporizer Location

With an out-of-system vaporizer, the anesthetic concentration within the circuit is dependent upon anesthetic uptake. Thus, during induction when uptake is great and ventilation is increased, fresh gas inflow is diluted by the gas within the circuit, and inspired concentration is lower than that delivered by the vaporizer; as uptake diminishes, the inspired concentration rises to equal that delivered by the vaporizer. This dilution effect of uptake upon the inspired concentration is countered clinically by increasing the fresh gas flow, as well as turning the vaporizer to a higher setting. At no time, however, with the out-of-system vaporizer is the inspired

concentration greater than that delivered by the vaporizer.

In contrast, when using the in-system vaporizer, particularly with low fresh gas inflow, the inspired concentration is *greater* than that associated with the particular setting of the vaporizer. In this situation, vaporization results from passing a mixture of fresh and expired gases through the vaporizer. Since in-system vaporizers are generally rather inefficient, recirculation of expired gases through the vaporizer enables the circuit concentration to rise. Thus, during controlled respiration, it is all too easy to raise the concentration in the circuit to dangerously high levels, especially with low fresh gas inflow. The use of the in-system vaporizer is less hazardous during spontaneous ventilation because the patient's ventilation is the motive force for the recirculation in the circuit; as anesthesia deepens, anesthetic-induced respiratory depression reduces gas flow through the vaporizer, and the anesthetic concentration within the circuit decreases. Increasing the fresh gas flow decreases the inspired concentration because fresh flow merely dilutes circuit gases; at high inflow rates, the circuit behaves as if it were a nonrebreathing system, and the in-system vaporizer no longer has a concentrating effect.

OVERVIEW

The advantages of the circle system relate principally to the presence of rebreathing: there is relative constancy of inspired concentration, and containment of anesthetic gases so that there is conservation of respiratory moisture and heat, diminished operating room pollution, and less risk of fires and explosions with flammable agents. The price paid includes increased resistance to respiration, increased difficulty in cleaning, greater bulk with loss of portability, and increased opportunity for malfunction of a more complex apparatus. Moisture may collect on the valve leaflets, causing them to stick and thereby increasing respiratory resistance further. Also, as a corollary of the stability of the circle concentration, inspired concentration changes slowly unless the fresh gas inflow (or anesthetic concentration delivered to the circle) is increased. An additional problem is the inability to predict the inspired oxygen concentration when using low flows (i.e., fresh gas inflow below 1.2 L), which necessitates the use of an oxygen analyzer in the circuit.[102]

CLOSED SYSTEMS

The semiclosed system becomes a closed system when the fresh gas inflow has decreased sufficiently so that the overflow valve remains closed. At that inflow, the closed system just satisfies the patient's metabolic oxygen requirement (e.g., 4 ml/kg/min) and the uptake of anesthetic agents.

THE TO-AND-FRO SYSTEM

This system, often called the Water's canister, resembles a Mapleson C system in which a carbon dioxide absorber has been placed just distal to the fresh gas inflow. Without valves interposed between the patient and the fresh gas, this system offers little resistance to respiration. Also, like the Mapleson systems, it is simple in design, sturdy, easy to assemble and clean, and conserves respiratory moisture and heat. In fact, because of the absorber's heat generation and moisture content, this system preserves respiratory moisture and heat optimally. Unfortunately, the canister can become *so* hot that the patient can become hyperthermic.[72] More common problems, however, have resulted in its disuse: the proximity of the absorber to the patient is inconvenient due to its bulk and heat and increases the likelihood of inhalation of the caustic dust, especially during assisted or controlled ventilation. With use, the absorbent nearest the patient becomes exhausted earliest, progressively increasing the apparatus dead space and, thus, rebreathing will result. (Fig. 5-19). This dead space may be minimized by reversing or changing the absorber periodically, but this is inconvenient, especially when it becomes hot; alternatively, the inflow rate can be increased and the overflow opened, but then the advantages of the closed system (economy of gases, conservation of heat and moisture) are lost. Even when the absorber is fresh, the system is inefficient because the alveolar gas is last to leave the patient but first to be inspired. This system enjoyed popularity for use with cyclopropane and especially in cases of pulmonary infection; typically, it was used as a semiclosed system during induction to denitrogenate the patient, then the flow was decreased to the metabolic oxygen requirement (e.g., 200 to 250 ml flow rate), with the anesthetic turned off intermittently. However, with the abandonment of flammable agents and the availability of bacterial filters and disposable circle systems, this system has

A. END-EXPIRATION WITH FRESH ABSORBER

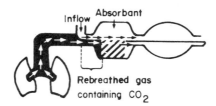

B. END-EXPIRATION WITH PARTIALLY EXHAUSTED ABSORBER

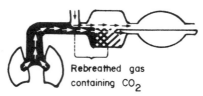

Fig. 5-19 To-and-fro breathing system before (A) and after (B) partial exhaustion of the carbon dioxide absorbent. (Redrawn from Eger EI II: Anesthetic Uptake and Action. Baltimore, Williams & Wilkins, 1974. © (1974) EI Eger II, M.D.)

been relegated to being one of theoretic interest.

THE CLOSED CIRCLE BREATHING SYSTEM

This is merely the circle system with very low flow rates (i.e., 500 to 600 ml/min). All of the advantages and disadvantages of the circle system discussed earlier apply here. The challenge imposed by the closed system is principally one of delivering a safe and appropriate inspired mixture.

Inspired Oxygen Concentration

The unpredictability of the inspired oxygen concentration when using the circle system with low flows[102] is also a problem with the closed system, especially during induction. It is at this time that the greatest variations in inspired concentrations occur, as anesthetic uptake is maximal, nitrogen is excreted into the lung in large volumes and

thereby dilutes the available oxygen,[103] and oxygen requirement is somewhat uncertain. The inspired oxygen concentration is particularly precarious when one of the gases is administered in large volumes, such as nitrous oxide, because even small changes in its uptake can have a large effect upon the concentrations of other gases in the circle, especially oxygen. Thus, the use of an oxygen analyzer in the *inspiratory* limb of the circle is mandatory during closed circle techniques to ensure that the patient is not receiving an hypoxic mixture.

Anesthetic Administration

The problem posed by the closed system upon the administration of the other gases, namely the anesthetics, is quite different. We need not know precisely *how much* we are administering because we monitor clinical signs of anesthesia and patients vary in their dose requirement, but rather the problem is *how* to administer the inhaled anesthetic agent safely. Clearly, one option is to induce anesthesia with the circle used as a semiclosed system with high flow (i.e., greater than 3 L/min) and to "close" the system after the patient is denitrogenated, perhaps 15 minutes later.[104] Thereafter, metabolic oxygen (e.g., 4 ml/kg/min) is supplied with sufficient nitrous oxide to result in a desired oxygen concentration on the oxygen analyzer; potent inhaled agent is added, as needed, from a bubble-through type of vaporizer. The alternative approach is a closed system from the very beginning of induction, with the administration of the potent agent based upon uptake models.[105, 106] In addition to monitoring the oxygen concentration, one must observe the fullness of the reservoir bag or an upward-travelling ventilator bellows to detect a leak in the system.

OVERVIEW

Beyond the advantages of the semiclosed circle system already cited, the closed circle system would appear to add improved humidification, less pollution, and economy in the use of anesthetics. The closed systems, particularly the to-and-fro system, conserve respiratory moisture better than any other. There is less pollution, but the need for a program to control waste anesthetics is not obviated; instead, the closed system is but one part of such a program (see next section). Closed system techniques also conserve anesthetics and, thus, save money, although the agents are not so expensive that this should be a primary reason for its choice.

CONTROLLING EXPOSURE TO WASTE ANESTHETIC GASES

THE PROBLEM

As early as 1920 "ether poisoning," characterized by gastrointestinal and central nervous system symptoms, occurred among those exposed to ether vapor while making gunpowder during World War I.[107] Anecdotal reports during the subsequent decades noted that personnel in poorly ventilated operating rooms experienced headaches, depression, anorexia, excessive fatigue, and memory loss, all of which disappeared with absence from the operating room or the installation of improved room ventilation. Since 1967, however, there has been a rapidly growing concern that chronic exposure to low levels of anesthetic gases constitutes a health hazard to operating room personnel.[108] The health hazard has been alleged to include an increased incidence of spontaneous abortion, congenital abnormalities, hepatic and renal diseases, and cancer, as well as changes in mood and intellectual function (see Ch. 14).

The validity of these allegations is uncertain due to methodologic flaws in the design of many of the surveys.[109-111] Given the problems inherent in studying such health problems, it is doubtful whether the existence of occupational hazards associated with chronic exposure to low levels of anesthetic gases can ever be proved, at least in the foreseeable future. Yet, even in the absence of unassailable proof, control of excess anesthetic gases ought to be undertaken because these gases do have offensive odors, there are sufficient similarities in the results of the surveys and laboratory studies to encourage a conservative approach, and, finally, many persons are at risk—approximately 70,000 in operating rooms, 100,000 in dental operatories, and 50,000 in veterinary settings.[112] Furthermore, in the future, regulatory agencies are likely to require control measures.[113] In particular, the general duty clause of the Occupational Safety and Health Act of 1970 mandates the Secretary of Labor to require each employer to maintain a workplace free from hazards. Even though the Occupational Safety and Health Administration (OSHA) is still reviewing recommended standards for control and other aspects of waste anesthetic gases,[112] OSHA personnel have already begun citing hospitals and anesthesiologists for alleged violations of the general duty clause.

QUANTITATING WASTE ANESTHETIC CONCENTRATION

Low concentrations of a gas are expressed on a volume/volume basis as parts per million (ppm). Thus, a sample composed of 100 percent of a gas is said to contain 1,000,000 ppm, and one containing 1 percent contains 10,000 ppm.

ANALYTIC METHODS AND SAMPLING APPROACHES

A variety of analytic methods can be used to determine concentrations of anesthetic gases, including manometry (e.g., Van Slyke), combustion, gas chromatography, and infrared spectrophotometry.[112] Gas chromatography and infrared analysis are most commonly used.

There are two general approaches to gas sampling, the simplest of which is the instantaneous, or "grab," sample. Using a gas syringe or other leak-free container, a single sample is obtained, and this can be repeated later during anesthesia to assess adequacy of excess gas control measures or after some intervention such as changing the room ventilation rate. A time-weighted sample is more representative of the average concentration to which personnel are exposed because it is obtained by pumping ambient air continuously into an inert bag at a constant, low flow rate.

TYPICAL AMBIENT CONCENTRATIONS

In the absence of specific control measures, the average concentrations of nitrous oxide in the operating room have been 130 to 6,800 ppm, and those of halothane, from 1 to 85 ppm; nitrous oxide concentrations in dental operatories are generally considerably higher.[112] The higher values were obtained in the breathing zone of the anesthesiologist when nonrebreathing or high-flow circle systems in poorly ventilated rooms were used. With control measures, nitrous oxide concentrations below 180 ppm[112, 114] and halothane below 2 ppm[112] can be achieved. Unfortunately, the proposed National Institute of Occupational Safety and Health (NIOSH) standards require nitrous oxide concentrations to be less than 25 ppm and halogenated agents used simultaneously to be less than 0.5 ppm (2 ppm when halogenated agents are used alone). It is doubtful that levels so low can be achieved consistently in the clinical setting.

SOURCES OF WASTE ANESTHETIC GASES

HIGH PRESSURE SYSTEM LEAKAGE

The high pressure system extends from the nitrous oxide sources—the tanks (5,180 kN/m or 750 lb/in) attached to the anesthesia machine and the central gas system (345 kN/m or 50 lb/in^2)—to the flow meters of the anesthesia machine. Even when *no* anesthesia is being administered, leakage from any portion of this system can give rise to background nitrous oxide concentrations substantially above the NIOSH standard of 25 ppm. Moreover, a recirculating room ventilation system can spread the pollution throughout the operating suite. Particularly likely leakage sites are the quick coupler (e.g., Shrader) at the delivery end of the flexible hose of the central nitrous oxide system and the tank yokes on the anesthesia machine.

LOW PRESSURE SYSTEM LEAKAGE

The low pressure system extends from the flow meters to the patient. Leakage can be so great that an otherwise effective control program is negated. Although myriad leakage sites exist (Table 5-7), one of the most com-

Table 5-7. Common Sites of Gas Leakage from the Low Pressure System

Gas delivery outlet at anesthesia machine
Gas delivery tubing from anesthesia machine
One-way valve domes
Carbon dioxide canister gasket seal
Carbon dioxide canister bypass tubing
Carbon dioxide canister drain cock
Breathing system tubing
Y connector joints

mon ones is the gasket seal of the carbon dioxide canister. The gasket may become worn and cracked, or granules of soda lime may prevent a tight seal.

ANESTHETIC TECHNIQUE

By definition, open-drop and insufflation techniques constitute unopposed spillage of large volumes of anesthetic into the operating room and thereby rapidly lead to concentrations considerably in excess of the NIOSH standards. At the other extreme is the closed system technique which, once established, should prevent clinically significant anesthetic spillage. For example, one study found the nitrous oxide concentration in the anesthesiologist's breathing zone to be below 31 ppm with a closed system nitrous oxide flow rate of 500 ml/min, and even less pollution with lower flows; the institution of a control program, including the removal of excess breathing system gases (scavenging), resulted in concentrations below 8 ppm.[115] Other anesthetic techniques result in levels of pollution between these extremes.[112]

CONTROL MEASURES

An effective program for the control of excess anesthetic gases requires the elimination of leakage from anesthetic equipment, alteration of anesthetic technique, and use of equipment to collect and remove excess breathing system gases (scavenging).[112,116] Such a program should not detract from pa-

tient care, which should continue to be the anesthesiologist's principal concern.

IMPROVED MACHINE MAINTENANCE

Four times a year, anesthesia machines should be serviced by factory-trained personnel, with particular attention focused upon correcting leakage in both the high and low pressure systems. Leakage, however, can develop between service visits and can even continue despite periodic servicing. Hence, those who use this equipment must be familiar with the rudiments of testing for leakage.

Leakage in the high pressure system requires disconnecting the anesthesia machine from the central gas supply, closing the flow meter valves, and opening a tank of nitrous oxide, closing that tank, and noting the pressure. If more than a minimal decrease in pressure occurs within an hour and the leakage site is not found to be the tank yoke or quick coupler (see below), the leak is within the machine and the service representative should be called.

Unlike leakage testing of the high pressure system, testing the low pressure system requires the flow of anesthetic gas. The presence and amount of leakage in the commonly used semiclosed circle system can be determined by closing the overflow (relief, or "popoff") valve, occluding the Y-piece at the patient end of the system, and noting the oxygen inflow required to maintain a pressure of 30 cm H_2O. Since leakage varies linearly with pressure and pressure in the breathing system during controlled ventilation averages about 10 cm H_2O, a 150 ml/min leakage rate at 30 cm H_2O represents leakage of about 50 ml/min during controlled ventilation. Although leakage of this magnitude contributes less than 5 ppm to the average operating room, greater leakage requires correction. Monitoring for specific leakage sites can be as simple as applying a 20 percent soap solution in water to components (e.g., gaskets of the carbon dioxide absorber) of and connections (e.g., quick couplers in the central nitrous oxide supply hose) in the high and low pressure systems and observing for bubbles. Correction of leakage often involves such simple maneuvers as replacing a torn canister gasket or removing a deformed washer on a tank yoke.

SCAVENGING

In an otherwise leak-free breathing system, the only site of spillage of anesthetic gases is the overflow valve, through which excess gases normally exit. *Scavenging* is the term applied to the collection and removal of this effluent. A system that accomplishes this has a gas-capturing assembly, a disposal route, and, between them, an interface.

The Gas-Capturing Assembly

The gas-capturing assembly collects gases from the breathing system—broadly defined to include the ventilator and extracorporeal pump oxygenator—and conducts the potential pollutant to the disposal route. Because effluent volumes vary greatly, especially when a ventilator is used, particular attention must be directed to matching a scavenging system of sufficient capacity (e.g., in L/min flow) to the given breathing system. An interface prevents pressure variations in the breathing system, which might otherwise affect system dynamics or delivered gas concentrations, consequent to scavenging. Although gas-capturing assemblies are readily available for the overflow valves of the breathing system and the ventilator, those for pump oxygenators are in the developmental stage.[117-119]

The Disposal System

Once collected, the waste gases can be directed into the exhaust grille of a *non*recirculating room ventilation system. Air flow into the exhaust grille is sufficient to entrain the waste gases. Because a nonrecirculating system is relatively expensive to operate, especially in very warm or cold climates, a recirculating system is encountered more frequently. If the waste gases do not enter this system distal to the recirculation point, all operating rooms ventilated from a common manifold will be polluted. An alternate disposal route is the central vacuum system; however, National Fire Protection Association regulations prohibit disposal of flammable anesthetic agents into such a system. Another alternate disposal system is an independent ("dedicated") vacuum system that is vented so that personnel exposure is avoided. Before any vacuum system is used, the hospital engineer should verify that the system has sufficient capacity and is resistant to corrosive materials. Waste gases can also be directed passively through the wall of the operating room. Finally, activated charcoal adsorbers can remove halogenated anesthetic agents but are relatively expensive, have a short life span, and do not adsorb nitrous oxide.

The Interface

Scavenging risks establishing marked pressure differences between the breathing system and the waste gas disposal system. Attaching any of the vacuum systems directly to the overflow valve of the breathing system threatens removal of substantial gas volumes from the breathing system, unless the fresh gas inflow is greater than the suction rate. The hazard of an excessive rate of suction commonly manifests itself by collapse of the breathing bag and consequent inability to ventilate the patient. On the other hand, if the disposal route becomes occluded (e.g., stepping on the tubing), the gases that normally exit via the overflow valve are effectively contained within the breathing system, and the pressure rises within the system, impeding pulmonary ventilation and eventually leading to pulmonary barotrauma. The interface is a pressure-balancing device that thereby prevents the development of negative and positive pressure in the breathing system. Although designs vary, the typical interface consists of two components: a reservoir contains the waste gases that collect, often intermittently, when outflow from the overflow valve exceeds the disposal rate; a unidirectional valve with a negative pressure relief mechanism at the overflow valve permits gases to leave the breathing system passively when a threshold pressure (e.g., 5 torr) is reached, but prevents gas flow into or active removal (i.e., suction) of gas from the breathing system. The negative pressure relief mechanism in the latter can be as simple as several holes that permit the disposal system to communicate with the atmosphere; thus, room air is entrained, protecting the breathing system (and the patient's lungs) from the negative pressure. The holes also allow the escape of waste gases into the room should the disposal route be occluded. Thoughtful design nonwithstanding, pressure differentials can still be established as a result of malfunction, with potential harm to the patient.[120-125] The addition of a second negative pressure relief mechanism, perhaps having a dissimilar design, has been suggested as a possible remedy.[126]

ALTERATION OF ANESTHETIC TECHNIQUE

Altering anesthetic technique and general work habits is also an important aspect of an effective control program. Poor fit of the face mask, as well as allowing anesthetic gases to flow prior to application of the mask and during tracheal intubation and suctioning, can result in the spillage of substantial amounts of gases into the room. Administering 100 percent oxygen for as long as practical at the end of an anesthetic can also diminish gas spillage because this washes out the breathing system and the patient's lungs. The use of low flow or closed system techniques can also diminish the level of waste gas con-

tamination in the operating room; however, scavenging is not obviated. Particular care should be taken when filling vaporizers, since each ml of anesthetic liquid vaporizes to approximately 200 ml of gas (e.g., 212 ml for halothane, 184 ml for enflurane and isoflurane) at room temperature. If halothane spillage is detectable by smell, the level of contamination is likely to be at least 33 ppm.[127] Assuming even gas mixing, spilling just *1 ml* of liquid halothane in a box 6 m on a side and 3 m tall, approximately the dimensions of an operating room, results in a concentration of 2 ppm, *four times* the upper NIOSH limit for a halogenated agent used with nitrous oxide!

EFFICIENT ROOM VENTILATION

A nonrecirculating ventilation system offers the advantage of providing a simple disposal route for scavenging but requires that all of the air must be heated or cooled, which is costly in cold or warm climates. While having a lower operating cost, the recirculating system can unfortunately redistribute excess anesthetic gases throughout the operating suite, to all rooms served by the same ventilation system. Redistribution, however, tends to lower the excess gas concentrations that might otherwise exist in a room in which anesthesia is being administered. In each room periodically the efficiency of ventilation (in terms of room air turnovers per hour) should be determined and ventilation filters should be checked for debris by the hospital engineer to ensure that the rooms are ventilated evenly.

ENVIRONMENTAL MONITORING

Several times a year excess anesthetic concentrations should be determined in each operating room after it has been out of service for at least 8 hours, using either an instantaneous ("grab") sample or infrared analysis. Another sample should be obtained in the breathing zone of the anesthesiologist 30 minutes after induction of anesthesia. There is no firm basis at this time for considering particular concentrations "dangerous" or "toxic." Particularly high concentrations (e.g., nitrous oxide in excess of 180 ppm), however, should alert personnel to search for leaks and consider modifications in the anesthetic technique and work habits.

PERSONNEL INVOLVEMENT

An otherwise excellent control program cannot be effective in reducing the concentrations of excess anesthetic gases without the active participation of all personnel in the anesthesia department. Results of the quarterly environmental monitoring can serve as the focus for reminding personnel of the need to check equipment for leaks and modifying techniques and habits to minimize contaminant levels. In addition, periodically *all* operating room personnel ought to be informed of the status of knowledge regarding the possible hazards resulting from chronic exposure to anesthetics.[128]

REFERENCES

1. Thomas KB: The Development of Anaesthetic Apparatus. Oxford, Blackwell, 1975
2. Macintosh R, Mushim WW, Epstein HG: Physics for the Anaesthetist. 3rd edition. Oxford, Blackwell, 1963
3. Hill DW: Physics Applied to Anaesthesia. 4th edition. London, Butterworths, 1980
4. Dorsch JA, Dorsch SE: Understanding Anesthetic Equipment: Construction, Care and Complications. Baltimore, Williams & Wilkins, 1975
5. Schreiber P: Anaesthetic Equipment: Performance, Classification and Safety. Berlin, Springer-Verlag, 1972
6. Wyant GM: Mechanical Misadventures in Anaesthesia. Toronto, University of Toronto Press, 1978
7. Phillips O: Historical perspective and results of early studies, Health Care Delivery in Anesthesia. Edited by Hirsh RA, Forrest WH Jr, Orkin FK, et al. Philadelphia, George F. Stickley, 1980, p 5
8. Edwards G, Morton HJV, Pask EA, et al: Deaths associated with anaesthesia: Report on 1000 cases. Anaesthesia 11:194, 1956
9. Dripps RD, Lamont A, Eckenhoff JE: The role of anesthesia in surgical mortality. JAMA 178:261, 1961
10. Clifton BS, Hotten WIT: Deaths associated with anaesthesia. Br J Anaesth 35:250, 1963
11. Marx GF, Mateo CV, Orkin LR: Computer analysis of postanesthetic deaths. Anesthesiology 39:54, 1973
12. Wylie WD: There, but for the grace of God . . . Ann Roy Coll Surg 56:171, 1975
13. Utting JE, Gray TC, Shelley FC: Human misadventure in anaesthesia. Can Anaesth Soc J 26:472, 1979
14. Cooper JB, Newbower RD, Long CD, et al: Preventable anesthesia mishaps: A study of human factors. Anesthesiology 49:399, 1978
15. Taylor G, Larson CP, Prestwich R: Unexpected cardiac arrest during anesthesia and surgery. JAMA 236:2758, 1976
16. Gaensler EA, Maloney JV, Bjork VO: Bronchospirometry. II. Experimental observations and theoretical considerations of resistance breathing. J Lab Clin Med 39:935, 1952
17. Orkin LR, Siegel M, Rovenstine EA: Resistance to breathing by apparatus used in anesthesia. Anesth Analg 33:217, 1954
18. Proctor DF: Studies of respiratory air flow. IV. Resistance to air flow through anesthesia apparatus. Bull Johns Hopkins Hosp 96:49, 1955
19. Hinforomi BK: The resistance of air flow of tracheostomy tubes, connections and heat and moisture exchangers. Br J Anaesth 37:454, 1965
20. Brown ES, Hustead RF: Resistance of pediatric breathing systems. Anesth Analg 48:842, 1969
21. Sullivan M, Paliotta J, Saklad M: The endotracheal tube as a factor in the measurement of respiratory mechanics. J Appl Physiol 41:590, 1976
22. Conway CM: Anaesthetic circuits, Scientific Foundations of Anaesthesia. 2nd edition. Edited by Scurr C, Feldman S. London, William Heinemann, 1974, p 509
23. Smith WDA: The effects of external resis-

tance to respiration. Part I. General review. Br J Anaesth 33:549, 1961

24. Smith WDA: The effects of external resistance to respiration. Part II. Resistance to respiration due to anaesthetic apparatus. Br J Anaesth 33:610, 1961

25. Graff TD, Sewall K, Lim HS, et al: The ventilatory response of infants to airway resistance. Anesthesiology 27:168, 1966

26. Nunn JF, Ezi–Ashi TI: The respiratory effects of resistance to breathing in anesthetized man. Anesthesiology 22:174, 1961

27. Duncan PG: Efficacy of helium-oxygen mixtures in the management of severe viral and post-intubation croup. Can Anaesth Soc J 26:206, 1979

28. Sykes MK: Rebreathing circuits: A review. Br J Anaesth 40:666, 1968

29. Wilson RE: Soda lime as absorbent for industrial purposes. Ind Eng Chem 12:1000, 1920

30. Adriani J, Rovenstine EA: Experimental studies on carbon dioxide absorption for anesthesia. Anesthesiology 2:1, 1941

31. Adriani J: Disposal of carbon dioxide from devices used for inhalation anesthesia. Anesthesiology 21:742, 1960

32. Brown ES, Bakamjian V, Seniff AM: Performance of absorbents: Effects of moisture. Anesthesiology 20:613, 1959

33. Grodin WK, Epstein RA: Halothane adsorption by soda lime. Anesthesiology (suppl) 51:S317, 1979

34. Adriani J: Soda lime containing indicators. Anesthesiology 5:45, 1944

35. Ten Pas RH, Brown ES, Elam JO: Carbon dioxide absorption. Anesthesiology 29:231, 1958

36. Brown ES: Performance of absorbents: Continuous flow. Anesthesiology 20:41, 1959

37. Kelley JM: Cranial nerve injury following trichloroethylene, Complications in Anesthesiology. Edited by Cooperman LH, Orkin FK. Philadelphia, JB Lippincott, 1981, Chapter 22 (in press)

38. Case history No. 39: Accidental use of trichloroethylene (Trilene, Trimar) in a closed system. Anesth Analg 43:740, 1964

39. Debban DG, Bedford RF: Overdistention of the rebreathing bag, a hazardous test for circle-system integrity. Anesthesiology 42:365, 1975

40. Lauria JI: Soda-lime dust contamination of breathing circuits. Anesthesiology 42:628, 1975

41. Adriani J, Batten DH: The efficiency of mixtures of barium and calcium hydroxides in the absorption of CO_2 in rebreathing appliances. Anesthesiology 3:1, 1942

42. Adriani J: Rebreathing in anesthesia. South Med J 35:798, 1942

43. Rogers RC, Hill GE: Equations for vapour pressure versus temperature: Derivation and usage of the Antoine equation on a hand-held programmable calculator. Br J Anaesth 50:415, 1978

44. Munson WM: Cardiac arrest: Hazard of tipping a vaporizer. Anesthesiology 26:235, 1965

45. Mark LC, Marx GF, Erlanger H, et al: Improper filling of kettle-type vaporizers. N Y State J Med 65:1151, 1965

46. Kopriva LJ, Lowenstein E: An anesthetic accident: Cardiovascular collapse from liquid halothane delivery. Anesthesiology 30:246, 1969

47. Keasling HH, Pittinger CB: Fluotec performance. Anesthesiology 29:682, 1958

48. Munson ES: Hazards of agent-specific vaporizers. Anesthesiology 34:393, 1971

49. Epstein HG, Macintosh R: An anaesthetic inhaler with automatic thermo-compensation. Anaesthesia 11:83, 1956

50. Morris LE: A new vaporizer for liquid anesthetic agents. Anesthesiology 13:587, 1952

51. Farmati O, Quinn JR, Fennell RM: Exfoliative cytology of the intubated larynx in children. Can Anaesth Soc J 14:321, 1967

52. Chalon J, Loew DAY, Malebranche J: Effect of dry anesthetic gases on tracheobronchial ciliated epithelium. Anesthesiology 37:338, 1972

53. Rashad KF, Wilson K, Hurt HH Jr, et al: Effect of humidification of anesthetic gases on static compliance. Anesth Analg 46:127, 1967

54. Knudsen J, Lomholt N, Wisborg K: Postoperative pulmonary complications using dry and humidified anaesthetic gases. Br J Anaesth 45:636, 1973

55. Radford EP: Ventilation standards for use in artificial respiration. J Appl Physiol 7:451, 1955

56. Nunn JF: Prediction of carbon dioxide tension during anaesthesia. Anaesthesia 15:123, 1960

57. Nunn JF: Predictors for oxygen and carbon dioxide levels during anaesthesia. Anaesthesia 17:182, 1962

58. Dery R: Water balance of the respiratory tract during ventilation with a gas mixture saturated at body temperature. Can Anaesth Soc J 20:719, 1973

59. Tausk HC, Miller I, Roberts RB: Maintenance of body temperature by heated humidification. Anesth Analg 55:719, 1976

60. Chalon J, Patel C, Ramanathan S, et al: Humidification of the circle absorber system. Anesthesiology 48:142, 1978

61. Chase HF, Trotta R, Kilmore MA: Simple methods for humidifying non-rebreathing anesthesia gas systems. Anesth Analg 41:249, 1962

62. Chalon J, Ramanathan S: Water vaporizer heated by the reaction of neutralization by carbon dioxide. Anesthesiology 41:400, 1974

63. Chalon J, Simon R, Patel C, et al: An infant circuit with a water vaporizer warmed by carbon dioxide neutralization. Anesth Analg 57:307, 1978

64. Mapleson WW, Morgan JG, Hilard EK: Assessment of condenser-humidifiers with special reference to a multiple-gauze model. Br Med J 1:300, 1963

65. Joseph JM: Disease transmission by insufficiently sanitized anesthesiology apparatus. JAMA 149:1196, 1952

66. Stark DCC, Green CA, Pask EA: Anaesthetic machines and cross-infection. Anaesthesia 17:12, 1962

67. Philips I, Spencer G: Pseudomonas aeruginosa cross-infection due to contaminated respiratory apparatus. Lancet 2:1325, 1965

68. Pundit SK, Mehta S, Agarwal SC: Risk of cross-infection from inhalation anaesthesia. Br J Anaesth 39:839, 1967

69. Grieble HG, Colton FR, Bird TJ, et al: Fine-particle humidifiers: Source of *Pseudomonas aeruginosa* infections in a respiratory-disease unit. N Engl J Med 282:531, 1970

70. Avery ME, Galina M, Nachman R: Mist therapy. Pediatrics 39:160, 1967

71. Cheney FW, Butler J: The effects of ultrasonically produced aerosols on airway resistance in man. Anesthesiology 29:1099, 1968

72. Clark RE, Orkin LR, Rovenstine EA: Body temperature studies in anesthetized man: Effect of environmental temperature, humidity, and anesthesia system. JAMA 154:311, 1954

73. Moyers J: A nomenclature for methods of inhalation anesthesia. Anesthesiology 14:609, 1953

74. Dorsch JA, Dorsch SE: Understanding Anesthesia Equipment: Construction, Care and Complications. Baltimore, Williams & Wilkins Company, 1975, pp 151–155

75. Hamilton WK: Nomenclature of inhalation anesthetic systems. Anesthesiology 25:3, 1964

76. Munson ES, Farnham M, Hamilton WK: Studies of respiratory gas flows. A comparison using different anesthetic agents. Anesthesiology 24:61, 1963

77. Sykes MK: Non-rebreathing valves. Br J Anaesth 31:450, 1959

78. Orkin LR, Siegal M, Rovenstine EA: Resistance to breathing by apparatus used in anesthesia. II. Valves and machines. Anesth Analg 36:19, 1957

79. Mapleson WW: The elimination of rebreathing in various semiclosed anaesthetic systems. Br J Anaesth 26:323, 1954

80. Kain ML, Nunn JF: Fresh gas economies of the Magill circuit. Anesthesiology 29:964, 1968

81. Norman J, Adams AP, Sykes MK: Rebreathing with the Magill attachment. Anaesthesia 23:75, 1968

82. Sykes MK: Rebreathing during controlled respiration with the Magill attachment. Anaesthesia 31:247, 1959

83. Bain JA, Spoerel WE: A streamlined anaesthetic system. Can Anaesth Soc J 19:426, 1972

84. Weeks DB: Provision of endogenous and exogenous humidity for the Bain breathing circuit. Can Anaesth Soc J 23:185, 1976

85. Bain JA, Spoerel WE: Flow requirements for a modified Mapleson D system during controlled ventilation. Can Anaesth Soc J 20:629, 1973

86. Henville JD, Adams AP: The Bain anaesthetic system: An assessment during controlled ventilation. Anaesthesia 31:247, 1976

87. Ungerer MJ: A comparison between the Bain and Magill anaesthetic systems during spontaneous breathing. Can Anaesth Soc J 25:122, 1978

88. Rose DK, Byrick RJ, Froese AB: Carbon

dioxide elimination during spontaneous ventilation with a modified Mapleson D system: Studies in a lung model. Can Anaesth Soc J 25:353, 1978

89. Chu YK, Rah KH, Boyan CP: Is the Bain circuit the future anesthesia system? An evaluation. Anesth Analg 56:84, 1977

90. Hannallah R, Rosales JK: A hazard connected with re-use of the Bain's circuit: A case report. Can Anaesth Soc J 21:511, 1974

91. Paterson JG, Vanhooydonk V: A hazard associated with improper connection of the Bain breathing circuit. Can Anaesth Soc J 22:373, 1975

92. Mansell WH: Bain circuit: "The Hazard of the Hidden Tube." Can Anaesth Soc J 23:227, 1976

93. Mansell WH: Spontaneous breathing with the Bain circuit at low flow rates: A case report. Can Anaesth Soc J 23:432, 1976

94. Ayre P: Anaesthesia for intracranial operation: New technique. Lancet 1:561, 1937

95. Ayre P: Endotracheal anesthesia for babies, with special reference to hare-lip and cleft-palate operations. Anesth Analg 16:331, 1937

96. Ayre P: The T-piece technique. Br J Anaesth 28:520, 1956

97. Jackson-Rees G: Anaesthesia in the newborn. Br Med J 2:1419, 1950

98. Waters DJ, Mapleson WW: Rebreathing during controlled respiration with various semiclosed anaesthetic systems. Br J Anaesth 33:374, 1961

99. Eger EI II: Anesthetic systems: Construction and function, Anesthetic Uptake and Action. Baltimore, Williams & Wilkins Company, 1974, pp 206–227

100. Brown ES, Seniff AM, Elam JO: Carbon dioxide elimination in semiclosed systems. Anesthesiology 25:31, 1964

101. Eger EI II, Ethans CT: The effects of inflow, overflow and valve placement of economy of the circle system. Anesthesiology 29:93, 1968

102. Smith TC: Nitrous oxide and low inflow circle systems. Anesthesiology 27:266, 1966

103. Hamilton WK, Eastwood DW: A study of denitrogenation with some inhalation anesthetic systems. Anesthesiology 16:864, 1955

104. Gorsky BH, Hall RL, Redford JE: A compromise for closed system anesthesia. Anesth Analg 57:18, 1978

105. Mapleson WW: The rate of uptake of halo

thane vapour in man. Br J Anaesth 34:11, 1962

106. Lowe HJ: The anesthetic continuum, Low Flow and Closed System Anesthesia. Edited by Aldrete JA, Lowe HJ, Virtue RW. New York, Grune & Stratton, 1979, pp 11–37

107. Hamilton A, Minot GR: Ether poisoning in the manufacture of smokeless powder. J Indust Hyg 2:41, 1920

108. Cohen EN (editor): Anesthetic Exposure in the Workplace. Littleton, MA, PSG Publishing Company, 1980

109. Vessey MP: Epidemiological studies of the occupational hazards of anaesthesia—a review. Anaesthesia 33:430, 1978

110. Cohen EN: Inhalation anesthetics may cause genetic defects, abortions, and miscarriages in operating room personnel, Controversy in Anesthesiology. Edited by Eckenhoff JE. Philadelphia, WB Saunders, 1980, pp 47–57

111. Ferstandig LL: Trace concentrations of anesthetics are not proved health hazards, Controversy in Anesthesiology. Edited by Eckenhoff JE. Philadelphia, WB Saunders, 1980, pp 60–69

112. National Institute for Occupational Safety and Health: Criteria for a Recommended Standard—Occupational Exposure to Waste Anesthetic Gases and Vapors. DHEW Pub No. (NIOSH) 77–140. Cleveland, National Institute for Occupational Safety and Health, US Department of Health, Education, and Welfare, 1977

113. Mazze RI: Waste anesthetic gases and the regulatory agencies. Anesthesiology 52:248, 1980

114. Whitcher C: Occupational exposure, education and sampling methods. Anesthesiology (suppl) 51:S336, 1979

115. Virtue RW, Escobar A, Modell J: Nitrous oxide levels in operating room air with various gas flows. Can Anaesth Soc J 26:313, 1979

116. Lecky JH: The mechanical aspects of anesthetic pollution control. Anesth Analg 56:769, 1977

117. Miller JD: A device for the removal of waste anesthetic gases from the extracorporeal oxygenator. Anesthesiolopgy 44:181, 1976

118. Annis JP, Carlson DA, Simmons DH: Scavenging system for the Harvey blood oxygenator. Anesthesiology 45:359, 1976

119. Muravchick S: Scavenging enflurane from extracorporeal pump oxygenators. Anesthesiology 47:468, 1977

120. Sharrock NE, Leith DE: Potential pulmonary barotrauma when venting anesthetic gases to suction. Anesthesiology 46:152, 1977

121. Mor ZF, Stein ED, Orkin LR: A possible hazard in the use of a scavenging system. Anesthesiology 47:302, 1977

122. Hagerdal M, Lecky JH: Anesthetic death of an experimental animal related to a scavenging system malfunction. Anesthesiology 47:522, 1977

123. Tavakoli M, Habeeb A: Two hazards of gas scavenging. Anesth Analg 57:286, 1978

124. Sharrock NE, Gabel RA: Inadvertent anesthetic overdose obscured by scavenging. Anesthesiology 49:137, 1978

125. Patel KD, Dalal FY: A potential hazard of the Drager scavenging interface system for wall suction. Anesth Analg 58:327, 1979

126. Milliken RA: Hazards of scavenging systems. Anesth Analg 59:162, 1980

127. Flemming DC, Johnstone RE: Recognition thresholds for diethyl ether and halothane. Anesthesiology 46:68, 1977

128. Lecky JH: Anesthetic pollution in the operating room: A notice to operating room personnel. Anesthesiology 52:157, 1980

Further Reading

Dorsch JA, Dorsch SE: Understanding Anesthetic Equipment: Construction, Care and Complications. Baltimore, Williams & Wilkins, 1975.

6

Monitoring

Carl C. Hug, Jr., M.D., Ph.D.

INTRODUCTION

A definition of the verb *to monitor* is, "to watch, observe, or check, especially for a special purpose," and a definition of the noun *monitor* is, "that which warns or instructs." There are several important implications of both definitions: (1) a person is involved in establishing the process and in responding to its results; (2) mere data collection alone is insufficient, since rules and logic must accompany data in order for it to warn; (3) a special purpose exists, that is, monitoring is focused on a specific objective and goes beyond the generalized, noncritical collection of data. It fits with the adage, "you see what you look for."

In the practice of anesthesiology we have a special concern about monitoring. Ideally anesthesia is a totally reversible process. The patient's primary objective is to have an examination or surgery, not to have anesthesia for its own sake. This by no means diminishes the importance of the anesthesiologist; rather his importance is all the greater because of the nature of anesthetics. Not only are they potent drugs with great potential for producing toxicity, but the anesthesiologist is more and more frequently called upon to administer them to critically ill patients with little capacity to tolerate any kind of stress. Beyond providing anesthesia, the anesthesiologist is responsible for the support of life itself during the procedure. It is no wonder then, that the anesthesiologist is the *monitor* of drug effects and of vital functions intraoperatively and beyond, at least until the effects of anesthetic drugs and procedures are fully reversed. Although he uses monitoring devices to accomplish his objectives, the anesthesiologist is the *monitor*.

Because the modern anesthesiologist is faced with challenges by potent drugs and by severe disease, a more sophisticated and precise evaluation of the status of the patient and of his responses to anesthetic drugs and surgery is required now than in the past. Monitoring devices have become correspondingly more complex and expensive in terms of money and, in some cases, in terms of risk to the patient. The anesthesiologist must, therefore, use carefully considered judgment in deciding which monitoring techniques to be used in each patient.

Monitoring of patients during anesthesia and surgery has three important objectives: diagnosis of a problem or recognition of a deleterious trend; estimation of the severity of the situation; and evaluation of the response to therapy, including both its effectiveness and side effects or toxicity. Monitoring can be performed at several levels.

Routine monitoring—applicable to all patients regardless of their pathophysiologic status.

Specialized monitoring for a particular

pathologic problem (e.g., serum glucose determinations in the diabetic patient) or for the use of a specialized technique (e.g., controlled hypotension).

Extensive monitoring of all major systems in the critically ill patient and in those undergoing extensive surgery potentially affecting all organ and tissue functions (e.g., cardiac surgery with cardiopulmonary bypass).

SCOPE OF THE CHAPTER

This chapter surveys monitoring techniques that are or potentially will become useful in the anesthetic management of adult patients undergoing surgery. Emphasis is placed on monitoring of the central nervous system, ventilation, hemodynamics, and body temperature because these are important in every case. The reader is referred to other chapters for discussions of the monitoring of blood volume (Chs. 27 and 28), coagulation (Ch. 28), hepatic and renal function (Ch. 24), and neuromuscular transmission (Ch. 17); and since monitoring techniques have become specialized just as the practice of anesthesiology has, the reader should consult the chapters dealing with pediatric (Ch. 36) and obstetric (Ch. 34) patients and with anesthesia for neurologic (Ch. 33) and cardiac (Ch. 30) surgery.

A number of reviews on the subject of monitoring surgical patients in the operating room and intensive care unit have been published in recent years.[1-4] They clearly indicate the potential for new developments in the monitoring of patients by anesthesiologists.

ROUTINE MONITORING

Basic monitoring of the patient under anesthesia is an extension of the basic elements of physical diagnosis including inspection, palpation, percussion, and auscultation (Table 6-1). Some of the individual

Table 6-1. Physical Diagnosis in Monitoring of Anesthetized Patients

Inspection
 Skin—color, capillary refill, rash, edema, hematoma
 Nail beds—color, capillary refill
 Mucous membrane—color, moisture, edema
 Surgical field—color of tissues and blood, rate of blood loss, muscular relaxation
 Blood loss—surgical drapes, gowns, sponges, suction bottles
 Position—potential for trauma (joints, nerves, circulation)
 Movement—purposeful or reflex (nonparalyzed patient), ventilation
 Eyes—conjunctive (color, edema), pupils (size, direct and consensual reactivity, change with stimulation)

Palpation
 Skin—temperature, texture (e.g., papular rash), edema, hematoma, subcutaneous emphysema (crepitation)
 Pulses—fullness, rate and rhythm
 Muscle tone

Percussion
 Urinary bladder distention—urine
 Gastric distention—air
 Pneumothorax

Auscultation
 Ventilation—breath sounds (normal, pathologic, absent; distribution over lung fields)
 Heart sounds—rate, rhythm, extrasounds, murmurs
 Blood pressure—sphygmomanometry
 Location of nasogastric tube

items provide information about the function of several organ systems. For example, normal skin color is indicative of normal circulation, ventilation, and body temperature. If the skin is pale, abnormalities can exist in one or more organ systems and further investigation is necessary to diagnose the cause or causes.

This level of monitoring may seem simple and obvious, and its value may be overlooked in this highly technical age to the detriment of the patient. The value of physical diagnosis lies in its use to corroborate data, especially that which is unexpected, from monitoring devices; as a back-up measure when the devices fail; and to extend the usefulness of some monitoring devices. For example: (1) a sphygmomanometer can be used in conjunction with direct arterial blood pressure monitoring to verify the accuracy of systolic pressure measurements by the transducer system; (2) palpation of a full and regular pulse indicates the fibrillation-like pattern in the electrocardiogram is artifact; and (3) the use of an esophageal stethoscope in combination with central venous pressure (CVP) monitoring allows more reliable adjustment of fluid and blood replacement; auscultation of abnormal breath (rales) and heart sounds (S_3) will herald the development of left heart failure even if the CVP remains within normal limits.

Routine monitoring of the anesthetized patient involves the physical diagnostic items listed in Table 6-1, including the use of a precordial or esophageal stethoscope to listen to breath and heart sounds continuously and a sphygmomanometer to measure blood pressure regularly. In addition, many anesthesiologists routinely monitor the electrocardiogram and body temperature because the risks and costs of doing so are minimal and the potential benefits are substantial. The frequency of dysrhythmias under anesthesia is considerable, and it is necessary to distinguish innocuous premature beats and dysrhythmias from those that are or may progress to a life-threatening type. Also, the high incidence of coronary artery disease in the adult patient population makes it worthwhile to be on the lookout for electrocardiographic (ECG) signs of myocardial ischemia in the anesthetized patient, who cannot complain of angina pectoris. Changes in body temperature are common during anesthesia and surgery and can affect organ function as well as the interpretation of certain monitoring data (e.g., blood-gas values). Malignant hyperpyrexia is a life-threatening consequence of anesthesia. Hence, the routine monitoring of body temperature is not only justified but is considered to be mandatory by many anesthesiologists.

A peripheral nerve stimulator to determine the degree of neurosmuscular junction blockade is used routinely by many anesthesiologists in any patient who receives a muscle relaxant. Some anesthesiologists believe it to be essential that a ventilator-anesthetic circuit-patient disconnect alarm system be used routinely in patients whose ventilation is supported mechanically in the operating room. Monitoring of the oxygen concentration in the inspired gas mixture and of anesthetic contamination of the operating room is routinely done under the direction of the anesthesiologists in some hospitals.

There are reasons to go beyond the routine monitoring described above even in fairly healthy patients undergoing common types of anesthesia and surgery. It may be worthwhile to verify the adequacy of ventilation by analysis of arterial blood gases. If a particular item is needed for one purpose, why not take advantage of it for monitoring purposes? For example, one can measure urine flow if an indwelling urinary catheter is used, measure central venous pressure if an external jugular vein is to be cannulated, and measure arterial blood pressure directly if an arterial cannula is inserted for blood-gas analysis.

Specialized monitoring is indicated for rapid detection of trends, precision of measurement, specific diagnosis of abnormalities that exist or are likely to develop, and to free the hands of the anesthesiologist for other tasks. The methods most frequently used by the anesthesiologist are discussed below and in other chapters of this book.

MONITORING PATIENT SAFETY

Ensuring patient safety and comfort should be considered as part of the routine monitoring of all patients undergoing anesthesia. Mechanisms of self-protection including warning signs (e.g., pain) and escape or withdrawal movements are lost with the induction of anesthesia. The anesthesiologist and others caring for the patient in this vulnerable state must act on the patient's behalf to prevent injury. The first step is to remain keenly

Table 6-2. Body Sites Especially Vulnerable to Injury in the Anesthetized Patient

Region	Part	Consequences
Head	Eyes	Corneal abrasion; retinal damage by pressure on globe (especially with glaucoma)
	Ears	Tympanic membrane perforation by foreign objects; cauliflower ear from folding the pinna
	Lips and tongue	Lacerations and bruising from teeth, airway devices, and instruments
	Teeth	Cracking, chipping, dislodgment by airway devices
	Airway	Silent aspiration of stomach contents, teeth, and other objects loose in the pharynx
Neck	Vasculature	Impairment of cerebral blood flow by rotation of the neck
	Brachial plexus	Neuropathy from stretching of plexus by neck rotation and arm abduction
Extremities	Nerves	Pressure on ulnar nerve at elbow (olecranon fossa), peroneal nerve lateral to the fibula
	Joints	Overextension, especially arthritic joints
	Vasculature	Distal ischemia and edema from circulatory occlusion
Skin		Burns from antiseptic solutions, warming blankets, electrocautery, improper grounding of electrical equipment

aware of the potential for harm. The second is to recognize the body areas most susceptible to injury, and the third is to monitor these sites for breakdown of protection and early signs of injury.

The areas of particular concern are listed in Table 6-2. Some suggestions for protection follow.

Positioning (see Ch. 4). Have the patient assume a position as close as possible to that required for surgery. Apply protective padding to vulnerable sites at risk from pressure and other types of injury. When moving the head and extremities of an anesthetized patient follow the usual direction and range of motion and do not force any movement (e.g., arthritic joints).

Monitoring devices and connecting lines should be arranged in anticipation of positional changes that will be made later in the procedure—this is done to minimize the difficulties of moving the patient, to avoid accidental disruption or distortion of monitoring, and to prevent complications related to dislodgment of cannulae and other devices from the patient.

Eyes. The eyes must be protected from corneal abrasion, pressure, and other injuries. Eyelids should be taped securely in the closed position without the tape exerting pressure on the cornea. If the head is covered under surgical drapes, the anesthesiologist should monitor the actions of others to avoid any pressure being exerted on the eyes or any part of the face (e.g., surgeon's elbow, instruments).

Infection. The anesthesiologist and others should be alert to any breakdown in sterile technique that may lead to the introduction of infectious organisms through percutaneous vascular cannulation sites, urinary bladder catheter, airway, or surgical wound.

Medication and blood administration errors. Obviously, labels should be read carefully. When practical, drugs packaged in containers that are distinctively shaped and labeled should be chosen over those that closely resemble one another.

Electrical burns.[5] An alarm mechanism, preferably both audible and visible, should be incorporated into the electrical cautery unit to indicate the lack of appropriate grounding of the patient. The cause triggering any electrical malfunction alarm in the operating room or piece of equipment should be identified.

Other sources of injury. Any small or dangerous objects should not be left lying loosely around the patient (e.g., needles, bottle caps). Of course, proper procedures including the use of restraints should be employed to prevent self-inflicted injuries by the delerious, semicomatose patient. Bed rails and safety straps should be utilized even for the fully conscious patient, who should never be left unattended or unobserved in the operating or recovery rooms.

DEPTH OF ANESTHESIA

There is need to assess the depth of general anesthesia in order to avoid the patient's being aware of the surgical environment as well as to minimize the risks associated with greater than necessary doses of anesthetic drugs.* Yet the anesthesiologist is often limited in estimating the adequacy of anesthesia, the primary objective of his work, his *raison d'etre*. First of all, movement or other skeletal muscle responses to stimulation are the only objective signs equally applicable to all general anesthetic drugs and the common use of muscle relaxants precludes the use of muscular movement as an indicator of anesthetic depth in many cases. Muscle relaxant–induced paralysis also eliminates changes in ventilation as a sign of changing levels of anesthesia, as does the need to control ventilation in many situations.

Secondly, while it is true that anesthetic depth is proportional to anesthetic concentration, the measurement of concentration has not proven very helpful under clinical conditions for several reasons. Rapid determination of anesthetic levels is currently feasible only for the inhalational drugs. The

---

* Except for hemodynamic changes with certain anesthetic drugs, acute toxicity is seldom a problem intraoperatively. However, risks of toxicity extend beyond the operative period when ventilatory depression may occur as a result of residual anesthetic drugs, especially the narcotic analgesics, and when metabolites of anesthetic drugs (e.g., flouride ion from methoxyflurane) may accumulate and impair organ function.

equipment is expensive and the relationships of concentration to depth may vary depending on where in the patient the sample is obtained. Anesthetic concentration in the anesthetic system varies considerably from anesthetic levels in the patient, especially during induction and emergence. Anesthetic concentrations in end-tidal gas are more closely related to the partial pressure of the anesthetic in the patient's blood but even here there can be subtle discrepancies related to the ventilatory pattern (e.g., tidal volume) and pulmonary function (e.g., dead space, shunt, disease states). More importantly, a number of factors other than anesthetic concentration determine the intensity of anesthetic effects in different patients (e.g., age, premedication) as well as in the same patient under different conditions (e.g., body temperature, intensity of stimulation).

The solution to this problem is for the anesthesiologist to develop clinical skills in assessing anesthetic depth from signs that are unique to each class of anesthetic drugs (e.g., volatile halogenated hydrocarbons, narcotic analgesics, ketamine). Such signs are discussed in the chapters dealing with specific anesthetic drugs.

Objective measures of anesthetic depth based on simplified analysis of the electroencephalogram appear to offer some promise. Presently they have some drawbacks: limited cost-effectiveness; the fact that each anesthetic alters the EEG differently; and the nonspecificity of the patterns (i.e., changes in oxygen and carbon dioxide tensions in blood may produce the same EEG patterns as alterations in anesthetic depth).

THE CENTRAL NERVOUS SYSTEM

The functional status of the central nervous system (also see Ch. 33) is of interest to the anesthesiologist not only because it is probably the primary target organ of anesthetic drugs, but also because it is the organ system

Table 6-3. Central Nervous System Monitoring in the Operating Room

Nervous system activity
    Electroencephalography
    Evoked potentials
    Oxygen consumption

Cerebral blood flow
    Tracer washout techniques

Intracranial pressure
    Intraventricular cannula
    Subarachnoid bolt

most vulnerable to hypoxia. Oxygen delivery to the brain is dependent on oxygen content of arterial blood and cerebral blood flow. In the absence of certain types of central nervous system disease, cerebral blood flow is dependent on cerebral perfusion pressure. Cerebral perfusion pressure is determined by the difference between mean arterial blood pressure and central venous pressure unless intracranial pressure is abnormally elevated. Thus, the usual monitoring and control of ventilation and hemodynamics is satisfactory for most patients undergoing anesthesia.

However, certain patients are at unusual risk of CNS complications either because of their disease (e.g., intracranial mass, hydrocephalus, cerebral vascular disease) or the type of surgery (e.g., neurosurgery, carotid endarterectomy, cardiac surgery). In these patients, direct indicators of CNS integrity are desirable for several reasons: blood flow to all areas of the CNS may not be closely related to mean arterial pressure; anesthetic and surgical techniques may compromise cerebral blood flow without changing the overall hemodynamic status of the patient; and intracerebral damage can develop without any reliable diagnostic signs in the anesthetized and paralyzed patient, and the brief opportunity for cerebral resuscitation and preservation may be missed.

Currently available techniques for CNS monitoring in the clinical setting of anesthesia and surgery (Table 6-3) operate on a relatively gross level and are limited in their application by cost, complexity, interfering factors, and problems of interpretation. Those with general applicability are discussed here; monitoring problems unique to the neurosurgical patient are presented in Chapter 33.

ELECTROENCEPHALOGRAPHY[7]

The most direct monitor of central nervous system function in the anesthetized or comatose patient is the electroencephalogram (EEG). It is a rapid and sensitive indicator of inadequate cerebral oxygenation. Depending on the number and location of electrodes, it can be used to detect relatively localized and specific problems.

For purposes of evaluating generalized changes in cerebral function it is sufficient to use a pair of low impedance, electrically matched leads (bipolar lead). The leads can be either chlorided-silver or tin discs cemented or otherwise secured to the scalp, or platinum or gold needles can be inserted into the scalp and stabilized. Needles have the disadvantages of producing hematoma, edema, and inflammation, and these conditions can change the electrical impedance of the electrode.

One lead is placed over the frontal cortex (forehead) and the other over the occipital cortex (behind the ear) on the same side of the head. The choice of sides is not crucial unless one or the other side is at higher risk because of disease-related or surgical factors. Bilateral leads are useful in detecting asymmetrical changes (e.g., during carotid endarterectomy). The usual EEG frequency ranges (delta < 4 Hz, theta 4 to 7 Hz, alpha 8 to 13 Hz, beta > 13 Hz) are seldom meaningful in the anesthetized patient, in whom there is a continuum of rapidly shifting frequencies. Rather, the patterns may be defined as "activated," characterized by low voltage and high frequency; "depressed," high voltage and low frequency; or "isoelectric," which occurs with ischemia, hypothermia, and death.

There are a number of disadvantages to the

Table 6-4. Factors Altering the Electroencephalogram

Anesthetic and premedicant drugs
Different EEG patterns for different drugs, even within the same pharmacologic class; activation and suppression of EEG activity can occur at different doses of the same drug.

Sensory stimulation
Stimulates the ascending reticular activating system and increases EEG activity; the EEG pattern reflects the net effect of sensory stimulation and anesthesia.

Oxygenation of tissue
Determined by both oxygen content of blood and cerebral perfusion rate; hypoxia may initially produce EEG activation through peripheral chemoreceptor activation of the ascending reticular activating system; persistent hypoxia will lead first to EEG slowing and then to an isoelectric EEG.

Carbon dioxide
Hypocarbia causes EEG slowing; mild hypercarbia activates the EEG through stimulation of the ascending reticular activating system; marked hypercarbia causes narcosis and reduces EEG activity.

Body temperature
Progressively greater degrees of hypothermia produce progressive EEG slowing

Serum glucose
Hypoglycemia produces coma and EEG slowing due to inadequate substrate availability for metabolic energy production; hyperglycemia (>600mg/dl) produces hyperosmolar coma and EEG slowing due to brain dehydration.

Electrolytes
Hyponatremia (<120mEq/L) results in progressive obtundation and EEG slowing; hypernatremia (>150mEq/L) produces hyperosmolar coma.

Convulsions
Variable EEG patterns depending on the factor precipitating convulsions; seizure is followed by postictal depression characterized by reduced EEG activity.

EEG as a monitor. There is a generally poor correlation of even extreme and persistent EEG changes with the ultimate neurologic outcome. It is subject to a large number of artifacts including skeletal muscular activity, gross movement of the patient, faulty leads, and electronic interference.* There is no practical display of unprocessed EEG data meaningful to the anesthesiologist in the usual clinical setting. Various types of electronic processing of the EEG are being investigated for their applicability to the operating room setting. Such processing is designed to reject artifacts, to provide quantitative data, and to allow continuous monitoring with easy recognition of trends. The only commercially available instrument is the Cerebral Function Monitor,[8] which can indicate grossly abnormal cerebral perfusion, seizure activity, and death. More sophisticated devices employing computers are being studied enthusiastically (e.g., spectral array techniques[9, 10]). Their role in intraoperative monitoring remains to be determined, especially in view of the large number of factors that can influence EEG activity (Table 6-4).

Another attempt to increase the usefulness of monitoring CNS electrical activity is the measurement of evoked potentials.[11] Various types of stimuli (e.g., visual, auditory, and somatosensory) produce an electrical response in corresponding areas of the cerebral cortex. The response occurs with a latency of 15 msec and consists of a specific primary wave (10 to 15 msec positive wave followed

---

* Distinguishing the low energy signals (10 to 200 μV) of nervous activity from all other electrical signals (e.g., heart 1,000 μV, electrical equipment 120 V) present in the operating room is the most challenging obstacle. Screening and other isolation techniques are impractical in the clinical operating room.

by a brief negative wave) and a nonspecific secondary wave (up to 100 msec of small positive-negative fluctuations). The disappearance and recovery of the early specific wave correlates well with focal neuropathology and is unaffected by general anesthetic drugs. The nonspecific, later waves are altered by anesthetic drugs as well as other factors. Again, the practical applications of evoked potentials in the clinical operating room remains to be determined.

CEREBRAL BLOOD FLOW

Currently available methods for estimating cerebral blood flow (CBF) have the same kinds of limitations as the EEG. That is, they measure overall CBF and do not identify localized problems without complex and expensive equipment, and there is a lack of rapid presentation of data meaningful to the anesthesiologist. The Kety-Schmidt method[12] based on the rate of uptake or release of an inert tracer substance provides a measurement of average blood flow and metabolism but is impractical in the clinical setting because of the requirements of jugular venous bulb cannulation and prolonged sampling periods.

The Lassen-Ingar method of administering a gamma-emitting radioisotope (^{133}Xe) and detecting its concentration in various brain regions through the use of external scintillation probes can determine regional changes in cerebral blood flow with a sufficient number of probes.[13, 14] In addition to the general limitations noted above, this technique has limitations related to radiation safety and also to cannulation of a carotid artery for injection of the isotope or to the use of computers to correct for recirculation of the isotope if it is administered systemically (e.g., by inhalation). Its one practical application at the present time is to determine the need for insertion of a shunting tube during carotid endarterectomy.[15] The isotope is injected into the exposed carotid artery immediately prior to clamping it and the rate of xenon clearance from the ipsilateral cerebral cortex is measured after the clamp is applied. By noting the time required for the radioactivity (measured by a single probe applied to the scalp) to decrease by one-half, it is easy to calculate xenon clearance, which is directly proportional to blood flow. If the clearance is below the acceptable level, the use of an intracarotid shunt is indicated. This technique is currently used only at a few university medical centers, but there is every reason to believe that its use will spread to other centers where carotid endarterectomy surgery is done frequently. Certainly, this method is the only reliable one currently available. Other measurements (e.g., carotid artery stump pressure) are known to be misleading.[16]

INTRACRANIAL PRESSURE[17]

Pressure within the cranial vault is usually low (5 to 15 torr) and elevations caused by coughing, etc. are mild and transient because of the rapid adjustments in cerebrospinal fluid (CSF) volume. CNS pathology can produce elevations of intracranial pressure (ICP) and compromise the mechanisms of CSF production and elimination. Sustained elevations of ICP disturb CNS function and reduce cerebral blood flow. Changes in ICP are common during anesthesia and surgery in patients with head trauma and with certain diseases of the central nervous system. Careful monitoring of ICP facilitates the maintenance of low ICP and optimal cerebral perfusion in such circumstances (see Ch. 33).

Monitoring problems related to neurosurgery are discussed in Chapter 33. Some of these problems are not unique to neurosurgery and are only mentioned here. *Air embolism* can occur from any site in which venous channels are open to air at a level above the central venous pressure level. The diagnosis, therapy, and complications are the same as for the patient undergoing a craniotomy in the sitting position. *Positional changes* of the

Table 6-5. Signs of Hypoxemia and Hypercarbia in the Normal, Awake Patient

Ventilation
   Increased ventilatory effort, frequency, and tidal volume in response to chemoreceptor stimulation by hypoxia (carotid body) and by hypercarbia (medullary respiratory centers).

Circulation
   Sympathetic nervous system stimulation by hypoxia and/or hypercarbia leads to increased heart rate and blood pressure.

   Direct effects of hypoxia on the heart lead to slowing of the rate, dysrhythmias, ECG signs of ischemia, and progressive impairment of myocardial contractility.

   Carbon dioxide acts directly on vascular smooth muscle to produce vasodilation; respiratory acidosis leads to cardiac dysrhythmias.

Skin, mucous membranes, conjunctiva
   Hypoxemia produces cyanosis in the absence of cutaneous vasoconstriction and anemia.

Surgical site
   Hypoxemia darkens the color of blood.

   Hypercarbia increases bleeding.

Central nervous system
   Hypercarbia may produce muscular twitching and convulsions prior to the onset of coma ($PaCO_2 > 250$ torr); halothane MAC is reduced progressively at $PaCO_2 > 90$ torr.

   Hypoxia produces coma.

patient can create problems related to monitoring. The zero level for arterial and venous pressure measurement should remain at the level of the right atrium and transducers should be moved accordingly with changes in the patient's position. It should be noted that there is a 10 torr gradient of hydrostatic (blood) pressure for every 13 cm difference between the zero level and the organ of interest. That is, the arterial and venous pressures will be 10 torr higher at the zero level than they are in the brain, which is positioned 13 cm higher than the right atrium.

VENTILATION

Ventilation is a vital function that is altered to some degree by most anesthetic techniques and by many surgical procedures (see Ch. 22). Patients requiring surgery may have pulmonary disease, and this may increase the difficulty of achieving satisfactory ventilation during and after anesthesia and surgery. The anesthesiologist assumes responsibility for the adequacy of the patient's ventilation intraoperatively and in many cases finds it necessary to assist or to support ventilation completely. Monitoring the effectiveness of ventilation is essential under these conditions, especially since most causes of ventilatory insufficiency in the perioperative period are avoidable and correctable.

Ventilation has as its primary purpose the provision of oxygen to and the removal of carbon dioxide from blood. The single, definitive monitor of the adequacy of ventilation is the analysis of oxygen and carbon dioxide partial pressures in arterial blood, and these laboratory tests are being used more commonly for patients in the operating room. There are other measures of ventilatory function that may be especially useful in diagnosing the cause of ventilatory insufficiency; and there are a number of early warning signs and devices that can alert the anesthesiologist to problems before they result in ventilatory insufficiency and its consequences.

There are a number of signs of hypoxemia and hypercarbia in the normal, awake subject (Table 6-5). These signs may prove to be unreliable in the anesthetized surgical patient under some circumstances. For example, the presence of anemia or cutaneous vasoconstriction may mask cyanosis. Certain anesthetic drugs (e.g., halothane) and techniques (e.g., spinal anesthesia) may obtund the hemodynamic manifestations of sympathetic stimulation produced by hypercarbia and/or hypoxemia. Also, these signs and symptoms are not useful in quantifying the severity of ventilatory insufficiency and often cannot be used to distinguish between ventilatory and circulatory problems. Hence, there is the need for accurate and reliable monitoring of ventilation during anesthesia and surgery, especially in patients who have a high risk of ventilatory insufficiency as a result of their disease state, type of surgery, or both.

Problems with ventilation during anesthesia can be classified in terms of the following: inspired gas mixture, ventilation of the lungs, and pulmonary blood flow and gas exchange. Monitoring techniques and devices can also be considered in relation to these aspects of ventilation. Techniques and devices limited to one aspect of ventilation are particularly useful in identifying the cause of ventilatory insufficiency; but accurate assessment of the degree of ventilatory failure can be accomplished only with analysis of arterial blood gases.

ANALYSIS OF BLOOD GASES

Routine analysis of blood gases in the clinical laboratory involves measurement of pH and of the partial pressures of oxygen and carbon dioxide. It is customary to determine the hematocrit (or hemoglobin content*) simultaneously in order to calculate the oxygen content of the blood and to estimate the base deficit or excess. The reader is referred elsewhere for a discussion of the methods of these analyses.[18] Physiological and pathologic changes in arterial blood gases are sum-

---

* The hemoglobin concentration in g/dl of blood is approximately one third of the hematocrit in percent.

Table 6-6. Normal Blood-Gas Values

		Arterial	Mixed Venous
pH		7.40	7.36
$PaCO_2$		40.0	46.0
PaO_2	*years of age**		40.0
	20–29	84–104	
	30–39	81–101	
	40–49	78–98	
	50–59	74–94	
	60–69	71–91	

* Mean $PaO_2 = 100 - \dfrac{\text{years of age}}{3}$

marized in Chapter 26, Acid-Base Balance and Blood-Gas Measurement. The discussion below focuses on the pitfalls in interpretation of the results of blood-gas analysis.

SAMPLE COLLECTION

Blood-gas analysis is usually performed on arterial blood in order to evaluate the adequacy of ventilation. When it is impractical to obtain an arterial sample (e.g., newborn infant), capillary blood from a finger or toe on a warmed and well-perfused extremity may provide a close approximation of arterial blood. Venous blood-gas analysis does *not* provide an estimate of pulmonary function in terms of oxygenation of blood, but it can give indications of the degree of oxygen extraction by peripheral tissues, of hypercarbia or hypocarbia (assuming the usual arteriovenous differences of 4 to 6 torr in PCO_2), and of acid-base balance. Obviously, it is important to recognize the differences between arterial and venous blood (Table 6-6) in interpreting the results of blood-gas analysis.

Certain precautions are necessary in collecting and preserving the blood sample in order to ensure that it accurately represents the circulating blood:

1. The syringe should be air-tight, rinsed with heparin (1000 units/ml), and the plunger depressed completely to expel the excess heparin from the syringe. Fifteen μl of a 1000 units/ml solution contain 15 units of

heparin, which is sufficient to anticoagulate 3 ml of whole blood.

2. If the blood sample is to be drawn from an indwelling cannula, old blood and flush solution contained in the cannula should be withdrawn and discarded before the sample is collected in order to ensure that the sample will be representative of the blood circulating at the time of collection.

3. Air bubbles should be eliminated from the sample, and the syringe should be immediately sealed and placed in ice to prevent uptake or loss of gases (i.e., from the ambient air, by metabolism in blood cells).

4. The temperature of the patient should be noted so that appropriate corrections can be made; typically, blood-gas analysis is performed in vitro at 37 °C. Temperature deviations alter the solubility of gases in blood and hence their partial pressures. Nomograms and slide rules are available to correct blood PO_2, PCO_2 and pH for temperature differences between the patient and electrode system.[19,20]

INTERPRETATION

Oxygen has a very limited solubility in blood; most of the oxygen is carried in combination with hemoglobin (Hgb), which is essentially saturated at an oxygen partial pressure of 100 torr. The total oxygen content of blood can be calculated as follows:

1. Determine the Hgb saturation by actual measurement or by reference to the appropriate oxyhemoglobin dissociation curve.*

2. Multiply the oxygen content of saturated Hgb (1.3 cc O_2/g Hgb) by the percentage saturation to determine the amount of oxygen carried by Hgb in blood. Hgb concentrations

in whole blood are usually expressed as g/dl. (One dl is 100 ml. Volume percent is the volume of gas (cc) in 100 ml or 1 dl.)

3. Multiply the oxygen solubility factor (0.003 ml O_2/dl blood/mm Hg) by the PaO_2 to determine the amount of oxygen carried in physical solution in blood.

4. Sum the values of steps 2 and 3 to determine the total oxygen content of blood.

For example: Hgb 15 g/dl blood, PaO_2 = 100 torr

1. Hgb 100% saturated at PaO_2 of 100 torr.

2. 15 g/dl × 100% × 1.3 cc O_2/g Hgb = 19.5 cc O_2/dl blood.

3. 100 torr × 0.003 ml/dl/torr = 0.3 cc O_2/dl blood.

4. 19.5 + 0.3 = 19.8 cc O_2/dl blood.

Carbon dioxide is hydrated to carbonic acid, which dissociates to bicarbonate and hydrogen ions. Thus, there is a relationship between PCO_2 and pH, which can be summarized on a nomogram[19] or Severinghaus slide rule.[20] Deviations from this relationship are due to the presence of other (metabolic or fixed) acids and bases and are expressed in terms of a base deficit or excess. Dripps et al. have summarized the relationships in two tables designed for memorization (Table 6-7).[22]

INDWELLING AND CUTANEOUS PROBES

Oxygen, carbon dioxide, and pH sensitive probes have been developed for insertion in peripheral arteries for continuous monitoring of these variables in blood. Their place in intraoperative monitoring has not yet been determined in relation to their cost and to their relative advantages and disadvantages over current practices of intermittent sampling of blood for in vitro analysis of gases.

Cutaneous oximetry is an indirect method of estimating arterial oxygen levels from the percentage oxygen saturation of hemoglobin passing through capillaries or veins of the

---

* The relationship between Hgb saturation and PaO_2 is affected by temperature, pH and base excess, ionic strength, type of hemoglobin, and the concentration of 2,3-diphosphoglycerate in the erythrocyte.[21]

Table 6-7. Relationships Between PaCO₂, pH, and Base Excess or Deficit

A. Predicted pH at different PaCO₂ levels
(No metabolic acid-base abnormality)

PaCO₂(torr)	pH	
70	7.25	
60	7.30	$\}$ −.05 pH units/10 torr PCO_2
50	7.35	
40	7.40	
30	7.5	
20	7.6	$\}$ +0.1 pH units/10 torr PCO_2
10	7.7	

B. Predicted pH at different levels of metabolic acidosis or alkalosis
($PaCO_2$ = 40 torr)

pH	Base (mEq/L)	
7.1	−21	
7.2	−14	
7.3	− 7	
7.4	− 0	± 7 mEq/0.1 pH unit
7.5	+ 7	
7.6	+14	
7.7	+21	

C. To estimate a base deficit or excess at a given pH and PCO_2
   1. Adjust the pH for the contribution by respiratory acidosis or alkalosis by the amount corresponding to the difference between the given PCO_2 and 40 torr (part A)
   2. Estimate the base deficit or excess from part B
e.g.: Given a pH = 7.25 and a PCO_2 = 50
   (1) PCO_2 50 → 40
       pH 7.25 → 7.30
   (2) 7.30 corresponds to a base of −7 mEq/L
       (i.e., a base deficit)

(Modified from Dripps RD, Eckenhoff JE, Vandam LD: Introduction to Anesthesia. Philadelphia, WB Saunders, 1977.)

skin of the ear lobe.[23] Accuracy of the device depends on the maintenance of a brisk blood flow through the skin and on proper calibration of the apparatus. Obviously, the device is less reliable than direct measurement of arterial blood gases, especially in the hemodynamically unstable patient. In the healthy patient it may be no more reliable than the watchful eyes of the anesthesiologist and surgeon viewing the color of the blood in the surgical wound.

INSPIRED GAS MIXTURE

The formulation of the inspired mixture of gases in the operating room is usually accomplished by the anesthesia machine, the function of which should be evaluated prior to the induction of anesthesia, and preferably before the patient arrives at the anesthetizing location.* (See Ch. 4.) Despite the best preparations, malfunction of the anesthesia machine can occur, and there are four potential problems related to the inspired gas mixture: inadequate oxygen content, presence of carbon dioxide (rebreathing), inappropriately high or low anesthetic concentrations, and contamination of the mixture with irritating or toxic volatile substances. Precise analysis of the components of the inspired gaseous mixture is becoming a reality with the use of mass spectrometers and other sophisticated and expensive devices (e.g., infrared analyz-

---

* The patient's anxiety can only increase when he hears comments such as "That doesn't work!" or "What's wrong with this?" and observes last-minute repairs that suggest the imperfect functioning of equipment upon which his life will depend.

Table 6-8. Normal Values of Ventilatory Variables for Adult Males at Rest

Variable	Abbreviation	Normal, Average Values
Frequency	f	12 breaths per min
Tidal volume	V_T	500 cc (3–4 cc/lb body weight)
Expired minute ventilation (total)	$\dot{V}_E$	6,000 cc/min
Anatomic dead space	V_D	150 cc (1 cc/lb body weight)
Alveolar minute ventilation	$\dot{V}_A$	4,200 cc/min
Vital capacity	VC	4,800 cc
Compliance of lung and thorax	C	0.1 L/cm H_2O

ers for carbon dioxide, halothane, and enflurane). However, most anesthesiologists do not have access to such equipment and are required to use other means of evaluating the gas mixture they administer to their patients.

The single most important constituent of any anesthetic mixture is oxygen. Oxygen analyzers (e.g., paramagnetic, fuel-cell, and polarographic) are relatively inexpensive (less than $500) and provide the only reliable means of quantifying the oxygen content in the inspired mixture.[24] An oxygen analyzer is absolutely required for low-flow or closed-circuit administration of anesthetic mixtures containing nitrous oxide. Oxygen analyzers measure the percentage oxygen in the gas mixture; nitrous oxide concentrations can be estimated as the difference between oxygen percentage and 100 percent.

The presence of carbon dioxide in the inspired gas (rebreathing) cannot be detected without relatively expensive equipment. The risk of rebreathing can be reduced by maintaining high flows of fresh gas mixture (with the disadvantages of wasting anesthetic gases and pollution of the operating room atmosphere) or by using a carbon dioxide absorber in a low-flow system. Function of the absorber can be checked by feeling its surface (CO_2 absorption produces heat) and by incorporating an indicator that turns a different color when the absorbent is exhausted. Of course, the anesthesiologist should be alert to physiological changes suggestive of hypercarbia.

The presence of inappropriate concentrations of volatile anesthetics or of irritating contaminants can often be detected by the anesthesiologist himself inhaling the anesthetic mixture for one or two breaths ("sniff test"). This practice is condemned by some because it is not a very sensitive test and it repeatedly exposes the anesthesiologist to anesthetics with the risk of their accumulation and toxicity. An ultraviolet analyzer for halothane (Cavitron) is available at a moderate cost and is adequate for clinical use. The Narkotest meter (Drager) is inexpensive and sensitive to all volatile anesthetics. However, it is not particularly accurate and has the disadvantages of a very slow response-time and of being affected by water vapor.[25] All the other commercially available devices, (i.e., infrared analyzer, gas chromatograph, mass spectrograph) offer specificity and precision of gas analysis, but currently they are so expensive as to be impractical for routine clinical practice. The anesthesiologist and patient are probably best served by regular inspection and maintenance of the anesthesia machine including the anesthetic vaporizers.

LUNG VENTILATION

Ventilation of the lungs is measured in terms of the volume of gas inspired (I) or exhaled (E) in a single breath (tidal volume, V_T) or over a minute's time (minute ventilation $\dot{V}$). Minute ventilation is the product of tidal volume and frequency (f) of breaths per minute:

$$\dot{V}_E = V_T \times f$$

Normal values for these ventilatory variables are shown in Table 6-8. The focus of this discussion is on monitoring the effectiveness of

Table 6-9. Monitors of Lung Ventilation

Visual
 Regular, normal movement of the diaphragm, chest and anesthesia reservoir bag; alternate condensation and vaporization of water in the endotracheal tube; rise and fall of anesthesia circuit pressure gauge.

Auditory
 Breath sounds through an esophageal or precordial stethoscope, at the lips, or in the anesthesia circuit.

Volume measurement
 Bellows of the ventilator (e.g., Ventimeter), spirometers, pneumotachograph.

Carbon dioxide measurement
 Rise and fall of carbon dioxide concentration in airway gases with ventilation by fresh gas (i.e., nonrebreathing or CO_2 absorber systems).

Apnea monitor
 Sounds an alarm when pressures within the anesthesia system do not change over a 15 to 20 second interval.

ventilation regardless of the particular mode of ventilation that is being used. Again, the definitive test of ventilation is the analysis of arterial blood gases. But there are other means of monitoring ventilatory variables that may be especially useful in diagnosing the causes of hypoxemia, hypercarbia, and acidosis (Table 6-9); and there are useful alarms for early warnings of impending or existing problems (e.g., apnea alarms).

Apnea alarms respond to the failure of airway or anesthetic circuit pressure to rise within a set period of time. Such alarms are probably indicated anytime the anesthesiologist is not directly in touch with the patient and especially when a mechanical ventilator is being used. Early detection of a disconnection between the patient and the breathing circuit is obviously necessary if the development of hypoxemia and hypercarbia are to be avoided.

The measurement of inspired or exhaled gas volumes is most accurately done with a water-sealed bell spirometer. However, this instrument is too bulky and cumbersome for routine clinical use. There are a number of more portable though less accurate devices (e.g., gas meters, anemometers, and pneumotachograph) that can adequately fill clinical needs providing they are calibrated regularly and handled carefully to avoid damage to their relatively delicate mechanisms. Probably the most widely used instrument is the Wright respirometer. Its performance is affected by the composition of the gas, humidity, and instantaneous rates of gas flow. Nevertheless, its use is justified for clinical purposes.[21]

Another aspect of lung ventilation that changes with anesthesia, surgery, and disease states is the compliance of the lungs and chest wall. Compliance is the volume change per unit change of the transmural pressure gradient and can be defined as follows:[21]

$$\text{Total compliance} = \frac{\text{change in lung volume}}{\text{change in alveolar-ambient pressure gradient}}$$

$$\text{Lung compliance} = \frac{\text{change in lung volume}}{\text{change in alveolar-intrathoracic pressure gradient}}$$

$$\text{Chest wall compliance} = \frac{\text{change in lung volume}}{\text{change in ambient-intrathoracic pressure gradient}}$$

The total compliance of the lungs plus the chest wall is related to their individual compliances:[21]

$$\frac{1}{\text{total compliance}} = \frac{1}{\text{lung compliance}} + \frac{1}{\text{thoracic cage compliance}}$$

In the usual clinical setting of the anesthetized patient, the anesthesiologist may utilize the pressure gauge in the anesthesia breathing system to monitor the lung inflation pressure produced by a given volume of ventilation. (Alternatively, the volume of inspired or exhaled gas can be measured for a given inflation pressure.) High inflation pressures indicate low compliance and may signify changes in skeletal muscle tone (intercostal, diaphragmatic, abdominal) as a result of a lessening of anesthetic depth or muscular paralysis, changes in lung compliance (e.g., interstitial edema), or the presence of airway obstruction from any of a large number of causes. Besides signifying alterations in the above, a reduced compliance affects the volume of ventilation delivered by a pressure-driven ventilator.

More precise determinations of compliance, both static and dynamic, are required for research purposes that add little to the clinical management of patients. Similarly, measurements of airway resistance are largely a research tool.

The prompt diagnosis of airway obstruction is of obvious vital importance. Causes of airway obstruction are listed in Table 6-10.

Airway obstruction can be partial or complete. Complete airway obstruction is more obvious, because there is no exchange of gas between the lungs and the anesthesia system or ambient air. It can be recognized most directly by the absence of breath sounds. Other signs of airway obstruction are listed in Table 6-11. If the location of the obstruction is in the trachea or upper airway, the cause obviously must be identified and remedied promptly. In the setting of anesthesia and surgery four possibilities should be considered:

1. Upper airway obstruction due to the tongue; usually corrected by proper positioning of the head and mandible and by insertion of an oral airway or endotracheal tube.

2. Foreign object in the airway from the patient (e.g., dental work, tobacco), the anes-

Table 6-10. Causes of Airway Obstruction

Lips
Tongue
Epiglottis
Edematous tissue
Secretions
Laryngospasm
Bronchospasm
Clamping of trachea or bronchus by surgeon
Low lung compliance
    Pulmonary edema
    Emphysema
Low thoracic compliance
    Muscular rigidity
    Circumferential bandaging of trunk
    Surgeon leaning on patient's chest and/or abdomen
Hemothorax, pleural effusion
Tension pneumothorax
Herniation of abdominal structures into thorax
Ascites, obesity
Foreign objects in airway

Endotracheal tube
    Kinking
    Balloon cuff overlying tip
    Overinflation of balloon cuff with invagination of endotracheal tube
    Single lumen occluded against mucosa
    Plugged with secretions or blood
    Endobronchial position

Table 6-11. Signs of Airway Obstruction

Spontaneous Ventilation
    Increasing ventilatory effort (reflex due to hypercarbia, hypoxia)
    Retraction of intercostal, supraclavicular, and abdominal tissues
    Reduced or absent breath sounds over lung fields
    Abnormal breath sounds due to turbulence especially in upper airway
    Reduced or absent exchange of gas (i.e., absence of sound; temperature change; moisture condensation at lips or in endotracheal tube; reduced or absent movement of reservoir bag; spirometer records low or no tidal volume)
    Signs of hypoxemia and hypercarbia

Positive Pressure Ventilation
    High lung inflation pressure
    Reservoir bag does not empty (i.e. inspiratory obstruction) or does not refill normally (i.e. expiratory obstruction)
    Absence of condensation in endotracheal tube
    Reduced or absent breath sounds over lung fields and in breathing circuit
    Little or no movement of thorax or abdominal wall with application and release of positive pressure
    Signs of hypoxemia and hypercarbia

thesiologist (e.g., improperly positioned airway device), or the surgeon (e.g., pharyngeal packing). Examination of the airway and possibly laryngoscopy or bronchoscopy assists in making the diagnosis and offers the means of removal of the obstructing object. An emergency tracheotomy may be necessary.

3. Laryngospasm is almost always associated with airway manipulation by the anesthesiologist or with the presence of foreign material in the larynx of a lightly anesthetized patient. The diagnosis is often obvious; laryngoscopy makes it definitive but is not often indicated or appropriate (wastes time and further stimulates the airway). Therapy involves maximal cephalad displacement of the mandible,[26] maintenance of positive airway pressure with pure oxygen, and, if necessary, administration of a muscle relaxant (e.g., 10 to 20 mg of succinylcholine intravenously).

4. Obstruction of the endotracheal tube is most easily ruled out by the passage of a lubricated suction catheter completely through the length of the tube. If the catheter cannot be passed, the endotracheal tube must be manipulated (e.g., deflation of the balloon or elimination of kinking) or removed for inspection (e.g., occlusion by clotted blood). When surgery involves the neck or upper mediastinum, the possibility of the surgeon obstructing the trachea should be considered.

Partial airway obstruction presents more subtle signs than does complete obstruction (Table 6-11). The exchange of gases continues through a partial obstruction and results in sounds that are useful in identifying the cause and location of the obstruction. Partial obstruction by the tongue creates rough, irregular stertorous (snoring) sounds that are loudest over the neck. Fluid in the pharynx is associated with a gurgling type of noise. Laryngospasm produces a high-pitched whistle or squeak. Foreign objects produce a variety of noises depending on the degree of the obstruction (pitch) and on their mobility in the airway (e .g., rattling or fluttering sounds). Bronchiolar constriction among other factors produces wheezing, bronchiolar secretions result in rhonchi, and alveolar fluid (edema) causes rales. Absent or distant breath sounds over a portion of the lung may signify bronchial obstruction, atelectasis, or pneumothorax.

In addition to sounds, partial airway obstruction can be evaluated in more quantitative terms of tidal volume, duration of inspiration or expiration, compliance, and arterial blood gases.

The measurement of lung volumes is not done by the anesthesiologist in the usual clinical setting except for the occasional estimation of functional residual capacity (FRC) during mechanical ventilation of patients under intensive care for acute respiratory failure. The closed-circuit helium dilution technique is the simplest, most accurate method.[27]

Estimates of wasted ventilation, that is dead space ventilation as a fraction of total ventilation (V_D/V_T), involves the measurements of the partial pressure of cabon dioxide in arterial blood and in mixed expired gas collected for several minutes in a large gas-tight bag (30 liters). The ratio can then be calculated:

$$\frac{V_D}{V_T} = \frac{PaCO_2 - PECO_2}{PaCO_2}$$

Again these measurements by the anesthesiologist are usually confined to the clinical setting of the intensive care unit and are made in an attempt to explain discrepancies between $PaCO_2$ and minute ventilation.

PULMONARY BLOOD FLOW AND GAS EXCHANGE

The uptake of oxygen by and elimination of carbon dioxide from venous blood occurs at the alveolar-capillary membrane. This exchange obviously depends on ventilation and perfusion of the alveoli and on the condition of the membrane. Even under normal conditions in healthy persons, some of the pulmonary blood flow is not exposed to ventilated alveoli and the mismatch of ventilation and perfusion tends to increase under conditions of anesthesia, surgery, and disease (see Ch. 22). Disease can also affect the condition of the alveolar-capillary membrane.

The effectiveness of the lungs in converting venous blood to arterial is most conveniently measured in terms of oxygenation.* Pulmonary blood flow through unventilated alveoli and right-to-left shunts represents wasted blood flow (Qs), which is usually expressed as a fraction of total pulmonary blood flow ($\dot{Q}_T$). Calculation of the fraction requires determinations of the partial pressure of oxygen in mixed venous (pulmonary artery) blood (PvO_2), in systemic arterial blood (PaO_2), and in the inspired (PiO_2) and expired gas ($P\bar{E}O_2$) along with the measurements of hemoglobin concentration and $PaCO_2$. From these data the oxygen content of mixed venous (CvO_2), arterial (CaO_2), and pulmonary end-capillary blood ($Cc'O_2$) can be calculated** and then the shunt fraction estimated:

$$\frac{\dot{Q}s}{\dot{Q}_T} = \frac{Cc'O_2 - CaO_2}{Cc'O_2 - CvO_2}$$

Making such measurements and calculations

---

* Increased minute ventilation can compensate for a large right to left shunting of pulmonary blood flow in terms of carbon dioxide elimination. Oxygen uptake by blood perfusing ventilated alveoli is limited in amount by hemoglobin saturation, since very little oxygen is carried by physical solution in blood. When arterial blood mixes with shunted venous blood, the PaO_2 and hemoglobin saturation fall as oxygen is taken up by the unsaturated hemoglobin in the shunted venous blood.

** Calculation of oxygen content is discussed and illustrated on page 167, and is readily done for CaO_2 and CvO_2. The estimation of $Cc'O_2$ involves a number of assumptions and is based on the alveolar air equation:

$$Pc'O_2 = \text{ideal alveolar } PO_2$$
$$= PiO_2 - PaCO_2 \left(\frac{PiO_2 - P\bar{E}O_2}{P\bar{E}O_2} \right)$$

is still limited in clinical practice, but they may probably be done more frequently with the increased availability of blood-gas analysis, pulmonary artery catheters, and inexpensive, programmable calculators.

In the usual clinical situation, the difference between alveolar (PAO_2) and arterial (PaO_2) oxygen tension is taken as an indication of "virtual" shunting. This A-a gradient is subject to considerable misinterpretation.[21] For example, the A-a gradient and the apparent magnitude of shunting will be less when the patient is receiving less than 100 percent oxygen in the inspired gas (Fig. 6-1). Nevertheless, the concept of "virtual" shunt and the use of an iso-shunt diagram in clinical practice is justified for estimating oxygen concentrations required to achieve a certain PaO_2, (verification of the accuracy of the estimate by blood-gas analysis is mandatory) for indicating progress in the patient's recovery, and for demonstrating the presence of problems other than shunting that may be contributing to the inadequate oxygenation of arterial blood.

THE CARDIOVASCULAR SYSTEM*

The cardiovascular system functions as a means of transporting substances from one organ to another in the body. For example, it is essential for the constant, continuous delivery of oxygen from the lung to all body tissues and for the conveyance of carbon dioxide from those tissues to the lung where it is eliminated. Probably the most precise indicator of satisfactory cardiovascular performance is the maintenance of efficient, effective, and integrated function of body organs and tissues (Table 6-12). For the most part, evaluation of individual organ function during anesthesia under clinical conditions has proven to be less practical and informative than the

---

* Electrocardiographic monitoring is discussed in Chapter 7.

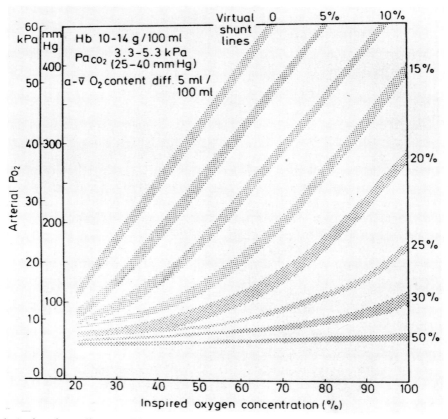

Fig. 6-1 An iso-shunt diagram. The relationships between inspired oxygen concentration (abscissa) and arterial PO_2 (ordinate) are shown for different percentages of right-to-left pulmonary shunting. If the degree of shunting is estimated, an inspired oxygen concentration can be chosen to produce a given PaO_2. If the relationship between the inspired oxygen concentration and PaO_2 is determined, the percentage of shunting can be estimated from this graph. (Redrawn by Nunn[21] from Benater SR, Hewlett AM, Nunn JF: The use of iso-shunt lines for control of oxygen therapy. Br J Anaesth 45:711, 1973).

monitoring of various aspects of cardiovascular performance.

Monitoring of hemodynamics in the patient undergoing anesthesia and surgery is indicated for several reasons:

1. Anesthetic drugs alter cardiovascular functions.

2. Surgery can result in acute and marked changes in hemodynamics as a result of body position, surgical manipulation, blood loss, and fluid loss and redistribution.

3. There is a prevalence of cardiovascular disease and of diseases affecting hemodynamics among surgical patients. The interactions of these disease states with anesthetic drugs and surgical procedures is not always predictable. Appropriate monitoring techniques can indicate inappropriate or unexpected trends that often can be corrected.

4. Therapy of adverse hemodynamic changes often involves potent drugs with specific actions on the cardiovascular system. Monitoring techniques are essential for the selection of the most appropriate therapy and for the evaluation of its effectiveness and safety.

Hemodynamic monitoring of the patient in the perioperative period encompasses a large number of techniques differing in their degree of precision, accuracy, complexity,

Table 6-12. Monitoring Organ Function and Perfusion

Organ or System	Monitor
Central nervous system	
Unanesthetized patient	Mentation, motor function
Anesthetized or comatose patient	EEG, reflexes, pupils
Heart	ECG—ischemia, dysrhythmias
	Cardiac output—pumping function
Kidney	Urine volume and composition
Skin	Color, capillary refill, temperature
Lung	Arterial blood gases, shunt

safety, and cost. The appropriateness and effectiveness of individual techniques will vary with the anesthesiologist and the clinical circumstances. Seldom is there only one right way to monitor a particular patient at a particular time in the perioperative course of events. In all cases, however, the objectives are the same. That is, to provide sufficient information in a form that can be collated and comprehended with sufficient speed by the anesthesiologist so that he can make a decision to act or to withhold action.

The following discussion summarizes the indications and limitations of techniques currently used in clinical practice. Technical information underlying the instrumentation, descriptions of specific steps in the application of techniques (e.g., vascular cannulation), and interpretation of the data are omitted because they are well described elsewhere.[28]

ARTERIAL BLOOD PRESSURE

Arterial blood pressure remains the focal point of cardiovascular monitoring for a number of reasons. It is one of the traditional vital signs that can provide an indication of cardiovascular problems. It is easily and frequently measured along with heart rate and can be used to characterize the "usual state" of the patient against which alterations can be compared. It represents the potential for perfusion of all tissues. In the case of the brain and the heart, blood pressure along with local metabolic activity (i.e., autoregulation) are the primary determinants of cerebral and coronary blood flow.

But there are two important points to be emphasized and remembered: blood *pressure* is *not* equivalent to blood *flow;* blood pressure may be normal when cardiovascular function is very abnormal.

INDIRECT MEASUREMENT

Indirect measurement of arterial blood pressure is done with a sphygmomanometer, which measures the pressure required to occlude a major artery in an extremity. A pneumatic bladder enclosed in a cuff is positioned over the artery and inflated to a pressure greater than systolic blood pressure. The air in the bladder is slowly released and one of four basic techniques is used to detect the systolic (and in some cases the diastolic) blood pressure: oscillation of the cuff pressure; auscultation of Korotkoff sounds; ultrasonic detection of arterial wall motion under the cuff; or detection of blood flow distal to the sphygmomanometer cuff by palpation of a pulse, Doppler ultrasound, photoelectric plethysmography, or other means. The physical basis of each of these techniques is discussed elsewhere.[29] Auscultation of Korotkoff sounds is the most commonly used and the others are substituted when Korotkoff sounds are not easily heard or for purposes of convenience.

A number of factors affect the accuracy of indirect blood pressure determinations

Table 6-13. Factors Affecting the Accuracy of Indirect Blood Pressure Measurements

Factor	Consequence
Hearing	Variable sensitivity to Korotkoff sounds
Touch	Variable sensitivity to pulse palpation
Cuff size	Falsely high BP—too small or loose fitting cuff
	Falsely low BP—too large a cuff
Aneroid manometer	Inaccurate BP with improper calibration
Deflation of sphyg-momanometer	Falsely low BP—too rapid deflation
Stethoscope	Malpositioning—variable sensitivity to Korotkoff sounds
Oscillometry	Imprecise detection of first and last oscillations indicating systolic and diastolic pressures respectively

(Table 6-13). The most common are the inaccuracy of aneroid manometers and of the size and positioning of the blood pressure cuff. Aneroid manometers should be calibrated regularly against a mercury manometer. The width of the blood pressure cuff should be greater than one third of the circumference of the limb; a cuff that is too wide relative to circumference of the arm will give falsely low pressures, and one that is too narrow will give incorrectly high estimates. The bladder should cover at least half of the circumference. The middle of the bladder should be positioned directly over the pulsating artery. In the auscultatory method, the stethoscope should be positioned directly over the pulsating artery under the most distal portion or just beyond the pneumatic cuff.

Even with meticulous attention to details, considerable discrepancy can be observed between indirect and direct methods of blood pressure measurement. The greatest discrepancies have been noted in hypertension, obesity, hypothermia, and shock. Both methods have their limitations as far as blood pressure measurements, but the direct method can provide other information that is useful in evaluating the overall hemodynamic status of the patient. Indirect measurement of blood pressure is usually sufficient for the patient who is hemodynamically stable in the preoperative period and who is not expected to experience marked instability for any reason during anesthesia and surgery.

DIRECT MEASUREMENT

Direct measurement of arterial blood pressure offers a number of advantages over sphygmomanometry that are especially valuable to the anesthesiologist caring for hemodynamically unstable patients. Information is provided continuously and very conveniently on a beat-by-beat basis that facilitates the earliest possible recognition of adverse hemodynamic responses and unfavorable trends. Modern equipment for direct pressure measurement affords reliability and sustained accuracy over the full range of blood pressures encountered clinically. Visual analysis of the pulse-pressure versus time wave form on an oscilloscope or recorder can yield additional information about cardiovascular function (Table 6-14).

Direct measurement of arterial blood pressure requires arterial cannulation and the use of a pressure measuring system. Both can affect the overall accuracy of the data and at least certain features of each should be familiar to the anesthesiologist.

ARTERIAL CANNULATION

Arterial cannulation is an invasive technique that can be readily justified by its high yield of information and minimal discomfort and risk to the patient if properly done. Arterial cannulation not only offers the advan-

Table 6-14. Information Derived from Visual Analysis of the Arterial Pressure

Myocardial contractility
    The upstroke of the pulse pressure wave is dependent on left ventricular dP/dt
    A steep upstroke indicates strong left ventricular contraction

Stroke volume
    The area under the systolic ejection phase of the pulse pressure tracing (i.e., upstroke to dicrotic notch) is
        proportional to stroke volume

Systemic vascular resistance
    A low dicrotic notch and a steep downstroke indicates rapid diastolic runoff and a low SVR

Hemodynamic significance of dysrhythmias
    The blood pressure and pulse contour following abnormal beats indicate the degree of impairment of cardiac
        pumping

Circulating blood volume
    Exaggerated beat-by-beat changes in blood pressure in relation to ventilation can indicate hypovolemia
    During a single cycle of ventilation:
        Positive pressure ventilation increases the stroke volume of the first beat or two and then decreases the
            stroke volume of subsequent beats
        Spontaneous ventilation decreases the stroke volume of the first beat or two and increases stroke volume
            during expiration

tages of direct measurement of arterial blood pressure and pulse wave form analysis, but it facilitates the collection of arterial blood samples for gas, electrolyte, glucose, coagulation, and other types of analyses. When multiple samples are required for patient care, a single arterial cannulation is obviously preferable to multiple needle punctures in terms of greater reliability and convenience and less trauma and discomfort. Indications for arterial cannulation in the surgical patient are listed in Table 6-15.

In most patients, arteries accessible for percutaneous cannulation include the radial, ulnar , brachial, axillary, dorsalis pedis, femoral, and superficial temporal. The radial artery is probably the most frequently used for intraoperative purposes because it is readily accessible, can be easily cannulated, supplies the hand (which normally has a collateral supply through the ulnar artery), and has been used with few long-term, functionally significant complications when properly cared for.[30, 31, 32] Also, it is usually convenient to position the arm of the patient so that the arterial cannulation site is in the view of and accessible to the anesthesiologist intraoperatively. Contraindications to the use of a particular radial artery include the presence of an inadequate circulation to the hand and

fingers (e.g., Raynaud's phenomenon), the lack of collateral circulation through the ulnar artery (abnormal Allen's test), the presence of infection in the proximity of the cannulation site, and recent cannulation of the same radial artery or the brachial artery above it. Previous cannulation may have resulted in changes in the artery (e.g., thrombus formation, scarring with narrowing of the vessel) that may increase the risk of complications and may increase the discrepancy between arterial pressures measured at that site and central aortic pressure.

Should the radial arteries in both forearms prove unsatisfactory, alternative sites can be considered. The ulnar artery has the same relative contraindications and precautions as the radial. It may be the preferred vessel when the palmar arch is supplied primarily by the radial artery as indicated by a rapid flush when compression of the radial artery is released after finding an abnormal Allen's test (i.e., lack of a palmar flush when the ulnar artery occlusion is released). The brachial artery is a larger diameter vessel and able to accommodate indwelling blood gas analyzing probes. Although some have reported few complications from brachial artery cannulation,[33, 34] there is reluctance to use this vessel because there is no collateral artery to pro-

Table 6-15. Indications for Arterial Cannulation in the Surgical Patient

Direct measurement of arterial pressure
  Cardiac surgery, especially with cardiopulmonary bypass
  Deliberate hypothermia
  Deliberate hypotension
  Intracranial operations
  Major vascular surgery—aorta, carotid, iliac, femoral arteries, vena cava
  Extensive surgery with prospect of sudden blood loss or marked shifts of body fluids
  Extensive trauma, especially with uncontrolled hemorrhage
  Thoracic or abdominal surgery with compression of the great vessels
  Noncardiac surgery in patients with significant cardiovascular disease and hemodynamic instability
  Cardiopulmonary resuscitation
  Inability to measure blood pressure indirectly (obesity, burns of the extremities)

Arterial blood sampling (repetitive)
  Blood gas analysis
    Pulmonary disease
    Lung surgery (one-lung ventilation)
    Airway surgery (apneic oxygenation)
    Major surgery (neural, cardiac, vascular, thoracic, abdominal)
  Severe metabolic derangements
    Acid-base evaluation
    Electrolyte determinations
    Glucose analysis
    Serum osmolarity measurement
  Heparin anticoagulation and protamine antagonism
    Cardiopulmonary bypass
    Arterial shunts (Gott shunt)

vide circulation should the brachial artery become occluded. The axillary artery is of still larger diameter and has been used especially for placement of a central aortic cannula and for long-term cannulation (6 to 21 days).[34, 35]

Cannulation of the dorsalis pedis artery is easy and a relatively safe alternative to the radial artery because of collateral circulation through the plantar vessels to the distal portions of the foot.[36] Plantar collateral circulation can be evaluated by occluding the dorsalis pedis artery, compressing the nail of the largest toe to blanch the nailbed, and observing capillary filling in the nailbed when pressure on the nail is released. The dorsalis pedis probably should not be used in patients with diabetes mellitus or peripheral vascular disease.

The femoral artery can be cannulated easily and there apparently has been a relatively low incidence of complications.[37] Cannulation of a femoral artery for monitoring purposes is indicated when it is necessary to evaluate arterial circulation to the lower half of the body (e.g., the use of circulatory bypass techniques while the descending aorta is clamped).

The superficial temporal artery has been cannulated for monitoring purposes, primarily in infants and children.

Techniques for cannulation of the radial artery and others are best learned from an experienced tutor and are well described elsewhere.[28] Skill is best developed by cannulating the arteries of patients with normal hemodynamics under circumstances of elective surgery. Certainly, well-developed skills are essential if the techniques are to be applied in emergency situations and in patients with impaired cardiovascular function.

The anesthesiologist should be aware of the potential complications of arterial cannulation and of the precautions to be taken. The principal complications at all sites are pain, trauma to the artery (e.g., dissection of the intima) and surrounding tissues (e.g., nerve), hematoma, infection, thrombosis, and distal embolization of air, clot, pieces of the cannula, and other debris. (Central or proximal embolization is possible with a rapid flushing of the cannula with a large volume of fluid under high pressure.[38]) Preventive measures for most of these complications are obvious, but a few deserve special mention. Skillful arterial cannulation obviously requires practice, but it is developed most rapidly and maintained at a high level by a thoughtful and deliberate approach. The accumulation of clot along the cannula can be minimized but not eliminated by using those made of the least thrombogenic material (e.g., Teflon), by using a nontapered, narrow diameter cannula, by maintaining a continuous flushing of the cannula with an isotonic salt (no sugar) solution containing heparin (2 units/ml), and by limiting manipulation and movement of the cannula that can traumatize the arterial endothelium. Thrombosis of the more distal vessels (i.e., radial, ulnar, dorsalis pedis) is more common the longer the period of cannulation, but they almost always recannulize within a few weeks. Extreme care should be used in reinserting the metal needle stylet through a flexible cannula so that the cannula is not punctured or sheared off in the artery. Meticulous care of the puncture site in the skin and of the stopcocks, etc. is required to prevent infection. The lines, connectors, stopcocks, and flush solution must all be kept free of air bubbles.

Erroneous data and mistaken interpretations of data can be associated with the use of techniques involving arterial cannulation. Simultaneous direct blood pressure measurements will differ according to the site of measurement, degree of arterial constriction, and diameter of the cannula. For example, systolic pressure is higher and diastolic pressure lower in the dorsalis pedis than in the brachial or radial arteries. Arterial spasm due to the use of vasoconstrictor drugs reduces the systolic pressure in the radial artery compared to the aorta. In general, the more distal the artery, the greater the vascular resistance in the vessels leading to the artery. The smaller the cannula, the greater the distortion of the pulse-pressure wave form and pressure measurements.

Blood sampling from an indwelling arterial cannula may yield erroneous data because of technical failures. Sufficient blood should be withdrawn and discarded before taking a sample in order to minimize its contamination by old blood in the cannula and by the heparinized flush solution. Air bubbles must be eliminated promptly from samples intended for blood gas analysis, and the samples should be placed in ice until they are analyzed in order to reduce blood cell metabolism and gas diffusion through the walls of plastic syringes and liquid seals in glass syringes.

PRESSURE MEASURING SYSTEMS

Pressure measuring systems consist of a mechanical coupling of a pressure transducer, to an amplifier and signal processing unit, and one or more means of displaying the data. The anesthesiologist should understand the principles underlying the function of each system, should be able to calibrate the system both internally and against a mercury manometer, and should recognize the limitations and potential for inaccuracy in each system. Discussions of general principles of pressure measurement are available elsewhere,[39] and the manufacturer's representative should be consulted about the specific details of operation and features of any particular device.

Obviously, the most important feature of the electromechanical system is how accurately it reflects the actual pressures and pulse wave occurring in the vascular system. The pressures displayed by the system can be compared with those simultaneously measured by a sphygmomanometer in the same patient. One method is to determine the "return-to-flow" pressure. The blood pressure cuff is placed above the site of arterial cannulation on an extremity and inflated until the pulse wave is eliminated. The cuff pressure is released slowly while watching for the return of the first sign of a pulse wave at which point the cuff pressure is noted as the "return-to-flow" systolic pressure. In most cases, there will be close agreement of systolic pressure determined by return-to-flow and by Korotkoff sounds, the latter being the most widely used clinically to describe the patient's blood pressure.

Direct pressure reading is commonly 10 to 20 torr greater than that measured by return-to-flow, especially at higher blood pressures associated with systolic hypertension and atherosclerotic vascular disease. Usually discrepancies of this sort are attributable to the characteristics of the pressure transducer. Directly measured systolic pressures lower than those determined by sphygmomanometry and Korotkoff sounds are attributable to the use of compliant rather than rigid tubing to connect the arterial cannula to the transducer, to the presence of air bubbles in the connecting tubing or transducer dome, or to marked peripheral vascular constriction produced by intense sympathetic stimulation or vasopressor drugs.

CENTRAL VENOUS PRESSURE

An anatomic definition of central venous pressure (CVP) is that pressure of blood measured in the vena cavae at their junction with the right atrium. In the normal subject lying in a supine position in the horizontal plane, the same mean pressure will exist in the right atrium, superior vena cava, and the inferior vena cava above the diaphragm. Phasic changes in the CVP occur normally as a result of the right atrial contraction, opening and closing of the tricuspid valve, and as a result of ventilation. In the absence of certain disease states, phasic changes in the CVP are inconsequential and the mean CVP provides useful information about the hemodynamic status of the patient providing that factors affecting it are recognized and its limitations understood.

In the normal individual, CVP reflects the balances between blood volume, venous capacitance, and cardiac function. The CVP is elevated by increases in the circulating blood volume and decreases in venous capacitance or cardiac output. In the patient with normal cardiovascular and pulmonary function, the CVP is a useful monitor that should be used by the anesthesiologist in the following circumstances:

1. Surgical procedures in which large fluctuations of blood volume are anticipated (e.g., blood loss, transudation of fluid).

2. Hypovolemic or potentially hypovolemic patients (e.g., bowel obstruction, ascites, chronic hypertension).

3. Patients in shock (i.e., from hemorrhage, anaphylaxis).

4. Massively traumatized patients.

In the above circumstances, the trend of change in the CVP may be more significant than the absolute pressure. Moreover, the CVP should be interpreted in the light of other indicators of cardiovascular function. For example, a declining arterial blood pressure and urine output may indicate cardiac failure in the presence of a rising CVP or they may reflect hypovolemia with a low or falling CVP. In the latter case, a rapid infusion of fluid or blood may be given until a satisfactory arterial blood pressure is established or until the CVP rises to an abnormally high level (> 15 torr), at which point an inotropic drug may be indicated.

In patients with cardiac disease and abnormal ventricular function, the use of a Swan-Ganz catheter is usually indicated to monitor *both* right and left heart filling pressures. In the face of vena caval obstruction, pulmonary embolism, pulmonary hypertension, right ventricular failure, or cardiac tamponade, it may be equally or more important to monitor the CVP than the left-sided filling pressures, and in some cases the Swan-Ganz catheter may be contraindicated. Obviously, the less expensive CVP catheter with its lesser risk of complications is preferable to the Swan-Ganz catheter when the latter is not indicated.

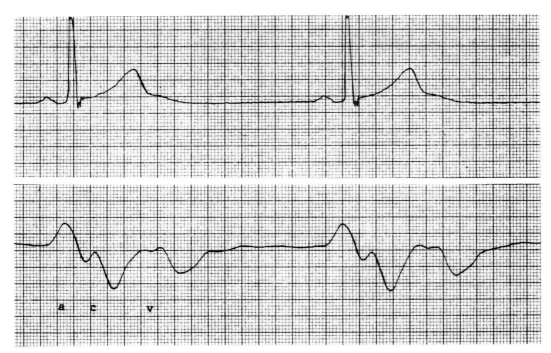

Fig. 6-2 Central venous pressure waves and the corresponding electrocardiogram. The *a* wave is produced by atrial contraction. The *c* wave is the result of bulging of the tricuspid valve into the atrium at the beginning of ventricular contraction. The *v* wave occurs as the atrium fills with the tricuspid valve closed. The transient decrease (*y* descent) in pressure following the *v* wave occurs when the tricuspid valve opens and the atrium is partially emptied by the flow of blood into the ventricle, and lasts until the continued return of blood to the heart restores the filling of the atrium. (Kaplan, JA: Hemodynamic monitoring, Cardiac Anesthesia. Edited by Kaplan JA. New York, Grune & Stratton, 1979, pp 71-115, by permission.)

Observation of venous pressure waves (Fig. 6-2) on an oscilloscope or recorder is sometimes useful in the patient with cardiac disease. The *a* wave is absent in atrial fibrillation, is inconstant in the presence of atrioventricular conduction block, and is very large (Cannon wave) if the atrium contracts against a closed tricuspid valve (e.g., junctional rhythm). Large *a* waves are also seen in the presence of tricuspid stenosis, right ventricular hypertophy, pulmonic stenosis, and pulmonary hypertension. A large *v* wave is seen when there is tricuspid regurgitation. Similar changes are present in left atrial and pulmonary capillary wedge pressures associated with comparable functional derangements of the left atrium and ventricle.

It must be remembered that the CVP reflects primarily right heart function and is not a reliable indicator of left ventricular performance. Left ventricular failure and pulmonary edema can be present, especially on an acute basis, and the CVP may remain well within the normal range.[40]

Central venous cannulation is indicated for CVP monitoring and for a variety of other reasons (Table 6-16). It can be accomplished by way of a number of venous routes, and the techniques for each are best learned from a tutor and are well described elsewhere.[28,41,42] The choice of a particular site for central venous cannulation is determined by accessiblity, convenience, success rate in directing the catheter to the central venous

Table 6-16. Indications for Central Venous Cannulation

Central venous pressure monitoring (see text)
Lack of peripheral veins for cannulation
Intravenous administration of vasopressors, potassium and other drugs likely to injure peripheral veins and tissues
Rapid infusion of blood and fluids
Removal of autologous blood
Frequent blood sampling
Aspiration of air emboli
Hyperalimentation
Transvenous insertion of temporary pacing leads
Right heart catheterization studies
Insertion of a pulmonary artery catheter (Swan-Ganz)
    Pressure measurements
    Cardiac output determinations by thermodilution
Pulmonary angiography
    Reduction of pulmonary vascular and left atrial pressures by removal of blood during cardiopulmonary bypass

circulation, risk to the patient, and probable duration of use. Cannulation at any particular site is contraindicated by the presence of infection at the site and by the inclusion of that site in the surgical field.

The highest success rate of localizing the catheter in the superior vena cava or right atrium is achieved through the internal jugular vein, which is a convenient and accessible route in most patients. There is a risk of cannulating the carotid artery, although this can be reduced to a minimum by careful adherence to proven techniques and especially the utilization of a small caliber needle (22 gauge, 1.5 inch length) to localize the internal jugular vein prior to insertion of the larger bore catheter (Table 6-17 and Fig. 6-3). Relative contraindications to using the internal jugular route include heparinization of the patient at the time of cannulation, previous surgery of the neck (e.g., thyroidectomy, carotid endarterectomy), distortion of anatomic relationships by tumor or trauma, and the inability to position the patient's head properly. Complications associated with internal jugular cannulation are those of any other route plus some specific ones (Table 6-18).

The availability of the "J-wire" guide for directing catheters past bends and branching

of vessels has increased the success rate of localizing the catheter tip in the central circulation by way of the external jugular veins.[41,42] Cannulation of an external jugular vein avoids the risks of inserting a needle deep into the neck. The high incidence of major complications has reduced the use of the subclavian vein by anesthesiologists. There is a low rate of success in reaching the central venous circulation by way of basilic and cephalic arm veins.[43] The femoral vein can be used providing the catheter is sufficiently long to reach the mediastinal level of the vena cava; the possibility of cannulating branches of the inferior vena cava is present.

Measurement of venous pressures can be done with a simple manometer filled with isotonic aqueous solution or with a pressure transducer system similar to that described for direct arterial pressure measurement (but with a higher gain to measure smaller changes and lower pressures). The recording of venous pressure waves requires a pressure transducer with a high frequency response. Several technical points should be remembered:

1. Different units of pressure may be used; 1.36 cm H_2O equals 1 mm Hg or 0.74 mm Hg equals 1 cm H_2O. One kilopascal (kPa) equals 7.5 mm Hg or 10.2 cm H_2O.

2. The zero point of the manometer or transducer must be positioned exactly if low venous pressures are to be measured accurately and reproducibly; the right atrium is usually considered as the zero level and it corresponds to the midaxillary line in the supine patient who has normal anatomy of the spine and thorax.

3. Changes in the CVP occur with ventilation because changes in intrathoracic pressure are readily transmitted through the relatively thin-walled atrium and vena cavae. During spontaneous ventilation, inspiration lowers the CVP. Positive pressure ventilation and all forms of positive airway pressure raise the CVP as does coughing or any Valsalva maneuver. (These CVP changes provide an indication of the central location of the CVP

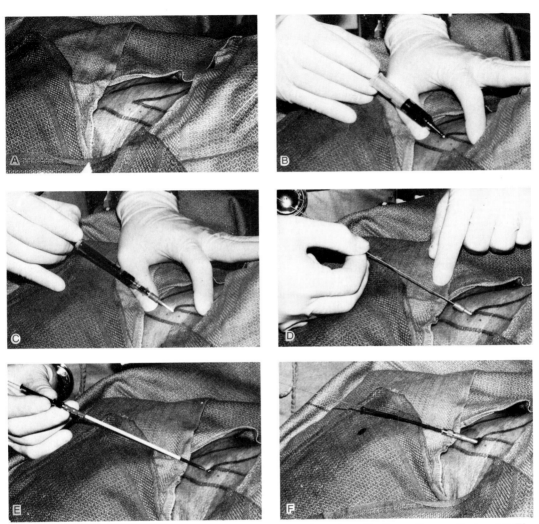

Fig. 6-3 Cannulation of the right internal jugular vein for insertion of a Swan-Ganz catheter. (*A*) The borders of the medial and lateral heads of the sternocleidomastoid muscle have been marked, the skin prepared with antiseptic, and the field draped with sterile towels. (*B*) The right internal jugular vein has been identified with a 1½ inch 21 gauge needle on a 5cc syringe. Venous blood has been withdrawn into the syringe. (*C*) A 1¾ inch 18 gauge Jelco Teflon catheter-over-needle unit is inserted into the right internal jugular vein while withdrawing venous blood into a 3 cc syringe. (*D*) A 0.9 mm x 40 cm flexible guide wire is inserted through the Jelco catheter into the right internal jugular vein and advanced into the superior vena cava. (*E*) After making a 3 mm slit in the skin, the 8-French dilator-sheath unit is about to be inserted over the guide wire and through the skin and subcutaneous tissues into the right internal jugular vein. (*F*) The 8-French sheath has been advanced into the right jugular vein and the guide wire and dilator have been partially withdrawn. They will subsequently be removed completely and the Swan-Ganz catheter will be inserted through the sheath. (Photographs provided by J. A. Kaplan, of Emory University Medical School. Figures C, D, and E are from Kaplan JA: Hemodynamic monitoring, Cardiac Anesthesia. Edited by Kaplan JA. New York, Grune & Stratton, 1979, pp 71-115, by permission.)

Table 6-17. Sequence of Steps in Cannulating the Right Internal Jugular Vein

1. Patient's head lying flat and rotated completely to left.

2. Palpate lateral aspect of the medial head and medial aspect of the lateral head of the sternocleidomastoid muscle as it divides to insert on the sternum and clavicle. Mark these borders on the overlying skin with a felt-tipped pen. A triangle will be formed with the clavicle as its base and the apex located approximately 6 cm (3 average-sized fingerbreadths) above the clavicle. The presence of arterial pulsation within the triangle may contraindicate an attempt to cannulate the internal jugular vein.

3. Prepare the area with antiseptic (e.g., povidone-iodine, Betadine).

4. Infiltrate the skin and subcutaneous tissue at the apex of the triangle with a local anesthetic (½ or 1 percent lidocaine HC1).

5. Cover the surrounding area with a sterile drape and follow sterile technique until the procedure is completed.

6. Place the patient in an appropriate degree of a head-down, legs-up position.

7. Using a 21 gauge 1.5 inch needle on a 5 ml syringe containing 1 cc of ½ or 1 percent lidocaine HC1, identify the internal jugular vein. Verify the medial location of the carotid artery and the absence of arterial pulsations within the triangle. Starting at the apex, direct the needle toward the middle third of the clavicle at a 30 degree angle to the skin and advance the needle while maintaining a slight negative pressure with the syringe plunger. Normally two "pops" will be felt: the first the carotid sheath and the second the vein wall.

   If the vein is not identified when the full length of the needle is inserted, gradually withdraw it while maintaining negative pressure in the syringe; sometimes the needle will have penetrated the back wall of the vein. A Valsalva maneuver by the patient will distend the vein. If unsuccessful, redirect the needle more laterally; if unsuccessful, try a more medial direction with cautious awareness of the carotid artery.

   The color of the blood drawn into the syringe provides a clue to whether it is venous or arterial as long as two points are remembered:
   (a)   The local anesthetic remaining in the syringe will make the original blood entering the syringe appear brighter red, but venous-colored blood will be evident as additional blood is withdrawn.
   (b)   The PvO_2 may be elevated if the patient is breathing oxygen-enriched gases.

   The vein diameter is approximately the same as the patient's thumb; it should be possible to maintain a withdrawal of blood while advancing or withdrawing the needle a distance of 1.5 to 2.5 cm in a normal size adult male.

   If there is doubt about arterial puncture, three steps can be considered:
   (a)   Remove the syringe from the needle and see if there is a spurting flow of blood, from the needle left in the vessel, indicating arterial puncture.
   (b)   Determine the PO_2 of the blood.
   (c)   Remove the needle, compress the vessel, and start over or choose an alternate site for venipuncture and cannulation.

8. If the vein is properly located, inject the local anesthetic–blood solution as the needle is withdrawn in order to anesthetize the track that will be followed when the larger cannula is inserted.

9. Insert the CVP-size cannula in exactly the same direction that was followed by the localizing needle. Two methods are used to insert the CVP cannula:
   (a)   the large bore cannula of at least 5 inches in length, is inserted directly. The cannula can be over the needle or within the needle.
   (b)   An 18 gauge 1¾ inch cannula is inserted, a guide wire passed, the 1¾ inch cannula removed, and then the CVP cannula is passed over the guide wire into the vein (Seldinger technique). This technique requires that a dilator or dilating type cannula be used to penetrate the subcutaneous tissues and vein wall *after* a small 2 to 3 mm puncture of the skin has been made with a scalpel blade inserted right up against the guide wire. The Seldinger approach is used for insertion of a Swan-Ganz type catheter (see Table 6-22).

(Continued)

Table 6-17. (*Continued*)

10. The success of central venous cannulation can be verified by: (a) the lack of a spurting flow of blood, (b) easy withdrawal of venous-colored blood, and (c) appropriate pressures and pressure wave forms for a CVP.

11. The cannula should be secured in place and the puncture site in the skin dressed with a sterile bandage. The site should be inspected periodically to detect evidence of hematoma formation and any change in the position of the cannula (i.e., to prevent dislodgement, kinking).

12. The patient should be returned to a normal position *only after* connecting the cannula to the pressure transducer manometer in order to avoid the aspiration of air emboli through the cannula. It is also helpful to have the patient hold his breath in inspiration while the cannula is open to air.

Table 6-18. Complications of Central Venous Cannulation

General
  Infection—local and systemic
  Tissue trauma—nerve, artery, vein injuries
  Hematoma and extravasation of infused substances
  Thrombophlebitis
  Catheter shearing and embolization
  Air embolism
  Perforation of vena cava or right atrium by catheter
    Mediastinal infusion of fluids
    Pericardial tamponade
    Hydrothorax, hemothorax

Specific sites
  Internal jugular cannulation
    Carotid artery puncture (hematoma, airway compression, arteriorvenous fistula)
    Brachial plexus injury
    Thoracic duct perforation (left internal jugular)
    Pneumothorax
  Subclavian cannulation
    Subclavian artery puncture (hemothorax)
    Pneumothorax
  Femoral cannulation
    Femoral artery puncture (retroperitoneal hemorrhage)
    Femoral nerve injury
    Inferior vena cava perforation (retroperitoneal infusion of substances)
    Venous thrombosis and emboli

catheter tip, but do not prove it.) Changes in thoracic and mediastinal pressures as a result o) the accumulation of air, fluid, and blood are also reflected in the CVP.

PULMONARY ARTERY PRESSURE

Availability of the balloon-tipped, flow-directed catheter (Swan-Ganz[44]) provides the anesthesiologist with an easy method of measuring pulmonary artery and left heart filling pressures in almost any patient. Swan-Ganz catheters are now produced with features allowing the measurement of central venous pressure (CVP) and pulmonary artery pressures (PAP) including diastolic (PAdP), systolic (PAsP), mean ($\overline{\text{PAP}}$), and occluded (PAoP) or pulmonary capillary wedge pressures (PCWP). It is feasible to obtain samples of mixed venous blood from the pulmonary artery (e.g., for measurements of PvO_2 and intrapulmonary shunt) and to administer drugs into the central venous circulation or directly into the pulmonary artery (e.g., vasodilators). In addition, the inclusion of a thermistor permits the measurement of cardiac output (CO) by thermodilution, and the incorporation of bipolar electrical lead wires makes it possible either to monitor the electrocardiogram or to pace the heart temporarily with an external pacemaker. Catheters are also made for angiographic studies, oxyhemoglobin measurements, and right-sided cardiac catheterization of pediatric patients. These features can be utilized to great advantage by the anesthesiologist in the operating room and intensive care unit for diagnostic, monitoring, therapeutic, and investigational purposes.

Data obtained with the aid of the Swan-Ganz catheter can be used to calculate hemodynamic variables of importance to the anethesiologist. For example, systemic and pulmonary vascular resistances, stroke volume, subendocardial coronary perfusion pressure, and several indices of cardiovascular performance can be estimated.

Indications for the preoperative insertion (intraoperative use) of a particular Swan-Ganz catheter are still evolving and differ among individual anesthesiologists. They are summarized in Table 6-19. Its potential usefulness to the anesthesiologist intraoperatively is illustrated in terms of differential diagnosis (e.g., see Table 6-20) and as a guide to therapy (e.g., see Fig. 30-8 in Ch. 30).

Interpretation and application of information obtained with a Swan-Ganz catheter requires a good understanding of normal physiology (Ch. 23) as well as of individual disease states (e.g., Chs. 29–31, 42). There are some generalizations and specific limitations that should be remembered.

Normal hemodynamic values are shown in Table 6-21. In *normal* individuals the following are true (~approximates; = equals; ∞ is proportional to):

LAP ~ PCWP ~ PAdP~CVP
LAP ~ LVEDP
LVEDP ∞ LVEDV
LV performance ∞ LVEDV (See Fig. 30-2)
LV output = RV output

Some of these generalizations are also true in patients with certain cardiovascular diseases, but they often must be verified in the particular patient; and it may prove to be worthwhile to do so. For example, it may be useful to record the PCWP and the PAdP simultaneously over the range of pressures encountered as time passes. If there is a close correlation, the PAdP can be used in place of the PCWP should it become impossible to obtain wedge pressures because of balloon malfunction or a change in the location of the catheter tip.

The generalizations clearly do not apply in certain disease states. For example, pulmonary diastolic hypertension distorts the relationship between PAdP and PCWP and LAP. The presence of mitral stenosis or of a mitral valvular prosthesis creates a gradient between LAP and LVEDP. Any left to right shunt (e.g., atrial or ventricular septal defect, patent ductus arteriosus) will increase right ventricular output and thermodilution measurements of cardiac output while reducing left ventricular output. The application of positive pressure to the airway alters the intracardiac and pulmonary artery pressures. It is customary to make pressure measurements at end-expiration to provide consistency. The use of positive end-expiratory pressure (PEEP) or continuous airway pressure (CPAP) alters the pressure readings (e.g., PCWP may not correlate with LAP when PEEP > 10 cm H_2O). This has led to some controversy about the interpretation of pressure measurements. It would appear that a workable compromise involves: following trends of pressure in relation to other hemodynamic and ventilatory variables rather than concentrating on the absolute values; assuming that measurements made under the actual clinical conditions are influencing cardiovascular performance in the manner expected; and most importantly, recognizing that changes in respiratory function and therapy will alter the measurements and probably cardiovascular function as well. Obviously, the effects of sudden large changes must be monitored closely and dealt with appropriately.

Techniques for insertion of the Swan-Ganz catheter are best learned from an experienced tutor and are well described elsewhere.[28] A few points are emphasized below in relation to minimizing the complications associated with the use of these catheters. Possible sites for insertion are the same as those for central venous cannulation, and again, the highest success rates are associated with the internal jugular route—especially the right internal jugular vein, which provides a straight path into the superior vena cava (Table 6-22 and Fig. 6-3). The limitations, complications, and contraindications related to each percutaneous cannulation site are essentially the same as described for central venous cannulation.

The curved tip containing an inflatable balloon can be used to advantage in directing

Table 6-19. Indications for the Preoperative Insertion of a Swan-Ganz Catheter

*Non-Cardiac Surgery**
  Heart disease
    With suspicion or evidence of impaired left ventricular function (e.g., heart failure)
    Severe coronary artery disease
    Severe, uncontrolled arterial hypertension
    Valvular disease
    Pericardial disease with evidence of tamponade
  Unstable circulation
    Massive trauma
    Extensive burns
    Hypotensive shock
    Sepsis

  Suspected or diagnosed pulmonary emboli

  Aortic surgery with anticipation of cross-clamping

  Portal systemic shunt surgery; severe portal hypertension with cirrhosis

  Severe respiratory failure

Cardiac Surgery
  Coronary artery revascularization† with
    Poor, left ventricular function: ejection fraction < 0.4, left ventricular end-diastolic pressure (LVEDP)> 18 torr
    Recent myocardial infarction
    Complication of myocardial infarction (e.g., ventricular aneurysm, septal rupture, mitral valvular insufficiency)
    Extensive coronary obstruction (e.g., triple vessel disease) with evidence of impaired ventricular performance during ischemia (e.g., LVEDP increases by more than 10 torr or is greater than 18 torr after injection of contrast media into coronary arteries)
    Diffuse coronary atherosclerosis especially in distal vessels (anticipate impaired ventricular function after cardiopulmonary bypass due to poor myocardial preservation by cold hyperkalemic perfusion of coronary arteries)
    Valvular heart disease

  Mitral or aortic valvular replacement

  Pulmonary hypertension

  Idiopathic hypertrophic subaortic stenosis (IHSS)

  Pericardiectomy with evidence of tamponade

* While major surgery involving significant blood and fluid replacement provides the strongest indication for use of the Swan-Ganz catheter in patients with the diseases listed, its use is also advisable for patients undergoing minor surgery while receiving a major anesthetic.
† The Swan-Ganz catheter is useful during cardiopulmonary bypass to detect elevations of pulmonary capillary pressure caused by the accumulation of blood in the absence of a functioning left ventricular vent. Elevated capillary hydrostatic pressure coupled with reduced oncotic pressure can lead to pulmonary edema.

Table 6-20. The Swan-Ganz Catheter in the Differential Diagnosis of Low Cardiac Output

Etiology of Low Cardiac Output	Right Atrial or Central Venous Pressure	PCWP	Pulmonary Artery Diastolic (PAdP) vs PCWP Pressures
Hypovolemia	Low	Low	PADP = PCWP
Left ventricular failure	Normal or high	High	PADP = PCWP
Right ventricular failure	High	Normal	PADP = PCWP
Pulmonary embolism	High	Normal	PADP > PCWP
Chronic pulmonary hypertension	High	Normal*	PADP > PCWP
Cardiac tamponade	High =	High =	PADP = PCWP

* In the absence of valvular disease.

Table 6-21. Normal Pressures in the Cardiovascular System of Recumbent Adults

Location	Abbreviation	Pressure (torr)	
		Mean	Range
Central venous	CVP	6	1–10
Right atrium	RAP	4	−1–+8
Right ventricle			
Systolic	—	24	15–28
End-diastolic	RVEDP	4	0–8
Pulmonary artery			
Systolic	PAsP	24	15–28
Diastolic	PAdP	10	5–16
Mean	$\overline{PAP}$	16	10–22
Pulmonary capillary wedge	PCWP	9	5–16
Left atrium	LAP	7	4–12
Left ventricle			
Systolic	—	130	90–140
End-diastolic	LVEDP	7	4–12
Brachial artery			
Systolic	s	130	90–140
Diastolic	dBP	70	60–90
Mean	$\overline{BP}$	85	70–105

(Modified from Schlant RC: Normal physiology of the cardiovascular system, The Heart .4th edition. Edited by Hurst, JW. New York, McGraw Hill, pp. 71–100.)

the catheter to the right atrium (e.g., from a femoral vein) but adds the possibility of damaging veins, especially peripheral ones and those branching from the vena cava if it is inflated carelessly and inappropriately in relation to the anatomy of the venous system. The balloon should always be inflated slowly and easily; no attempt should be made to inflate it against higher than normal resistance (as determined by the feel of inflating the balloon prior to its insertion into the body).

Complications related to the insertion and maintenance of pulmonary artery catheters include the following:

1. Complications related to central venous cannulation (see Table 6-18).

2. Perforation of the right atrium, right ventricle, or a pulmonary artery resulting in hemopericardium, hemothorax, hemoptysis, or frank bleeding into the airway. Perforation of the right side of the heart and of the pulmonary artery is very unlikely to occur if the catheter is advanced gradually with the balloon inflated and without forcing its insertion. Coiling of the catheter in the heart or vessels should be avoided because its repeated abra-

sion of the endothelium could lead to erosion of the wall. Coiling is suspected when an unusually long length of catheter is inserted (i.e., greater than 60 cm from the internal jugular puncture site to the wedge position, see Table 6-23) and it can be verified by a standard anterior-posterior chest x-ray. Other clues to coiling are the recurrence of dysrhythmias and the apparent flipping of the catheter tip in and out of the right ventricle as indicated by pressure changes. Perforation of a small pulmonary artery can occur especially if the catheter tip is maintained in a continuous wedge position or if the vessel is ruptured by improper inflation of the balloon (i.e., overinflation or inflation against higher than normal resistance).

3. Cardiac dysrhythmias of all types due to contact of any part of the catheter with the wall of the heart, especially the intraventricular septum in the area of the conducting system. Precautions include (a) electrocardiographic and continuous systemic arterial blood pressure monitoring during insertion of the catheter; (b) complete inflation of the balloon to cover the catheter tip when it

Table 6-22. Sequence of Steps in the Insertion of a Swan-Ganz Catheter via the Right Internal Jugular Vein of an Average-Size Adult Patient

1. Place an 18 gauge 1¾ inch cannula into the right internal jugular vein as described in Table 6-17 (steps 1 to 9b). Verify the proper location of the cannula by the easy withdrawal of venous blood and the absence of spurting arterial blood. This verification step is very important in minimizing the inadvertent insertion of the guide wire and introducer into extravascular tissues or the carotid artery.

2. Insert a 0.9 mm × 40 cm guide wire flexible or J-end first through the cannula. It should advance easily to a total distance of approximately 20 cm.

3. Remove the 1¾ inch cannula and with a No. 11 scalpel blade enlarge the cutaneous hole around the wire to a 3 mm slit to facilitate introduction of the dilator and sheath. It is important to insert the scalpel blade directly against the wire so that no strand of skin will obstruct the insertion of the dilator and sheath.

4. Place the dilator-sheath set over the wire but do not advance it into the skin until the external tip of the guide wire extends back beyond the length of the dilator where it can be grasped as needed to withdraw it from the patient.

5. Insert the dilator-sheath set through the skin and subcutaneous tissues and into the vein while twisting (rotating) it back and forth to facilitate its penetration of the tissues. As the dilator-sheath set is advanced, withdraw the guide wire progressively to avoid its internal tip being advanced into the heart. When the sheath is inserted to an appropriate length (9 to 10 cm), remove both the guide-wire and dilator together and place a syringe directly on the sheath to verify its proper placement by the easy withdrawl of venous blood and to avoid the aspiration of air into the venous circulation. Aspiration of air is minimized by keeping the patient in a head-down position and by asking the patient to hold his breath at maximum inspiration.

6. Prepare the Swan-Ganz catheter for insertion by (a) inflating the 1.5 cc capacity balloon to check for leaks, (b) filling the CVP and PA channels with heparinized saline, and (c) checking the integrity of the electrical leads for the thermister and pacing functions if these are in the catheter. With the pressure transducer open to the fluid-filled PA channel, the pressure tracing on the oscilloscope screen or writer should reflect motion of the catheter tip.

7. Insert the Swan-Ganz catheter as follows (Fig. 6-4):
   (a) the curved tip of the catheter should be pointed to 11 to 12 o'clock as the catheter is inserted into the introducer sheath and internal jugular vein;
   (b) once the 20 cm mark reaches the hub of the sheath, the balloon should be inflated with 1 cc of air and a CVP tracing should be evident on the screen or writer;
   (c) the catheter should then be advanced gradually as it passes through the right atrium (RA tracing usually evident after 25 to 30 cm of the catheter has been inserted) and into the right ventricle (RV tracing at 35 to 40 cm);
   (d) as soon as an RV tracing is seen, the volume of the balloon should be inflated to 1.5 cc, and then the catheter advanced into the pulmonary artery (PA tracing at 45 to 50 cm);
   (e) once a PA tracing is observed, the catheter should be advanced slowly to the wedge position (PCWP tracing 50 to 60 cm). Proper placement is indicated by a PA tracing when the balloon is deflated and a PCWP tracing when it is inflated. Frequently, the catheter will advance into a continuous wedge position as it becomes more compliant at body temperature and is subjected to the continuous drag of flowing blood. Obviously, it will have to be withdrawn to the proper position.

8. With satisfactory positioning of the catheter, the introducer sheath can be connected to a side-arm port adapter to allow the infusion of substances via the internal jugular vein or it can be withdrawn from the vein. If it is to be withdrawn from the vein, it is useful to maintain the tip of the sheath in the subcutaneous tissues temporarily (1 to 2 hours) to provide a sterile channel for adjustments of the catheter's position.

9. The site of skin puncture should then be covered with a sterile dressing and the catheter secured so as to avoid kinking and dislodgment.

10. Some of the commonly encountered problems include:
    (a) catheter enters the inferior vena cava instead of the right atrium (continuous CVP tracing as it is advanced)—withdraw the introducer sheath by 1 to 1.5 cm and repeat steps listed in item 7.
    (b) catheter enters right atrium and ventricle but fails to enter pulmonary artery—often remedied by orienting curved tip of catheter toward 11 to 12 o'clock on insertion; may require different orientation; often facilitated by advancing the catheter from the right ventricle as the patient takes a deep inspiration, which increases the blood flow into the pulmonary artery.
    (c) an excessive length of catheter is inserted (i.e., > 60 cm in adult)—coiling is likely and this can be confirmed by portable anterior-posterior chest x-ray; the catheter should be withdrawn carefully and another attempt to insert it correctly should be made.

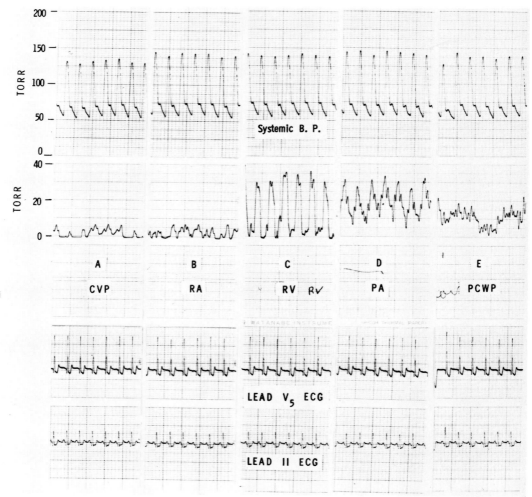

Fig. 6-4 Pressure tracings recorded during the insertion of a balloon-tipped, flow-directed pulmonary artery catheter (Swan-Ganz). The top tracing shows systemic blood pressure, the tracing beneath it shows pressures measured at the tip of the Swan-Ganz catheter as it passed through the superior vena cava, CVP; right atrium, RA; right ventricle, RV; pulmonary artery, PA; and into a wedge position, PCWP. The transient decrease in the PCWP occurred with spontaneous inspiration by the patient. Refer to Table 6.22 for details of catheter insertion.

enters the right ventricle; (c) efficient passage of the catheter through the ventricle and into the pulmonary artery (facilitated by orienting the curved tip of the catheter to 11 or 12 o'clock before inserting it into the right internal jugular vein and by having the patient take a deep inspiration as the catheter is advanced from the ventricle); (d) withdrawing the catheter from the ventricle should dys-rhythmias persist; (e) having intravenous lidocaine ready to administer rapidly; (f) having a functional defibrillator close at hand; (g) using a Swan-Ganz catheter with pacing leads in a patient with a high risk of developing complete heart block (e.g., right and posterior left bifasicular conduction block); and (h) having an assistant experienced in cardiopulmonary resuscitation in the imme-

Table 6-23. Usual Distances from the Site of Percutaneous Venous Insertion of a Swan-Ganz Catheter to Various Locations in Adults

Location	Range of Distances in cm from Vein Puncture Site			
	Right Internal Jugular	Right Femoral	Right Antecubital	Left Antecubital
Junction vena cavae and right atrium	15–20	30	40	50
Right atrium	25–35	+10–15*	+20–25	+30–35
Right ventricle	35–45	+10–15	+20–25	+30–35
Pulmonary artery	45–55	+10–15	+20–25	+30–35
Pulmonary artery wedge position	50–60	+10–15	+20–25	+30–35

* The distance from the right femoral vein to the right atrium is 35 to 50 cm (i.e., 25 to 35 + 10 to 15 cm).

diate vicinity. Dysrhythmias may also occur during withdrawal of the catheter after it has been used for some time. A smooth, steady withdrawal avoiding sudden forceful motions is probably best.

4. Pulmonary infarction can result from maintaining the catheter in a continuous wedge position. This can be prevented by limiting continuous inflation of the balloon to less than a few minutes; continous monitoring of the PAP and immediately withdrawing the catheter should the pressure tracing change to that of the PCWP (the presence of a *v* wave in the PCWP tracing may lead to its being mistaken for a PAP tracing [Fig. 6-5]); (c) avoiding the insertion of excessive lengths of catheter and coiling; and obtaining an anterior-posterior chest x-ray as soon as possible after insertion of the catheter (at least in the immediate postoperative period) and daily thereafter to rule out coiling and malpositioning of the catheter.

5. Thrombus formation begins to occur along the catheter immediately after its insertion. This appears to be of little consequence in the short term use of the catheter and is a reason to avoid using it any longer than necessary. It results in a utilization of platelets[45] and theoretically could lead to embolization of the thrombus while the catheter is in position or during its removal.

6. Infection along the length of the catheter can lead to thrombophlebitis, endocar-ditis, pulmonary vasculitis, and interstitial infection. For this reason, insertion of the catheter should be done under sterile conditions and prophylactic antibiotics may be indicated.

7. Trauma to cardiac and vascular structures can occur during insertion and withdrawal of the catheter as a result of knotting of the catheter or retained air in the balloon. This is best prevented by avoiding coiling of the catheter and by avoiding kinking, which can obstruct the return of air from the balloon. Any unusual resistance encountered during removal of the catheter should be investigated (e.g., chest roentgenogram) before any further attempt to withdraw the catheter is made.[46]

8. Improper therapy based on misinterpretation of data obtained with the Swan-Ganz catheter. To minimize the incidence of obtaining incorrect data or of misinterpreting data the following procedures, among others, should be done: regular checking of the function of the catheter and the pressure measuring system; making therapeutic decisions in the light of an evaluation of the total patient and not just relying on a single monitoring device; and careful observation of the responses to therapy.

Contraindications to the insertion of a Swan-Ganz catheter (Table 6-24) are mostly relative to the benefits that may be derived from its use.

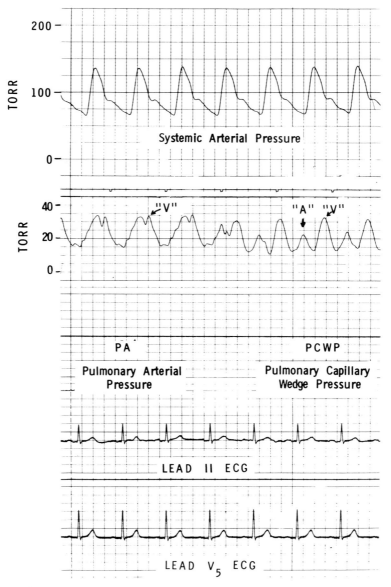

Fig. 6-5 An example of the occurrence of a *v* wave ("V") in both the pulmonary artery and pulmonary capillary wedge pressure tracings from a patient with impaired left ventricular function due to coronary artery disease. Notice that the *v* wave in the PCWP tracing could be mistaken for a pulmonary arterial pressure tracing with the catheter in a continuous wedge position.

CARDIAC OUTPUT

Cardiac output is the volume of blood pumped into the systemic circulation each minute. It summarizes the overall perform-ance of the cardiovascular system, but partic-ularly the pumping function of the heart. It is the volume of blood available for tissue per-fusion, although the actual blood flow to any specific tissue is regulated by several factors

Table 6-24. Relative Contraindications to the Insertion of a Swan-Ganz Catheter

Lack of experienced personnel
Lack of suitable pressure monitoring equipment
Presence of a recently inserted transvenous pacemaker*
Tricuspid or pulmonic valvular stenosis or prosthetic valve
Frequent ventricular dysrhythmias uncontrolled by antiarrhythmic drugs
Coagulopathy (relative contraindication to the use of internal jugular, subclavian, or femoral vein for insertion)
Bifasicular heart block. Use Swan-Ganz catheter with bipolar pacing leads.
Inability to insert catheter into pulmonary artery because of pulmonary hypertension, pulmonic or tricuspid regurgitation, right to left shunt†

* There is less risk of dislodging permanent pacing wires or entangling them with the Swan-Ganz catheter after the wires have been covered with tissue (scar, endothelium). The Swan-Ganz catheter should be inserted cautiously to avoid its coiling within the ventricle, and it should be removed as soon as possible when the patient's condition no longer warrants its use.
† The catheter tip should not be left in the right ventricle where it can contact the septum and cause dysrhythmias. A catheter coiled in the ventricle should be withdrawn as soon as the coiling is discovered or suspected and as carefully as possible to avoid entangling the chordae tendinae and papillary muscles.

controlling resistance in the arterioles conveying blood to that tissue. As such, cardiac output is a useful clinical measure to help assess the overall status of the circulatory system.

Blood pressure, the most widely measured hemodynamic variable, is determined by two factors, cardiac output and systemic vascular resistance:

$$BP = CO \times SVR$$

This relationship is important on two counts: if cardiac output and blood pressure are known, the systemic vascular resistance can be calculated (Table 6-25); and it is apparent that blood pressure can be in the normal range even with a very low cardiac output, if vascular resistance is sufficiently high. A patient with a very high vascular resistance and an abnormally low cardiac output does not survive very long in that state because his tissues and organs are not being perfused adequately even if his blood pressure is normal. On that basis, determinations of cardiac output have considerable clinical significance.

Indications for measurements of cardiac output in patients undergoing anesthesia and surgery are currently defined more by the circumstances encountered than by the particular type of disease or surgery. It is important to note the disturbing frequency at which unexpectedly low cardiac outputs and high vascular resistances are found when inciden-

tal measurements are made in patients whose hemodynamic status otherwise appears to be satisfactory. The significance of such unexpected findings awaits greater clinical experience and formal studies of the impact of such measurements on the overall results of patient care.

Clearly, cardiac output determinations have become a mainstay in the therapeutic management of hemodynamically unstable patients in the operating room, especially those undergoing cardiac surgery.[47-50] The analysis of cardiovascular function, and particularly left ventricular performance, in relation to cardiac filling pressures, cardiac output, and systemic vascular resistance, has simplified the therapeutic management of such patients. For example: Is hypotension following cardiopulmonary bypass a result of inadequate blood volume, poor myocardial contractility, or low systemic vascular resistance? Under anesthesia produced by nitrous oxide and narcotic analgesics, is a hypertensive episode better treated with a myocardial depressant such as halothane or with a vasodilating drug such as sodium nitroprusside? In the treatment of cardiac failure with an infusion of a catecholamine, is there an undesirable increase in vascular resistance that will impede the pumping of blood by the heart and limit perfusion of vital organs such as the kidney and liver?

Methods of measuring cardiac output in-

Table 6-25. Hemodynamic Values for Normal Recumbent Adults

Variable Cardiac Performance	Abbreviation		Formula	Units	Range
Cardiac output (70 kg, 1.7 m², male)	CO		*	L/min	5–6
Cardiac index	CI	=	$\dfrac{CO}{BSA\dagger}$	L/min/m²	2.8–4.2
Heart rate	HR		*	bpm	60–90
Stroke volume	SV	=	$\dfrac{CO}{HR} \times 1000$	ml/beat	60–90
Stroke index	SI	=	$\dfrac{SV}{BSA\dagger}$	ml/beat/m²	40–60
LV stroke work index	LVSWI	=	$\dfrac{1.36 \ \overline{BP} - PCWP}{100} \times SI$	gram-meters/m²	45–60
RV stroke work index	RVSWI	=	$\dfrac{1.36 \ \overline{PAP} - CVP}{100} \times SI$	gram-meters/m²	5–10
Vascular Resistance					
Systemic (total peripheral)	SVR(TPR)	=	$\dfrac{\overline{BP} - CVP}{CO} \times 80$	dynes-sec/cm⁻⁵	900–1500
Pulmonary	PVR	=	$\dfrac{\overline{PAP} - PCWP}{CO} \times 80$	dynes-sec/cm⁻⁵	150–250

* Determine by measurement.
† BSA = body surface area in square meters (m²).

clude thermodilution, dye dilution, the Fick technique, and analysis of the aortic pulse contour.[51-53] The principles underlying each of these techniques are discussed in the references cited along with the details of their application.

Thermodilution has become the most widely used technique in clinical practice for a number of reasons. It can be accomplished with the thermodilution-type Swan-Ganz catheter, and the catheter is usually needed for pressure measurements in the same patients who would benefit from cardiac output determinations. Multiple determinations can be made at frequent intervals. The indicator is a small volume of 5 percent dextrose in water at room temperature or chilled in ice. There is no need for the withdrawal and reinfusion of arterial blood. There is no recirculation of the indicator to confound computations of cardiac output. The measurement is easily made with a portable and compact, though expensive computer. (Computer costs will probably lessen as catheter

sales increase.) With good technique, the measurements by thermodilution are reproducible and correlate closely with those obtained by more traditional methods.

There are several limitations of the thermodilution technique. It measures right heart output and therefore is invalid in the presence of intracardiac and pulmonary-systemic shunts (e.g., atrial and ventricular septal defects, patent ductus arteriosus); it requires the insertion of a Swan-Ganz catheter, which is not always possible or desirable; and the speed of injection and the temperature of the thermal indicator solution should be constant for reproducible results.

The principle of cardiac output determination by thermodilution is similar to that of other indicator dilution techniques. That is, a known quantity of the indicator is injected at one point and its concentration is measured at a more distant point after it has been thoroughly mixed with the blood volume that dilutes it. Knowing the initial quantity and measuring the final concentration permits calculation of the dilution volume. In the case of thermodilution, a cold solution is diluted by warm blood; the amount of "cold" injection is known and the change of temperature over time in the blood passing from the injection site (CVP port of the Swan-Ganz catheter) to the catheter-thermistor site in the pulmonary artery is a measure of the dilution of the "cold" bolus.

DERIVED HEMODYNAMIC VARIABLE AND INDICES

With pressure measurements and cardiac output determinations in hand, it is possible to calculate a number of other estimates of cardiovascular performance. These are summarized in Table 6-25. Calculations can be facilitated with a slide rule, pocket calculator, or a computer (programmable calculator). Computers are becoming more common in the operating suite and intensive care units, and they can easily be programmed to perform these simple calculations.[47]

OTHER MEASURES OF CARDIOVASCULAR FUNCTION

A number of other techniques for assessing cardiac function are employed in clinical research. Their use in patient care outside of the investigational setting is currently very limited, but with further refinements, clinical applications will likely develop, especially for those that are noninvasive. Systolic time intervals,[54] echocardiography,[55] and radioisotopes in combination with scanning devices[56] are examples of noninvasive methods.[29, 57]

In addition to new techniques, there are modifications and new uses of existing methods that may prove useful to the anesthesiologist in the operating room. As for most of the modern sophisticated monitoring techniques, new developments are likely to occur primarily in the care of patients undergoing anesthesia and surgery for heart disease. Of current interest is the estimation of myocardial oxygen supply and demand.

Direct measurements of total and regional coronary blood flow (CBF) are largely confined to the research setting. Recognition of the important factors determining CBF has led to the development of some indicators of the potential for coronary perfusion, although each index has its limitations.[58] For example, CBF depends on the coronary perfusion pressure (CPP). Also, coronary perfusion, especially in the subendocardium, occurs mostly during diastole when the intracavitary pressure transmitted to the coronary capillaries is lowest. Thus, two indices of the potential for coronary perfusion are:

$$CPP = dBP - LVEDP$$

where CPP = coronary perfusion pressure, dBP = diastolic arterial blood pressure, and LVEDP = left ventricular diastolic pressure, which can be estimated by the PCWP in the absence of certain congenital and valvular heart diseases; and

$$DPTI = (dBP - LAP) \times d_t$$

where DPTI = diastolic pressure time index, dBP = diastolic arterial blood pressure, LAP = left atrial pressure for which the PCWP can be substituted, and d_t = the diastolic time

It should be noted that increases in left ventricular filling pressures (LVEDP, LAP, PCWP) will decrease CPP and DPTI and at the same time increase myocardial oxygen demand. Similarly, tachycardia reduces the diastolic time and the DPTI and increases oxygen utilization by the heart. Most importantly, it has to be recognized that coronary perfusion in the presence of coronary artery obstruction is determined primarily by the resistance at the individual obstructions rather than by the LVEDP. Thus, the above indices represent the potential for total coronary perfusion and do not indicate the sufficiency of perfusion of any particular areas of the myocardium, especially those dependent on blood flow through partially obstructed vessels.

Estimates of myocardial oxygen demand are also based on the knowledge of the most important factors that determine it: systolic blood pressure (sBP), LVEDP, heart rate, and contractility. A series of indices of demand have been proposed because no one index has been developed to include all four factors.[28]

The rate pressure product (RPP) is the product of heart rate and systolic blood pressure:

$$RPP = sBP \times HR$$

The RPP correlates with myocardial oxygen consumption during exercise and bears a fairly constant relationship to the onset of angina pectoris in any one patient with ischemic heart disease. If the RPP for the development of angina or ischemic changes in the ECG is known for a particular patient, the anesthesiologist should attempt to maintain a lower RPP during the perioperative period. In the absence of specific information, it is desirable to keep the RPP at less than 15,000 (e.g., HR < 100, sBP < 150). There is some controversy about the usefulness of the RPP because it is fairly obvious that the increase in heart rate may be more detrimental than an increase in blood pressure. Increased heart rate increases oxygen demand and reduces its supply (i.e., less diastolic perfusion time). Increased systolic blood increases oxygen demand but also increases mean and often diastolic blood pressure so that coronary perfusion pressure and oxygen supply tend to increase.

A triple index has been suggested as a means of including three of the four major determinants of myocardial oxygen demand.

$$TI = sBP \times HR \times PCWP$$

A somewhat arbitrary upper limit of 150,000 is suggested but no correlations with symptoms and signs of ischemia have been made.

The tension time index (TTI) is the product of heart rate and area under the systolic portion of the aortic blood pressure curve. It can be calculated as:

$$TTI = sBP \times Ts$$

where sBP = mean *systolic* blood pressure, and Ts = duration of systole. The mean *systolic* blood pressure is not readily determined, and the correlation of TTI with direct measurements of oxygen consumption is not uniformly consistent.

The endocardial viability ratio (EVR) has been suggested as an index of subendocardial ischemia under certain conditions. It can be represented as:

$$EVR = \frac{DPTI}{TTI} = \frac{\text{oxygen supply}}{\text{oxygen demand}}$$

A normal EVR is above 1.0. Its usefulness in patients with coronary artery obstructions is questionable, since perfusion through the obstructed vessel is determined primarily by resistance at the site of partial obstruction.

RENAL FAILURE

Monitoring renal function intraoperatively is important for two reasons: renal function is intimately linked to the hemodynamic status of the patient and the volume and composition of urine are sensitive indicators of hypovolemia and deficiencies of cardiovascular performance; and the kidneys are vulnerable to damage from a variety of causes and renal failure accounts for a significant portion of the postoperative morbidity and mortality in critically ill patients.

The primary means of monitoring renal function intraoperatively involves the collection of urine, which usually necessitates the insertion of a urinary bladder catheter. As with almost any other monitoring device, there are risks associated with bladder catheterization, especially the risk of a urinary tract infection and the associated fever, which can pose the difficult problems of differential diagnosis and antibacterial therapy in the postoperative period. Obviously, the decision to insert a catheter should be justified by the benefits of monitoring renal function (and by the potential risks of failing to do so). Indi-

Table 6-26. Indications for the Preoperative Insertion of Urinary Bladder Catheter and Monitoring of Urine Volume and Composition

Hypovolemia (e.g., dehydration, hemorrhage)
Major trauma
Anticipation of the need for transfusion of large volumes of blood
Cardiopulmonary bypass
Aortic or renal vascular surgery
Renal disease
Obstructive jaundice, major biliary tract surgery
Sepsis and therapy with nephrotoxic antibiotics
Lengthy or extensive surgery especially in elderly and critically ill patients
Complicated obstetrics (e.g., abruptio placentae)

(Modified from Mazze, RI. Critical care of the patient with acute renal failure. Anesthesiology 47:138, 1977.)

cations for urinary bladder catheterization prior to surgery are listed in Table 6-26.[59]

The major problem faced by the anesthesiologist in terms of renal function is oliguria. It is widely held that a urine flow rate of less than 0.5 ml/kg/hr in the perioperative period represents oliguria and should be investigated. It is essential first to rule out mechanical problems in the transfer of urine from the bladder to the urometer (e.g., obstruction of the catheter by mucus plugs, tissue, clots; kinking or disconnection of the tubing; and impairment of gravity drainage by a steep head-down position). Once mechanical problems have been eliminated as the cause of a low recovery of urine, the anesthesiologist is faced with the differential diagnosis of oliguria. This is discussed in detail in Chapter 24. However, it is worth noting here that the differential diagnosis is facilitated by laboratory analysis of the composition of urine, especially in relation to plasma (e.g., see Table 6-27). Determination of the differential diagnosis is also aided by the use of hemodynamic monitoring techniques to evaluate the adequacy of fluid and blood replacement and to determine the level of cardiovascular performance.[59,60]

The anesthesiologist may gain some useful information about nonrenal disorders by observing the appearance of the urine and by making some simple tests of its composition.

For example, a pink to port-wine coloration of urine is indicative of the degree of hemolysis that may result from cardiopulmonary bypass or from the transfusion of incompatible blood. Testing the urine from a diabetic patient for glucose and ketones is one way to evaluate his need for insulin. Cloudy urine may indicate a high protein content reflecting myoglobinuria in the traumatized patient, renal damage in the patient with acute tubular necrosis, or the presence of bacteria from a urinary tract infection. Appropriate testing of the urine at the direction of the anesthesiologist can lead to the early initiation of the appropriate therapy and enhance the possibilities of preserving renal function.

BODY TEMPERATURE

It is common for body temperature to change during anesthesia and surgery for many reasons (Table 6-28). A decrease of 2 or 3 °C is usually tolerated without serious adverse consequences except for postoperative shivering, which increases oxygen demand and patient discomfort. There is greater concern about body temperature 2 or 3 °C above normal and about temperatures below 34 °C (Table 6-29). Because of its high risk of morbidity and mortality and because it is induced by certain anesthetic drugs, the detection of malignant hyperthermia is of special importance to anesthesiologists. For these reasons, it has become the standard of practice to monitor body temperature in all patients undergoing general anesthesia except for the briefest minor surgical procedures.

It should be noted that certain patients are especially at risk for significant changes in body temperature. Infants and young children have a large body surface relative to their body mass; as a result they are vulnerable to both hypothermia and hyperthermia from external causes. Their relatively high minute ventilation adds to this vulnerability. Patients with a personal or family history of malignant hyperpyrexia are obviously at un-

Table 6-27. Differential Diagnosis of Oliguria

Measure	Physiological Oliguria*	Prerenal Oliguria†	Acute Tubular Necrosis
Urinary sodium	< 10 mEq/L	< 25 mEq/L	> 25 mEq/L
Urinary specific gravity	> 1.024	> 1.015	1.010–1.015
Urine/Plasma osmolality	> 2.5	> 1.8	< 1.1
Urine/Plasma urea	> 100	> 20	< 10
Urine/Plasma creatinine	> 60	> 30	< 10

* Due to the action of antidiuretic hormone.
† Due to poor perfusion of the kidneys.
(Modified from Mazze, RI. Critical care of the patient with acute renal failure. Anesthesiology 47:138, 1977.)

Table 6-28. Causes of Body Temperature Changes Intraoperatively

Exposure (skin, surgical site)
Humidification and warming of inspired gases
Intravenously administered fluids, blood products
Irrigating solutions, wet packs
Chemical reactions (e.g., polymerization of bone cement, methylmethacrylate)
Alterations of body temperature regulation (e.g., anesthetic effects on the hypothalamus, muscle relaxants prevent shivering)
Disease states (e.g., malignant hyperthermia, thyrotoxicosis, infection)
Mechanical devices (e.g., thermal blankets, cardiopulmonary heat exchangers, heat lamps)

Table 6-29. Consequences of Hyperthermia and Hypothermia

Hyperthermia (Fever)	Hypothermia
Increased oxygen demand	Decreased oxygen availability
Respiratory and metabolic acidosis	Slowing of metabolically dependent process
Increased ventilatory work	Decreased drug biotransformation
Increased cardiac work	Impaired renal transport processes
Hypovolemia due to evaporation	Altered membrane excitability
Hypoglycemia	Cardiac rate and rhythm changes
	CNS depression, coma
Malignant hyperthermia	Shivering
Death	Sympathetic nervous system stimulation
	Hyperglycemia

usual risk, perhaps even when the indicted drugs (i.e., succinylcholine, halothane) are avoided. Patients undergoing prolonged operations are at risk of hypothermia because of their prolonged ventilation with dry gases through an endotracheal tube; and patients having extensive abdominal or thoracic surgery easily become hypothermic because of the exposure of large surface areas in the operative field and because of the inefficiency of warming blankets placed under them.

There are a number of body sites at which body temperature can be monitored (Table 6-30).[29] They differ in the precision with which they reflect the temperature of the body core and in the complications of im-

proper placement of the temperature probe. In most cases, however, it is the direction and rate of change rather than the precise degree of temperature that is of concern to the anesthesiologist.

There are a number of devices including the standard thermometer to measure body temperature. The temperature probes most commonly used in modern operating rooms are based on the change in the electrical resistance of certain metals.[61] Although they are relatively sophisticated and sturdy devices, they occasionally malfunction. The wise anesthesiologist regularly evaluates their function in order to minimize the occurrence of spurious readings.

Table 6-30. Sites of Body Temperature Monitoring

Sites	Comments
Skin	Varies with subcutaneous blood flow, sweating, radiation and conduction of heat to/from extracorporeal objects
Axilla	Varies with blood flow
Muscle	Requires special probe; varies with blood flow
Rectum	Varies with blood flow, fecal mass acts as an insulator
Pharyngeal and upper esophagus	Reflects temperature of respiratory gases; nasal probes have the risk of producing epistaxis
Tympanic membrane	Closely approximates temperature of blood perfusing the brain when probe is against tympanic membrane; discrepancies arise when probe is located away from membrane or impacted in cerumen, which acts as an insulator; risks of membrane perforation and hemorrhage
Lower esophagus (20 cm below pharyngoesophageal junction)	Closely approximates temperature of aortic blood (core temperature)
Pulmonary artery (Swan-Ganz thermodilution catheter)	Not the primary purpose of the Swan-Ganz catheter, but it can be used to measure the temperature of blood in the body core

THE ANESTHESIA LABORATORY[62]

It is becoming more common for anesthesia departments to operate a clinical biochemistry-type laboratory in close proximity to the operating rooms for determinations of blood gases, hematocrit and hemoglobin, electrolytes (K^+, Na^+, Ca^{++}), glucose, osmolality, coagulation studies, etc. The information provided by these analyses can be invaluable to the management of anesthetized and critically ill patients. It is essential that the anesthesiologist understand the laboratory procedures and methods so that he can recognize the potential sources of errors. It is important for the laboratory to function efficiently; accurate results should be produced in a minimum time so that the anesthesiologist can identify problems and recognize trends in time to take corrective actions that will minimize the morbidity and mortality of patients under his care. Needless to state, the accuracy of the results is of primary importance. The anesthesiologist should be alert to the possibility of technical errors, equipment malfunction, and spurious results (e.g., the interchange of samples from different patients). He should always attempt to correlate the biochemical data with that derived from physiological monitoring.

REFERENCES

1. Gravenstein JS, Newbower RS, Ream AK, et al (Editors): *Monitoring Surgical Patients in the Operating Room.* Springfield, Ill, Charles C Thomas, 1979
2. Gravenstein JS, Newbower RS, Ream AK et al (Editors): Essential Noninvasive Monitoring. New York, Grune and Stratton, 1980
3. Laver MB (Editor): Symposium on Monitoring. Anesthesiology, 45:113, 1976
4. Saidman LJ, Smith NT (Editors): Monitoring in Anesthesia, New York, John Wiley and Sons, 1978
5. Bruner JMR: Fundamental concepts of electrical safety. ASA Refresher Courses in Anesthesiology 2:11, 1974
6. Eger EI II: Anesthetic Uptake and Action. Baltimore, Williams and Wilkins, 1974
7. Shapiro HM: Monitoring in neurosurgical anesthesia, Monitoring in Anesthesia. Edited by Saidman LJ and Smith NT. New York, John Wiley and Sons, 1978, pp 171–204
8. Cucchiara RF, Sharbrough FW, Messick JM, et al: An electroencephalographic filter-processor as an indicator of cerebral ischemia during carotid endarterectomy. Anesthesiology 51:77, 1979
9. Fleming RA, Smith NT: An inexpensive device for analyzing and monitoring the electroencephalogram. Anesthesiology 50:456, 1979; also see Letters to Editor, Anesthesiology 52:101, 1980
10. Myers RR, Stockard JJ, Saidman LJ: Moni-

toring of cerebral perfusion during anesthesia by time-compressed Fourier analysis of the electroencephalogram. Stroke 8:331, 1977

11. Clark DL, Rosner BS: Neurophysiologic effects of general anesthetics: I. Electroencephalogram and sensory evoked responses in man. Anesthesiology 38:564, 1973

12. Kety SS, Schmidt CF: Determination of cerebral blood flow in man by the use of nitrous oxide in low concentrations. Am J Physiol 143:53, 1945

13. Hoedt-Rasmussen K, Sveinsdottir E, Lassen NA: Regional cerebral blood flow in man determined by intraarterial injection of radioactive inert gas. Circ Res 18:237, 1966

14. Obrist WD, Thompson HK, Wang HS, et al: Regional cerebral blood flow estimated by ^{133}Xe inhalation. Stroke 6:245, 1975

15. Sharbrough FW, Messick JM, Sundt TM: Correlation of continuous electroencephalograms with cerebral blood flow measurements during carotid endarterectomy. Stroke 4:674, 1973

16. Geevarghese KP, Patel TC: Anesthesia and surgical treatment of cerebrovascular insufficiency. Int Anesthesiol Clin 15:57, 1977

17. Shapiro HM: Intracranial hypertension: Therapeutic and Anesthetic considerations. Anesthesiology 43:445, 1975

18. Hill DW: Electrode systems for the measurement of blood-gas tensions content and saturation, The Scientific Foundations of Anaesthesia, 2nd edition. Edited by Scurr C and Feldman S. Chicago, Year Book Medical Publishers, 1974, pp 98–107

19. Kelman GR, Nunn JF: Nomograms for correction of blood PO_2, P_{CO_2}, pH and base excess for time and temperature. J Appl Physiol 21:1484, 1966

20. Severinghaus JW: Blood gas calculator. J Appl Physiol 21:1108, 1966

21. Nunn JF: Applied Respiratory Physiology. 2nd edition. London, Butterworths, 1977

22. Dripps RD, Eckenhoff JE, Vandam LD: Introduction to Anesthesia. Philadelphia, WB Saunders, 1977

23. Messner JT, Loux PC, Grossman LB: Intraoperative transcutaneous pO_2 monitoring in infants. Anesthesiology 51:S319, 1979

24. Mazze RI: Therapeutic misadventures with oxygen delivery systems: The need for continuous in-line oxygen monitors. Anesth Analg 51:787, 1972

25. Benumof JL: Monitoring respiratory function during anesthesia, Monitoring in Anesthesia. Edited by Saidman LJ and Smith NT. New York, John Wiley and Sons, 1978, pp 31-51

26. Fink BR: The Human Larynx: A functional study. New York, Raven Press, 1975

27. Suter PM, Schlobohm RM: Determination of functional residual capacity during mechanical ventilation. Anesthesiology 41:605, 1974

28. Kaplan JA: Hemodynamic monitoring, Cardiac Anesthesia. Edited by Kaplan JA. New York, Grune and Stratton, 1979, pp 71-115

29. Reitan JA: Noninvasive monitoring, Monitoring in Anesthesia. Edited by Saidman LJ and Smith NT. New York, John Wiley and Sons, 1978, pp 85-125

30. Bedford RF: Wrist circumference predicts the risk of radial-arterial occlusion after cannulation. Anesthesiology 48:377, 1978

31. Bedford RF: Long-term radial artery cannulation: Effects on subsequent vessel function. Crit Care Med 6:64, 1978

32. Mangano DT, Hickey RF: Ischemic injury following umcomplicated radial artery catheterization. Anesth Analg 58:55, 1979

33. Barnes RW, Foster EJ, Janssen GA, et al: Safety of brachial artery catheters as monitors in the intensive care unit—Prospective evaluation with the Doppler ultrasonic velocity detector. Anesthesiology 44:260, 1976

34. Prys-Roberts C: Monitoring of the cardiovascular system, Monitoring in Anesthesia. Edited by Saidman LJ and Smith NT. New York, John Wiley and Sons, 1978, pp 53-83

35. Adler DC, Byron-Brown CW: Use of the axillary artery for intravascular monitoring. Crit Care Med 1:148, 1973

36. Youngberg JA, Miller ED: Evaluation of percutaneous cannulation of the dorsalis pedis artery. Anesthesiology 44:80, 1976

37. Ersoz CJ, Hedden M. Lain L: Prolonged femoral artery catheterization for intensive care. Anesth Analg 49:160, 1970

38. Lowenstein E, Little JW, Lo HH: Prevention of cerebral embolization from flushing radial-artery cannulas. N Engl J Med 285:1414, 1971

39. Cliffe P: Transducers for the measurement of pressure, The Scientific Foundations of Anaesthesia. 2nd edition. Edited by Scurr C and Feldman S. Chicago, Year Book Medical Publishers, 1974, pp 42-52

40. Buchbinder N, Ganz W: Hemodynamic

monitoring: Invasive Techniques. Anesthesiology 45:146, 1976

41. Blitt CD, Wright WA, Petty WC, et al: Central venous catheterization via the external jugular vein: A technique employing the J-wire. JAMA 229:817, 1974

42. Blitt CD: Monitoring the cardiovascular system during anesthesia, *Anesthesia and the Patient with Heart Disease.* Edited by Brown BR Jr. Philadelphia, FA Davis Co, 1980, pp 19-37

43. Webre DR, Arens JF: Use of cephalic and basilic veins for introduction of central venous catheters. Anesthesiology 38:389, 1973

44. Swan HJC, Ganz W, Forrester JS, et al: Catheterization of the heart in man with the use of a flow directed balloon tipped catheter. N Engl J Med 283:447, 1970

45. Richman KA, Kim YL, Marshall BE: Thrombocytopenia induced by Swan-Ganz catheters. Anesthesiology 51:S161, 1979

46. Fibuch EE, Tuohy GF: Intracardiac knotting of a flow-directed balloon-tipped catheter. Anesth Analg 59:217, 1980

47. Barash PG, Chen Y, Kitahata LM, et al: The hemodynamic tracking system: A method of data management and guide for cardiovascular therapy. Anesth Analg 59:169, 1980

48. Forrester JS, Diamond G, Chatterjee K, et al: Medical therapy of acute myocardial infarction by application of hemodynamic subsets. N Engl J Med 295:1356, and 1404, 1976

49. Lappas DG, Powell WMJ, Daggett WM: Cardiac dysfunction in the perioperative period: Pathophysiology, diagnosis, and treatment. Anesthesiology 47:117, 1977

50. Lappas DG, and Gayes JM: Intraoperative monitoring. Int Anesthesiol Clin 17:157, 1979

51. English JB, Hodges MR, Sentker C, et al: Comparison of aortic pulse-wave contour analysis and thermodilution methods of measuring cardiac output during anesthesia in the dog. Anesthesiology 52:56, 1980

52. Ganz W, Swan HJC: Measurement of blood flow by thermodilution. Am J Cardiol 29:241, 1972

53. Guyton AC, Jones CE, Colman TG: Circulatory Physiology: Cardiac Output and Its Regulation. 2nd edition. Philadelphia, WB Saunders, 1973

54. Lewis RP, Rittgers SE, Forrester WF, et al. A critical review of the systolic time intervals. Circulation 56:146, 1977

55. Gerson JI, Gianaris CG: Echocardiographic analysis of human left ventricular diastolic volume and cardiac performance during halothane anesthesia. Anesth Analg 58:23, 1979

56. Pitt B, Strauss HW: Evaluation of ventricular function by radioisotopic techniques. N Engl J Med 296:1097, 1977

57. Wexler LF, Pohost GM: Hemodynamic monitoring: Noninvasive techniques. Anesthesiology 45:156, 1976

58. Klocke FJ, Ellis AK, Orlick AE: Sympathetic influences on coronary perfusion and evolving concepts of driving pressure, resistance, and transmural flow regulation. Anesthesiology 52:1, 1980

59. Mazze RI: Critical care of the patient with acute renal failure. Anesthesiology 47:138, 1977

60. Bastron RD, Deutsch S: Anesthesia and the Kidney. New York, Grune and Stratton, 1976

61. Cliffe P: The measurement of temperature, The Scientific Foundations of Anaesthesia. 2nd edition. Edited by Scurr C and Feldman S. Chicago, Year Book Medical Publishers, 1974, pp 79-84

62. Gabel JC: Monitoring of body chemistry during anesthesia, Monitoring in Anesthesia. Edited by Saidman LJ and Smith NT. New York, John Wiley and Sons, 1978, pp 15-29

7

The Electrocardiogram and Anesthesia*

Joel A. Kaplan, M.D.

INTRODUCTION

The electrocardiogram (ECG) is presently used as a routine monitor during anesthesia and surgery. Cannard and Dripps showed the value of the ECG in diagnosing rhythm disturbances during anesthesia back in 1960.[1] Standard limb lead II was used at that time and is still often used to diagnose dysrhythmias, since its electrical axis parallels the electrical axis of the heart and the P wave is usually easily observed. In recent years, coronary artery disease has become the number one health problem in the United States. Patients coming for all types of surgical procedures have significant coronary artery disease and in these patients, the ECG should be used to identify myocardial ischemia as well as for dysrhythmias. Many patients are now coming for surgery with pacemakers in place and the ECG also is necessary in order to enable the physician to evaluate the function of the pacemaker during the surgical procedure.

The major uses of the ECG in the perioperative period may be broken down into its role in the preoperative, intraoperative, and postoperative periods.

Preoperative Diagnostic Use

1. Rate and rhythm disturbances[2]—bradycardias and tachycardias can be diagnosed as to their site of origin, possible etiologies, and seriousness. Supraventricular rhythms can be separated from ventricular rhythms and decisions about therapeutic interventions made preoperatively.

2. Ischemic heart disease[3]—previous myocardial infarction or myocardial ischemia can be diagnosed from the QRS complex and the ST segments of the ECG. Acute changes indicating ischemia must always be sought in the preoperative period.

3. Chamber enlargement[4]—atrial and ventricular hypertrophy can easily be diagnosed from the preoperative ECG. Specific chamber enlargements tend to be associated with certain diseases, e.g., left ventricular hypertrophy with hypertension and left atrial hypertrophy with mitral stenosis.

4. Heart block[5]—both sinoatrial and atrioventricular conduction blocks can be diagnosed. Especially important are combinations of bundle branch blocks of the conduction system. First degree, second degree, and third degree heart block, as well as different types of hemiblocks, can be diagnosed and may even lead to the institution of pacemaker therapy in the preoperative period.

5. Electrolyte and/or drug effects[6,7] can

* Parts of this chapter are reproduced with modification from Kaplan JA (Editor): Cardiac Anesthesia. New York, Grune & Stratton, 1979, by permission of the publisher.

frequently be diagnosed from the preoperative ECG. For example, a tentative diagnosis of hypokalemia and digitalis effect may be important in the anesthetic management of the patient.

6. Pericardial disease[8] occasionally may be diagnosed from the preoperative ECG. Pericarditis and pericardial effusions have characteristic ECG abnormalities associated with them.

Intraoperative Uses

1. Dysrhythmia detection[9] is still the most important use of the intraoperative ECG. The ability to separate supraventricular from ventricular dysrhythmias and to be able to assess therapeutic interventions are extremely important uses of the ECG. Common dysrhythmias, such as wandering atrial pacemaker or AV dissociation under halogenated anesthetics, may explain hemodynamic changes occurring during the anesthetic procedure.

2. Ischemia detection[10] has become much more important, since we now often anesthetize patients with severe coronary artery disease. Differentiation of inferior wall from anterior or lateral wall ischemia is now possible in the intraoperative period.

3. Electrolyte changes frequently occur during anesthesia and mechanical ventilation.[11] Significant changes in potassium as well as calcium levels occur and can be diagnosed with the ECG.

4. Pacemaker function needs to be continuously evaluated during surgical procedures in patients with permanent pacemakers.[12] This is especially important when the surgical procedure will be carried out near the pacemaker wires or pacemaker unit, or the electrocautery will be used during surgery.

Postoperative Use

1. To detect significant dysrhythmias with associated changes in blood gases or electrolytes which may be a result of the anesthetic procedure.[13]

2. To detect myocardial ischemia or infarction which may occur in the postoperative period.[14]

DYSRHYTHMIA DETECTION

Dysrhythmia detection has been and still is the most important use of the ECG during and after surgery. Intraoperative dysrhythmias were reported in the early 1900's, but the first large series of ECG studies during anesthesia was reported in 1936 by Kurtz.[15] In over 100 patients, he found that sinus dysrhythmias, premature ventricular contractions, and downward displacement of the pacemaker site predominated. More recent studies by Katz, et al, have found the incidence of intraoperative dysrhythmias to vary from 16 to 62 percent.[9] Bertrand studied 100 patients, using continuous electromagnetic tape recording during surgery and reported an 84 percent incidence of supraventricular and ventricular dysrhythmias when *continuous* ECG monitoring was used.[16] Dysrhythmias were most common at times of endotracheal intubation and extubation. Patients with preexisting cardiac disease had a higher incidence of ventricular dysrhythmias than patients without known heart disease (60 percent versus 37 percent). Twenty-four of 25 patients with heart disease had a rhythm disturbance during surgery. In a further study of patients undergoing cardiac surgery, Angelini reported that 29 of 50 patients (58 percent) having valve surgery and 35 to 78 patients (45 percent) having coronary revascularization developed significant postoperative dysrhythmias.[13] These dysrhythmias tended to correlate with the severity of the heart disease, led to a prolonged hospital stay, and were responsible for up to 80 percent of the surgical mortality in their series.

During surgery, the ECG is read off the oscilloscope and may be recorded if indicated. All operating rooms where cardiac surgery is performed should have ECG recording capabilities and portable recorders should be available to all other operating rooms for interesting diagnostic problems. It would be ideal to have a single-channel ECG recorder on *all* operating room oscilloscope monitors. The recorder is needed to make an accurate

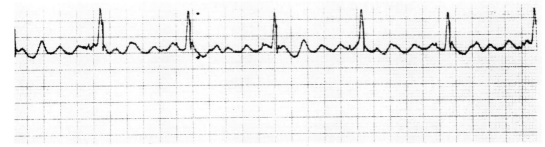

Fig. 7-1 The electrocardiogram of the patient shortly after he was placed on cardiopulmonary bypass. He is in a regular sinus rhythm; however, the ECG appears to show atrial flutter because of an artifact created by the roller pump on the heart-lung machine.

diagnosis of complex dysrhythmias as well as to precisely evaluate changes in the P wave, QRS complex, ST segment, and T wave. In addition, the recorder is frequently needed to assure that artifacts are not being seen on the oscilloscope. It is preferable to have the recorder make the tracing directly from the patient without going through the oscilloscope's additional filtering circuits. The presence of a written record of the dysrhythmia is far preferable to storage, nonfade oscilloscopes that have been employed on some operating room monitors. The ability to store the tracing on the oscilloscope adds little to our capability of diagnosis in the operating room. It certainly does not provide written documentation and a legal record, both of which a written ECG trace provides because the latter tracing can be added to the patient's hospital record. The ECG recorders in the operating room should meet all the standards of accepted cardiology ECG recorders, including types of paper, paper speeds, and markers.

Artifacts on the oscilloscope can be a major problem and lead to incorrect diagnosis in the intraoperative period. The ECG may simulate dysrhythmias under the following conditions:

1. tremors of various types, as when the patient is awake and shivering in the operating room;

2. hiccoughing or movements of the diaphragm;

3. artifacts in the ECG machine;

4. poor ECG connections;

5. interference from other electrical apparatus, especially the electrocautery or heart lung machine; and

6. interference from contact with other persons.

The ECG may produce several types of artifacts either as a result of malfunction or improper adjustment.[17] Loose electrodes may simulate many types of arrhythmias. Broken electrode wires, as well as hypothermia with shivering, have been reported to produce an ECG pattern easily mistaken for atrial flutter.[18] Artifacts produced by the roller pumps on the heart-lung machine can also create an ECG pattern that resembles atrial flutter (Fig. 7-1).

The biggest electrical problem with ECG monitoring in the operating room is the electrocautery. When the cautery is used, the standard ECG is totally lost as a result of electrical interference. This interference is a combination of radio frequency current (800 to 2,000 kHz), AC line frequency (60 Hz), and low frequency current (0.1 to 10 Hz). Doss has shown that it is possible to modify the ECG preamplifiers so that they will function well in the presence of the electrocautery.[19] It is *surprising* that this has not been done to more monitoring units designed for use in the operating room.

In addition to the above causes of ECG changes that may occur during surgery, there

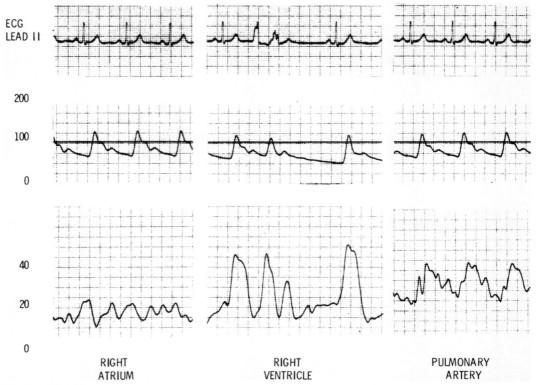

ECG
LEAD II

200

100

0

40

20

0

RIGHT
ATRIUM

RIGHT
VENTRICLE

PULMONARY
ARTERY

Fig. 7-2 Multifocal premature ventricular contractions are demonstrated on lead II of the ECG. These occurred with passage of the catheter from the right atrium into the right ventricle and then disappeared upon placement of the catheter into the pulmonary artery. The arterial tracing demonstrates the systemic hemodynamic effects of these premature contractions.

are purely mechanical factors that can also affect the ECG.[20] Respiratory variation can affect the height of the QRS complex, which is most marked in leads III and AVF. This is due to either a shift of the mediastinum with respirations or to a change in volume of the heart with the respiratory effects of venous return. Studies have shown that increases in the ventricular end-diastolic volume lead to increased height of the QRS complex and hemorrhage leads to a decreased height of the QRS complex.[21] Catheters or wires in the heart may lead to dysrhythmias; this is seen with the placement of the Swan-Ganz catheter often leading to premature ventricular contractions (Fig. 7-2). There is also decreasing amplitude of the QRS complex and T

waves with increasing age as well as an increased incidence of premature ventricular contractions in patients over the age of 40 years.[22]

The use of ECG telemetry has been tried in a few institutions up to the present time. Most authorities feel that it is not necessary in the modern operating room setting. The advantages of having no hard wires are balanced against disadvantages with technical problems and limitations in capabilities and modifications. However, there are some instances in which it could be extremely useful such as during neurodiagnostic radiologic procedures, e.g., pneumoencephalography or computer axial tomography (CT scan). In these cases, access to the patient is not very

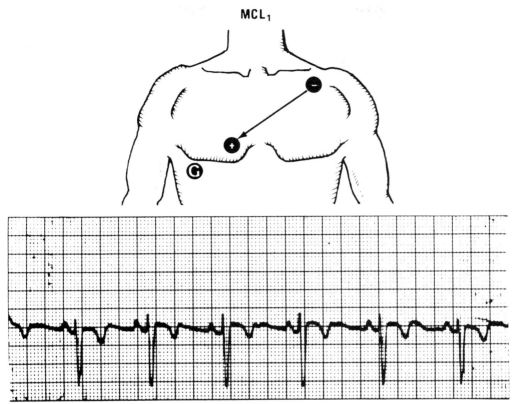

Fig. 7-3 The electrode position and ECG tracing of a typical MCL$_1$ lead are demonstrated. (Hampton AG: Monitoring and dysrhythmia recognition in advanced life support. American Heart Association. Advanced Life Support Course.)

good, wires are totally in the way, easily twisted and dislodged, and telemetery may be a useful method of monitoring.

The computer has been increasingly employed in the ECG diagnosis of dysrhythmias by cardiologists.[23] However, its intraoperative use as part of a routine monitoring system is still in the future. There are many difficulties with electronic interpretation of the ECG, especially in the area of dysrhythmia analysis when external interference is a common event. The P wave is especially difficult to analyze, since in most leads it has a low amplitude that may be only 50 to 70 percent of the level of external noise. Short periods of time, such as 5 to 10 seconds, are usually sampled; and complex dysrhythmias usually detected with long rhythm strips may be misdiagnosed. The present availability and economics of this computer technology make it primarily a research tool. However, developments in computer design and refinements of programming during the next decade may enable us to use these techniques in the operating room.

The usual ECG lead systems used intraoperatively consist of either three, four, or five electrodes. In all systems there is one electrode on each arm and one on the left leg. In the four wire system an additional electrode which serves as the ground is placed on the right leg. In a five wire system, the extra electrode is placed on the precordium and is used specifically in the diagnosis of ischemia.

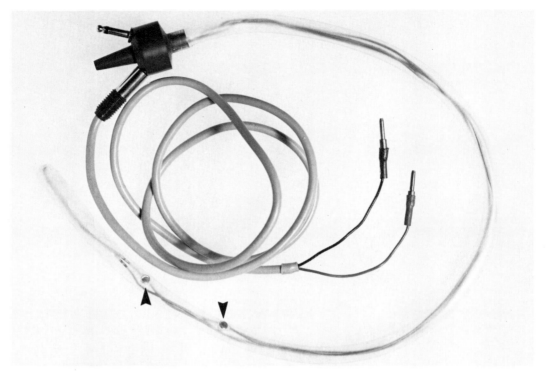

Fig. 7-4 An esophageal stethoscope is demonstrated in which there are two electrodes. These can be used to obtain a unipolar or bipolar esophageal ECG to aid in the diagnosis of dysrhythmias.

The following are the best leads for diagnosing dysrhythmias:[24]

1. V_1 uses the four limb electrodes and the fifth V electrode is placed in the fourth intercostal space to the right of the sternum. This lead shows a good atrial deflection and QRS complex and is probably the best lead from which to make specific rhythm diagnoses.

2. MCL_1 (modified chest lead I) is a popular lead for cardiac monitoring, dysrhythmia detection, and conduction disturbance monitoring in coronary care units.[25] The MCL_1 lead is really a modified lead V_1. However, this is a bipolar lead with the positive electrode to the right of the sternum in the fourth intercostal space (V_1 position), while the negative electrode is placed near the left shoulder or under the left clavicle (Fig. 7-3). This lead system can be set up by placing the left arm electrode under the left clavicle and the left leg electrode in the V_1 position and setting the lead selector switch on lead III.

3. Lead II is the third choice for dysrhythmia detection. It shows a good atrial deflection, but not necessarily a good QRS complex. Overall, this is probably the most useful lead intraoperatively. It allows not only for dysrhythmia detection, but also for the observation of inferior wall myocardial ischemia.

4. Unipolar esophageal leads have also been used to record atrial complexes and diagnose dysrhythmias.[26] The active electrode is placed in the esophagus (and can be part of an esophageal stethoscope arrangement) and thus the posterior surface of the left ventricle and atrioventricular junction can be explored. (Fig. 7-4).

5. Intracardiac electrocardiography has also been used for diagnostic purposes, since

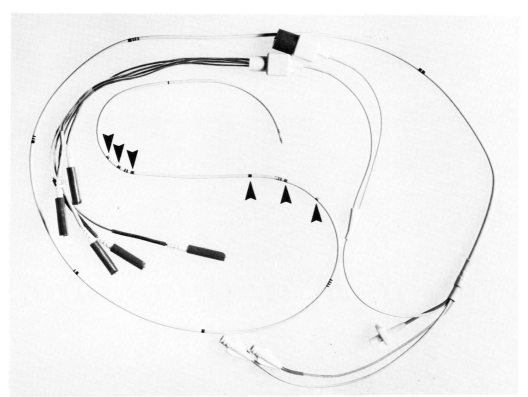

Fig. 7-5 A multipurpose Swan-Ganz catheter with both atrial and ventricular ECG or pacing electrodes is demonstrated. There are three atrial electrodes and two ventricular electrodes (see arrows). This catheter can be used to diagnose complex dysrhythmias or for atrial, ventricular, or atrioventricular sequential pacing.

it is relatively easy to obtain these traces. In the past, a long central venous pressure catheter was filled with hypertonic saline and advanced into the cardiac chambers. The catheter was attached to the V lead of the ECG by an alligator clip in order to read the tracing. When the catheter reached the superior vena cava, the ECG tracing looked like a normal lead AVR with inverted P, QRS, and T waves. In the high right atrium, the P wave was large and deeply inverted; in midatrium, the P was biphasic; and in the low atrium it was upright. When the ventricle was entered, the QRS complex became very large. Recently, multipurpose pulmonary artery catheters with both atrial and ventricular ECG and/or pacing electrodes have become available.[27] These catheters permit monitoring of bipolar atrial or ventricular electrograms and diagnosis of complex dysrhythmias using any of the five electrodes placed on the catheter (Fig. 7-5).

6. A further diagnostic ECG step is to record the bundle of His electrogram using an intracardiac catheter.[28] This part of electrical conduction in the heart is so rapid that it does not appear on the standard ECG. This technique may be used to localize heart blocks to certain areas of the conduction system or to diagnose the mechanism of complex dysrhythmias (Fig. 7-6).

The following factors have been shown to be possible contributors to the etiology of dysrhythmias in the perioperative period:

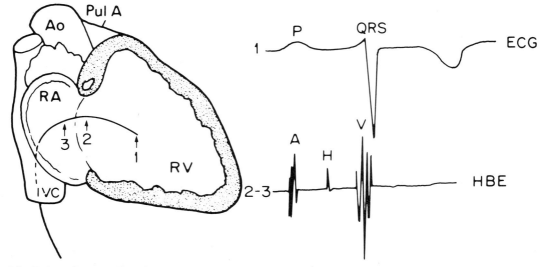

Fig. 7-6 An intracardiac electrocardiographic lead is shown coming through the inferior vena cava, the right atrium, and across the tricuspid valve with the tip in the right ventricle. A normal ECG is shown as well as the intracavitary His bundle electrograph. The His bundle electrograph (HBE) demonstrates normal A, H, and V waves. (Akhtar M: Clinical use of His bundle electrocardiography. Am Heart J 91:520, 1976.)

1. Anesthetic agents—halogenated hydrocarbons such as halothane or enflurane have been shown to produce dysrhythmias, probably by a reentrant mechanism.[29] In addition, these agents, especially halothane, have been shown to sensitize the myocardium to both endogenous and exogenous catecholamines. Drugs, such as cocaine and ketamine, that block the reuptake of norepinephrine can facilitate the development of epinephrine-induced dysrhythmias.[30]

2. Abnormal arterial blood gases or electrolytes—Edwards showed that hyperventilation to a $PaCO_2$ of 30 or 20 torr lowered a normal serum potassium to 3.64 or 3.12 mEq/L, respectively.[11] If serum and total body potassium start at low levels, it is possible to decrease the serum potassium into the 2 mEq/L range by hyperventilation, and thus precipitate severe cardiac dysrhythmias. Alterations of blood gases or electrolytes may lead to dysrhythmias either by producing reentrant mechanisms or by altering phase 4 depolarization of conduction fibers.

3. Endotracheal intubation—this may be the most common cause of dysrhythmias during surgery. These dysrhythmias occasionally can be associated with severe hypertension.[31] Several authors have emphasized the hemodynamic alterations which may occur during endotracheal intubation (see Ch. 8).[32]

4. Reflexes—vagal stimulation may produce sinus bradycardias and allow for ventricular escape mechanisms to occur. In addition, specific reflexes such as the occulocardiac reflex can produce severe rhythm disturbances during surgery.[9]

5. Central nervous system stimulation[33]—many ECG abnormalities have been reported with intracranial pathology, especially subarachnoid hemorrhage, including changes in QT intervals, development of Q waves, ST segment changes, and the occurrence of U waves. The mechanism of dysrhythmias appears to be due to changes in the autonomic nervous system.

6. Location of surgery—dental surgery is often associated with dysrhythmias, since profound stimulation of both the sympathetic

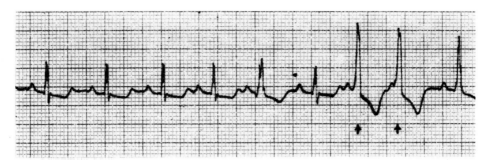

Fig. 7-7 An ECG tracing with multiple premature atrial contractions is demonstrated. The fourth beat shows no aberration, while the fifth beat shows partial aberration and the seventh and eighth beats, with arrows, show marked aberration.

and parasympathetic nervous systems often occurs.[34] Junctional rhythms commonly occur and may be due to stimulation of the autonomic nervous system via the 5th cranial nerve.

7. Preexisting cardiac disease—studies by Angilini et al. have shown that patients with known cardiac disease have a much higher incidence of dysrhythmias during anesthesia than patients without known cardiac disease.[13]

Arrhythmias may also be attenuated or eliminated by general anesthesia.[35] This could be due to the relief of anxiety and loss of sympathetic stimulation; due to an antiarrhythmic property of the anesthetic agent itself; or due to the correction of abnormalities of respiration, blood gases, and electrolytes.

The diagnosis and treatment of important intraoperative dysrhythmias can be managed by using the following six questions when looking at a rhythm and attempting to decide whether treatment is necessary:[36]

1. What is the heart rate?
2. Is the rhythm regular?
3. Is there one P wave for each QRS complex?
4. Is the QRS complex normal?
5. Is the rhythm dangerous?
6. Does the rhythm require treatment?

The following are common intraoperative dysrhythmias which require diagnosis and treatment and to which the six key questions can be applied.

Premature Atrial Contractions (PACs)

These arise from an atrial focus other than the SA node, making them ectopic. They are recognized by a premature, abnormally shaped P wave, and usually a normal QRS complex. They tend to reset the SA node and cause a slight pause, but not a full compensatory pause. Occasionally, the PAC may find part of the ventricular conduction system refractory. Then it will travel down an aberrant pathway and create an abnormal QRS complex. This is called a premature atrial contraction with ventricular aberration and can very easily be confused with a premature ventricular contraction. Helpful points in separating a PAC with aberration from a PVC are (1) there is a preceding P wave, usually abnormally shaped; (2) the complex is often of a right bundle branch block configuration; (3) there is an rSR^1 in V_1; and (4) the initial vector forces are identical with the preceding beat, but are usually the opposite with a PVC (Fig. 7-7). Other characteristics are:

1. Heart rate—variable, depending on frequency of PACs.
2. Rhythm—irregular.
3. P:QRS—usually 1:1; the P waves have various shapes and may even be lost in the QRS or T waves. Occasionally, the P wave will be so early as to find the ventricle refractory and a nonconducted beat will then occur.
4. QRS complex—usually normal unless

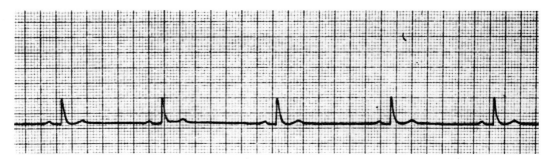

Fig. 7-8 A sinus bradycardia with an intrinsic rate of about 45 beats/min is demonstrated. It can also be noticed that the patient has a mild sinus arrhythmia with variations in heart rate associated with respirations.

there is ventricular aberration as mentioned above.

5. Significance—usually not dangerous, but very frequent PACs can lead to other supraventricular tachyarrhythmias or be a sign of digitalis intoxication.

6. Treatment—usually none. Rarely, digitalis or propranolol can be given if the dysrhythmia is causing poor hemodynamic function.

Sinus Bradycadia

The discharge site is the SA node but at a slower than normal rate (Fig. 7-8). Occasionally, other pacemaker sites will try to take over and cause escape beats, e.g., PVCs. The characteristics of sinus bradycardia are:

1. Heart rate—40 to 60 beats/min. In patients receiving propranolol chronically, this dysrhythmia should be redefined to be a heart rate less than 50 beats/min.[37]

2. Rhythm—regular, except for premature ventricular escape beats which occasionally occur.

3. P:QRS 1:1

4. QRS complex—normal.

5. Significance—this is the goal for patients treated with beta-blockers for ischemic heart disease. It may also be seen with acute inferior myocardial infarction and many drugs such as morphine or neostigmine. It is of little significance unless peripheral perfusion is decreased, and it is associated with hypotension or premature escape beats. A sinus bradycardia may be part of the so-called sick sinus syndrome in which sinus node dysfunction can precipitate bradycardias, heart block, tachyarrhythmias, or alternating bradytachyarrhythmias.[38]

6. Treatment—usually none. Atropine is indicated if the bradycardia is associated with hypotension or escape beats. Rarely, isoproterenol or a pacemaker will be necessary.

Sinus Tachycardia

Discharge site is the SA node, but at a faster than normal rate (Fig. 7-9). This is a very common dysrhythmia during and after surgery. Determining its etiology is frequently a problem, since there are many diverse etiologies such as pain, light anesthesia, hypovolemia, fever, emotion, heart failure, and hyperthyroidism to name just a few. Its characteristics are:

1. Heart rate—above 100 beats/min. The top sinus node rate, is 150 to 170 beats/min, which may be seen with a severe episode of hyperpyrexia.

2. Rhythm—regular.

3. P:QRS—1:1.

4. QRS complex—normal. There may be associated ST segment depression with severe increases in heart rate and resulting myocardial ischemia.

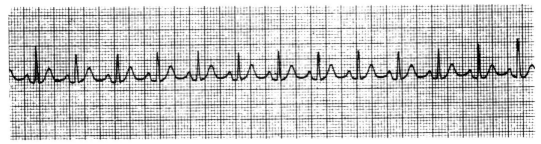

Fig. 7-9 A sinus tachycardia is demonstrated with an intrinsic heart rate of 100 beats/min.

5. Significance—prolonged tachycardias in patients with underlying heart disease can precipitate congestive heart failure due to the increased myocardial work required. The tachycardia decreases coronary perfusion time, which can cause secondary ST-T wave changes and can precipitate angina pectoris in patients with coronary disease.

A major diagnostic problem is encountered when the heart rate is 150 beats/min, since this is a common rate for either a sinus tachycardia, a paroxysmal atrial tachycardia (PAT), or atrial flutter with a 2:1 block.[39] These three dysrhythmias can sometimes be separated by using carotid sinus massage, intravenous administration of edrophonium, or atrial or esophageal ECG leads in order to get a better look at the P waves on the ECG.

6. Treatment—the underlying disorder should be treated. If necessary while determining the cause propranolol may be used in patients with ischemic heart disease who de-velop ST segment changes in order to prevent further myocardial ischemia.

Paroxysmal Atrial Tachycardia (PAT)

This is a run of rapidly repeated supraventricular premature beats arising from a site other than the SA node. This dysrhythmia is frequently seen in patients with Wolff-Parkinson-White (WPW) syndrome, in which an abnormal conduction pathway is present through the bundle of Kent (Fig. 7-10). The characteristics of PAT are:

1. Heart rate—150 to 250 beats/min.
2. Rhythm—usually regular.
3. P:QRS—1:1; P waves often abnormal and may be difficult to see.
4. QRS complex—normal; ST-T wave depression is common.
5. Significance—may occur under anesthesia when precipitated by changes in the

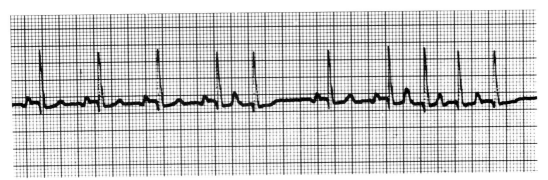

Fig. 7-10 A short run of paroxysmal atrial tachycardia is demonstrated on the right of the tracing in a patient with an underlying normal sinus rhythm. The heart rate during the tachycardia is about 150 beats/min. The P waves are difficult to see, since they are buried in the previous T wave.

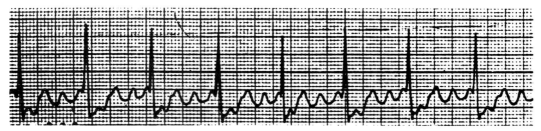

Fig. 7-11 Classical saw-toothed flutter waves (F waves) are seen in this patient with atrial flutter.

autonomic nervous system, drug effects, or volume shifts and can produce severe hemodynamic deterioration.[40] It can be seen in 5 percent of normal young adults and in many patients with WPW. At times, the PAT may be associated with atrioventricular block due to the fast atrial rate and slow AV conduction. PAT with 2:1 block represents digitalis intoxication in many patients.

6. Treatment—this dysrhythmia often must be treated due to its rapid rate and associated poor hemodynamic function. The following steps can be taken to treat this dysrhythmia:[41]

a. carotid sinus massage, which should only be applied to one side;

b. edrophonium (Tensilon) in 5 to 10 mg IV bolus doses;

c. phenylephrine—if the patient is hypotensive, 100 μg IV bolus doses can be used in an effort to increase the blood pressure and achieve a reflex vagal slowing of the heart rate;

d. propranolol in 0.5 mg IV bolus doses.

e. rapid overdrive pacing,[42] in an effort to capture the ectopic focus;

g. cardioversion[43] with appropriate synchronization.

Atrial Flutter

This represents a faster discharge from an irritable focus in the atria than does a rapid atrial tachycardia. Since it is so fast, it is usually associated with atrioventricular block. Classical saw-toothed flutter waves (F waves) are usually present. (Fig. 7-11). The characteristics of atrial flutter are:

1. Heart rate—atrial rate 250 to 350 beats/min; with a ventricular rate of about 150 beats/min.

2. Rhythm—atrial rhythm is regular, but the ventricular rhythm may be regular if a fixed block or irregular if a variable block exists.

3. P:QRS—usually 2:1 block with an atrial rate of 300 and ventricular rate of 150, but may vary between 2:1 and 8:1. F waves are best seen in leads V_1 and II.

4. QRS complex—normal; T waves are lost in the F waves.

5. Significance—associated with severe heart disease.

6. Treatment—pharmacologic treatment can be used when the rhythm is being tolerated by the patient and usually consists of digitalis and propranolol. In situations of acute hemodynamic deterioration, cardioversion using very low voltage (10 to 40 watt/seconds) is effective in more than 90 percent of cases.[44]

Atrial Fibrillation

This is an excessively rapid and irregular atrial focus with no P waves appearing on the ECG but instead, a fine fibrillatory activity called "f" waves. This is the most irregular rhythm and is thus called irregularly irregular and may be associated with a pulse deficit (Fig. 7-12). The characteristics are:

1. Heart rate—atrial rate 350 to 500

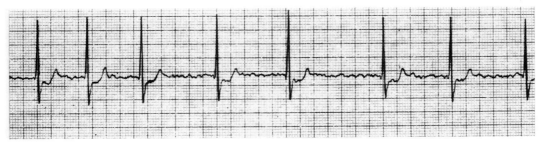

Fig. 7-12 Atrial fibrillation with fine fibrillatory activity is demonstrated in this patient. The irregularly irregular pattern of the QRS complexes should be noted.

beats/min and a ventricular rate between 60 and 170 beats/min.

2. Rhythm—irregularly irregular.

3. P:QRS—P wave is absent and replaced by "f" waves or no obvious atrial activity at all.

4. QRS complex—normal.

5. Significance—associated with severe heart disease.

6. Treatment—digitalis is usually used to slow the ventricular response and propranolol may be added if necessary. Cardioversion may be used to reestablish sinus rhythm in cases of recent onset of atrial fibrillation.

Premature Ventricular Contractions (PVC)

These are premature ectopic beats arising from a focus below the atrioventricular junction and are one of the most common dys-

rhythmias seen in anesthesia and in patients with cardiac disease. These are identified by being premature, having a wide QRS complex, an ST segment that slopes in the opposite direction, and a compensatory pause. Usually there is no P wave associated with these beats (Fig. 7-13). PVCs are characterized by:

1. Heart rate—depends on the frequency of PVCs.

2. Rhythm—irregular.

3. P:QRS—no P waves are seen.

4. QRS complex—wide and bizarre with a width of over 0.12 seconds.

5. Significance—potentially a very dangerous dysrhythmia which can procede to ventricular tachycardia or fibrillation. The most dangerous forms are multiple PVCs, multifocal PVCs, coupled PVCs, short runs of PVCs (more than 3 in a row is usually considered ventricular tachycardia), or the R-on-T phenomenon where the PVCs are near the

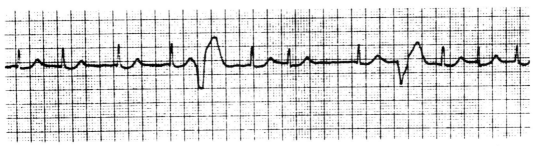

Fig. 7-13 Premature ventricular contractions are identified by the fact that they are premature, have a wide QRS complex, and an ST-segment that slopes in the opposite direction. They may also have a compensatory pause.

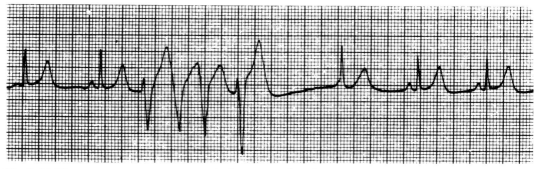

Fig. 7-14 Three or more premature ventricular contractions in a row is defined by most as a run of ventricular tachycardia. If a fusion beat, capture beat, or AV dissociation can be diagnosed on the trace it helps make the specific diagnosis of ventricular tachycardia.

vulnerable period on the electrocardiogram.[45]

6. Treatment—the first step is to correct any underlying abnormalities such as a low potassium or arterial oxygen tension. Then lidocaine is usually the treatment of choice with an initial bolus dose of 1.5 mg/kg intravenously. Recurrent PVCs can be treated with a lidocaine infusion of 1 to 4 mg/min or additional therapy can be supplied with propranolol, bretylium, procainamide, quinidine, or disopyramide.

Ventricular Tachycardia

These are a run of rapidly repeated ectopic beats arising from the ventricle and can be life-threatening. Diagnostic criteria include the presence of fusion beats, capture beats, and AV dissociation (Fig. 7-14).[46] The characteristics of ventricular tachycardia are:

1. Heart rate—100 to 200 beats/min.
2. Rhythm—usually regular but may be irregular if the ventricular tachycardia is paroxysmal.
3. P:QRS—no fixed relationship, since ventricular tachycardia is a form of atrioventricular dissociation in which the P waves can be seen marching through the QRS complex.
4. QRS complex—wide, over 0.12 seconds in width.

5. Significance—Acute onset is life-threatening and requires immediate treatment.
6. Treatment—lidocaine or cardioversion is usually required.

Ventricular Fibrillation

The ventricle is discharged in a completely chaotic asynchronus fashion without effective cardiac output. There is no clear-cut ventricular complex seen on the ECG (Fig. 7-15). The characteristics are:

1. Heart rate—rapid and grossly disorganized.
2. Rhythm—totally irregular.
3. P:QRS—none are seen.
4. QRS complex—not present.
5. Significance—there is no effective cardiac output and life must be sustained by artificial means, such as external cardiac massage.
6. Treatment—cardiopulmonary resuscitation must be initiated immediately and then defibrillation performed as rapidly as possible. External defibrillation should be performed with a DC defibrillator using between 200 and 400 watt-seconds.[47] Supportive pharmacologic therapy may include propranolol, bretylium, or lidocaine. In some instances, epinephrine is used to coarsen the fibrillation in an attempt to be able to defibrillate the patient.[45]

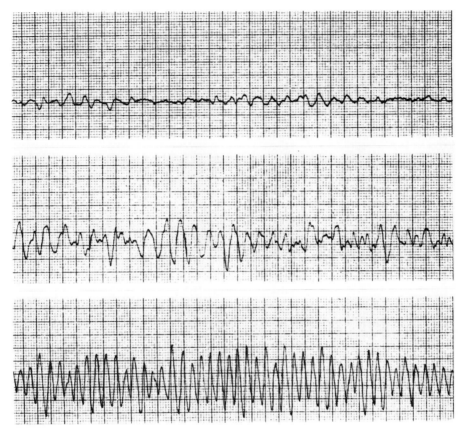

Fig. 7-15 Ventricular fibrillation can occur in a very fine, moderate, or coarse pattern as is demonstrated on the ECGs.

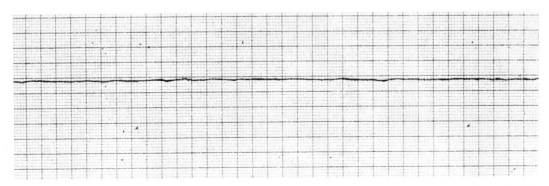

Fig. 7-16 Asystole is diagnosed by the straight-line activity on the ECG. It must be ascertained that this is not an ECG strip taken from a disconnected cable to the patient.

Asystole

During asystole, no ventricular activity is present (Fig. 7-16). Asystole is the second most common rhythm disorder (after ventricular fibrillation) during cardiac arrests. The characteristics are:

1. Heart rate—none present.
2. Rhythm—straight-line on the ECG.
3. P:QRS—none present.
4. QRS complex—absent.
5. Significance—difficult to treat and an attempt should be made to convert it to ventricular fibrillation.
6. Treatment—maintain cardiopulmonary resuscitation while administering calcium chloride, isoproterenol, epinephrine, sodium bicarbonate, and if necessary inserting a transvenous pacemaker.

CONDUCTION ABNORMALITIES

Three types of conduction system block are possible: sinoatrial block, intraventricular conduction block, and atrioventricular heart block.

Bundle of His electrograms have greatly improved our understanding of conduction through the heart.[48] In sinoatrial block, the block occurs at the sinus node. Since atrial excitation is not initiated, P waves are not found on the ECG. The next beat can be a normal sinus beat, a nodal escape beat, or a ventricular escape beat.

The second type of block is intraventricular conduction disturbances, which are usually classified as either left bundle branch blocks, right bundle branch blocks or hemiblocks.[49]

The left bundle branch block is the most serious of these conduction disturbances. Impulses reach the ventricles exclusively through the right bundle branch and therefore, there is a wide QRS complex of more than O.12 seconds and a wide-noticed R wave seen in leads I, AVL, and V_6. The most important leads to study in bundle branch blocks are I, V_1, and V_6. The pattern of left bundle branch block in V_6 is similar to left ventricular hypertrophy, but exaggerated. A left bundle branch block pattern is always associated with significant cardiac disease (Fig. 7-17).

In a right bundle branch block, the QRS complex exceeds O.11 seconds, and leads V_1 to V_3 have broad rSR' complexes, while leads I and V_6 have wide S waves. A right bundle branch block may be of no clinical significance as opposed to the left bundle branch block. However, it is frequently associated with chronic lung disease or atrial-septal defects (Fig. 7-18).

Hemiblock is the term used when one of two divisions of the left bundle is blocked, since if both divisions are blocked a complete left bundle branch block exists. Even though hemiblocks are a form of intraventricular block, the QRS complex is not prolonged. Marriott's criteria for a left anterior hemiblock are: (1) a left axis deviation greater than −60 degrees; (2) a small Q in lead I, an R in lead III; and (3) a normal QRS duration. On the other hand, the criteria for a left posterior hemiblock are: (1) right axis deviation greater than +120 degrees; (2) a small R in lead I, small Q in lead III; (3) normal QRS duration; and (4) no right ventricular hypertrophy.[49] The hemiblocks can occur by themselves, but are often associated with a right bundle branch block to form a bilateral bundle branch block. Patients with right bundle branch block and a left anterior hemiblock progress to complete heart block only 10 percent of the time, while patients with right bundle branch block and a left posterior hemiblock usually proceed to complete heart block (Fig. 7-19).

The third type of heart block is atrioventricular heart block, or AV block, which may be either incomplete or complete.[50] First and second degree AV blocks are usually considered incomplete, while a third degree AV block is considered to be complete heart block. First degree atrioventricular block is often found in normal hearts but is also associated with coronary artery disease or digi-

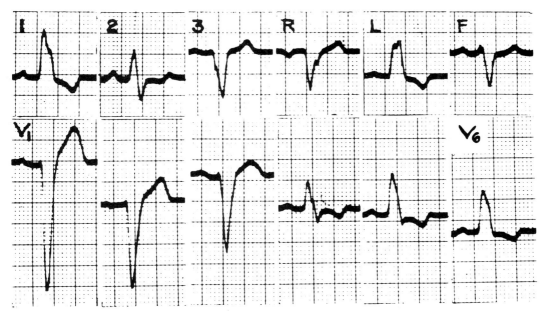

Fig. 7-17 A left bundle branch block can be diagnosed from the above ECG. It is important to note the wide QRS complex and wide-notched R waves in leads I, AVL, and V_6. (Marriott HJL: Practical Electrocardiography. 6th edition. © (1977) The Williams & Wilkins Co., Baltimore.)

talis administration. It is characterized by a PR interval longer than 0.21 seconds. All atrial impulses progress through the atrioventricular node to the Purkinje system. This form of heart block ordinarily requires no treatment (Fig. 7-20).

Second degree atrioventricular block is associated with the conduction of some, but not all, of the atrial impulses to the AV node and into the Purkinje system. It is further subdivided into two specific types.[51] Mobitz type 1, or Wenckebach block, is characterized by progressive lengthening of the PR interval until an impulse is not conducted and the beat is dropped (Fig. 7-21) This form of block is relatively benign, often reversible, and does not require a pacemaker. It may be caused by digitalis toxicity or myocardial infarction and

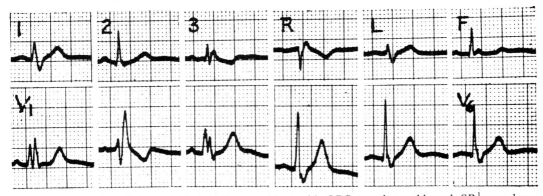

Fig. 7-18 A right bundle branch block is diagnosed by a wide QRS complex and broad rSR^1 complexes in leads V_1 to V_3. Leads I and V_6 have wide S waves. (Marriott HJL: Practical Electrocardiography. 6th edition. © (1977) The Williams & Wilkins Co., Baltimore.)

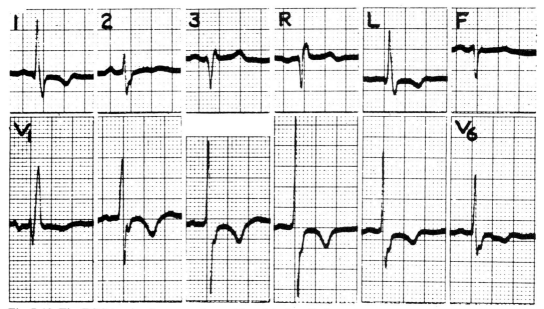

Fig. 7-19 The ECG tracing from a patient with a right bundle branch block and left anterior hemiblock is seen. There is a left axis deviation greater than −60° on the tracing. (Marriott HJL: Practical Electrocardiography. 6th edition. © (1977) The Williams & Wilkins Co., Baltimore.)

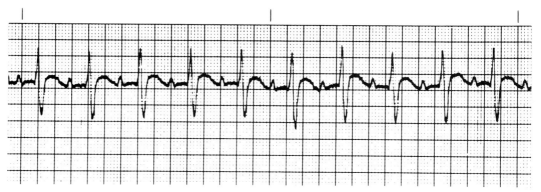

Fig. 7-20 First degree heart block is diagnosed by the presence of a PR interval of longer than 0.21 seconds.

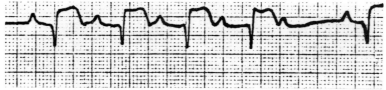

Fig. 7-21 Mobitz type 1 or Wenckebach block is diagnosed by the progressive lengthening of the PR interval until an impulse is not conducted and a dropped beat occurs.

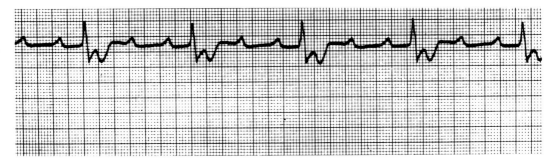

Fig. 7-22 Mobitz type 2 second degree heart block is demonstrated in which dropped beats occur without a progressive lengthening of the PR interval.

is usually transient in nature. The Mobitz type 1 block reflects disease of the atrioventricular node. The other form of second degree heart block is a Mobitz type 2 block, which reflects disease of the His bundle Purkinje tissues. In this, the less common and more serious form of second degree heart block, dropped beats occur without any progressive lengthening of the PR interval. This type of block has a serious prognosis, since it frequently progresses to complete heart block and may require pacemaker insertion prior to major surgical procedures (Fig. 7-22).

Third degree atrioventricular block, also called complete heart block, occurs when all electrical activity from the atria fails to progress into the Purkinje system. The atrial and ventricular contractions have no relationship to each other, although each can regularly contract. The ventricular rate will be approximately 40 beats/min. The QRS complex may be normal if the pacemaker site is in the AV node, but is usually widened to longer than 0.12 seconds when the pacer site is located in the ventricle. The heart rate is usually too slow to maintain adequate cardiac output and syncope or Stokes-Adams syndrome may occur as well as heart failure. These patients usually require the insertion of either a transvenous endocardial or an epicardial pacemaker to increase their heart rate and cardiac output (Fig. 7-23).

MYOCARDIAL ISCHEMIA

Electrocardiographic monitoring of myocardial ischemia is a relatively new technique in the operating room. Early studies of intraoperative ECG monitoring did not even mention the use of the ECG to diagnose isch-

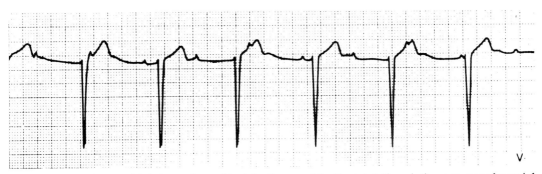

Fig. 7-23 Complete or third degree heart block is diagnosed by the total dissociation between the atrial and the ventricular complexes with a ventricular rate of about 40 beats/min.

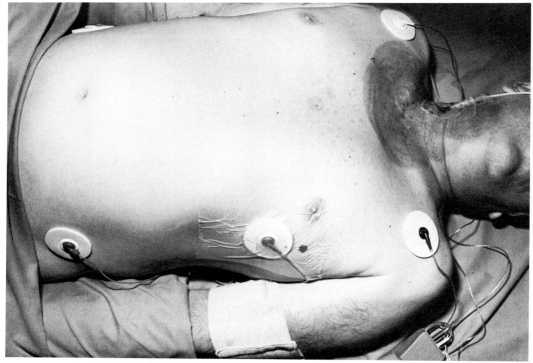

Fig. 7-24 The five disposable ECG pads are demonstrated. One pad is placed on each extremity and the fifth pad is placed in the V_5 position and covered with a small piece of Steri-drape.

emia but only for diagnosis of dysrhythmias.[1] In recent years, coronary artery disease has become the number one health problem in the United States. Patients coming for all types of surgical procedures have significant coronary artery disease, and many have histories of acute myocardial infarctions or angina pectoris. In these patients, the ECG should be used to identify myocardial ischemia during the stresses of anesthesia and surgery, as well as for dysrhythmia detection. Until recently, the older ECG lead systems and monitors designed primarily for dysrhythmia detection have been the only ones available in the operating room. These are frequently totally inadequate for the diagnosis and recording of subtle ST segment changes which may occur with early myocardial ischemia. The most obvious deficiency has been the lack of flexibility in se-

lecting the appropriate leads for diagnosing myocardial ischemia.

In 1931, precordial leads had been noted to have a greater sensitivity in detecting ST segment depression of ischemic origin than the standard leads. Since then a number of lead systems have been developed to monitor myocardial ischemia and have been studied extensively during exercise stress testing. Blackburn has done many studies of the lead systems and found the most sensitive exploring electrode was at the V_5 chest position.[52] He showed that 89 percent of the ST segment information contained in a conventional 12-lead ECG was found in lead V_5. It was not until 1976 that any information on the use of precordial leads for monitoring of ischemia during anesthesia first appeared. Dalton recommended placing a sterile spinal needle in the V_4 or V_5 position after the skin was pre-

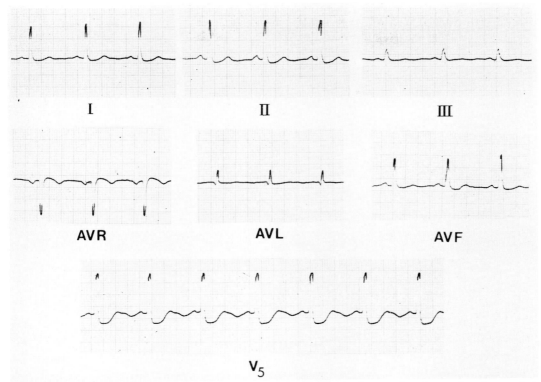

I   II   III

AVR   AVL   AVF

V_5

Fig. 7-25 This figure demonstrates the seven different ECG leads that can be observed and recorded during surgery when using the five electrode system. (Kaplan JA: The precordial electrocardiographic lead (V_5) in patients with coronary artery disease. Anesthesiology 45:570, 1976.)

pared for cardiac surgery.[53] I reported that a multiple ECG lead system, including a V_5 lead, can be used for patients with coronary artery disease.[10] Since then I have used four disposable electrocardiographic pads placed on the extremities and a fifth pad placed in the V_5 position and covered with a small piece of Steri-drape (Fig. 7-24). This lead does not interfere with the majority of surgery and can be placed before the induction of anesthesia and monitored during the entire operative procedure. Using the five electrodes, seven different ECG leads can be selected to be observed (I, II, III, AVR, AVL, AVF, and V_5) (Fig. 7-25). All seven leads are observed prior to the start of anesthesia and *recorded* for later reference. In patients with known cardiac disease, we record all seven leads

and *simultaneously display two leads* (V_5, II) using two different ECG amplifier circuits (Fig. 7-26). This allows us to look at the anterior lateral wall (V_5 lead) and the inferior wall (lead II) of the heart at the same time. Robertson has shown that there is good correlation between the site of the coronary artery obstruction and the lead in which ischemia is detected.[54] ST segment changes in leads II, III, and AVF correspond to disease of the right coronary artery; and ischemic changes in V_4 to V_6 indicate disease of the left anterior descending or circumflex coronary artery (Fig. 7-27).[55]

We prefer the five electrode system discussed above, including the true V_5 lead. However, some operating room ECG systems still have only three or four electrode wires. A

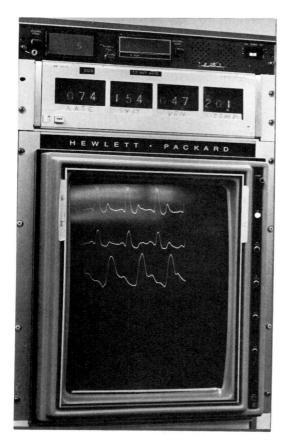

Fig. 7-26 A simultaneous display of leads V_5 (top) and lead II (bottom) are shown. Also demonstrated are the arterial trace, and digital readouts.

modification of the V_5 lead can be readily used in those cases as is frequently done during exercise stress testing.[56, 57] The most popular modified leads during stress testing have been the CM_5 or CS_5 bipolar leads in which the negative electrode is at the upper sternum in CM_5 or under the right clavicle in CS_5, with the positive electrode at the V_5 position. These leads are more convenient than V_5 because they require fewer wires. They are good leads for the detection of ischemia, but Frohlicher has recently shown they are not as good as V_5.[58] In the operating room, the right arm electrode can be placed just under the clavicle on the right shoulder and the left arm electrode placed in the V_5 position while the left leg lead is left in its usual place. Then lead I can be selected to observe the anterior heart wall (a modified CS_5) and lead II for the inferior wall (Fig. 7-28).

Myocardial ischemia is diagnosed by changes in the ST segment and T wave of the ECG.[59] Significant myocardial ischemia is defined as greater than 1 mm of horizontal or downsloping ST segment depression measured from a point 0.06 seconds from the J point. Increased magnitude of ST segment depression probably denotes an increased degree of ischemia. All ST segment elevations of greater than 1 mm are considered significant transmural myocardial ischemia (Fig. 7-29). It is extremely important that the electrocardiographic monitor or oscilloscope not introduce any type of artifacts or distortions to the ST segments or the T waves of the ECG when it is being used for the diagnosis of myocardial ischemia. This has been a problem with many of the present oscilloscopes in operating rooms.[17] The low frequency filters of the ECG circuitry have been the main

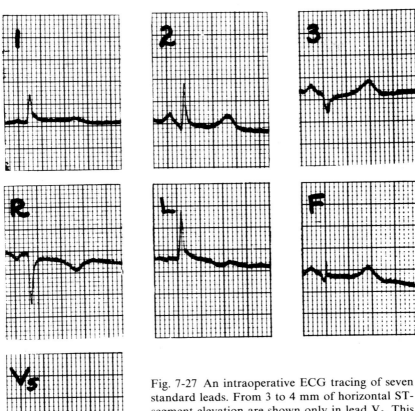

Fig. 7-27 An intraoperative ECG tracing of seven standard leads. From 3 to 4 mm of horizontal ST-segment elevation are shown only in lead V_5. This patient had an acutely obstructed circumflex coronary artery graft that had to be repaired. (Kaplan JA: Diagnostic value of the V_5 precordial lead. Anesth Analg 57:364, 1978.)

source of the problem. The *diagnostic* mode on some monitors filters frequencies below 0.1 Hz. A second mode frequently available is called the *monitor* mode and this filters all frequencies below 4 Hz. The diagnostic mode should be used when trying to diagnose ST segment changes, but unfortunately, it is susceptible to baseline wandering caused by respirations and movement. As more filtration is added, up to 4 Hz, the baseline becomes more stable, but the ECG complex becomes more distorted. The P and T waves may decrease in amplitude, but the main problem is changes in the ST segment. An isoelectric ST segment may be elevated or depressed, resembling ischemic changes. In addition, elevated or depressed ST segments may also be shifted towards the isoelectric line, hiding ongoing myocardial ischemia (Fig. 7-30).

The ST segments and T waves can be affected by many factors other than myocardial ischemia. These other factors produce the "non-specific ST-T wave changes." Drugs that can affect the ST segments include digitalis, diuretics, and reserpine.[6] Hypokalemia or glucose can affect the ST segment by altering the membrane-potassium relationship. The ST segments may appear to be depressed

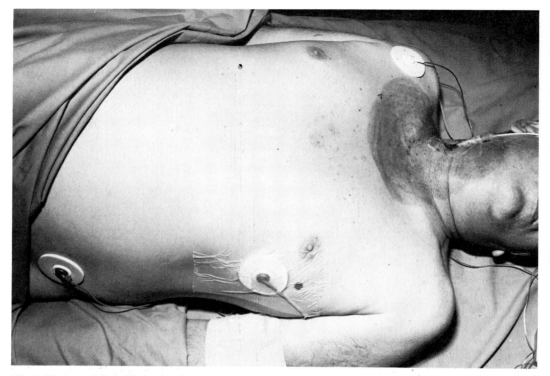

Fig. 7-28 A modified CS$_5$ lead is demonstrated in which the left arm lead has been moved down to the V$_5$ position. Lead I can then be turned on to measure from the right arm to the V$_5$ position (CS$_5$) and lead II can be used to look at the inferior wall.

by the T$_a$ wave of atrial repolarization and altered by conduction disturbances such as left bundle branch block or Wolff-Parkinson-White syndrome.

Another problem has been that when the size of the oscilloscope tracing is increased on some monitoring equipment, an obvious resolution problem appears. As the size of the tracing is increased, the stair-step effect of the electronic beam on the oscilloscope is much more obvious and can even look like horizontal ST segment changes of myocardial ischemia. Manufacturers will have to be made more aware of the fact that the ST segments are critical and should be kept entirely normal when making their electronic modifications on modern operating room monitors.

Computerized ST-segment analyzers are now available for use during exercise stress testing.[60, 61] They can analyze 10 to 20 heart beats and produce a histogram and digital readout of ST segment level, ST index, ST slope, and ST interval. These computations are still controversial with regard to their usefulness in diagnosing myocardial ischemia. I have tried these instruments in the cardiac surgical operating rooms and have found them to be useful, at times. However, they are useless when the electrocautery is switched on, since they must then reset themselves and count 10 to 20 beats to give the next reading.

ECG mapping techniques have been developed in an effort to define the size of the area of ischemia that has occurred in a patient or animal. This is important since the concept has been put forth that an ischemic area or even a necrotic area is not fixed in size at its

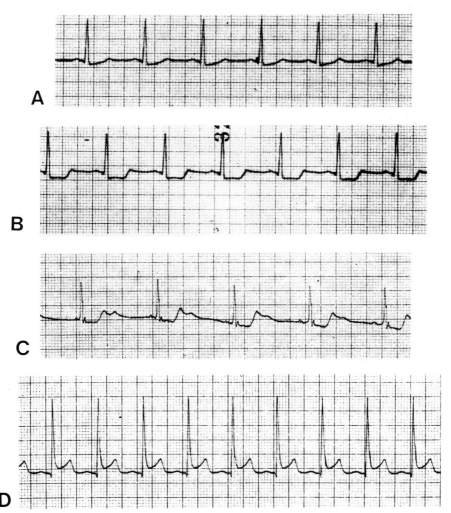

Fig. 7-29 Significant myocardial ischemia is defined as greater than 1 mm of horizontal or downsloping ST-segment depression or any ST-segment elevation greater than 1 mm. ST-segment changes of myocardial ischemia are demonstrated. (*A*) shows J-point depression and upsloping ST-segment depression; (*B*) shows horizontal ST-segment depression of ischemia; (*C*) shows downsloping ST-segment depression of ischemia; and (*D*) shows ST-segment elevation of the ischemia.

initial onset but that its size may in fact be modified by therapeutic interventions in either a positive or negative direction. In order to measure the areas of ischemia and evaluate therapeutic interventions, Muller, Maroko, and Braunwald[62, 63] have developed a series of mapping techniques. These techniques have evolved from epicardial ST segment mapping to epicardial QRS mapping, to precordial ST mapping and, finally, to precordial QRS mapping. The epicardial techniques were first used in animals and then precordial techniques were compared to them in animals and are now being applied in patients. A good correlation has been shown between the epicardial and precordial map-

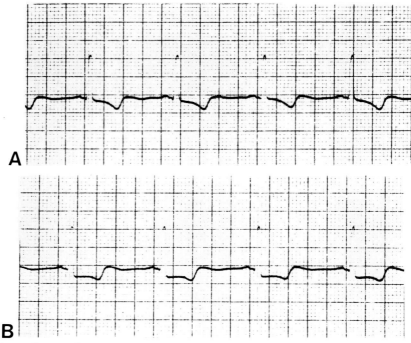

Fig. 7-30 An artifact on the ECG can be demonstrated by switching from (*A*) the diagnostic filter mode to (*B*) the monitoring filter mode. Significant changes in the ST-segments can be produced by altering these filters as is demonstrated in the figure.

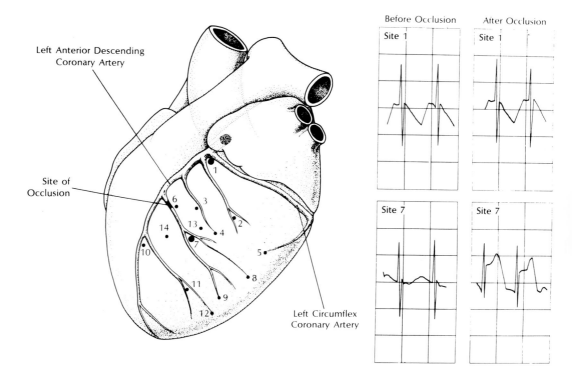

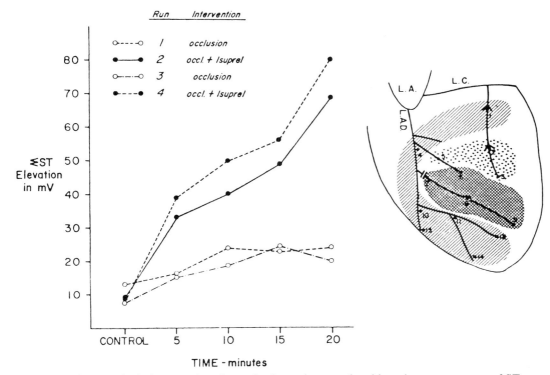

Fig. 7-32 Pharmacologic interventions have also been shown to be able to increase an area of ST-segment elevation. Infusion of isoproterenol increased the severity of myocardial ischemia as reflected in the sum of the ST-segment elevation recorded after coronary occlusion. After occlusion, the sum ranged from 15 to 25 mV, while, after occlusion and Isuprel, it ranged from 40 to 80 mV. (Figure by R. Ingle from Braunwald E, Maroko R: Protection of the ischemic myocardium, The Myocardium: Failure and Infarction. Edited by Braunwald E. New York, HP Publishing Co., 1974. Reproduced with permission.)

ping techniques. Epicardial ST segment mapping has been used to evaluate most potential therapeutic interventions in dogs with acute myocardial ischemia. In this model, known as the Maroko dog model, an occlusion is placed on the left anterior descending coronary artery of the dog and the ST segment elevation at multiple epicardial sites is determined after the occlusion (Fig. 7-31).[64] The procedure is then repeated in the presence of the specific intervention under study and the mean ST segment elevations compared in the treatment and control groups, Hillis and Braunwald have recently summarized all the data on interventions that have been obtained by this technique. They divided therapeutic interventions into those that increased myocardial injury either by increasing MVO_2 or decreasing myocardial oxygen supply and those that decreased myocardial injury either by decreasing MVO_2 or increasing myocardial oxygen supply.[65]

◀Fig. 7-31 The Maroko dog model is demonstrated. A branch of the left anterior descending coronary artery is occluded and epicardial ST-segment mapping is performed. An affected site, Site 7, which became ischemic, is demonstrated as well as an unaffected site, Site 1. (Figure by R. Ingle from Braunwald E, Maroko R: Protection of the ischemic myocardium, The Myocardium: Failure and Infarction. Edited by Braunwald E. New York, HP Publishing Co., 1974. Reproduced with permission.)

Precordial ST segment mapping has had the greatest clinical application of these techniques. A 35-lead electrode blanket was developed by Maroko to record precordial maps in patients with acute infarctions. Interventions such as propranolol, aortic counterpulsation, nitroglycerin, and oxygen have been shown to reduce ST segment elevation (Fig. 7-32).[66]

There are many limitations and controversies associated with ST segment mapping techniques. The greatest limitation is that they can only be used in patients with anterior or lateral wall ischemia. In addition, they cannot be used in patients with intraventricular conduction defects, since these markedly affect the ST segment. The areas of controversy involve validation of this method in relation to other techniques measuring infarct size, and questions about the technical limitations and electrophysiology involved in the technique.[67-69]

REFERENCES

1. Cannard TH, Dripps RD, Helwig J, et al: The ECG during anesthesia and surgery. Anesthesiology 21:194, 1960
2. Cranefield PF, Wit AL, Hoffman BF: Genesis of cardiac arrhythmias. Circulation 47:109, 1973
3. Benchimol A, Harris CL, Desser KB, et al: Resting ECG in major coronary artery disease. JAMA 224:1489, 1973
4. Hurst JW: The Heart. 4th edition. New York, McGraw Hill, 1978
5. Rooney S, Goldiner P, Muss E: Relationship of right bundle branch block and marked left axis deviation to complete heart block during general anesthesia. Anesthesiology 44:64, 1976
6. Surawicz B., Lasseter KC: Effect of drugs on the ECG. Prog Cardiovasc Dis 13:26, 1970
7. Surawicz B: Relationship between ECG and electrolytes. Am Heart J 73:814, 1967
8. Spodick DH: Acute pericardial tamponade, pathologic physiology, diagnosis and management. Prog Cardiovasc Dis 10:64, 1967
9. Katz RL, Bigger JT: Cardiac arrhythmias during anesthesia and operation. Anesthesiology 33:193, 1970
10. Kaplan JA, King SB: The precordial electrocardiographic lead (V_5) in patients who have coronary artery disease. Anesthesiology 45:570, 1976
11. Edwards R, Winnie AL, Ramamurthy S: Acute hypocapnic hypokalemia: An iatrogenic anesthetic complication. Anesth Analg 56:786, 1977
12. Simon A: Perioperative management of the pacemaker patient. Anesthesiology 46:127, 1977
13. Angelini L, Feldman MI, Lufschonowski R, et al: Cardiac arrhythmias during and after heart surgery: Diagnosis and management. Prog Cardiovasc Dis 16:469, 1974
14. Kennedy FB, Ticzon AR, Duffy FC, et al: Disappearance of ECG pattern of inferior wall myocardial infarction after aortocoronary bypass surgery. J Thorac Cardiovasc Surg 74:585, 1977
15. Kurtz CM, Bennett JH, Shapiro HH: ECG studies during surgical anesthesia. JAMA 106:434, 1936
16. Bertrand CA, Steiner NV, Jameson AG, et al: Disturbances of cardiac rhythm during anesthesia and surgery. JAMA 216:1615, 1971
17. Arbeit SR, Rubin IL, Gross H: Dangers in interpreting the ECG from the oscilloscope monitor. JAMA 211:453, 1970
18. Borrello G: ECG artifacts stimulating atrial flutter. JAMA 223:439, 1973
19. Doss JD, McCabe CW, Weiss GK: Noise free ECG data during electrosurgical procedures. Anesth Analg 52:156, 1973
20. Goldberg E: Mechanical factors and the ECG. Am Heart J 93:629, 1977
21. Voukydis PC: Effect of intracardiac blood on the ECG. N Engl J Med 291:612, 1974
22. Simonson E: The effect of age on the ECG. Am J Cardiol 29:64, 1972
23. Caceres CA, Hochberg HM: Performance of the computer and physician in the analysis of the electrocardiogram. Am Heart J 79:439, 1970
24. Schamroth L: How to approach an arrhythmia. Circulation 47:420, 1973
25. Hamptom AG: Monitoring and dysrhythmia recognition in advanced life support. American Heart Association. Advanced Life Support Course.
26. Kistin AD, Bruce JC: Simultaneous esopha-

geal and standard ECG leads for the study of cardiac arrhythmias. Am Heart J 53:65, 1957

27. Mantel JA, Massing GK, James TN, et al: A multipurpose catheter for electrocardiographic and hemodynamic monitoring plus atrial pacing. Chest 72:285, 1977

28. Aktar M, Damato AN: Clinical uses of His bundle electrocardiography. Part I. Am Heart J 91:520, 1976

29. Atlee JL, Rusy BF: Ventricular conduction times and AV nodal conductivity during enflurane anesthesia in dogs. Anesthesiology 47:498, 1977

30. Koehntop DE, Liao JC, Van Bergen FH: Effects of pharmacologic alterations of adrenergic mechanisms by cocaine, tropolone, aminophylline, and ketamine on epinephrine-induced arrhythmias during halothane-nitrous oxide anesthesia. Anesthesiology 46:83, 1977

31. Fox EJ, Sklar GS, Hill CH, et al: Complications related to the pressor response to endotracheal intubation. Anesthesiology 47:524, 1977

32. Stoelting RK: Circulatory changes during direct laryngoscopy and tracheal intubation: Influence of duration of laryngoscopy with and without prior lidocaine. Anesthesiology 47:381, 1977

33. Smith M, Ray CT: Cardiac arrhythmias, increased intracranial pressure, and the autonomic nervous system. Chest 61:125, 1972

34. Alexander JP: Dysrhythmia and oral surgery. Br J Anaesth 43:773, 1971

35. Borg DE: Paradox of cardiac arrhythmias in anaesthesia. Br J Anaesth 41:709, 1969

36. Kaplan JA: Electrocardiographic monitoring, Cardiac Anesthesia. Edited by Kaplan JA. New York, Grune & Stratton, 1979, pp 117-166

37. Kaplan JA, Dunbar RW, Bland JW, et al: Propranolol and cardiac surgery: A problem for the anesthesiologist? Anesth Analg 54:571, 1975

38. Slapa WJ: The sick sinus syndrome. Am Heart J 92:648, 1976

39. Moe GK, Mendez C: Physiologic basis of premature beats and sustained tachycardia. N Engl J Med 288:250, 1973

40. Sprague DH, Mandel SD: Paroxysmal supraventricular tachycardia during anesthesia. Anesthesiology 46:75, 1977

41. Chung EK: Tachyarrhythmias in Wolff-Parkinson-White syndrome: Antiarrhythmia therapy. JAMA 237:376, 1977

42. Escher DJW, Furman S: Emergency treatment of cardiac arrhythmias: Emphasis on use of electrical pacing. JAMA 214:2028, 1970

43. Kleiger RE: Cardioversion of paroxysmal arrhythmias. JAMA 213:107, 1970

44. Glassman E: Direct current cardioversion. Am Heart J 82:128, 1971

45. Cranefield PF: Ventricular fibrillation. N Engl J Med 289:732, 1973

46. Pietras RJ, Mautner R, Denes P, et al: Chronic recurrent right and left ventricular tachycardia: Comparison of clinical and hemodynamic and angiographic findings. Am J Cardiol 40:32, 1977

47. Geddes LA, Tacker WA, Rosborough J, et al: The electrical dose for ventricular defibrillation with electrodes applied directly to the heart. J Thorac Cardiovasc Surg 68:593, 1974

48. Hecht HH, Kossman EC, Childers RW, et al: Atrioventricular and intraventricular conduction: Revised nomenclature and concepts. Am J Cardiol 31:232, 1973

49. Marriott HJL: Practical Electrocardiology. 6th edition. Baltimore, Williams & Wilkins, 1977

50. Kastor JA: Atrioventricular block. N Engl J Med 292:462, 572, 1976

51. Wynands JE: Anesthesia for patients with heart block and artificial cardiac pacemakers. Anesth Analg 55:626, 1976

52. Blackburn H: The exercise electrocardiogram: Technological, procedural, and conceptual development, Measurements in Exercise Electrocardiography. Edited by Blackburn H. Springfield, Ill, Charles C Thomas, 1967

53. Dalton B: A precordial ECG lead for chest operations. Anesth Analg 55:740, 1976

54. Robertson D, Kostuk WJ, Ahuja SP: The localization of coronary artery stenosis by 12 lead ECG response to graded exercise test. Am Heart J 91:437, 1976

55. Kaplan JA, Dunbar RW, Hatcher CR: Diagnostic value of the V_5 precordial electrocardiographic lead. Anesth Analg 57:364, 1978

56. Ellestad MH: Stresss-testing: Principles and Practice. Philadelphia, FA Davis, 1975

57. Fortuin NJ, Weiss JL: Exercise stress testing. Circulation 56:699, 1976

58. Froelicher VF, Wolthius R, Keiser N, et al: A comparison of two bipolar exercise ECG leads to lead V_5. Chest 70:611, 1976

59. Kattus AA: Exercise ECG: Recognition of the ischemic response, false positive and negative pattern. Am J Cardiol 33:721, 1976

60. Scheffield GT, Holt JH, Lester FM: On-line analysis of the exercise electrocardiogram. Circulation 40:935, 1969

61. Roy WL, Edelist G, Gilbert B: Myocardial ischemia during non-cardiac surgical procedures in patients with coronary artery disease. Anesthesiology 51:393, 1979

62. Muller JE, Maroko PR, Braunwald E: Precordial ECG mapping: A technique to assess the efficacy of interventions designed to limit infact size. Circulation 57:1, 1978

63. Muller JE, Maroko PR, Braunwald E: Evaluation of precordial ECG mapping as a means of assessing change in myocardial ischemic injury. Circulation 52:16, 1975

64. Maroko PR, Kjekshus JK, Sobel BE, et al: Factors influencing infarct size following experimental coronary artery occlusion. Circulation 43:67, 1971

65. Hillis LD, Braunwald E: Myocardial ischemia. N Engl J Med 296:971, 1977

66. Madias JE, Madias NE, Hood WB: Precordial S-T segment mapping: Effects of oxygen inhalation on ischemic injury in patients with acute myocardial infarction. Circulation 53:411, 1976

67. Holland RP, Brooks H: TQ-ST segment mapping critical review and analysis of current concepts. Am J Cardiol 40:110, 1977

68. Surawicz B: The disputed S-T segment mapping: Is the technique ready for wide application in practice? Am J Cardiol 40:137, 1977

69. Fozzard HA, Das Gupta DS: S-T segment potential and mapping: Theory and experiment. Circulation 54:533, 1976

8

Endotracheal Intubation

Robert K. Stoelting, M.D.

INTRODUCTION

Endotracheal intubation (placement of a catheter in the trachea) is an integral part of the anesthesiologist's contribution to patient care. Continued improvement in equipment and use of neurosmuscular blockers combined with the technical skills of the anesthesiologist have made endotracheal intubation a safe and common practice in modern-day anesthesia.

PREOPERATIVE EVALUATION OF THE PATIENT

Preoperative patient evaluation determines the route (oral or nasal) and method (awake or anesthetized) for endotracheal intubation. Examination includes an assessment of anatomic or pathologic factors which may make endotracheal intubation difficult, a thorough dental inspection, and an evaluation of temporomandibular joint function and cervical spine mobility. A written note in the patient's medical record documents pertinent findings related to anesthesia management of the airway.

If nasotracheal intubation is planned, the patency of the nares can be evaluated by asking the patient to breath through each naris while the examiner occludes the other. This is supplemented by direct questioning about previous nasal trauma, pathology, or difficulty breathing through the nose.

Anatomic characteristics that impair alignment of the oral, pharyngeal, and laryngeal axes (Fig. 8-1) and make visualization of the glottis by direct laryngoscopy difficult include the following: a short muscular neck with a full set of teeth; a receding mandible; protruding maxillary incisor teeth; poor mandibular mobility; and a long high arched palate associated with a long narrow mouth.[1]

A dental examination should be performed before direct laryngoscopy is attempted. If orotracheal intubation may involve a high chance of dental injury, the patient should be advised of such risk preoperatively or the anesthesiologists should consider nasotracheal intubation—either blind or with the aid of a fiberoptic laryngoscope. The important observations and steps in the preoperative dental examination include the following:[2]

Presence of loose teeth. Newly erupted deciduous teeth or permanent teeth initially have little support because the roots are only partially formed. Deciduous teeth begin to erupt at about 6 months of age and permanent teeth start at about 6 years of age. As a permanent tooth erupts the root portion of the overlying deciduous tooth undergoes resolution such that just before exfoliation it may be held in place only by fibrous tissue. Children 6 to 12 years old are considered to be in the mixed dentition stage. Peridontal

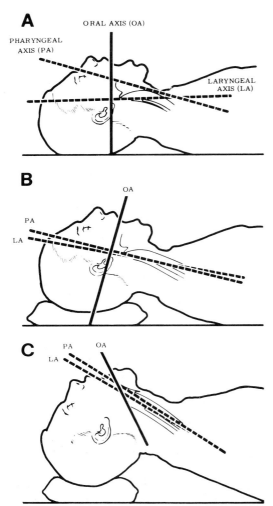

Fig. 8-1 Schematic diagram demonstrating head position for endotracheal intubation. (*A*) Successful direct laryngoscopy requires alignment of the oral, pharyngeal, and laryngeal axes. (*B*) Elevation of the head about 10 cm with pads under the occiput with the shoulders remaining on the table aligns the laryngeal and pharyngeal axes (*C*) Subsequent head extension at the atlanto-occipital joint serves to create the shortest distance and most nearly straight line from the incisor teeth to glottic opening.

disease results in loss of bony support and loosening of teeth.

Existence and position of dental crowns and

bridges. An individual crown (cap) is affixed to an underlying natural tooth and is difficult to detect particularly if it is porcelain. A fixed bridge fills a gap between one or more missing permanent teeth and prosthetic (often porcelain) appliances are attached to the bridge. Crowns and fixed bridges are not removable and are vulnerable to injury by a laryngoscope blade or bite block.

Removable bridges or dentures. These prostheses may be removed preoperatively or left in place until after anesthesia induction so as to facilitate a mask fit.

Preexisting dental abnormalities. The position of missing teeth and chips or fractures (especially on maxillary incisors) must be noted.

Proclination. Loosening and fracture of anterior maxillary teeth is an ever present danger during orotracheal intubation. Protruding maxillary incisors are particularly susceptible to levering effects of the laryngoscope blade.

Mandibular opening can be evaluated by having the patient open his mouth as widely as possible. Normal opening in an adult is in the range of 40 mm (at least 2 fingerbreadths).[3] Any form of arthritis (degenerative or rheumatoid) may limit mandibular mobility. The temporomandibular joint can be evaluated by placing the index finger just anterior to the targus and instructing the patient to open the mouth maximally. One should feel the initial rotational (hinge action) and secondary transitional movement (forward gliding) of the condylar head. Arthritis usually interferes with the forward gliding of the condylar head. If only the first phase of opening is present, difficulty may be experienced in opening the mouth wide enough to accomplish direct laryngoscopy for endotracheal intubation.

Motility of cervical vertebrae, as demonstrated by flexion and extension of the head, is essential for proper positioning and ease of nasal or orotracheal intubation. The normal range of flexion-extension of the head varies from 165 to 90 degrees, with range decreasing

Table 8-1. Indications for Orotracheal Intubation

Prevent aspiration

Facilitate tracheal suctioning

Positive pressure ventilation
  Thoracotomy
  Neuromuscular blockade
  Prolonged need for controlled ventilation

Adverse operative position
  Sitting
  Prone
  Lateral
  Extreme lithotomy or head down

Operative site near or involving upper airway

Airway maintenance by mask difficult

Disease involving upper airway

approximately 20 percent by 75 years of age.[4] Patients may be unaware preoperatively of impaired motion of their cervical vertebrae, since the head may be extended to some degree at the lower cervical vertebrae with the aid of bending the back in the lumbar area.

INDICATIONS FOR OROTRACHEAL INTUBATION

Orotracheal intubation may be considered for every patient receiving general anesthesia. Specific indications for tracheal intubation in the surgical patient receiving general anesthesia are several (Table 8-1).

Aspiration of vomitus, blood, or secretions into the lungs is minimized by placement of a tube in the trachea and inflation of the cuff to provide a seal between the tracheal wall and tube. Protection of the lungs with a cuffed tracheal tube is mandatory in patients who have recently ingested food or in whom intestinal obstruction is present. Although tubes less than 5.0 mm internal diameter rarely have cuffs, selection of a proper sized uncuffed tube for pediatric patients with small tracheas usually results in a sufficient seal to provide acceptable protection against aspiration. Any patient requiring frequent tracheal suction can be best managed with an endotracheal tube in place.

Operations in which positive pressure ventilation is required (thoracotomy, neuromuscular blockade) or in which prolonged controlled ventilation is necessary are most reliably managed with the aid of an endotracheal tube. Without an endotracheal tube, upper airway pressure greater than 25 cm H_2O may force air through a relaxed cricopharyngeal sphincter. When neurosmuscular blockade is incomplete or partial airway obstruction exists, even less pressure may force some gas into the stomach. Gastric distension from air may impede spontaneous ventilation and increases the incidence of regurgitation or vomiting.

Operations performed in other than the supine position may require an endotracheal tube. Maintenance of a patent upper airway or delivery of positive pressure ventilation usually is not reliable without an endotracheal tube when the patient is in the prone, lateral, or sitting position. Steep head-down or lithotomy position may displace abdominal contents against the diaphragm resulting in compromised ventilation or an increased hazard of aspiration. Operations about the head, neck, or upper airway require a tracheal tube for both airway maintenance and/or removal of anesthetic equipment from the operative site.

Prolonged application of a mask on the face may result in tissue ischemia. Although maintenence of an acceptable mask fit on an edentulous patient can be difficult, tracheal intubation usually is technically easy. Various anatomic characteristics (receding mandible, large tongue, short neck, large facial features) make mask placement difficult and airway obstruction likely. Although tracheal intubation is indicated, exposure of the glottic opening may be technically difficult due to the adverse anatomic characteristics.

The presence of a paralyzed vocal cord, supraglottic or subglottic tumor, or external compression of the airway requires insertion of a tracheal tube to insure a patent airway during anesthesia and operation.

TECHNIQUE FOR
OROTRACHEAL INTUBATION

Orotracheal intubation under direct vision in an anesthetized patient is routinely chosen unless specific circumstances dictate otherwise. This is a technique that requires training and experience to make it safe, effective, and atraumatic. Equipment for endotracheal intubation varies and often depends on personal preferences, but always includes a proper sized endotracheal tube or tubes, functioning laryngoscope, appropriate anesthetic drugs and neuromuscular blockers, suction, and facilities to provide positive pressure ventilation with oxygen. If a cuffed endotracheal tube is chosen, the cuff should be checked for air-tightness.

Anesthesia for Endotracheal Intubation

A popular and safe approach in the majority of patients is to produce anesthesia with an intravenous injection of barbiturate followed by succinylcholine to provide skeletal muscle relaxation. With the use of this drug combination direct laryngoscopy may be initiated about 60 seconds following administration of succinylcholine. Oxygen administration prior to laryngoscopy (preoxygenation) minimizes the hazard of hypoxemia developing during the apneic period required for insertion of the tracheal tube. An alternative approach is administration of an inhalation anesthetic for several minutes to achieve an anesthetic depth for laryngoscopy similar to that which will be necessary for surgery. Intubation of the trachea may then be accomplished utilizing the muscle relaxation produced by the inhalation anesthetic but most often succinylcholine is also administered. In some cases, intubation of the trachea is accomplished using a longer-acting nondepolarizing muscle relaxant.

Head Position for Orotracheal Intubation

Successful direct laryngoscopy requires aligning the oral, pharyngeal, and laryngeal axes such that the passageway from the incisor teeth to glottis is most nearly a straight line (Fig. 8-1). Elevating the head about 10 cm with pads under the occiput (shoulders remaining on the table) and head extension at the atlanto-occipital joint serves to align these axes most nearly into a straight line. This posture is described as the "sniffing position." Full extension of the head, without elevation of the occiput, increases the lips to glottis distance, rotates the larynx anteriorly, and may necessitate leverage on the maxillary teeth or gums with the laryngoscope blade to expose the larynx. A frequently forgotten but important element in successful intubation of the trachea is adjustment of the table to a height such that the patient's face is at the level of the laryngoscopist's xiphoid cartilage. If not opened by head extension, the mouth may be manually opened by depressing the mandible with the right thumb while stabilizing the head by counter pressure on the maxillary teeth. Simultaneously, the lower lip can be rolled away with the right index finger.

Use of the Laryngoscope

The laryngoscope is held in the left hand (near the junction between the handle and blade) whether the laryngoscopist is right or left handed and is inserted on the right side of the patient's mouth so as to avoid the incisor teeth and deflect the tongue away from the lumen of the blade. The laryngoscope handle must be maintained perpendicular to the plane of the patient's body after placing the blade in the mouth. Gentleness and avoidance of pressure on the teeth or gums are essential—a protective shield over the maxillary incisors may prevent damage. The laryngoscopist should never lever the handle

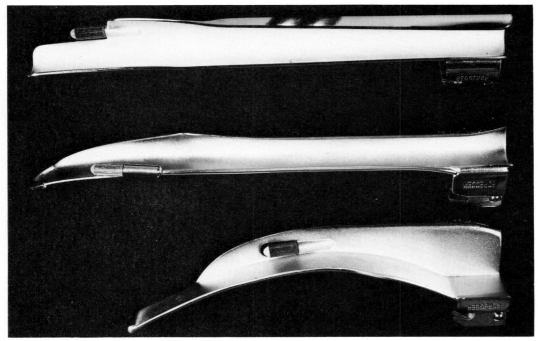

Fig. 8-2 Examples of the most frequently used laryngoscope blades. The uppermost blade is the straight or Jackson-Wisconsin design. The middle blade incorporates a curved distal tip (Miller). The lowermost blade is the curved or MacIntosh blade. All three blades are available in lengths appropriate for neonates and adults.

toward himself. The epiglottis is visualized. The next step depends on the type of laryngoscope blade used (Fig. 8-2).

Curved blade (MacIntosh).[5] The tip of the blade is advanced into the space between the base of the tongue and the pharyngeal surface of the epiglottis (vallecula) (Fig. 8-3*A*). Forward and upward movement of the blade, exerted along the axis of the handle but not by pulling back on the handle, stretches the hypoepiglottic ligament causing the epiglottis to move upward. The glottic opening is then exposed. Insertion of the blade too far in the mouth prevents elevation of the epiglottis and subsequent exposure of the glottis may be limited.

Straight blade (Jackson-Wisconsin) or straight blade with curved tip (Miller).[6] The tip of the blade is passed beneath the laryngeal surface of the epiglottis (Fig. 8-3*B*). Subsequent forward and upward movement of the blade (exerted along the axis of the handle—not by pulling back on the handle) elevates the epiglottis and exposes the glottic opening. Depression or lateral movement of the thyroid cartilage externally on the neck with the right hand may facilitate exposure of the glottis. This maneuver is especially helpful when the epiglottis is floppy and tends to double back on itself. Too deep insertion of the blade may result in elevation of the entire larynx and exposure of the esophagus.

Choice of laryngoscope blade. The choice of laryngoscope blade is often based on personal preference. Advantages cited for the straight blade include greater exposure of the glottic opening permitting observation of the tube as it passes through the glottis and less need for a stylet to direct the tube into an anterior larynx. Some recommend routine use of a stylet when a curved blade is used. Advantages cited for the curved blade include less trauma

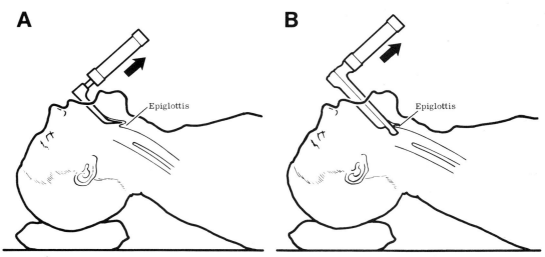

A **B**

Epiglottis Epiglottis

Fig. 8-3 Schematic diagram depicting proper position of the laryngoscope blade during direct laryngo-scopy. (*A*) The distal end of the curved blade is advanced into the space between the base of the tongue and pharyngeal surface of the epiglottis (vallecula). (*B*) The distal end of the straight blade (Jackson-Wisconsin or Miller) is advanced beneath the laryngeal surface of the epiglottis. Regardless of blade design, forward and upward movement exerted along the axis of the laryngoscope blade, as denoted by the arrows, serves to elevate the epiglottis and expose the glottic opening.

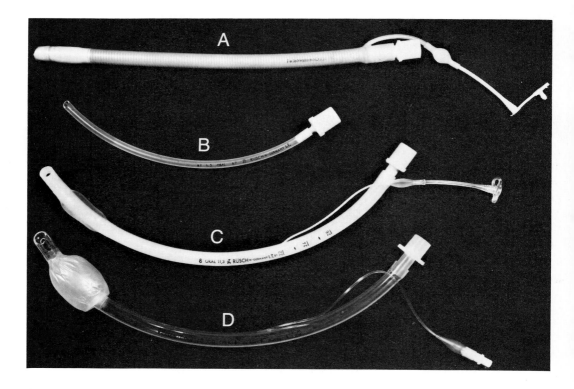

A

B

C

D

Table 8-2. Average Dimensions of Endotracheal Tubes Based on Patient Age

Age	Internal Diameter (mm)	French Unit	Distance Inserted From Lips to Place Distal End in the Midtrachea (cm*)
Premature	2.5	10–12	10
Full Term	3.0	12–14	11
1–6 months	3.5	16	11
6–12 months	4.0	18	12
2 years	4.5	20	13
4 years	5.0	22	14
6 years	5.5	24	15–16
8 years	6.5	26	16–17
10 years	7.0	28	17–18
12 years	7.5	30	18–20
14 years and over	8.0–9.0	32–36	20–24

* Add 2 to 3 cm for nasal tubes.

to teeth and more room for passage of the tube, less bruising of the epiglottis because the blade tip should not touch this structure, and decreased incidence of coughing and laryngospasm. The last theoretic advantage relates to the sensory innervation of the laryngeal surface of the epiglottis by the superior laryngeal nerve and the pharyngeal surface by the glossopharyngeal nerve. Stimulation of the laryngeal surface of the epiglottis is alleged to predispose to laryngospasm and coughing. The frequent use of neuromuscular blockers during endotracheal intubation largely negates this potential advantage.

Endotracheal Tube Size, Length, and Design

Various types of endotracheal tubes are shown in Figure 8-4. Endotracheal tube sizes (Table 8-2) are specified according to internal diameter (ID), which is marked on each tube. Tubes are available in 0.5 mm internal diameter increments. Tube size may also be designated in French units (external diameter in mm times 3, which approximates the external tube circumference). Most adult tracheas readily accept a cuffed 8.0 to 9.0 mm internal diameter tube. The tube also has lengthwise cm markings starting at the distal tracheal end to permit accurate determination of tube length inserted past the nares or lips. The letters I.T. (implantation tested) or Z-79 (Committee Z-79 on Anesthesia Equipment of the USA Standards Institute) on a tube indicate that the tube material has been determined to be free of any tissue irritant or toxicity properties. Tube material should also be radiopaque to demonstrate position of the tube in vivo and transparent to permit visualization of secretions or blockage of air flow as by cessation of breath fogging.

◄Fig. 8-4 Various types of endotracheal tubes. Tube A is an armored or anode tube with a built-in spiral wire to minimize the opportunity of collapse or kinking. Tubes B, C, and D are made of smooth plastic and are recommended for single use. Tube B is uncuffed and is a size appropriate for a child. Tubes C and D are appropriate for adult patients. Tube C is equipped with a built-in high pressure, low residual volume cuff. Tube D is constructed to incorporate a low pressure, high residual volume cuff. Numbers and letters visible on Tubes B, C, and D denote tube diameter, length from tracheal end, and confirmation the tubes have been tested for tissue compatibility (I.T. or Z-79).

Endotracheal Tube Cuff

Cuffs or balloons near the tracheal end of the tube are built into the structure of the tube. The cuff is inflated with air to create a seal against the underlying tracheal mucosa. This seal facilitates positive pressure ventilation and prevents pulmonary aspiration. Cuffs are classified as low residual volume (high pressure) or high residual volume (low pressure).[7] Residual volume is the volume of air that can be withdrawn from the cuff after it has been inflated to just produce a no-leak seal againt the tracheal wall.

Low residual volume cuffs must be inflated to high intraluminal cuff pressures (180 to 250 torr) before they expand sufficiently to create a seal between the tube and tracheal wall. This high cuff pressure is partially transmitted to the underlying tracheal mucosa. Sensing devices placed in the anterior tracheal wall reveal tracheal wall pressure may exceed 100 to 200 torr.[8] Ischemia may occur whenever the pressure on the tracheal mucosa (tracheal wall pressure) exceeds capillary arteriolar pressure (about 32 torr). Small increments of air (1 ml) added to the cuff above that necessary to achieve a no-leak seal may result in further increases in tracheal wall pressure. These cuffs may also inflate asymmetrically, deforming the trachea and eventually producing tracheal dilation.

Tracheal wall changes at low residual volume cuff sites show a consistent pattern of damage.[9] Initially, mucosa beneath the cuff becomes inflamed followed after 3 to 5 days by ulcers overlying cartilaginous rings. Ulcers usually develop first on the more rigid anterior tracheal wall. The exposed cartilaginous rings may subsequently become infected contributing to destruction of the tracheal wall. With continued cuff inflation the infected cartilaginous rings may soften and disappear. This is accompanied by expansion of the trachea at the cuff site visible on standard roentgenography or tantalum tracheograms.[10] Continued pressure from the inflated cuff may result in posterior erosion into the esophagus or anterior erosion into the innominate artery. Following extubation, the tracheal segment may persist as an area of tracheomalacia or become a circumferential cicatricial scar with resulting tracheal stenosis.[11]

High residual volume cuffs inflate symmetrically adapting to the contour of the tracheal wall and developing low intraluminal cuff pressure at no-leak inflation volumes. The resulting tracheal wall pressure has been found to equal peak airway pressure (15 to 30 torr) during positive pressure ventilation.[12] Furthermore, additional air (1 ml) added to these cuffs after the minimal occlusive volume is reached results in small (6 to 25 torr) increases in tracheal wall pressure providing some margin of safety with inadvertent cuff overinflation. Thus, tracheal mucosa ischemia and tracheal dilation would seem less likely with high residual volume cuffs. Indeed, high residual volume cuffs decrease but do not prevent tracheal injury observed at the cuff site.[12]

The intracuff pressure should be controlled at a level sufficient to prevent aspiration yet low enough to allow capillary blood flow in the area contacted by the cuff. Maintaining intracuff pressure in high residual volume thin-walled cuffs (cuff thickness 0.1 mm or less) between 17 and 23 torr during either spontaneous or controlled ventilation prevents aspiration and should still allow adequate capillary mucosal blood flow.[13] Compared with thin cuffs, thick-walled cuffs (0.25 mm and greater) form larger channels or folds when inflated in the trachea and may not prevent aspiration with intracuff pressures in this range. For this reason high residual volume thin-walled cuffs are recommended.

The intraluminal pressure of both high and low residual volume cuffs may be increased by temperature changes as the air used to inflate the cuffs warms to body temperature and by diffusion of anesthetic gases (particularly nitrous oxide) into the air-filled cuff.[14] Inflation of the cuff with the gas mixture delivered from the anesthesia machine negates this latter effect.

Periodic monitoring of the intraluminal cuff pressure and readjustments to prevent excessive pressures may be achieved with an aneroid pressure gauge and a syringe connected to the endotracheal tube cuff via a standard three-way stopcock. Intracuff pressure at no-leak or minimal occlusive volume in high residual volume cuffs is a reasonable guide to tracheal wall pressure. However, similar measurements may not reliably reflect tracheal wall pressure exerted by low residual volume cuffs. Nevertheless there is probably no period of tracheal intubation that does not produce some laryngotracheal damage. Ciliary denudation has been found to occur predominantly over the tracheal rings and underlying cuff site with only 2 hours of intubation and tracheal wall pressures less than 25 torr.[12] Tracheal intubation with cuff inflation for 72 hours was often sufficient to cause wide exposure of several cartilage rings.

Lubricants and Tracheal Spray

Lubricants containing a local anesthetic are often placed on the tracheal end of the tube. However, such lubrication is probably not essential for easy passage of the tube through the already mucus-lubricated glottis. The hazards of an allergic or irritant response to the local anesthetic and/or lubricant must be considered. Tracheal spray of local anesthetic (lidocaine) just before intubation decreases the duration of circulatory responses to tracheal intubation and permits early toleration of the tube with less general anesthetic drug.[15]

Placement of the Endotracheal Tube

The glottis is recognized by its triangular shape and the pale-white vocal cords. The endotracheal tube is held in the right hand like a pencil and introduced on the right side of the mouth with the built-in curve directed anteriorly. Attempts to insert the tube in the midline of the mouth and then down the lumen of the laryngoscope blade usually obscure vision of the glottis. The tube is then advanced past the vocal cords until the cuff just disappears or with an uncuffed tube a distance predicted to place the distal end of the tube midway between the vocal cords and carina (Table 8-2). At this point the laryngoscope blade is withdrawn or readjusted to facilitate placement of an esophageal stethoscope. Then the high residual volume cuff should be inflated with air to just a no-leak volume during positive pressure ventilation, the tube secured with tape, and a bite block inserted between the premolar and molar teeth. Central placement of the bite block may result in impaction or dislodgement of monorooted incisor teeth if forceful closure occurs. Distension of the small pilot balloon attached to the inflation tube leading to the cuff confirms cuff inflation. Distension of the pilot balloon, however, may be misleading if the inflating tube between the balloon and the cuff is obstructed. Insertion of the tube in the trachea can be confirmed by equal chest and air movement bilaterally. Noting the depth of insertion as determined by the cm markings on the endotracheal tube at the lips helps predict a midtracheal position of the distal end of the tube (Table 8-2). Also, if a cuffed tube is properly placed in the midtrachea one can easily detect inflation and deflation of the cuff by palpation in the suprasternal notch.

Anatomic problems leading to difficult visualization of the glottis may be overcome occasionally with a stylet placed in the tube to facilitate directing the tube anteriorly. When properly shaped the tracheal end of the tube should resemble a "hockey stick." Rotating the head to the left, retracting the mouth to the right and placing the laryngoscope blade between the molar teeth provides the shortest distance to the glottis and may be an effective solution to mechanical problems.

When orotracheal intubation during general anesthesia is impossible or unsafe under direct vision, other approaches may be considered—awake intubation, nasotracheal intubation, intubation using a fiberoptic laryngoscope, or retrograde intubation.

AWAKE ENDOTRACHEAL INTUBATION

Local analgesia for awake endotracheal intubation may include topical spray, superior laryngeal nerve block, and transtracheal injection of local anesthetics. This combination permits painless direct laryngoscopy and endotracheal intubation without coughing. When vomiting is a hazard, only topical spray is usually recommended thus avoiding anesthetization of either the larynx or trachea.[16]

The lips, tongue, palate, and pharynx should be sprayed with 3 to 5 ml of 2 to 4 percent lidocaine. It is helpful to reduce secretions with an anticholinergic drug. When nasotracheal intubation is planned, cocaine (1 to 2 ml of a 4 to 5 percent solution) is also used to constrict and anesthetize the nasal mucosa. This is accomplished by inserting into the selected naris cocaine-containing pledgets attached to applicators. Spray devices are usually less satisfactory, since they may provide topical anesthesia for only the anterior portion of the nasal cavity. Furthermore, advancement of the pledgets into the nasopharynx confirms patency and illustrates the direction the nasotracheal tube should follow through the naris.

The superior laryngeal nerve may be blocked as it penetrates the thyrohyoid membrane near the cornu of the hyoid bone. The needle is inserted caudad to the hyoid and 2 to 3 ml of 2 percent lidocaine deposited just below the greater cornu.[17] Injection of 2 to 3 ml of 2 to 4 percent lidocaine into the lumen of the trachea will anesthetize the trachea and larynx below the vocal cords. The cricothyroid or cricotracheal membrane is pierced with a needle attached to a syringe, correct placement confirmed by aspiration of

air, and the lidocaine injected rapidly at end-expiration to enable subsequent inspiration and cough to distribute the local anesthetic along the trachea and against the inferior aspects of the vocal cords.

NASOTRACHEAL INTUBATION

Nasotracheal intubation may be performed electively for intraoral operations, when anatomic abnormalities or disease of the upper airway make direct laryngoscopy difficult or impossible, and occasionally when long-term mechanical ventilation is anticipated. Advantages cited for nasotracheal intubation include more stable tube fixation, less chance for tube kinking, greater comfort in an awake patient, and fewer oropharyngeal secretions. Awake blind nasotracheal intubation is usually reserved for situations in which laryngoscopy or ventilation would be impossible or induction of anesthesia before endotracheal intubation would be hazardous. When vomiting is not a hazard and ventilation can be maintained by means of a mask, but laryngoscopy is impossible, anethesia may be safely produced before blind nasotracheal intubation. Otherwise, nasotracheal intubation is accomplished under direct laryngoscopy with anesthesia and frequently neuromuscular blockade.

Technique for Awake Blind Nasotracheal Intubation

To insure maximum patient comfort and nasal patency and to minimize the chance of epistaxis the nasal mucosa should be anesthetized and constricted with cocaine. Topical anesthesia of the tongue and pharynx, superior laryngeal nerve block, and transtracheal anesthesia may be performed to improve patient comfort. Conversely, local anesthesia of the upper airway, larynx, and trachea may be distressing to an awake patient and impair protective reflexes should vomiting occur.

Either naris may be chosen depending on history and examination but the right is preferable because the bevel of most nasotracheal tubes when introduced through the right naris will face the flat nasal septum reducing damage to the turbinates. In an adult a 7.0 to 7.5 mm internal diameter tube is usually adequate. Nasal and oral tubes may be used interchangeably.

The occiput should be elevated about 10 cm and a well-curved and generously lubricated nasotracheal tube introduced into the selected naris. Extension of the head at the atlanto-occipital joint helps lift the epiglottis away from the posterior pharyngeal wall. The tube is then advanced along the floor of the nose (in the direction determined earlier with cocaine-soaked pledgets) into the oropharynx and aligned with the glottic opening by listening to the air passing through the tube. The tube is advanced as long as breath sounds are maximal. The anesthesiologist must have his ear close to the tube connector to readily detect change in breath sounds. Ideally, the tube is swiftly passed through the glottis just before inspiration because the vocal cords are most open during inspiration and the risk of vocal cord trauma is thus minimized. The technique of passing the tube at the moment of an explosive cough is often successful. Successful placement in the trachea is confirmed by continued breathing through the tube.

Blind Nasotracheal Intubation During Anesthesia

Cocaine is applied to the nasal mucosa. No additional anesthesia is necessary but transtracheal anesthesia may be performed to prevent coughing. Anesthesia is produced with intravenous or inhalation drugs taking care to avoid deep anesthesia, as maintenance of spontaneous ventilation is essential to identifying the glottic opening. Occasionally, carbon dioxide or doxapram may be used to stimulate ventilation. Anesthesia with intra-venous ketamine (2 to 3 mg/kg) followed by transtracheal anesthesia may also be used, advantages being that the airway and spontaneous ventilation are maintained.[18] After appropriate anesthesia, the tube is introduced through the nose and directed to the glottic opening in the same manner as described for awake blind nasotracheal intubation.

Diagnosis and Corrective Maneuvers When the Nasotracheal Tube Does Not Enter the Larynx

A common problem is for the tube to impinge in the sulcus between the base of the tongue and epiglottis or on the anterior commissure of the glottic opening. Observation of the neck reveals a bulge in the midline just above the thyroid cartilage. The remedy is to divert the tube more posterior by increased flexion of the head. Conversely, passage into the esophagus, manifested by easy advancement to the full length of the tube, loss of breath sounds, and continued phonation in the awake patient is corrected by diverting the tube more anterior by increased extension of the head. Lateral displacement into the pyriform sinus is manifested by loss of breath sounds, resistance to further tube advancement, and bulging in the neck lateral to the laryngeal prominence. Withdrawing the tube 2 to 3 cm and rotation 45 to 90 degrees in the opposite direction serves to orient the tube to the midline. Alternatively, the thyroid cartilage may be manually and externally displaced to align the glottic opening with the tube. Excessive force should never be used to pass a tube through the nasopharynx. If the nasotracheal tube has an excessive curve, advancement beyond the level of the vocal cords may be impossible because the tip impinges against the anterior wall of the larynx. If hyperflexion of the head does not resolve this problem, a less curved tube may be substituted. Nasotracheal intubation under direct vision demonstrates the maneuvers that are necessary to produce appropriate deflec-

Table 8-3. Complications Peculiar to Nasotracheal Intubation

Epistaxis
Trauma to posterior pharyngeal wall
Dislodgement of pharyngeal tonsils (adenoids)
Pressure necrosis
Eustachian tube obstruction
Maxillary sinusitis
Bacteremia

tions of the tube when blind endotracheal intubation is necessary.

Nasotracheal Intubation with Direct Vision of the Glottis

After application of cocaine to the nasal mucosa, anesthesia is produced with intravenous or inhalation anesthetic drugs most often combined with succinylcholine to produce skeletal muscle relaxation. After the nasotracheal tube has entered the oropharynx, the glottis is visualized by direct laryngoscopy. The tube is guided into the larynx under vision by manually advancing it at the nasal end or the tube may be grasped in the oropharynx with intubating forceps (Magill type) and directed so that pressure on the nasal end causes the tube to pass between the vocal cords. Again, the right naris is usually preferred because a left nasotracheal tube is clumsy to advance under direct vision with the left hand holding the laryngoscope.

Complications Peculiar to Nasotracheal Intubation

A summary of these complications is shown in Table 8-3. Epistaxis may follow avulsion of nasal mucosa covering the turbinates. Proper shrinkage of the nasal mucosa with cocaine and use of small generously lubricated tubes should minimize this complication. Should bleeding occur, the nasotracheal tube should be left in place to provide a tamponade effect. In some instances the tube may be withdrawn so that only the cuff re-

mains in the naris and subsequent inflation of the cuff tamponades the bleeding site. Perforation and dissection of the posterior pharyngeal wall creating a false passage may occur especially if force is used to advance the tube through the nasopharynx. Pharyngeal tonsils (adenoids) may be prominent, especially in children, producing resistance to passage through the nasopharynx or bleeding if the tonsils are traumatized. Again, gentle advancement and avoidance of excessive force should minimize this hazard. It is preferable, when pharyngeal tonsils are prominent, to perform all nasotracheal intubations under direct vision so as to prevent carrying a dislodged piece of tonsil into the trachea with the tube.

Necrosis of the external naris reflects excessive pressure from the nasotracheal tube and may be minimized by proper fixation of the tube and, obviously, the earliest extubation possible consistent with patient safety.[19] Eustachian tube obstruction by the nasotracheal tube may impair hearing. Maxillary sinusitis resulting from impaired drainage due to obstruction by the nasotracheal tube may be manifested by facial pain, nasal stuffiness, purulent secretions, or fever.[20]

Bacteremia may occur following nasotracheal intubation, reflecting the entrance of normal upper airway flora into the circulation via traumatized nasal mucosa or the transport of flora from the nose into the trachea by the tube and the subsequent entrance into the circulation via the vascular tracheal mucosa.[21] When nasotracheal intubation is necessary in patients with heart disease, prophylactic antibiotics may be indicated.

TECHNIQUE FOR FIBEROPTIC LARYNGOSCOPY

Endotracheal intubation using a flexible fiberoptic laryngoscope (fiberscope) has been described.[22, 23] The fiberscope is lubricated to allow easy passage through an appropriate-sized endotracheal tube (about 8 mm internal diameter) and the tip is treated with an antifogging solution to assure a clear view during laryngoscopy. After topical anesthesia as described for awake blind nasotracheal intubation, with or without intravenous analgesia, the endotracheal tube is passed through the naris into the oropharynx. The fiberscope is advanced through the endotracheal tube until the epiglottis is visualized. After the fiberscope is passed between the vocal cords, the endotracheal tube is advanced using the fiberscope as a guide. The endotracheal tube is positioned proximal to the carina by direct vision. Oral intubation is accomplished in a similar manner by placing the fiberscope behind the base of the tongue with the fingers or with limited traction using a laryngoscope blade.

Appreciation of the following will increase success with the fiberscope:[23]

1. Secretions obscure the view, therefore an anticholinergic drug in the preoperative medication is helpful.

2. The epiglottis is surprisingly high in the oropharynx.

3. In contrast to the stretched appearance with direct laryngoscopy the pyriform sinuses are relaxed and can resemble the pathway to the glottis.

4. It is essential that the fiberscope be kept in the midline to avoid entering the pyriform sinus.

5. The optics of the fiberscope exaggerate the depth of the vocal cords, which may not be seen until the false vocal cords are passed.

6. A helpful sign that the fiberscope is properly positioned is the glow seen over the anterior neck from transillumination of the larynx and trachea as the fiberscope tip passes through the glottis. This is not seen when the fiberscope is passed posteriorly into the esophagus.

In addition to its use in difficult endotracheal intubations, the fiberscope may be passed through an endotracheal tube to diagnose accidental endobronchial intubation or the cause of endotracheal tube obstruction (kinks, secretions) during anesthesia. Also,

proper placement of double-lumen endobronchial tubes may be confirmed if the tube lumen is sufficient to allow passage of the fiberscope. The diameter of most fiberscopes prevents passage through tube lumens with an internal diameter less than 6 mm.

RETROGRADE INTUBATION

Retrograde intubation is accomplished by passing a plastic catheter through a needle (17 gauge intracath) previously placed through the cricothyroid membrane.[24] The catheter is directed cephalad and brought out the mouth or naris. An endotracheal tube is threaded over the plastic catheter and directed through the glottis using the catheter as a guide. This technique is probably best considered only when others such as nasotracheal intubation or use of the fiberoptic laryngoscope have been unsuccessful.

ENDOTRACHEAL INTUBATION IN CHILDREN

Anatomic Differences From Adults

Because newborns and children are anatomically different from adults, their tracheas may be more difficult to intubate than those of adults.[25] These differences result in difficulty aligning the oral, pharyngeal, and tracheal axes and elevating the epiglottis to expose the anterior glottic opening. For example, the newborn head and tongue are large and the neck is short. The larynx is more cephalad than in the adult—the lower border of the cricoid cartilage is opposite the 4th cervical vertebra at birth and opposite the 5th cervical vertebra at age 6. The epiglottis is U-shaped and stiff. Furthermore, the cricoid cartilage is the narrowest point in the larynx, and a tube that passes through the glottis may resist advancement at this site. Also, excessive traction with the laryngoscope blade may angulate the trachea producing the same problem.

Endotracheal Tube Size and Length

Selection of the appropriate endotracheal tube size and length is critical in children as the margin for error is small. Excessive tube size is responsible for unnecessary laryngotracheal trauma which may be manifest as laryngeal edema when the tube is removed. Likewise, the short glottis to carina distance in children necessitates careful calculation of correct length of the tube. Ideally, the tip of the tube should be located midway between the glottis and carina to minimize the hazards of accidental endobronchial intubation or extubation. One must be aware that head flexion or change from the supine to head down position may shift the carina upward converting a tracheal tube placement to an endobronchial intubation and that head extension may place the tube in the pharynx.

Recommended tube size and distance of insertion are summarized in Table 8-2. In children 2 to 14 years old, proper tube size may be predicted using the following formulas, recognizing that these provide only a guide:

Internal diameter (mm)
= (age in years/4) + 4.5 (Ref. 26)
French catheter size (units)
= 18 + age in years (Ref. 27)

An endotracheal tube one size above and below the calculated size should be available with the final choice made when the glottis is visualized and the tube is inserted into the trachea. Cuffed tubes are probably not necessary before 5 years of age because the narrow subglottic tracheal diameter insures an adequate seal until this time.

A formula may be used as a guide to predict proper tube length for ideal tube placement in the trachea. This formula may be useful until about 14 years of age. Nasotracheal tubes should be about 20 percent longer.

Orotracheal tube length for midtrachea placement (cm)
= (age in years/2) + 12 (Ref. 28)

Resistance to breathing is a consideration for the small lumen tubes and connectors necessary in children. Narrow curved endotracheal tube connectors should be avoided because they increase airway resistance and impede passage of a suction catheter. A connector with a lumen as large as or larger than the endotracheal tube should always be employed. When increased airway resistance is a concern the best approach is placement of a proper (not the largest possible) sized tube and controlled ventilation to prevent increased work of breathing.

Method of Endotracheal Intubation

Complications of endotracheal intubation in children have been minimized by employing single use polyvinylchloride sterile tubes of appropriate size that have been inserted with minimal trauma. Orotracheal intubation is routinely chosen for short-term endotracheal tube placement. Awake intubation in the newborn is preferable. This is accomplished with the head elevated on a padded ring while an assistant immobilizes and extends the head and depresses the shoulders. Two-week-old healthy infants are sufficiently strong to vigorously resist awake intubation and anesthesia may be produced before direct laryngoscopy. A straight laryngoscope blade may provide better exposure of the glottis than the curved blade especially in children less than 3 years of age.

The route of tube placement when the intubation is likely to be prolonged beyond 12 hours is unsettled. Orotracheal intubation permits use of a large internal diameter tube and easier suctioning; however, nasotracheal intubation allows more stable tube fixation with decreased chance of accidental extubation.

The tube must be securely fixed to prevent tube movement, which may result in accidental slippage of the tube into a mainstem bronchus or into the pharynx. Benzoin applied to the skin and tube at the lips or nose facilitates fixation with tape. For prolonged intubation, covering the benzoin-prepared skin with Elastoplast and then suturing the tube to the Elastoplast may be considered. A sandbag behind the head may help maintain it in a neutral position.

EXTUBATION

Extubation of the trachea following general anesthesia is ideally accomplished while the patient is still adequately anesthetized to diminish coughing and laryngospasm. This assumes that adequate ventilation is present or can be maintained without the endotracheal tube and vomiting is not a likely hazard. Suctioning of the pharynx should be performed prior to extubation of the trachea so that secretions proximal to the cuff do not drain into the trachea when the cuff is deflated. Unless secretions are audible in the endotracheal tube or the lungs, aspiration through the tube is not advised because of the risk of introducing bacteria into the trachea. The cuff is then deflated and the tube removed. Some prefer pressure on the reservoir bag as the tube is removed so the lungs will be inflated and initial gas flow is outward. This maneuver may also facilitate a cough and expulsion of any aspirated material. Laryngospasm and vomiting are the most serious immediate hazards; therefore, oxygen, succinylcholine, equipment for reintubation, and suction must be immediately available.

When vomiting is a hazard at the conclusion of anesthesia, the endotracheal tube should not be removed until protective laryngeal reflexes have returned. However, patients occasionally "cough" vigorously when allowed to awaken with an endotracheal tube in place. This response is often referred to as "bucking" and represents a modified cough as the glottis cannot close. Coughing and associated contraction of abdominal and chest muscles, if allowed to persist, may strain recently placed sutures, produce hypoxemia if breath holding occurs, and increase intracranial pressure. Furthermore, laryngeal trauma is more likely when the arytenoid cartilages attempt to close forcibly around the endotracheal tube. Vigorous reaction to the tracheal tube (bucking) signals the return of the cough reflex and at this point either the tube must be removed or further sedation instituted to permit tolerance of the tube. Lidocaine 1 mg/kg intravenously 2 minutes before extubation may prevent coughing, hypertension, and tachycardia associated with extubation of the trachea.[29]

COMPLICATIONS OF ENDOTRACHEAL INTUBATION

The complications of endotracheal intubation (Table 8-4) rarely occur. Even this low incidence may be reduced by skillful technique, appropriate use of anesthetic drugs and neuromuscular blockers, and an understanding of the causes of these complications. Certainly the benefits of a properly placed and patent endotracheal tube far exceed the risks of intubation. Complications may be categorized as those occurring during direct laryngoscopy and endotracheal intubation, while the endotracheal tube is in place, and following extubation—either immediately or after a delay.[30]

Complications During Direct Laryngoscopy and Endotracheal Intubation

Trauma related to direct laryngoscopy may occur anywhere from the lips to glottis but dental trauma is most serious and frequent.

Table 8-4. Complications of Endotracheal Intubation

Complications During Direct Laryngoscopy and Endotracheal Intubation
Trauma—teeth most vulnerable
Hypertension and tachycardia
Dysrhythmias
Aspiration

Complications While the Endotracheal Tube is in Place
Tracheal tube obstruction
Endobronchial intubation
Esophageal intubation
Accidental extubation
Increased resistance to breathing
Aspiration
"Bucking"
Bronchospasm
Tracheal mucosa ischemia

Immediate and Delayed Complications Following Extubation
Laryngospasm
Aspiration
Pharyngitis (sore throat)
Laryngitis
Laryngeal or subglottic edema
Laryngeal ulceration with or without granuloma formation
Tracheitis
Tracheal stenosis
Introduction of bacteria into the lungs
Vocal cord paralysis—unilateral or bilateral
Arytenoid cartilage dislocation

Avoidance of pressure on teeth from the laryngoscopy blade will minimize the hazard of dental trauma. Tooth protectors may protect vulnerable natural teeth (maxillary incisors) or fragile dental prostheses from chipping or fracture by the laryngoscopy blade. Should injury occur, immediate expert dental advice is necessary and a notation describing the circumstances surrounding the injury should be placed in the patient's record. A dislodged tooth must be recovered and if the search is unsuccessful appropriate thoracic and abdominal roentgenograms should be taken. A displaced tooth should be placed in saline as reimplantation may be possible.

Hypertension and tachycardia frequently accompany laryngoscopy and endotracheal intubation. Similar changes accompany the use of either a straight or curved laryngoscope blade.[31] Limiting the duration of direct laryngoscopy to about 15 seconds and immediately preceding placement of the tube in the trachea with laryngotracheal lidocaine spray (2 mg/kg of a 4 percent solution) minimizes the magnitude and duration of these responses.[32] Laryngotracheal lidocaine produces almost immediate topical anesthesia such that a 3 to 5 minute delay between application and insertion of the tracheal tube is not necessary.

The transient circulatory responses to direct laryngoscopy and endotracheal intubation are probably innocuous in patients with a normal circulatory system. Overzealous use of deep anesthesia, topical anesthesia, depressant drugs, or vasodilators in an attempt to prevent changes caused by laryngoscopy and intubation may ultimately introduce more hazard than the response it was intended to attenuate. However, the responses to direct laryngoscopy may be exaggerated in patients with preexisting hypertension. Furthermore, these responses may jeopardize tissue viability in patients with coronary artery disease or valvular heart disease. In these patients when laryngoscopy and tracheal intubation cannot be predictably accomplished in a rapid manner, intravenous nitroprusside 1 to 2 μg/kg 15 seconds before starting direct laryngoscopy will attenuate the blood pressure response.[33]

Cardiac dysrhythmias apart from sinus tachycardia or bradycardia occur in 5 to 15 percent of patients during endotracheal intubation under light anesthesia.[34] These dysrhythmias are rarely serious or prolonged especially if adequate oxygenation is maintained. Ventilation with oxygen for 1 minute before initiating laryngoscopy maintains arterial oxygen partial pressure above awake levels for at least 2 to 3 minutes of apnea in most adults.[35]

Complications While the Endotracheal Tube is in Place

Obstruction of the endotracheal tube may result from secretions, blood, or a foreign body in the tube; kinking; inward collapse of the tube lumen by pressure on the inflated cuff; migration of a slip-on cuff over the tip of the tube; and asymmetrical inflation of the cuff forcing the tube against the tracheal wall. Passage of a fiberoptic laryngoscope through the endotracheal tube may facilitate rapid diagnosis when obstruction is not relieved by deflating the cuff or passing a suction catheter through the tube.

Inadvertent endobronchial intubation will be minimized by calculating the proper tube length for every patient and then noting the cm marking on the tube at the point of fixation (Table 8-2). Ideally, the tip of the tube should be midway between the glottis and carina. Since the suprasternal notch is midway between the glottis and carina, proper tube position may be confirmed by external palpation in the suprasternal notch and detection of cuff distension during rapid inflation. Auscultation to determine equal air entry, visual confirmation of equal and bilateral chest movement (particularly upper chest), and chest roentgenograms are also helpful in confirming proper tube placement. The trachea may move cephalad with head flexion, lateral rotation, or the head-down positioning converting a tracheal tube to an endobronchial tube especially if the tube was placed near the carina with the head in a neutral position. Hyperextension of the head may place the distal end of the tracheal tube in the pharynx. Accurate interpretation of tube placement on chest roentgenograms requires a knowledge of head position when the picture was taken. Roentgenograms of adult patients demonstrated an average 1.9 cm movement of the tracheal tube with both flexion and extension of the head.[36] Lateral head rotation moved the tube 0.7 cm away from the carina.

Esophageal placement of the endotracheal tube is accompanied by a characteristic "bubbly" sound and auscultation of gastric air entry with positive pressure. Should esophageal intubation occur, the tube should be disconnected from the anesthetic system to avoid further gastric distension. If regurgitation is a consideration, one may leave the tube in the esophagus and inflate the cuff. Following tracheal intubation, the stomach should be decompressed and the esophageal tube removed.

Accidental extubation, which is most likely in young patients, may be minimized by proper fixation of the endotracheal tube and maintenance of the head in a neutral position. Narrow endotracheal tubes and connectors cause turbulent air flow increasing the work of breathing and, in the extreme, hypoxemia and hypercarbia. Secretions or blood may pool above the endotracheal tube cuff only to enter the trachea if the cuff is deflated. Vigorous attempts (bucking) by the patient to dislodge the tracheal tube may decrease lung volumes with subsequent hypoxemia. Bronchospasm has been attributed to placement of the tracheal tube in a lightly anesthetized patient.

The inflated tracheal tube cuff may transmit excessive pressure to tracheal mucosa and impair capillary blood flow. As described previously, ischemia of the trachea mucosa is minimal with high residual volume cuffs, but even low residual volume cuffs may exert tracheal wall pressures above 100 torr.[7]

Immediate and Delayed Complications Following Endotracheal Extubation (also see Chs. 39 and 43)

Laryngospasm is unlikely if anesthetic depth is sufficient during extubation or the patient is allowed to awaken before extubation. It is the patient who is lightly anesthetized at the time of extubation who is most at risk. Adequate pharyngeal suctioning before extubation is important. If laryngospasm occurs, oxygen under positive pressure with a face mask or forward displacement of the mandible using the index fingers to apply pressure at the temporomandibular joint may be sufficient treatment. Administration of succinylcholine (intravenous or intramuscular) may be given if spasm persists.

Aspiration is most likely to occur in the debilitated patient or in the presence of gastrointestinal obstruction. Laryngeal competence may be decreased immediately following removal of the tracheal tube predisposing patients to the hazards of aspiration. The ability of the larynx to sense foreign material does not return to normal until 4 to 8 hours following extubation.[37]

Some denudation of pharyngeal and laryngeal epithelium is inevitable with endotracheal intubation. A number of studies have attempted to determine the incidence of pharyngitis (sore throat) after endotracheal intubation. The incidence ranges from 5.7 percent[38] to nearly 40 percent.[39] The higher incidence occurred when patients were asked specifically about symptoms of sore throat rather than when based on complaints volunteered by the patient. The incidence of sore throat was more frequent following intubation with tubes having a large cuff-tracheal contact area.[40] Females manifest sore throat more often than males, possibly because of the thinner mucosal covering over the posterior vocal cords. Sore throat disappears within 48 to 72 hours without any specific therapy. This side-effect is so minor it should not influence the decision to perform endotracheal intubation.

Laryngitis occurs in about 3 percent of patients and is manifested by hoarseness and a tight feeling in the throat.[41] Recovery is usually spontaneous without any treatment.

Symptomatic laryngeal or subglottic edema is most likely in children because a small amount of laryngeal swelling greatly reduces the lumen of the larynx.[42] For example, 1 mm of edema in a newborn reduces the cross-sectional area of the larynx by 65 percent. The same amount of edema produces only slight hoarseness in an adult. In addition, the cricoid cartilage prevents any external expansion when edema occurs. The most likely causes of edema in children are mechanical injury (traumatic intubation, oversized tube) or infection (unsterile endotracheal tube or a recent or preexisting upper re-

spiratory infection). However, even with adequate precautions and flawless technique, edema may still occur.

Laryngeal ulceration, with or without granuloma formation, typically occurs on the posterior portion of the vocal cords underlying the rigid projection of the arytenoid cartilage known as the vocal process.[43] This initial contact ulcer is most likely produced by the endotracheal tube moving on the thin mucoperichondrial covering underlying the vocal processes. Hyperextension of the neck, as during thyroid operations, may increase the pressure exerted on the vocal processes by the tracheal tube. Excessive head movement or inadequate depression of laryngeal reflexes may also accentuate damage when the arytenoid cartilages scrape the endotracheal tube. Often the cause of ulceration is unrelated to the endotracheal tube and remains unknown. Preoperative respiratory infections seem to exacerbate the laryngeal reaction by constantly bathing the ulcerated mucosa with bacteria. Granulation tissue tends to cover the ulcerated area, resulting in a sessile granuloma. Subsequently, the ulcer base narrows by fibrosis until pedunculation occurs.

Granuloma of the larynx following endotracheal intubation is rare (1 in every 10,000 to 20,000 intubations) and has been described only in adults.[44] The greater incidence in females may reflect the fact that the mucosal layer covering the vocal processes of the arytenoid cartilages is twice as thick in males as in females. Granulomas are bilateral in about half the reported cases. Bilateral ulcerations may heal by side to side adhesions resulting in a laryngeal web. Postintubation granulomas usually require 14 to 21 days to develop but may appear in as little as 72 hours.[45] Persistent hoarseness is the most common symptom and alone or in combination with sore throat, pain or fullness in the laryngotracheal area, or unexplained upper airway obstruction is an indication for indirect laryngoscopy. If an ulceration is observed strict vocal rest should allow healing without granuloma formation. Surgical removal of the pedunculated granuloma under direct laryngoscopy followed by absolute vocal rest may be required.

During prolonged endotracheal intubation, the route used for tracheal tube insertion may influence the incidence and type of laryngeal injury. In patients intubated an average 6.7 days, laryngeal injury (vocal cord ulceration and cratering) following extubation was more frequent and severe after oral than nasal tracheal intubation.[46] This may reflect the use of smaller tracheal tubes for nasal intubation and better stability so that nasotracheal tube movement is less likely with changes in head position.

Ulceration of the tracheal mucosa may occur at the anterior tracheal wall where the tip of the endotracheal tube has abraded the epithelium. The resulting tracheitis is manifested as substernal discomfort and coughing.

The endotracheal tube cuff may exert excessive pressure on the tracheal wall (capillary pressure at the arterial end is about 30 torr) and thus produce mucosa ischemia. This may progress to destruction of cartilaginous rings and subsequent circumferential cicatricial scar formation and tracheal stenosis. Other causative factors to consider include duration of intubation (greater than 48 hours), high ventilator pressures with tube movement, bacterial infection, and persistent systemic hypotension. Stenosis becomes symptomatic when the adult tracheal lumen is reduced to less than 5 mm. Some patients may be managed with dilatation, but surgical resection of the stenotic segment may be necessary. These hazards are minimized by use of high residual volume cuffs which, when properly used, do not produce excessive tracheal wall pressures.

A relation between endotracheal intubation and pulmonary complications (pneumonia) has never been proven. More important are the preoperative pulmonary status and the operative procedure. Nevertheless, oropharyngeal bacteria not ordinarily present in the trachea may be introduced into the trachea with an endotracheal tube and bacteremia has been shown after nasotracheal (not orotracheal) intubation.[21] Good oral hygiene may reduce tracheal contamination especially in patients with carious teeth.

Unilateral[47] and bilateral[41] vocal cord paralyses have been reported after short-term endotracheal intubation for operations not about the larynx. The mechanism is unknown. Irregular cuff inflation compressing a branch of the recurrent laryngeal nerve between the cuff and thyroid cartilage has been implicated.[48] When paralysis is unilateral the left vocal cord is affected twice as frequently as the right. Males are affected approximately seven times more frequently than females.[49] Asymptomatic laryngeal nerve palsy may even predate tracheal intubation. In such patients any edema from instrumentation might produce hoarseness with a subsequent diagnosis of recurrent laryngeal nerve palsy and wrongful implication of the tracheal tube as the etiology.[50]

Arytenoid cartilage dislocation is a rare complication that has been attributed to inserting the laryngoscope blade too far behind the cricoid cartilage with resulting arytenoid cartilage dislocation during elevation of the blade.[51] A weak voice following extubation after prolonged intubation has been reported due to unilateral arytenoid cartilage dislocation.[52] Treatment is reduction and cricoarytenoid arthrodesis.

DELIBERATE ENDOBRONCHIAL INTUBATION

Endobronchial intubation (also see Ch. 29) serves to provide separate airways to the healthy and diseased lung or to improve intrathoracic operating conditions by providing a nonventilated quiet lung. Specific indications for selective lung ventilation or suction include lung abscess, bronchiectasis, or bronchopleural fistula. Selective lung ventilation may be accomplished with a double-lumen endobronchial tube, which permits isolated but simultaneous ventilation of both

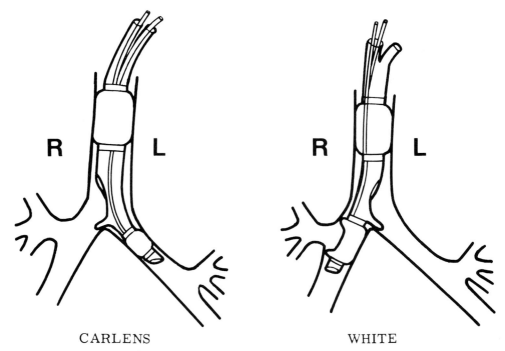

CARLENS   WHITE

Fig. 8-5 The Carlens double-lumen endotracheal tube is advanced down the trachea with the tip directed to enter the left mainstem bronchus until the rubber hook engages the carina. Inflation of the tracheal and left mainstem bronchus cuffs effectively isolates the lungs and permits selective ventilation. The White tube is advanced with the distal end directed to enter the right mainstem bronchus until the hook engages the carina. Inflation of the cuffs isolates the lungs. Ventilation of the right upper lobe is accomplished via an opening in the portion of the tube opposite the right mainstem bronchus.

lungs. It should be remembered that the carina to right upper lobe bronchus distance is about 1.5 cm compared with about 5 cm on the left. Proper endobronchial tube position is confirmed by auscultation, by chest roentgenogram, or by passing a fiberoptic laryngoscope through the tube.

The need for one-lung ventilation must be weighed against the hazard of hypoxemia. Intrapulmonary shunting occurs regardless of ventilation patterns, and efforts to improve arterial oxygenation by raising intraalveolar pressure in the ventilated lung may act to divert blood flow to the unventilated lung.[53] Arterial hypoxemia, not corrected by high inspired oxygen concentrations, has been documented during anesthesia delivered through a double-lumen tube with collapse of the nondependent (operated) lung.[54] Patients

undergoing similar operations with conventional endotracheal tubes manifested less intrapulmonary shunting and maintained satisfactory arterial oxygen partial pressures breathing high inspired oxygen concentrations. This suggests that the partially inflated upper lung contributed to their oxygenation during the surgical procedure. Arterial oxygenation would be best maintained by deferring unilateral ventilation until the circulation to the nonventilated lung has been surgically interrupted. Arterial carbon dioxide partial pressures do not change greatly during one-lung ventilation.[55]

The Carlens double-lumen tube (Fig. 8-5) is introduced under direct vision using a rotational motion and advanced down the trachea with the tip pointed to enter the left mainstem bronchus until the rubber hook engages the carina.[56] The left lung is ventilated through the tube lumen that lies in the bronchus and the right lung through the lumen that opens above the carina. Disadvantages of the Carlens tube include increased airway resistance and difficulty suctioning thick secretions through the small lumens (6 to 8 mm). The small lumen size may make it difficult or impossible to pass a fiberoptic laryngoscope to confirm proper tube placement. Furthermore, this tube must be withdrawn into the trachea during a left pneumonectomy.

The White double-lumen tube (Fig. 8-5) is designed for introduction into the right mainstem bronchus.[57] The lumen of the tube in the bronchus carries a cuff surrounding a rectangular slot in the tube so that the right upper lobe bronchus can be ventilated. A rubber hook on the tube engages the carina.

The Robertshaw double-lumen tube was designed for maximum lumen size to offset the disadvantages of the Carlens tube.[58] Both left- and right-sided bronchial models are available. Left-sided tubes have a tip angled at 45 degrees to enter the left mainstem bronchus, while the tip of the right-sided tube is angled at 20 degrees to enter the right mainstem bronchus. Neither tube has a carinal hook.

REFERENCES

1. Cass NM, James NR, Lines V: Difficult direct laryngoscopy complicating intubation for anesthesia. Br Med J 1:488, 1956
2. Wright RB, Manfield FFV: Damage to teeth during the administration of general anesthesia. Anesth Analg 53:405, 1974
3. Block C, Brechner VL: Unusual problems in airway management II: The influence of the temporomandibular joint, the mandible, and associated structures on endotracheal intubation. Anesth Analg 50:114, 1971
4. Brechner VL: Unusual problems in the management of airways: I. Flexion-extension mobility of the cervical vertebrae. Anesth Analg 47:363, 1968
5. MacIntosh RR: New laryngoscope. Lancet 1:205, 1943
6. Miller RA: A new laryngoscope. Anesthesiology 2:317, 1941
7. Carroll R, Hedden M, Safar P: Intratracheal cuffs: Performance characteristics. Anesthesiology 31:275, 1969
8. Knowlson GTG, Bassett HFM: The pressures exerted on the trachea by endotracheal inflatable cuffs. Br J Anaesth 42:824, 1970
9. Cooper JD, Grillo HC: Analysis of problems related to cuffs on intratracheal tubes. Chest 62:215, 1972
10. Dunn CR, Dunn DL, Moser KM: Determinants of tracheal injury by cuffed tracheostomy tubes. Chest 65:128, 1974
11. Andrews MJ, Pearson FG: Incidence and pathogenesis of tracheal injury following cuffed tube tracheostomy and assisted ventilation: Analysis of a two year prospective study. Ann Surg 173:249, 1971
12. Klainer AS, Turndorf H, Wen-Hsien WU et al: Surface alterations due to endotracheal intubation. Am J Med 58:674, 1975
13. Bernard AV, Cottrell JE, Sivakumaran C et al: Adjustment of intracuff pressure to prevent aspiration. Anesthesiology 50:363, 1979
14. Stanley TH: Effects of anesthetic gases on endotracheal tube cuff gas volumes. Anesth Analg 53:480, 1974
15. Stoelting RK, Peterson C: Circulatory changes during anesthetic induction: Impact of d-tubocurarine pretreatment, thiamylal, succinylcholine, laryngoscope and tracheal lidocaine. Anesth Analg 55:77, 1976
16. Walts LF: Anesthesia of the larynx in the patient with a full stomach. JAMA 192:121, 1965
17. Wycoff CC: Aspiration during induction of anesthesia. Anesth Analg 38:5, 1959
18. Defalque RJ: Ketamine for blind nasal intubation. Anesth Analg 50:984, 1971
19. Zwillich C, Pierson DJ: Nasal necrosis: A complication of nasotracheal intubation. Chest 64:376, 1973
20. Arens JF, LeJeune FE, Webre DR: Maxillary sinusitis, a complication of nasotracheal intubation. Anesthesiology 40:415, 1974
21. Berry FA, Blankenbaker WL, Ball CG: A comparison of bacteremia occurring with nasotracheal and orotracheal intubation. Anesth Analg 52:873, 1973
22. Davis NJ: A new fiberoptic laryngoscope for nasal intubation. Anesth Analg 52:807, 1973

23. Raj PP, Forestner J, Watson TD et al: Techniques for fiberoptic laryngoscopy in anesthesia. Anesth Analg 53:708, 1974
24. Powell WF, Ozdil T: A translaryngeal guide for tracheal intubation. Anesth Analg 46:231, 1967
25. Eckenhoff JE: Some anatomic considerations of the infant larynx influencing endotracheal anesthesia. Anesthesiology 12:401, 1951
26. Webster AC: Anesthesia for operations on the upper airway. Int Anes Cl 10:61, 1972
27. Cole F: Correspondence. Anesthesiology 14:506, 1953
28. Levine J: Endotracheal tube in children. Anesthesia 13:40, 1958
29. Bidwai AV, Bidwai VA, Rogers CR et al: Blood pressure and pulse rate responses to endotracheal extubation with and without prior injection of lidocaine. Anesthesiology 51:171, 1979
30. Blanc VF, Tremblay NAG: The complications of tracheal intubation: A new classification with a review of the literature. Anesth Analg 53:202, 1974
31. Takeshima K, Noda K, Higaki M: Cardiovascular response to rapid anesthesia induction and endotracheal intubation. Anesth Analg 43:201, 1964
32. Stoelting RK: Blood pressure and heart rate changes during short duration laryngoscopy for tracheal intubation. Influence of viscous or intravenous lidocaine. Anesth Analg 57:197, 1978
33. Stoelting RK: Attenuation of blood pressure response to laryngoscope and tracheal intubation with sodium nitroprusside. Anesth Analg 58:116, 1979
34. Gibbs JM: The effects of endotracheal intubation on cardiac rate and rhythm. New Zel Med J 66:465, 1967
35. Cole WL, Stoelting VK: Blood gases during intubation following two types of oxygenation. Anesth Analg 50:68, 1971
36. Conrardy PA, Goodman LR, Lainge F et al: Alteration of endotracheal tube position. Flexion and extension of the neck. Crit Care Med 4:8, 1976
37. Burgess GE, Cooper JR, Marino RJ et al: Laryngeal competence after tracheal extubation. Anesthesiology 51:73, 1979
38. Hartsell CJ, Stephen CR: Incidence of sore throat following endotracheal intubation. Canad Anaesth Soc J 11:307, 1964
39. Winkel E, Knudsen J: Effect on the incidence of postoperative sore throat of 1 percent cinchocaine jelly for endotracheal intubation. Anesth Analg 50:92, 1971
40. Loeser EA, Machin R, Colley J et al: Postoperative sore throat—importance of endotracheal tube conformity versus cuff design. Anesthesiology 49:430, 1978
41. Holley HS, Gildea JE: Vocal cord paralysis after tracheal intubation. JAMA 215:281, 1971
42. Holinger P, Johnston K: Factors responsible for laryngeal obstruction in infants. JAMA 143:1229, 1950
43. Jackson C: Contact ulcer granuloma and other laryngeal complications of endotracheal anesthesia. Anesthesiology 14:425, 1953
44. Snow JC, Harano M, Balogy K: Postintubation granuloma of the larynx. Anesth Analg 45:425, 1966
45. Fine J. Finestone SC: An unusual complication of endotracheal intubation: Report of a case. Anesth Analg 52:204, 1973
46. Dubick MN, Wright BD: Comparison of laryngeal pathology following long term oral and nasal endotracheal intubations. Anesth Analg 57:663, 1978
47. Hahn FW, Martin JT, Lillie JC: Vocal cord paralysis with endotracheal intubation. Arch Otolaryngol 92:226, 1970
48. Ellis PDM, Pallister WK: Recurrent laryngeal nerve palsy and endotracheal intubation. J Laryngol Otol 89:823, 1975
49. Cook WR: A comparison of idiopathic laryngeal paralysis in man and horse. J Laryngol 84:819, 1970
50. Ellis PDM: Letter to the editor. Anesthesiology 16:374, 1977
51. Jaffe BF: Postoperative hoarseness. Am J Surg 123:432, 1972
52. Prasertwanitch Y, Schwartz JJH, Vandam LD: Arytenoid cartilage dislocation following prolonged endotracheal intubation. Anesthesiology 41:516, 1974
53. Khanam T, Branthwaite MA: Arterial oxygenation during one-lung anesthesia (2). Anaesthesia 28:280, 1973
54. Tarhan S, Lundborg RO: Carlens endobronchial catheter versus regular endotracheal tube during thoracic surgery. A comparison of blood gas tensions and pulmonary shunting. Canad Anaesth Soc J 18:594, 1971
55. Kerr J, Smith AC, Prys-Roberts C et al: Observations during endobronchial anesthesia I:

Ventilation and carbon dioxide clearance. Br J Anaesth 45:159, 1973

56. Bjork VO, Carlens E: The prevention of spread during pulmonary resection by the use of a double lumen catheter. J Thorac Surg 20:151, 1950

57. White GMJ: A new double-lumen tube. Brit J Anaesth 32:232, 1960

58. Robertshaw FL: Low resistance double lumen endobronchial tubes. Brit J Anaesth 34:576, 1962

9

MAC

Arthur L. Quasha, M.D.
Edmond I. Eger II, M.D.

INTRODUCTION

Attempts to assess anesthetic depth and potency appear as early as 1847 in the monograph on ether by John Snow.[1] Snow and others who followed him analyzed the inspired,[2] mixed expired,[3] arterial,[4] and even venous anesthetic concentrations that produced specific manifestations of CNS depression. These manifestations varied from abolition of movement in response to surgical stimulation;[1–3] to loss of the righting reflex;[2] to attainment of a given level of electroencephalographic suppression;[4] to achievement of certain changes in pupillary diameter, eye movement, respiration, and muscle tone.[5]

In 1963 Merkel and Eger[6] established MAC (minimum alveolar concentration of anesthetic required to abolish movement in response to a noxious stimulus) as an index of anesthetic equipotency which allowed comparison of the pharmacologic properties of two anesthetic agents. Unlike previous estimates of anesthetic potency, MAC emphasized measurement of anesthetic partial pressure in the alveolus at equilibrium. The advantage of this approach lay in the equality of alveolar and brain partial pressures at equilibrium. Therefore, MAC represents anesthetic activity at the anesthetic site of action. Unlike clinical signs, which rely on side effects and vary from drug to drug, MAC can

be applied to all inhalation anesthetics.[7] For these and other reasons, MAC has become the most widely accepted measure by which potencies of different anesthetics are compared.

DEFINITION

MAC 1.0 was initially defined as the "minimal anesthetic concentration in the alveolus required to keep a dog from responding by gross purposeful movement to a painful stimulus."[6] Anesthetic dose could then be expressed as MAC multiples, e.g., 1.5 MAC or 3.0 MAC. MAC for humans was defined as the alveolar anesthetic concentration at which 50 percent of the patients moved in response to a surgical incision.[8] These early studies revealed two facts: first, that MAC was remarkably consistent, both in animals and in humans; and second, that beyond a certain point, an increase in stimulus intensity (supramaximal stimulation) did not increase MAC.

MAC is defined in terms of percent of one atmosphere, and therefore is an alveolar anesthetic partial pressure (i.e., MAC would be the same at sea level or at the top of Mount Everest). Because partial pressures of anesthetics will be equal in all body tissues (e.g., alveolus, blood, and brain) at equilibrium,

MAC should, at equilibrium, represent the anesthetic partial pressure (not the concentration) at the anesthetic site of action (the brain). The constancy of MAC for animals and man, the relative ease of its measurement, and its predictable relationship with the partial pressure at the anesthetic site of action have made MAC the most widely accepted measure of anesthetic potency in our literature during the past 15 years.[9]

TECHNICAL ASPECTS OF OBTAINING MAC IN ANIMALS AND HUMANS

The determination of MAC differs slightly for animals and man. An animal is anesthetized with the anesthetic to be studied in oxygen, and the trachea is intubated usually without succinylcholine. A predetermined end-tidal anesthetic concentration is obtained and held constant for at least 15 min to achieve equilibrium among alveolus, blood, and brain. The animal is then stimulated with either a tail clamp (full-length hemostat applied close to the base of the tail and clamped to full ratchet lock) or subcutaneous electrical current (50 volts at 50 cycles/sec for 10 msec). If no movement occurs in response to stimulation, then the end-tidal ("alveolar") anesthetic concentration is lowered to 80 or 90 percent of the initial concentration and the stimulus is repeated after allowing 15 min for reequilibration. If a positive response to stimulation is obtained initially, then the end-tidal anesthetic concentration is increased 10 to 20 percent, and the process of reequilibration for 15 minutes (followed by stimulus application) is repeated. MAC 1.0 is the concentration midway between that which allows and that which prevents movement. The narrower the brackets (e.g., 10 percent step changes in anesthetic concentration versus 20 percent changes), the more precise (and time-consuming) will be the determination.

The usual stimulus applied to man is the skin incision, although electrical currents passed through subcutaneous tissues have also been used[8] (application, via 20-gauge needles in the forearm, of 30 to 45 volts AC with a 1.2-msec pulse at 50 cycles/sec for less than 60 sec). Since a patient normally is subjected to only one incision, the "bracketing" technique used in animals cannot be applied to a single subject. In all other respects the determination of MAC is the same. Anesthesia is induced with the anesthetic in oxygen. No premedication is given and no other anesthetic agents are administered. A preselected end-tidal anesthetic concentration is held constant for 15 min prior to skin incision. During and immediately after incision the patient is observed for movement or lack of movement. Several such patient studies are accomplished over a range of end-tidal anesthetic concentrations that permit and prevent movement. The patients may then be taken in groups of four or more starting with the ones having the lowest end-tidal ("alveolar") concentration (Fig. 9-1). The percentage of patients moving within each group is plotted against the average end-tidal concentration for the group. A visual line of best-fit through these points yields the concentration at which 50 percent of patients respond, i.e., MAC (Fig. 9-2). A more rigorous analysis (Waud,[10] Litchfield and Wilcoxon[11]) yields the same value for MAC and adds one element: these approaches also estimate the variance of MAC (i.e., they give a standard deviation). Thus, the determination of MAC has three components: an applied noxious stimulus, a defined response, and the measurement of end-tidal anesthetic concentration.

In early animal studies, variability in MAC was found to decrease as stimulus intensity increased, and certain stimuli appeared to be supramaximal.[12] Simultaneous application of two different supramaximal stimuli did not increase MAC above that seen with a single supramaximal stimulus. A skin incision was not quite a supramaximal stimulus in dogs. Because the tail clamp was simply applied and because MAC did not change with the application of a more intense stimulus, tail-clamping was chosen as the noxious stimulus

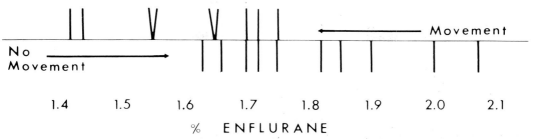

Fig. 9-1 End-tidal enflurane concentrations are plotted on the horizontal axis. Patient response (movement) to surgical incision is expressed as an upward deflection, and lack of response (no movement), as a downward deflection. (Gion H, Saidman LJ: The minimum alveolar concentration of enflurane in man. Anesthesiology 35:361, 1971.)

required for determination of MAC. Skin incision remains the standard stimulus in humans.

A positive response is considered to be "gross purposeful muscular movement,"[12]

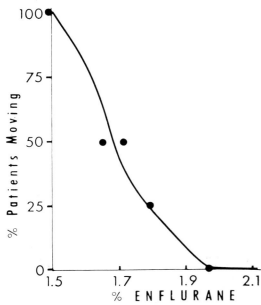

Fig. 9-2 MAC determined from data in Figure 9-1. Starting with the lowest end-tidal enflurane concentrations, subjects were taken in groups of four. The percentage of patients moving within each group was plotted against that group's mean end-tidal enflurane concentration. MAC is the enflurane concentration corresponding to the 50 percent point on the vertical axis, i.e., 1.68 percent. (Gion H, Saidman LJ: The minimum alveolar concentration of enflurane in man. Anesthesiology 35:361, 1971.)

usually of the head or extremities. Head movement does not include a twitch or grimace, but only a "jerking or twisting"[12] motion. Extremity movements are most common; motion of the torso without motion of the head or extremity is rare. Coughing, swallowing, and chewing are not considered positive responses.

The concept of MAC assumes that end-tidal, alveolar, arterial, and brain anesthetic partial pressures are equal after 15 min of equilibration. This assumption may be incorrect, but dysequilibrium is usually small. End-tidal gas partial pressure in normal unanesthetized man reasonably approximates the "ideal" alveolar partial pressure.[13] Anesthesia may enhance the ventilation/perfusion ratio inequalities that exist even in normal patients, and thus some degree of alveolar-to-arterial partial pressure gradient must result.[14, 15] Decreasing the inspired-to-alveolar (end-tidal) anesthetic partial pressure difference minimizes this potential error[15] (i.e., with poorly soluble anesthetics, with normal ventilation (V) and cardiac output (Q) as opposed to hypoventilation or increased cardiac output, and/or after prior equilibration at a higher anesthetic partial pressure) (Fig. 9-3).

Several factors may produce a difference between the end-tidal and arterial anesthetic partial pressures.[16] Contamination of end-tidal samples by gas from nonperfused alveoli (alveolar deadspace) or poorly perfused alveoli (severe V/Q abnormalities) increase the end-tidal partial pressure by contributing anesthetic partial pressures that approach those

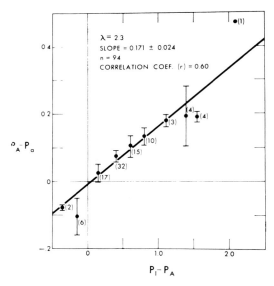

λ = 2 3
SLOPE = 0.171 ± 0.024
n = 94
CORRELATION COEF. (r) = 0.60

Fig. 9-3 The relationship between halothane end-tidal (P_A) to arterial (P_a) partial pressure difference and inspired (P_I) to end-tidal difference is depicted. The halothane blood/gas partition coefficient is assumed to equal 2.3. Differences are expressed in percent of one atmosphere. Data are from 94 sets of samples (i.e., 3 × 94 values) in 17 young, healthy human volunteers. Values were grouped by 0.25 percent segments of the P_A-P_I difference. Bars indicate standard errors of the mean. The data suggest that there is a five-to-one relationship between P_I-P_A and P_A-P_a; that is, if $P_I = 2$ percent and $P_A = 1$ percent, then $P_a = 0.8$ percent. (Eger EI II, Bahlman SH: Is the end-tidal anesthetic partial pressure an accurate measure of the arterial anesthetic partial pressure? Anesthesiology 35:301, 1971.)

in inspired gas. The greater the difference between inspired and "true" alveolar (normally ventilated and perfused alveoli) partial pressures, the greater the error introduced by this contamination. A slower emptying of the ventilated, nonperfused portion of the lung exaggerates the error (the difference between end-tidal and arterial partial pressures). Finally, significant amounts of very soluble gases will dissolve in the airway tissues during inhalation and are released during expiration. The contribution of this gas to the end-tidal sample will erroneously increase the

estimate of the arterial anesthetic partial pressure.

The technique for determination of MAC described above also assumes that equilibration for 15 minutes produces equality of arterial and brain partial pressures. This is based on the following equation:[17]

$$t = \frac{\lambda \cdot VT}{CBF} \cdot \log_e \frac{1}{0.05}$$

t = time to 95 percent blood-brain equilibration in minutes

λ = anesthetic brain-blood partition coefficient

CBF = cerebral blood flow (44 ml/100 g tissue/min)

VT = volume of brain tissue

A lower tissue solubility or a greater tissue blood flow (as achieved by hypoventilation or anesthesia itself[18]) will accelerate equilibration.[19,20] Hypoventilation, particularly with relatively insoluble agents, may slightly delay equilibration.[21] In any case, the time to equilibration is probably shorter than that implied above because grey matter (presumably the part of the brain important to the anesthetic process) has a blood flow one and one-half to two times mean cerebral blood flow.[18]

WHAT AFFECTS MAC

Type of Stimulation

MAC is unaffected by type of stimulation, provided a supramaximal stimulus is applied.[12]

Duration of Anesthesia

Gregory[22] and Eger[23] found no difference in MAC in humans for the separate stimuli of two herniorrhaphy incisions performed at different times during the same anesthesia. Halothane MAC in dogs is constant for up to 500 min of anesthesia.[12] Acute[24] and chronic[25,26] tolerance to nitrous-oxide-induced analgesia have been described, however. Mice can be made tolerant to nitrous oxide with cross-tolerance to cyclopropane and isoflurane.[27,28] These changes in murine anesthetic requirement are generally small, i.e., 10 to 20 percent. In addition, the development of acute tolerance is complete after 10 min of anesthesia,[27] while chronic tolerance does not develop for several days.[28]

Circadian Rhythms

MAC varies slightly ($\pm$ 10 percent) in the same animal when measured at different times.[12] Circadian rhythms may play some role in this observed variation.[29–31] MAC increases 10 to 14 percent from the mean during the "dark" phase of circadian cycle in the rat, which is the period of greatest metabolic activity in that species.[31]

Intraspecies and Interspecies Variation

The standard deviation obtained from analysis of MAC values from several animals of a given species is usually less than 10 percent of the MAC value itself.[12] This variation is only slightly greater than that observed (7 percent) for different determinations in a single animal.[12] Different species or classes of animals (for example, amphibians versus mammals) do not show large variations in MAC; MAC values for a given anesthetic remain within a two-fold range (Table 9-1).[23,32–37]

Sex

Unpublished data from two laboratories indicate that MAC is not different between the sexes in humans or rats.[23] However, unpublished work in our laboratory suggests that MAC in female mice may be slightly higher than MAC in male mice.

Hypocarbia and Hypercarbia

Reducing $PaCO_2$ from 42 to 14 torr (pH 7.7) does not alter halothane MAC in dogs.[12] Bridges and Eger[38] reported no difference in halothane MAC in man with normocapnia ($PaCO_2$ = 38 torr) versus hypocapnia ($PaCO_2$ = 21 torr). Extreme hypocapnia ($PaCO_2$ = 10 torr) in dogs does not affect MAC for halothane administered in oxygen but slightly (10 percent) reduces MAC for halothane in air.[39] The authors postulated that the MAC reduction in the halothane-plus-air group was due to cerebral hypoxia secondary to cerebral vasoconstriction in the presence of a reduced blood-oxygen content. Increasing $PaCO_2$ from 15 to 95 torr (arterial and cerebrospinal fluid pH = 7.6 to 7.10) does not affect halothane MAC in dogs. $PaCO_2$ levels greater than 95 torr—associated with arterial and cerebrospinal fluid pH less than 7.10—are, however, increasingly narcotic.[40] "Anesthesia" (i.e., 1.0 MAC) is produced by a $PaCO_2$ of approximately 245 torr (cerebrospinal fluid pH less than 6.90) (Fig. 9-4). The degree of CO_2 narcosis correlates with cisternal cerebrospinal fluid pH, but not with pHa, $PaCO_2$, or $PcsfCO_2$.

Metabolic Acidosis

In dogs, intravenous infusion of 60 to 80 mEq of ammonium chloride[12] decreased halothane MAC from 0.90 percent to 0.73 percent. End-tidal PCO_2 was held constant while at the same time arterial pH fell from 7.38 to 7.20. This modest change in MAC cannot be attributed to such a small pH change and may have resulted from the increase in ammonia.[12] Infusion of hydrochloric acid in dogs sufficient to lower pHa from 7.34 to 6.90 was associated with a decrease in halothane MAC of less than 15 percent.[40] An alternative explanation for the small decrease in MAC following ammonium chloride infusion is that such an infusion may have decreased cerebrospinal fluid sodium. A decrease in cerebrospinal fluid sodium

Table 9-1. Anesthetic Potency (MAC) of Various Anesthetics in Different Species (and Classes) of Animals*

Anesthetic	Man	Monkey Java	Monkey Stump-tail	Dog	Horse	Cat	Rabbit	Rat	Mouse	Toad	Newt	Goldfish
Halothane	0.73[107] 0.74[8,38] 0.77[108]	1.15[158]	0.89[34]	0.86[69] 0.87[34,70]	0.88[159]	0.82[154] 1.14[34]	0.82[35]	1.11†[32] 1.13†[62] 1.17†[160]		0.67[45]		0.76[68]
Enflurane	1.68[33]	1.84[158]		2.2[161] 2.06[36]	2.12[159]	1.2[154]						
Isoflurane	1.15[67]	1.28[158]		1.28[162]	1.31[159]	1.63[162]		1.38†[32]				
Methoxyflurane	0.16[108]			0.23[163] 0.24[70]		0.23[154]		0.27†[160]		0.22[45]		0.13[68]
Cyclopropane	9.2[108]			15.9[70] 17.5[163] 20.6[69]		19.7[154]		20.5†[62]		9.0[45]		
Fluroxene	3.4[102]			6.0[163] 6.57[70]				4.22[143]				
Ethylene	67[107]							132[143]				

Anesthetic	Man	Monkey Java	Monkey Stump-tail	Dog	Horse	Cat	Rabbit	Rat	Mouse	Toad	Newt	Goldfish
Diethyl ether	1.92[108]			3.04[163] 3.29[70]		2.1[154]			3.2[2]	1.64[45]		2.20[68]
Nitrous oxide	105[144]		200[34]	188[163] 222[34]		255[34]		136[143]	150[164] 146[139]	82.2[45]		
Chloroform				0.77[161]					0.78[2]			0.63[68]
Sulfur hexafluoride				490[161]					530[139] 540[164]		193[139]	
Carbon tetrafluoride				2600[161]					2290[139]			
Xenon	71[140]			119[163]					95[164]			
Argon									1520[164] 1640[139]		1690[139]	

* All values are expressed as a percentage of one atmosphere. The observed variance in MAC among species is in part due to variations in the technique used in measuring MAC, as well as to some variability in the ages, temperatures, and circadian cyles of the subjects tested. The stimulus used to obtain MAC in man was either a surgical incision or electrical pulse; and in the dog and horse, either a tail clamp or electrical pulse. Monkeys, cats, rabbits, and rats were tested with a tail clamp. The stimulus in mice and newts was a rotating chamber, and the end point was loss of righting reflex. Toads were stimulated with a clamp to the lower extremity. Goldfish were electrically stimulated. End-tidal anesthetic concentrations were measured in man, monkey, dog, horse, cat, rabbit, and rat where indicated (†); while in all other subjects, inspired anesthetic concentration was used. References are given as superscripts.

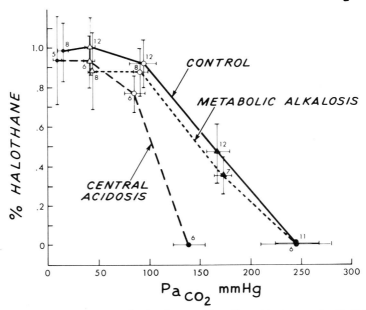

Fig. 9-4 Halothane requirement (MAC) in the dog may be affected by increasing $PaCO_2$. Three groups were studied. All dogs were anesthetized with some combination of carbon dioxide and halothane in oxygen. The control group received no other treatment. The central acidosis group was hyperventilated prior to the experiment for several hours ($PaCO_2 \leq 10$ mm Hg) and received intravenous hydrochloric acid to reduce cerebrospinal fluid bicarbonate from 23 to 13 mEq/L. The metabolic alkalosis group received 30 mEq/kg sodium bicarbonate intravenously. Number of dogs is given beside each point. Note that at a $PaCO_2$ of 245 torr, carbon dioxide becomes "anesthetizing," and that by reducing the cerebrospinal fluid buffer, base $PaCO_2$ becomes "anesthetizing" at 130 torr. In both instances, cerebrospinal fluid pH is about 6.80. Note also the lack of effect of bicarbonate administration (metabolic alkalosis). (Eisele JH, Eger EI II, Muallem M: Narcotic properties of carbon dioxide in the dog. Anesthesiology 28:856, 1967.)

concentration may decrease the magnitude of nerve action potential and thereby decrease MAC (see below under "electrolytes").

Metabolic Alkalosis

Eisele et al.[40] determined halothane MAC in dogs and then concomitantly increased $PaCO_2$ and infused 30 mEq/kg of sodium bicarbonate. The infusion of bicarbonate limited the decrease in pHa, which at the highest $PaCO_2$ ranged from 7.1 to 7.4. Because carbon dioxide and not bicarbonate readily crosses the blood-brain barrier, the cerebro-

spinal fluid pH was far more affected. The associated changes in MAC with changes in cerebrospinal fluid pH were identical to those seen in the absence of bicarbonate infusion, suggesting that metabolic alkalosis should not influence MAC.

Hypoxia and Hyperoxia

The lower limit of PaO_2 in normal man compatible with consciousness lies between 25 and 35 torr.[41] The mechanism by which such severe hypoxia produces narcosis is unknown. Halothane MAC in dogs is affected until PaO$_2$ falls below 30 torr.[12] Cullen et al.[42–44] demonstrated that halothane MAC in dogs was unaffected by a PaO$_2$ between 38 and 500 torr. Below 38 torr, hypoxia induced progressive narcosis.[42] At a PaO$_2$ of 38 torr, MAC was still 80 percent of control, whereas a PaO$_2$ of approximately 28 torr decreased MAC to 40 percent of control. A metabolic acidosis indicating anaerobic metabolism always accompanied this decrease in arterial oxygen content and MAC.[42] A decrease in oxygen content during normocapnic hypoxia (pHa = 7.29) decreased MAC more than during hypocapnic hypoxia (pHa = 7.39), possibly because the Bohr effect produced a higher oxygen content at the same PaO$_2$ during hypocapnia. The effects of acidosis could not be differentiated from those of decreased oxygen content.[42] This finding differed from the data reported by Eisele et al.[40] for severe metabolic acidosis without hypoxemia. This apparent conflict may be related to the differing effects of endogenously produced metabolic acidosis (secondary to hypoxia) and endogenously produced acidosis (hydrochloric acid administration). The former would likely reduce cerebrospinal fluid pH whereas the latter would not. However, in a subsequent study, Cullen et al.[43] did not find a consistent correlation between hypoxia-induced decreases in halothane MAC in dogs and cerebral extracellular fluid PO$_2$, PCO$_2$, or pH obtained with cortical surface electrodes. Shim and Andersen[45] noted increased anesthetic requirements for halothane and methoxyflurane, but not ether or cyclopropane, in toads breathing 100 percent oxygen. These animals were hyperventilated (pHa 7.6) and hypothermic, and the contribution of these variables is uncertain. In mice the ED$_{50}$ of oxygen alone is approximately 5.3 atm.[46]

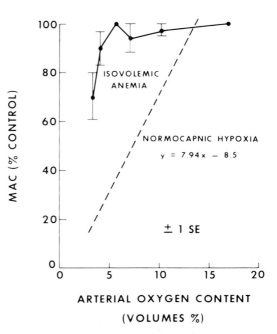

Fig. 9-5 The decrease in MAC with hypoxemia-induced decreasing oxygen content (dashed regression line) in dogs does not occur with anemia-induced decreasing oxygen content (solid line) until the oxygen content is decreased to levels that are nearly fatal. (Cullen DJ, Eger EI II: The effects of hypoxia and isovolemic anemia on the halothane requirement (MAC) of dogs. III. The effects of acute isovolemic anemia. Anesthesiology 32:46, 1970.)

these possibilities, Cullen and Eger[44] measured MAC before and after imposition of graded isovolemic anemia in dogs. Halothane MAC was unchanged until arterial oxygen content decreased below 4.3 cc of oxygen/100 cc of blood (hematocrit 10 percent). In this model, unlike the hypoxic models, there was no evidence of metabolic acidosis indicating impaired tissue oxygenation or perfusion (Fig. 9-5).

Anemia

The effect of hypoxia on MAC might relate to a decrease in either PaO$_2$ or arterial oxygen content (or both). To distinguish between

Hypotension

That hypotension may reduce anesthetic requirement was evaluated by Tanifuji and Eger[47] in three groups of dogs. In the first

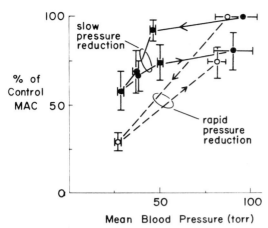

Fig. 9-6 Halothane requirement in dogs is expressed as a percentage of control MAC with a stepwise reduction of mean arterial pressure (filled circles, continuous lines) or an immediate reduction to that same pressure (open circles, dashed lines). Arrows indicate the sequence of pressure changes. The decrease in MAC was significantly greater ($P < 0.05$) with rapidly established hypotension. (Tanifuji Y, Eger EI II: Effect of arterial hypotension on anesthetic requirement in dogs. Br J Anaesth 48:947, 1976.)

group, mean arterial pressure (MAP) was reduced to 40 to 50 torr. Halothane MAC decreased by 20 percent after the first hr; no further MAC reduction occurred during the ensuing 3 hr of similar hypotension. Neither arterial nor cerebrospinal fluid lactate and pyruvate concentrations were affected, and arterial pH declined minimally. In the second group, MAP was gradually and successively reduced to 40 to 50 torr, 30 to 40 torr, and 20 to 30 torr. MAC decreased by 30 to 50 percent at the lower two pressure ranges (Fig. 9-6). In the third group, MAP was rapidly decreased to 20 to 30 torr. MAC decreased by 75 to 85 percent, a significantly greater decrease than occurred with the slower three-stage pressure reduction imposed in the second group. MAC returned to control levels (i.e., there was hysteresis) when blood pressure was restored to normal in group I but not in groups II and III (Fig. 9-6). The implication of the hysteresis is that neural function is impaired and

not readily reversible by profound hypotension. Perhaps a MAP below 40 to 50 torr should be deliberately sought (induced hypotension) only in essential situations.

Hypertension

Over 25 years ago investigators reported potentiation of chloral-induced and barbiturate-induced CNS depression following administration of large doses of epinephrine.[48,49] Conversely, Westfall[50] had found that epinephrine antagonized pentobarbital anesthesia. The effects of various inotropes and vasopressors on halothane MAC have been evaluated in dogs.[12,51] Only infusion of ephedrine increased MAC significantly (50 percent), although the increase with mephentermine (21 percent) approached statistical significance. Phenylephrine, metaraminol, methoxamine, norepinephrine, and epinephrine did not alter MAC. MAP was increased 50 to 100 percent in all cases. These results support the hypothesis that anesthetic requirement is increased by release of CNS catecholamines: ephedrine and mephentermine cause a central release of norepinephrine (ephedrine to a greater degree than mephentermine); whereas metaraminol, phenylephrine, methoxamine, norepinephrine, and epinephrine cause only a peripheral release and therefore exert only peripheral effects in the doses administered. These results also indicate that arterial hypertension per se does not affect MAC.

Neurotransmitter Release

Drugs that interfere with central neurotransmitter release may decrease MAC. A dose-related reduction in halothane MAC in dogs has been demonstrated after acute and chronic administration of α-methyldopa and reserpine, drugs that reduce both central and peripheral catecholamines and serotonin.[52] Guanethidine reduces norepinephrine pe-

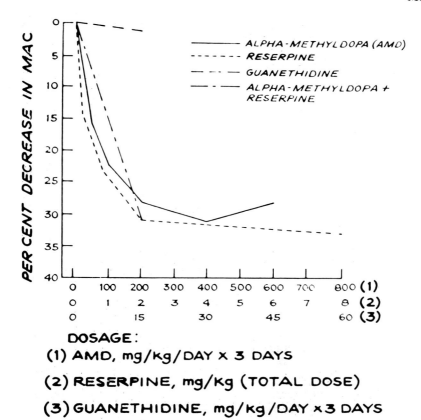

DOSAGE:
(1) AMD, mg/kg/DAY x 3 DAYS
(2) RESERPINE, mg/kg (TOTAL DOSE)
(3) GUANETHIDINE, mg/kg/DAY x 3 DAYS

Fig. 9-7 Halothane requirement (MAC) in dogs is decreased with alpha-methyldopa or reserpine alone or in combination. Note that guanethidine, which does not enter the CNS, had no effect on MAC. (Miller RD, Way WL, Eger EI II: The effects of alpha-methyldopa, reserpine, guanethidine, and iproniazid on minimum alveolar anesthetic requirement (MAC). Anesthesiology 29:1153, 1968.)

ripherally but not centrally and does not affect MAC (Fig. 9-7). Conversely, pretreatment with a monoamine oxidase inhibitor (iproniazid) slightly but significantly increases cyclopropane requirement in rats.[52] Iproniazid increases intracellular levels of catecholamines and serotonin by interfering with their degradation. Selective blockade of nerve terminals containing catecholamine and serotonin in rat brain slightly decreases halothane requirement.[53] Acute intravenous administration of *d*-amphetamine in dogs during halothane anesthesia increases MAC up to 96 percent.[54] In contrast, chronic treatment with *d*-amphetamine decreases halothane MAC by 22 percent.[54] The fact that

acute administration of *d*-amphetamine increases norepinephrine release in CNS nerve terminals, whereas chronic administration depletes CNS norepinephrine, further supports the hypothesis that increases in the release of CNS catecholamines cause anesthetic requirement to increase.[55] This hypothesis is still further supported by the finding that the increase in halothane MAC in dogs secondary to acute *d*-amphetamine administration could be partially blocked by pretreatment with large doses of reserpine or α-methyl-*p*-tyrosine (an inhibitor of norepinephrine synthesis).[55] Pretreatment with parachlorophenylalanine, a serotonin depleter, did not affect halothane MAC.[55] This result conflicts with an earlier finding in rats by Mueller et al.[53]

Halothane MAC in dogs increases in a dose-dependent fashion following administration of 2 or 4 mg/kg of cocaine.[56] Cocaine inhibits catecholamine reuptake in CNS nerve terminals, thereby increasing extracellular catecholamine concentrations.

Moderate intravenous doses of *l*-dopa reduce halothane MAC in dogs.[57] Larger doses (50 mg/kg) transiently increase requirement but cause a reduction 3 hr after injection.[57] Chronic pretreatment with *l*-dopa does not consistently alter anesthetic requirement.[57] Levodopa is a precursor of CNS dopamine and norepinephrine. The increase in dopamine is greater than that of norepinephrine.[58] Because dopamine is an inhibitory neurotransmitter[59] (as opposed to norepinephrine, which is excitatory), smaller does of *l*-dopa may reduce MAC by increasing central dopamine concentrations, and larger doses of *l*-dopa may cause central excitement by displacing norepinephrine.

Both cyclopropane and halothane selectively increase catecholamines[60] and serotonin[61] in discrete areas of rat brain, suggesting that these anesthetics depress neurotransmitter release at highly specific CNS sites. Stereotactic electrolytic destruction of these specific brain sites in rats decreases MAC for both halothane and cyclopropane by up to 35 percent.[62]

Age

In 1937 Guedel[63] observed that anesthetic requirement decreases with age. Fifteen years later Deming[64] demonstrated that infants require higher blood cyclopropane concentrations than adults to achieve a similar level of electroencephalographic suppression. Gregory et al.[22] determined MAC for halothane in eight groups of patients defined by age. MAC was greatest (1.1 percent) in the newborn (0 to 6 months) and smallest (0.64 percent) in the elderly (72 to 91 years). This decrease in anesthetic requirement with age parallels several

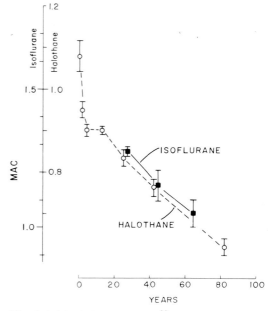

Fig. 9-8 MAC for halothane[22] and isoflurane decreases with increasing age. (Modified from Stevens WC, Dolan WM, Giffons RT et al: Minimum alveolar concentrations (MAC) of isoflurane with and without nitrous oxide in patients of various ages. Anesthesiology 42:197, 1975.)

physiological variables that also decrease with age, namely, cerebral blood flow, cerebral oxygen consumption, and neuronal density.[22,65] Nicodemus et al.[66] measured MAC in three groups of pediatric patients. They used the log dose-probit transformation described by Litchfield and Wilcoxon[11] to analyze their data and concluded that halothane requirement decreased with increasing age: i.e., MAC for infants less than 24 months old was 1.18 percent; for children 25 to 48 months old, 1.07 percent; and for adults, 0.94 percent. Hypotension was more frequent at MAC in infants than in adults, implying a smaller cardiovascular margin of safety in the infant group. Stevens et al.[67] determined isoflurane MAC with and without nitrous oxide in three patient populations grouped by age (Fig. 9-8). Their results agree with those of both Gregory et al.[22] and Nicodemus et al.,[66] i.e., isoflurane requirement decreases with age.

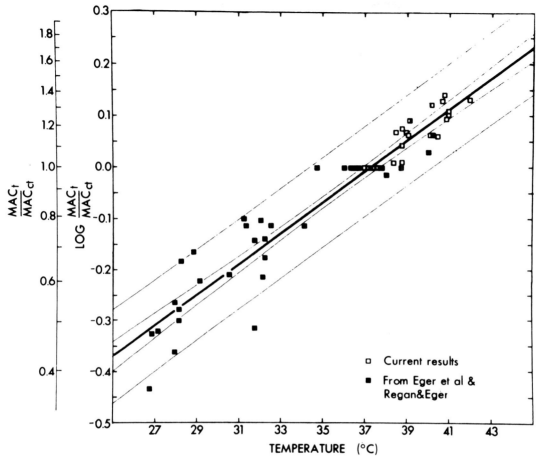

Fig. 9-9 An increase in esophageal temperatures from 26 to 42 °C causes a rectilinear increase in halothane MAC in dogs. Hypothermic data are from Eger et al.[69] and Regan and Eger,[70] while hyperthermic data are from Steffey and Eger.[72] MAC values are plotted as fractional changes from normothermic values (control or MAC CT) on logarithmic (right y axis) and arithmetic (left y axis) coordinates. Ninety-five percent confidence limits are shown. (Steffey EP, Eger EI II: Hyperthermia and halothane MAC in the dog. Anesthesiology 41:392, 1974.)

Addition of 70 percent nitrous oxide decreased isoflurane requirement by 57 to 65 percent regardless of age.

Temperature

Hypothermia decreases MAC in a rectilinear fashion.[68-71] The absolute decrease may differ among anesthetics as a function of their lipid solubilities or the change in lipid solubility with temperature. MACs for halothane, methoxyflurane, and isoflurane decrease by about 50 percent when temperature is reduced from 37 to 27 °C,[69-71] while the decrease with cyclopropane is only about 20 percent[69-70] for the same temperature change.

Steffey and Eger[72] evaluated the effect of hyperthermia on halothane requirement in dogs. As would be predicted from the above results with hypothermia, MAC increased linearly at 8 percent per degree centigrade (from 37.3 to 40.7 °C). At temperatures greater than 42 °C, MAC decreased (Fig. 9-9).

Death occurred at a mean temperature of 45 °C.

Electrolytes

In 1906 Meltzer and Auer[73] reported that intravenous administration of magnesium salt in animals produced sedation followed by paralysis and respiratory arrest. Peck and Meltzer[74] proposed in 1916 that magnesium had a definite, albeit limited, role as an adjunct to general anesthesia. Subsequently, however, the "anesthetic effect" of magnesium was shown to be cerebral hypoxia due to progressive cardiac and respiratory depression.[75] Magnesium-induced peripheral neuromuscular blockade occurs at lower serum magnesium concentration than does the central sedative effect, and humans remain conscious when skeletal muscular function is depressed.[76,77] Aldrete[78] concluded that although magnesium does depress nervous tissue, the amount of magnesium that crosses the blood-brain barrier is insufficient to produce narcosis.

Mannisto and Saarnivaara[79] reported that lithium enhanced morphine analgesia in mice. Tanifuji and Eger (unpublished data) have found that administration of lithium decreases MAC.

The anesthetic potency of halothane and cyclopropane in cats varies directly with cerebrospinal fluid calcium ion concentrations.[80] Very high cerebrospinal fluid calcium ion concentrations may alone produce a state resembling general anesthesia.[81]

The production of bromine by halothane biodegradation may result in postoperative sedation.[82,83] Sedation from bromine alone can occur at serum levels of 6 mEq/L, and toxicity may occur at concentrations greater than 10 mEq/L.[82] Increases in serum bromide concentrations (2.4 to 4.2 mEq/L) were found for 9 days following anesthesia in seven volunteers given 6 MAC-hr of halothane.[82] The findings of Tinker et al.[83] in patients given halothane are in agreement. However, bromine pro-

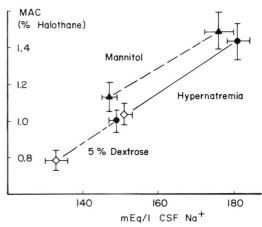

Fig. 9-10 Cerebrospinal fluid sodium concentration was altered by intravenous administration of mannitol, hypertonic saline, or 5 percent dextrose. Halothane requirement (MAC) in dogs increased with increasing cerebrospinal fluid sodium and decreased with decreasing sodium. (Tanifuji Y, Eger EI II: Brain sodium, potassium, and osmolality: Effects on anesthetic requirement. Anesth Analg 57:404, 1978.)

duction probably does not significantly affect halothane MAC. Although the half-life is long (12 to 25 days), the peak serum bromine levels require 2 days to develop.[82,83] Bromine levels at the end of anesthesia average only 0.5 mEq/L.[82]

Tanifuji and Eger[84] studied the effects of hyperkalemia, hypernatremia, and hyperosmolality and hypo-osmolality on halothane MAC in dogs. Hyperkalemia neither altered cerebrospinal fluid potassium concentration nor affected MAC. Hypernatremia proportionally increased cerebrospinal fluid sodium concentration and osmolality, and increased halothane MAC by 43 percent. Serum hyperosmolality increased cerebrospinal fluid osmolality without consistently altering cerebrospinal fluid sodium concentration or MAC. Serum and cerebrospinal fluid hypo-osmolality diluted cerebrospinal fluid sodium and reduced halothane MAC by 24 percent. Thus, changes in serum electrolytes or osmolality appear to alter anesthetic requirement if associated changes in sodium concentrations of the brain occur (Fig. 9-10).

Alcohol

Standard textbooks[85] and clinical reports[86] since 1937 have suggested that alcoholic subjects require larger doses of inhalation anesthetics than nonalcoholic subjects. Animal[87-90] and human [91-93] studies have provided qualitative and quantitative evidence that support these clinical impressions. Chronic ingestion of alcohol produces a 30- to 45-percent increase in MAC for isoflurane[89] or halothane.[90-93] As might be expected from its depressant effects, the acute administration of alcohol decreases anesthetic requirement.[89, 90, 94]

Thyroid Function

Guedel[63, 95] believed that anesthetic requirement correlated with metabolic activity. As noted, MAC and cerebral oxygen consumption ($CMRO_2$) decrease with increasing age or decreasing body temperature. Anesthetic requirement is not proportional to whole-body oxygen consumption ($\dot{V}O_2$). Doubling whole-body $\dot{V}O_2$ (grossly hypothyroid to hyperthyroid) in dogs causes only a 20 percent increase in halothane MAC.[96] Similarly, Munson et al.[97] could not demonstrate a significant effect of hypothyroidism or hyperthyroidism on cyclopropane MAC in rats, despite marked alterations in basal metabolic requirements. Whole-body metabolic changes induced by changes in thryroid function may have less effect on MAC than age or temperature because $CMRO_2$ is not affected by thryroid function.[97]

Narcotics

Narcotics reduce anesthetic requirement. Seevers et al.[98] reported in 1934 that dogs premedicated with morphine and scopolamine required far less cyclopropane to achieve a given plane of anesthesia. Subsequent investigations in animals[99, 100] have confirmed this conclusion. Hoffman and DiFazio[99] demonstrated a log dose-related reduction in cyclopropane requirement for morphine and meperidine in rats. Unlike morphine and meperidine, pentazocine demonstrated a "ceiling effect," i.e., above 20 mg/kg little additional reduction in anesthetic requirement occurred (Fig. 9-11). In 1957, Taylor et al.[101] administered 10 mg of morphine intravenously to patients 10 min before induction of ether anesthesia: the arterial blood ether concentration necessary to produce a predetermined level of electroencephalographic suppression decreased approximately 15 percent. Numerous clinical studies since 1957 have had similar results.[8, 102-104]

Tolerance to morphine occurs with chronic use, and this tolerance extends to other depressants. Han et al.[100] studied morphine-addicted dogs and found that halothane MAC increased linearly during the course of addiction. Also, morphine had a decreasing effect on halothane MAC as the animals became tolerant. Similarly, rats made tolerant to morphine exhibit a decreased analgesic response to nitrous oxide.[105]

Sedatives and Tranquilizers

Nonnarcotic premedicants also decrease anesthetic requirement. Barbital (150 mg/kg) given to dogs 30 min prior to anesthesia decreases cyclopropane requirement 49 to 67 percent, while 250 mg/kg decreases anesthetic requirement 66 to 77 percent. Premedication with 30 mg/kg amobarbital decreases cyclopropane requirement in dogs 42 to 59 percent, while 45 mg/kg causes a 66 to 70 percent reduction. Chlorpromazine, 50 mg intramuscularly 1 hr before anesthesia, decreases by 13 percent the ether concentration needed to produce a specific level of electroencephalographic suppression in patients, while the intravenous administration of pentobarbital 200 mg 10 min prior to anesthesia causes a 27 percent reduction.[101] Halothane MAC in man is only 0.43 to 0.48 percent 15 to 30 min after the intravenous administration

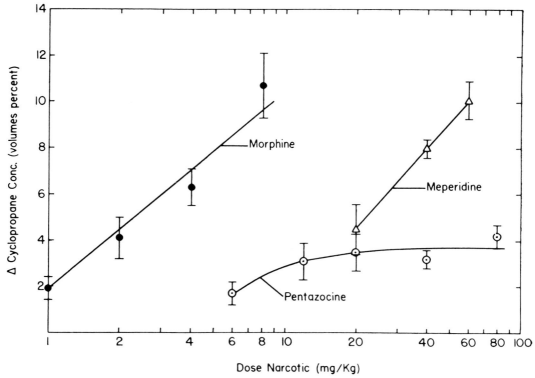

Fig. 9-11 Morphine and meperidine each produce a progressive, log dose-related reduction of cyclo-propane requirement in rats. A ceiling effect is demonstrated for pentazocine. Brackets show the standard error of the differences. (Hoffman JC, DiFazio CA: The anesthesia-sparing effect of pentazocine, meperidine, and morphine. Arch Int Pharmacodyn 186:261, 1970.)

of diazepam 0.2 to 0.5 mg/kg.[103, 106] Since halothane MAC in unpremedicated patients is approximately 0.75 percent,[8, 38, 107, 108] this represents a significant reduction in anesthetic requirement. The higher dose of diazepam significantly depressed ventilation without causing an additional decrease in MAC.[104] Hydroxyzine, 2 mg/kg intravenously, reduces halothane MAC in volunteers by 24 percent (0.95 to 0.72 percent).[103]

Miscellaneous Drugs

Delta-9-tetrahydrocannabinol, 1.0 and 2.0 mg/kg injected intraperitoneally 2 hr prior to cyclopropane anesthesia in rats, decreases MAC by 15 and 25 percent, respectively.[109] Neither acute (2 or 10 mg/kg intravenously)

nor chronic (10 mg/kg/day orally for 10 days) administration of propranolol or isoproterenol affects halothane MAC in dogs.[110] Intramuscular injection of ketamine, 50 mg/kg, decreases halothane MAC in rats by 56 percent 1 to 2 hr after injection, and 14 percent after 5 to 6 hr.[111]

Naloxone

Studies in mice and rats suggested that naloxone antagonized both analgesia induced by nitrous oxide[25, 112, 113] and anesthesia produced by cyclopropane, enflurane, halothane,[114] or barbiturate.[115] However, studies by other investigators failed to confirm a significant effect of naloxone on anesthesia with halothane in rats,[116, 117] nitrous oxide in mice,[118] and barbiturates in patients.[119] The importance of these findings lies in the hypothesis that anesthesia in part might be attributable to the release of endogenous morphine-like substances.[112] Therefore, although the analgesia component of general anesthesia might result from release of endogenous morphine-like substances, the failure to demonstrate a significant increase in halothane MAC by naloxone suggested that the analgesic component is not vital to production of general anesthesia.[120] In opposition to this view, Arndt and Freye[121] found that continuous perfusion of the fourth cerebral ventricle of the dog with naloxone antagonized the hypnotic effects of halothane, as evidenced by reversal of electroencephalographic suppression and by an increase in responsiveness to stimulation.[121] Nitrous-oxide-induced analgesia has been reversed with naloxone in man.[122] The above reports are thus conflicting, and the importance of endogenous morphine-like receptors in the maintenance of the analgesic and hypnotic components of general anesthesia remains unsettled.

Cholinesterase Inhibitors

Physostigmine and neostigmine decrease halothane MAC in dogs in a dose-dependent fashion.[123] Physostigmine, unlike neostigmine, transiently (within the first 30 min after intravenous injection) increases anesthetic requirement. The clinical significance of these findings is unclear because the effect on MAC was small and the doses used were at least ten times greater than those used clinically.

Local Anesthetics

Local anesthetics have been used systemically to supplement general anesthesia for over 25 years.[124–126] Lidocaine linearly reduces cyclopropane MAC in rats up to blood lidocaine concentrations of 1.0 μg/ml.[127] Higher concentrations decrease anesthetic requirement slightly more, with a maximal reduction of 42 percent.[127] In humans, a plasma lidocaine concentration of 3.2 μg/ml plus 70 percent nitrous oxide equals 1.0 MAC.[128] In dogs, plasma lidocaine concentrations of less than 1.0 μg/ml cause little or no decrease in halothane MAC.[128, 129] Higher concentrations decrease MAC; a 45-percent reduction occurs at a lidocaine level of 11.6 μg/ml.[128] Lidocaine arterial plasma concentrations in dogs of 1.0 to 3.5 μg/ml produce dose-related decreases in enflurane MAC of up to 37 percent[129] (Fig. 9-12). These alterations in anesthetic requirement may result from blockade of nociceptive impulses by suppression of spinal cord neurons.[130]

Pregnancy

Selye[131] was the first to note that steroids such as progesterone possessed anesthetic activity. Large daily intravenous doses of progesterone can induce sleep in women.[132] Pregnancy in sheep is associated with reductions in MAC of 32 percent for methoxyflurane, 25 percent for halothane, and 40 percent for isoflurane, possibly as a result of hormonal alterations.[133] Plasma progesterone increases 10- to 20-fold during late pregnancy in ewes.[134] Pregnancy in rats also decreases halothane MAC,[135] but the reductions do not correlate with changes in progesterone levels.[136] It thus appears that progesterone changes are not entirely responsible for pregnancy-associated reductions in MAC.

Effects of Other Inhalational Anesthetics

The effects of combinations of inhalation anesthetics are cumulative[4, 8, 67, 102, 137–139] and in general appear to be simply additive (Fig. 9-13),[107, 140] although some combinations are synergistic[141] or even antagonistic.[142, 143] In

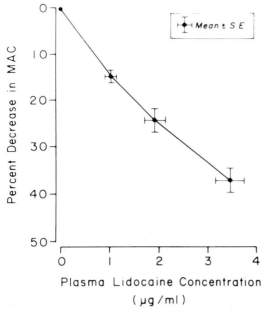

Fig. 9-12 Enflurane MAC in dogs decreases as a function of plasma lidocaine concentration. (Himes RS Jr, Munson ES, Embro WJ: Enflurane requirement and ventilatory response to carbon dioxide during lidocaine infusion in dogs. Anesthesiology 51:131, 1979.)

patients, nitrous oxide lowers the blood concentration of diethyl ether required to produce a given level of electroencephalographic suppression.[4] Similarly, 70 percent nitrous oxide decreases halothane MAC by 61 percent[8] and enflurane MAC by 60 percent.[67] Seventy-seven percent nitrous oxide decreases fluroxene requirement from 3.4 to 0.8 percent, a 76 percent reduction.[102] Sixty percent nitrous oxide decreases methoxyflurane MAC by 56 percent.[137] Enflurane MAC in the presence of 30 percent nitrous oxide is 1.17 percent and is only 0.5 percent when 70 percent nitrous oxide is concomitantly administered.[138] Presuming additivity, these data consistently suggest that MAC for nitrous oxide equals 105 to 110 percent of one atmosphere. Under hyperbaric conditions, nitrous oxide MAC in man has been determined to be 105 percent of one atmosphere, supporting the data obtained by extrapolation.[144]

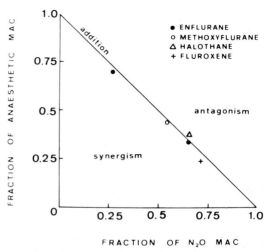

Fig. 9-13 The vertical axis represents the fraction of MAC in patients for four anesthetics. The value 1.0 represents 1 MAC of 1.68 percent enflurane, 0.76 percent halothane, 0.16 percent methoxyflurane, or 3.4 percent fluroxene. The horizontal axis represents MAC fraction of nitrous oxide; in this case, 1 MAC represents 101 percent nitrous oxide. The straight line connecting the 1.0 MAC points represents the line of simple addition. Points falling to the left of the line would represent synergism, while those to the right, antagonism. Note that the values obtained with all four anesthetics fall very near the line of simple addition. (Torri G, Damia G, Fabiani ML: Effect of nitrous oxide on the anesthetic requirement of enflurane. Br J Anaesth 46:468, 1974.)

The combination of halothane plus xenon[140] or halothane plus ethylene[107] also appears to be additive. However, not all inhalational anesthetics may be additive. Low concentrations of nitrous oxide or ethylene plus cyclopropane appear to produce antagonistic effects,[142,143] whereas cyclopropane plus isoflurane are synergistic.[141] Sulfur hexafluoride (SF6) plus nitrous oxide and argon plus nitrous oxide are additive in mice, but Ar plus SF6 are less than additive (i.e., exhibit antagonism).[139] We could not explain these results, but concluded that such anomalies are insufficient to cast serious doubts about theories of anesthetic action that suggest a critical effect in a lipid-like membrane phase.

MAC AND PHARMACOLOGIC PRINCIPLES

MAC is defined by a quantal dose (concentration)-response curve. As such, it differs from the two other kinds of dose-response curves, namely graded and ordered.[10, 145–147] Graded responses are those that can be measured precisely on a continuous scale, e.g., body temperature, pulse rate, and intravascular pressure. Ordered responses are qualitative in nature, wherein x is known to be greater than y and y greater than z, but the difference cannot be quantitated, i.e., the exact scale is in doubt. Guedel's signs of anesthetic depth are an example of ordered responses. Quantal responses are counts of the number of "yes" or "no" observations, wherein the subject may only respond in one of two ways. Thus, a quantal "dose-response curve" is in fact a cumulative frequency distribution. MAC fits this description.

MAC provides one measure of anesthetic potency. The quantal dose-response relationships that define MAC are not "depth-of-anesthesia" dose-response curves. MAC represents one point in a presumed continuum of anesthetic depth. Other endpoints define different levels of anesthetic depth—for example, "MAC awake"[148] in the sub-MAC range for "MAC for endotracheal intubation"[149, 150] in the supra-MAC range. These additional responses generally occur at constant percentages of MAC for various anesthetics. The constant relationship of the concentrations associated with these indices of anesthetic depth to MAC suggests that the dose (alveolar concentration)-response (anesthetic depth) curves for different anesthetics are parallel. The importance of such a parallel relationship lies in the fact that a shift of one point (e.g., MAC) may be used to indicate a shift in the whole curve (rather than an alteration in the slope of the curve).[145] Comparisons between anesthetics that are defined only by MAC also assume greater significance, since the comparisons apply equally to other indices of depth.[145]

The use of MAC fractions or MAC multiples for purposes of comparing physiological "side effects" of anesthetics (e.g., circulatory depression, respiratory depression, and neuromuscular block) has been generally accepted.[151-156] By determining the concentration required to produce unacceptable circulatory or respiratory depression and by relating those concentrations to MAC, one can define the "margin of safety" of any anesthetic.[6, 69, 157]

SUMMARY

From the discovery of the first anesthetics, the need for measurement of potency was apparent. Early concepts emphasized inspired anesthetic concentrations or concentrations in arterial or venous blood. Perhaps the major contribution of MAC was the emphasis of "alveolar" (end-tidal) anesthetic partial pressure, which at equilibrium represents the partial pressure at the anesthetic site of action (the brain). MAC gained wide acceptance and has become the primary index of anesthetic potency. There are several reasons for this. First, the endpoint of abolition of movement in response to a surgical incision is the basic element of clinical anesthesia and as such is of obvious interest to all clinicians. Second, MAC applies equally to all inhaled anesthetics, unlike "clinical signs" of anesthesia such as pupillary dilatation or respiratory depression, which vary from drug to drug. Third, MAC is remarkably and easily reproducible in the laboratory, making it attractive to those involved in research.

The uses of MAC are many. It permits a definition of the therapeutic index of various agents with respect to vital organ depression. It may be used to determine quantitatively the effect of age, body temperature, drugs, and other factors on anesthetic requirement; and thereby may serve as a clinical guide to the delivery of anesthesia. Finally, it may be used to increase our understanding of how anesthetics act.

REFERENCES

1. Snow J: On the Inhalation of the Vapour of Ether in Surgical Operations: Containing a Description of the Various Stages of Etherization and a Statement of the Result of Nearly Eight Operations in which Ether has been Employed in St. George's and University College Hospitals. London, John Churchill, 1847

2. Robbins BH: Preliminary studies of the anesthetic activity of fluorinated hydrocarbons. J Pharmacol Exp Ther 86:197, 1946

3. Haggard HW: The absorption, distribution, and elimination of ethyl ether. J Biol Chem 59:783, 1924

4. Faulconer A: Correlation of concentrations of ether in arterial blood with electroencephalographic patterns occurring during ether-oxygen and during nitrous oxide, oxygen and ether anesthesia of human surgical patients. Anesthesiology 13:361, 1952

5. Guedel AE: Inhalation Anesthesia: A Fundamental Guide. New York, MacMillan, 1937, pp 14-60

6. Merkel G, Eger EI II: A comparative study of halothane and halopropane anesthesia. Anesthesiology 24:346, 1963

7. Cullen DJ, Eger EI II, Stevens WC, et al: Clinical signs of anesthesia. Anesthesiology 36:21, 1972

8. Saidman LJ, Eger EI II: Effect of nitrous oxide and of narcotic premedication on the alveolar concentration of halothane required for anesthesia. Anesthesiology 25:302, 1964

9. De Jong RH, Eger EI II: MAC expanded: AD_{50} and AD_{95} values of common inhalation anesthetics in man. Anesthesiology 42:384, 1975

10. Waud DR: On biological assays involving quantal responses. J Pharmacol Exp Ther 183:577, 1972

11. Litchfield JT, Wilcoxon F: A simplified method of evaluating dose-effect experiments. J Pharmacol Exp Ther 96:99 1949

12. Eger EI II, Saidman LJ, Brandstater B: Minimum alveolar anesthetic concentration: A standard of anesthetic potency. Anesthesiology 26:756, 1965

13. Nunn JF: Applied Respiratory Physiology. Second edition. London, Butterworths, 1977, p 214

14. Eger EI II, Babad, AA, Regan MJ, et al: Delayed approach of arterial to alveolar nitrous oxide partial pressures in dog and in man. Anesthesiology 27:288, 1966

15. Eger EI II, Bahlman SH: Is the end-tidal anesthetic partial pressure an accurate measure of the arterial anesthetic partial pressure? Anesthesiology 35:301, 1971

16. Eger EI II, Severinghaus JW: Effect of uneven pulmonary distribution of blood and gas on induction with inhalation anesthetics. Anesthesiology 25:620, 1964

17. Larson CP, Eger EI II, Severinghaus JW: The solubility of halothane in blood and tissue homogenates. Anesthesiology 23:349, 1962

18. Smith AL, Wollman H: Cerebral blood flow and metabolism: Effects of anesthetic drugs and techniques. Anesthesiology 36:378, 1972

19. Eger EI II: Anesthetic Uptake and Action. Baltimore, Williams and Wilkins, 1974, pp 122-123

20. Eger EI II, Larson CP: Anesthetic solubility in blood and tissues: Values and significance. Br J Anaesth 36:140, 1964

21. Munson ES, Bowers DL: Effects of hyperventilation on the rate of cerebral anesthetic equilibration. Anesthesiology 28:377, 1967

22. Gregory GA, Eger EI II, Munson ES: The relationship between age and halothane requirement in man. Anesthesiology 30:488, 1969

23. Eger EI II: Anesthetic Uptake and Action. Baltimore, Williams and Wilkins, 1974, p 5

24. Whitwam JG, Morgan M, Hall GM, et al: Pain during continuous nitrous oxide administration. Br J Anaesth 48:425, 1976

25. Berkowitz BA, Finck AD, Ngai SH: Nitrous oxide analgesia: Reversal by naloxone and development of tolerance. J Pharmacol Exp Ther 203:539, 1977

26. Kripke BJ, Hechtman HB: Nitrous oxide for pentazocine addiction and for intractable pain: Report of case. Anesth Analg 51:520, 1972

27. Smith RA, Winter PM, Smith M, et al: Rapidly developing tolerance to acute exposures to anesthetic agents. Anesthesiology 50:496, 1979

28. Smith RA, Winter PM, Smith M, et al: Tolerance to and dependence on inhalational anesthetics. Anesthesiology 50:505, 1979

29. Matthews JH, Marte E, Halberg F: A circadian susceptibility-resistance cycle to

Fluothane in male B_1 mice. Can Anaesth Soc J 11:280, 1964

30. Matthews JH, Marte E, Halbert F: Fluothane toxicity in mice studied by indirect periodicity analysis, Toxicity of Anesthetics. Edited by Fink BR. Baltimore, Williams and Wilkins, 1968, pp 197-208

31. Munson ES, Martucci RW, Smith RE: Circadian variations in anesthetic requirement and toxicity in rats. Anesthesiology 32:507, 1970

32. White PF, Johnston RR, Eger EI II: Determination of anesthetic requirement in rats. Anesthesiology 40:52, 1974

33. Gion H, Saidman LJ: The minimum alveolar concentration of enflurane in man. Anesthesiology 35:361, 1971

34. Steffey EP, Gillespie Jr, Berry JD, et al: Anesthetic potency (MAC) of nitrous oxide in the dog, cat, and stump-tail monkey. J Appl Physiol 36:530, 1974

35. Davis NL, Nunnally RL, Malinin TI: Determination of the minimum alveolar concentration (MAC) of halothane in the white New Zealand rabbit. Br J Anaesth 47:341, 1975

36. Steffey EP, Howland D: Potency of enflurane in dogs: Comparison with halothane and isoflurane. Am J Vet Res 39:573, 1978

37. Steffey EP: Enflurane and isoflurane anesthesia: A summary of laboratory and clinical investigations in horses. J Am Vet Med Assoc 172:367, 1978

38. Bridges BE, Eger EI II: The effect of hypocapnia on the level of halothane anesthesia in man. Anesthesiology 27:634, 1966

39. Cullen DJ, Eger EI II: The effect of extreme hypocapnia on the anesthetic requirement (MAC) of dogs. Br J Anaesth 43:339, 1971

40. Eisele JH, Eger EI II, Muallem M: Narcotic properties of carbon dioxide in the dog. Anesthesiology 28:856, 1967

41. Nunn JF: Applied Respiratory Physiology. 2nd edition. London, Butterworths, 1977, pp 416-419

42. Cullen DJ, Eger EI II: The effects of hypoxia and isovolemic anemia on the halothane requirement (MAC) of dogs. I. The effect of hypoxia. Anesthesiology 32:28, 1970

43. Cullen DJ, Cotev S, Severinghaus JW, et al: The effects of hypoxia and isovolemic anemia on the halothane requirement (MAC) of dogs. II. The effects of acute hypoxia on halothane requirement and cerebral-surface PO_2, PCO_2, pH and HCO_3^-. Anesthesiology 32:35, 1970

44. Cullen DJ, Eger EI II: The effects of hypoxia and isovolemic anemia on the halothane requirement (MAC) of dogs. III. The effects of acute isovolemic anema. Anesthesiology 32:46, 1970

45. Shim CY, Andersen NB: The effects of oxygen on minimal anesthetic requirements in the toad. Anesthesiology 34:333, 1971

46. Smith RA, Paton WD: The anesthetic effect of oxygen. Anesth Analg 55:734, 1976

47. Tanifuji Y, Eger EI II: Effect of arterial hypotension on anesthetic requirement in dogs. Br J Anaesth 48:947, 1976

48. Lamson PD, Greig ME, Williams L: Potentiation by epinephrine of the anesthetic effect in chloral and barbiturate anesthesia. J Pharmacol Exp Ther 100:219, 1952

49. Milosevic MP: The action of sympathomimetic amines on intravenous anesthesia in rats. Arch Int Pharmacodyn 106:437, 1956

50. Westfall BA: Pyruvic acid antagonism to barbiturate depression. J Pharmacol Exp Ther 87:33, 1946

51. Steffey EP, Eger EI II: The effect of seven vasopressors on halothane MAC in dogs. Br J Anaesth 47:435, 1975

52. Miller RD, Way WL, Eger EI II: The effects of alpha-methyldopa, reserpine, guanethidine, and iproniazid on minimum alveolar anesthetic requirement (MAC). Anesthesiology 29:1153, 1968

53. Mueller RA, Smith RD, Spruill WA, et al: Central monaminergic neuronal effects on minimum alveolar concentrations (MAC) of halothane and cyclopropane in rats. Anesthesiology 42:143, 1975

54. Johnston RR, Way WL, Miller RD: Alteration of anesthetic requirement by amphetamine. Anesthesiology 36:357, 1972

55. Johnston RR, Way WL, Miller RD: The effect of CNS catecholamine-depleting drugs on dextroamphetamine-induced elevation of halothane MAC. Anesthesiology 41:57, 1974

56. Stoelting RK, Creasser CW, Martz RC: Effect of cocaine administration on halothane MAC in dogs. Anesth Analg 54:422, 1975

57. Johnston RR, White PF, Way WL, et al: The effect of levodopa on halothane anesthetic requirements. Anesth Analg 54:178, 1975

58. Everett GM, Borcherding JW: L-dopa: Ef-

fect on concentrations of dopamine, norepinephrine, and serotonin in brains of mice. Science 168:849, 1970

59. Hornykiewicz O: Dopamine (3-hydroxytyramine) and brain function. Pharmacol Rev 18:925, 1966

60. Roizen MF, Kopin IJ, Thoa NB, et al: The effect of two anesthetic agents on norepinephrine and dopamine in discrete brain nuclei, fiber tracts and terminal regions of the rat. Brain Res 110:515, 1976

61. Roizen MF, Kopin IJ, Palkovits M, et al: The effect of two diverse inhalation anesthetic agents on serotonin in discrete regions of the rat brain. Exp Brain Res 24:203, 1975

62. Roizen MF, White PF, Eger EI II, et al: Effects of ablation of serotonin or norepinephrine brain-stem areas on halothane and cyclopropane MACs in rats. Anesthesiology 49:252, 1978

63. Guedel AE: Inhalation Anesthesia: A Fundamental Guide. New York, Macmillan, 1937, pp 61-62

64. Deming MN: Agents and techniques for induction of anesthesia in infants and young children. Anesth Analg 31:113, 1952

65. Kety SS: Human cerebral blood flow and oxygen consumption as related to aging. J Chronic Dis 3:478, 1956

66. Nicodemus HF, Nassiri-Rahimi C, Bachman L, et al: Median effective doses (ED_{50}) of halothane in adults and children. Anesthesiology 31:344, 1969

67. Stevens WC, Dolan WM, Gibbons RT, et al: Minimum alveolar concentrations (MAC) of isoflurane with and without nitrous oxide in patients of various ages. Anesthesiology 42:197, 1975

68. Cherkin A, Catchpool JF: Temperature dependence of anesthesia in goldfish. Science 144:1460, 1964

69. Eger EI II, Saidman LJ, Brandstater B: Temperature dependence of halothane and cyclopropane anesthesia in dogs: Correlation with some theories of anesthetic action. Anesthesiology 26:764, 1965

70. Regan MJ, Eger EI II: Effect of hypothermia in dogs on anesthetizing and apneic doses of inhalation agents. Determination of the anesthetic index (apnea/MAC). Anesthesiology 28:689, 1967

71. Vitez TS, White PF, Eger EI II: Effects of hypothermia on halothane MAC and iso-flurane MAC in the rat. Anesthesiology 41:80, 1974

72. Steffey EP, Eger EI II: Hyperthermia and halothane MAC in the dog. Anesthesiology 41:392, 1974

73. Meltzer SJ, Auer J: Physiological and pharmacological studies of magnesium salts. Am J Physiol 15:387, 1906

74. Peck CH, Meltzer SJ: Anesthesia in human beings by intravenous injection of magnesium sulphate. JAMA 67:1131, 1916

75. Aldrete JA, Barnes DR, Aikawa JK: Does magnesium produce anesthesia. Anesth Analg 47:428, 1968

76. Somjen G, Hilmy M, Stephen CR: Failure to anesthetize human subjects by intravenous administration of magnesium sulfate. J Pharmacol Exp Ther 154:652, 1966

77. Hilmy MI, Somjen GG: Distribution and tissue uptake of magnesium related to its pharmacological effects. Am J Physiol 214:406, 1968

78. Aldrete JA: Clinical implications of magnesium therapy, The Anesthesiologist, Mother and Newborn. Edited by Shnider SM, Moya F. Baltimore, Williams and Wilkins, 1974, pp 128-135

79. Mannisto PT, Saarnivaara L: Effect of lithium and rubidium on the sleeping time caused by various intravenous anesthetics in the mouse. Br J Anaesth 48:185, 1976

80. Johnson ER, Crout JR: Calcium ion concentration in cerebrospinal fluid and anesthetic potency. Abstracts of Scientific Papers, Annual Meeting of the American Society of Anesthesiologists, 1970, p 1

81. Feldberg W, Sherwood SL: Effects of calcium and psotassium injected into the cerebral ventricles of the cat. J Physiol (Lond) 139:409, 1957

82. Johnstone RE, Kennell EM, Behar MG, et al: Increased serum bromide concentration after halothane anesthesia in man. Anesthesiology 42:598, 1975

83. Tinker JH, Gandolfi AJ, Van Dyke RA: Elevation of plasma bromide levels in patients following halothane anesthesia: Time correlation with total halothane dosage. Anesthesiology 44:194, 1976

84. Tanifuji Y, Eger EI II: Brain sodium, potassium, and osmolality: Effects on anesthetic requirement. Anesth Analg 57:404, 1978

85. Sollman T: A Manual of Pharmacology and

Its Applications to Therapeutics and Toxicology. Philadelphia, WB Saunders, 1937

86. Keilty SR: Anesthesia for the alcoholic patient. Anesth Analg 48:659, 1969

87. Abreu BE, Emerson GA: Susceptibility to ether anesthesia of mice habituated to alcohol, morphin or cocain. Anesth Analg 18:294, 1939

88. Lee PK, Cho MH, Dobkin AB: Effects of alcoholism, morphinism, and barbiturate resistance on induction and maintenance of general anesthesia. Can Anaesth Soc J 11:354, 1964

89. Johnstone RE, Kulp RA, Smith TC: Effects of acute and chronic ethanol administration on isoflurane requirement in mice. Anesth Analg 54:277, 1975

90. Orkin LR, Chen CH: Effect of alcohol on the MAC with halothane in the cat. Abstracts of Scientific Papers, Annual Meeting of the American Society of Anesthesiologists, 1977, pp 735-736

91. Tammisto T, Takki S: Nitrous oxide-oxygen-relaxant anesthesia in alcoholics: A retrospective study. Acta Anaesthesiol Scand (suppl) 53:68, 1973

92. Han YH: Why do chronic alcoholics require more anesthesia? Anesthesiology 30:341, 1969

93. Barber RE: Anesthetic requirement in alcoholic patients. Abstracts of Scientific Papers, Annual Meeting of the American Society of Anesthesiologists, 1978, pp 623-624

94. Parikh RK: Effect of acute alcohol administration on halothane requirement in rats. Br J Anaesth 48:1126, 1976

95. Guedel AE: Metabolism and reflex irritability in anesthesia. JAMA 83:1736, 1924

96. Babad AA, Eger EI II: The effects of hyperthyroidism and hypothyroidism on halothane and oxygen requirements in dogs. Anesthesiology 29:1087, 1968

97. Munson ES, Hoffman JC, DiFazio CA: The effects of acute hypothyroidism and hyperthyroidism on cyclopropane requirement (MAC) in rats. Anesthesiology 29:1094, 1968

98. Seevers MH, Meek WJ, Rovenstine EA, et al: A study of cyclopropane anesthesia with especial reference to gas concentrations, respiratory and electrocardiographic changes. J Pharmacol Exp Ther 51:1, 1934

99. Hoffman JC, DiFazio CA: The anesthesia-sparing effect of pentazocine, meperidine, and morphine. Arch Int Pharmacodyn 186:261, 1970

100. Han YH, Shiwaku Y, Deery A, et al: Effects of chronic morphine addiction and naloxone on halothane MAC in dogs. Abstracts of Scientific Papers, Annual Meeting of the American Society of Anesthesiologists, 1977, pp 739-740

101. Taylor HE, Doerr JC, Gharib A, et al: Effect of preanesthetic medication on ether content of arterial blood required for surgical anesthesia. Anesthesiology 18:849, 1957

102. Munson ES, Saidman LJ, Eger EI II: Effect of nitrous oxide and morphine on the minimum anesthetic concentration of fluroxene. Anesthesiology 26:134, 1965

103. Tsunoda Y, Hattori Y, Takatsuka E, et al: Effects of hydroxyzine, diazepam, and pentazocine on halothane minimum alveolar anesthetic concentration. Anesth Analg 52:390, 1973

104. Woodruff RE, Bartee RM, Steffenson JL: The effect of fentanyl, droperidol and Innovar[R] on MAC and respiratory depression. Abstracts of Scientific Papers, Annual Meeting of the American Society of Anesthesiologists, 1977, pp 739-740

105. Berkowitz BA, Finck AD, Hynes MD, et al: Tolerance to nitrous oxide anesthesia in rats and mice. Anesthesiology 51:309, 1979

106. Perisho JA, Beuchel DR, Miller RD: The effect of diazepam (Valium[R]) on minimum alveolar anaesthetic requirement (MAC) in man. Can Anaesth Soc J 18:536, 1971

107 Miller RD, Wahrenbrock EA, Schroeder CF, et al: Ethylene-halothane anesthesia: Addition or synergism? Anesthesiology 31:301, 1969

108. Saidman LJ, Eger EI II, Munson ES, et al: Minimum alveolar concentrations of methoxyflurane, halothane, ether and cyclopropane in man: Correlation with theories of anesthesia. Anesthesiology 28:994, 1967

109. Vitez TS, Way WL, Miller RD, et al: Effects of delta-9-tetrahydrocannabinol on cyclopropane MAC in the rat. Anesthesiology 38:525, 1973

110. Tanifuji Y, Eger EI II: Effect of isoproterenol and propranolol on halothane MAC in dogs. Anesth Analg 55:383, 1976

111. White PF, Johnston RR, Pudwill CR: Interaction of ketamine and halothane in rats. Anesthesiology 42:179, 1975

112. Berkowitz BA, Finck AD, Ngai SH: Nitrous oxide analgesia and its reversal by narcotic antagonists. Pharmacologist 18:177, 1976

113. Berkowitz BA, Ngai SH, Finck AD: Nitrous oxide "analgesia": Resemblance to opiate action. Science 194:967, 1976

114. Finck AD, Ngai SH, Berkowitz BA: Antagonism of general anesthesia by naloxone in the rat. Anesthesiology 46:241, 1977

115. Furst Z, Foldes FF, Knoll J: The influence of naloxone on barbiturate anesthesia and toxicity in the rat. Life Sci 20:921, 1977

116. Harper MH, Winter PM, Johnson BH, et al: Naloxone does not antagonize general anesthesia in the rat. Anesthesiology 49:3, 1978

117. Bennett PB: Naloxone fails to antagonize the righting response in rats anesthetized with halothane. Anesthesiology 49:9, 1978

118. Smith RA, Wilson M, Miller KW: Naloxone has no effect on nitrous oxide anesthesia. Anesthesiology 49:6, 1978

119. Duncalf D, Nagashima H, Duncalf RM: Naloxone fails to antagonize thiopental anesthesia. Anesth Analg 57:558, 1978

120. Goldstein A: Enkephalins, opiate receptors, and general anesthesia (editorial). Anesthesiology 49:1, 1978

121. Arndt JO, Freye E: Perfusion of naloxone through the fourth cerebral ventricle reverses the circulatory and hypnotic effects of halothane in dogs. Anesthesiology 51:58, 1979

122. Chapman CR, Benedetti C: Nitrous oxide effects on cerebral evoked potential to pain: Partial reversal with a narcotic antagonist. Anesthesiology 51:135, 1979

123. Horrigan RW: Physostigmine and anesthetic requirement for halothane in dogs. Anesth Analg 57:180, 1978

124. De Clive-Lowe SG, Desmond J, North J: Intravenous lignocaine anaesthesia. Anaesthesia 13:138, 1954

125. Steinhaus JE, Howland DE: Intravenously administered lidocaine as a supplement to nitrous oxide-thiobarbiturate anesthesia. Anesth Analg 37:40, 1958

126. Phillips OC, Lyons WB, Harris LC, et al: Intravenous lidocaine as an adjunct to general anesthesia: A clinical evaluation. Anesth Analg 39:317, 1960

127. DiFazio CA, Niederlehner JR, Burney RG: The anesthetic potency of lidocaine in the rat. Anesth Analg 55:818, 1976

128. Himes RS, DiFazio CA, Burney RG: Effects of lidocaine on the anesthetic requirements for nitrous oxide and halothane. Anesthesiology 47:437, 1977

129. Himes RS Jr, Munson ES, Embro WJ: Enflurane requirement and ventilatory response to carbon dioxide during lidocaine infusion in dogs. Anesthesiology 51:131, 1979

130. Dohi S, Kitahata LM, Toyooka H, et al: An analgesic action of intravenously administered lidocaine on dorsal-horn neurons responding to noxious thermal stimulation. Anesthesiology 51:123, 1979

131. Selye H: Studies concerning the anesthetic action of steroid hormones. J Pharmacol Exp Ther 73:127, 1941

132. Merryman W, Boiman R, Barnes L, et al: Progesterone "anesthesia" in human subjects (correspondence). J Clin Endocrinol Metab 14:1567, 1954

133. Palahniuk RJ, Shnider SM, Eger EI II: Pregnancy decreases the requirement for inhaled anesthetic agents. Anesthesiology 41:82, 1974

134. Stabenfeldt GH, Drost M, Franti CE: Peripheral plasma progesterone levels in the ewe during pregnancy and parturition. Endocrinology 90:144, 1972

135. Strout CD, Nahrwold ML, Wolf JW, et al: Halothane requirement during pregnancy and lactation in rats. Abstracts of Scientific Papers, Annual Meeting of the American Society of Anesthesiologists, 1977, pp 547-548

136. Grota LJ, Eik-Nes KB: Plasma progesterone concentrations during pregnancy and lactation in the rat. J Reprod Fertil 13:83, 1967

137. Stoelting RK: The effect of nitrous oxide on the minimum alveolar concentration of methoxyflurane needed for anesthesia. Anesthesiology 34:353, 1971

138. Torri G, Damia G, Fabiani ML: Effect of nitrous oxide on the anesthetic requirement of enflurane. Br J Anaesth 46:468, 1974

139. Clarke RF, Daniels S, Harrison CB, et al: Potency of mixtures of general anesthetic agents. Br J Anaesth 50:979, 1978

140. Cullen SC, Eger EI II, Cullen BF, et al: Observations on the anesthetic effect of the combination of xenon and halothane. Anesthesiology 31:305, 1969

141. DiFazio CA, Hurt D, Burney RG, et al: Unusual observations in anesthetic additivity.

Abstracts of Scientific Papers, Annual Meeting of the American Society of Anesthesiologists, 1977, pp 619-620

142. DiFazio CA, Brown RE: Additive effects of combined anesthetics (abstract). Fed Proc 28:475, 1969

143. DiFazio CA, Brown RE, Ball CG, et al: Additive effects of anesthetics and theories of anesthesia. Anesthesiology 36:57, 1972

144. Winter PM, Hornbein TF, Smith G, et al: Hyperbaric nitrous oxide anesthesia in man: Determination of anesthetic potency (MAC) and cardiorespiratory effects. Abstracts of Scientific Papers, Annual Meeting of the American Society of Anesthesiologists, 1972, pp 103-104

145. Waud BE, Waud DR: On dose-response curves and anesthetics (editorial). Anesthesiology 33:1, 1970

146. Eger EI II: MAC and dose-response curves (correspondence). Anesthesiology 34:202, 1971

147. Waud BE, Waud DR: MAC and dose-dependent curves (correspondence). Anesthesiology 34:203, 1971

148. Stoelting RK, Longnecker DE, Eger EI II: Minimum alveolar concentrations in man on awakening from methoxyflurane, halothane, ether and fluoroxene anesthesia: MAC awake. Anesthesiology 33:5, 1970

149. Yakaitis RW, Blitt CD, Angiulo JP: End-tidal halothane concentration for Endotracheal intubation. Anesthesiology 47:386, 1977

150. Yakaitis RW, Blitt CD, Angiulo JP: End-tidal enflurane concentration for endotracheal intubation. Anesthesiology 50:59, 1979

151. Munson ES, Larson CP, Babad AA, et al: The effects of halothane, fluroxene and cyclopropane on ventilation: A comparative study in man. Anesthesiology 27:716, 1966

152. Larson CP, Eger EI II, Muallem M, et al: Effects of diethyl ether and methoxyflurane on ventilation. II. A comparative study in man. Anesthesiology 30:174, 1969

153. Eger EI II, Smith NT, Cullen DJ, et al: A comparison of the cardiovascular effects of halothane, fluroxene, ether and cyclopropane in man: A resume. Anesthesiology 34:25, 1971

154. Brown BR, Crout JR: A comparative study of the effects of five general anesthetics on myocardial contractility. I. Isometric conditions. Anesthesiology 34:236, 1971

155. Merin RG, Kumazawa T, Luka NL: Enflurane depresses myocardial function, perfusion, and metabolism in the dog. Anesthesiology 45:501, 1976

156. Miller RD, Way WL, Dolan WM, et al: Comparative neuromuscular effects of pancuronium, gallamine, and succinylcholine during Forane and halothane anesthesia in man. Anesthesiology 35:509, 1971

157. Wolfson B, Hetrick WD, Lake CL et al: Anesthetic indices—further data. Anesthesiology 48:187, 1978

158. Tinker JH, Sharbrough FW, Michenfelder JD: Anterior shift of the dominant EEG rhythm during anesthesia in the JaVa monkey: Correlation with anesthetic potency. Anesthesiology 46:252, 1977

159. Steffey EP, Howland D Jr, Giri S, et al: Enflurane, halothane, and isoflurane potency in horses. Am J Vet Res 38:1037, 1977

160. Waizer PR, Baez S, Orkin LR: A method for determining minimum alveolar concentration of anesthetic in the rat. Anesthesiology 39:394, 1973

161. Eger EI II, Lundgren C, Miller SL, et al: Anesthetic potencies of sulfur hexafluoride, carbon tetrafluoride, chloroform and Ethrane in dogs: Correlation with the hydrate and lipid theories of anesthetic action. Anesthesiology 30:129, 1969

162. Steffey EP, Howland D Jr: Isoflurane potency in the dog and cat. Am J Vet Res 38:1833, 1977

163. Eger EI II, Brandstater B, Saidman LJ, et al: Equipotent alveolar concentrations of methoxyflurane, halothane, diethyl ether, fluroxene, cyclopropane, xenon and nitrous oxide in the dog. Anesthesiology 26:771, 1965

164. Miller KW, Paton WDM, Smith EB, et al: Physiochemical approaches to the mode of action of general anesthetics. Anesthesiology 36:339, 1972

10

How Do Inhaled Anesthetics Work?

Donald D. Koblin, Ph.D.
Edmond I. Eger II, M.D.

INTRODUCTION

A variety of inhaled agents can produce general anesthesia. These include hydrogen (H_2), argon (Ar), xenon (Xe), nitrous oxide (N_2O), cyclopropane (C_3H_6), diethyl ether ($C_2H_5OC_2H_5$), halothane ($CF_3CHBrCl$), and methoxyflurane ($CHCl_2CF_2OCH_3$). Some of the properties of these agents may vary considerably. For example, xenon and argon are essentially inert, while halothane possesses a permanent dipole moment, can form hydrogen bonds, and is metabolized by the liver. The molecular size of the inhaled agents differs by a factor of about 10.

The structural diversity of the inhaled anesthetics suggests that they do not interact directly with a single specific receptor site. However, some of the correlations of the potencies of anesthetics with their physiochemical properties do suggest a common (unitary) mechanism of general anesthetic action. An example is the striking relationship between anesthetic potency and lipid solubility. Although these relationships do not provide a detailed mechanism of anesthesia, such correlations have been helpful in defining the environment in which anesthetics act.

Any molecular hypothesis of anesthesia must be consistent with the effects of anesthetics on the whole organism. For instance, since anesthetic administration can rapidly induce unconsciousness, and since awakening can quickly occur following the discontinuation of anesthesia, physical or biochemical changes important to the mechanism of anesthetic action must occur within seconds. Similarly, physical or biochemical alterations caused by anesthetics are meaningful only at clinical doses and not at high anesthetic levels. High levels may produce toxic effects unrelated to the mechanism by which inhaled anesthetics act. Finally anesthetic requirement does not change with increasing duration of anesthesia,[1] except, perhaps, for a small, hyperacute tolerance that is complete within 10 to 30 minutes following the start of anesthesia.[2] Thus any physical or biochemical change causally related to anesthesia should be stable for a period of hours to days.

MEASUREMENT OF ANESTHETIC POTENCIES

An exploration of the mechanism by which anesthetics act requires a knowledge of relative anesthetic potencies for each of the agents. The best estimate of anesthetic potency is MAC—the minimum alveolar concentration of an agent that produces immobility in 50 percent of those subjects exposed to a noxious stimulus (see Ch. 8). For determination of MAC in humans, the stimulus is a surgical skin incision. In animals, the painful stimulus is produced by clamping the tail or by passing electric current through subcutaneous electrodes. The advantage of measuring the alveolar concentration is that following a short equilibration period it directly represents the partial pressure of the anesthetic in the central nervous system and is independent of the uptake and distribution of the agent to other tissues.[3] Another advantage of MAC is its consistancy in a given animal or species or between different species or classes of animals.[3] This consistancy makes it possible to discern small changes in anesthetic requirement which may provide a clue to how anesthetics act.

The anesthetic concentration that abolishes the righting reflex in 50 percent of the animals is often used to measure anesthetic potencies in smaller animals (i.e., an anesthetic ED_{50}).[4] Since the inspired rather than alveolar concentrations are measured, the method applies best to rapidly equilibrating (poorly blood-soluble) agents. Only with equilibration can it be assumed that the partial pressure of the inspired gas equals that at the site of action. The use of small animals and inspired concentrations facilitates work with agents at very high pressures (i.e. tens or hundreds of atmospheres). The anesthetic ED_{50} in the mouse determined by the rolling response (i.e. the righting reflex) correlates closely with MAC in humans over a 300-fold range in anesthetic requirements (Fig. 10-1).

ALTERATIONS IN ANESTHETIC REQUIREMENT PERTINENT TO THEORIES OF NARCOSIS

Any theory of narcosis must account for the effect of temperature and pressure on anesthetic requirement. In mammals, MAC decreases with decreasing body temperatures

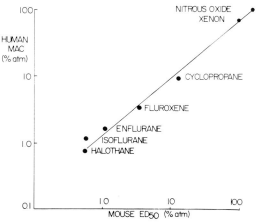

Fig. 10-1 The minimum alveolar concentrations (MAC) of various anesthetics required to prevent a response to surgical incision in humans and the inspired dose of an anesthetic (ED_{50}) required to abolish the righting reflex in the mouse are closely correlated. That is, the values obtained in mice may be used to predict those in man and vice versa. Values are taken from Eger[3] and Smith et al.[188]

(from 41 °C to 26 °C) for all anesthetics, but the reduction per degree decrease in body temperature varies from agent to agent.[5-7] The decrease in MAC varies from 2 percent per degree for cyclopropane to 5 percent per degree for halothane. Similar decreases in requirement with decreasing temperature are seen in fishes[8] and toads.[9]

Application of increasing hydrostatic pressures progressively increases the anesthetic dose required to bring about unresponsiveness, a phenomenon termed the "pressure reversal of anesthesia."[10-13] In experiments with mammals, pressure increases are brought about by the addition of helium, since helium does not produce anesthesia.[14] At a total pressure of 100 atmospheres, a 30 to 60 percent increase in the partial pressure of nitrous oxide, isoflurane, argon, or nitrogen is required to abolish the righting reflex.[12, 13, 15, 16] These effects of pressure and temperature may be used to test the various models of general anesthetic action and we will refer to them repeatedly in later parts of the chapter.

WHERE DO INHALED ANESTHETICS ACT IN THE CENTRAL NERVOUS SYSTEM?

General anesthetics may act by altering neuronal activity in selected regions of the central nervous system. Since the brainstem reticular formation plays a role in altering the state of consciousness and alertness and in regulating motor activity,[17] this structure is thought to be an important site of anesthetic action. French et al.[18] found that ether blocked conduction of auditory-evoked potentials in the ascending reticular activating system but not in the lemniscal system. They suggested that the multisynaptic interneuronal organization of the reticular activating system made it more susceptible to anesthetic blockade than the paucisynaptic lateral pathways. Later experiments confirmed the reversible disruption of the midbrain reticular system with anesthetizing concentrations of various inhaled agents (reviewed by Rosner and Clark[19] and Winters[20]). However, other studies showed that the effect of anesthesia on evoked and spontaneous nervous activity in the reticular formation is variable and can be increased, unaltered, or decreased depending upon the agent and the neuronal unit examined.[21,22] These experiments suggest that the anesthetic-induced disruption of reticular formation nervous activity depends on the specific interaction of a general anesthetic with specific structures within each neuronal unit.

General anesthetics interrupt transmission in the central nervous system at sites other than the reticular formation. Anesthetizing doses of inhaled agents depress excitatory transmission in the cerebral cortex,[21] olfactory cortex,[23] cuneate nucleus,[24] and hippocampus.[25] General anesthetics reduce the sensitivity of neurons in several brain regions to iontophoretically applied putative neurotransmitters. The excitatory effects of iontophoretically applied acetylcholine are depressed by ether in the caudate nucleus[26] and by halothane but not methoxyflurane in single cortical neurons.[27] Ether and methoxyflurane depress the excitatory effects of *l*-glutamate applied to olfactory cortex neurons.[28] In addition to blocking excitatory effects, halothane prolongs the gamma-aminobutyric acid-induced inhibition of mitral cells in the olfactory cortex.[29] Inhaled agents may also enhance excitation. Halothane potentiates the efficiency of synaptic transmission through the cuneate nucleus,[30] and acetylcholine-induced firing in the olfactory cortex is augmented by ether, methoxyflurane, and halothane.[31]

Transmission through the spinal cord is depressed by general anesthetics. Ether, halothane, methoxyflurane, cyclopropane, chloroform, and nitrous oxide block monosynaptic excitatory postsynaptic potentials recorded in the ventral root.[32-35] The effect may be on a specific region of the spinal cord. In the lumbar spinal cord, halothane depresses the spontaneous firing frequency of cells in lamina I, V, and VI and the evoked firing frequency of cells in I and V but has no effect on transmission through lamina IV.[36]

Thus, inhaled anesthetics interrupt transmission in many areas of the central nervous system, and anesthesia may not selectively influence one specific region. The most common action of anesthetics is a depression of excitatory transmission, but instances are known where clinical concentrations of anesthetics have essentially no effect, prolong inhibitory transmission, or even potentiate excitatory transmission. Considering the complexity of the human brain, composed of approximately 20 billion neurons with each neuron forming thousands of synapses,[37] the variable nature of general anesthetic effects is perhaps not surprising. Attempts to reduce this complexity and to increase understanding of general anesthetic action have led to experiments on isolated neuronal preparations.

ANESTHETIC BLOCKADE OF SYNAPTIC AND AXONAL TRANSMISSION

Anesthetizing concentrations of inhaled agents block synaptic transmission but have little or no effect on peripheral receptors or axonal transmission. The concentration of ether or chloroform which halves the amplitude of the action potential in sympathetic nerve axons is three to five times that which halves synaptic transmission.[38] Anesthetizing concentrations of ether, halothane, and methoxyflurane do not alter compound action potentials recorded from the saphenous branch of the femoral nerve and cutaneous receptor responses to touch and movement of hair.[39] Anesthetic concentrations close to MAC do not alter the compound action potential of lateral olfactory tract fibers[23] nor the electrical excitability of afferent fibers to the hippocampus,[25] whereas they do produce a 50 to 100 percent blockade of postsynaptic potentials. Compound action potentials in presynaptic fibers are not affected until concentrations of approximately twice MAC are obtained. Similarly, concentrations of gaseous and volatile agents well in excess of those producing anesthesia are required to alter action potentials in frog sciatic and rabbit vagus nerve.[40] These findings suggest that general anesthetics selectively block synaptic transmission in the central nervous system.

If anesthetics act by blocking synaptic transmission, polysynaptic pathways may be assumed to be more susceptible to anesthetic blockade than monosynaptic pathways, since the probability of blockade could increase with the number of synaptic connections. However, inhaled agents equally depress monosynaptic and polysynaptic responses recorded from the ventral root of the spinal cord.[33, 35] Thus, the safety factor for transmission during anesthesia along a chain of

neurons does not seem to be a function of synaptic chain length. This finding may be due to the variable sensitivities of different synapses to anesthetics or from a combination of the depressing effects of anesthetics on excitatory and inhibitory pathways. In addition, the output of a given neuron depends upon the input received from hundreds or thousands of other neurons. Anesthetics could disrupt normal synaptic transmission by altering the summation of the potential changes produced by these converging inputs.

Synaptic blockade by anesthetics usually results from an interference with neurotransmitter release or from an interference with binding or activation of the neurotransmitter on the postsynaptic membrane. However, several investigators suggest that anesthetics partially or completely block impulse conduction in small diameter terminal branches of afferent axons. Even partial blockade might interfere with transmission by decreasing transmitter release. A 15 mV increase in the nerve action potential can produce a 10-fold increase in transmitter output.[41] Anesthetic blocking concentrations in bullfrog single myelinated fibers that are 18 μ in diameter are about four times higher than in 3 μ fibers.[42] Similarly, concentrations that block rat phrenic nerve axons (11 μ in diameter) are two to twenty times lower than those that block rat and frog sciatic nerve axons (16 μ in diameter).[43] Inhaled anesthetics at just above clinical concentrations partially block compound action potentials in small diameter axons of preganglionic sympathetic nerves of the rat[44] and crayfish.[45] However, this relationship between axon size and anesthetic sensitivity may not hold for all axons.[46] Other factors, such as internodal length or degree of myelination, may be important determinants of the differential blockade of axons.[47]

As mentioned previously, high pressures antagonize anesthesia in the intact animal. Therefore, the effects of pressure on axonal conduction and synaptic transmission in the

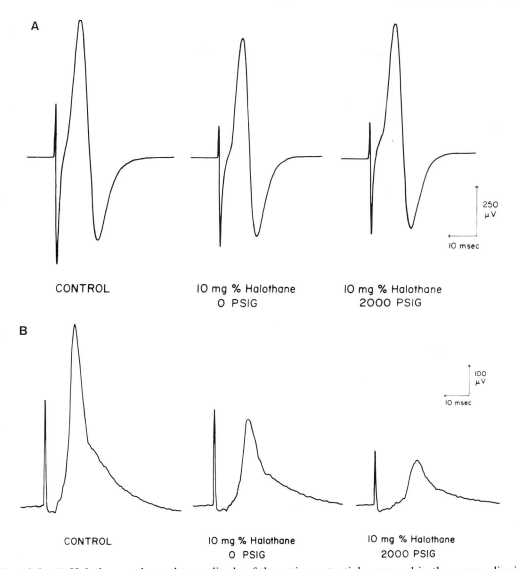

Fig. 10-2 (*A*) Halothane reduces the amplitude of the action potential measured in the preganglionic nerve from the superior cervical ganglion of the rat. The effect is reversed by the application of 2,000 PSIG (136 atm). (*B*) Recordings of the postganglionic action potential show that halothane depresses synaptic transmission and that high pressures add to this depressant effect. (Kendig JJ, Trudell JR, Cohen EN: Effects of pressure and anesthetics on conduction and synaptic transmission. J Pharmacol Exp Ther 195:216, 1975, © 1979 The Williams & Wilkins Co., Baltimore.)

presence of anesthetics may provide a clue concerning the cellular site of anesthetic action. Compression to approximately 100 atmospheres reverses the depression of the compound action potential amplitudes in rat preganglionic sympathetic nerves treated with halothane or methoxyflurane at concentrations greater than MAC[48] (Fig. 10-2*A*). In contrast, pressure alone depresses synaptic transmission[49] and adds to the depressant effects of anesthetics[48,50] (Fig. 10-2*B*). These results in isolated model systems imply conduction blockade as a possible mechanism of anesthesia and not blockade of excitatory synaptic transmission. This assumes, however, that pressure produces its antagonism by acting at the same site as the anesthetics—an assumption that may be in error (see section on Critical Volume Hypothesis).

Presynaptic and Postsynaptic Actions of Inhaled Anesthetics and the Role of Neurotransmitters

Anesthetics may disrupt normal synaptic transmissions by interfering with release of neurotransmitters from the presynaptic nerve terminals into the synaptic cleft, by altering the binding of the transmitter to receptor sites on the postsynaptic membrane, or by influencing the ionic conductance change that follows the activation of the postsynaptic receptor by neurotransmitter.[51] Since research on identifying transmitters in the central nervous system and assigning them to specific neuronal pathways has just started,[52-54] only limited information is available on the ability of inhaled anesthetics to influence presynaptic transmitter release and postsynaptic receptor activation.

Intracellular recordings from lumbosacral motoneurons suggest a presynaptic site of diethyl ether action.[33] Diethyl ether decreases monosynaptic excitatory postsynaptic potentials evoked by impulses in single Ia afferent fibers but does not affect the postsynaptic potential change produced by one transmitter quantum.[33] This implies that diethyl ether depresses excitatory transmitter release presynaptically, while not altering the chemosensitivity of the postsynaptic membrane. Similarly, halothane decreases the release of norepinephrine from the guinea-pig vas deferens secondary to hypogastric nerve stimulation.[55] Halothane depresses the electrically stimulated, but not the norepinephrine-induced, contractile response of the saphenous vein of the dog.[56] Halothane inhibits norepinephrine output evoked by activation of sympathetic nerve terminals in the heart[57] and adrenal medulla,[58] and decreases the release of dopamine from rat striatal slices following the application of a nicotinic agonist.[59] These alterations in release of catecholamines imply a presynaptic effect.

Inhaled anesthetics also decrease acetylcholine release from the brain,[60] but it is unknown whether this results from a direct presynaptic action or a general decrease in activity. In the isolated guinea-pig ileum preparation, diethyl ether and chloroform decrease acetylcholine output at all rates of stimulation,[61] whereas the gaseous anesthetics increase both spontaneous and electrically evoked acetylcholine release.[62, 63] These increases in release of acetylcholine do not parallel the anesthetic potencies of the gaseous agents.[63] These increases in acetylcholine output are not reversed by adding helium to a total pressure of 136 atm (Fig. 10-3), a pressure that reverses their anesthetic effect in vivo.

The above results show presynaptic effects of anesthetics in certain isolated preparations, but evidence is also available for postsynaptic anesthetic effects in other preparations. Postsynaptic sites of anesthetic action may be studied by iontophoretic application of putative neurotransmitters that are thought to act directly on postsynaptic membrane receptors. Concentrations of methoxyflurane or ether, but not halothane, that depress synaptic transmission in the olfactory cortex also depress the sensitivity of the cortical neurons to *l*-glutamate.[28] An opposite, yet still postsynaptic, effect on cortical neurons is produced by these same volatile agents: the anesthetics augment, in a dose-related fashion, the cortical neuron firing induced by iontophoretic application of acetylcholine.[31] A postsynaptic anesthetic action may be implied by the ability of halothane to block discharges elicited by the application of a nicotinic agonist to the hamster stellate ganglion,[64] although halothane does not block the discharges elicited by a muscarinic agonist.[64] General anesthetics can alter the postsynaptic response at the

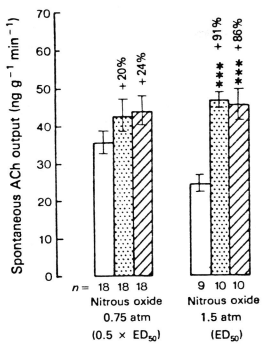

$n =$ 18 18 18   9 10 10

Nitrous oxide   Nitrous oxide

0.75 atm   1.5 atm

$(0.5 \times ED_{50})$ (ED_{50})

Fig. 10-3 Nitrous oxide increases spontaneous acetylcholine output from the guinea-pig ileum, and these effects of nitrous oxide are not reversed by the application of high pressures. Open columns = controls; stippled columns = effects of nitrous oxide; hatched columns = effects of nitrous oxide plus helium up to 136 atm. Mean values are shown, ± S.E. Gaseous agents also increase the electrically evoked acetylcholine output. *** = P < .01. (Halliday DJX, Little HJ, Paton WDM: The effects of inert gases and other general anesthetics on the release of acetylcholine from the guinea pig ileum. Br J Pharmac 67:229, 1979.)

neuromuscular junction. The ability of volatile anesthetics to depress the carbachol-induced depolarization of the end-plate region of guinea-pig lumbrical muscles correlates closely with their anesthetic potencies in man.[65] At the neuromuscular junction, a spontaneously secreted quantum of acetylcholine generates a miniature end-plate current, and the rate of the miniature end-plate current decay is increased by halothane, enflurane, diethyl ether, and chloroform[66,67] (Fig. 10-4). The time constant of the miniature end-plate current decay and its ampli-

tude essentially are determined by the number of ions and the amount of charge transferred across the postsynaptic membrane. The increase in the rate of channel closing caused by the volatile agents[68] decreases the amplitude of the postsynaptic response (the miniature end-place potential) and thereby depresses synaptic transmission (Fig. 10-4). In sum, inhaled anesthetics apparently depress the postsynaptic response to some (but not all) neurotransmitters and may alter the decay of the postsynaptic response.

Anesthetics do not affect synaptic transmission by depleting neurotransmitters. However, although neither halothane nor enflurane alter acetylcholine concentrations in several brain structures, they do decrease the acetylcholine turnover rate.[69] This decrease in turnover rate may result from an inhibition of acetylcholine release or simply a decrease in activity. Halothane and cyclopropane do not alter norepinephrine or dopamine levels in most brain regions, but may increase norepinephrine content in the nucleus accumbens, locus coeruleus, and central gray catecholamine areas.[70] Whole brain levels of serotonin and dopamine increase during enflurane anesthesia.[71] Halothane treatment of rat cerebral cortex slices increases production of the inhibitory transmitter gamma-aminobutyric acid (GABA).[72] If this accumulation of GABA in inhibitory neurons were associated with an increase in inhibitory activity, the resulting decrease in synaptic transmission could create the anesthetic state (the GABA theory of anesthesia).[73]

Although anesthesia does not deplete brain neurotransmitters, a change in neurotransmitter availability significantly influences the anesthetic requirement. Drugs that decrease central levels of norepinephrine and dopamine produce a dose-related decrease in halothane MAC,[9,74-76] whereas drugs that elevate central norepinephrine levels increase the anesthetic requirement.[74,76] The ablation of certain norepinephrine-rich and serotonin-rich brain stem areas decreases MAC in

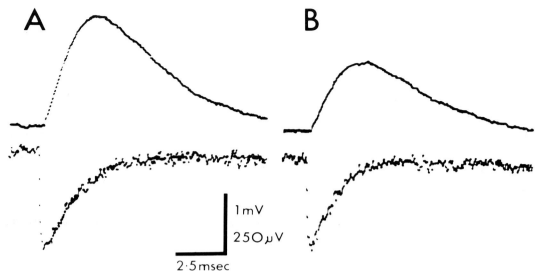

Fig.10-4 Halothane (1 mM) reduces the amplitude of miniature end-plate potentials (upper traces) by reducing the time constant of decay of miniature end-plate currents (lower traces). Records are shown in control solution (*A*) and in 1 mM halothane (*B*). (Gage PW, Hamill OP: Effects of several inhalation anesthetics on the kinetics of postsynaptic conductance changes in mouse diaphragm. Br J Pharmacol 57:263, 1976.)

rats when compared to sham-operated littermate controls.[77] However, since gross depletions in central monoamine levels cause at most a 35 percent reduction in MAC, other factors besides central monoamine levels must be the primary determinants of anesthetic requirement.

In summary, inhaled anesthetics probably act on synaptic regions including small diameter afferent axons at the nerve terminal. General anesthetics depress synaptic transmission in isolated neuronal systems and may have both a presynaptic and postsynaptic action. Clinical concentrations of inhaled agents can depress, leave unchanged, or enhance presynaptic transmitter release and postsynaptic membrane excitation depending upon the preparation, the particular neurotransmitter, and the anesthetic examined. However, since high pressure further depresses synaptic transmission, synaptic regions may not be the site of pressure-anesthetic antagonism. Anesthetizing concentrations of inhaled agents have little or no effect on peripheral receptors or transmission in large axons, but partially block conduction in small diameter axons. This partial conduction block is antagonized by high pressure.

PHYSICOCHEMICAL NATURE OF THE SITE OF ANESTHETIC ACTION

The preceeding sections suggested that anesthetics may act at several gross (e.g., spinal cord versus reticular activating system) or microscopic (e.g., presynaptic versus postsynaptic) sites to produce the anesthetic state. The varied nature of these sites, however, does not preclude a unique action at a molecular level. For instance, depression of transmitter release presynaptically and blockade of current flow through the postsynaptic membrane may arise from an anesthetic perturbation at an identical molecular site, even though the geographic locations of these sites differ. The theory that all inhaled anesthetics

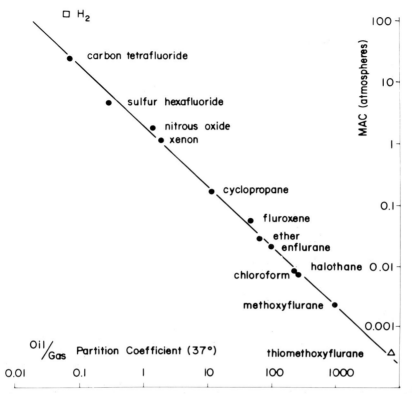

Fig. 10-5 MAC may be correlated with lipid solubility (i.e. the oil/gas partition coeffecient) over a 74,300-fold difference in potency from 0.00035 atm (thiomethoxyflurane) to 26 atm (carbon tetrafluoride). The line drawn through the points corresponds to the equation MAC × oil/gas partition coefficient = 2.17 atm. (Tanifuji Y, Eger EI II, Terrell RC: Some characteristics of an exceptionally potent inhaled anesthetic: Thiomethoxyflurane. Anesth Analg 56:387, 1977.)

have a common mode of action on a specific molecular structure is called the "unitary theory of narcosis." The nature of this presumed common site has been explored by correlating the physical properties of anesthetics with their potencies. The rationale behind this approach is that the best correlation between anesthetic potency and a physical parameter will suggest the nature of the site of action. For example, the correlation of MAC and lipid solubility (see below) indicates that the site of action is hydrophobic. However, correlations that depend upon the forces exerted between anesthetic molecules (e.g., the boiling point of an anesthetic) are not important to the study of anesthetic mechanisms, since such intermolecular forces cannot be repre-

sentative of a single site of action. That is, such correlations are defined by the interaction of each anesthetic with itself rather than with a common site.

The physical parameter that correlates best with anesthetic potency is that of lipid solubility[78-81] (Fig. 10-5). This correlation is termed the Meyer-Overton rule, after its two discoverers. The product of the anesthetizing partial pressure of an inhaled agent and its olive oil/gas partition coefficient varies less than twofold over a 70,000-fold range of anesthetizing partial pressures[82] (Fig. 10-5). The amazing closeness of this correlation implies a unitary molecular site of action and suggests that anesthesia results when a specific number of anesthetic molecules occupy a crucial hydrophobic region in the central nervous system. No other correlation employing the complete spectrum of inhaled agents approaches the excellent fit of that observed between anesthetic potency and lipid solubility.[83-87] This finding has led most recent investigators to look for the molecular basis of anesthetic action in cellular hydrophobic regions.

Nonetheless, some investigators believe that the anesthetic site of action is not necessarily hydrophobic in nature.[88-93] For example, Pauling[88] and Miller[89] independently suggested that anesthesia may be caused by the formation of hydrates (the hydrate theory of anesthesia). However, correlation between the ability of anesthetics to form hydrates and their potency is relatively poor[79,80]; the failure of this correlation has led to the abandonment of the hydrate theory.

The correlation of potency to solubililty in olive oil (Fig. 10-5) suggests that olive oil closely mimics the anesthetic site of action and that anesthesia occurs when a critical anesthetic concentration is attained at that site. However, since olive oil is a mixture of oils and is not very well characterized from a physicochemical point of view, anesthetic solubility has been examined in simpler solvents in order to better define the nature of where anesthetics act. A pure solvent may be characterized by its solubility parameter, which is a measure of the intermolecular forces in that solvent.[80] Anesthetic potency correlates best with solubility in solvents having solubility parameters of 8 to 10 (calories $cm^{-3})^{1/2}$.[80,94,95] These values are representative of a solvent such as benzene and again imply a hydrophobic site of anesthetic action.

The Meyer-Overton rule predicts that it is the number of molecules dissolved at the site of anesthetic action and not the type of molecules present that causes the development of anesthesia. Thus, half MAC of one agent plus half MAC of another agent should have the same effect as one MAC of either agent. In general, this prediction has been confirmed,[96-99] with only two minor exceptions.

A slight antagonism is reported for ethylene-nitrous oxide and cyclopropane-nitrous oxide mixtures in rats. However, this antagonism may arise from errors in the extrapolations made to estimate the potencies of nitrous oxide and ethylene.[98] The slight antagonism also noted for mixtures of sulfur hexafluoride with carbon tetrafluoride or argon, may be due to specific pulmonary effects associated with the breathing of sulfur hexafluoride at high pressures.[99] Thus, the evidence to date is consistent with an additive effect of anesthetics.

Although most evidence favors a unitary hydrophobic site of anesthetic action, the observation that not all lipid soluble molecules are anesthetics indicates that this simplified view may be misleading. For example, n-decane is a highly lipid soluble compound yet is nonanesthetic,[100] even though lower paraffin homologs such as n-pentane do cause anesthesia. Any unitary theory of narcosis involving a single hydrophobic site of action must eventually explain why such lipid soluble compounds are not anesthetics.

The Critical Volume Hypothesis

The Meyer-Overton rule indicates that anesthesia occurs when a sufficient number of anesthetic molecules dissolve as a certain site, but does not explain why anesthesia results. Mullins[95] took the lipid solubility correlation one step further and postulated that anesthesia occurs when the absorption of anesthetic molecules expands the volume of a hydrophobic region beyond a critical amount (critical volume hypothesis). Such an expansion might produce anesthesia by obstructing ion channels. An expansion might also alter the electrical properties of a membrane by increasing the thickness and decreasing the membrane capacitance.

The volume expansion hypothesis of anesthetic action suggested several experiments. One prediction of the hypothesis was that anesthetizing partial pressures of inhaled agents should produce a consistent volume expansion in a model hydrophobic system. Indeed, anesthetizing doses of several agents cause olive oil to undergo approximately a 0.4 percent increase in volume.[101] The hypothesis also predicts that anesthesia should be reversed by compression of the volume of the expanded hydrophobic region. High pressures do reverse anesthetic effects in vivo.[10-16,94,102] In addition, the critical volume theory is consistent with the observations that helium and neon, agents with low lipid solubilities, are not anesthetics and also explains why hydrogen is not as potent as predicted from the lipid solubility anesthetic potency correlation (Fig. 10-5). The explanation is that the expansion caused by these agents is counterbalanced by the compression resulting from their high pressures.[102] Pressure does not act by simply ejecting anesthetic molecules from their site of action, since the theoretic predictions indicate that the displacement is too small to explain the experimental data.[102] The finding that hyperbaric pressures have little effect on the partitioning of anesthetics into hydrophobic model systems supports this prediction.[103]

The critical volume model also suggests that a decrease in body temperature should antagonize the effect of anesthesia by contracting the volume of the expanded hydrophobic region. However, as mentioned previously, MAC does not increase but rather decreases with decreasing temperature.[5-7] Although this seemingly contradicts the critical volume hypothesis, this prediction probably is complicated by the increased partitioning of anesthetics into nonpolar solvents at decreased temperatures[104] and the uncertainty of the effects of temperature per se on the organism.

Several arguments may be raised against the critical volume hypothesis. If MAC levels of all inhaled agents do cause an equal increase in volume, then the degree of pressure reversal for a given total pressure should be the same for all agents and the increase in anesthetic requirement should be rectilinearly

related to the total pressure. However, the degree of pressure reversal differs for different agents. Also the anesthetic requirements of argon and nitrogen increase in a curvilinear fashion with increases in pressure.[16] Although the degree of this nonlinearity is questionable,[94] a nonlinear pressure antagonism suggests that anesthetics and pressure may act at different sites. Thus the main effect of pressure may be to increase the general level of central nervous system excitability. Indeed, in the absence of anesthetics, high pressures produce tremors and convulsions.[105,106] Since all lipid soluble compounds are not anesthetics, the critical volume hypothesis is even more suspect. There is no immediate explanation of why these nonanesthetics should not expand the suspected crucial hydrophobic sites. In summary, the critical volume hypothesis is probably an oversimplified view of the way anesthetics act.

The Membrane as the Site of Anesthetic Action

The activity immediately underlying transmission of nervous impulses principally occurs at the surface of nerves. Since inhaled agents disrupt this transmission, synaptic or axonal membranes are assumed to be the primary sites of anesthetic action. Since cellular membranes largely consist of hydrophobic components, a membrane site of action is also consistent with the hydrophobic theories of anesthesia.

Cytoplasmic sites of anesthetic action seem unlikely, since the cytoplasm is thought to play a relatively minor role in the short-term conduction of nervous impulses. Nevertheless, anesthetics could act indirectly at a cytoplasmic membrane site. For example, anesthetics might depress the ion-accumulating activity of mitochondria, thus altering the cytoplasmic levels of free ions which could in turn influence the conductance properties of excitable membranes.[107] Indeed, inhaled agents do inhibit mitochondrial activity and brain metabolism, but usually higher than clinical doses are required to inhibit mitochondrial function.[108, 109]

Reversible depolymerization of cytoplasmic microtubules and microfilaments has been suggested as a mechanism of anesthetic action (microtubular theory of anesthesia). Although some inhaled agents depolymerize microtubules,[110] others do not.[111] The disruption of microtubules by colchicine also does not block membrane excitation.[112] Moreover, high pressures also deploymerize microtubules.[113] Thus if microtubules were the site of anesthetic action, high pressure should augment rather than antagonize the effect of anesthesia.

The above discussion suggests that it is the association of inhaled agents with plasma membranes of nerves that produces anesthesia. The question then arises as to which membrane components are altered by the anesthetics. Biologic membranes are generally thought to consist of a phospholipid-cholesterol bilayer matrix with peripheral proteins weakly bound to the hydrophilic membrane exterior and integral proteins deeply imbedded into or even passing through the lipid bilayer[114] (Fig. 10-6*A*). Although neuronal membranes are difficult to biochemically isolate completely free from other cellular contaminants, synaptic plasma membrane preparations of reasonable purity have been obtained. They are approximately 50 percent protein and 50 percent lipid by weight.[115] Anesthetic action at a hydrophobic site in these membranes could be on the nonpolar interior of the lipid bilayer, at hydrophobic pockets in membrane proteins, or at the hydrophobic interface between the intrinsic membrane proteins and the lipid matrix (Fig. 10-6*A*).

Attempts to better understand the penetration of inhaled agents into and their interaction with membrane sites have led to an examination of isolated membrane components. These experiments were greatly aided by the discovery that when phospholipids are dispersed in an aqueous medium, they spontaneously form bilayers that comprise the surface of spherical structures (liposomes). These phospholipid bilayers act as a permeability barrier to ions and are similar to those found in biomembranes.[116] Liposomes have been extensively employed as model systems in which the interaction of anesthetics with membrane lipids has been studied. In contrast, membrane proteins are difficult to isolate and purify, especially those protein ionophores thought to permit the passage (tunneling) of ions through membranes during excitation.[117] Thus, most investigators who examine anesthetic-protein interactions employ soluble proteins as model systems. Such proteins are easy to prepare in reasonable quantities but may not precisely mimic the natural proteins responsible for ion translocation.

The Interaction of Inhaled Anesthetics with Membrane Lipids

When liposomes are prepared in a salt solution containing radioactive ions, the untrapped ions exterior to the liposomes can be removed and the subsequent flux of ions from the interior to the exterior of the liposomes may be measured. Inhaled agents increase the cation permeability of liposomes in a dose-related manner.[116, 118, 119] These anesthetic-induced increases in cation permeability are found both in the presence of ionophores that facilitate the transport of ions through membranes and in the absence of ionophores.[118, 119] All agents increase cation permeability, but the magnitude of the increase depends upon the lipid composition of the liposome and the anesthetic examined.[118] Furthermore, the anesthetic-induced increases in cation permeability are reversed by the application of high pressures (approximately 100 atmospheres),[118] and these results parallel the antagonism observed between pressure and anesthesia in vivo.

To learn more about the nature of this proposed perturbation, several investigators

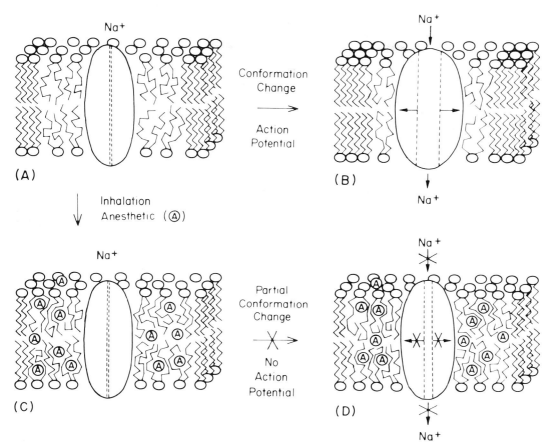

Fig. 10-6 (*A*) This representation of a neuronal membrane contains an integral membrane protein (the oval structure) which spans the phospholipid bilayer. The membrane protein has an ionic channel in the closed configuration. The small circles depict the hydrophilic phosphate head groups and the zigzag lines depict fatty acid chains. On the left and right edges of the bilayer segment there are regions in which the fatty acid chains are highly ordered. The phospholipids surrounding the intrinsic protein are disordered. (*B*) Following a stimulus, the membrane protein expands (i.e. undergoes a conformational change) in a fashion which allows passage of ions through the channel. The expansion is accomplished by converting some high-volume fluid-phase lipids into the low-volume solid phase. (*C*) Anesthetic molecules invade both solid and fluid phases and convert much of the solid to a fluid phase. (*D*) Following a stimulus, the membrane protein is unable to expand in conformation and open its channel, since the high-volume fluid-phase lipids cannot be converted into the low-volume solid phase lipids in the presence of the anesthetic and the compression of the fluid phase without conversion requires more lateral pressure than is immediately available. (Trudell JR: A unitary theory of anesthesia based on lateral phase separations in nerve membranes. Anesthesiology 46:5, 1977.)

have examined how anesthetics influence the dimensions of model lipid systems. Inhaled agents increase the lateral pressure of lipid monolayers in a manner that parallels their anesthetic potency.[120, 121] This finding is consistent with the notion that anesthetics may exert pressure on the ionic channels needed for impulse transmission and thereby inhibit their opening or accelerate their closure (a variation of the volume expansion theory of anesthesia). Such an expansion may also explain the ability of inhaled agents to protect erythrocytes from hypotonic hemolysis.[122] Alternatively, an expansion may result in the thickening of a membrane lipid bilayer and thereby reduce the stability of ionic channels formed during excitation.[123] Indeed the conductance of one model lipid membrane system is inversely related to membrane thickness,[124] and pentane has been shown to cause a thickening in the myelin membrane.[125]

Attempts to further define the molecular changes that occur upon the insertion of anesthetic molecules into lipid membranes led to studies concerning the influence of anesthetics on the mobility of membrane components (the fluidization theory of anesthesia). Inhaled agents cause a dose-related increase in the mobility of fatty acid chains in a phospholipid bilayler.[126-130] This "fluidization" of the lipid bilayer is reversed by the application of high pressures,[131, 132] a finding consistant with the previously described pressure reversal of anesthesia. Inhaled agents apparently produce this fluidization by interacting at all depths within the lipid bilayer, since anesthetic molecules are found along the entire length of the fatty acid chains.[133] The ability of an anesthetic to fluidize a lipid bilayer depends upon the structure of the agent examined and upon the bilayer lipid composition. Fluidization is most readily accomplished by a given anesthetic partial pressure when liposomes contain about 30 percent cholesterol and about 10 percent of an acidic phospholipid.[134] Although whether this fluidization of liposomal membranes occurs at clinical concentrations is debateable,[92, 135] all cholesterol containing lipid bilayers appear to be fluidized by anesthetizing doses of agents.[136] However, the same may not be true for neuronal membranes. Indeed, the fluidity of synaptic plasma membranes is decreased at clinical concentrations of halothane.[137]

Even a small change in lipid fluidity may produce a profound change in membrane function: a 20 percent change in liposome cation permeability is associated with a 2 percent change in the fluidity structural parameter.[119] Anesthesia might result from such changes in permeability. The permeability

changes might be induced by an indirect action of anesthetics on the physiological ionophores, since the ion-transporting properties of several membrane proteins depend upon the physical state of their neighboring lipids.[138] The increased decay rate of postsynaptic currents in the presence of inhaled agents may be caused by an increased fluidity of the postsynaptic membrane, allowing for a more rapid relaxation of the proteins involved in the conductance change that occurs following acetylcholine activation.[66, 67]

Liposomes consisting of a single type of phospholipid undergo a "phase transition" at a critical temperature.[139] This phase transition is characterized by a sudden conversion of the lipids from a "solid" or "gel" phase to a "liquid" or "fluid" phase as the temperature slowly increases. For example, dipalmitoyl-phosphatidylcholine (DPPC) (a lecithin molecule possessing two saturated fatty acid chains, 16 carbon atoms in length), undergoes a major transition at $41°C$,[139] and inhaled agents decrease the phase transition temperature of this molecule.[140-143] This effect is reversed by the application of high pressures.[142-143] These results have led to a hypothesis that lipids surrounding an excitable membrane channel normally are exclusively in the more rigid gel phase, thereby helping to maintain patency of the channel. Upon anesthetic addition these lipids become fluidized and loss of the surrounding structural support allows the channel to close (the phase transition theory of anesthesia).[144]

Since neuronal membranes consist of several types of phospholipids each with a different fatty acid composition, a "lateral phase separation" may exist and neuronal membrane lipids may be in both fluid and gel forms. The conversion of one form to another may permit the expansion or contraction of the membrane with greater ease than would be required if the membrane were purely fluid or gel.[145] The importance of this concept to the effect of an anesthetic on nerve transmission is illustrated in Figure 10-6. The resting neuronal membrane has a globular protein that spans the lipid bilayer region and possesses a closed ionic channel. The lipids immediately surrounding this protein are depicted as being in a disordered (fluid) state (Fig. 10-6*A*). During membrane excitation, a change in the protein conformation opens the channel. This volume expansion of the protein is accomplished by converting a fraction of the high-volume fluid phase lipids to low-volume solid phase lipids (Fig. 10-6*B*). If anesthetic molecules are introduced into the membrane (Fig. 10-6*C*) the low-volume solid phase cannot form and the protein cannot change its conformation to the open channel state (Fig. 10-6*D*). Support for this hypothesis comes from the finding that general anesthetics disrupt lateral phase separations in model membranes composed of two types of phospholipids, and that these effects are partially reversed by pressure.[146]

The presence of lateral phase separations is generally thought to permit an energy "cheap" way to expand or contract membranes. That is, less energy may be required to reduce membrane lipid volume by going through a phase change and converting fluid lipids to solid lipids, than by compressing the lipids without a phase change. However, some simple calculations do not support this idea. If one *assumes* an ideal compression, *less* energy is required to alter the volume of DPPC by compressing it than by going through a phase change.* However, correc-

tion for nonideality may give an opposite result, a result that may confirm the original thought that reducing volume by compression is more "expensive" than by causing a phase change. In addition, since we are considering a lateral compression, the energy required to compress the lipids should be calculated on the two-dimensional level, a calculation that has not been performed.

Both the "fluidization" and "lateral phase transition" theories suggest that anesthetics may act by making membranes more disordered or fluid, and that this anesthetic perturbation is accompanied by an expansion in the membrane that can be counterbalanced by the application of high pressures. These theories are compromised by the fact that an increase in temperature also increases membrane fluidity and therefore should augment anesthesia. However, as previously mentioned an increase in body temperature consistently decreases anesthetic potency.[5-7]

Another difficulty in relating the above work on artificial lipid membranes to anesthetic action is that such membranes may differ significantly from neuronal membranes. In fact, halothane may have a biphasic effect on the structure of mammalian synaptic plasma membranes, increasing the ordering (decreasing fluidity) of these membranes at low (anesthetizing) halothane concentrations and increasing the fluidity at higher concentrations.[137, 147] Furthermore, low halothane concentrations only cause an ordering in

---

* For DPPC, the measured volume change (ΔV) that occurs by going through the phase transition is 0.035 ml/g, and the measured energy change associated with the transition is 8,400 cal/mole.[142]

The energy required to compress DPPC by 0.035 ml/g may be approximated. It is assumed that the compressibility for DPPC is about the same as for olive oil, 6×10^{-5} atm^{-1} (i.e., the volume decreases by 6×10^{-5} of the original volume for each atm increase in pressure). It is also assumed that 1 g of DPPC occupies about 1 ml. The pressure (P) needed to be applied to this 1 ml (1 g) of DPPC to change the volume by 0.035 ml is:

$$P = \frac{0.035}{6 \times 10^{-5} \text{atm}^{-1}} = 583 \text{ atm}$$

Assuming ideality, the energy involved in this process is $P\Delta V$:

$$
\begin{aligned}
P\Delta V &= (583 \text{ atm}) (0.035 \text{ ml}) \\
&= 20.4 \text{ atm-cm}^3 \left(\frac{10^6 \text{dynes/cm}^2}{\text{atm}} \right) \\
&= 2.04 \times 10^7 \text{ dynes-cm} \\
&= 2.04 \times 10^7 \text{ erg} \left(\frac{1 \text{ cal}}{4.2 \times 10^7 \text{ erg}} \right) \\
&= \frac{0.49 \text{ cal}}{\text{g DPPC}} \left(\frac{750 \text{ g DPPC}}{\text{mole DPPC}} \right) \\
&= 367 \text{ cal/mole DPPC}
\end{aligned}
$$

From these calculations it would appear that 23 times less energy is required to change the volume of DPPC by compressing it, than by going through the phase change.

synaptic plasma membranes and not in myelin or mitochondrial membranes.[147] This finding is more consistant with the effect of temperature on anesthetic requirement but implies that at very high anesthetic concentrations patients should awaken! Future detailed studies with purified neuronal membrane preparations will reveal more about the importance of anesthetic perturbations in the membrane lipid bilayer.

The Interaction of Inhaled Agents with Proteins

Only a few of the neuronal membrane proteins, which permit the translocation of ions during membrane excitation, have been isolated. Therefore, little information is available on the interaction of anesthetics with these membrane proteins; most experiments have employed other soluble proteins as model systems for the study of anesthetic effects.

Distinct anesthetic binding sites have been identified for myoglobin,[148] hemoglobin,[149-151] β-lactoglobulin,[152, 153] adenylate kinase,[154] serum albumin,[153] and serum lipoproteins.[155] A binding site may be occupied by more than one anesthetic molecule.[152] Not all nonpolar regions of a protein may act as binding sites.[154] The binding of inhaled agents to hemoglobin and β-lactoglobulin gives rise to conformational changes in these proteins,[149, 151, 153] and these perturbations may be transmitted to a part of the protein molecule relatively distant from the anesthetic binding site.[151] The perturbation of β-lactoglobulin[153] and hemoglobin[151] caused by an anesthetic parallels the lipid solubility and potency of that anesthetic.

The interaction of inhaled agents with proteins may be indirectly monitored by examining the change in enzyme activity induced by the anesthetic. Anesthetics inhibit the enzyme-induced luminescence output of light-emitting organisms and this inhibition can be reversed by application of high pressures.[156] Anesthetics probably depress luminescence by binding to areas near the active site of the enzyme luciferase, thus interfering with the normal association of the substrate or cofactor with the enzyme.[157-158] The ability of inhaled agents to depress luminescence intensity parallels their lipid solubility,[159] and thermodynamic arguments suggest that anesthetic binding to a hydrophobic site results in inactivation by inducing a major conformational change of the enzyme structure.[159]

Not all enzyme systems are affected. The activities of glycolytic enzymes are not influenced even by high doses of anesthetics,[160] and activities of Na^+ and K^+ ATPase isolated from brain tissue are only altered by concentrations much higher than MAC.[161, 162] Serum cholinesterase activity is unchanged by saturated solutions of volatile agents.[163] High anesthetic concentrations are required to inhibit acetylcholinesterase activity,[161, 163] and the effect of an agent on acetylcholinesterase activity does not parallel its anesthetic potency.[163]

Inhaled anesthetics affect various enzymes in different ways. The anesthetic inhibition of glutamate dehydrogenase activity is related to the lipid solubility of the anesthetic. This decreased activity probably results from a conformational change that prevents the enzyme subunits from associating into an active form.[160] Inhaled agents may influence the amount of an enzyme in its soluble and particular forms: anesthetics may inhibit glucose phosphorylation in brain by solubilizing the more active mitochondrial hexokinase.[164] The activity of neuronal membrane-bound neuraminidase is enhanced by anesthetics,[165-167] as is the activity of dopamine-sensitive adenylate cyclase in the caudate nucleus.[168] However, it is uncertain whether the effect of an anesthetic on a membrane-bound enzyme is due to a direct interaction with the enzyme, or an indirect alteration due to perturbation of the membrane lipids surrounding the enzyme.

Young et al.[169] examined the influence of

anesthetics on the properties of a receptor-ionophore complex known to be involved in the membrane translocation of ions. Clinical concentrations of halothane, diethyl ether and chloroform greatly facilitate the agonist-induced structural transition of the acetylcholine receptor and decrease the half-time of the agonist-induced conformational change to 10 percent of the value seen in the absence of anesthetics. The structural change promoted by the anesthetics is associated with a desensitized and inactive state of the acetylcholine receptor–ionophore complex.

These observations on isolated proteins have led to the postulate that general anesthetics inactivate proteins essential for central nervous system function by combining with hydrophobic regions of protein molecules and inducing a conformational change in the molecules that makes them less active.[170] This conformational change is thought to be due to an unfolding of the molecule, accompanied by an increase in volume.[170] Although some convincing thermodynamic arguments are given for this protein perturbation hypothesis, the hypothesis does not offer a distinct mechanism by which anesthetics produce inactivation. A clearer picture may develop with an increased understanding of the structure and function of membrane proteins.

The Action of Inhaled Anesthetics at the Opiate Receptor

Several reports state that naloxone, a narcotic antagonist, partially reverses the action of inhaled anesthetics either when the former is given intravenously[171] or when perfused through the fourth (but not the third) cerebral ventricle.[172] These studies suggest that anesthetics may act by releasing endogenous opiate-like substances (the endorphin-release theory of anesthesia). However, replication of these studies showed that the antagonistic effect of naloxone could be explained by an insignificant shift in the anesthetic dose-response curve,[173-176] and that the anesthetic

requirement (as measured by lack of response to a painful stimulus or ability to abolish the righting reflex) is altered at most a few percent by naloxone, even at doses as high as 250 mg/kg.[173] Furthermore, naloxone does not antagonize the depressant effects of halothane on the longitudinal muscle of the guinea-pig ileum.[177] Nevertheless, naloxone partially antagonizes the analgesic effects of nitrous oxide in mice (as measured by the "writhing" response[178]), in rats (as measured by the "tail flick" test[179]) and in humans (as measured by cerebral evoked potential response to painful tooth-pulp electric shocks[180]). Naloxone also antagonizes, at relatively high doses, the nitrous oxide stimulation of locomotor activity in mice.[181] Thus, although anesthetics may produce analgesia by release of endogenous opiate-like compounds, the current consensus is that they do not produce anesthesia by this mechanism.[182]

FUTURE STUDIES

Two observations that merit further study are that apparently not all lipid soluble compounds produce anesthesia, and that certain inhaled agents may act as convulsants (e.g., flurothyl [$CF_3CH_2OCH_2CF_3$]). Convulsant halogenated ethers may have different physical properties from the anesthetic halogenated ethers, since the convulsants are characterized by a low solubility parameter.[183] For example, flurothyl has a solubility parameter of 6.9 compared to values of around 8 for the anesthetic halogenated ethers.[183] Furthermore, halogenated compounds that are both anesthetics and convulsants have different effects on synaptic transmission. Anesthetic agents block excitatory but not inhibitory transmission at the crab neuromuscular junction, whereas convulsant agents block inhibitory but not excitatory transmission.[184] An explanation of why slight structural changes in the halogenated ethers alters the convulsant or anesthetic properties of these compounds may give a clue as to how anesthetics act.

Another future approach to the mechanism of anesthetic action relates alterations in anesthetic requirement with biochemical and biophysical changes occurring in the central nervous system. A correlation between anesthetic requirement and a structural change in the nervous system might indicate the critical properties of the anesthetic site of action and how anesthetics affect that site.

A prerequisite for such studies is the production of sustained alterations in anesthetic requirement. General anesthetic requirement can be increased by chronically exposing mice to subanesthetic levels of nitrous oxide.[185-186] We examined the possibility that such mice adapted to the subanesthetic N_2O exposure by altering their synaptic plasma membrane lipid composition. However, no significant alterations in synaptic membrane fatty acid, phospholipid, or cholesterol compositions occurred in the N_2O-tolerant animals.[186]

Another method of producing two groups of animals with different anesthetic requirements is to make use of the fact that anesthetic requirement varies slightly among animals of a given species and that members resistant to and vulnerable to anesthesia may be found in a normal population. Mice with consistently high and consistently low nitrous oxide requirements were selected from a normal population. Offspring from parents with consistently high requirements also had high requirements, while offspring from parents with low requirements similarly had low requirements. By selecting the offspring with the highest and lowest nitrous oxide requirements and by repeating the process of breeding, testing for nitrous oxide requirement, and selection through five generations, two lines of mice have been obtained that are separated by approximately 0.5 atm in nitrous oxide requirement[187] (Fig. 10-7). No detectable differences in the synaptic plasma membrane lipid compositions were found between the two lines of mice.[187] The discovery of the

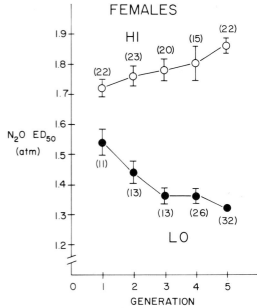

Fig. 10-7 Nitrous oxide righting reflex ED_{50}s ± S.E. in the female offspring of mice which were selectively bred for their resistance to (HI group) or susceptibility to (LO group) nitrous oxide anesthesia for five generations become progressively more separated in terms of their anesthetic requirement. Numbers in parentheses indicate the number of mice tested for each ED_{50} value. (Koblin DD, Dong DE, Deady JE, Eger EI II: Selective breeding alters mouse resistance to nitrous oxide without alteration in synaptic membrane lipid composition. Anesthesiology 52:401, 1980.)

structural changes in the central nervous system that produce these differences in nitrous oxide requirement could provide an important insight into the mechanism of anesthetic action.

CONCLUSIONS

Inhaled anesthetics disrupt neuronal transmission in many areas of the central nervous system. They act by either enhancing inhibitory effects or depressing excitatory transmission through synaptic regions or small diameter axons at the nerve terminal. Both presynaptic and postsynaptic actions have been found. Regardless of the macroscopic site of action, anesthetics almost certainly exert their effect by interacting with neuronal membranes. The excellent correlation between lipid solubility and anesthetic potency suggests that anesthetics have a hydrophobic site of action. Anesthetics cause conformational perturbations in both membrane lipids and proteins, but it is presently uncertain how these perturbations might lead to the anesthetic state. Future advances in anesthetic mechanisms will be associated with an increased knowledge of synaptic transmission in selective regions of the central nervous system, a better understanding of membrane proteins and membrane lipids in synaptic processes, and an ability to relate biophysical and biochemical changes in synaptic regions to alterations in anesthetic requirement.

REFERENCES

1. Eger EI II, Saidman LJ, Brandstater B: Minimum alveolar anesthetic concentration: A standard of anesthetic potency. Anesthesiology 26:756, 1965
2. Smith RA, Winter PM, Smith M, et al: Rapidly developing tolerance to acute exposures to anesthetic agents. Anesthesiology 50:496, 1979
3. Eger EI II: Anesthetic Uptake and Action. Baltimore, Williams and Wilkins, 1974
4. Miller KW, Paton, WDM, Smith EB: The anesthetic pressures of certain fluorine-containing gases. Br J Anaesth 39:910, 1967
5. Regan MJ, Eger EI II: Effect of hypothermia in dogs on anesthetizing and apneic doses of inhalation agents. Anesthesiology 28:689, 1967
6. Steffey EP, Eger EI II: Hyperthermia and halothane MAC in the dog. Anesthesiology 41:392, 1974
7. Vitez TS, White PF, Eger EI II: Effects of hypothermia on halothane MAC and isoflurane MAC in the rat. Anesthesiology 41:80, 1974
8. Cherkin A, Catchpool JF: Temperature dependence of anesthesia in goldfish. Science 144:1460, 1964
9. Shim CY, Andersen NB: The effect of oxygen on minimal anesthetic requirements in the toad. Anesthesiology 34:333, 1971
10. Lever MJ, Miller KW, Paton WDM, et al: Pressure reversal of anesthesia. Nature 231:368, 1971
11. Halsey MJ, Wardley-Smith B: Pressure reversal of narcosis produced by anesthetics, narcotics and tranquilizers. Nature 257:811, 1975
12. Kent DW, Halsey MJ, Eger EI II, et al: Isoflurane anesthesia and pressure antagonism in mice. Anesth Analg 56:97, 1977
13. Miller KW, Wilson MW: The pressure reversal of a variety of anesthetic agents in mice. Anesthesiology 48:104, 1978
14. Miller KW: The pressure reversal of anesthesia and the critical volume hypothesis, Progress in Anesthesiology, vol 1. Edited by Fink BR. New York, Raven Press, 1975, pp 341-351
15. Halsey MJ, Eger EI II, Kent DW, et al: High-pressure studies of anesthesia, Progress in Anesthesiology, vol 1. Edited by Fink BR. New York, Raven Press, 1975, pp. 353-361
16. Smith RA, Smith M, Eger EI II, et al: Nonlinear antagonism of anesthesia in mice by pressure. Anesth Analg 58:19, 1979
17. Truex RC, Carpenter MB: Human Neuroanatomy. Baltimore, Williams and Wilkins, 1969
18. French JD, Verzeano M, Magoun HW: A neural basis of the anesthetic state. Arch Neurol Psychiat 69:519, 1953
19. Rosner BS, Clark DL: Neurophysiologic effects of general anesthetics: II. Sequential regional actions in the brain. Anesthesiology 39:59, 1973
20. Winters WD: Effects of drugs on the electrical activity of the brain: Anesthetics. Ann Rev Pharmacol Toxicol 16:413, 1976
21. Darbinjan TM, Golovchinsky VB, Plehotkina SI: The effects of anesthetics on reticular and cortical activity. Anesthesiology 34:219, 1971
22. Shimoji K, Matsuki M, Shimizu H, et al: Dishabituation of mesencephalic reticular neurons by anesthetics. Anesthesiology 47:349, 1977
23. Richards CD, Russell WJ, Smaje JC: The action of ether and methoxyflurane on synaptic transmission in isolated preparations of

the mammalian cortex. J Physiol (Lond) 248:121, 1975

24. Galindo A: Effects of procaine, pentobarbital and halothane on synaptic transmission in the central nervous system. J Pharmacol Exp Ther 169:185, 1969

25. Richards CD, White AE: Actions of volatile anesthetics on synaptic transmission in the dentate gyrus. J Physiol (Lond) 252:241, 1975

26. Bloom FE, Costa E, Salmoiraghi GC: Anesthesia and the responsiveness of individual neurons of the caudate nucleus of the cat to acetylcholine, norepinephrine and dopamine administered by microelectrophoresis. J Pharmacol Exp Ther 150:244, 1965

27. Crawford JM: Anesthetic agents and the chemical sensitivity of cortical neurones. Neuropharmacology 9:31, 1970

28. Richards CD, Smaje JC: Anesthetics depress the sensitivity of cortical neurones to L-glutamate. Br J Pharmacol 58:347, 1976

29. Nicoll RA: The effects of anesthetics on synaptic excitation and inhibition in the olfactory bulb. J Physiol (Lond) 223:803, 1972

30. Morris ME: Facilitation of synaptic transmission by general anesthetics. J Physiol (Lond) 284:307, 1978

31. Smaje JC: General anesthetics and the acetylcholine-sensitivity of cortical neurones. Br J Pharmacol 58:359, 1976

32. Somjen G: Effects of anesthetics on spinal cord of mammals. Anesthesiology 28:135, 1967

33. Zorychta E, Capek R: Depression of spinal monosynaptic transmission by diethyl ether: Quantal analysis of unitary synaptic potentials. J Pharmacol Exp Ther 207:825, 1978

34. Freund FG, Martin WE, Hornbein TF: The H-reflex as a measure of anesthetic potency in man. Anesthesiology 38:642, 1969

35. De Jong RH, Robles R, Corbin RW, et al: Effect of inhalation anesthetics on monosynaptic and polysynaptic transmission in the spinal cord. J Pharmacol Exp Ther 162:326, 1968

36. Kitahata LM, Ghazi-Saidi K, Yamashita M, et al: The depressant effect of halothane and sodium thiopental on the spontaneous and evoked activity of dorsal horn cells: Lamina specificity, time course and dose dependence. J Pharmacol Exp Ther 195:515, 1975

37. Eccles JC: The Understanding of the Brain. New York, McGraw-Hill, 1977

38. Larrabee MG, Posternak JM: Selective action of anesthetics on synapses and axons in mammalian sympathetic ganglia. J Neurophys 15:91, 1952

39. De Jong RH, Nace RA: Nerve impulse conduction and cutaneous receptor responses during general anesthesia. Anesthesiology 28:851, 1967

40. Roth SH, Smith RA, Paton WDM: Pressure antagonism of anesthetic-induced conduction failure in frog peripheral nerve. Br J Anaesth 48:621, 1976

41. Katz B: The transmission of impulse from nerve to muscle, and the subcellular unit of synaptic action. Proc Roy Soc Lond [B] 155:455, 1962

42. Staiman A, Seeman P: Conduction blocking concentrations of anesthetics increase with nerve axon diameter: Studies with alcohol, lidocaine, and tetrodotoxin on single myelinated fibers. J Pharmacol Exp Ther 201:304, 1977

43. Staiman A, Seeman P: The impulse-blocking concentrations of anesthetics, alcohols, anticonvulsants, barbiturates, and narcotics on phrenic and sciatic nerves. Can J Physiol Pharmacol 52:535, 1974

44. Kendig JJ, Cohen EN: Pressure antagonism to nerve conduction block by anesthetic agents. Anesthesiology 47:6, 1977

45. Kendig JJ, Schneider TM, Cohen EN: Anesthetics inhibit pressure-induced repetitive impulse generation. J Appl Physiol 45:747, 1978

46. Heavner JE, de Jong RH: Lidocaine blocking concentrations for B- and C-nerve fibers. Anesthesiology 40:228, 1974

47. Franz DN, Perry RS: Mechanisms for differential block among single myelinated and nonmyelinated axons by procaine. J Physiol (Lond) 236:193, 1974

48. Kendig JJ, Trudell JR, and Cohen EN: Effects of pressure and anesthetics on conduction and synaptic transmission. J Pharmacol Exp Ther 195:216, 1975

49. Campenot RB: The effects of high hydrostatic pressure on transmission at the crustacean neuromuscular junction. Comp Biochem Physiol 52B:133, 1975

50. Kendig JJ, Cohen EN: Neuromuscular function at hyperbaric pressures: Pressure-anesthetic interactions. Am J Physiol 230:1244, 1976

51. Richards CD: The action of anesthetics on synaptic transmission. Gen Pharmacol 9:287, 1978

52. Krnjevic K: Chemical nature of synaptic transmission in vertebrates. Physiol Rev 54:418, 1974

53. Orrego F: Criteria for the identification of central neurotransmitters, and their application to studies with some nerve tissue preparations *in vitro*. Neuroscience 4:137, 1979

54. Moore RY, Bloom FE: Central catecholamine neuron systems: Anatomy and physiology of the norepinephrine and epinephrine systems. Ann Rev Neurosci 2:113, 1979

55. Roizen MF, Thoa NB, Moss J. et al: Inhibition by halothane of release of norepinephrine, but not of dopamine-β-hydroxylase, from guinea pig vas deferens. Eur J Pharmacol 31:313, 1975

56. Muldoon SM, Vanhoutte PM, Lorenz RR, et al: Venomotor changes caused by halothane acting on sympathetic nerves. Anesthesiology 43:41, 1975

57. Gothert M: Effects of halothane on the sympathetic nerve terminals of the rabbit heart. Naunyn-Schmiedebergs Arch Pharmacol 286:125, 1974

58. Gothert M, Dorn W. Loewenstein I: Inhibition of catecholamine release from the adrenal medulla by halothane. Naunyn-Schmiedebergs Arch Pharmacol 294:239, 1976

59. Westfall TC, DiFazio CA, Saunders J: Local anesthetic- and halothane-induced release of ^{3}H-dopamine from rat striatal slices. Anesthesiology 48:118, 1978

60. Pepeu G: The release of acetylcholine from the brain: An approach to the study of the central cholinergic mechanisms. Prog Neurobiol 2:257, 1973

61. Speden RN: The effect of some volatile anesthetics on the transmurally stimulated guinea-pig ileum. Br J Pharmacol Chemother 25:104, 1965

62. Little HJ, Paton WDM: The effects of high pressure helium and nitrogen on the release of acetylcholine from the guinea-pig ileum. Br J Pharmacol 67:221, 1979

63. Halliday DJX, Little JH, Paton WDM: The effects of inert gases and other general anesthetics on the release of acetylcholine from the guinea-pig ileum. Br J Pharmacol 67:229, 1979

64. Christ D: Effects of halothane on ganglionic discharges. J Pharmacol Exp Ther 200:336, 1977

65. Waud BE, Waud DR: Comparison of the effects of general anesthetics on the end-plate of skeletal muscle. Anesthesiology 43:540, 1975

66. Gage PW, Hamill OP: General anesthetics: Depression consistent with increased membrane fluidity. Neurosci Letts 1:61, 1975

67. Gage PW, Hamill OP: Effects of several inhalation anesthetics on the kinetic of postsynaptic conductance changes in mouse diaphragm. Brit J Pharmacol 57:263, 1976

68. Gage PW, Hamill OP, Van Helden D: Dual effects of ether on end-plate currents. J Physiol (Lond) 287:353, 1979

69. Ngai SH, Cheney DL, Finck DL: Acetylcholine concentrations and turnover in rat brain structures during anesthesia with halothane, enflurane, and ketamine. Anesthesiology 48:4, 1978

70. Roizen MF, Kopin IJ, Thoa NB, et al: The effect of two anesthetic agents on norepinephrine and dopamine in discrete brain nuclei, fiber tracts, and terminal regions of the rat. Brain Res 110:515, 1976

71. Rosenberg PH, Klinge E: Some effects of enflurane anesthesia on biogenic monoamines in the brain and plasma of rats. Br J Anaesth 46:708, 1974

72. Cheng SC, Brunner EA: Alteration of tricarboxylic acid cycle metabolism in rat brain slices by halothane. J Neurochem 30:1421, 1978

73. Cheng SC, Brunner EA: A neurochemical hypothesis for halothane anesthesia. Anesth Analg 54:242, 1975

74. Miller RD, Way WL, Eger EI II: The effects of alpha-methyldopa, reserpine, guanethidine, and iproniazid on minimum alveolar anesthetic requirement (MAC). Anesthesiology 29:1153, 1968

75. Mueller RA, Smith RD, Spruill WA, et al: Central monoaminergic neuronal effects on minimum alveolar concentrations (MAC) of halothane and cyclopropane in rats. Anesthesiology 42:143, 1975

76. Johnston RR, Way WL, Miller RD: The effect of CNS catecholamine-depleting drugs on dextroamphetamine-induced elevation of halothane MAC. Anesthesiology 41:57, 1974

77. Roizen MF, White PF, Eger EI II, et al: Effects of ablation of serotonin or norepineph-

rine brainstem areas on halothane and cyclopropane MACs in rats. Anesthesiology 49:252, 1978

78. Meyer KH: Contributions to the theory of narcosis. Trans Faraday Soc 33:1062, 1937

79. Eger EI II, Lundgren C, Miller SL, et al: Anesthetic potencies of sulfur hexafluoride, carbon tetrafluoride, chloroform and Ethrane in dogs. Anesthesiology 30:129, 1969

80. Miller KW, Paton WDM, Smith EB, et al: Physiochemical approaches to the mode of action of general anesthetics. Anesthesiology 36:339, 1972

81. Seeman P: The membrane actions of anesthetics and tranquilizers. Pharmacol Rev 24:583, 1972

82. Tanifuji Y, Eger EI II, Terrell RC: Some characteristics of an exceptionally potent inhaled anesthetic: Thiomethoxyflurane. Anesth Analg 56:387, 1977

83. Halsey MJ: Mechanisms of general anesthesia, Anesthetic Uptake and Action. Edited by Eger EI II. Baltimore, Williams and Wilkins 1974, pp 45-76

84. Miller JC, Miller KW: Approaches to the mechanisms of action of general anesthetics, MTP International Review of Science, Biochemistry, series 1, vol 12. Edited by Blaschko HKF. London, Butterworth, 1975, pp 33-76

85. Kaufman RD: Biophysical mechanisms of anesthetic action. Anesthesiology 46:49, 1977

86. Richards CD: Anesthetics and membranes. Int Rev Biochem 19:157, 1978

87. Wardley-Smith B, Halsey MJ: Recent molecular theories of general anesthesia. Br J Anaesth 51:619, 1979

88. Pauling L: A molecular theory of general anesthesia. Science 134:15, 1961

89. Miller SL: Effects of anesthetics on water structure. Fed Proc 27:879, 1968

90. Hansch C, Vittoria A, Silipo C, et al: Partition coefficients and the structure-activity relationship of the anesthetic gases. J Med Chem 18:546, 1975

91. Sandorfy C: Intermolecular interactions and anesthesia. Anesthesiology 48:357, 1978

92. Franks NP, Lieb WR: Where do general anesthetics act? Nature 274:339, 1978

93. Katz Y, Simon SA: Physical parameters of the anesthetic site. Biochim Biophys Acta 471:1, 1977

94. Miller KW, Wilson MW, Smith RA: Pressure resolves two sites of action of inert gases. Molec Pharmacol 14:950, 1978.

95. Mullins LJ: Some physical mechanisms in narcosis. Chem Rev 54:289, 1954

96. Cullen SC, Eger EI, Cullen BF, et al: Observations on the anesthetic effect of the combination of xenon and halothane. Anesthesiology 31:305, 1969

97. Miller RD, Wahrenbrock EA, Schroeder CF, et al: Ethylene-halothane anesthesia. Anesthesiology 31:301, 1969

98. DiFazio CA, Brown RE, Ball CG, et al: Additive effects of anesthetics and theories of anesthesia. Anesthesiology 36:57, 1972

99. Clarke RF, Daniels S, Harrison CB, et al: Potency of mixtures of general anesthetic agents. Br J Anaesth 50:979, 1978

100. Mullins LJ: Anesthetics, Handbooks of Neurochemistry, vol 6. Edited by Lajtha A. New York, Plenum, 1971, pp 395-421

101. Miller KW: Inert gas narcosis, the high pressure neurological syndrome, and the critical volume hypothesis. Science 185:867, 1974

102. Miller KW, Paton WDM, Smith RA, et al: The pressure reversal of anesthesia and the critical volume hypothesis. Mol Pharmacol 9:131, 1973

103. Miller KW, Yu SCT: The dependence of the lipid bilayer membrane: buffer partition coefficient of pentobarbitone on pH and lipid composition. Br J Pharmacol 51:57, 1977

104. Allott PR, Steward A, Flook V, et al: Variation with temperature of the solubilities of inhaled anesthetics in water, oil, and biological media. Br J Anaesth 45:294, 1973

105. Brauer RW: The high pressure nervous syndrome: animals, The Physiology of Medicine and Diving. Edited by Bennett PB, Elliott DH. Baltimore, Williams and Wilkins, 1975, pp 221-247

106. Bennett PB: The high pressure nervous syndrome: man, The Physiology of Medicine and Diving. Edited by Bennett PB, Elliott DH. Baltimore, Williams and Wilkins, 1975, pp 248-263

107. Krnjevic K: Central actions of general anesthetics, Molecular Mechanisms in General Anesthesia. Edited by Halsey MJ, Millar RA, Sutton JA. Edinburgh, Churchill Livingstone, 1974, pp 65-89

108. Brunner EA, Cheng SC, Berman ML: Effects of anesthesia on intermediary metabolism. Ann Rev Med 26:391, 1975

109. Nahrwold ML, Rapiejko JA, Cohen PJ: The mitochondrian as a model of the anesthetic receptor site, Progress in Anesthesiology, vol 1. Edited by Fink BR. New York, Raven Press, 1975, pp 431-438

110. Allilson AC, Nunn JF: Effects of general anesthetics on microtubules. Lancet 2:1326, 1968

111. Saubermann AJ, Gallagher ML: Mechanisms of general anesthesia: Failure of pentobarbital and halothane to depolymerize microtubules in mouse optic nerve. Anesthesiology 38:25, 1973

112. Hinkley RE, Green LS: Effects of halothane and colchicine on microtubules and electrical activity of rabbit vagus nerves. J Neurobiol 2:97, 1971

113. Salmon ED: Pressure-induced depolymerization of brain microtubules *in vitro.* Science 189:884, 1975

114. Singer SJ: The molecular organization of membranes. Ann Rev Biochem 43:805, 1974

115. Breckenridge WC, Gombos G, Morgan IG: The lipid composition of adult rat brain synaptosomal plasma membranes. Biochim Biophys Acta 266:695, 1972

116. Bangham AD, Standish MM, Miller N: Cation permeability of phospholipid model membranes: Effect of narcotics. Nature 208:1295, 1965

117. Hucho F, Schiebler W: Biochemical investigations of ionic channels in excitable membranes. Molec Cell Biochem 18:151, 1977

118. Johnson SM, Miller KW, Bangham AD: The opposing effects of pressure and general anaesthetics on the cation permeability of liposomes of varying lipid composition. Biochim Biophys Acta 307:42, 1973

119. Pang KY, Chang TL, Miller KW: On the coupling between anesthetic-induced membrane lipid fluidization and cation permeability in lipid vesicles. Molec Pharmacol 15:729, 1979

120. Clements JA, Wilson KM: The affinity of narcotic agents for interfacial films. Proc Natl Acad Sci USA 48:1008, 1962

121. Ueda I, Shieh DD, Eyring H: Anesthetic interactions with a model cell membrane. Anesthesiology 41:217, 1974

122. Seeman P, Roth SH: General anesthetics expand cell membranes at surgical concentrations. Biochim Biophys Acta 255:171, 1972

123. Haydon DA, Hendry BM, Levinson SR, et al: Anesthesia by the n-alkanes. Biochim Biophys Acta 470:17, 1977

124. Hendry BM, Urban BW, Haydon DA: The depression of the electrical conductance in a pore-containing membrane by the n-alkanes. Biochim Biophys Acta 513:106, 1978

125. Padron R, Mateu L, Requena J: A dynamic X-ray diffraction study of anesthetic action. Thickening of the myelin membrane by n-pentane. Biochim Biophys Acta 552:535-539, 1979

126. Trudell JR, Hubbell WL, Cohen EN: The effect of two inhalation anesthetics on the order of spin-labeled phospholipid vesicles. Biochim Biophys Acta 291:321, 1973

127. Kendig JJ, Trudell JR, Cohen EN: Halothane stereoisomers: Lack of stereospecificity in two model systems. Anesthesiology 39:518, 1973

128. Vanderkooi JM, Landesberg R, Selick H, et al: Interaction of general anesthetics with phospholipid vesicles and biological membranes. Biochim Biophys Acta 464:1, 1977

129. Chin JH, Trudell JR, Cohen EN: The compression-ordering and solubility-disordering effects of high pressure gases on phospholipid bilayers. Life Sci 18:489, 1976

130. Puskin JS, Martin T: Effects of anesthetics on divalent cation binding and fluidity of phosphatidylserine vesicles. Molec Pharmac 14:454, 1978

131. Trudell JR, Hubbell WL, Cohen EN: Pressure reversal of inhalation anesthetic-induced disorder in spin-labeled phospholipid vesicles. Biochim Biophys Acta 291:328, 1973

132. Mastrangelo CJ, Trudell JR, Cohen EN: Antagonism of membrane compression effects by high pressure gas mixtures in a phospholipid bilayer system. Life Sci 22:239, 1978

133. Trudell JR, Hubbell WL: Localization of molecular halothane in phospholipid bilayer model nerve membranes. Anesthesiology 44:202, 1976

134. Miller KW, Pang KY: General anesthetics can selectively perturb lipid bilayer membranes. Nature 263:253, 1976

135. Boggs JM, Yoong T, Hsia JC: Site and mechanism of anesthetic action. I. Effects of anes-

thetics and pressure on fluidity of spin-labeled lipid vesicles. Molec Pharmacol 12:127, 1976

136. Mastrangelo CJ, Trudell JR, Edmunds HN, et al: Effect of clinical concentrations of halothane on phospholipid cholesterol membrane fluidity. Molec Pharmacol 14:463, 1978

137. Rosenberg PH, Jannson S, Gripenberg J: Effects of halothane, thiopental, and lidocaine on fluidity of synaptic plasma membranes and artificial phospholipid membranes. Anesthesiology 46:322, 1977

138. Korenbrot JI: Ion transport in membranes: Incorporation of biological ion-translocating proteins in model membrane systems. Ann Rev Physiol 39: 19, 1977

139. Chapman D: Phase transitions and fluidity characteristics of lipids and cell membranes. Quart Rev Biophys 8:185, 1975

140. Hill MW: The effect of anesthetic-like molecules on the phase transition in smectic mesophases of dipalmitoyllecithin. I. The normal alcohols up to C=9 and three inhalation anesthetics. Biochim Biophys Acta 356:117, 1974

141. Jain MK, Wu NY, Wray LV: Drug-induced phase change in bilayer as possible mode of action of membrane expanding drugs. Nature 255:494, 1975

142. MacDonald AG: A dilatometric investigation of the effects of general anesthetics, alcohols, and hydrostatic pressure on the phase transition in smectic mesophases of dipalmitoyl phosphatidylcholine. Biochim Biophys Acta 507:26, 1978

143. Mountcastle DB, Biltonen RL, Halsey MJ: Effects of anesthetics and pressure on the thermotropic behavior of multilamellar dipalmitoyl phosphatidylcholine liposomes. Proc Natl Acad Sci USA 75:4906, 1978

144. Lee AG: Model for action of local anesthetics. Nature 262:545, 1976

145. Trudell JR: A unitary theory of anesthesia based on lateral phase separations in nerve membranes. Anesthesiology 46:5, 1977

146. Trudell JR, Payan DG, Chin JH, et al: The antagonistic effect of an inhalational anesthetic and high pressure on the phase diagram of mixed dipalmitoyl-dimyristoylphosphatidylcholine bilayers. Proc Natl Acad Sci (USA) 72:210, 1975

147. Rosenberg PH: Effects of halothane, lidocaine, and 5-hydroxytryptamine on fluidity of synaptic membranes, myelin membranes and synaptic mitochondrial membranes. Naunyn-Schmiedebergs Arch Pharmacol 307:199, 1979

148. Schoenborn BP: Binding of anesthetics to protein: An X-ray crystallographic investigation. Fed Proc 27:888, 1968

149. Laasberg LH, Hedley-Whyte J: Optical rotary dispersion of hemoglobin and polypeptides. Effects of halothane. J Biol Chem 246:4886, 1971

150. Brown FF, Halsey MJ, Richards RE: Halothane interactions with hemoglobin. Proc R Soc Lond [B] 193:387, 1976

151. Halsey MJ, Brown FF, Richards RE: Perturbations of model protein systems as a basis for the central and peripheral mechanisms of general anesthesia, Molecular Interactions and Activity in Proteins, CIBA Foundation Symposium 60. Excerpta Medica, 1978, pp 123-136

152. Wishnia A, Pinder TW: Hydrophobic interactions in proteins. The alkane binding site of β-lactoglobulins A and B. Biochemistry 5:1534, 1966

153. Balasubramanian D, Wetlaufer DB: Reversible alteration of the structure of globular proteins by anesthetic agents. Proc Natl Acad Sci USA 55:762, 1966

154. Sachsenheimer W, Pai EF, Schulz GE, et al: Halothane binds in the adenine-specific niche of crystalline adenylate kinase. FEBS Letts 79:310, 1977

155. Stone WL: Hydrophobic interactions of alkanes with liposomes and lipoproteins. J Biol Chem 250:4368, 1975

156. Johnson FH, Eyring H, Stover BJ: Reaction rate theory in bioluminescence and other life phenomena. Ann Rev Biophys Bioeng 6:111, 1977

157. White DC, Wardley-Smith B, Adey G: The site of action of anesthetics on bacterial luminescence. Life Sci 12:453, 1973

158. Middleton AJ, Smith EB: General anesthetics and bacterial luminescence. II. The effect of diethyl ether on the *in vitro* light emission of *Vibrio fisheri*. Proc R Soc London [B] 193:173, 1976

159. Ueda I, Kamaya H: Kinetic and thermodynamic aspects of the mechanism of general anesthesia in a model system of firefly lu-

minescence *in vitro.* Anesthesiology 38:425, 1973

160. Brammall A, Beard DJ, Hulands GH: Inhalation anesthetics and their interaction *in vitro* with glutamate dehydrogenase and other enzymes. Br J Anaesth 46:643, 1974

161. Maheshwari UR, Chan SL, Trevor AJ: Reversible inhibition of mammalian brain acetylcholinesterase and sodium potassium-stimulated adenosine triphosphatase by cyclopropane. Biochem Pharmacol 24:663, 1975

162. Levitt JD: The effects of halothane and enflurane on rat brain synaptosomal sodium-potassium-activated adenosine triphosphatase. Anesthesiology 42:267, 1975

163. Braswell LM, Kitz RJ: The effect *in vitro* of volatile anesthetics on the activity of cholinesterases. J Neurochem 29:665, 1977

164. Bielicki L, Krieglestein J: The effect of anesthesia on brain mitochondrial hexokinase. Naunyn-Schmiedebergs Arch Pharmacol 298:229, 1977

165. Sandhoff K, Pallmann B: Membrane-bound neuraminidase from calf-brain: Regulation of oligosialoganglioside degradation by membrane fluidity and membrane components. Proc Natl Acad Sci USA 75:122, 1978

166. Sandhoff K, Schraven J, Nowoczek G: Effect of xenon, nitrous oxide and halothane on membrane-bound sialidase from calf brain. FEBS Letts 62:284, 1976

167. Knight PR, Nahrwold ML, Rosenberg A: Sialic acid release by *Vibrio cholerae* sialidase (neuraminidase) from the outer surface of neural cells is greatly raised by halothane. J Neurochem 30:1645, 1978

168. Woo SY, Verosky M, Vulliemoz Y, et al: Dopamine-sensitive adenylate cyclase activity in the rat caudate nucleus during exposure to halothane and enflurane. Anesthesiology 51:27, 1979

169. Young AP, Brown FF, Halsey MJ, et al: Volatile anesthetic facilitation of *in vitro* desensitization of membrane-bound acetylcholine receptor from *Torpedo Californica.* Proc Natl Acad Sci USA 75:4563, 1978

170. Eyring H, Woodbury JW, D'Arrigo JS: A molecular mechanism of general anesthesia. Anesthesiology 38:415, 1973

171. Finck AD, Ngai SH, Berkowitz BA: Antagonism of general anesthesia by naloxone in the rat. Anesthesiology 46:241, 1977

172. Arndt JO, Freye E: Perfusion of naloxone through the fourth cerebral ventricle reverses the circulatory and hypnotic effect of halothane in dogs. Anesthesiology 51:58, 1979

173. Harper MH, Winter PM, Johnson BH, et al: Naloxone does not antagonize general anesthesia in the rat. Anesthesiology 49:3, 1978

174. Smith RA, Wilson M, Miller KW: Naloxone has no effect on nitrous oxide anesthesia. Anesthesiology 49:6, 1978

175. Bennett PB: Naloxone fails to antagonize the righting response in rats anesthetized with halothane. Anesthesiology 49:9, 1978

176. Pace NL, Wong KC: Failure of naloxone and naltrexone to antagonize halothane anesthesia in the dog. Anesth Analg 58:36, 1979

177. Shiwaku S, Nagashima H, Duncalf RM, et al: Naloxone fails to antagonize halothane-induced depression of the longitudinal muscle of the guinea pig ileum. Anesth Analg 58:93, 1979

178. Berkowitz BA, Ngai SH, Finck AD: Nitrous oxide "analgesia": Resemblance to opiate action. Science 194:967, 1976

179. Berkowitz BA, Finck AD, Ngai SH: Nitrous oxide analgesia: Reversal by naloxone and development of tolerance. J Pharmacol Exp Ther 203:539, 1977

180. Chapman CR, Benedetti C: Nitrous oxide effects on cerebral evoked potential to pain: Partial reversal with a narcotic antagonist. Anesthesiology 51:135, 1979

181. Hynes MD, Berkowitz BA: Nitrous oxide stimulation of locomotor activity: Evidence for an opiate-like behavior effect. J Pharmacol Exp Ther 209:304, 1979

182. Goldstein A: Enkephalins, opiate receptors, and general anesthesia. Anesthesiology 49:1, 1978

183. Cohen S, Goldschmid A, Shtacher G, et al: The inhalation convulsants: A pharmacodynamic approach. Mol Pharmacol 11:379, 1975

184. Richter J, Landau EM, Cohen S: Anesthetic and convulsant ethers act on different sites at the crab neuromuscular junction *in vitro.* Nature 266:70, 1977

185. Smith RA, Winter PM, Smith M, et al: Tolerance to and dependence on inhalational anesthetics. Anesthesiology 50:505, 1979

186. Koblin DD, Dong DE, Eger EI II: Tolerance of mice to nitrous oxide. J Pharmacol Exp Ther 211:317, 1979

187. Koblin DD, Dong DE, Deady JE, et al: Selective breeding alters mouse resistance to nitrous oxide without alteration in synaptic membrane lipid composition. Anesthesiology 52:401, 1980

188. Smith RA, Koblin DD, Smith M, et al: The anesthetic portency of volatile agents in mice. American Society of Anesthesiologists, Abstracts, pp 741-742, 1977

11

Uptake and Distribution of Inhaled Anesthetics

Edmond I. Eger II, M.D.

INTRODUCTION

To produce a brain anesthetic concentration sufficient for surgery requires proper manipulation of anesthetic delivery to the patient. Proper manipulation also requires that the delivered concentration not produce excessive depression. Thus, knowledge of the factors that govern the relationship between the delivered and brain (or heart or muscle) concentrations is indispensable to the optimum conduct of anesthesia. It is these factors that are the substance of anesthetic uptake and distribution.

THE INSPIRED TO ALVEOLAR ANESTHETIC RELATIONSHIP

Of the steps between delivered and brain anesthetic partial pressures, none is more pivotal than that between the inspired and alveolar gases. By use of high inflow rates (and hence conversion to a nonrebreathing system), the anesthetist can precisely control the partial pressure of anesthetic that is inspired. The alveolar partial pressure governs the partial pressure of anesthetic in all body tissues: all must approach and ultimately equal the alveolar partial pressure.

THE EFFECT OF VENTILATION

Two factors determine the rate at which the alveolar concentration of anesthetic (F_A) rises towards the concentration being inspired (F_I): the inspired concentration (to be discussed in the section on the concentration effect) and the alveolar ventilation. The effect of ventilation is a powerful one. If unopposed, ventilation produces a rapid change in alveolar concentration (i.e., F_A/F_I quickly approaches 1). This is seen with preoxygenation to achieve nitrogen washout: normally 2 minutes or less are required to cause a 95 percent or greater washout of nitrogen when a nonrebreathing (or high inflow rate) system is used.

The rapid washout of nitrogen or washin of oxygen is not mimicked by the inhaled anesthetics. The far higher solubility of anesthetics causes the transfer of substantial quantities of anesthetic to the blood passing through the lung. This uptake opposes the effect of ventilation to increase the alveolar anesthetic concentration. At low inspired concentrations, the F_A/F_I ratio ultimately is determined by the balance between the delivery of anesthetic by ventilation and its removal by uptake. The relationship is a simple one. For example, if uptake removes $\frac{1}{3}$ of the inspired anesthetic molecules then the F_A/F_I ratio will equal ⅔; if uptake removes ¾ of the inspired molecules then Fᴀ to Fɪ ratio will equal ¼.

ANESTHETIC UPTAKE FACTORS

Anesthesic uptake itself is the product of 3 factors: solubility (λ), cardiac output (Q), and the alveolar to venous partial pressure difference (Pᴀ−Pv).[1] That is:

$$\text{Uptake} = \lambda \cdot Q \cdot (\text{Pᴀ}-\text{Pv}) / \text{BP} \qquad (1)$$

BP is the barometric pressure. Being a product rather than a sum means that if any component of uptake approaches zero, then uptake must approach zero and the effect of ventilation to rapidly drive the alveolar concentration upwards will be unopposed. Thus if the solubility is small (as in the case of nitrogen), the cardiac output approaches zero (profound myocardial depression or death), or the alveolar to venous difference becomes inconsequential (as might occur after a very long anesthetic) then uptake would be minimal and Fᴀ/Fɪ would equal 1.

Solubility

The blood/gas partition coefficient (or "blood solubility") describes the relative affinity of anesthetic for two phases and hence how the anesthetic will *partition* itself between the two phases when equilibrium has been achieved. For example, enflurane has a blood/gas partition coefficient of 1.9 indicating that at equilibrium the concentration in blood will be 1.9 times the concentration in the gas (alveolar) phase. Remember that "equilibrium" means that no difference in partial pressure exists—that is, the blood/gas partition coefficient of 1.9 does *not* indicate that the partial pressure in blood will be 1.9 times that in the gas phase. The partition coefficient may be thought of in one other way: it indicates the relative capacity of the two phases. Thus a value of 1.9 means that each ml of blood can hold 1.9 times as much enflurane as a ml of alveolar gas.

A larger blood/gas partition coefficient will produce a greater uptake and hence a lower Fᴀ/Fɪ ratio. Since the anesthetic partial pressure in all tissues approaches that in the alveoli, the development of an adequate brain anesthetic partial pressure may be delayed in the case of highly blood soluble agents such as ether or methoxyflurane (Table 11-1). Even the moderate solubility of enflurane or halothane would slow induction of anesthesia with these agents were it not for our use of "anesthetic overpressure." That is, we compensate for the uptake of anesthetic by delivering a far higher concentration than we hope to achieve in the alveoli. For example, on induction of anesthesia, we may use 3 to 4 percent halothane to produce an alveolar concentration of 1 percent.

Cardiac Output

The effect of altering cardiac output is intuitively obvious. The passage of more blood through the lungs will remove more anesthetic and thereby lower the alveolar anesthetic concentration. To the beginning student of uptake and distribution this may appear to produce a conflict. It would seem that if more agent were taken up and delivered more rapidly to the tissues, then the tissue anesthetic partial pressure should rise more rapidly. In one sense this *is* true: an increase in cardiac output does hasten the equilibration of tissue anesthetic partial pressure with the partial pressure in arterial blood. What this reasoning ignores is the fact that the anesthetic partial pressure in arterial blood is lower than it would be if cardiac output were normal.

The effect of a change in cardiac output is analogous to the effect of a change in solubility. As already noted, doubling solubility doubled the capacity of the same volume of blood to hold anesthetic. Doubling cardiac output also would double capacity—but in this case by increasing the volume of blood exposed to anesthetic.

Table 11-1. Partition Coefficients at 37°C

Anesthetic	Blood / Gas	Brain / Blood	Liver / Blood	Kidney / Blood	Muscle / Blood	Fat / Blood
Cyclopropane	0.4–0.6	1.1	1.2	0.6	1.2	13
Nitrous oxide	0.47	1.1	0.8	—	1.2	2.3
Isoflurane	1.4	2.6	2.5	—	4.0	45
Enflurane	1.8	1.4	2.1	—	1.7	36
Halothane	2.3	2.9	2.6	1.6	3.5	60
Diethyl ether	12	1.1	1.0	1.1	1.0	3.7
Methoxyflurane	12	2.0	1.9	0.9	1.3	49

(Adapted from Eger, EI II: Anesthetic Uptake and Action. Baltimore, Williams & Wilkins, 1974. © (1974) EI Eger II, M.D.)

The Alveolar to Venous Anesthetic Gradient

The alveolar to venous anesthetic partial pressure difference results from tissue uptake of anesthetic. Were there no tissue uptake then the venous blood returning to the lungs would contain as much anesthetic as it had when it left the lungs as arterial blood. That is, the alveolar (equals arterial) to venous partial pressure difference would be zero. The presumption that alveolar and arterial anesthetic partial pressures are equal is reasonable in normal patients who have no barrier to diffusion of anesthetic from alveoli to pulmonary capillary blood and who do not have ventilation/perfusion ratio abnormalities. Later we shall consider the effect of ventilation/perfusion ratio abnormalities on anesthetic uptake.

The factors that determine the fraction of anesthetic removed from blood traversing a given tissue parallel those factors that govern uptake at the lungs: tissue solubility, tissue blood flow, and arterial to tissue anesthetic partial pressure difference. Again, uptake is the product of these three factors. If any one factor approaches zero then uptake by that tissue becomes inconsequential. The succeeding paragraphs will discuss the characteristics of each of these factors and then how uptake by individual tissues can be summed to give the venous component of the alveolar to venous anesthetic partial pressure difference.

Blood/gas partition coefficients span a range of values extending from 0.4 for cyclopropane or nitrous oxide to 12 for methoxyflurane (Table 11-1). In contrast, tissue/blood partition coefficients (i.e., tissue solubility) for lean tissues are close to 1, ranging from slightly less than 1 to a maximum of 4 (Table 11-1). That is, different lean tissues do not have greatly different capacities per ml of tissue. Put another way, a given anesthetic has roughly the same affinity for lean tissues and blood. As with blood/gas partition coefficients, tissue/blood partition coefficients define the concentration ratio of anesthetic at equilibrium. For example, a halothane brain/blood partition coefficient of 2.9 means that a ml of brain can hold 2.9 times more halothane than a ml of blood having the same halothane partial pressure.

Lean tissues differ in terms of their perfusion per gram—i.e., the volume of tissue relative to the blood passing that tissue. A larger volume of tissue relative to flow confers a greater capacity to hold anesthetic. This has two implications. First, the large tissue capacity increases the transfer of anesthetic from blood to tissue. Second, it takes longer to fill up a tissue with a large capacity—i.e., it will take longer for the tissue to equilibrate with the anesthetic partial pressure being delivered in arterial blood. That is, a large tissue volume relative to blood flow will sustain the arterial to tissue anesthetic partial pressure difference (and hence uptake) for a longer time. Brain with its high perfusion per gram will equilibrate rapidly. Muscle with about one twentieth the perfusion of brain will take

Table 11-2. Tissue Group Characteristics

	VRG (Vessel Rich)	MG (Muscle)	FG (Fat)	VPG (Vessel Poor)
Percent body mass	10	50	20	20
Perfusion as percent of cardiac output	75	19	6	0

(Adapted from Eger EI II: Anesthetic Uptake and Action. Baltimore, Williams & Wilkins, 1974. © (1974) EI Eger II, M.D.)

about 20 times longer to equilibrate. Uptake of anesthetic by muscle will continue long after uptake by brain has ceased.

Fat has a tissue/blood coefficient that is significantly greater than 1 (Table 11-1). Fat/blood coefficients range from 2.3 (nitrous oxide) to 60 (halothane). That is, each ml of fat tissue will contain 2.3 times more nitrous oxide or 60 times more halothane than a ml of blood having the same nitrous oxide or halothane partial pressure. This enormous capacity of fat for anesthetic means that most of the anesthetic contained in the blood perfusing fat will be transferred to the fat. Although most of the anesthetic will move from the blood perfusing fat into the fat, the anesthetic partial pressure in that tissue will rise very slowly. Both the large capacity of fat and the low perfusion per ml of tissue prolong the time required to narrow the anesthetic partial pressure difference between arterial blood and fat.

Tissue Groups. The algebraic sum of uptake by individual tissues determines the alveolar to venous partial pressure difference and hence uptake at the lungs. It is not necessary to analyze the effect of individual tissues to arrive at the algebraic sum. Instead, we can group tissues in terms of their perfusion and solubility characteristics—i.e., in terms of those features that define the duration of a substantial arterial to tissue anesthetic partial pressure difference. Four tissue groups are the result of such an analysis (Table 11-2).

The vessel rich group (VRG) is composed of the brain, heart, splanchnic bed (including liver), kidney, and endocrine glands. These organs make up less than 10 percent of the body weight but receive 75 percent of the cardiac output. This high perfusion confers several features. Access to a large flow of blood permits the VRG to take up a relatively large volume of anesthetic in the earliest moments of induction. However, the small volume of tissue relative to perfusion produces a rapid equilibration of this tissue group with the anesthetic delivered in arterial blood. The time to half equilibration (i.e., the time where the VRG anesthetic partial pressure equals half that in arterial blood) varies from about 1 minute for nitrous oxide to 3 minutes for halothane or enflurane. The longer time to equilibration with halothane or enflurane results from their higher tissue/blood partition coefficients (Table 11-1). Equilibration of the VRG with the anesthetic partial pressure in arterial blood is over 90 percent complete in 3 to 10 minutes. Thus, after 10 minutes, uptake by the VRG is too small (i.e., the arterial to VRG anesthetic partial pressure difference is too small) to significantly influence the alveolar concentration. Uptake after 10 minutes is principally determined by the muscle group.

Muscle and skin, which make up the muscle group (MG), have similar blood flow and solubility (lean tissue) characteristics. The lower perfusion (about 3 ml blood per 100 ml tissue per minute) sets this group apart from the VRG (75 ml per 100 ml per minute). Although about half of the body bulk is muscle and skin, this volume receives only 1 liter per minute blood flow at rest. The large bulk relative to perfusion means that during induction, most of the anesthetic delivered to the MG is removed from the MG blood flow. The time to half equilibration ranges from 20 to 25 minutes (nitrous oxide) to 70 to 90 minutes (enflurane or halothane). Thus, long after equilibration of the VRG has taken place, muscle continues to take up substantial amounts of anesthetic. This tissue approaches equilibration in 1 to 4 hours.

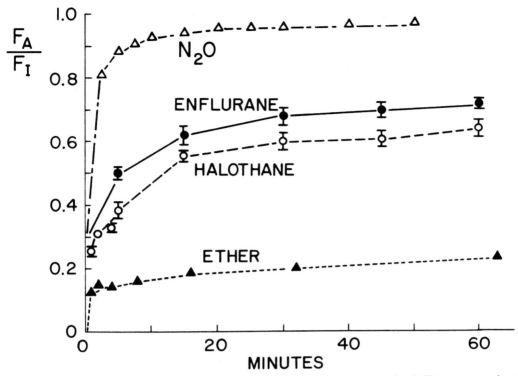

Fig. 11-1 The rise in alveolar (F_A) anesthetic concentration towards the inspired (F_I) concentration is most rapid with the least soluble anesthetic, nitrous oxide, and slowest with the most soluble anesthetic, diethyl ether. All data are from human studies.[2,3,4]

Once equilibration of muscle is complete only fat (i.e., the fat group or FG) continues to serve as an effective depot for uptake. Fat occupies a fifth of the body bulk and receives a blood flow of about 300 ml per minute. That is, the perfusion per 100 ml of fat nearly equals the perfusion per 100 ml of resting muscle. Fat differs from muscle in its higher affinity for anesthetic, a property which greatly lengthens the time over which it absorbs anesthetic. The half time to equilibration of fat ranges from 70 to 80 minutes for nitrous oxide to 19 to 32 *hours* for enflurane and halothane respectively. It is apparent that equilibration with fat will not occur in the course of an ordinary halothane or enflurane anesthetic.

One tissue group, the vessel poor group (VPG), remains to be defined. This group is composed of ligaments, tendons, bone, and cartilage—that is, those lean tissues which have little or no perfusion. The absence of a significant blood flow means that this group does not participate in the uptake process despite the fact that it makes up a fifth of the body mass.

A SYNTHESIS OF THE FACTORS GOVERNING THE RISE OF THE F_A/F_I RATIO

We now may consider the combined impact of ventilation, solubility, and the distribution of blood flow on the development of the alveolar anesthetic partial pressure. The initial rate of rise of F_A/F_I is rapid for all agents regardless of their solubility (Fig. 11-1). The rapidity of this upswing results from the absence of an alveolar to venous anesthetic partial pressure difference (there is no anesthetic present in the lung to create a gradient) and hence the absence of uptake in the first moment of induction. Thus, the effect of ventilation to generate a sudden rise in FA/FI is unopposed. Obviously, the delivery of more and more anesthetic to the alveoli by ventilation produces a progressively greater alveolar to venous partial pressure difference. The increasing uptake that ensues will increasingly oppose the effect of ventilation to drive the alveolar concentration upwards. Ultimately a rough balance is struck between the input by ventilation and removal by uptake. The height of the FA/FI ratio at which the balance is struck depends upon the solubility factor in the uptake equation (equation 1). A higher solubility produces a greater uptake for a given alveolar to venous partial pressure difference. Hence the initial rapid rise in FA/FI will be halted at a lower level with a more soluble agent. This results in the first "knee" in the curve—higher for nitrous oxide than enflurane, higher for enflurane than halothane, and higher for halothane than ether.

The balance struck between ventilation and uptake does not remain constant. FA/FI continues to rise, albeit at a slower rate than seen in the first minute. This rise results from the progressive decrease in uptake by the vessel rich group, a decrease to an inconsequential amount after 10 minutes. Thus, by about 10 minutes the three quarters of the cardiac output returning to the lungs from the vessel rich group contains nearly as much anesthetic as it had when it left the lungs. The consequent rise in venous anesthetic partial pressure decreases the alveolar to venous partial pressure difference and hence uptake—allowing ventilation to drive the alveolar concentration upward to the second knee at 10 to 15 minutes.

With the termination of effective uptake by the vessel rich group, muscle and fat become the principal determinants of tissue uptake. The slow rate of change of the anesthetic partial pressure difference between arterial blood and muscle or fat produces the rela-

tively stable terminal portion of each curve in Figure 11-1. In fact this terminal portion gradually ascends as muscle, and to a lesser extent fat, progressively equilibrate with the arterial anesthetic partial pressure. Were the graphs extended for several hours, a third knee would be found indicating equilibration of the muscle group. Uptake after that time would principally depend on the partial pressure gradient between arterial blood and fat.

THE CONCENTRATION EFFECT

The above analysis ignores the impact of the "concentration effect" on FA/FI. The inspired anesthetic concentration influences both the alveolar concentration that may be attained and the *rate* at which that concentration may be attained.[5,6] Increasing the inspired concentration accelerates the rate of rise. At an inspired concentration of 100 percent the rate of rise is extremely rapid, since it is dictated solely by the rate at which ventilation washes gas into the lung. That is, at 100 percent inspired concentration, uptake no longer limits the level to which FA/FI may rise. The cause of this extreme effect is readily perceived. At 100 percent inspired concentration the uptake of anesthetic creates a void that draws gas down the trachea. This additional "inspiration" replaces the gas taken up. Since the concentration of the replacement gas is 100 percent, uptake cannot modify the alveolar concentration.

The concentration effect results from two factors: a concentrating effect and an augmentation of inspired ventilation.[7] Both are illustrated in Figure 11-2. The first rectangle represents a lung containing 80 percent nitrous oxide. If half of this gas is taken up, the residual 40 volumes of nitrous oxide exists in a total of 60 volumes yielding a concentration of 67 percent (Fig. 11-2A). That is, uptake of half the nitrous oxide did not halve the concentration because the remaining gases were "concentrated" in a smaller volume. If the void created by uptake is filled by drawing

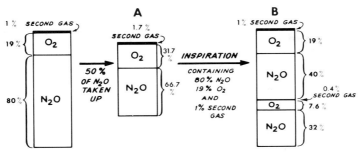

Fig. 11-2 The rectangle to the left represents a lung filled with 80 percent nitrous oxide plus 1 percent of a second gas. Uptake of half the nitrous oxide (A) does not halve the concentration of nitrous oxide and the reduction in volume concentrates and thereby increases the concentration of the second gas. Restoration of the lung volume (B) by addition of gas at the same concentration as that contained in the left-most rectangle will increase the nitrous oxide concentration and will add to the amount of the second gas present in the lung. (Stoelting RK and Eger EI II: An additional explanation for the second gas effect: A concentrating effect. Anesthesiology 30:273, 1969.)

more gas into the lungs (an augmentation of inspired ventilation), then the final concentration equals 72 percent (Fig. 11-2B).

The impact of the concentration effect on F_A/F_I may be thought of as identical to the impact of a change in solubility.[8] As the inspired concentration increases, the effective solubility decreases. That is, at 50 percent inspired nitrous oxide, F_A/F_I rises as rapidly as the F_A/F_I of an anesthetic that equals half the solubility of nitrous oxide. Seventy-five percent inspired nitrous oxide acts like an anesthetic with one quarter the solubility.

THE SECOND GAS EFFECT

The factors that govern the concentration effect also influence the concentration of any gas given concomitantly.[7,9] This second gas effect applies to halothane or enflurane when administered with nitrous oxide. The loss of volume associated with the uptake of nitrous oxide concentrates the halothane or enflurane (Fig. 11-2A). Replacement of the gas taken up by an increase in inspired ventilation will augment the amount of halothane or enflurane present in the lung (Fig. 11-2B).

Both the concentration effect and second gas effect were demonstrated by the following experiments.[9] Dogs were given 0.5 percent halothane in either 10 percent nitrous oxide

or 70 percent nitrous oxide. The F_A/F_I ratio rose more rapidly when 70 percent nitrous oxide was inspired than when 10 percent was inspired (concentration effect—Fig. 11-3). Similarly, the F_A/F_I ratio for halothane rose more rapidly when 70 percent nitrous oxide was inspired than when 10 percent was inspired (second gas effect).

FACTORS MODIFYING THE RATE OF RISE OF F_A/F_I

Alteration of those factors that govern the rate of delivery of anesthetic to the lungs or its removal from the lungs will alter the alveolar concentration of anesthetic. We have seen the importance of differences in solubility (Fig. 11-1). The succeeding sections examine the impact of differences in ventilation and circulation and the interaction of these differences with factors such as solubility.

THE EFFECT OF VENTILATORY CHANGES

By augmenting the delivery of anesthetic to the lungs, an increase in ventilation accelerates the rate of rise of F_A/F_I (Fig. 11-4).[1,10] A change in ventilation produces a greater relative change in F_A/F_I with a more soluble an-

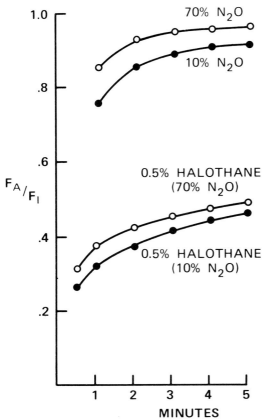

Fig. 11-3 In dogs, administration of 70 percent nitrous oxide produces a more rapid rise in F_A/F_I of nitrous oxide than administration of 10 percent (concentration effect, upper 2 curves). The F_A/F_I for 0.5 percent halothane rises more rapidly when given with 70 percent nitrous oxide than when given with 10 percent (second gas effect, lower 2 curves). (Epstein RM, Rackow H, Salanitre E, et al: Influence of the concentration effect on the uptake of gas mixtures: The second gas effect. Anesthesiology 25:364, 1964.)

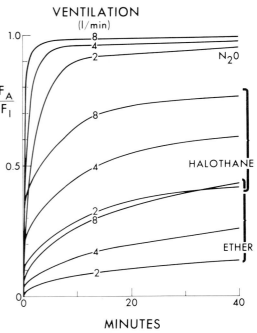

Fig. 11-4 The F_A/F_I ratio rises more rapidly if ventilation is increased. Solubility modifies this impact of ventilation: the effect on the anesthetizing partial pressure is greatest with the most soluble anesthetic (ether) and least with the least soluble anesthetic (nitrous oxide). (Eger EI II: Anesthetic Uptake and Action. Baltimore, Williams & Wilkins, 1974. © (1974) EI Eger II, M.D.)

esthetic. In Figure 11-4, an increase in ventilation from 2 to 8 L/min triples the ether concentration at 10 minutes, only doubles the halothane concentration, and scarcely affects the nitrous oxide concentration.

The impact of solubility may be explained as follows. With a poorly soluble agent such as nitrous oxide, the rate of rise of F_A/F_I is rapid even with hypoventilation. Since F_A normally cannot exceed F_I, there is little room for an augmentation of ventilation to increase F_A/F_I. With a highly soluble agent such as ether or methoxyflurane, most of the anesthetic delivered to the lungs is taken up. That is, if the uptake at 2 L/min ventilation equalled "X", then the uptake at 4 L/min would approach "2 X." Thus if cardiac output is held constant, ventilation of 4 L/min produces an arterial ether concentration that is nearly twice the concentration produced by a ventilation of 2 L/min. Since arterial and alveolar concentrations are in equilibrium, our example suggests that doubling ventilation must nearly double the anesthetic concentration in lung or blood.

These observations imply that imposed alterations in ventilation (e.g., an increase pro-

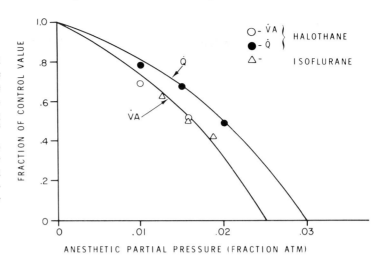

Fig. 11-5 Alveolar ventilation ($\dot{V}_A$) and cardiac output ($\dot{Q}$) are expressed as a percent of awake values. These data for halothane and isoflurane are taken from human studies.[12,13] (Munson ES, Eger EI II, Bowers DL: Effects of anesthetic-depressed ventilation and cardiac output on anesthetic uptake. Anesthesiology 38:251, 1973.)

duced by conversion from spontaneous to controlled ventilation) will produce greater changes in anesthetic effect with more soluble agents. Since such effects include both anesthetic depth and depression of circulation, greater caution must be exercised when ventilation is augmented during anesthesia produced with a highly soluble agent.

Anesthetics themselves may alter ventilation and thereby alter their own uptake.[11] Modern potent agents such as halothane, enflurane, or isoflurane all are profound respiratory depressants whose depression of ventilation is inversely related to anesthetic dose (Fig. 11-5).[12–14] At some dose, all the inhaled anesthetics probably produce apnea—a feature that must limit the maximum alveolar concentration that can be obtained if ventilation is spontaneous.

Thus, administration of an anesthetic concentration that can produce significant respiratory depression will progressively decrease delivery of anesthetic to the alveoli.[15,16] That is, doubling the inspired concentration does not double the alveolar concentration attained at a given point in time. At high inspired concentrations, further increases in inspired concentration produce little absolute change in the alveolar concentration (Fig. 11-6). Anesthetics thereby can exert a negative feedback

effect on their own alveolar concentration, an effect that increases the safety of spontaneous ventilation by limiting the maximum concentration that is attained in the alveoli.

THE EFFECT OF CHANGES IN CARDIAC OUTPUT

The discussion in the previous section involved circulation being held constant while ventilation was modified. In this section the reverse process is discussed. An increase in cardiac output augments uptake and thereby hinders the rise in F_A/F_I.[1,17] As with a change in ventilation, a change in cardiac output scarcely affects the alveolar concentration of a poorly soluble agent; the alveolar concentration of a highly soluble agent will be much more influenced (Fig. 11-7). The reason for the impact of a change in solubility is similar to that which explains the effect of a change in ventilation. A decrease in cardiac output can do little to increase the F_A/F_I ratio of a poorly soluble agent, since the rate of rise is rapid at any cardiac output. In contrast, nearly all of a highly soluble agent will be taken up and a halving of blood flow through the lungs must concentrate the arterial (equals alveolar) anesthetic (partial

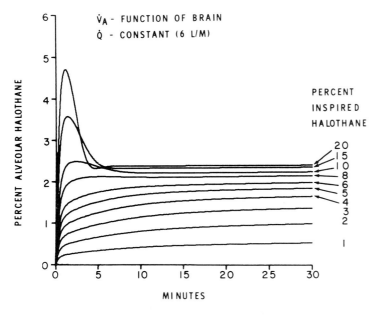

Fig. 11-6 An increase in inspired halothane concentration does not produce a proportional increase in the alveolar concentration because of the progressively greater depression of ventilation which occurs as alveolar halothane is increased. The initial "overshoot" seen with 10 to 20 percent inspired halothane results from the delay in the transfer of alveolar halothane partial pressure to the brain. (Munson ES, Eger EI II, Bowers DL: Effects of anesthetic-depressed ventilation and cardiac output on anesthetic uptake. Anesthesiology 38:251, 1973).

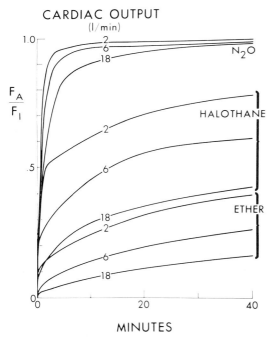

Fig. 11-7 If unopposed by a concomitant increase in ventilation, an increase in cardiac output will decrease alveolar anesthetic concentration by augmenting uptake. The resulting alveolar anesthetic change is greatest with the most soluble anesthetic. (Eger EI II: Anesthetic Uptake and Action. Baltimore, Williams & Wilkins, 1974. © (1974) EI Eger II, M.D.)

pressure), nearly doubling it in the case of an extremely soluble agent.

This effect of solubility suggests that conditions that lower cardiac output (e.g., shock) may produce unexpectedly high alveolar anesthetic concentrations if highly soluble agents are used. The higher F_A/F_I ratio should be anticipated and the inspired anesthetic concentration lowered accordingly to avoid further depression of circulation. Shock presents a two pronged problem: an increase in ventilation usually accompanies the circulatory depression. Both factors accelerate the rise in F_A/F_I. Perhaps this is why such heavy reliance is placed on the use of nitrous oxide in patients in shock. In contrast to methoxyflurane or halothane, the alveolar concentration of nitrous oxide would be little influenced by the associated cardiorespiratory changes.

Anesthetics also affect circulation. Usually they depress cardiac output (Fig. 11-5),[18, 19] although stimulation may occur with some agents (e.g., ether or fluroxene). In contrast to the negative feedback that results from respiratory depression, circulatory depression produces a positive feedback: depression decreases uptake, and this increases the alveolar concentration, which in turn further de-

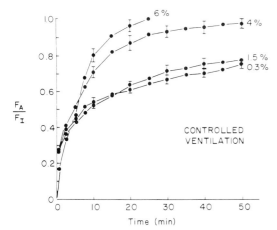

Fig. 11-8 Dogs given a constant ventilation demonstrate different rates of rise of F_A/F_I. The rates of rise depend upon the inspired halothane concentration. The two higher concentrations caused a depression of cardiac output which through a reduction in uptake accelerate the rate of rise. (Gibbons RT, Steffey EP, Eger EI II: The effect of spontaneous versus controlled ventilation on the rate of rise of alveolar halothane concentration in dogs. Anesth Analg 56:32, 1977.)

creases uptake. The result is a potentially lethal acceleration of the rise in F_A/F_I (Fig. 11-8).[15, 16] The impact of this acceleration increases in importance with increasing anesthetic solubility. Thus, high inspired concentrations of agents such as enflurane or halothane should be administered with considerable caution, particularly if ventilation is controlled.

THE EFFECT OF CONCOMITANT CHANGES IN VENTILATION AND PERFUSION

Consideration of the effects of ventilatory and circulatory alterations usually presumed that only one of these variables was changed while the other was held constant. In fact, both may change concomitantly. If both ventilation and cardiac output increase proportionately an intuitive expectation might be that F_A/F_I would be little altered. After all, uptake equals the product of solubility,

cardiac output, and the alveolar to venous anesthetic partial pressure difference (equation 1). In the absence of other changes, doubling cardiac output will double uptake and this should exactly balance the influence of doubling of ventilation on F_A/F_I. That is, a doubling of both delivery of anesthetic to the lungs and removal of anesthetic from the lungs should produce no net change in the alveolar concentration.

The above reasoning ignores one other factor in the equation that defines uptake. By accelerating the rate at which tissue equilibration occurs, an increase in cardiac output accelerates the narrowing of the alveolar to venous partial pressure difference.[20] This accelerated narrowing of the alveolar to venous partial pressure difference reduces the impact of the increase in cardiac output on uptake. Thus, a proportional increase in ventilation and cardiac output will increase the rate of rise of F_A/F_I.

The magnitude of the acceleration of rise in F_A/F_I will depend in part on distribution of the increase in cardiac output. If the increase is distributed proportionately to all tissues (i.e. if a doubling of output doubles flow to all tissues) then the increase is fairly small (Fig. 11-9).[4, 20] Thus, conditions such as hyperthermia or thyrotoxicosis would not be expected to influence the development of an anesthetizing anesthetic concentration through their influence on F_A/F_I. However, if the increase in cardiac output is diverted to the vessel rich group then a greater effect is seen.[20, 21] Perfusion of the vessel rich group already is high and results in equilibration. Further increases in perfusion only hasten the rate of equilibration. Since blood returning from the vessel rich group soon has the same partial pressure as it had when it left the lungs, it cannot remove more anesthetic from the lungs. Thus the increase in ventilation will not be matched, even in part, by an increase in uptake. The result will be a considerable acceleration in the rise in F_A/F_I. This effect may be seen in a comparison of the F_A/F_I curves for children and adults (Fig. 11-10). Children (especially infants) have a

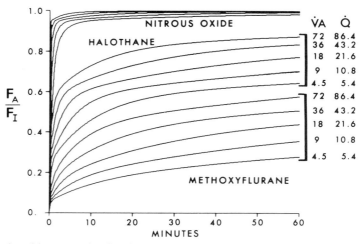

Fig. 11-9 Proportional increases in alveolar ventilation (VA) and cardiac output (Q) will increase the rate at which F_A/F_I rises. As indicated in the illustration, the effect is relatively small if the increase in cardiac output is distributed proportionately to all tissues (i.e. if Q is doubled then all tissue blood flows are doubled). The greatest effect occurs with the most soluble anesthetic. (Eger EI II, Bahlman SH, Munson ES: Effect of age on the rate of increase of alveolar anesthetic concentration. Anesthesiology 35:365, 1971.)

relatively greater perfusion of the vessel rich group and consequently show a significantly faster rise in F_A/F_I.[21] A clinical result of this accelerated rise is the more rapid development of anesthesia in young patients.

VENTILATION/PERFUSION RATIO ABNORMALITIES

To this point I have assumed that alveolar and arterial anesthetic partial pressures are equal, i.e., that the alveolar gases completely equilibrate with the blood passing through the lungs. In some extent this assumption is incorrect, but the usual deviation from complete equilibration is small. Diseases such as emphysema, atelectasis, or congenital cardiac defects will increase the deviation. The associated ventilation/perfusion ratio abnormality will do two things: increase the alveolar (end-tidal) anesthetic partial pressure; and decrease the arterial anesthetic partial pressure (i.e., a partial pressure difference will appear between alveolar gas and arterial

blood). The relative change depends on the solubility of the anesthetic. With a poorly soluble agent, the end-tidal concentration is slightly increased but the arterial partial pressure is significantly reduced. The opposite occurs with a highly soluble anesthetic.[22]

The considerable decrease in the arterial anesthetic partial pressure that occurs with poorly soluble agents may be explained as follows. Ventilation/perfusion ratio abnormalities of some alveoli increase ventilation relative to their perfusion while in other alveoli the reverse occurs. With a poorly soluble anesthetic, an increase in ventilation relative to perfusion does not appreciably increase alveolar or arterial anesthetic partial pressure issuing from those alveoli (see effect for nitrous oxide in Fig. 11-4). However, when ventilation decreases relative to perfusion, a significant effect can occur—particularly when ventilation is absent as in a segment of atelectatic lung. Blood emerges from that segment with no additional anesthetic. Such anesthetic deficient blood then mixes with the blood from the ventilated segments contain-

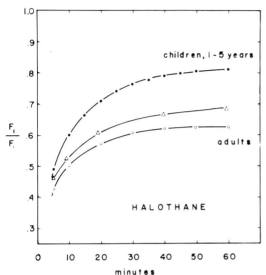

Fig. 11-10 The alveolar rate of rise of halothane is more rapid in children (uppermost curve) than adults (lower two curves, each from separate studies). The difference probably results from the greater ventilation and perfusion per kg of tissue in children *and* the fact that a disproportionate amount of the increased perfusion is devoted to the vessel rich group. (Salanitre E, Rackow H: The pulmonary exchange of nitrous oxide and halothane in infants and children. Anesthesiology 30:388, 1969.)

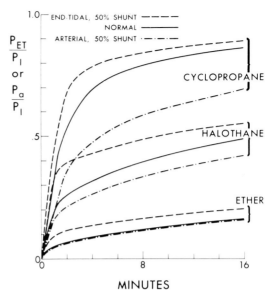

Fig. 11-11 When no ventilation/perfusion abnormalities exist then the alveolar (P_A or P_{ET}) and arterial (P_a) anesthetic partial pressures rise together (continuous lines) toward the inspired partial pressure (P_I). When 50 percent of the cardiac output is shunted through the lungs then the rate of rise of the end-tidal partial pressure (dashed lines) is accelerated while the rate of rise of the arterial partial pressure (dot-dashed lines) is retarded. The greatest retardation is found with the least soluble anesthetic, cyclopropane. (Eger EI II: Anesthetic Uptake and Action. Baltimore, Williams & Wilkins, 1974. © (1974) EI Eger II, M.D.)

ing a normal compliment of anesthetic. The mixture produces an arterial anesthetic partial pressure considerably below normal.

With highly soluble agents, a different situation results from similar ventilation/perfusion ratio abnormalities. In alveoli receiving more ventilation relative to perfusion, the anesthetic partial pressure rises to a higher level than usual (see Fig. 11-4 for the effect on diethyl ether). That is, blood issuing from these alveoli has an increased anesthetic content which is nearly proportional to the increased ventilation. Assuming that overall (total) ventilation remains normal, this increase in the anesthetic contained by blood from the relatively hyperventilated alveoli will compensate for the lack of anesthetic uptake in unventilated alveoli.

These effects are illustrated in Figure 11-11 for a condition that may be iatrogenically produced: endobronchial intubation. Since all ventilation now is directed to the intubated lung, this lung will be hyperventilated relative to perfusion. FA/FI for this lung will be slightly increased with the poorly soluble cyclopropane and greatly increased with the highly soluble ether. As indicated earlier, the increase with ether will compensate for the absence of uptake from the unventilated lung—a compensatory mechanism not available with cyclopropane. The result is that the cyclopropane arterial partial pressure is well below normal while the ether arterial partial pressure is scarcely changed.

These concepts have been confirmed experimentally by comparing the rate of arterial anesthetic rise with and without endobron-

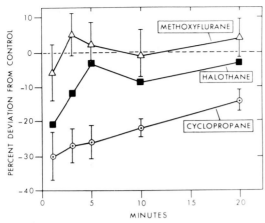

Fig. 11-12 In dogs when only the right lung was ventilated, the rise of the very soluble anesthetic, methoxyflurane, in arterial blood was normal (i.e., did not deviate from control) while the rise for the poorly soluble anesthetic, cyclopropane, was significantly slowed. (Stoelting RK, Longnecker DE: Effect of right-to-left shunt on rate of increase in arterial anesthetic concentration. Anesthesiology 36:352, 1972.)

chial intubation in dogs.[23] Endobronchial intubation significantly slowed the arterial rate of rise of cyclopropane but did not influence the rise with methoxyflurane. An intermediate result was obtained with halothane (Fig. 11-12). These data suggest that in the presence of ventilation/perfusion ratio abnormalities, the anesthetic effect of agents such as cyclopropane or nitrous oxide may be delayed whereas the effect of ether or methoxyflurane will be unaffected.

PERCUTANEOUS ANESTHETIC LOSS

I have ignored two possible avenues by which anesthetics may be lost: transcutaneous movement and metabolism. Probably neither is a major determinant of anesthetic uptake during the course of a clinical anesthetic. Although transcutaneous movement occurs, the movement is small.[24, 25] The greatest loss per alveolar anesthetic percent occurs

with nitrous oxide. Loss of nitrous oxide might equal 5 to 10 ml/min with an alveolar concentration of 70 percent.

METABOLISM OF ANESTHETIC

Loss of anesthesic by biodegradation is also probably limited. However, some evidence suggests that anesthetic metabolism may be important with agents that undergo extensive biodegradation. Berman et al. found that phenobarbital pretreatment in rats decreased the arterial level of methoxyflurane.[26] However three reasons suggest that agents such as halothane, isoflurane, or enflurane are less likely to be affected. First, they are not metabolized as readily as methoxyflurane.[27] Second, anesthetizing concentrations appear to saturate the enzymes responsible for anesthetic metabolism.[28] Third, halothane, enflurane, and isoflurane are less soluble than methoxyflurane. The lower solubility means that relatively fewer molecules of halothane or enflurane or isoflurane reach the liver. The combined effect of these factors remains to be determined but it appears that metabolism is not a major determinant of F_A/F_I during anesthesia.

THE EFFECT OF NITROUS OXIDE ON CLOSED GAS SPACES

VOLUME CHANGES IN HIGHLY COMPLIANT SPACES

I have not discussed a third avenue for gas transfer, movement of nitrous oxide into closed gas spaces. Although this transfer does not influence F_A/F_I, it may have important functional consequences. There are two types of closed gas spaces in the body, compliant and noncompliant. Compliant spaces, such as bowel gas, pneumothorax, or pneumoperitoneum, are subject to changes in volume secondary to the transfer of nitrous oxide.[29] These spaces normally contain nitrogen

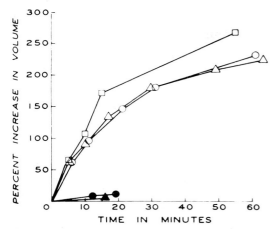

Fig. 11-13 The volume of a pneumothorax created by air injection is little affected when oxygen subsequently is breathed (filled triangle and circles). However, if 75 percent nitrous oxide is breathed, the volume doubles in 10 minutes and triples in a half hour (open circles, squares, and triangles). (Eger EI II, Saidman LJ: Hazards of nitrous oxide anesthesia in bowel obstruction and pneumothorax. Anesthesiology 26:61, 1965.)

(from air), a gas whose low solubility (blood/gas partition coefficient = 0.015) limits its removal by blood. Thus, the entrance of nitrous oxide (whose solubility permits it to be carried by blood in substantial quantities) is not countered by an equal loss. The result is an increase in volume. The theoretic limit to the increase in volume is a function of the alveolar nitrous oxide concentration, since it is this concentration that ultimately is achieved in the closed gas space. That is, at equilibrium the partial pressure of nitrous oxide in the closed gas space must equal its partial pressure in the alveoli. An alveolar concentration of 50 percent might double the gas space volume while a 75 percent concentration might produce a fourfold increase.

These theoretic limits may be approached where equilibrium is rapidly achieved. Two examples are pneumothorax and gas emboli. The administration of 75 percent nitrous oxide in the presence of a pneumothorax may double the pneumothorax volume in

10 minutes and triple it by 30 minutes (Fig. 11-13).[29] This increase in volume may seriously impair cardiorespiratory function [30] and the use of nitrous oxide is contraindicated in the presence of a significant pneumothorax.

A still more rapid expansion of volume occurs when air inadvertantly enters the blood stream in a patient anesthetized with nitrous oxide. Expansion may be complete in seconds rather than minutes. Munson and Merrick demonstrated that the lethal volume of an air embolus was decreased in animals breathing nitrous oxide as opposed to air (Fig. 11-14).[31] The difference could be entirely explained by expansion of the embolus in the animals breathing nitrous oxide—i.e., the predicted total volume of air plus nitrous oxide in the embolus equaled the volume of air needed to produce death in animals breathing only air. These studies suggest

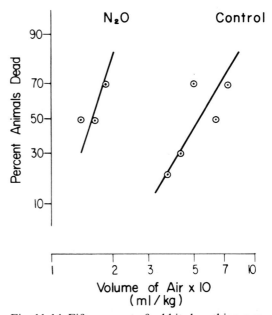

Fig. 11-14 Fifty percent of rabbits breathing oxygen were killed by an air embolus equalling 0.55 ml/kg. If the inspired gas mixture contained 75 percent nitrous oxide then only 0.16 ml/kg were required to kill half the animals. (Munson ES, Merrick HC: Effect of nitrous oxide on venous air embolism. Anesthesiology 27:783, 1966.)

caution in the use of nitrous oxide for procedures where air embolization is a risk (e.g., posterior fossae craniotomies, laparoscopy). They also suggest that if air embolization is suspected, an immediate part of therapy should be the discontinuation of nitrous oxide.

The endotracheal tube cuff normally is filled with air. It, too, is susceptible to expansion by nitrous oxide.[32] The presence of 75 percent nitrous oxide surrounding such a cuff can double or triple its volume. The result may be an unwanted increase in pressure exerted on the tracheal mucosa.

PRESSURE CHANGES IN POORLY COMPLIANT SPACES

Pressure can be produced by the entrance of nitrous oxide into gas cavities surrounded by poorly compliant walls. Examples include the gas space created by pneumoencephalography and the natural gas space in the middle ear. Pressures in either case may rise by 20 to 50 torr due to the ingress of nitrous oxide at a faster rate than air can be removed.[33, 34] Recognition of this problem has decreased the use of nitrous oxide for pneumoencephalography or for tympanoplasty. In the latter case, the increased pressure may displace the graft. Increase in middle ear pressure also may cause adverse postoperative effects on hearing.[35]

ANESTHETIC CIRCUITRY

The previous discussions generally have considered that the alveolar anesthetic concentration (FA) was moving towards a constant inspired anesthetic concentration (FI). In practice, the inspired concentration usually is not constant because a nonrebreathing system is not used. The interposition of an anesthetic circuit between the anesthetic source and the patient causes the inspired concentration to be less than that in the gas delivered from the anesthetic machine.

WASHIN OF THE CIRCUIT

To begin anesthesia, anesthetic must be "washed into" the volume of the circuit. At inflow rates of 1 to 5 L/min and a circuit volume of 7 L (3 L bag, 2 L carbon dioxide absorber, and 2 L in corrugated hoses and fittings) the washin of the circuit is 75 to 100 percent complete in 10 minutes (Fig. 11-15). Higher inflow rates produce a more rapid rise in the inspired concentration, suggesting that induction can be accelerated and made more predictable by use of high flow rates.

ANESTHETIC LOSS TO PLASTIC AND SODA LIME

Uptake of anesthetic by several depots also constitutes a hindrance to the development of an adequate inspired anesthetic concentration. The rubber or plastic components of the circuit may remove agent.[36] This is a significant problem in the case of methoxyflurane (rubber/gas partition coefficient of 630), but has a relatively minor influence on halothane (a coefficient of 120), enflurane (74), isoflurane (62), or nitrous oxide (1.2).[37] Similarly, uptake by soda lime is small unless the soda lime becomes dry in which case substantial amounts may be absorbed.[38]

THE EFFECT OF REBREATHING

Inspired gas actually is two gases: that delivered from the anesthetic machine and that previously exhaled by the patient and subsequently rebreathed. Since the patient has removed (taken up) anesthetic from the rebreathed gas, the amount taken up *and* the amount rebreathed will influence the inspired anesthetic concentration. An increase in uptake or rebreathing will lower the inspired

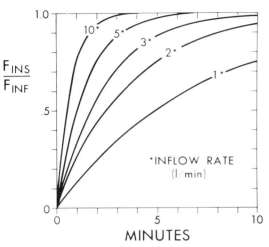

$$\frac{F_{INS}}{F_{INF}}$$

*INFLOW RATE
(l/min)

MINUTES

Fig. 11-15 The rate at which the inspired anesthetic concentration (F_{INS}) rises toward the inflowing concentration (F_{INF}) is determined by the inflow rate and circuit volume. In the case illustrated here, the circuit volume is 7 liters. (Eger EI II: Anesthetic Uptake and Action. Baltimore, Williams & Wilkins, 1974. © (1974) EI Eger II, M.D.)

concentration of a highly soluble gas more than the inspired concentration of a poorly soluble gas. This effect of uptake can be diminished by decreasing rebreathing. Rebreathing is reduced by increasing the inflow rate. With a ventilation of 5 L/min, rebreathing can be essentially abolished by the use of a 5 L/min inflow rate.[39]

High inflow rates (i.e., 5 L/min or greater) have the advantage of increasing the predictability of the inspired anesthetic concentration. They have the disadvantage of being wasteful and of increasing the tendency towards atmospheric pollution. They also may result in drier inspired gas and greater difficulty in estimating ventilation from excursions of the rebreathing bag.

THE LOW FLOW OR CLOSED CIRCLE TECHNIQUE

These disadvantages of high inflow rates have led to a small but increasing application of closed circuit anesthesia.[40] Administration

of closed circuit anesthesia has two requirements. First, if nitrous oxide is used, oxygen concentration must be measured and inflow adjusted to ensure adequacy of the inspired oxygen partial pressure. Second, there must be some gauge by which anesthetic is delivered from the machine. Ultimately this delivery is dictated by the response of the patient; but an initial estimate of the amount of anesthetic needed may be made from the "square root of time" formula (originally noted by Severinghaus[41]), which suggests that uptake decreases as a function of the square root of time. Application of this formula requires that anesthetic uptake for the first minute of anesthesia (U_1) be calculated. Uptake at subsequent times (U_t) is obtained as:

$$U_t = U_1 / (t)^{1/2} \qquad (2)$$

Uptake during the first minute may be estimated from the formula for uptake given earlier (equation 1). Thus:

$$U_1 = \lambda \cdot Q \cdot (A-v) / BP \qquad (3)$$

The individual components are either known or can be easily estimated. For example, blood solubility (λ) for enflurane is 1.9. Cardiac output (Q) in a normal adult is about 5,000 ml/min. During the first minute of anesthesia the venous anesthetic partial pressure (v) is zero or low so that (A−v) / BP reduces to A/BP. We may assume that A/BP is the alveolar concentration that we *want* to achieve. Since enflurane MAC with 60 percent nitrous oxide is about 0.8 percent enflurane and since we need something modestly in excess of MAC—say 1.2 percent—then A/BP equals 0.012. Thus U_1 = 1.9•5000•0.012 or 114 ml/min. After 9 minutes of anesthesia this reduces to 114/3 = 38 ml/min; after 25 minutes it is 114/5 = 23 ml/min etc. Flow through the vaporizer then must be adjusted to give the above output—e.g., a 23 ml/min enflurane output at 20°C and one atmosphere pressure would require a flow through a copper kettle of 78 ml/min (about 3⅓ times as much as the amount of vapor desired; for halothane or insoflurane the factor is about 2 times). It should be remembered that this estimate should be modified by a knowledge of any factors that might alter anesthetic requirement: for example, the amount of anesthetic needed would be reduced by hypothermia, advanced age, or shock. It should also be remembered that the patient's response ultimately must govern the amount of anesthetic delivered; movement, hypertension, or tachycardia might indicate an increased need.

RECOVERY FROM ANESTHESIA

GENERAL PRINCIPALS

Nearly all of the factors that governed the rate at which the alveolar anesthetic concentration rose on induction apply to recovery. Thus, the immediate decline is extremely rapid, since the washout of the functional residual capacity by ventilation is as rapid as the washin. It should be recalled that only 2 minutes are required to eliminate 95 to 98 percent of nitrogen from the lungs when pure oxygen is breathed.

Nitrogen, however, is a poorly soluble gas relative to the inhaled anesthetics. As ventilation sweeps anesthetic from the alveoli, an anesthetic partial pressure gradient develops from the returning venous blood to that in the alveoli. This gradient drives anesthetic into the alveoli, thereby opposing the tendency of ventilation to lower the alveolar concentration. The effectiveness of the venous to alveolar gradient in opposing the tendency of ventilation to decrease the alveolar anesthetic partial pressure is in part determined by the solubility of the anesthetic. A highly soluble agent, such as methoxyflurane, will be more effective than a poorly soluble agent, such as nitrous oxide, because a greater blood reserve exists for the highly soluble agent. That is, far more methoxyflurane is available at a given partial pressure for transfer to the alveoli. Thus the fall in the alveolar partial pressure of methoxyflurane is slower than the fall with halothane and the latter in turn decreases less rapidly than nitrous oxide. The rate at which recovery occurs is similarly affected: it is rapid with nitrous oxide and may be slow with methoxyflurane.

DIFFERENCES BETWEEN INDUCTION AND RECOVERY

Recovery differs from induction in two crucial ways. First, on induction, the effect of solubility to hinder the rise in alveolar anesthetic concentration could be overcome by increasing the inspired anesthetic concentration (i.e., by the application of "overpressure"). No such luxury is available during recovery: the inspired concentration cannot be reduced below zero. Second, on induction all the tissues initially have the same anesthetic partial pressure—zero. On recovery the tissue partial pressures are variable. The vessel rich group has a pressure that usually equals that required for anesthesia. That is, the vessel rich group has come to equilibrium with the alveolar anesthetic partial pressure. The muscle group may or may not have the same partial pressure as that found in the alveoli. A long anesthetic (2 to 4 hours) might permit equilibrium to be approached but a shorter case would not. The high capacity of fat for all anesthetics except nitrous oxide precludes equilibration of the fat group with the alveolar anesthetic partial pressure with hours or even days of anesthesia.

The failure of muscle and fat to equilibrate with the alveolar anesthetic partial pressure means that these tissues initially cannot contribute to the transfer of anesthetic back to the lungs. In fact, as long as an anesthetic partial pressure gradient exists between arterial blood and that in a tissue, that tissue will continue to *take up* anesthetic. Thus for the first several hours of recovery from halothane anesthesia, fat continues to take up halothane and by so doing accelerates the rate of recovery. Only after the alveolar (equals arterial) anesthetic partial pressure falls below that in a tissue can the tissue contribute anesthetic to the alveoli.

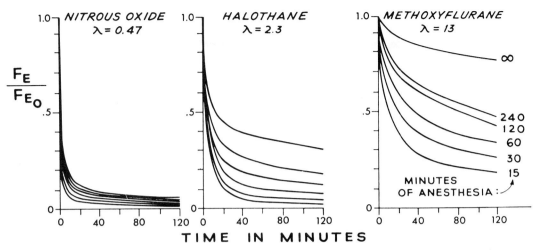

Fig. 11-16 Both solubility and duration of anesthesia affect the fall of the alveolar concentration (F_E) from the alveolar concentration immediately preceding the cessation of anesthetic administration (F_{E_O}). A longer anesthetic slows the fall as does a greater solubililty. (Stoelting RK, Eger EI II: The efects of ventilation and anesthetic solubility on recovery from anesthesia: An *in vivo* and analog analysis before and after equilibration. Anesthesiology 30:290, 1969.)

The failure of several tissues to reach equilibration with the alveolar anesthetic partial pressure means that the rate of decrease of alveolar anesthetic on recovery is more rapid than the rate of increase on induction. The difference between the rates for induction and recovery depends in part on the duration of anesthesia (Fig. 11-16).[42,43] A longer anesthetic puts more anesthetic into the slowly filling muscle and fat depots. Obviously, these reservoirs can supply more anesthetic to the blood returning to the lungs when they are filled than when they are empty.

Solubility influences the effect of duration of anesthesia on the rate at which the alveolar anesthetic partial pressure declines.[43] The decline of the partial pressure of a poorly soluble agent such as nitrous oxide is rapid in any anesthetic, and thus the acceleration imparted by a less-than-complete tissue equilibration cannot significantly alter the rate of recovery. The approach to equilibration becomes important with halothane and even more important with methoxyflurane (Fig. 11-16). A rapid recovery may follow a short methoxyflurane anesthetic but may occur slowly after a prolonged anesthetic. This is one of the reasons why nitrous oxide is usually a component of an inhaled (or for that matter, an injected) anesthetic regimen. The rapid elimination of this component permits at least a portion of recovery to be rapid.

METABOLISM

The saturation of the enzymes responsible for the metabolism of anesthetics prevented metabolism from significantly altering the rate at which the alveolar anesthetic partial pressure rose. This limitation does not exist on recovery and metabolism may be an important determinant of the rate at which the alveolar anesthetic partial pressure declines. The importance of metabolism to recovery is implied by results from Munson et al. who showed that contrary to what might be predicted from their respective solubilities, the alveolar washout of halothane is more rapid than that of enflurane.[44] This agrees with the relative ease with which these two agents are metabolized: 15 to 20 percent of the halothane taken up during the course of an ordi-

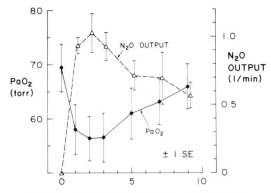

MINUTES AFTER END OF N₂O ANESTHESIA

Fig. 11-17 At time zero the inspired gas was changed from 21 percent oxygen/79 percent nitrous oxide to 21 percent/79 percent nitrogen. Arterial oxygen subsequently fell in association with the outpouring of nitrous oxide. (Adapted from Sheffer L, Steffenson JL, Birch AA: Nitrous oxide-induced diffusion hypoxia in patients breathing spontaneously. Anesthesiology 37:436, 1972.)

nary anesthetic can be recovered as urinary metabolites.[45] Only 2 to 3 percent of enflurane can similarly be recovered.[46] Thus there are two major routes by which halothane can be eliminated: the lung and the liver. With enflurane, elimination via the liver is relatively minor and explains why Munson et al. found a more rapid fall in alveolar halothane.[44]

DIFFUSION HYPOXIA

The uptake of large volumes of nitrous oxide on induction of anesthesia gives rise to the concentration and second gas effects. On recovery from anesthesia, the outpouring of large volumes of nitrous oxide can produce what Fink called "diffusion anoxia."[47] These volumes may cause hypoxia (Fig. 11-17) in two ways. First, they may directly affect oxygenation by displacing oxygen.[47-49] Second, by diluting alveolar carbon dioxide they may decrease respiratory drive and hence ventilation.[49] Both of these effects require that large

volumes of nitrous oxide be released into the alveoli. Since large volumes of nitrous oxide are released only during the first 5 to 10 minutes of recovery, this is the period of greatest concern. This concern is enhanced by the fact that the first 5 to 10 minutes of recovery also may be the time of greatest respiratory depression. For these reasons many anesthetists administer 100 percent oxygen for the first 5 to 10 minutes of recovery. This procedure may be particularly indicated in patients with preexisting lung disease or when postoperative respiratory depression is anticipated (e.g., after a nitrous oxide–narcotic anesthetic).

THE ANESTHETIC CIRCUIT

The anesthetic circuit may limit the rate of recovery just as it limited induction. If the patient is not disconnected from the circuit on cessation of anesthetic delivery, the patient may continue to inspire anesthetic. To reduce the inspired level to zero or near zero, several factors must be taken into account. The anesthetic within the circuit must be washed out. In addition, the rubber or plastic components of the circuit and the soda lime within the circuit will have absorbed anesthetic that can be released back into the gas phase,[50] and this too must be washed out. Finally, the patient's exhaled air contains anesthetic that cannot be rebreathed if the inspired anesthetic concentration is to approach zero. The effect of each of these factors to raise the inspired anesthetic concentration can be negated by the use of high inflow rates of oxygen, i.e., 5 L/min or greater.

REFERENCES

1. Eger EI II: Anesthetic Uptake and Action. Baltimore, Williams and Wilkins, 1974
2. Salanitre E, Rackow H, Greene LT et al: Uptake and excretion of subanesthetic concentrations of nitrous oxide in man. Anesthesiology 23:814, 1962

3. Torri G, Damia G, Fabiani ML et al: Uptake and elimination of enflurane in man. Br J Anaesth 44:789, 1972

4. Wahrenbrock EA, Eger EI II, Laravuso RB et al: Anesthetic uptake of mice and men (and whales). Anesthesiology 40:19, 1974

5. Eger EI II: Application of a mathematical model of gas uptake, Uptake and Distribution of Anesthetic Agents. Edited by Papper EM and Kitz RJ. McGraw-Hill, New York, 1963, pp 88-103

6. Eger EI II: Effect of inspired anesthetic concentration on the rate of rise of alveolar concentration. Anesthesiology 24:153, 1963

7. Stoelting RK, Eger EI II: An additional explanation for the second gas effect: A concentrating effect. Anesthesiology 30:273, 1969

8. Eger EI II, Smith RA, Koblin DD: The concentration effect can be mimicked by a decrease in blood solubility. Anesthesiology 49:282, 1978

9. Epstein RM, Rackow H, Salanitre E, et al: Influence of the concentration effect on the uptake of anesthetic mixtures: The second gas effect. Anesthesiology 25:364, 1964

10. Yamamura H, Wakasugi B, Okuma Y, et al: The effects of ventilation on the absorption and elimination of inhalation anesthetics. Anaesthesia 18:427, 1963

11. Munson ES, Eger EI II, Bowers DL: Effects of anesthetic-depressed ventilation and cardiac output on anesthetic uptake. Anesthesiology 38:251, 1973

12. Munson ES, Larson CP Jr, Babad AA, et al: The effects of halothane, fluroxene and cyclopropane on ventilation: A comparative study in man. Anesthesiology 27:716, 1966

13. Fourcade HE, Stevens WC, Larson CP Jr, et al: Ventilatory effects of Forane—a new inhaled anesthetic. Anesthesiology 35:26, 1971

14. Calverley RK, Smith NT, Jones CW, et al: Ventilatory and cardiovascular effects of enflurane anesthesia during spontaneous ventilation in man. Anesth Analg 57:610, 1978

15. Munson ES, Eger EI II, Bowers DL: Effects of anesthetic-depressed ventilation and cardiac output on anesthetic uptake. Anesthesiology 38:251, 1973

16. Gibbons RT, Steffey EP, Eger EI II: The effect of spontaneous versus controlled ventilation on the rate of rise of alveolar halothane concentration in dogs. Anesth Analg 56:32, 1977

17. Yamamura H: The effect of ventilation and blood volume on the uptake and elimination of inhalation anesthetic agents, Progress in Anaesthesiology. Proceedings of the Fourth World Congress of Anesthesiologists. Excerpta Medica International Congress Series 200, Amsterdam, 1968, pp 394-399

18. Eger EI II, Smith NT, Stoelting RK, et al: Cardiovascular effects of halothane in man. Anesthesiology 32:396, 1970

19. Calverley RK, Smith NT, Eger EI II: Cardiovascular effects of enflurane anesthesia during controlled ventilation in man. Anesth Analg 57:619, 1978

20. Eger EI II, Bahlman SH, Munson ES: Effect of age on the rate of increase of alveolar anesthetic concentration. Anesthesiology 35:365, 1971

21. Salanitre E, Rackow H: The pulmonary exchange of nitrous oxide and halothane in infants and children. Anesthesiology 30:388, 1969

22. Eger EI II, Severinghaus JW: Effect of uneven pulmonary distribution of blood and gas on induction with inhalation anesthetics. Anesthesiology 25:620, 1964

23. Stoelting RK, Longnecker DE: Effect of right-to-left shunt on rate of increase in arterial anesthetic concentration. Anesthesiology 36:352, 1972

24. Stoelting RK, Eger EI II: Percutaneous loss of nitrous oxide, cyclopropane, ether and halothane in man. Anesthesiology 30:278, 1969

25. Cullen BG, Eger EI II: Diffusion of nitrous oxide, cyclopropane, and halothane through human skin and amniotic membrane. Anesthesiology 36:168, 1972

26. Berman ML, Lowe HJ, Hagler KT, et al: Uptake and elimination of methoxyflurane as influenced by enzyme induction in the rat. Anesthesiology 38:352, 1973

27. Halsey MJ, Sawyer DC, Eger EI II, et al: Hepatic metabolism of halothane, methoxyflurane, cyclopropane, Ethrane and Forane in miniature swine. Anesthesiology 35:43, 1971

28. Sawyer DC, Eger EI II, Bahlman SH, et al: Concentration dependence of hepatic halothane metabolism. Anesthesiology 34:230, 1971

29. Eger EI II, Saidman LJ: Hazards of nitrous oxide anesthesia in bowel obstruction and pneumothorax. Anesthesiology 26:61, 1965

30. Hunter AR: Problems of anesthesia in artifi-

cial pneumothorax. Proc R Soc Med 48:765, 1955

31. Munson ES, Merrick HC: Effect of nitrous oxide on venous air embolism. Anesthesiology 27:783, 1966

32. Stanley TH, Kawamura R, Graves C: Effects of nitrous oxide on volume and pressure of endotracheal tube cuffs. Anesthesiology 41:256, 1974

33. Thomsen KA, Terkildsen LK, Arnfred J: Middle ear pressure variations during anesthesia. Arch Otolaryng 82:609, 1965

34. Saidman LJ, Eger EI II: Change in cerebrospinal fluid pressure during pneumoencephalography under nitrous oxide anesthesia. Anesthesiology 26:67, 1965

35. Waun JE, Sweitzer RS, Hamilton WK: Effect of nitrous oxide in middle ear mechanics and hearing acuity. Anesthesiology 28:846, 1967

36. Eger EI II, Larson CP Jr, Severinghaus JW: The solubility of halothane in rubber, soda lime and various plastics. Anesthesiology 23:365, 1962

37. Titel JH, Lowe HJ: Rubber-gas partition coefficients. Anesthesiology 29:1215, 1968

38. Titel JH, Lowe HJ, Elam JO, et al: Quantitative closed-circuit halothane anesthesia. Anaesth Analg 47:560, 1968

39. Harper M, Eger EI II: A comparison of the efficiency of three anesthesia circle systems. Anesth Analg 55:724, 1976

40. Aldrete JA, Lowe HJ, Virtue RW: Low Flow and Closed System Anesthesia. Grune and Stratton, New York, 1979

41. Severinghaus JW: The rate of uptake of nitrous oxide in man. J Clin Invest 33:1183, 1954

42. Mapleson WW: Quantitative prediction of anesthetic concentrations, Uptake and Distribution of Anesthetic Agents. Edited by Papper EM and Kitz RJ. McGraw-Hill, New York, 1963, pp 104-119

43. Stoelting RK, Eger EI II: The effects of ventilation and anesthetic solubility on recovery from anesthesia: An *in vivo* and analog analysis before and after equilibration. Anesthesiology 30:290, 1969

44. Munson ES, Eger EI II, Tham MK, et al: Increase in anesthetic uptake, excretion and blood solubility in man after eating. Anesth Analg 57:224, 1978

45. Rehder K, Forbes J, Alter H, et al: Halothane biotransformation in man: A quantitative study. Anesthesiology 28:711, 1967

46. Chase RE, Holaday DA, Fiserova-Bergerova V, et al: The biotransformation of Ethrane in man. Anesthesiology 35:262, 1971

47. Fink BR: Diffusion anoxia. Anesthesiology 16:511, 1955

48. Sheffer L, Steffenson JL, Birch AA: Nitrous-oxide-induced diffusion hypoxia in patients breathing spontaneously. Anesthesiology 37:436, 1972

49. Rackow H, Salanitre E, Frumin MH: Dilution of alveolar gases during nitrous oxide excretion in man. J Appl Physiol 16:723, 1961

50. Eger EI II, Brandstater B: Solubility of methoxyflurane in rubber. Anesthesiology 24:679, 1963

12

Circulatory Pharmacology of Inhaled Anesthetics

Robert F. Hickey, M.D.
Edmond I. Eger II, M.D.

INTRODUCTION

The search for the ideal inhaled anesthetic has led to the development of agents with properties that differ markedly from those possessed by older agents. Included in these differences are the circulatory effects of modern anesthetics. Older agents, such as nitrous oxide, ether, and cyclopropane, tended to support the circulation by causing sympathetic stimulation, by less directly depressing the heart, and/or by producing contraction of peripheral vessels. As anesthesiologists took a more active role in controlling the circulation through pharmacologic or physiological means they became progressively less fearful of the cardiovascular depression inherent in anesthesia and in fact have made use of it. The modern anesthetics both engendered and reflect this attitude. In the present chapter we contrast the circulatory properties of old with new inhaled agents. These contrasts provide insights into the breadth and limitations imposed by anesthesia.

HUMAN VOLUNTEER STUDIES

Studies in volunteers permit the isolation of anesthetic effects from those of disease, surgery, and concomitant pharmacologic and physiological interventions. They therefore are more likely to reveal the untainted effects of anesthesia but it must be remembered that these effects may be modified by the milieu of clinical practice. That modification is explored in a later section of this chapter. First, we consider the circulatory changes that result from anesthesia when $PaCO_2$ is maintained normal by controlled ventilation.

ARTERIAL PRESSURE (Fig. 12-1)

The modern anesthetics, halothane,[1,2] enflurane,[3] and isoflurane,[4] all decrease mean arterial pressure in direct proportion to their concentration. At 2.0 MAC, mean arterial pressure is approximately 50 percent of the control (awake) value. By contrast, the older agents (diethyl ether,[5] fluroxene,[6] and cyclopropane[7,8]) have little effect on pressure even at concentrations above 3.0 MAC.

CARDIAC OUTPUT (Fig. 12-2)

Halothane[1,2] and enflurane[3] reduce cardiac output and this effect parallels their effect on arterial pressure. Similarly, the older agents, cyclopropane,[7,8] diethyl ether,[5] and fluroxene,[6] which do not reduce arterial

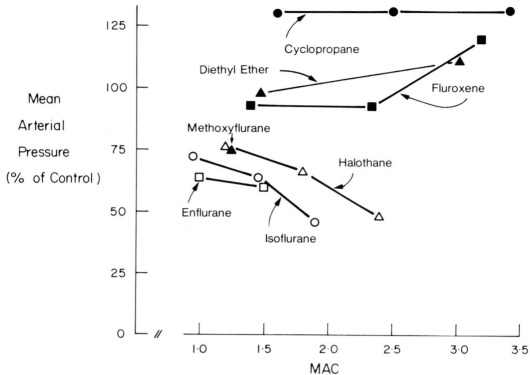

Fig. 12-1 Halothane, isoflurane, enflurane, and methoxyflurane decrease mean arterial pressure in a dose-related fashion. Arterial pressure is unchanged with diethyl ether and lower concentrations of fluroxene. It is increased with cycloproprane and at the highest concentration of fluroxene studied. In this figure and subsequent ones, control values are those obtained prior to induction of anesthesia. Ventilation is controlled and $PaCO_2$ is normal.

pressure also do not change cardiac output. The exception to this dichotomy is isoflurane, which has little affect on cardiac output but profoundly reduces mean arterial pressure.

Figure 12-2 provides somewhat misleading information. Enflurane appears similar to halothane in its effect upon cardiac output but in fact differs significantly. In volunteers given 2.0 MAC enflurane, a progressive decrease in cardiac output and blood pressure to unacceptable levels occurred but no such progression is evident with halothane even at 2.4 MAC. In the steady state, fluroxene either does not change or increase cardiac output.[6] However, an acute increase in fluroxene concentration temporarily decreases cardiac

output. A similar effect is seen with diethyl ether.[5] This response indicates an underlying capacity of these agents to cause cardiovascular depression; it also suggests that in the steady state these agents permit or cause a compensatory circulatory stimulation that masks the underlying depressant effect.

SYSTEMIC VASCULAR RESISTANCE (Fig. 12-3)

This calculated variable is obtained by dividing systemic perfusion pressure (mean arterial minus right atrial pressure) by cardiac output. The modern agents, halothane[1,2] and

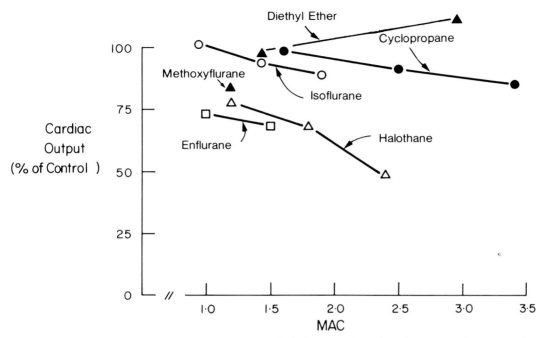

Fig. 12-2 Cardiac output is depressed by enflurane, halothane, and methoxyflurane. Isoflurane, cyclopropane, and diethyl ether have little effect on cardiac output.

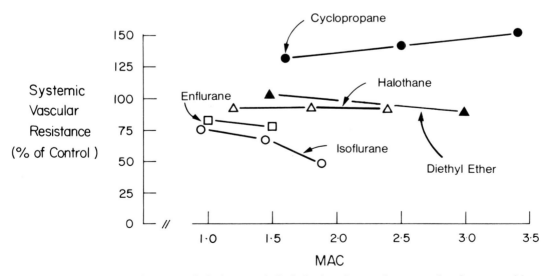

Fig. 12-3 Cyclopropane increases, halothane and diethyl ether do not change, and enflurane and isoflurane reduce systemic vascular resistance.

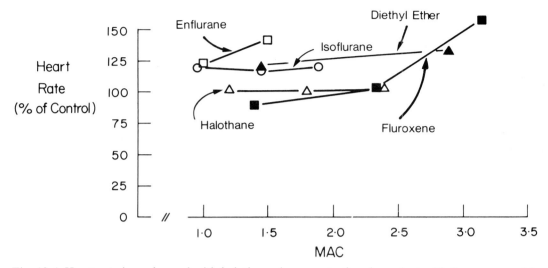

Fig. 12-4 Heart rate is unchanged with halothane, is concentration-dependent with fluroxene, and is increased with enflurane, isoflurane, and diethyl ether.

enflurane,[3] modestly reduce systemic vascular resistance (SVR). The older ethers, fluroxene[6] and diethyl ether,[5] share this property. Isoflurane[4] profoundly reduces SVR (50 percent reduction at 1.9 MAC) in part by dilatation of skeletal muscle vasculature.

All inhaled anesthetics reduce resistance to flow to the brain and the skin. An earlier impression that halothane is a profound vasodilator resulted from studies done during spontaneous ventilation. The associated respiratory depression and consequently elevated $PaCO_2$ contributed significantly to the vasodilation. Cyclopropane is the only potent inhaled anesthetic that significantly increases SVR at all anesthetic levels. Cyclopropane increases resistance by several mechanisms: it directly causes contraction of vessels; it increases the sensitivity of vessel musculature to norepinephrine; and it also increases sympathetic outflow.[9]

HEART RATE (Fig. 12-4)

Inhaled anesthetics change heart rate by altering rate of sinus node depolarization, by changing myocardial conduction times, or by shifting autonomic nervous system activity. The bradycardia sometimes seen with halothane may result from a direct depression of atrial rate. Halothane at 0.5 to 1.5 MAC decreases the contractile rate of isolated rat atria.[10] In contrast, methoxyflurane, diethyl ether, and enflurane each increase the rate of contraction of isolated atria and fluroxene causes a slight depression.[10]

Fluroxene, diethyl ether, methoxyflurane, isoflurane, and enflurane all increase heart rate in human volunteers. An anesthetic-induced reduction in arterial pressure would tend to increase heart rate by withdrawal of baroreceptor stimulation. The increase in heart rate seen with methoxyflurane and enflurane can be partially attributed to a baroreceptor mechanism. By contrast, halothane has profound baroreceptor blocking activity.[11] Baroreceptor blockade plus the direct effect of halothane on atrial contraction rate explains why heart rate remains constant during halothane anesthesia.

The effect of anesthesia on heart rate and blood pressure also must be considered in the context of preanesthesia values for these variables. Excitement and concomitant tachycardia, hypertension, and increased

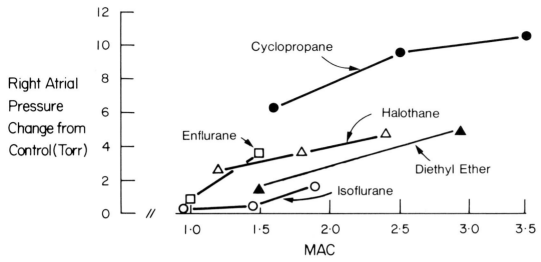

Fig. 12-5 All anesthetics depicted increase right atrial pressure in a dose-dependent fashion. Cyclopropane, enflurane, and halothane induce the greatest increases.

cardiac output will be altered by anesthesia; excitement is ultimately abolished and heart rate, pressure, and output decreases to more normal levels. In contrast, if preanesthetic parasympathetic activity is enhanced, anesthesia may increase pulse rate and pressure. These notions have been documented by Roizen and Horrigan (unpublished data).

RIGHT ATRIAL PRESSURE

All inhalation anesthetics tend to increase right atrial pressures in a dose-related fashion (Fig. 12-5). The changes are both related to a depression of myocardial function and to the anesthetic effect on peripheral vasculature. In vitro studies of myocardial depression indicate that right atrial pressure should be increased similarly by halothane, enflurane, and isoflurane; yet at similar doses right atrial pressure is less with isoflurane and enflurane. Vasodilation by these two drugs may account for these findings. Certainly the right atrial pressure increases produced by cyclopropane are in part explained by cyclopropane's direct constriction of veins.

MYOCARDIAL FUNCTION

At some concentration all inhaled anesthetics depress myocardial function. This is most clearly seen in vitro studies where direct myocardial depressant properties of the anesthetics are not obscured by homeostatic mechanisms and/or the capacity of the anesthetics to cause peripheral vasodilation or stimulate sympathetic activity. Brown and Crout[12] found that five anesthetics produce a linear, dose-dependent depression of isolated cat papillary muscle (Fig. 12-6). However, the amount of depression differed with enflurane > halothane > methoxyflurane > cyclopropane > diethyl ether. Itwatsuki and Shimosoto[13] in similar in vitro studies using the cat papillary muscle confirmed the dose-dependent linear depression of the same five inhalation anesthetics. However, they found that enflurane was not the most depressant drug but similar to diethyl ether and less depressant than either halothane or methoxyflurane. Slight differences in technique (temperature, use of peer groups) may account for the different order of depression found in these two in vitro studies.

The cardiac depression seen in vitro does

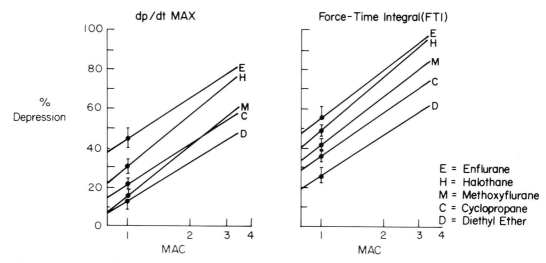

Fig. 12-6 In vitro effects of five anesthetics demonstrate a dose-dependent depression of myocardial contractility. The ordering of depression from most to least is enflurane > halothane > methoxyflurane > cyclopropane > diethyl ether. (Brown BR and Crout JR: A comparative study of the effect of five general anesthetics on myocardial contractility. Anesthesiology 34: 236, 1971.)

not appear to exist in intact animals or man. For example neither isoflurane nor fluroxene causes myocardial depression, as indicated by the sustained amplitude of the ballistocardiogram (BCG) in volunteers anesthetized with 1.0 to 2.0 MAC of these agents (Fig. 12-7). Both 1.25 MAC methoxyflurane[14] and halothane[15] decrease right ventricular dP/dt by 15 to 20 percent of the values obtained prior to anesthesia, but this depression is less than that produced by comparable anesthetic doses in vitro. Moreover, with continuing anesthesia in humans, dP/dt returns to awake values whereas in vitro values remain depressed.[14, 15] These data imply that in vivo compensatory mechanisms counter the depressant effects of inhaled agents and, further, that the effect of these compensatory mechanisms increases with the passage of time.

The most extensive studies of myocardial function in anesthetized man are those reported by Sonntag et al.[16] They measured left ventricular function awake and at 1.1 and 2.1 MAC halothane. As halothane increased, stroke volume, mean arterial pressure, and left ventricular dP/dt (max) progressively decreased. Left ventricular end-diastolic pressure increased with values being 11 torr in the nonanesthetized volunteers and 12 and 14 torr respectively at 1.1 and 2.1 MAC halothane. Systemic vascular resistance remained constant. These findings of decreased contractility at increased preload while systemic vascular resistance and heart rate remain constant document the negative inotropic effect of halothane in man.

During controlled ventilation, halothane increases left ventricular volume in dogs[17–19] and in humans[20] in a dose-related fashion even though afterload (systemic blood pressure) decreases. Both diastolic and systolic volumes increase, and in one study,[19] increases occurred despite a concomitant increase in heart rate. A rise in heart rate should increase contractility and thereby reduce ventricular volume. In contrast to the above studies with controlled ventilation, in spontaneously breathing man Rathod et al.[21] found that 1.1 MAC halothane reduced a left ventricular dimension to 93 percent of that measured in the same subjects before anesthesia.

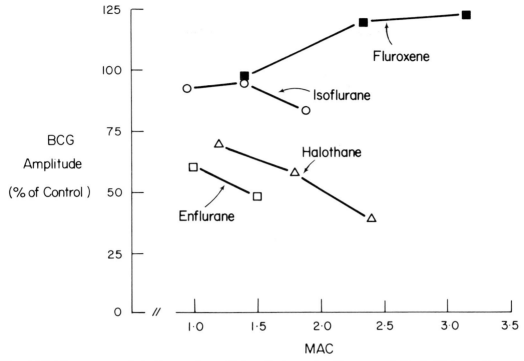

Fig. 12-7 Fluroxene and isoflurane have little effect on the IJ wave of the ballistrocardiogram. Halothane and enflurane both show dose-dependent depression.

Enflurane anesthesia produced a similar effect although it like halothane is known to be a myocardial depressant. The reduced heart size in the patients of Rathod et al.[21] may have resulted from a decreased preload, a decreased afterload (systemic pressure was reduced), an increased heart rate, and an increase in sympathetic activity associated with an increase in $PaCO_2$.

MYOCARDIAL OXYGEN CONSUMPTION

Inhaled anesthetics reduce myocardial oxygen consumption (MVO_2) primarily by decreasing those variables that control oxygen demand. In dogs[22,23] and humans[24] 1.5 to 2.0 MAC halothane decreases myocardial oxygen consumption by 40 to 60 percent. Isoflurane causes a similar decrease in dogs.[25]

CORONARY BLOOD FLOW

Halothane decreases coronary blood flow (CBF). Coronary vascular resistance either increases or remains constant depending on halothane's effect on MVO_2 and systemic arterial pressure. Lactate extraction remains constant suggesting adequacy of coronary artery perfusion.[23,24] If autoregulation is present during halothane anesthesia, a reduction in MVO_2 should result in an increase in coronary artery resistance (i.e., an increase in resistance does not imply that halothane is a coronary vasoconstrictor). However, halothane lowers systemic arterial pressure, which should decrease coronary artery blood flow and invite a decrease in resistance. The two opposing effects, reduction of both demand and supply, tend to balance. However, the balance is only partial since coronary arteriovenous oxygen difference decreases (i.e., the tendency for a decrease in resistance to occur appears to be predominant and implies, in fact, that halothane acts as a coronary artery vasodilator).

Wolff et al.[26] demonstrated that some element of autoregulation exists during halothane anesthesia. They cannulated and perfused the left coronary arteries of dogs to maintain a constant coronary artery blood pressure. With administration of halothane to both the whole animal and the coronary artery, the coronary artery blood flow decreased indicating an increase in coronary artery resistance. Such an increase in resistance should occur with autoregulation, since the administration of halothane also decreased systemic pressure and hence heart work and oxygen consumption.

In summary, the effect of inhalation anesthetic on coronary blood flow is determined primarily in part by the effect of the anesthetic on those variables that control oxygen supply and demand, in part by a direct effect on the coronary arteries, and in part by the "control" state. Apropos of the last of these factors, tachycardia and hypertension may accompany apprehension in an awake volunteer or a "light basal" anesthetic in an animal. Such humans or animals will demonstrate much greater decreases in CBF and MVO$_2$ on administration of a general anesthetic.

EFFECT OF NITROUS OXIDE

The most frequently administered inhalation anesthetic is nitrous oxide. At one time nitrous oxide was considered to be an impotent vehicle for the administration of more potent inhaled anesthetics. It has become clear that nitrous oxide has significant effects of its own and may appreciably alter the actions of potent agents given concomitantly.

Nitrous oxide directly depresses the myocardium. It produces a dose-dependent depression of the dog myocardium in a heart-lung preparation that is less than that produced by more potent agents.[27] Similarly, it

depresses peak developed isometric depression and the maximum rate of tension development in cat heart muscle strips maintained at 37 °C.[28] However, at 37 °C depression is also produced by lowering oxygen partial pressure with nitrogen by an amount equal to that lowering achieved with nitrous oxide. Although this suggests that depression from nitrous oxide results from hypoxia, an experiment by Price[29] argues otherwise. Cat papillary muscle maintained at 25 °C is depressed more by 50 percent nitrous oxide than by 50 percent nitrogen. The use of a lower temperature avoids the hypoxia that may develop in the deeper layers of muscle. That is, diffusion of oxygen to those deeper layers can keep pace with the lower metabolic rate at 25 °C but not the higher rate at 37 °C. It is noteworthy that the depression produced by nitrous oxide is less than that produced by a comparable concentration of halothane.

In man breathing 40 percent nitrous oxide, Eisele and Smith[30] found a 10 percent reduction of the amplitude of the ballistocardiogram. This was considered to indicate direct myocardial depression. To study nitrous oxide at anesthetic concentrations requires the use of hyperbaric pressure. Winter et al.[31] anesthetized nine normal volunteers at 1.55 and 1.10 atmospheres of nitrous oxide. At 1.55 atmospheres of nitrous oxide, arterial pressure and heart rate increased 6 and 10 percent respectively while cardiac output and systemic vascular resistance remained unchanged (Fig. 12-8). No evidence of myocardial depression was found. However, sympathetic stimulation was suggested by sweating, dilated pupils, and increased serum catecholamines and corticosteroids. This stimulation could have obscured any direct evidence of myocardial depression.

Mean arterial blood pressure and dP/dt decrease and left ventricular end-diastolic pressure increases in patients suffering from coronary artery disease who are given 40 percent nitrous oxide.[32] Similarly, cardiac output and blood pressure decrease when 60 percent nitrous oxide is added to the anes-

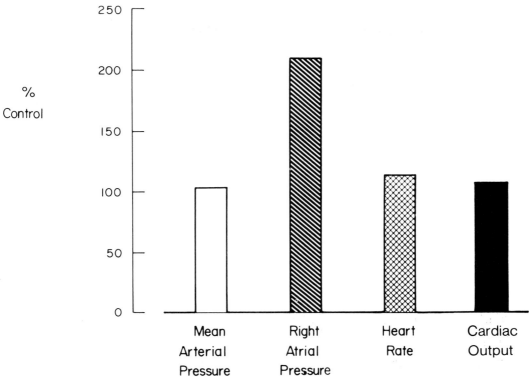

Fig. 12-8 Administration of 1.5 MAC nitrous oxide results in little change in arterial pressure, heart rate, or cardiac output. (See text for details.)

thetic regimen of patients who already have received 1 mg/kg of morphine.[33] Such studies indicate that nitrous oxide does have cardiodepressant properties.

Results from studies of the combination of nitrous oxide with potent inhaled anesthetics also indicate that nitrous oxide is sympathomimetic and has mild cardiac depressant effects. Smith et al.[34] added 70 percent nitrous oxide to either 1 to 1.5 MAC or 2 to 2.5 MAC halothane anesthesia. In the first 10 to 20 minutes after addition of the nitrous oxide, systemic vascular resistance, arterial and right atrial pressure, and pupil diameter and plasma norepinephrine all increased whereas heart rate, cardiac output, and the amplitude of the ballistocardiogram remained constant. Hill et al.[35] added 20, 40, and 60 percent nitrous oxide to 0.95, 1.4, and 1.9 MAC halothane. Addition of 60 percent nitrous oxide

increased right atrial pressure at all halothane concentrations. Other cardiovascular changes depended on the concentrations of halothane. Subjects at 0.95, 1.4, and 1.9 MAC halothane responded to the addition of 60 percent nitrous oxide by decreasing, not changing, and increasing their systemic vascular resistance. Systemic vascular resistance changes were associated with opposite (inverse) changes in stroke volume.

Bahlman et al.[36] compared nitrous oxide plus halothane anesthesia to halothane anesthesia alone at 1.2, 1.8, and 2.4 MAC in human volunteers (Fig. 12-9). To have comparable concentrations of anesthetics the subjects received a greater concentration of halothane when not receiving nitrous oxide. At 1.2 and 2.4 MAC anesthesia, IJ wave amplitude of the ballistocardiogram, cardiac output, right atrial pressure, and arterial

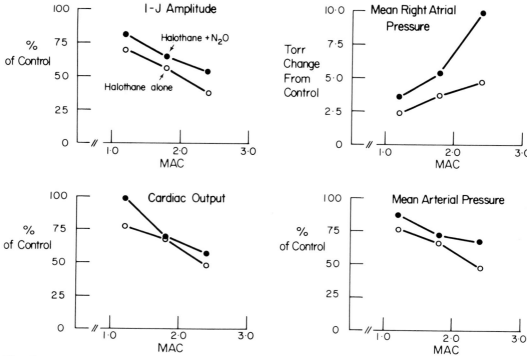

Fig. 12-9 Nitrous oxide plus halothane has less circulatory depression than does halothane at similar anesthetic concentrations. ● = Halothane + nitrous oxide; ○ = halothane alone. (Bahlman SH, Eger EI II, Smith NT, et al: The cardiovascular effects of nitrous oxide-halothane anestheia in man. Anesthesiology 35: 274, 1971.)

pressure were higher in subjects anesthetized with halothane plus nitrous oxide. At 1.8 MAC no significant differences existed. Thus the substitution of nitrous oxide for halothane either produced no change in or lessened the cardiovascular depression.

In a similar study with nitrous oxide and isoflurane, Dolan et al.[37] found that at 1.0 and 2.0 MAC, mean arterial pressure and peripheral vascular resistance were 27 and 12 percent greater respectively in volunteers receiving nitrous oxide. No other variable differed between these two groups.

Smith and co-workers[38] also examined the effects of enflurane with and without nitrous oxide during controlled ventilation. The administration of nitrous oxide with enflurane at 1.5 MAC resulted in less decrease in cardiac output, stroke volume, IJ wave ampli-

tude, and aortic dP/dt than did the administration of enflurane alone.

In summary, nitrous oxide alone or in combination with potent inhaled agents produces sympathetic stimulation. Such stimulation may obscure any cardiac depressant effects. The combination of nitrous oxide plus halothane or enflurane appears to produce less depression at a given MAC level than either potent agent given alone.

EFFECT OF TIME

The cardiovascular effect of several inhaled agents appears to change with the duration of anesthesia. Longer anesthesia is associated with an increase in β-sympathetic activity. Heart rate, cardiac output, myocar-

Table 12-1. Directional Change in Some Circulatory Values on Changing from Controlled to Spontaneous Ventilation

Measure	Halothane	Enflurane	Isoflurane
Cardiac output	↑	↑	↑
Arterial pressure	↑	±	±
Heart rate	↑	↑	↑
Systemic vascular resistance	↓	↓	↓
IJ wave amplitude ballistocardiogram	↑	↑	±
Mean right atrial pressure	±	↓	±

dial function, and mean right atrial pressure all reflect such an increased activity; function and rate increase while atrial pressure decreases. Systemic vascular resistance falls; thus despite an increase in cardiac output, blood pressure does not change. Cyclopropane,[8] isoflurane,[4] enflurane,[3] methoxyflurane,[14] halothane,[2] diethyl ether,[5] and fluroxene[6] each demonstrate some if not all of these temporally related changes. The largest changes are seen with diethyl ether, fluroxene, and halothane. In contrast to these in vivo changes, in vitro depression of cat papillary at a constant concentration of halothane remains unchanged over a three-hour period, indicating that recovery with time is not based on improved myocardial function.[39] Volunteers anesthetized with halothane do not demonstrate the temporally related stimulation if they are given propranolol prior to anesthesia.[15] These findings suggest that the effect of time is the result of an increase in sympathetic nervous activity.

SPONTANEOUS VENTILATION

Studies of the circulatory changes produced by anesthetics during spontaneous ventilation introduce $PaCO_2$ as a variable that at equipotent concentrations differs between anesthetics because of the different capacity of each agent to depress respiration.[41-43] Carbon dioxide has three predominant actions: dilation of smooth muscle, stimulation of the sympathetic nervous system, and direct depression of the

heart by acidosis. These circulatory effects of carbon dioxide may add to or oppose the action of the anesthetics.

Administration of CO_2 to awake man produces cardiac stimulation and decreases systemic vascular resistance.[44] Similar but attenuated results are seen during anesthesia. The attenuation is directly related to anesthetic dose.[45] (Table 12-1).

In addition to affecting the circulation by altering carbon dioxide levels, spontaneous as opposed to controlled positive pressure ventilation favors the return of venous blood to the heart. The venoconstrictive reflex response to positive intrathoracic pressure increases peripheral venous pressure and tends to restore venous return towards normal. The inhaled anesthetics limit this compensatory venoconstriction and thereby exaggerate the depressant influence of positive pressure ventilation. During halothane anesthesia in volunteers, a change from spontaneous to controlled ventilation decreases cardiac output, heart rate and arterial pressure.[45] Systemic vascular resistance is increased (Fig. 12-10). Similar differences are seen with other agents.[3,43]

THE EFFECT OF DISEASE

The presence of heart disease increases the chance of complications during or following anesthesia. For example, one study reported a 0.33 percent incidence of myocardial infarction following general anesthesia in patients who had not had a prior myocardial infarct,

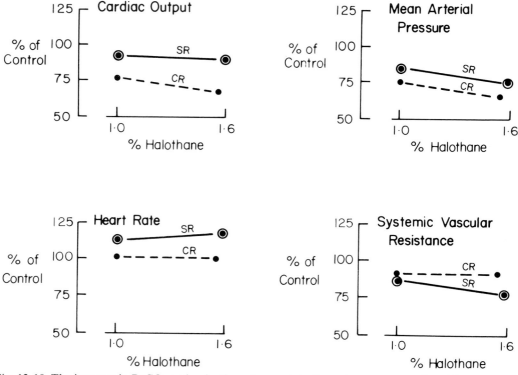

Fig. 12-10 The increase in PaCO$_2$ and reduction of mean intrathoracic pressure produced by spontaneous ventilation result in increases in cardiac output, heart rate, and mean arterial pressure and decreases in systemic vascular resistance. (Bahlman SH, Eger EI II, Halsey MJ, et al: The cardiovascular effects of halothane in man during spontaneous ventilation. Anesthesiology 36: 494, 1972.)

but a 6.6 percent incidence in those who had had a prior myocardial infarction.[46] Other indices of myocardial disease may be more important than a history of infarction as a predictor of perioperative complications.[47] In any case, cardiovascular disease contributes significantly to anesthesia-surgery risk (see Ch. 2).

The quantitative estimation of cardiac disease and cardiovascular reserve is not easily accomplished. Serious ailments are often associated with normal indices of circulatory function at rest. For example, blood pressure, heart rate, cardiac output, myocardial contractility, filling pressures, and electrocardiogram all may be normal in the patient with coronary artery disease. Exercise stress testing frequently is used to assess coronary artery disease, but recent studies suggest this test is of limited value.[48] Since atherosclerosis is the most frequent cause of coronary artery disease, the extent of obstruction is best measured by coronary angiogram—a procedure requiring some skill and not without risk.

Other cardiac diseases, such as aortic stenosis, also may present with few specific findings but may nearly eliminate the circulatory reserve needed to compensate for perioperative stress. A reduced reserve may relate both to the disease and to the treatment of that disease. For example, patients with valvular heart disease undergoing open heart surgery may be hypovolemic and may react adversely to the vasodilation produced by anesthetic agents because of this hypovolemia. The hypovolemia is secondary to salt and water depletion induced by diuretics given, by necessity, to treat congestive heart failure.[49]

Diseases such as myocardial infarction and rheumatic heart disease directly affect the amount of functioning myocardium; diseases such as ventricular hypertrophy reduce reserve by decreasing perfusion per gram of heart muscle.[50]

Right ventricular hypertrophy or congestive heart failure can be produced in cats by pulmonary artery obstruction. Papillary muscle from these cats has a 30 to 55 percent decrease in maximum velocity of contraction. The addition of halothane to that already compromised muscle produces proportionately the same depression as in normal muscle but the degree of depression is greater, since the diseased muscle starts from a lower baseline.[51] These studies provide insight into the sensitivity of patients with congestive heart failure or ventricular hypertrophy to anesthetic concentrations that in normal patients usually are well tolerated.

The study reported by Eisele et al.[32] illustrates the interaction between disease and anesthesia. In nine patients with two vessel coronary artery disease and reduced left ventricular ejection fractions, the inhalation of 40 percent nitrous oxide significantly decreased mean arterial pressure and dP/dt and increased left ventricular end diastolic pressure. In four patients without angiographic evidence of coronary disease, breathing 40 percent nitrous oxide produced no myocardial depression. Similarly, administration of 1.5 percent halothane increased the preinjection period (PEP) and decreased left ventricular ejection time (LVET) to a greater extent in patients with heart disease than in those without heart disease.[52]

The drug therapy used to treat hypertension and ischemic heart disease (propranolol, α-methyldopa, reserpine) may attenuate the normal responses of the sympathetic nervous system. This may augment the cardiovascular depression induced by anesthesia and has led in the past to the preoperative discontinua-

tion of these medications. One report linked the preoperative administration of propranolol with the inability to wean a patient from cardiopulmonary bypass following open heart surgery.[53]

The interaction between propranolol and the volatile anesthetics produces effects that may depend on the specific anesthetic and on patient disease. Anesthetics that normally stimulate the sympathetic nervous system may produce cardiac depression when β blockade is present. In humans anesthetized with diethyl ether, 5 mg of intravenous propranolol decreases heart rate, mean arterial pressure, cardiac output, and stroke volume and increases central venous pressure and systemic vascular resistance.[54] In dogs anesthetized with cyclopropane, 0.3 mg/kg of propranolol decreases cardiac output, stroke volume, and myocardial contractility and increases systemic vascular resistance.[55] Both ether and cyclopropane are thought to increase sympathetic activity. In contrast, methoxyflurane, trichloroethylene, and enflurane do not, and dogs anesthetized with these agents exhibit minor to moderate cardiac depression on administration of β blockers.[56-58] However, when subjected to graded hemorrhage, the animals who receive the blockers have more severe circulatory depression than similarly bled animals maintained at the same anesthetic concentration who do not receive the β blockers.[56-58]

Circulatory depression consequent to administration of β-blockers appears to be least with halothane and isoflurane.[59-63] Similarly, the addition of stresses such as graded hemorrhage[62,63] and hypoxemia[60] appear better tolerated with these anesthetics than with enflurane, methoxyflurane, or trichloroethylene. In general, with any potent inhalation anesthetic there is an additive depressant effect produced by β blockers. Safe anesthetic management in patients receiving β blockers may require both judicious selection of the agent and/or reduction in anesthetic concentration. However, the earlier notion that β blockers should be discontinued prior to anesthesia largely has been discarded. Such discontinuation has been found to produce excessive complications related to the patient's underlying disease (e.g., hypertension, angina, arrhythmias).

Valvular heart disease places narrow constraints on anesthetic choice and management. Aortic stenosis results in ventricular hypertrophy and the potential for a reduced coronary artery perfusion pressure. Induction of peripheral vasodilation by a drug such as isoflurane, when cardiac output is limited by the stenosis, could be particularly hazardous. By contrast, this same anesthetic could prove of benefit in mitral or aortic insufficiency. With insufficiency, reduction of systemic vascular resistance favors forward cardiac flow rather than regurgitation and has been demonstrated to improve circulatory indices.[64]

Obstructive coronary artery disease presents indications for anesthetic management and choice that depend on the facets of myocardial function most affected by the coronary artery disease. For example a patient with potential myocardial ischemia from a flow-limiting segment would theoretically benefit from a drug that reduced myocardial oxygen consumption but did not reduce systemic vascular resistance. Halothane is such a drug, and it favorably affects electrocardiographic signs of myocardial ischemia.[65] By contrast both enflurane and isoflurane increase heart rate and induce systemic vasodilation. Systemic vasodilation might be sought if the coronary artery disease had led to congestive heart failure and reduction of afterload was desirable. Isoflurane might then be considered the drug of choice. Another anesthetic consideration is indicated if hypoxia or injury of myocardial muscle has led to dysrhythmias. Fifty percent of patients receiving 2.1 $\mu g/kg$ of subcutaneously injected epinephrine develop ventricular extrasystoles when anesthetized with 1.25 MAC halothane. The epinephrine dose required to produce the same incidence in patients anesthetized with isoflurane is 6.4 $\mu g/kg$ and is greater than 10 $\mu g/kg$ when the anesthetic is enflurane.[66]

In general, the halogenated alkanes (halothane, chloroform, trichloroethylene) or cyclic hydrocarbons (cyclopropane) predispose to arrhythmias whereas the ethers (fluroxene, enflurane, isoflurane, methoxyflurane) do not (see Ch. 7) and are indicated in patients with significant arrhythmias.

Disease may decrease oxygen content in arterial blood by a decrease in hemoglobin or arterial PO_2. Hypoxemia or anemia may alter the circulatory responses to halothane. Hypoxic dogs given 1.0 to 1.25 MAC halothane have increased arterial pressure, heart rate, and cardiac output when compared to control dogs that are not hypoxic.[67] However, an increase in halothane dose kills hypoxic animals whereas control animals exhibit the expected increase in circulatory depression. By contrast, anemic dogs anesthetized with halothane have no difference in cardiac output, blood pressure, heart rate, left ventricular end-diastolic pressure, and arterial base excess than anesthetized control animals.[68] Anemia alters neither apneic nor lethal concentrations of halothane.[68] Thus a decrease of arterial oxygen content by anemia does not have the same effect on the response to halothane as does a similar decrease in content by hypoxemia.

THE EFFECT OF SURGERY

Surgery modifies the circulatory effects of the volatile anesthetic agents. Rarely does a surgical incision not produce an increase in blood pressure and heart rate. Surgical incision is a stress that produces stimulation of the sympathetic nervous system. Anesthesia opposes this response to surgical stress in a dose-dependent fashion. Roizen and Horrigan[69] demonstrated that as halothane or enflurane concentrations were increased, surgically induced increases in serum norepinephrine levels were decreased or prevented. The anesthetic doses for blocking adrenergic responses to skin incision in 50 percent of patients studied were 1.47 MAC halothane and 1.63 MAC enflurane. Thus surgery becomes a variable that the anesthesiologist may use and must allow for in anesthetic and anesthetic dose selection.

SUMMARY

In vitro studies demonstrate that all anesthetics produce a consistent dose-related cardiac depression. This clear evidence of depression by all anesthetics becomes less clear in vivo wherein homeostatic mechanisms come into play. Although halothane and enflurane depress myocardial contractility, neither diethyl ether, cyclopropane, nor isoflurane reduce cardiac output and cyclopropane actually raises arterial pressure. Nitrous oxide may stimulate the circulation. The circulatory actions of the inhaled anesthetics are modified by many of the variables that infringe on the patient in the clinical milieu. Such variables include an increase in $PaCO_2$, patient disease, surgical stress, and the presence of various drug therapies. The anesthesiologist must consider the impact of each of these factors in choosing the patient's anesthetic and the dosage to be used.

Duration of anesthesia and mode of ventilation are factors in determining circulatory depression. Halothane and methoxyflurane at 1.25 MAC both depress right ventricular dP/dt in man. At constant depth anesthesia, these values return to control with time. Controlled ventilation results in circulatory depression both through mechanical impairment of venous return and a decrease in the sympathetic nervous system stimulation provided by carbon dioxide.

Patients with cardiac disease have less reserve and are less tolerant of anesthetic agents than healthy patients. Excessive cardiac depression must be avoided, yet a high anesthetic dosage may be needed to avoid unwanted circulatory stimulation by surgery and endotracheal intubation. The severity and type of circulatory disease are major factors influencing anesthesia choice and surgical risk. For example, both congestive heart failure and asymetrical septal hypertrophy (ASH) are heart disease. Congestive heart failure may be treated by afterload reduction and cardiac stimulation. In treatment of ASH, cardiac depressants are administered; these patients tolerate afterload reduction poorly. Thus two types of cardiac disease will require different drugs or anesthetics. This interrelationship between cardiovascular disease and the circulatory effects of anesthetic agents is the area in which we have the least knowledge.

REFERENCES

1. Deutsch S, Linde HW, Dripps RD, et al: Circulatory and respiratory actions of halothane in normal man. Anesthesiology 23: 631, 1962
2. Eger EI II, Smith NT, Stoelting RK, et al: Cardiovascular effects of halothane in man. Anesthesiology 32: 396, 1970.
3. Calverley RK, Smith NT, Prys-Roberts C, et al: Cardiovascular effects of enflurane anesthesia during controlled ventilation in man. Anesth Analg 57: 619, 1978
4. Stevens WC, Cromwell TH, Halsey MJ, et al: The cardiovascular effects of a new inhalation anesthetic, Forane, in human volunteers at constant arterial carbon dioxide tension. Anesthesiology 35: 8, 1971
5. Gregory GA, Eger EI II, Smith NT, et al: The cardiovascular effects of diethyl ether in man. Anesthesiology 34: 19, 1971
6. Cullen BF, Eger EI II, Smith NT, et al: Cardiovascular effects of fluroxene in man. Anesthesiology 32: 218, 1970
7. Jones RE, Guldmann N, Linde HW, et al: Cyclopropane anesthesia III. Effects of cyclopropane on respiration and circulation in normal man. Anesthesiology 21: 380, 1960
8. Cullen DJ, Eger EI II, Gregory GA: The cardiovascular effects of cyclopropane in man. Anesthesiology 31: 398, 1969
9. Price ML, Price HL: Effects of general anesthesia on contractile responses of rabbit aortic strips. Anesthesiology 23: 16, 1962
10. Price HL, Linde HW, Jones RE, et al: Sympathoadrenal responses to cyclopropane in

man and their relation to hemodynamics. Anesthesiology 20: 563, 1959

11. Duke PC, Fownes D, Wade JG: Halothane depresses baroreflex control of heart rate in man. Anesthesiology 46: 184, 1977

12. Brown BR and Crout JR: A comparative study of the effects of five general anesthetics on myocardial contractility: I. Isometric conditions. Anesthesiology 34: 236, 1971

13. Iwatsuki N, Shimosato S: Diethyl ether and contractility of isolated cat heart muscle. Br J Anaesth 43: 420, 1971

14. Libonati M, Cooperman LH, Price HL: Time-dependent circulatory effects of methoxyflurane in man. Anesthesiology 34: 439, 1971

15. Price HL, Skovsted P, Pauca AW, et al: Evidence for β-receptor activation produced by halothane in normal man. Anesthesiology 32: 389, 1970

16. Sonntag H, Donath U, Hillebrand W, et al: Left ventricular function in conscious man and during halothane anesthesia. Anesthesiology 48: 320, 1978

17. Hamilton WK, Larson CP, Bristow JD, et al: Effect of cyclopropane and halothane on ventricular mechanics: A change in ventricular diastolic pressure-volume relationship. J Pharmacol Exp Ther 154: 566, 1966

18. Rusy BF, Moran JE, Vongvises P, et al: The effects of halothane and cyclopropane on left ventricular volume determined by high speed biplane cineradiography in dogs. Anesthesiology 36: 369, 1972

19. Vatner SF, Smith NT: Effects of halothane on left ventricular function and distribution of regional blood flow in dogs and primates. Circ Res 34: 155, 1974

20. Gerson JI, Gianaris CG: Echocardiographic analysis of human left ventricular diastolic volume and cardiac performance during halothane anesthesia. Anesth Analg 58: 23, 1979

21. Rathod R, Jacobs HK, Kramer NE, et al: Echocardiographic assessment of ventricular performance following induction with two anesthetics. Anesthesiology 49: 86, 1978

22. Theye RA: Myocardial and total oxygen consumption with halothane. Anesthesiology 28: 1042, 1967

23. Merin RG, Kumazawa T, Luka NL: Myocardial function and metabolism in the conscious dog and during halothane anesthesia. Anesthesiology 44: 402, 1976

24. Sonntag H, Merin RG, Donath U, et al: Myocardial metabolism and oxygenation in man awake and during halothane anesthesia. Anesthesiology 51: 204, 1979

25. Theye RA, Michenfelder JD: Individual organ contributions to the decrease in wholebody $\dot{V}O_2$ with isoflurane. Anesthesiology 42: 35, 1975

26. Wolff G, Claude B, Rist M, et al: Regulation of coronary blood flow during ether and halothane anesthesia. Br J Anaesth 44: 1139, 1972

27. Price HL, Helrich M: The effect of cyclopropane, diethyl ether, nitrous oxide, thiopental and hydrogen ion concentration on the myocardial function of the dog heart-lung preparation. J Pharmacol Ex Ther 115: 206, 1955

28. Goldberg AH, Sohn YZ, Phear WP: Direct myocardial effects of nitrous oxide. Anesthesiology 37: 373, 1972

29. Price HL: Myocardial depression by nitrous oxide and its reversal by Ca++. Anesthesiology 44: 211, 1976

30. Eisele JH, Smith NT: Cardiovascular effects of 40 percent nitrous oxide in man. Anesth Analg 51: 956, 1972

31. Winter PM, Hornbein TF, Smith G: Hyperbaric nitrous oxide anesthesia in man: Determination of anesthetic potency (MAC) and cardiorespiratory effects. Abstracts of Scientific Papers. 1972 ASA meeting, p 103

32. Eisele JH, Reitan JA, Massumi RA, et al: Myocardial performance and N_2O analgesia in coronary artery disease. Anesthesiology 44: 16, 1976

33. Stoelting RK, Gibbs PS: Hemodynamic effects of morphine and morphine-nitrous oxide in valvular heart disease and coronary artery disease. Anesthesiology 38: 45, 1973

34. Smith NT, Eger EI II, Stoelting RK, et al: The cardiovascular and sympathomemetic responses to the addition of nitrous oxide to halothane in man. Anesthesiology 32: 410, 1970

35. Hill GE, English JE, Lunn J, et al: Cardiovascular response to nitrous oxide during light, moderate and deep halothane anesthesia in man. Anesth Analg 57: 84, 1978

36. Bahlman SH, Eger EI II, Smith NT, et al: The cardiovascular effects of nitrous oxide-

halothane anesthesia in man. Anesthesiology 35: 274, 1971

37. Dolan WM, Stevens WC, Eger EI II, et al: The cardiovascular and respiratory effects of isoflurane—nitrous oxide anesthesia. Canad Anaesth Soc J 21: 557, 1974

38. Smith NT, Calverley RK, Prys-Roberts C, et al: Impact of nitrous oxide on the circulation during enflurane anesthesia in man. Anesthesiology 48: 345, 1978

39. Shimosato S, Yasuda I: Cardiac performance during prolonged halothane anesthesia in the cat. Br J Anaesth 50: 215, 1978

40. Severinghaus JW, Larson CP: Respiration in anesthesia, Handbook of Physiology-Respiration. Vol II. Edited by Fenn WO, Rahn H. Washington DC, American Physiologic Society, 1965, pp 1219–1264

41. Munson ES, Larson CP Jr, Babad AA: The effect of halothane, fluroxene and cyclopropane on ventilation: A comparative study in man. Anesthesiology 27: 716, 1966

42. Larson CP, Eger EI II, Muallenn M, et al: The effect of diethyl ether and methoxyflurane on ventilation. Anesthesiology 30: 174, 1969

43. Calverley RK, Smith NT, Jones CW, et al: Ventilatory and cardiovascular effects of enflurane anesthesia during spontaneous ventilation in man. Anesth Analg 57: 610, 1978

44. Cullen DJ, Eger EI II: Cardiovascular effects of carbon dioxide in man. Anesthesiology 41: 345, 1974

45. Bahlman SH, Eger EI II, Halsey MJ, et al: The cardiovascular effects of halothane in man during spontaneous ventilation. Anesthesiology 36: 494, 1972

46. Tarhan S, Moffitt EA, Taylor WF, et al: Myocardial infarction after general anesthesia. JAMA 220: 1451, 1972

47. Goldman L, Caldera DL, Nussbaum SR, et al: Multifactorial index of cardiac risk in non cardiac surgical procedures. N Engl J Med 297: 845, 1977

48. Weiner DA, Ryan TJ, McCable CH, et al: Correlations between history and exercise ECG with coronary arteriography. N Engl J Med 301: 230, 1979

49. Cohn JN, Franciosa JA: Vasodilator therapy of cardiac failure. N Engl J Med 297: 27, 1977

50. Ljundquist A, Unge S: The finer intramyocardial vasculature in various forms of ex-

perimental canine hypertrophy. Acta Path Microbiol Scand [A] 80: 329, 1972

51. Shimosato S, Yasuda I, Kemmotsu O, et al: Effect of halothane on altered contractility of isolated heart muscle obtained from cats with exerimentally produced ventricular hypertrophy and failure. Br J Anaesth 45: 2, 1973.

52. Dauchot PJ, Rasmussen JP, Nicholson DH, et al: On-line systolic time intervals during anesthesia in patients with and without heart disease. Anesthesiology 44: 472, 1976

53. Viljoen JF, Estafanous FG, Kellner GA: Propranolol and cardiac surgery. J Thorac Cardiovasc Surg 64: 826, 1972

54. Jorfeldt L, Lofstromm B, Moller J, et al: Cardiovascular pharmacodynamics of propranolol during ether anaesthesia in man. Acta Anaesthesiol Scand 11: 159, 1967

55. Craythorne NWB, Huffington PE: Effects of propranolol on the cardiovascular response to cyclopropane and halothane. Anesthesiology 27: 580, 1966

56. Horan BF, Prys-Roberts C, Hamilton WK, et al: Haemodynamic responses to enflurane anaesthesia and hypovolemia in the dog, and their modification by propranolol. Br J Anesth 49: 1189, 1977

57. Roberts JG, Föex P, Clarke TNS, et al: Haemodynamic interaction of high-dose propranolol pretreatment and anaesthesia in the dog. III. The effect of hemorrhage during halothane and trichloroethylene anaesthesia. Br J Anaesth 48: 411, 1976

58. Saner CA, Föex P, Roberts JG, et al: Methoxyflurane and practalol: A dangerous combination? Br J Anaesth 47: 1025, 1975

59. Roberts JG, Föex P, Clarke TNS, et al: Haemodynamic interactions of high dose propranolol pretreatment and anaesthesia in the dog. I: Halothane dose-response study. Br J Anaesth 48: 315, 1976

60. Roberts JG, Föex P, Clarke TNS, et al: Haemodynamic interactions of high-dose propranolol pretreatment and anaesthesia in the dog. II: The effect of acute arterial hypoxemia at increasing depth of halothane anesthesia. Br J Anaesth 48: 403, 1976

61. Philbin DM, Lowenstein E: Lack of Beta-adrenergic activity of isoflurane in the dog: A comparison of circulatory effects of halothane and isoflurane after propranolol administration. Br J Anaesth 48: 1165, 1976

62. Weis KH, Brackenbush HD: On the cardiovascular effect of propranolol during halothane anaesthesia in normovolemic and hypovolemic dogs. Br J Anaesth 42: 272, 1970

63. Horan BF, Prys-Roberts C, Roberts JG, et al: Haemodynamic responses to isoflurane anaesthesia and hypovolemia in the dog and their modification by propranolol. Br J Anaesth 49: 1179, 1977

64. Stone JG, Faltas AN, Hoar PF: Sodium nitroprusside therapy for cardiac failure in anesthetized patients with valvular insufficiency. Anesthesiology 49: 414, 1978

65. Bland JHL, Lowenstein E: Halothane-induced decreases in experimental myocardial ischemia in the non-failing canine heart. Anesthesiology 45: 287, 1976

66. Johnson RR, Eger EI II, Wilson C: A comparative interaction of epinephrine with enflurane, isoflurane, and halothane in man. Anesth Analg 55: 709, 1976

67. Cullen DJ, Eger EI II: The effects of halothane on respiratory and cardiovascular responses to hypoxia in dogs: A dose response study. Anesthesiology 33: 487, 1970

68. Loarie DJ, Wilkinson P, Tyberg J, et al: The hemodynamic effects of halothane in anemic dogs. Anesth Analg 58: 195, 1979

69. Roizen MF, Horrigan RW: Anesthetic dose that blocks adrenergic response to incision. Anesthesiology 51: S141, 1979

13

Respiratory Pharmacology of Inhaled Anesthetic Agents

Edward G. Pavlin, M.D.

INTRODUCTION

Lung function may be augmented or diminished by the administration of pharmacologic agents. When choosing the appropriate therapeutic agent for treatment of pulmonary disease, systemic side effects of drugs are of major importance in determining our choice of therapy. Similarly, the choice of anesthetic agents may frequently be determined by the known side effects of these agents on various organ systems in the body. Although seldom administered primarily as pulmonary therapeutic drugs, inhaled agents may act at various sites in the central nervous system, airways, alveoli, and pulmonary vasculature. Knowledge of these pulmonary effects of what are primarily cerebral depressants is important in that lung function can be monitored and preserved in the face of anesthetic depression. In some circumstances, a particular pharmacologic action may determine the choice of anesthetic agent. For example, halothane is considered by many clinicians to be the most appropriate anesthetic for the asthmatic patient because of its bronchodilating qualities.

Since inhaled anesthetics pervade the whole body, pulmonary function may be affected by both direct and indirect actions. The line between "physiological" and "phar-macologic" effects may be very thin indeed. To avoid repetition of later chapters dealing with anesthesia and the lung, this chapter describes the more direct methods by which anesthetic gases and vapors alter the activities of various anatomic components of the lung. To this end, sections deal with airway resistance, pulmonary vascular caliber, mucociliary function, and ventilatory control. Although the latter involves discussion of receptors and the nervous system anatomically removed from the lung, dose-related depression of ventilation caused by anesthesia obviously is one of the most potent and important pulmonary "side effects."

EFFECTS ON BRONCHOMOTOR TONE

The increase in airway resistance observed during an acute asthmatic attack may be both frightening and potentially lethal. Although a universally accepted definition of "asthma" is difficult to enunciate, in this discussion it is considered to be a transient state of increased airway resistance caused at least in part by an increase in bronchiolar smooth muscle tone. This increased muscle tone occurs in patients who exhibit clinical manifestations of extrinsic or intrinsic asthma as well as in those with a pharmacologically reversible component of chronic obstructive lung disease. Indeed, with the proper stimulus, bronchospasm can occur in normal subjects who have no underlying history of lung disease of any kind. A mainstay of treatment is the administration of bronchodilating drugs. An excellent review of the mechanisms of action and clinical role of bronchodilating drugs has recently been published.[1] Because of legitimate concerns regarding anesthesia in these patients, the pharmacology of inhaled agents with respect to their effects on bronchial smooth muscle is of great clinical importance.

PHARMACOLOGY OF BRONCHIAL MUSCLE

Some consideration must be given to the basic physiology and pharmacology of airways before the effects of inhaled agents or other types of bronchodilating agents can be predicted or evaluated. The autonomic nervous system plays a key role in the control of bronchomotor tone both in normal airways and in those of patients with bronchospastic disease (Fig. 13-1).

Airway smooth muscle, which extends as far distally as the terminal bronchioles, is under the influence of both parasympathetic and sympathetic nerves. Vagal innervation of the bronchial tree has been well documented, and sympathetic innervation, though less well defined, probably plays a role as well. The effects of the autonomic nervous system are thought to be mediated through their action on the stores of cyclic AMP and cyclic GMP in bronchial smooth muscle cells. Acetylcholine, or stimulation by the vagus nerve, is thought to provide an increase in the amounts of cyclic GMP relative to cyclic AMP, leading to smooth muscle contraction (Fig. 13-1). Release of histamine in the airway or various forms of mechanical or chemical stimulation can result in an increase in afferent vagal activity with subsequent reflex bronchocon-striction. This increase in bronchomotor tone can be attenuated by atropine.

Adrenergic receptors in bronchial smooth muscle are classified into α and β types according to the classic description of Ahlquist.[2] While α receptors are in the bronchial tree in man, their activity seems to be low and clinically unimportant. The β receptors have been further refined into β_1 and β_2 types; the latter play the most significant role in bronchial muscle, while β_1 receptors appear to be of greater importance in modifying cardiac inotropic and chronotropic activity. Stimulation of β_2 receptors in bronchial smooth muscle, either by stimulation of sympathetic nerves or by the use of circulatory or topically applied agents possessing β_2 activity (e.g., epinephrine and isoproterenol), causes relaxation of bronchial smooth muscle. This is probably mediated by an increase within muscle cells in levels of cyclic AMP relative to cyclic GMP (see also Chs. 2 and 18). The result of these findings has been an increased interest in the formulation of β_2-specific drugs with potent bronchodilatory properties and a minimum of cardiac side effects (e.g., isoetharine, metaproterenol, terbutaline, salbutamol).

SPECIFIC INHALED ANESTHETICS

Since its clinical introduction in 1956 halothane has been recommended as the anesthetic of choice in the presence of bronchospasm because of its bronchodilating characteristics. In a retrospective study Shnider and Papper[3] found that in 49 patients with preanesthetic wheezing, halothane was clearly superior to ether, cyclopropane, ethylene, and regional anesthetic in decreasing this audible manifestation of bronchospasm. This study suffers from its retrospective design and the fact that a clinical sign, rather than objective measurements, was used to gauge the efficacy of anesthetic agents. Nonetheless, this and other earlier clinical obser-

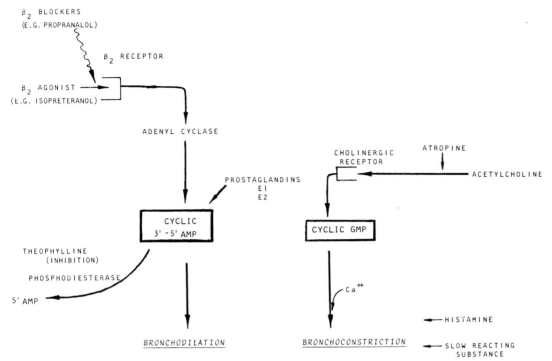

Fig. 13-1 Some aspects of sympathetic and parasympathetic control of bronchial smooth muscle tone. Not included are α-receptor mechanisms which may act by diminishing the level of cyclic 3'-5' AMP. Interference with Ca^{++} kinetics may be an important mechanism of bronchodilating action of some anesthetic agents.

vations[4] established halothane as the drug of choice for patients with either a history of asthma in the past or bronchospasm occurring during induction or maintenance of anesthesia.

The effects of inhaled agents on airway caliber have been studied in vivo. Colgan[5] noted a decrease in "bronchial distensibility" in dogs anesthetized with halothane, ether, methoxyflurane, or trichlorethylene, with halothane having the most pronounced effect. The effect of changes in functional residual capacity (FRC) during anesthesia and of unmeasured but probably varying levels of CO_2 on bronchomotor tone makes this study difficult to interpret. Subsequent to the Colgan study, it has been found that a reduction in PCO_2 in airways causes a reversible increase in airway resistance and that con-

versely, increasing levels of PCO_2 have a bronchodilating effect. Klide and Aviado[6] found a dose-dependent decrease in resting airway resistance with increasing concentrations of halothane in spontaneously ventilating dogs. Again, the possibility of bronchodilation secondary to an increased resting $PaCO_2$ with deeper planes of anesthesia was not taken into account. The authors showed that this apparent effect of halothane persisted in spite of attempts to decrease sympathetic nervous activity by sympathectomy, adrenalectomy, or treatment with reserpine, but was blocked by a β-blocking drug.

In isolated guinea-pig tracheal chains, halothane, diethyl ether, and thiopental caused relaxation of resting tone.[7] These drugs also attenuated tracheal muscle constriction induced by acetylcholine but only

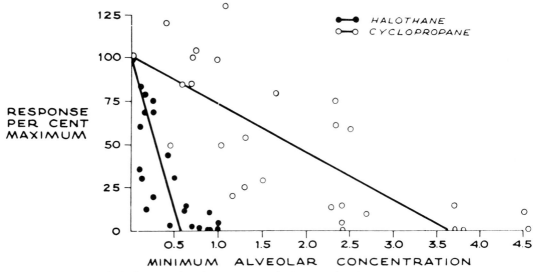

Fig. 13-2 Effects of halothane and cyclopropane on the increase in airway resistance produced by electrical stimulation of the vagus nerves of dogs. Closed circles are halothane; open circles represent cyclopropane. In the face of bronchial constriction produced by this particular stimulus, halothane appears to be a powerful bronchodilator and much more effective at equal anesthetic doses than cyclopropane. (Hickey RF, Graf PD, Nadel JA, et al: The effects of halothane and cyclopropane on total pulmonary resistance in the dog. Anesthesiology 31:334, 1969.)

halothane accomplished this in clinically relevant doses. In this instance, propranolol, a β-blocking drug, did not antagonize the relaxing properties of halothane on acetylcholine-induced bronchoconstriction, leading to a conclusion different from that of Klide and Aviado[6] regarding the β-receptor stimulating action of halothane.

Hickey et al.[8] demonstrated the importance of controlled levels of $PaCO_2$ in evaluating the effects of agents on bronchial smooth muscle tone. In anesthetized, intubated dogs whose ventilation was controlled to achieve a $PaCO_2$ of approximately 40 torr, increasing concentrations of halothane and cyclopropane produced no change in resistance in the resting unstimulated airway. In the unstimulated airway, resting tone may be minimal and therefore the bronchodilating properties of any drug may be masked because no additional relaxation of bronchial musculature can be effected. By inducing a state of increased bronchial tone by use of either hista-

mine administration or vagal stimulation, the superior bronchodilating qualities of halothane were well demonstrated when compared to cyclopropane at 1.5 minimal alveolar concentration (MAC) levels of anesthesia (Fig. 13-2). Halothane, enflurane, and methoxyflurane were found to reverse the bronchoconstricting effects of hypocapnia in vivo in the isolated left lower lobe of the dog,[9] with halothane again proving the most efficacious at lower doses. This effect was not blocked by propranolol. Again no change in unstimulated resting bronchial tone was detected after the administration of anesthetics or isoproterenol, a well-known β-agonist bronchodilator.

Bronchoconstriction produced by the methods described may not be directly comparable to that which occurs in the asthmatic patient. Recent investigations by Hirshman and Bergman[10] are exciting in that they have utilized dogs sensitized to ascaris antigen as an experimental testing model. Asthma was

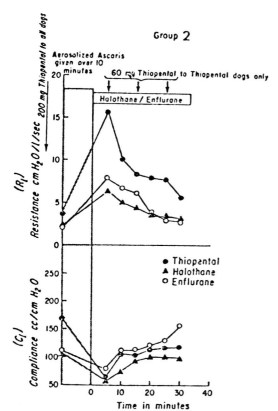

Fig. 13-3 The effect of halothane and enflurane on increased airway resistance in dogs; the airway resistance was triggered by prior administration of aerosolized ascaris. This is a model of extrinsic asthma. Although the allergic stimulus was not maintained throughout the experiment, both halothane and enflurane apear to lower airway resistance compared to the control thiopental-anesthetized animals. (Hirschman CA, Bergman NA: Halothane and enflurane protect against bronchospasm in an asthma dog model. Anesth Analg 57:629, 1978.)

induced by intratracheal administration of an aerosol of ascaris antigen. This model is perhaps more representative of the asthmatic patient with atopic bronchospasm.[11] These authors demonstrated attenuation of antigenically induced bronchospasm[10] by concentrations of approximately 1 MAC of either halothane or enflurane with no significant difference between the two agents (Fig. 13-3).

No attempt was made to describe a dose-response curve. The stimulus to bronchospasm was not continued throughout the administration of anesthetic gases, a condition that differs slightly from an "asthmatic" attack during anesthesia. Nonetheless, this is a useful model of the investigation of the bronchodilating qualities of these and other anesthetic agents.

Because of their bronchodilating effects, anesthetics, such as halothane, may be an effective method of treating status asthmaticus when other more conventional treatments have failed. However, documentation of this effectiveness is lacking. Gold and Helrich[12] evaluated the effect of halothane and tracheal intubation on six patients in status asthmaticus who had been treated for at least 72 hours with bronchodilators, steroids, and antibiotics. No significant change in airway resistance was recorded in either the anesthetic or immediate postanesthetic period. Cardiac arrhythmias proved to be of some concern during the halothane therapy. Although all six patients improved within 3 days after treatment, the lack of a similar control group makes interpretation difficult. The lack of any change in airway resistance and the appearance of ventricular arrhythmias indicate that halothane may not be effective in this patient group.

Patterson et al.[13] measured the resistive work of breathing during cardiopulmonary bypass and found that neither airway nor systemic administration of halothane caused significant changes in airway mechanics in the unstimulated state; however, the bronchoconstricting effects of low inhaled CO_2 mixtures were attenuated by inhaled halothane, but not by halothane administered via the blood. A similar experiment by Meloche et al.[14] demonstrated that administration of halothane did indeed decrease the bronchoconstriction produced by hypocapnia although not to the same extent as did the addition of 6.5 percent CO_2 to the inhaled mixture. That systemic administration of halothane via the bypass pump did not have

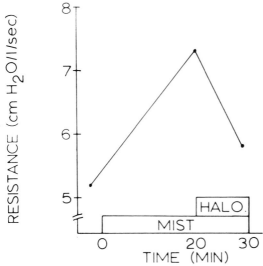

Fig. 13-4 The effect of halothane on increased respiratory resistance in man provoked by inhalation of ultrasonic mist. Halothane effectively decreased airway resistance triggered by the irritation of ultrasonic droplets. (Waltemath CL, Bergman NA: Effects of ketamine and halothane on increased respiratory resistance provoked by ultrasonic aerosols. Anesthesiology 41: 473, 1974.)

similar effects suggests that halothane acts directly on the airway musculature and/or local reflex arcs rather than via centrally controlled reflex pathways.

Measurements of resistances in normal man have generally failed to show a bronchodilatory effect of halothane.[15] This is perhaps not surprising, since some initial smooth muscle constriction would be necessary to subsequently demonstrate reversal by any pharmacologic agent. Provoking bronchoconstriction either by hypocapnia[16] or inhalation of ultrasonic aerosols[17] has allowed the demonstration of the potential of halothane and enflurane in reversing bronchoconstriction under some circumstances (Fig. 13-4). Since different stimuli may act on bronchomotor tone through different mechanisms, either centrally or directly, it does not necessarily follow that halothane will reverse bronchoconstriction from all causes. The value and effectiveness of enflurane relative

to halothane needs to be evaluated more thoroughly; the former agent offers the potential advantage of being less likely to induce cardiac arrhythmias in patients who frequently are receiving arrhythmia-provoking medications. Objective data showing decreases in airway resistance in asthmatic patients during inhalational anesthesia are lacking.

The use of more conventional bronchodilators in conjunction with anesthetics has not been extensively examined. Isoetharine was found to decrease severity of wheezing and peak airway pressure in 16 patients whose tracheas were intubated and who were anesthetized with different general anesthetics.[18] However, grading of the auscultatory changes was not done in a double-blind fashion. An excellent clinical study showed that a combination of subtoxic doses of aminophylline and isoetharine yielded greater relief of bronchospasm than either agent when used alone.[19] The risk of cardiac arrhythmias following bronchodilator administration simultaneously with inhaled anesthetic agents remains unknown for most agents.

MECHANISMS OF ACTION

The mechanisms by which various general anesthetics decrease bronchial smooth muscle tone have been reviewed by Aviado.[20] By far the most extensively examined agent has been halothane. Several sites of action have been proposed; reflex bronchoconstriction in response to airway irritants may be attenuated by the anesthetic state itself, either by a reduction in afferent nerve traffic or by central medullary depression of bronchoconstriction reflexes.

Klide and Aviado[6] suggested that halothane functions as a β-agonist in bronchial smooth muscle. They demonstrated a dose-related reduction in airway resistance in dogs anesthetized with halothane that was unaffected by reserpine, guanethidine, lung denervation, or adrenalectomy. They found that a β-blocking agent, sotalol, prevented halothane-induced bronchodilation, evidence that they felt supported the claim of a β-agonist activity of halothane. Conversely, Fletcher[7] found that perfusion with ether and halothane caused relaxation of guinea-pig tracheal smooth muscle stimulated by acetylcholine. Flecher[7] also found that propranolol had no effect on halothane's relaxant activity. Thus, halothane appears to have a direct relaxant effect that was effective against increases in muscle tension caused by either acetylcholine- or histamine-induced constriction. In other smooth muscle preparations with β-receptor sites, relaxation by halothane has not been attributed to β-adrenergic activity. Yang et al.[21] showed that halothane or epinephrine blocked acetylcholine-induced uterine smooth muscle contractions in an in vitro preparation. While addition of propranolol blocked the effect of epinephrine, the relaxant effect of halothane was unchanged. Halothane increased the tissue concentration of cyclic AMP, a substance known to cause smooth muscle relaxation. One possible mechanism of the salutory effects of halothane is through stimulation of adenylcyclase. Conversely, Klide et al.[22] found relaxation of rabbit uterine muscle induced by halothane was prevented by a β-blocking agent, sotalol. This work of Klide et al.[22] provides further evidence of β-agonist activity of halothane. However, solatol alone has been found to increase tone and motility of rabbit uterine muscle and lends some doubts to the validity of their conclusions. In a similar study, Sprague et al.[23] demonstrated that while halothane and isoflurane produced dose-dependent relaxation of rat aortic muscle strips, propanolol did not block this effect. Relaxation was associated with stimulation of cyclic AMP production in the absence of any change in phosphodiesterase activity.

In summary, inhaled anesthetics may act at several different sites in affecting bronchial smooth muscle relaxation. The direct action may involve the cyclic AMP mechanisms, although alternative actions on prostaglandins and Ca^{++} activity must be considered. While arguments for a specific β-agonist role of halothane exist, more recent data would suggest this is not the mechanism of halothane activity on smooth muscle mechanics.

CLINICAL IMPLICATIONS

The mechanisms by which increases in airway resistance may be stimulated have been summarized by Aviado.[20] Bronchospasm may occur in patients under conditions of disease other than asthma. Patients with chronic obstructive lung disease may present with elements of bronchospasm that contribute to their increased airway resistance, which may be discerned by demonstrating improvement in forced expiratory flow rates after administration of a bronchodilator. Normal healthy patients undergoing surgical stimulation of pulmonary arteries and parenchyma or trachea are known to be at risk of developing bronchospasm.[24] An isolated case report has described an episode of wheezing in a patient undergoing transurethral resection.[25] Indeed, in the lightly anesthetized patient clinically discernible bronchospasm is not an unusual event following surgical stimulation or irritation of the trachea by endotracheal tubes. In anticipating such events in patients with known reactive airway disease or in the unexpected episode of bronchospasm, the choice of preoperative medication, induction agent, muscle relaxant, and the type and dosage of anesthetic drug are important in minimizing clinical symptoms. The variety of studies previously described strongly suggest halothane as the anesthetic of choice. The high incidence of postanesthetic pulmonary complications in patients with chronic obstructive disease is well known. Studies of outcome with different anesthetic agents are not specific enough to evaluate the role of anesthetic drugs vis à vis effects on postoperative morbidity, airway resistance, or both. Thus, more objective studies are needed to evaluate effects of various inhaled agents in patients who are at high risk of developing bronchospasm in the perioperative period.

EFFECTS ON PULMONARY VASCULAR RESISTANCE

Interest in the pulmonary vasculature, sometimes referred to as "the lesser circulation," has increased geometrically over the past 15 years. Techniques for easy measurement of pulmonary blood flow (cardiac output) and pulmonary vascular pressures have become commonplace. The role of the pulmonary vasculature in various disease states and its reaction to drugs has spurred much interest.

DETERMINANTS OF PULMONARY VASCULAR RESISTANCE

The role of pharmacologic agents in determining pulmonary vascular pressures and resistances is a complicated one, since many vasoactive agents have both direct effects on pulmonary blood vessels as well as indirect effects through alterations of cardiac output and pulmonary blood flow. Changes in pulmonary vascular resistance (PVR) and pressure may have significant effects on gas or fluid exchange in the lung. Increased pulmonary vascular resistance may give rise to an increase in pulmonary artery pressure if cardiac output is maintained constant and thereby promote increased transudation of fluid into the interstitium of the lung. Conversely, increased resistance may cause sufficient impedance to the output of the right ventricle that cardiac output and pulmonary blood flow are reduced.

Regional changes in pulmonary vascular resistance may alter the relative distribution of blood flow within the lung leading to altered ventilation-perfusion relationships and accompanying changes in gas exchange. Thus, a localized increase in PVR in an area of atelectasis may cause a shift of blood flow away from the atelectic segment to better-ventilated regions of lung and therefore ultimately lead to improved gas exchange by decreasing blood flow to non-ventilated lung.

The increase in pulmonary vascular resistance in an area of atelectasis is believed to be partially due to localized tissue hypoxia. This phenomenon, termed hypoxic vasoconstriction, has been of considerable interest to pulmonary physiologists recently because of its importance in determining the magnitude of the effects of diseased and/or nonventilated areas of lung on gas exchange and $PaCO_2$. Hypoxic vasoconstriction appears to have protective value, and drugs that interfere with this "protective" mechanism may adversely affect gas exchange. Many of the commonly used agents in anesthesia are included in the list of offenders.

Pulmonary vascular resistance can be altered by several mechanisms. Passive changes in the diameter of the pulmonary blood vessels may be induced by increased cardiac output (increased pulmonary blood flow) or by elevations of left atrial pressure or by both. The increased vascular distending pressure may cause an increase in cross-sectional diameter of the pulmonary vascular bed and hence a fall in pulmonary vascular resistance. Similarly, changes in lung volume may alter the dimensions of the vasculature and hence affect resistance. Increases of lung volume above FRC caused by increased pressure in the airway are characteristically associated with passive increases in pulmonary vascular resistance; the latter are presumably caused by transmission of the higher alveolar pressures to blood vessels located in alveolar walls. On the other hand, reduction in lung volumes below normal FRC is also associated with passive increases in pulmonary vascular resistance. The latter are thought to be the result of a reduction in vascular dimensions as the lung shrinks. At low lung volumes, vessels are both shorter and narrower, apparently because of loss of a tethering effect of surrounding lung tissue. Additionally, vessels may become tortuous and crinkled at lower lung volumes. The net effect of these changes is a rise in pulmonary vascular resistance. It is of interest that resistance in the pulmonary circuit appears to be least at normal FRC.

Active changes in pulmonary vascular tone may also contribute to the level of resistance in the lesser circulation. These may be induced by changes in sympathetic tone, by local changes in PO_2 and/or PCO_2, or by changes in levels of catecholamines or other vasoactive substances released locally or in blood perfusing the lung. The pulmonary vasoconstrictor response to hypoxia, hypercarbia, or both is of interest in that it is opposite to that observed in most systemic vascular beds. Many anesthetic drugs tend to reduce lung volume[26] and, therefore, may have additional effects on pulmonary vascular resistance through this mechanism as well.

A complete description of the ways in which anesthetic agents may alter PVR is well beyond the scope of this chapter. We confine ourselves to the much narrower question of how anesthetic agents may alter pulmonary vascular resistance with particular emphasis on the direct effects of anesthetic agents on hypoxic vasoconstriction. The effect of inhaled anesthetic agents on pulmonary blood flow and pulmonary artery pressure in man without significant underlying pulmonary abnormality is small. In general, the more potent agents such as halothane and ethrane simultaneously produce a decrease in PVR and an increase in left atrial pressure.[27, 28] The net effect is usually little or no change in pulmonary artery pressure and a small decrease in pulmonary blood flow. Nitrous oxide and ether have less effect on cardiac output and, therefore, pulmonary blood flow is relatively unaffected. Overall, changes in PVR are small, tending to rise slightly during anesthetic administration.

HYPOXIC PULMONARY VASOCONSTRICTOR RESPONSE

The hypoxic pulmonary vasoconstrictor response is believed to be mediated locally. The demonstration of this response in isolated perfused lungs reflects the local nature of this reflex. Furthermore, a similar response may be elicited in animals whose catecholamines have been depleted by reserpine or following α-adrenergic blockade. The sympathetic nervous system may, however, play a role in augmenting the response in certain circumstances, particularly those in the presence of systemic hypoxemia. Sympathetic innervation of the pulmonary vasculature may play a role in mediating some types of pulmonary edema (e.g., neurogenic). Stimulation of the peripheral chemoreceptor by hypoxemia or hypercarbia produces reflex changes in the systemic circulation.[29] Increases of blood pressure and heart rate also stimulate a reflex sympathetic response. Similarly, pulmonary arterial pressure rises secondary to increased pulmonary vascular resistance, which is believed caused principally by increased pulmonary arteriolar tone. Pulmonary venular constriction may also occur but this has not been well established. Arteriolar constriction occurs in response to decreased oxygen tension in the alveolus. Acidosis also appears to be a pulmonary vasoconstrictor both in intact animals as well as in isolated perfused lungs.[30] With normal alveolar oxygen tensions, changes in pulmonary vascular resistance in response to acidosis are small, but in the presence of alveolar hypoxia they are greatly enhanced.[31] Thus, vasoconstriction may be augmented by elevations in arterial hydrogen ion concentration, alveolar PCO_2 or both. The local mediator of the response to hypoxia and acidosis has not been identified.

The vasoconstrictor response of the pulmonary circulation to hypoxemia and acidosis is different from that of the systemic vasculature and appears to be suited to matching of lung perfusion to ventilation. Thus hypoxic areas of the lung, because of local pulmonary vasoconstrictor reflexes, have reduced blood flow with a shift of blood flow to the better ventilated (less hypoxic and acidotic) areas of the lung. This selective redistribution of blood away from the poorly ventilated areas has been shown to decrease alveolar-arterial oxygen tension gradients $(P(A-a)O_2)$.[32] The obliteration of this response by infusion of a pulmonary vasodilator, such as nitroprusside, has been shown to decrease arterial PO_2 and increase pulmonary shunting in dogs with oleic acid–induced pulmonary edema.[33]

INHALED AGENTS AND HYPOXIC PULMONARY VASOCONSTRICTION

A decrease in PaO_2 and an increase in $P(A-a)O_2$ has been frequently described during general anesthesia. Many mechanisms exist by which this decrease in oxygenation may take place. Earlier explanations centered mostly on the effect of anesthesia on lung mechanics. Such effects as progressive pulmonary atelectasis, and diminishment of functional residual capacity relative to closing capacity of the lung have been just two of the mechanisms suggested. In 1964 Buckely et al.[34] suggested that the local pulmonary vasoconstriction in response to hypoxia might be attenuated by halothane anesthesia. Since that time the effect of numerous inhaled anesthetics on hypoxic vasoconstriction (HPV) have been examined in a variety of animals and experimental models. Many of the studies have produced conflicting results regarding the effects of certain anesthetic agents, particularly halothane. A summary of experiments and results in this area are shown in Table 13-1.

Sykes et al.[35] examined the effects of halothane and other anesthetic agents on the HPV response in isolated perfused cat lungs. The lungs of cats were surgically isolated and perfused with oxygen-saturated blood using a nonpulsatile continuous flow technique. At constant flow rate and left atrial pressure, a rise in mean pulmonary artery pressure occurred in response to ventilation with a hypoxic gas mixture; this response was attenuated by halothane. These experiments have been criticized because the control response of pulmonary artery pressure to alveolar hypoxia decreased with time to a degree similar to that occurring during halothane anesthesia. This deterioration of hypoxic vasoconstrictive response makes quantification of the effect of inhaled anesthetics a difficult task. The apparently dose-related effect of anesthetic agents studied is also difficult to evaluate since blood or alveolar levels of halothane, trichlorethylene, and ether were not measured. These experiments were repeated in cat lungs in which sympathetic nervous innervation was preserved.[36] Under these conditions, HPV was diminished by halothane only at inspired concentrations of 3 percent or greater. It is significant that in these latter experiments, there was no evidence that the hypoxic vasopressor response deteriorated with time as had been found by the previous investigations. Again, alveolar (end-expired) concentrations of anesthetic agent were not measured and, therefore, the true alveolar concentration of halothane was unknown. Thus, although the effect of halothane on hypoxic pulmonary constriction appeared to be attenuated in this model as compared to the isolated denervated cat lung, it is difficult to compare equianesthetic doses of anesthetic because the alveolar concentrations were unknown. However, in studies which used isolated rat lungs halothane also attenuated the response of pulmonary artery pressure to hypoxic alveolar gas mixtures.[37] Further conflicting experimental data exists in a series of studies performed on dogs.[38] Benumof and Wahrenbrock[39] tested the hypothesis that halogenated anesthetics and nitrous oxide cause local inhibition of hy-

Table 13-1. Effects of Inhaled Agents on Airway Resistance (Raw)

Anesthetic Agent	Reference	Model	Measurement	Effect*
Halothane	Shnider & Papper[3]	Human—(retrospective)	Wheezing	++
	Waltemath & Bergman[17]	Human—normal	Raw	0
	Brakensiek & Bergman[15]	Human—bronchospasm (aerosol)	Raw	++
	Hickey et al.[8]	Dog—bronchospasm (vagus, histamine)	Raw	++
	Coon & Kampine[9]	Dog—LL Lobe bronchoconstriction ($\downarrow CO_2$)	Raw	++
	Klide & Aviado[6]	Dog—normal	Raw	++
	Fletcher et al.[7]	G. Pig—isolated tracheal muscle	Length	++
	Gold & Helrich[12]	Human—status asthmaticus	Raw	0
	Meloche et al.[14]	Human—C.-P. Bypass bronchoconstriction ($\downarrow CO_2$)	Raw	0
	Colgan[5]	Dog—normal	"Bronchial distensibility"	0
	Hirshman & Bergman[10]	Dog—bronchospasm (ascaris)	Raw	++
Diethyl Ether	Shnider & Papper[3]	Human—(restrospective)	Wheezing	+
Cyclopropane	Hickey et al.[8]	Dog—bronchospasm (histamine, vagus)	Raw	+
	Colgan[5]	Dog—normal	"Bronchial distensibility"	0
Enflurane	Coon & Kampine[9]	Dog—LL Lobe bronchoconstriction ($\downarrow CO_2$)	Raw	+
	Hirshman & Bergman[10]	Dog—bronchospasm (ascaris)	Raw	++
Methoxyflurane	Coon & Kampine[9]	Dog—LL Lobe bronchoconstriction ($\downarrow CO_2$)	Raw	+

* Symbols used: + + = pronounced bronchodilation; + = bronchodilation; 0 = no effect.

poxic pulmonary vasoconstriction. Their experimental design consisted of isolating the left lower lobe of a dog and selectively ventilating this lobe with hypoxic gas mixtures containing MAC multiples of inhaled anesthetics. The remainder of the lung was ventilated with 100 percent oxygen. The effect on pulmonary vasculature resistance was assessed by the measurement of blood flow to the isolated lobe, by use of an electromagnetic flowmeter, and comparing it to total pulmonary blood flow. With constant pulmonary blood flow (cardiac output), pulmonary artery pressure, and left atrial pressure, a significant decrease in flow to the isolated left lower lobe was found in the presence of localized alveolar hypoxia. The administration of halothane or nitrous oxide did not diminish the magnitude of the hypoxic vasoconstrictive response (Fig. 13-5), although a profound dose related effect could be demonstrated in the presence of fluroxene and isoflurane (Fig.

13-6). The investigators then repeated these experiments[40] but administered the anesthetic agent to the whole animal as well as to the isolated lung segment. In this preparation, cardiac output was diminished by halothane, isoflurane, and enflurane but the effects on blood flow to the isolated segment were almost identical to those obtained when administration of anesthetic agent was confined to the isolated lobe alone. Halothane at levels up to 2 MAC did not significantly interfere with hypoxic vasoconstriction of the test lobe, while isoflurane, enflurane, and fluroxene did lessen the vasoconstrictive effect of hypoxemia.

Sykes et al.[38] examined the effects of alveolar hypoxia in one lung on the relative distribution of pulmonary blood flow between both lungs. Blood-flow distribution was measured using xenon 133 in dogs whose tracheas were intubated with a double lumen tube permitting independent ventilation of

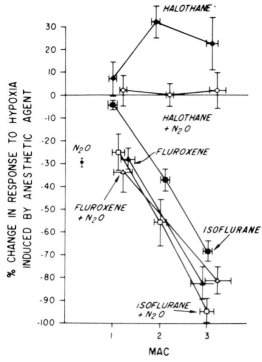

Fig. 13-5 The effect of anesthetic agents on the hypoxia-induced increase in pulmonary vascular resistance of an isolated left lower lobe of the dog. Zero on the vertical axis represents the normal distribution of pulmonary blood flow between the hypoxic left lower lobe and the remainder of the lung. A negative percentage change represents a decrease in the hypoxia-induced pulmonary vasoconstriction of the nitrogen-ventilated left lower lobe. In this preparation, halothane seems to have little effect on pulmonary vasoconstriction, but fluroxene, nitrous oxide, and isoflurane exhibit a dose dependent decrease in hypoxic vasoconstriction. (Benumof JL, Wahrenbrock, EA: Local effects of anesthetics on regional hypoxic pulmonary vasoconstriction. Anesthesiology 43:525, 1975.)

each lung. One lung was ventilated with nitrogen while the other lung was ventilated with 100 percent oxygen. The PaO$_2$ was greater than 100 torr. A significant redistribution of flow to the well-oxygenated lung was found, which is evidence of a brisk hypoxic vasoconstrictive response. This redistribution of pulmonary blood flow was pre-served in the presence of halothane at inspired concentrations of up to 3 percent. The preparation was substantially different, of course, from the isolated cat lung experiments, and this might account for the different results observed. However, substantial reduction in hypoxic vasoconstrictive responses have been demonstrated with other anesthetic agents. Indeed, Sykes et al.[41] in the same preparation demonstrated that ether profoundly affected the redistribution of pulmonary blood flow in response to hypoxia (Fig. 13-7). Fargas-Babjak and Forrest[42] also found that the increases in pulmonary vascular resistance in a nitrogen-ventilated lung were affected by inhalation of 1.5 percent halothane. Alveolar concentrations of halothane were not measured, however, and cardiac output was substantially reduced when compared to the unanesthetized state.

In the only study of the effects of anesthetic agents on the phenomenon in man, Bjertnaes[43] examined the effects of diethyl ether and halothane on the distribution of pulmonary blood flow. In these human subjects, the trachea was intubated with a Carlens double lumen tube. Each lung was then ventilated by use of a separate anesthetic machine. Distribution of blood flow was assessed by lung-perfusion scan on two separate occasions following the injection of macroaggregated serum albumin labelled with two different radioisotopes. While one lung was ventilated with oxygen the test lung was ventilated with nitrogen only; equal end-expiratory carbon dioxide concentrations were maintained in both lungs. Hypoxic vasoconstriction was demonstrated in the nitrogen-ventilated lung during intravenous anesthesia with barbiturates. This vasoconstrictive response disappeared with the inhalation of either halothane or diethyl ether in the N$_2$ ventilated lungs. Abolishment of the HPV response was accompanied in most patients by a decrease in PaO$_2$. The method of measurement precluded the ability to demonstrate a return of hypoxic vasoconstriction to its former level following the withdrawal of the inhaled anes-

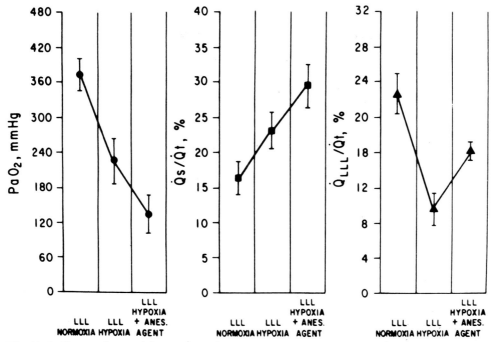

Fig. 13-6 Changes in arterial oxygen tension (PaO_2), physiological shunt ($\dot{Q}s/\dot{Q}t$), and the percentage of the cardiac output perfusing the left lower lobe ($\dot{Q}_{LLL}/\dot{Q}t$) during the ventilation of the left lower lobe with nitrogen which resulted in pulmonary artery vasoconstriction of the left lower lobe. The right hand box of each graph illustrates the effect of adding an anesthetic agent (2 to 3 MAC fluroxene or isoflurane) to the hypoxic left lower lobe. PaO_2 decreases with nitrogen ventilation of the left lower lobe but perfusion is decreased by the hypoxic vasoconstrictive response. The addition of fluroxane and isoflurane increases the relative perfusion of the hypoxic left lower lobe causing an increase in physiological shunting and a further decrease in PaO_2. (Benumof JL, Wahrenbrock EA: Local effects of anesthetics on regional hypoxic pulmonary vasoconstriction. Anesthesiology 43:525, 1975.)

thetic. In addition, pulmonary artery and left atrial pressures were not measured and it is known that changes in left atrial pressure may alter the pulmonary vascular response to hypoxia.[44]

The observed variations in response to administration of halothane may in part be due to species differences as well as to differences in experimental protocols. While diethyl ether has been found to have a profound effect on diminishing hypoxic pulmonary vasoconstriction in all models tested, the pulmonary vascular response to inhalation of nitrous oxide has been as varied as that measured during the administration of halothane.

Sykes demonstrated in isolated cat lung[45] and in dog lung[41] that nitrous oxide appeared to attenuate hypoxic pulmonary vasoconstriction. Other investigators have shown little or no effect from the addition of nitrous oxide to inhaled gas mixtures.[39] The effects of other less commonly used anesthetic agents are summarized in Table 13-2.

The mechanism by which some anesthetic agents appear to interfere with the pulmonary vasoconstrictor responses to hypoxia remains as yet a mystery. If in fact pulmonary vascular smooth muscle responds to locally accumulated tissue metabolites, then anesthetic agents may be acting by interfering with the

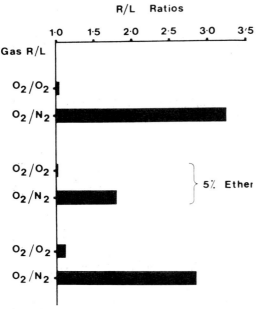

Fig. 13-7 The effect of diethyl ether anesthesia on the distribution of pulmonary blood flow between the right and left lungs of the dog. Ventilation of the left lung with nitrogen directs the blood flow to the opposite lung, thus increasing the right to left ratio of flow. This response is depressed during the administration of 5 percent diethyl ether. The hypoxic pulmonary vasoconstrictive response returns after the withdrawal of ether anesthesia. (Sykes MK, Hurtig JB, Tait, AR, et al: Reduction of hypoxic pulmonary vasoconstriction during diethyl ether anesthesia in the dog. Br J Anaesth 49:293, 1977.

metabolic production of these vasoactive substances. It is possible that anesthetics that have a direct relaxing effect on vascular smooth muscles may counteract locally or systemically mediated vasoconstrictive responses. Interference with calcium uptake by smooth muscle has also been suggested as one possible mechanism whereby anesthetics may interfere with smooth muscle constriction. Similarly, increases in vascular tone in healthy lung caused by specific anesthetic agents or methods of ventilation might in-

crease pulmonary vascular resistance in normal lung segments and thereby cause a redistribution of blood flow to the diseased lung.

One of the important factors involved in modulating the effects of hypoxic vasoconstriction may be the overall level of pulmonary artery pressure. Thus high pulmonary artery pressures, by increasing vascular distending pressure, may tend to cause passive distention of constricted vascular beds and thereby tend to reverse hypoxic vasoconstriction. Similarly, reflex pulmonary and systemic vasoconstriction in response to stimuli such as hypotension may increase pulmonary vascular resistance in healthy lung segments again leading to a shift of blood flow to the diseased or "hypoxic" areas of lung. The net effect of anesthetic agents on HPV obviously depends upon a number of other factors that commonly occur during surgery and anesthesia.

Clinically, despite some variation in experimental results, the effect of anesthetic agents on the pulmonary vasculature must be taken into account as one possible factor when considering the causes of hypoxemia under anesthesia. Although changes in distribution may account for some of these problems, attenuation of the hypoxic vasoconstrictor response may have a significant influence on PaO_2. In dogs with oleic acid–induced pulmonary edema, quite remarkable reversible increases in pulmonary shunting have been demonstrated by the administration of pulmonary vasodilators such as nitroprusside[33] and nitroglycerin.[46] Some anesthetic agents probably produce a similar response in patients with adult respiratory distress syndrome or with other types of pulmonary pathology associated with large right-to-left intrapulmonary shunts. The most likely effect of the various anesthetic agents in these patients remains to be defined. The selection of the appropriate type of anesthetic drugs may be of great importance in minimizing arterial hypoxemia in patients with wide alveolar to arterial oxygen tension

Table 13-2. Effects of Inhaled Agents on Hypoxic Pulmonary Vasoconstriction (HPV)

Anesthetic Agent	Reference	Model	Effect
Halothane	Buckley et al.[34]	Dog—5% O_2 whole lung	Inhibit
	Kaur et al.[98]	Dog—10% O_2 whole lung	None
	Benumof & Wahrenbrock[39]	Dog—N_2 LL Lobe	None
	Mathers et al.[40]	Dog—N_2 LL Lobe	None
	Sykes et al.[35]	Cat—3% O_2 isolated lung	Inhibit
	Bjertnaes et al.[37]	Rat—2% O_2 isolated lung	Inhibit
	Loh et al.[36]	Cat—3% O_2 innervated lung	Inhibit
	Sykes et al.[38]	Dog—whole lung	None
	Fargas-Babjak & Forrest[42]	Dog—8% O_2 whole lung	None
	Bjertnaes[43]	Human—N_2 one lung	Inhibit
Ether	Sykes et al.[35]	Cat—3% O_2 isolated lung	Inhibit
	Sykes et al.[41]	Dog—N_2 left lung	Inhibit
	Loh et al.[36]	Cat—3% O_2 innervated lung	Inhibit
	Bjertnaes[43]	Human—N_2 one lung	Inhibit
	Bjertnaes et al.[37]	Rat—2% O_2 isolated lung	Inhibit
Trichlorethylene	Sykes et al.[35]	Cat—3% O_2 isolated lung	Inhibit
	Sykes et al.[99]	Dog—N_2 one lung	Inhibit
Nitrous oxide	Buckley et al.[34]	Dog—5% O_2 whole lung	Enhanced
	Sykes et al.[41]	Dog—N_2 one lung	Inhibit
	Hurtig et al.[45]	Cat—3% O_2 isolated lung	Inhibit
	Mathers et al.[40]	Dog—N_2 LL Lobe	Inhibit (slight)
	Benumof & Wahrenbrock[39]	Dog—N_2 LL Lobe	None
	Bjertnaes et al.[37]	Rat—2% O_2 isolated lung	None
Fluroxene	Benumof & Wahrenbrock[39]	Dog—N_2 LL Lobe	Inhibit
	Mathers et al.[40]	Dog—N_2 LL Lobe	Inhibit
Methoxyflurane	Sykes et al.[35]	Cat—3% O_2 isolated lung	Inhibit
	Bjertnaes et al.[37]	Rat—2% O_2 isolated lung	Inhibit
Isoflurane	Benumof & Wahrenbrock[39]	Dog—N_2 LL Lobe	Inhibit
	Mathers et al.[40]	Dog—N_2 LL Lobe	Inhibit
Enflurane	Mathers et al.[40]	Dog—N_2 LL Lobe	None
Cyclopropane	Tait et al.[100]	Cat—3% O_2 isolated lung	None

differences. More work needs to be done, particularly in humans, before the effect of a particular anesthetic agent can be predicted.

EFFECTS ON MUCOCILIARY FUNCTION

NORMAL MUCOCILIARY FUNCTION

The clearance of mucus from the respiratory tract is an important defense mechanism of the lungs. Foreign particulate matter as well as the "debris" of pulmonary infection are removed by the upward and outward flow of mucus. Ciliated respiratory epithelium is located throughout the respiratory tract and extends distally as far as the terminal bronchioles,[47] although the density of such cells decreases from trachea to alveoli.[48] Mucus-producing cells (goblet and submucous glands) are similarly distributed.[49] The peculiar pattern of ciliary motion has been established for some time and is consistent through various kinds of species. A rapid stroke in a cephalad direction is followed by a slower recovery stroke in the opposite direction. The

Table 13-3. Effects of Inhaled Agents on Mucociliary Function

Function	Anesthetic Agent	Reference	Model	Effect*
Ciliary Function	Halothane	Nunn et al.[64]	Protozoa	−−
	Halothane	Manawadu et al[65]	Dog—tracheal culture	−
	Ether, Methoxyflurane	Nunn et al.[64]	Protozoa	−−
	Trichlorethylene	Nunn et al.[64]	Protozoa	−−
Mucociliary Flow	Halothane	Forbes[61]	Dog—intact	−−
	Halothane	Forbes & Horrigan[62]	Dog—intact	−−
	Halothane, Nitrous oxide	Lichtiger et al.[60]	Human	−−
	Enflurane	Forbes & Horrigan[62]	Dog—intact	−−
	Nitrous oxide, Morphine	Forbes & Horrigan[62]	Dog—intact	−
	Ether	Forbes & Horrigan[62]	Dog—intact	0
Mucociliary Clearance	Halothane	Forbes & Gamsu[63]	Dog—intact	−−
	Ether	Forbes & Gamsu[63]	Dog—intact	−−

* Symbols used: −− = pronounced depression; − = depression; 0 = no effect.

movement of cilia occurs in a coordinated fashion; movement of distal cilia are followed closely by like movements of those immediately proximal; the resulting wave of motion is referred to as metachromism.[50] The mechanism by which this coordination occurs has not been elucidated. In mammals, the sympathetic and parasympathetic nervous systems appear to play no role in the coordination of ciliary movement. The bending of individual cilia appears to be the result of an ATP-dependent sliding of two parallel fibers within the ciliary filament.

Mucus represents a mixture of water, electrolytes, and macromolecules (lipids, mucins, enzymes) secreted by goblet cells and mucosal glands. Mucous secretions appear to provide a medium for entrapping and carrying foreign material and dead cells as well as for influencing the movement of the cilia. The "blanket" of mucus interacts with cilia and influences the rate and efficiency of ciliary movement. For instance, thicker layers of mucus appear to slow the removal of surface articles from the airway. The rheologic properties of mucus are very important and influence mucociliary function with high elasticity and low viscosity appearing to be the characteristics required to promote the fastest trans-

port by cilia.[51] The presence and characteristics of the mucous layer may also promote the coordination of ciliary beats.

METHODS OF MEASUREMENT OF MUCOCILIARY FUNCTION

Various methods have been used experimentally to assess mucociliary function in both normal animals and in man and to examine the effect of airway disease and drugs (Table 13-3). Determination of the beat frequency of cilia is one such method. The movement of cilia are examined optically by uses of a microscope and high speed photography. This has usually been accomplished in vitro, using either single cilia or tissue cultures of respiratory epithelium. In vivo techniques in animals have made use of a tracheal window, but in vivo measurements in man would obviously pose some difficulty. The physical and chemical characteristics of mucus have also been studied extensively by Reed.[52] Since these studies have been done on expectorated specimens, the characteristics may differ from the situation in vivo because of contamination by salivary secretions and desiccation of expectorated secretions.

Techniques more applicable to man include the measurement of movement of markers placed in the airway. One type of measurement, that of mucus velocity, involves the placement of radioactive markers in the airway followed by a measurement (utilizing external scintillation counters) of the velocity of movement of these particles in a cephalad direction. This measurement is confined to the examination of mucus velocity in the trachea. Sackner et al.[53] have developed a method of determining mucus velocity through a fiberoptic bronchoscope. A second group of measurements assessing mucociliary clearance involves the deposition of radiopaque or radioactive particles throughout the lung fields followed by sequential radiographic examinations of clearance of these inhaled particles. This allows an examination of mucociliary function in both peripheral as well as central airways. Coughing may enhance the rate of removal thus contributing to errors in measurements.

SPECIFIC EFFECTS

Postoperative hypoxemia and atelectasis are common findings in patients who have undergone anesthesia and surgery. Although many physiological derangements may contribute to pulmonary complications (e.g., airway closure and decreased functional residual capacity), the role of inhibited mucociliary function has sparked some recent interest and investigation. Gamsu et al.[54] compared the rate of tantalum clearance from the lungs of two groups of postoperative patients who had received general anesthesia with that of a control group consisting of awake patients undergoing tracheography following topical application of local anesthetic to the pharynx and trachea. One group of patients, who underwent orthopedic procedures, showed no significant differences from the control group. In contrast, in patients following intra-abdominal vascular surgery, retention of tantalum was demonstrated for as long as 6 days, with an average retention time threefold greater than in the control group. Retention of tantalum was correlated with the retention of mucus demonstrated in areas of atelectasis. Disappearance of tantalum from these areas of atelectasis occurred only after reexpansion of collapsed segments of lung.

The role of anesthesia in mucus retention must be viewed with caution because many other factors may affect and diminish mucociliary function, particularly in the mechanically ventilated patient. Extensive literature exists demonstrating the importance of maintenance of a high relative humidity of inspired gases on optimum mucociliary transport. Thus, dry inspired gases may both decrease ciliary beat frequency as well as cause a drying out of the mucous layer. In dogs, mucus flow rates measured by the rate of movement of a radioactive marker in the trachea were found to be maintained at normal rates for a 40 minute period if inspired air temperature was greater than 32 °C with an inspired water vapor content of 33 mg/L.[55] A similar study demonstrated a complete cessation of flow of tracheal mucus after 3 hours of inhalation of dry air.[56] Mucus movement could be reinstituted by restoring inspired gases to a 100 percent relative humidity at 38 °C. Other factors diminishing the rate of mucus movement are high inspired oxygen concentration,[57] inflation of the endotracheal tube cuff,[58] and positive pressure ventilation.[59] One must take these factors into account in assessing any study examining the effects of anesthetics per se.

In a study of tracheal mucus velocity in young anesthetized women undergoing gynecological surgery, Lichtiger et al.[60] used a technique of placement of Teflon discs on the tracheal mucosa; the discs were then observed and filmed through the lens of a fiberoptic bronchoscope. Control values in awake volunteers had revealed a tracheal mucus velocity of 20 mm/min. Induction of anesthesia with halothane (1 to 2 percent) and nitrous oxide (60 percent) decreased the rate of

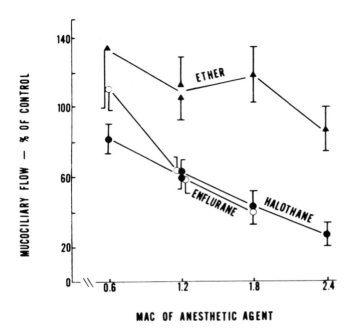

Fig. 13-8 Effects of various MAC levels of halothane, enflurane, and ether on mucociliary flow rates in dog tracheas. Each value is a mean ± SE expressed as a percentage of the thiopental control. Note the dose-dependent depression of mucus velocity with enflurane and halothane anesthesia. (Forbes AR, Horrigan RW: Mucociliary flow in the trachea during anesthesia with enflurane, ether, nitrous oxide, and morphine. Anesthesiology 46:319, 1977.)

mucus travel to 7.7 mm/min with little or no motion being seen by 90 minutes of anesthesia. Inspired gases were humidified but the presence of higher than normal FiO_2, the use of a cuffed endotracheal tube, and the maintenance of ventilation by use of positive pressure could all have contributed to this dysfunction as well as the anesthetic.

In a study in which temperature and humidity of inspired gases and endotracheal tube cuff pressure were well controlled, Forbes[61] measured the effect of halothane anesthesia on mucociliary flow. Utilizing external scintillation counters to measure the progression of radioactive droplets placed in the trachea, a dose-related depressant effect of halothane was found on this measurement of mucociliary function. Further studies showed a similar depressant effect in response to anesthesia with equipotent doses of enflurane and of nitrous oxide with halothane or nitrous oxide with narcotic anesthesia.[62] Conversely, ether anesthesia did not affect the velocity of mucus movement at concentrations of up to 2.4 MAC (Fig. 13-8).

Utilizing a different measure of mucociliary function—that of clearance of tantalum from the peripheral and central airways of anesthetized, intubated, mechanically ventilated dogs—Forbes and Gamsu[63] showed a delayed clearance of mucus both during and after 6 hours of anesthesia with halothane or ether at concentrations of 1.2 MAC. The dysfunction occurred in both peripheral and central airways and persisted for 6 hours or more after the cessation of anesthesia. It is not readily apparent why ether should cause slowing of tantalum clearance whereas mucus velocity in central airways was apparently not affected.[62] These same authors[62] have recently found that controlled ventilation with O_2 in barbiturate-anesthetized dogs decreased tantalum clearance to approximately 50 percent of rates in awake spontaneously ventilating controls. Since mechanical ventilation was utilized in the previously mentioned studies, its interaction with general anesthesia is unclear. Certainly the dose-related effects of halothane speak to a primary influence of halothane per se on mucus velocity.[62]

The mechanisms by which inhaled anesthetics diminish rates of mucous clearance are unknown. This could be accomplished by

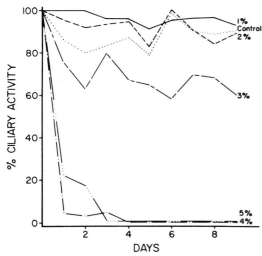

Fig. 13-9 In a culture of dog tracheal ring, ciliary activity is diminished by high doses of halothane. (Manawadu BR, Mostow SR, LaForce FM: Impairment of tracheal ring ciliary activity by halothane. Anesth Analg 58:500, 1979.)

diminishing ciliary beat frequency or by altering the characteristics or quantity of mucus produced during the anesthetized period. Nunn et al.[64] found dose-related decreases of ciliary activity and cellular mobility of the ciliated protozoan *Tetrahymena pyriformis* by exposure to six inhalational anesthetics including halothane. The ED_{50} for cessation of organism and ciliary movement corresponded closely to MAC values of the various anesthetics. The mechanism by which cilia were affected was not clear, although the rapidity and reversibility of the depression suggested that metabolic depression of ATP stores was not involved. Extrapolation from the protozoan to the airway epithelia of mammals is hazardous but offers a very plausible explanation of observed slowing of mucus clearance.

In a recent study utilizing in vitro cultures of ciliated epithelium of dogs, Manawadu et al.[65] showed a depression of ciliary movement by halothane, but only at doses of 3 percent or more (Fig. 13-9); these doses were well above that of usual clinical concentrations. These are substantially different sensitivities of cilia

to halothane than that found by Nunn in *Tytrahymena pyriformis*. The effects of anesthetics on ciliary beat frequency in humans have not been elucidated.

Ciliary metachromatism has not been studied with respect to anesthesia. Both adrenergic and cholinergic drugs involved in ciliary activity[66] have been shown to increase mucociliary clearance with the latter group of drugs affecting both ciliary frequency and volume of mucus production. The known reduction in sympathetic nervous activity caused by halothane and enflurane may be one mechanism by which mucus removal is compromised.

CLINICAL SIGNIFICANCE

Because many factors contribute to postoperative pulmonary complications, the role of depressed mucociliary function is not known. It would seem clear that prolonged anesthesia could lead to pooling of mucus and thus result in atelectasis and respiratory infections. The patients at greatest risk would be those with excessive or abnormal mucus production: that is, those with chronic bronchitis, asthma, respiratory tract infection, or cystic fibrosis. Some evidence exists that patients with chronic obstructive lung disease anesthetized by regional block techniques show a lesser incidence of respiratory failure than those anesthetized with general anesthetics,[67] while other studies have failed to demonstrate this advantage. Controlled studies of the effects of inhaled anesthetics on mucociliary function in these already compromised groups of patients have not been done nor has the role of general anesthesia on their rate of pulmonary complications been clearly delineated. In animals mucus pooling appears to occur in the intra-anesthetic and postanesthetic period; this suggests a need in the immediate postoperative period for vigorous pulmonary therapy directed toward enhancing clearance of secretions from the airways.

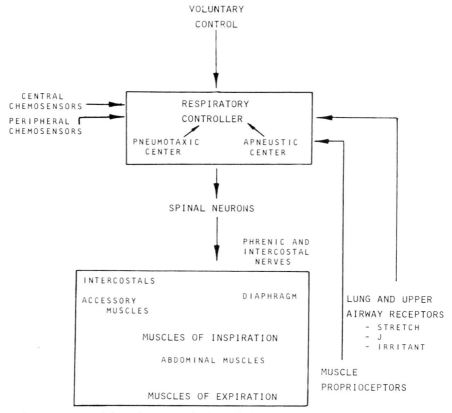

Fig. 13-10 Some aspects of the reflex control of ventilation. Input from many sources interact to alter ventilatory controller output and hence ventilation.

EFFECTS ON THE CONTROL OF VENTILATION

Of the many derangements of lung function caused by anesthetic agents, alterations of minute ventilation are the most obvious. Many different stimuli interact in a complex manner to determine the level of ventilation in man. The traditional approach to studying anesthetic effects on ventilation has been to measure ventilatory responsiveness before and after drug administration. The index of ventilatory response may be expired minute volume, frequency of respiration, or arterial carbon dioxide tension (a measure of alveolar ventilation). All of these offer some problem in interpretation of the effects on ventilatory control. Though an area of intense investiga-

tion, many aspects of ventilatory control are still unclear. Indeed, the precise origin of the normal respiratory pattern (the ventilatory "pacemaker") remains a mystery up to the present time. Investigations in man are frequently hampered by being limited to measurements of expired gas volumes as an indicator of respiratory drive. Obviously, alterations in lung mechanics, such as those occurring during airway obstruction, may alter minute ventilation in the face of constant nerve traffic to the muscles of respiration. Similarly, a sufficient dose of muscle relaxant such as pancuronium will negate any ventilatory response to inhalation of carbon dioxide, but this would hardly constitute evidence of depression of ventilatory control.

A complete description of ventilatory control is beyond the scope of this chapter. Several excellent reviews of this subject already exist.[68,69] However, some understanding of normal ventilatory responses is necessary to appreciate the effects of drugs and the methods by which these effects are measured.

CONTROL OF BREATHING

The volume of gas moving in and out of the lungs is matched to the requirements of the body for oxygen delivery and carbon dioxide elimination. Oxygen consumed and carbon dioxide produced vary widely in disease, during exercise, and with alterations in man's environment (including differences in the chemical composition of inspired gases). A control system that modulates ventilation is necessary therefore to maintain stability in blood gas tensions and acidity (Fig. 13-10). Furthermore, changes in the environment, in the mechanical properties of the lung, and in the work of ventilation necessitate the presence of receptors to detect changes and provide sufficient altered "drive" to the respiratory muscles such that body homeostasis is maintained. Frequency and tidal volume are integrated in such a manner as to minimize the work of breathing in response to variations in the total ventilatory requirements.

The system responsible for receiving and integrating the many input signals and ultimately producing movement of air in and out of the lungs is composed of:

Sensors, which may be chemical (peripheral and central chemoreceptors) or mechanical (distortion receptors located in airways, alveoli, and respiratory muscles);

A respiratory control system, which integrates the signal inputs from the receptor sites, centers of consciousness, and other influences (e.g., pain) and culminates in a level and pattern of nerve traffic to the muscles of respiration; and

The "motor system", composed of the chest wall and intercostal, diaphragmatic, and abdominal muscles, all of which respond to signals from the control center via the phrenic and spinal nerves.

For our purposes, discussion is more detailed in those areas in which the role of anesthetic agents has been most clearly delineated.

MEASUREMENT OF RESPIRATORY CONTROL CENTER OUTPUT

Detailed discussion of the respiratory control center may be found in the review of Berger et al.[68]

The "controller," located in the medulla and pons, consists of two groups of neurons: the dorsal respiratory group (DRG), composed of cells active during inspiration; and the ventral respiratory groups (VRG), containing both inspiratory and expiratory neurons. The DRG may be the source of respiratory rhythm, and the apneustic center (VRG) may determine frequency and depth of ventilation and function as the off switch for inspiration. The exact site for integration of afferent stimuli from pulmonary receptors is not clear, although the pneumotaxic center has been suggested.

The output of the respiratory control center may be assessed by measurement of cellular activity, phrenic nerve discharge, or various parameters of ventilation of which minute ventilation ($\dot{V}E$) is most commonly used clinically. $\dot{V}E$ is a useful measurement in normal man, but becomes a doubtful indicator of respiratory drive in patients with neuromuscular or mechanical impairment of breathing. Diaphragmatic electromyography is of some interest but is distressing to the subject and sometimes not readily reproducible.

The search for a method of quantifying respiratory controller output led Whitelaw et al.[70] to develop a method measuring the pressure developed in the first 0.1 second of inspiration during the time that the airway is acutely obstructed immediately prior to inspiration. These investigators found that this parameter (P_{100}) was independent of airway resistance and correlated well with phrenic nerve discharge. It was, however, sensitive to changes in lung functional residual capacity. A study involving the measurement of respiratory drive during methoxyflurane anesthesia showed an elevation of $PaCO_2$ but no change in P_{100}.[71] One interpretation was that methoxyflurane did not decrease ventilatory drive but that the hypercapnia was caused by mechanical alterations in the lung or chest wall. Obviously, more study is required to establish such a mechanism or the validity of P_{100} as a measure of controller output under anesthesia. This is, however, a step in separating controller output ("drive") from volume of gas ventilated by the lungs. Such a separation is necessary to answer such questions as: Is ventilatory drive decreased in patients with chronic lung disease? Is the effect of anesthetics on such patients a decreased response to chemical stimuli or secondary to airway mechanical abnormalities?

MECHANORECEPTORS AND BREATHING

In the resting patient, the total amount of alveolar ventilation is believed to be determined by the partial pressures of oxygen and carbon dioxide as well as by acidity in arterial blood. The pattern of ventilation by which this minute volume is attained is determined by input signals emanating from the upper airways, lungs, and chest wall and mediated by the vagus nerve.

LUNG AND AIRWAY RECEPTORS

Pulmonary receptors that may have some relevance to the effect of anesthetics include irritant receptors and pulmonary stretch receptors. Irritant receptors are believed to be situated between airway epithelial cells. Such a location may explain the rapid response of the airways to various kinds of stimuli such as

chemical irritants, smoke, and dust and to sudden mechanical deformation of the bronchial tree. These receptors are involved in coughing in response to many types of stimuli as well as in producing reflex tachypnea. They may also enhance the ventilatory response to inhaled carbon dioxide.

Pulmonary stretch receptors, located within the smooth muscle of small airways, respond to stretching or changes in lung volume. Increases in lung volume increase afferent nerve traffic via the vagus nerve to the respiratory control center, thereby inhibiting further inspiration; this phenomena is known as the Hering-Breuer reflex. This limitation of inspiration thereby determines the relationship between tidal volume and respiratory frequency. Thus, an attractive hypothesis is that although the level of alveolar ventilation is determined by chemical stimuli, the pattern of ventilation is determined by afferent mechanical signals from the lung and, to some extent, the chest wall. The pulmonary stretch receptors would therefore represent the off switch limiting tidal volume. This reflex has been demonstrated in animals at normal tidal volumes. In man, however, tidal volumes in excess of one liter are required to demonstrate an effect on ventilation. No change in normal breathing pattern has been observed in man following bilateral vagal blockade, although an increase in tidal volume with no change in respiratory rate has been observed following inhalation of carbon dioxide. The data available would suggest that in awake, adult man, many other factors in addition to pulmonary mechanoreceptors summate to determine the pattern of breathing.

The effects of common inhaled anesthetics on breathing patterns is depicted in Figures 13-11 and 13-12. With increasing depths of anesthesia, alveolar ventilation is progressively diminished; this is effected by a decrease in tidal volume with a simultaneous dose-related increase in breathing frequency. The rate of breathing is greatest with halothane anesthesia at higher MAC concentrations.[72]

The alteration in ventilatory pattern has

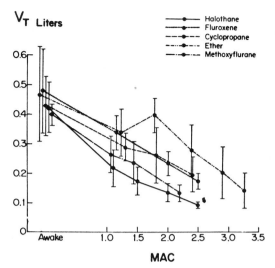

Fig. 13-11 Comparison of mean changes in tidal volume at multiples of MAC in patients anesthetized with one of five different anesthetic agents. Reduction of tidal volume was greatest for halothane and least for diethyl ether. (Larson CP, Eger EI II, Muallem M, et al: The effects of diethyl ether and methoxyflurane on ventilation. Anesthesiology 30:174, 1969.)

been attributed to sensitization of pulmonary stretch receptors leading to lower tidal volumes and tachypnea.[73] Vagal afferent activity was measured at various lung volumes in decerebrate cats with and without the intervention of various general anesthetics.[74] The presence of volatile anesthetics increased receptor discharge at any lung volume, that is, pulmonary stretch receptors did seem to be sensitized. Vagotomy in dogs produced a similar increase in tidal volume. During ether anesthesia[75] respiratory frequency decreased in dogs, although ventilatory responses to inhaled carbon dioxide were unchanged. Little evidence exists of such a mechanism in man. Paskin et al.[76] examined the effect of elevation of functional residual capacity in anesthetized man. The added volume and hence increased stimulus to pulmonary stretch receptors should have increased tachypnea. Instead, respiratory frequency decreased. Thus, the mechanism of production of tachypnea with decreased tidal volume in anesthetized man remains unclear.

MECHANORECEPTORS IN THE CHEST WALL

The force exerted by the muscles of inspiration is a function of afferent nerve traffic emanating from the control center. Although this may vary in response to chemical stimuli, mechanoreceptors in the chest wall also provide input to modify the pattern of breathing. Alteration in the position of the chest wall produces a change in afferent impulses from stretch receptors in tendons and intercostal muscle spindles. The effect of this input is to maintain tidal volume in the face of variations in inspiratory resistance. An increase in spindle discharge causes increased motor discharge to muscle fibers until muscle shortening relieves tension in the spindles. With increased inspiratory resistance, the muscle spindles detect a failure of shortening by the appropriate amount and therefore afferent signals are increased to the motor neuron pool. Accessory muscles of inspiration may

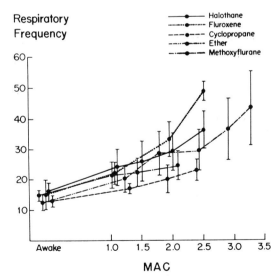

Fig. 13-12 Comparison of mean changes in respiratory frequency at multiples of MAC obtained in patients anesthetized with one of five different anesthetics. With all anesthetics, respiratory frequency increases as anesthesia is deepened. (Larson CP, Eger EI II, Muallem M, et al: The effects of diethyl ether and methoxyflurane on ventilation. Anesthesiology 30:174, 1969.)

be brought into use as well. This reflex increase in inspiratory effort results in sustained tidal volume and minute ventilation with increasing inspiratory resistive loading. These and other reflexes explain the ability of the body to maintain normal ventilation with different body positions, inspiratory resistance and, changes in compliance.

Anesthetics diminish but do not abolish ventilatory responsiveness to inspired resistance.[77] During halothane anesthesia, as inspiratory loading increases minute ventilation diminishes. An exact dose response relationship of halothane and attenuation of chest wall reflexes has not yet been established. Prolonged resistance may lead to retention of carbon dioxide. This has obvious clinical implications in anesthetized patients with partial upper airway obstruction or those breathing spontaneously through endotracheal tubes of small cross-sectional diameter.

During normal quiet breathing, expiration is passively effected by the recoil characteristics of the lung. Expiratory pressures up to 10 cm of water do not bring abdominal muscles into play. Instead, lung volume is increased until increased lung recoil pressure offsets the elevation of expiratory resistance. In anesthetized patients[78] the ventilatory response to expiratory resistance is diminished more than to inspiratory resistance. This is curious in light of the study by Freund et al.[79] demonstrating that the onset of anesthesia immediately produced activity of abdominal muscles during expiration (i.e., active muscular as well as passive lung recoil forces acted during the expiratory phase of ventilation).

Pietak et al.[80] found that patients with chronic obstructive lung disease who did *not* retain CO_2 while awake, hypoventilated to a greater degree than normal patients under halothane anesthesia. The resting $PaCO_2$ was directly proportional to the severity of the obstruction (Fig. 13-13). These data[80] demonstrate the potentially obtunded responses of

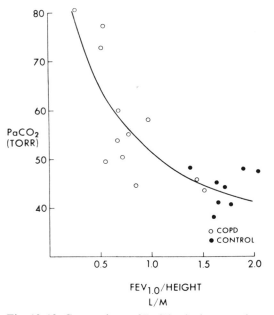

Fig. 13-13 Comparison of $PaCO_2$ during anesthesia during spontaneous ventilation relative to preoperative $FEV_{1.0}$. The COPD (chronic obstructive pulmonary disease) patients did not exhibit CO_2 retention prior to anesthesia, yet the degree of alveolar hypoventilation is much greater in the more severely obstructed patients. (Pietak S, Weenig CS, Hickey RF, et al: Anesthetic effects on ventilation in patients with chronic obstructive lung disease. Anesthesiology 42:160, 1975.)

patients with obstructive airway disease to anesthesia and clearly demonstrate the requirements for both close monitoring of alveolar ventilation and the use of mechanical ventilation in these patients.

EFFECTS ON VENTILATORY RESPONSE TO CHEMICAL STIMULI

Anesthetic agents and sedatives may exert potent depressant effects on the function of many organs including those involved in the control of ventilation. Depression of ventilatory drive has been quantitated utilizing the physiological principles of chemoreceptor function. These tests have usually involved varying of a chemical stimulus (arterial carbon dioxide or oxygen tension), measuring the ventilatory response to this variation, and then repeating this test after the administration of an anesthetic drug. The variation between the predrug and postdrug responses gives a measure of the depressant potential of the agent in question. Respiratory drive can thus be characterized by the ventilatory responsiveness to $PaCO_2$ (resting $PaCO_2$, apneic threshold, and ventilatory responses to an increase in CO_2 tension) or to a decrease in PaO_2. To obtain a more complete discussion of the basic elements of chemical ventilatory control, the reader is referred to other reviews.[68,81]

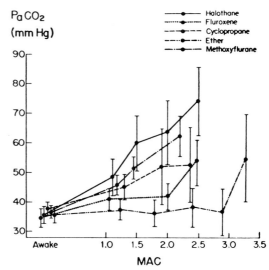

Fig. 13-14 Comparison of mean $PaCO_2$ values in patients anesthetized with one of five different agents. Patients were resting, spontaneously ventilating, and unstimulated. In this study halothane depressed $PaCO_2$ to the greatest degree at equipotent doses of anesthetic, while ether produced the least change in alveolar ventilation. (Larson CP, Eger EI II, Muallem M, et al: The effects of diethyl ether and methoxyflurane on ventilation. Anesthesiology 30:174, 1969.)

RESPONSES TO CARBON DIOXIDE

Changes in ventilation secondary to alterations in $PaCO_2$ are believed to be mediated chiefly via chemoreceptors located in the medulla. Patients whose peripheral chemoreceptor has been denervated by endarterectomy demonstrate approximately 85 percent of the increase in ventilation observed prior to carotid body denervation changes in $PaCO_2$.

The resting $PaCO_2$ is probably the most common index of ventilatory drive used clinically. Ventilation appears to be regulated in such a manner as to maintain $PaCO_2$ very close to 40 torr. Variation from this long-established normal value is interpreted as an indication of either interference with ventilatory drive or severe compromise of the mechanics of breathing. Indeed, elevation of the $PaCO_2$ is often used to define the presence of ventilatory failure. The effects of various concentrations of inhaled anesthetics on $PaCO_2$ are demonstrated in Figure 13-14.[72] Different anesthetics obviously depress resting ventilation to a different degree, with diethyl ether being least depressant and halothane being the most depressant agent. Other investigators examining the effect of en-

flurane (Ethrane) on $PaCO_2$ demonstrated a $PaCO_2$ of over 60 torr at 1.0 MAC enflurane.[82] These kinds of observations have established ether as the least depressant inhalational anesthetic agent, with little changes in $PaCO_2$ being demonstrated at concentrations as high as 3.0 MAC. An explanation of the difference between diethyl ether and other inhaled anesthetics is lacking. Resting $PaCO_2$ is unchanged in ether-anesthetized dogs following vagal denervation, high spinal anesthesia, or bilateral carotid body denervation.[75] The absence of ventilatory alterations after bilateral vagal denervation suggests that irritant receptors are not causally related to this remarkable maintenance of resting ventilation during ether anesthesia. The effects of surgical stimulation on ventilation in anesthetized patients has been noted by many clinical anesthesiologists

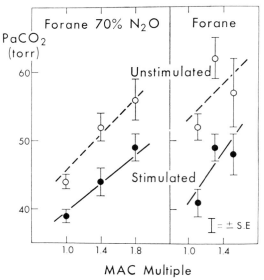

Fig. 13-15 The effect of surgical stimulation on the ventilatory depression of inhalational anesthesia with both nitrous oxide and Forane (isoflurane) or Forane alone. Surgical stimulation increased alveolar ventilation and decreased PaCO$_2$ at all depths of anesthesia examined. (Eger EI II, Dolan WM, Stevens WC, et al: Surgical stimulation antagonizes the respiratory depression produced by Forane. Anesthesiology 36:544, 1972.)

and was documented for the anesthetic isoflurane by Eger et al. (Fig. 13-15).[83] At various multiples of MAC, these investigators demonstrated that the stimulation of surgical incision brought about a decrease in resting PaCO$_2$ of as much as 10 torr. The duration of anesthesia also plays a role in the level of ventilation. For both halothane and enflurane, the resting PaCO$_2$ after 6 hours of anesthesia was less than that measured after induction or after 3 hours of anesthesia.[84] PaCO$_2$ decreased from 63 torr to 53 torr over 6 hours of enflurane anesthesia. The reason for this apparent recovery of ventilatory drive is not clear.

APNEIC THRESHOLDS

Apneic threshold is defined as the highest arterial or alveolar PCO$_2$ at which a hyperventilated subject will remain apneic. It is not usually possible to demonstrate an apneic threshold in a conscious, unmedicated subject, who hyperventilates presumably because of stimuli from the cerebrum. However, one study[85] reported apnea thresholds in

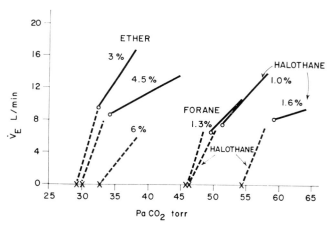

Fig. 13-16 Ventilatory responses to increased carbon dioxide and apneic thresholds during ether, Forane (isoflurane), and halothane anesthesia in patients. Note that apneic threshold in this study appeared to have a relative fixed relationship to resting PaCO$_2$. With an increase in ventilatory depression at increasing depths of anesthesia, resting PaCO$_2$ and apneic threshold increase approximately the same amount. (Hickey RF, Fourcade HE, Eger EI II, et al: The effects of ether, halothane and Forane on apneic threshold in man. Anesthesiology 35:32, 1971.)

awake man approximately 5 torr below resting $PaCO_2$. A study by Hickey et al.[86] on the effects of ether, halothane, and isoflurane on apnea thresholds in man demonstrated a similar relationship between apnea threshold and resting $PaCO_2$ for all three anesthetics and, remarkably enough, for various concentrations of the same anesthetics (Fig. 13-16). The difference between resting $PaCO_2$ and apnea threshold bore no relationship to the slope of CO_2 response curves or to the absolute level of resting $PaCO_2$. This phenomenon suggests that assisted ventilation under the influence of anesthetics is of little use in lowering $PaCO_2$. The effectiveness would be limited to a change of approximately 5 torr. Ventilation that lowered $PaCO_2$ below the apnea threshold would then in fact become "controlled" ventilation rather than "assisted" ventilation. Another clinically important aspect of this observation is in the reestablishment of spontaneous ventilation in the mechanically hyperventilated patient. On cessation of mechanical ventilation, CO_2 stores in the body must accumulate to raise the $PaCO_2$ level in the blood to the apnea threshold. The deeper the level of anesthesia, the longer the period of apnea necessary before the patient will commence spontaneous ventilation. An alternative method of management might be to decrease the anesthetic concentration by continuing mechanical ventilation so as to lower the apnea threshold toward the hyperventilated level of $PaCO_2$, thus diminishing the time of apnea required to initiate spontaneous ventilation.

CARBON DIOXIDE RESPONSE CURVES

Measuring the minute ventilation in response to varying levels of $PaCO_2$ is a common method of quantitating the effects of drugs on ventilatory drive. In the presence of a high inspired concentration of oxygen, $PaCO_2$ is elevated by the investigation increasing concentrations of inspired carbon dioxide inhaled by the subject. This response may be obtained either by the steady state technique in which $PaCO_2$ is elevated and maintained at various constant levels for approximately 10 minutes or by the rebreathing method of Read[87] in which a subject rebreathes from a 5 liter bag filled with 7 percent carbon dioxide in oxygen. In the latter method, exhalation of carbon dioxide into the bag gradually increases the inspired CO_2, hence elevating $PaCO_2$ continually. This test is both faster and simpler than the steady state method and yields approximately similar slopes of ventilation versus change in $PaCO_2$. In normal man, inspiration of CO_2 increases minute ventilation approximately 3 L/min/torr $PaCO_2$, demonstrating a high gain from a central chemoreceptor in response to variations in $PaCO_2$. Within physiological range, the response approximates a straight line. Thus, the slope of the plot is an index of ventilatory drive in response to carbon dioxide stimulus.

All inhaled agents generally depress the CO_2 response curve at anesthetic levels (Fig. 13-17).[72] The degree of ventilatory depression varies both with the anesthetic agent and with the expired anesthetic concentration. Ether diminished the ventilatory response to inhaled carbon dioxide at anesthetic depths at which $PaCO_2$ is maintained at normal levels. Thus, although ether has a lesser effect on CO_2 response than other anesthetic agents, it is clear that it too is a ventilatory depressant, a conclusion that is not apparent from examination of resting $PaCO_2$ levels alone. Although sedating concentrations of halothane and enflurane have little effect on CO_2 response slopes, 1 MAC halothane is a profound depressant of this measurement. Indeed, at levels of 2.5 MAC or more, no further increase in ventilation to altered inspired CO_2 is observed. Isoflurane produces a similar degree of depression.[88] The slope of the ventilatory response curve during halothane anesthesia (like the resting $PaCO_2$) returns toward normal after 6 hours of anesthesia, although ventilatory responsiveness to CO_2 is still profoundly depressed (Fig. 13-18).[84] In

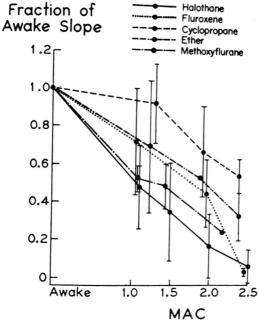

Fig. 13-17 Comparison of mean slopes of ventilatory response to inhaled CO_2 at multiples of MAC in an anesthetized patient. Values on the ordinate are expressed as a fraction of the awake slope. In this study halothane depressed the ventilatory response to CO_2 to the greatest degree and cyclopropane was the least depressant of this measure of ventilatory depression. In all cases increasing the depth of anesthesia diminished the ventilatory response to inhaled carbon dioxide. (Larson CP, Eger EI II, Muallem M, et al: The effects of diethyl ether and methoxyflurane on ventilation. Anesthesiology 30:174, 1969.)

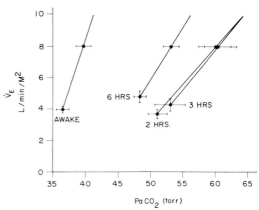

Fig. 13-18 Effects of time on the ventilatory response to inhaled carbon dioxide during constant depth halothane anesthesia. The increase in arterial PCO_2 with induction of anesthesia is diminished by 6 hours although not to the awake level of alveolar ventilation. No good explanation of this readustment is available. (Forcade HE, Larson CP, Hickey RF, et al: Effects of time on ventilation during halothane and cyclopropane anesthesia. Anesthesiology 36:83, 1972.)

contrast to halothane, enflurane, and isoflurane, two other potent inhaled agents, cyclopropane and methoxyflurane, produce much more modest depression. Nitrous oxide, a relatively weak inhaled agent, did not depress the ventilatory response to CO_2 at concentrations of 50 percent. Studies by Hornbein et al.[89] showed that equipotent doses of nitrous oxide and halothane depressed ventilation less than an equipotent dose of halothane alone. It is somewhat surprising that in the only study performed at anesthetic concentrations of nitrous oxide (which took place under hyperbaric conditions), 1.5 MAC concentrations of nitrous oxide proved to be a potent respiratory depressant, which lowered the CO_2 response slope to 15 percent of that of the control.[90]

Depression of ventilatory responsiveness to inhaled carbon dioxide has great clinical relevance. Accumulation of carbon dioxide and the ensuing arterial and tissue acidosis may cause dysfunction in several organs, including the heart, where this condition may cause potentially dangerous cardiac arrhythmias. The attenuation of the normal ventilatory responses to elevated $PaCO_2$ (tachypnea, increased tidal volume) makes clinical diagnosis of hypercarbia difficult and necessitates the measurement of either arterial, alveolar, or end-tidal CO_2 tensions. During anesthesia, the ventilatory system will be less likely to compensate for carbon dioxide elevations secondary to rebreathing of carbon dioxide from malfunctioning anesthetic circuits or from increased metabolic production of carbon dioxide.

In their study on the effect of anesthesia

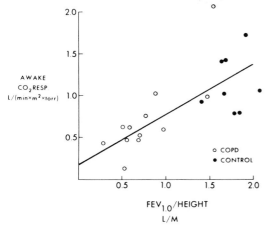

Fig. 13-19 Cabron dioxide response related to $FEV_{1.0}$ in awake patients breathing oxygen. Patients with COPD (chronic obstructive pulmonary disease) exhibit a diminished increase in ventilation to increases in inhaled carbon dioxide. The presence of airway obstruction makes the interpretation of "decreased ventilatory drive" difficult. (Pietak S, Weenig CS, Hickey RF, et al: Anesthetic effects on ventilation in patients with chronic obstructive pulmonary disease. Anesthesiology 42:160, 1975.)

on patients with chronic obstructive lung disease, Pietak et al.[80] clearly showed the decreased ability of these patients to respond to increased $PaCO_2$ (Fig. 13-19). This demonstrates the requirement for strict monitoring of arterial blood gases in these patients.

VENTILATORY RESPONSES TO HYPOXEMIA

Increased ventilation in response to progressively lowered PaO_2 is mediated entirely by the peripheral chemoreceptor. The hyperbolic response curve thus obtained rises most sharply at PaO_2 of approximately 40 torr. Various indices have been used to quantitate this response. Currently popular is the index "A" made popular by Weil and his associates.[91] This parameter describes the curvature of the hyperbola; a low value of "A" is con-

sistent with a flattened or lesser ventilatory response to progressive hypoxemia.

For some time the opinion was held that while the ventilatory responses to hypercarbia and acidosis were profoundly affected by anesthetic agents, the peripheral chemoreceptor was spared and the ventilatory response to hypoxemia preserved. It is now evident from the results of studies performed during the 1970's that this belief is erroneous. Weiskopf and colleagues[92] studied the ventilatory response to hypoxia in three dogs during halothane anesthesia (1.1 percent end-tidal halothane concentration) and at different levels of $PaCO_2$. Significant depression of ventilatory responsiveness to hypoxia was observed at 1 MAC levels of halothane. In addition, the usual synergistic effect of hypoxia and hypercarbia on ventilation was profoundly attenuated. This work has subsequently been confirmed in dogs by Hirshman et al.,[93] who extended the study to demonstrate similar ventilatory depression by both enflurane and isoflurane. Furthermore, a dose-related attenuation of the hypoxic response was demonstrated. In an important study, Knill and Gelb[94] showed a similar response in man to halothane anesthesia; however, the peripheral chemoreceptor function in man was even more sensitive to the effects of anesthetic agents than in the dog. At 1.1 MAC halothane, the ventilatory response to hypoxemia was completely absent (Fig. 13-20). Furthermore, at very low anesthetic concentrations (0.1 MAC halothane), ventilatory responsiveness was severely attenuated. At the same "sedative" levels of halothane, no change was seen in the CO_2 response curve (Fig. 13-21). This profound depression of hypoxic responsiveness is clinically very important in that it suggests that patients will manifest a diminished ventilatory response to hypoxemia for some time after cessation of an anesthetic and at the arterial concentrations of halothane one would expect in a patient in the recovery room. The implications of this in patients who depend to some degree on a hypoxic drive to set their

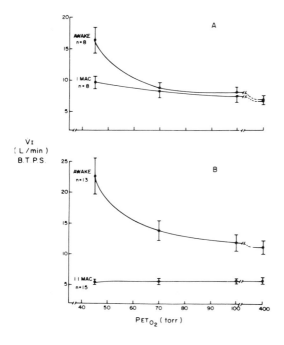

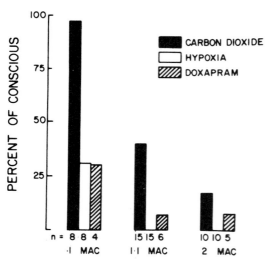

Fig. 13-20 Ventilatory response to hypoxia in human volunteers and patients anesthetized with halothane. (A) The ventilatory increase to hypoxia is severely attenuated at levels of only 0.1 MAC halothane and (B) completely absent in this experiment at the 1.1 MAC halothane anesthesia. This represents a more significant depression of this measure of ventilatory drive during inhaled anesthetics than that previously demonstrated in dogs. (Knill RL, Gelb AW: Ventilatory responses to hypoxia and hypercapnia during halothane sedation and anesthesia in man. Anesthesiology 49:244, 1978.)

Fig. 13-21 The effect of halothane anesthesia at different doses on three different tests of ventilatory drive in human subjects. The ventilatory drive to hypoxia seems to be depressed at much lower levels of halothane anesthetic than does the ventilatory increase to inhaled carbon dioxide. (Knill RL, Gelb AW: Ventilatory responses to hypoxia and hypercapnia during halothane sedation and anesthesia in man. Anesthesiology 49:244, 1978.)

level of ventilation is obvious. The impaired function of the peripheral chemoreceptor in the presence of low levels of halothane was also ingeniously demonstrated by a marked reduction in ventilatory responsiveness to doxapram or metabolic acidosis (Fig. 13-21), both of which normally have a significant stimulatory effect on the peripheral chemoreceptor. Both enflurane[95] and nitrous oxide[96] have also been shown to depress hypoxic responsiveness in man at low subanesthetic concentrations.

These studies demonstrate that, in contrast to previous beliefs, the peripheral chemoreceptor is remarkably sensitive to the depressant effects of inhaled anesthetics as well as to many intravenous agents, such as morphine and thiopental. The exact site of depression is not known. A systematic examination of the effects of anesthetic agents on nerve traffic from the peripheral chemoreceptor has not been done, although some studies have suggested that this may be one site of attenuation by halothane.[97] Thus, whether ventilatory depression is caused by depressed peripheral chemoreceptor responsiveness or by a depression of the central control mechanism or both is not known at the present time. It is clear that tachypnea and increased ventilation seen with hypoxia under normal conditions would be absent or severely decreased during even light levels of anesthesia. Lack of these clinical signs mandates the frequent assessment of arterial oxygen tensions. Patients with chronic respiratory failure in whom the level of PaO_2 may represent an important determinant of minute ventilation may be drastically affected by even low doses of inhaled anesthetics. Thus, the ability of these patients to maintain adequate ventilation while breathing spontaneously may be severely impaired.

REFERENCES

1. Paterson JW, Woolcock AJ, Shenfield GM: Bronchodilator drugs. Am Rev Respir Dis 120:1149, 1979
2. Ahlquist RP: A study of the adrenotropic receptors. Am J Physiol 153:586, 1948
3. Shnider WM, Papper EM: Anesthesia for the asthmatic patient. Anesthesiology 22:886, 1961
4. Brown D: Halothane-oxygen anesthesia for bronchoscopy, method suitable for children. Anaesthesia 14:135, 1959
5. Colgan FJ: Performance of lungs and bronchi during inhalation anesthesia. Anesthesiology 26:778, 1965
6. Klide AM, Aviado DM: Mechanism for the reduction in pulmonary resistance induced by halothane. J Pharmacol Ex Ther 158:28, 1967
7. Fletcher SW, Flacke W, Alper MH: The actions of general anesthetic agents on tracheal smooth muscle. Anesthesiology 29:517, 1969
8. Hickey RF, Graf PD, Nadel JA, et al: The effects of halothane and cyclopropane on total pulmonary resistance in the dog. Anesthesiology 31:334, 1969
9. Coon RL, Kampine JP: Hypocapnic bronchoconstriction and inhalation anesthetics. Anesthesiology 43:635, 1975
10. Hirshman CA, Bergman NA: Halothane and enflurane protect against bronchospasm in an asthma dog model. Anesth Analg 57:629, 1978
11. Gold WM, Kessler GF, Yu DYC, et al: Pulmonary physiologic abnormalities in experimental asthma in dogs. J Appl Physiol 33: 496, 1972
12. Gold MI, Helrich M: Pulmonary mechanics during general anesthesia: V. status asthmaticus. Anesthesiology 32:422, 1970
13. Patterson RW, Sullivan SF, Malm JR, et al: The effect of halothane on human airway mechanics. Anesthesiology 29:900, 1968
14. Meloche R, Norlander O, Norden I, Herzog P: Effects of carbon dioxide and halothane on compliance and pulmonary resistance during cardiopulmonary bypass. Scand J Thor Cardiovasc Surg 3:69, 1969
15. Brakensiek AL, Bergman JA: The effects of halothane and atropine on total respiratory resistance in anesthetized man. Anesthesiology 33:341, 1970
16. McAslan C, Mima M, Norden I, et al: Effects of halothane and methoxyflurane on pulmonary resistance to gas flow during lung bypass. Scand J Thorac Cardiovasc Surg 5:193, 1971
17. Waltemath CL, Bergman NA: Effects of ketamine and halothane on increased respiratory resistance provoked by ultrasonic aerosols. Anesthesiology 41:473, 1974
18. Sprague DH: Treatment of intraoperative bronchospasm with nebulized isoetharine. Anesthesiology 46:222, 1977
19. Wolfe JD, Tashkin DP, Calvares B, et al: Bronchodilator effects on terbutaline and aminophylline alone and in combination in asthmatic patients. N Engl J Med 298:363, 1978
20. Aviado DM: Regulation of bronchomotor tone during anesthesia. Anesthesiology 42:68, 1975
21. Yang JC, Triner L, Vulliemoz Y, et al: Effects of halothane on the cyclic 3'5'-adenosine monophosphate (cyclic AMP) system in rat uterine muscle. Anesthesiology 38:244, 1973
22. Klide AM, Penna M, Aviado DM: Stimulation of adrenergic beta receptors by halothane and its antagonism by two new drugs. Anesth and Analg 48:58, 1969
23. Sprague DH, Yang JC, Ngai SH: Effects of isoflurane and halothane on contractility and the cyclic 3'5'-adenosine monophosphate system in the rat aorta. Anesthesiology 40:162, 1974
24. Bennett DJ, Torda TA, Horton DA, et al: Severe bronchospasm complicating thoracotomy. Arch Surg 101:555, 1970

25. Bloch EC: Bronchospasm during anesthesia. Br J Anaesth 43:108, 1971

26. Nunn JF: Applied Respiratory Physiology. 2nd edition. Butterworth & Co. Ltd, London, 1977, p 68

27. Price HL, Cooperman LH, Warden JC, et al: Pulmonary hemodynamics during general anesthesia in man. Anesthesiology 30:629, 1969

28. Marshall BE, Cohen PJ, Klingenmaier CH, et al: Some pulmonary and cardiovascular effects of enflurane (Ethrane) anaesthesia with varying $PaCO_2$ in man. Br J Anaesth 43:996, 1971

29. Bergofsky EH: Mechanisms underlying vasomotor regulation of regional pulmonary blood flow in normal and disease states. Am J Med 57:378, 1974

30. Malik AB, Kidd BSL: Independent effects of changes in H^+ and CO_2 concentrations on hypoxic pulmonary vasoconstriction. J Appl Physiol 34:318, 1973

31. Enson Y, Giuntini C, Lewis ML, et al: The influence of hydrogen ion and hypoxia on the pulmonary circulation. J Clin Invest 43:1146, 1964

32. Haas F, Bergofsky EH: Effect of pulmonary vasoconstriction on balance between alveolar ventilation and perfusion. J Appl Physiol 24:491, 1968

33. Colley PS, Chency FW Jr, Hlastala MP: Ventilation-perfusion and gas exchange effects of sodium nitroprusside in dogs with normal and edematous lungs. Anesthesiology 50:489, 1979

34. Buckley MJ, McLaughlin JS, Fort L III, et al: Effects of anesthetic agents on pulmonary vascular resistance during hypoxia. Surg Forum 15:183, 1964

35. Sykes MK, Davies DM, Chakrabarti MK, et al: The effects of halothane, trichlorethylene and ether on the hypoxic pressor response and pulmonary vascular resistance in the isolated, perfused cat lung. Br J Anaesth 45:655, 1973

36. Loh L, Sykes MK, Chakrabarti MK: The effects of halothane and ether on the pulmonary circulation in the innervated perfused cat lung. Br J Anaesth 49:309, 1977

37. Bjertnaes LJ, Hauge A, Nakken KF, et al: Hypoxic pulmonary vasoconstriction: Inhibition due to anesthesia. Acta Physiol Scand 96:283, 1976

38. Sykes MK, Biggs JM, Loh L, et al: Preservation of the pulmonary vasoconstrictor response to alveolar hypoxia during the admin-

istration of halothane to dogs. Br J Anaesth 50:1185, 1978

39. Benumof JL, Wahrenbrock EA: Local effects of anesthetics on regional hypoxic pulmonary vasoconstriction. Anesthesiology 43:525, 1975

40. Mathers J, Benumof JL, Wahrenbrock EA: General anesthetics and regional hypoxic pulmonary vasoconstriction. Anesthesiology 46:111, 1977

41. Sykes MK, Hurtig JB, Tait AR, et al: Reduction of hypoxic pulmonary vasoconstriction during diethyl ether anaesthesia in the dog. Br J Anaesth 49:293, 1977

42. Fargas-Babjak A, Forrest JB: Effect of halothane on the pulmonary vascular response to hypoxia in dogs. Canad Anesth Soc J 26:6, 1979

43. Bjertnaes LJ: Hypoxia-induced pulmonary vasoconstriction in man: Inhibition due to diethyl ether and halothane anesthesia. Acta Anaesthesiol Scand 22:570, 1978

44. Benumof JL, Wahrenbrock EA: Local effects of anesthetics on regional hypoxic pulmonary vasoconstriction. Anesthesiology 43:525, 1975

45. Hurtig JB, Tait AR, Sykes MK: Reduction of hypoxic pulmonary vasoconstriction by diethyl ether in the isolated perfused cat lung: The effect of acidosis and alkalosis. Can Anaesth Soc J 24:433, 1977

46. Colley PS, Cheney FW, Hlastala MP: Ventilation-perfusion effects of nitroglycerine. Anesthesiology 51:S372, 1979

47. Delahnuty JE, Cherry J: The laryngeal saccule. J Laryngol Otol 83:803, 1969

48. Leeson TS, Leeson CR: A light and electron microscope study of developing respiratory tissue in the rat. J Anat 98:183, 1964

49. Sleigh MA: Some aspects of the comparative physiology of cilia. Am Rev Respir Dis 93:16, 1966

50. Kinosita H, Murakami A: Control of ciliary motion. Physiol Rev 47:53, 1967

51. Wanner A: Clinical aspects of mucociliary transport. Am Rev Resp Dis 116:73, 1977

52. Reid L: Natural history of mucous in the bronchial tree. Arch Environ Health 10:265, 1965

53. Sackner MA, Rosen MJ, Wanner A: Estimation of tracheal mucous velocity by bronchofiberoscopy. J Appl Physiol 34:495, 1973

54. Gamsu G, Singer MM, Vincent HH, et al: Postoperative impairment of mucous transport in the lung. Am Rev Respir Dis 114:673, 1976

55. Forbes AR: Temperature, humidity and mucous flow in the intubated trachea. Br J Anaesth 46:29, 1974

56. Hirsch JA, Tokayer JL, Robinson MJ, et al: Effects of dry air and subsequent humidification on tracheal mucous velocity in dogs. J Appl Physiol 39:242, 1975

57. Wolfe WG, Ebert PA, Sabiston DC: Effect of high oxygen tension on mucociliary function. Surgery 72:246, 1972

58. Sackner MA, Hirsch J, Epstein S: Effect of cuffed endotracheal tubes on tracheal mucous velocity. Chest 68:774, 1975

59. Forbes AR, Gamsu G: Lung mucociliary clearance after anesthesia with spontaneous and controlled ventilation. Am Rev Resp Dis 120:857, 1979

60. Lichtiger M, Landa JF, Hirsch JA: Velocity of tracheal mucus in anesthetized women undergoing gynecologic surgery. Anesthesiology 42:753, 1975

61. Forbes AR: Halothane depresses mucociliary flow in the trachea. Anesthesiology 45:59, 1976

62. Forbes AR, Horrigan RW: Mucociliary flow in the trachea during anesthesia with enflurane, ether, nitrous oxide, and morphine. Anesthesiology 46:319, 1977

63. Forbes AR, Gamsu G: Mucociliary clearance in the canine lung during and after general anesthesia. Anesthesiology 50:26, 1979

64. Nunn JF, Sturrock JE, Wills EJ, et al: The effect of inhalational anaesthetics on the swimming velocity of *Tetrahymena pyriformis.* J Cell Sci 15:537, 1974

65. Manawadu BR, Mostow SR, LaForce FM: Impairment of tracheal ring ciliary activity by halothane. Anesth Analg 58:500, 1979

66. Iravani J, Melville GN: Mucociliary function of the respiratory tract as influenced by drugs. Respiration 31:350, 1974

67. Tarhan S, Moffitt EA, Sessler AD, et al: Risk of anesthesia and surgery in patients with chronic bronchitis and chronic obstructive pulmonary disease. Surgery 74:720, 1973

68. Berger AJ, Mitchell RA, Severinghaus JW: Regulation of respiration. N Engl J Med 297:92, 138, 194, 1977

69. Hornbein TF, Sorensen SC: The chemical control of ventilation, Physiology and Biophysics. Twentieth edition. Edited by Ruch TC, Patton HD. Philadelphia, WB Saunders, 1974, pp 803–819

70. Whitelaw WA, Derenne JP, Milic-Émili J: Occlusion pressure as a measure of respiratory center output in conscious man. Respir Physiol 23:181, 1975

71. Dereen JP, Couture J, Iscoe S, et al: Occlusion pressures in man rebreathing CO_2 under methoxyflurane anesthesia. J Appl Physiol 40:805, 1976

72. Larson CP, Eger EI II, Muallem M, et al: The effects of diethyl ether and methoxyflurane on ventilation. Anesthesiology 30:174, 1969

73. Dundee JW, Drips RD: Effects of diethyl ether, trichloroethylene and trifluroethylvinyl ether on respiration. Anesthesiology 18:282, 1957

74. Whittenridge D, Bulbring E: Changes in the activity of pulmonary receptors in anesthesia and their influence on respiratory behavior. J Pharmacol Exp Ther 81:340, 1944

75. Muallem M, Larson CP Jr, Eger EI II: The effects of diethyl ether on $PaCO_2$ in dogs with and without vagal, somatic and sympathetic block. Anesthesiology 30:185, 1969

76. Paskin S, Skovsted P, Smith TC: Failure of the Hering-Breuer reflex to account for tachypnea in anesthetized man: A survey of halothane, fluroxene, methoxyflurane and cyclopropane. Anesthesiology 29:550, 1968

77. Freedman S, Campbell EJM: The ability of normal subjects to tolerate added inspiratory loads. Respir Physiol 10:213, 1970

78. Nunn JF, Ezi-Ashi TI: The respiratory effects of resistance to breathing in anesthetized man. Anesthesiology 22:174, 1961

79. Freund FG, Roos A, Dodd RB: Expiratory activity of the abdominal muscles in man during general anesthesia. J Appl Physiol 19:693, 1964

80. Pietak S, Weenig CS, Hickey RF, et al: Anesthetic effects on ventilation in patients with chronic obstructive pulmonary disease. Anesthesiology 42:160, 1975

81. Pavlin EG: Chemical control of ventilation, ASA Refresher Courses in Anesthesiology. Philadelphia, JB Lippincott, 1976, pp 63-74.

82. Caverley RK, Smith NT, Jones CW, et al: Ventilatory and cardiovascular effects of enflurane anesthesia during spontaneous ventilation in man. Anesth Analg 57:610, 1979

83. Eger EI, Dolan WM, Stevens WC, et al: Surgical stimulation antagonizes the respiratory depression produced by Forane. Anesthesiology 36:544, 1972

84. Fourcade HE, Larson CP, Hickey RF, et al: Effects of time on ventilation during halo-

thane and cyclopropane anesthesia. Anesthesiology 36:83, 1972

85. Bainton CR, Mitchell RA: Posthyperventilation apnea in awake man. J Appl Physiol 21:411, 1966

86. Hickey RF, Fourcade HE, Eger EI II, et al: The effects of ether, halothane and Forane on apneic threshold in man. Anesthesiology 35:32, 1971

87. Read DJC: A clinical method for assessing the ventilatory response to carbon dioxide. Aust Ann Med 16:20, 1967

88. Fourcade HE, Stevens WC, Larson CP, et al: The ventilatory effects of Forane, a new inhaled anesthetic. Anesthesiology 35:26, 1971

89. Hornbein TF, Martin WE, Bonica JJ, et al: Nitrous oxide effects on the circulatory and ventilatory responses to halothane. Anesthesiology 31:250, 1969

90. Winter PM, Hornbein TF, Smith G, et al: Hyperbaric nitrous oxide anesthesia in man, Abstracts of Scientific Papers. 1972 ASA Meeting, pp 103-104

91. Weil JV, McCullough RE, Kline JS, et al: Diminished ventilatory response to hypoxia and hypercapnia after morphine. N Engl J Med 292:1103, 1975

92. Weiskopf RB, Raymond LW, Severinghaus JW: Effects of halothane on canine respiratory responses to hypoxia with and without hypercarbia. Anesthesiology 41:350, 1974

93. Hirshman CA, McCullough RE, Cohen PJ, et al: Hypoxic ventilatory drive in dogs during thiopental, ketamine, or pentobarbital anesthesia. Anesthesiology 43:628, 1975

94. Knill RL, Gelb AW: Ventilatory responses to hypoxia and hypercapnia during halothane sedation and anesthesia in man. Anesthesiology 49:244, 1978

95. Knill RL, Manninen PH, Clement JL: Ventilation and chemoreflexes during enflurane sedation and anaesthesia in man. Can Anaesth Soc J 26:5, 1979

96. Yacoub O, Doell D, Kryger MH, et al: Depression of hypoxic ventilatory response by nitrous oxide. Anesthesiology 45:385, 1976

97. Biscoe TJ, Millar RA: Effects of inhalation anaesthetics on carotid body chemoreceptor activity. Br J Anaesth 40:2, 1968

98. Kaur AE, Mazzic VV, Bergofski CH: Effect of anesthesia and neuromuscular blockers on pulmonary vascular responses to hypoxia and hypercapnia. Anesth Analg 51:402, 1972

99. Sykes MK, Arnot RN, Jastrzebski J, et al: Reduction of hypoxic pulmonary vasoconstriction during trichloroethylene anesthesia. J Appl Physiol 39:103, 1975

100. Tait AR, Chakrabarti MK, Sykes MK: Effect of cyclopropane on pulmonary vascular resistance and hypoxic pulmonary vasoconstriction in the isolated perfused cat lung. Br J Anaesth 50:209, 1978

14

Metabolism and Toxicity of Inhaled Anesthetics

Jeffrey M. Baden, M.B., B.S.
Susan A. Rice, Ph.D.

INTRODUCTION

The inhaled anesthetics were considered for many years to be classic examples of biochemically inert drugs with therapeutic efficacy. The occasional toxicity following their administration was attributed to direct effects of the anesthetics on susceptible tissues or organs or secondary effects via unwanted physiological changes. It is now clear that these views are untenable. Not ony are the inhaled anesthetics metabolized in vivo, but their metabolites are responsible for the acute and chronic toxicities associated with their use.

This chapter discusses the metabolism and toxicity of inhaled anesthetics and explores their relationship.

METABOLISM

Early concepts of drug biotransformation were predicated on the assumption that metabolism resulted in deactivation or detoxification of drugs. Today it is known that drug metabolism may result in (1) deactivation of pharmacologic or toxic actions; (2) activation to a more potent pharmacologic or toxic compound; (3) alteration of the type of pharmacologic or toxic action; or (4) production of an equally active pharmacologic or toxic agent. Many factors, such as drug absorption, adsorption, excretion, secretion, and metabolism, affect drug efficacy and toxicity. These factors are themselves affected to various degrees by the chemical and physical properties of the drug. The following sections discuss these properties of drugs and cellular membranes and how they influence a drug's availability to the metabolizing machinery of the body.

PHYSICOCHEMICAL CONSIDERATIONS

PHYSICOCHEMICAL PROPERTIES OF DRUG MOLECULES

The three physicochemical properties of a drug molecule that primarily determine its distribution and availability for metabolism are: ionization, lipid solubility, and molecular dimensions.[1]

The degree to which a drug is ionized is dependent on its pKa and the pH of the solution in which it is dissolved. Most drugs are weak bases or weak acids and have one or more functional groups which are capable of ionizing. The pKa for weak acids is high while that for weak bases is low. The relationship between the degree of ionization, the pKa, and the pH of a solution is described by the Henderson-Hasselbalch equation:

$$pH = pKa + \log \frac{[\text{dissociated drug}]}{[\text{undissociated drug}]}$$

The lipid solubility of a drug is determined by the presence or absence of lipophilic (hydrophobic) or nonpolar groups in the structure of the molecule. Alkyl groups ($C_nH_{2n+1}-$), such as a methyl group (CH_3-), are nonpolar. The lipophilic property of the drug molecule increases as the length of the alkyl group increases. For example, the presence of an n-propyl group ($CH_3CH_2CH_2-$) makes the compound more lipophilic than does the presence of a methyl group. An increase in a compound's lipophilic properties are seen when an alkyl group is inserted in the molecule, whether the substitution occurs on a carbon, nitrogen, oxygen, or sulfur atom. Substitution of oxygen by sulfur often markedly increases the lipophilic properties of a drug. The lipophilic properties are decreased and the hydrophilic or polar properties are increased when the molecule contains structural elements that allow hydrogen bonding to water (e.g., –OH, –O–, –CHO, –COOH, –COOR, –Cl, and –Br). The presence of unsaturated bonds (e.g., –CH=CH–) further helps to promote hydropholicity.

The molecular dimensions, size, and shape, also determine a drug's distribution. Differences exist in the estimated pore sizes of various membranes and, correspondingly, the size molecule that can pass through these membranes. For example, molecules up to about the size of albumin (MW 69,000; major axis 150 Å; minor axis 35 Å) can appear in the glomerular filtrate, but molecules larger than 4 Å radius are excluded from the erythrocyte. All three of the above physicochemical factors influence the distribution of a drug and its ability to penetrate cellular membranes.

PROPERTIES OF CELLULAR MEMBRANES

Membranes are lipoid and are a matrix consisting of a phospholipid bilayer and intercalated functional proteins.[2,3] Various cellular and subcellular membranes contain large amounts of phospholipids, cholesterol, and neutral lipids in association with proteins. The phospholipids of the membrane are amphoteric (i.e., have distinct polar and nonpolar regions). The nonpolar hydrocarbon chains are directed toward the center of the bilayer, while the polar head groups remain in contact with the aqueous phase on the bilayer surface. Membrane proteins either penetrate the lipid structure completely or partially and bind to interior and exterior surfaces of the bilayer. These proteins are necessary not only for the maintenance of membrane integrity, but also for the specialized transport of endogenous (and structurally similar exogenous) molecules. These membrane properties, as well as drug properties, determine the ability of a drug to enter cells.

Very small molecules and ions (e.g., K^+, Cl^-) apparently diffuse through aqueous membrane channels, while lipid soluble molecules may diffuse freely through the membrane. Water soluble molecules and ions of moderate size, including the ionic form of most drugs, can only enter the cell by specialized transport. The relative lipophilic and hydrophilic properties (i.e., the lipid solubility) of the entire drug molecule determine whether the drug will readily cross the biologic membrane by a passive process. Membranes are generally permeable to the nonionized forms of lipid soluble drugs. Ionized groups on the molecule (e.g., $-COO^-$, which is almost completely ionized at pH 7.4) interact strongly with water dipoles and as a result penetrate the lipoidal cell membrane poorly or not at all. For practical purposes, the diffusion rate of a drug can best be described by the concentration gradient for the nonionized drug form. In general, the greater the lipid solubility, the greater the rate of a drug's transmembranal movement.[1]

THE FUNCTION OF THE LIVER IN DRUG METABOLISM

The inhaled anesthetics are primarily metabolized in the liver and, to a lesser extent, by other tissues (blood, gastrointestinal tract, kidneys, lungs, and skin). We have limited discussion of anesthetic metabolism to that which occurs in the liver because the principles of drug metabolism are common to all tissues.

Hepatic physiology is fully discussed in Chapter 24; however, a brief description is included in this discussion to aid in understanding the relationship between drug metabolism and toxicity. The liver is the largest organ in the body, weighing up to 1,500 g in man. It is a unique organ in that it has a double blood supply: 70 percent from the portal vein and 30 percent from the hepatic artery. Blood in the portal vein comes from the alimentary canal, pancreas, and the spleen. This is important because any toxic material absorbed from the alimentary canal is handled by the liver before it enters the systemic circulation. The hepatic arterial blood supply presumably insures adequate oxygenation of the liver. Portal veins and hepatic arteries are distributed in such a way as to define the periphery of a roughly hexagonal zone of tissue, histologically defined as the hepatic lobule. The lobule is comprised of two cell types, the Kupffer cell and the liver cell (hepatocyte). The phagocytic Kupffer cell is part of the reticuloendothelial system, while the hepatocyte is primarily concerned with homeostatic synthesis and metabolism. The cuboidal hepatic cells are arranged in one-cell-thick interconnecting sheets that are separated by sinusoidal capillaries (sinusoids). Blood flows through these sinusoids from the periphery of the lobule, fed by portal veins and hepatic arteries, to a centrally lo-

cated terminal hepatic venule (central vein). The hepatocyte has several intracellular components intimately involved in intermediary and drug metabolism. The most important is the endoplasmic reticulum. This membranous matrix of lipoprotein is the major site of protein synthesis, electron transfer, lipid metabolism, and hormone and drug oxidation, reduction, hydroxylation, and conjugation. It is also the main center for the synthesis of cellular structural components for the endoplasmic reticulum as well as of the lipid and protein components for other organelles. Microscopically, the endoplasmic reticulum appears as a series of vesicles and tubules suspended within the cytoplasm. Both the parallel arrays of rough membranes and the maze of smooth membranes, rough and smooth endoplasmic reticululm, are part of one interconnected system. This complex is the channel for the passive intracellular transport of proteins (including enzymes), lipids, and other compounds and the intracellular storage of some. Under normal (nonenzyme-induced) conditions, the area of rough endoplasmic reticulum is about 25,000 μ^2 while the smooth endoplasmic reticulum is less, 15,000 to 20,000 μ^2. The rough endoplasmic reticulum is the site of protein synthesis and is identified by the presence of ribosomes (particles of ribonucleic acid) adjacent to the tubular membrane. It is extensively developed in protein-secreting cells. The smooth endoplasmic reticulum contains no granules and is the site of drug metabolism, bilirubin conjugation, and synthesis of steroids and some enzymes. It appears extensively in steroid-secreting cells.

In hepatocytes, both smooth and rough endoplasmic reticulum are involved in drug metabolism. Many in vitro studies of endoplasmic reticulum, its components, and some types of drug metabolism have been performed on microsomes resulting from cell fractionation. Microsomes, as they are referred to in drug metabolism studies, are not naturally occurring organelles but are vesi-

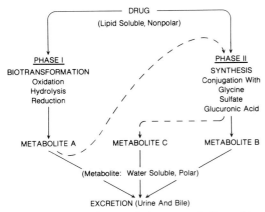

Fig. 14-1 Two phases of drug metabolism (biotransformation and synthesis) generally result in the formation of more water soluble metabolites, which are readily excreted in the urine and bile.

cles that arise from breakage of cisternal and tubular systems of the endoplasmic reticulum.[4]

DRUG METABOLISM

Drug metabolism requires the interaction of substrate and enzyme. An enzyme-catalyzed chemical reaction proceeds at a rate approximately 10^9 times faster than a non-catalyzed reaction. The enzyme molecule and the substrate (drug) molecule form a complex as the result of intermolecular forces (Van der Walls, ionic, etc.) The complex reacts to alter the substrate. The complex then decomposes, regenerating the enzyme and liberating a product different from the substrate.

$$\text{Enzyzme + Substrate} \rightarrow \text{Enzyme-Substrate Complex} \rightarrow \text{Enzyme + Product}$$

The metabolism of a drug is important in determining its therapeutic activity and toxicity. Many factors affect drug biotransformation: route of administration, species, sex, age, strain, diet, temperature, time of day, season, chronic drug administration, and previous or concurrent administration of other drugs or chemicals. Unlike most drugs, the inhaled anesthetics are administered in great excess of the amount metabolized. For this reason biotransformation of the anesthetics plays a significant role in determining toxicity but has little affect on pharmacologic activity.

The major pathways of drug metabolism involve oxidation, reduction, hydrolysis, and conjugation. A drug may simultaneously undergo several forms of metabolism because of enzyme competition for substrate (drug). The ratio of end products (metabolites) to each other and the unchanged drug depends on enzymatic reaction rates, drug concentration near an enzyme, and physicochemical reactions between metabolites and enzymes.

The general pattern of drug metabolism is common to all animal species; it is biphasic in nature and consists of stepwise biotransformation and synthesis reactions. Figure 14-1 shows the general scheme of drug metabolism. Phase I (biotransformation) consists of oxidation (hydroxylation), reduction, or hydrolysis of a lipid soluble or nonpolar drug. Phase II (synthesis) consists of the conjugation of drug or metabolite with an endogenous compound (predominantly glycine, sulfate, or glucuronic acid). Generally, the net result of either phase is the production of compounds that are more easily excreted in the bile or urine. The two phases of metabolism are controlled by tissue enzymes that may be present in plasma, cytoplasm, mitochondria, or endoplasmic reticulum. The variations in metabolism, both quantitative and qualitative, seen with different species lie mainly in the nature of these enzymes.

Phase I metabolism occurs primarily in the environment of the endoplasmic reticulum while phase II metabolism occurs generally in the more aqueous environment of the cytoplasm. Usually, but not necessarily, substrates for phase I reactions are not substrates of phase II reactions. However, a product of phase I metabolism may be a substrate for phase II reactions.

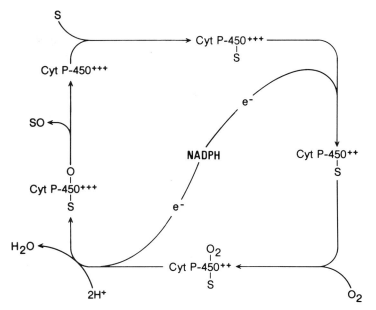

Fig. 14-2 A drug substrate (S) of the hepatic mixed-function oxidase system interacts with cytochrome P-450 and is biotransformed to a hydroxylated product (SO).

PHASE I REACTIONS

Microsomal Drug-Metabolizing Enzymes

The cytochrome P-450-mediated mono-oxygenases are a collective example of phase I enzymes. This hydroxylating enzyme system is called a mixed-function oxidase or mono-oxygenase because one of the two atoms of molecular oxygen (O_2) is incorporated into cellular water (H_2O). Reactions of the mono-oxygenase system have been extensively studied in vitro using microsomes and reconstituted systems. The overall hydroxylation reaction can be represented as:

$$RH + NADPH + H^+ + O_2 \rightarrow ROH + NADP^+ + H_2O$$

RH is the substrate, ROH is the hydroxylated product, and NADPH is the reduced form of nicotinamide-adenine dinucleotide phosphate (NADP). The membrane-bound multicomponent enzyme system requires molecular oxygen (O_2) and NADPH. The key enzyme components of the mono-oxygenase system are cytochrome P-450 and NADPH-cytochrome P-450 reductase.

The overall flow of electrons proceeds from NADPH to the flavoprotein (NADPH-cytochrome P-450) to molecular oxygen. Under some circumstances, reduced nicotinamide-adenine dinucleotide (NADH) can contribute an electron instead of NADPH. The intermediate electron carrier for NADH is microsomal cytochrome b_5. The role of cytochrome b_5 and NADH in microsomal drug metabolism is not known at this time.

Figure 14-2 demonstrates the steps in cytochrome P-450-mediated drug hydroxylation. Cytochrome P-450 is shown as Cyt P-450^{+++} (the valence state of iron in the hemoprotein is indicated); S is the drug (substrate); and SO is the hydroxylated drug metabolite. The first step of the hydroxylation reaction is assumed to be the formation of a ferric (Fe^{+++}) cytochrome P-450-substrate complex by a reversible reaction of substrate with the oxidized hemoprotein. This complex accepts one electron (e^-) from NADPH (via NADPH-cytochrome P-450 reductase) to form a ferrous (Fe^{++}) cytochrome P-450-

substrate complex that subsequently combines with molecular oxygen to yield an oxygenated drug complex (SO). Upon introduction of a second electron from NADPH, an internal electronic rearrangement takes place and the complex undergoes decomposition, via an intermediate, leading to the liberation of the hydroxylated product and regeneration of ferric cytochrome P-450.

The cytochrome P-450 containing mixed-function oxidases, along with other metabolically linked enzymes, provide an important pathway whereby the cell may metabolize and thus eliminate xenobiotics. These enzyme systems are responsible not only for deactivation of toxic compounds but also for activation of drugs, chemicals, and environmental pollutants to toxic, mutagenic, and carcinogenic forms. These mixed-function oxidases catalyze the oxidation of a variety of substrates. The enzyme systems of the endoplasmic membranes participating in hydroxylations and other processes are distributed in a specific pattern to allow coordinated and side-directed reactions.

Numerous factors affect the performance of the endoplasmic reticulum and its drug-metabolizing complex, predominantly genetic and environmental factors (including chemicals and drugs). Since the microsomal membrane is not formed and degraded as a unit, but is formed by the random insertion of newly synthetized protein molecules into existing membranes, membrane proteins of liver microsomes are heterogenous in their turnover rates.[5] Various microsomal enzymes are not tightly coupled with one another but behave rather independently in their synthesis and degradation. The turnover rates of cytochrome P-450 and NADPH-cytochrome P-450 reductase are different from each other; so are the turnover rates of cytochrome b_5 and NADH-cytochrome b_5 reductase, which also are functionally intimately associated.

The human liver contains less cytochrome P-450 than other species (10 to 20 nmoles/g of liver tissue). Rat liver contains approximately 30 to 50 nmoles/g of liver. Likewise, human liver is 2 percent of body weight and rat liver is aproximately 4 percent. These differences in the total cytochrome P-450 seem to account for the fact that man metabolizes drugs in vivo at rates 10 to 20 times slower than rat.[6]

Microsomal cytochrome P-450 is not a single component, but rather a mixture of molecular species having different substrate specificities. Along with species and interindividual differences in the hepatic content of cytochrome P-450, differences in the cytochrome species themselves may be responsible for observed differences between man and laboratory animals in rates and pathways of anesthetic metabolism in vivo and in vitro. Experimental studies show that this may be especially true with regard to cytochrome P-450-mediated dehalogenation and dealkylation of the inhaled anesthetics.[7,8] The difference in metabolism of man and animals must seriously be considered when determining potential toxicity.

Reactions Relevant to Anesthetic Biotransformation

Reactions that can be classified as oxidations, reductions, and hydrolyses are many and varied. They are carried out by two kinds of enzymes. The first consists of enzymes primarily involved in the metabolism of natural substrates of the body. These enzymes, however, will also metabolize foreign substrates. The second group consists of the so-called drug metabolizing enzymes, the cytochrome P-450-mediated mono-oxygenases, which appear primarily to utilize foreign compounds as substrates. These enzymes are located mainly in the endoplasmic reticulum of the liver cell. The inhaled anesthetics are metabolized by enzymes in this second group, primarily by oxidation reactions.[9] Two types of oxidations, dehalogenation and O-dealkylation, are responsible for the greatest proportion of anesthetic metabolism.[9] One additional type of oxidation, epoxidation, represents a minor metabolic route for a few anesthetics; it is important, however, because of the toxic potential of epoxides. Only one anesthetic, halothane, is known to undergo reductive metabolism.[10] None is metabolized via hydrolysis because none possesses the necessary ester linkage. Examples of these reactions are shown below.

O-dealkylation. Dealkylation is the result of the hydroxylation of an alkyl group. The resulting hemiacetyl is a relatively unstable intermediate, which rapidly decomposes to an alcohol and an aldehyde. The rate of the O-dealkylation reaction decreases as the length of the alkyl chain increases.

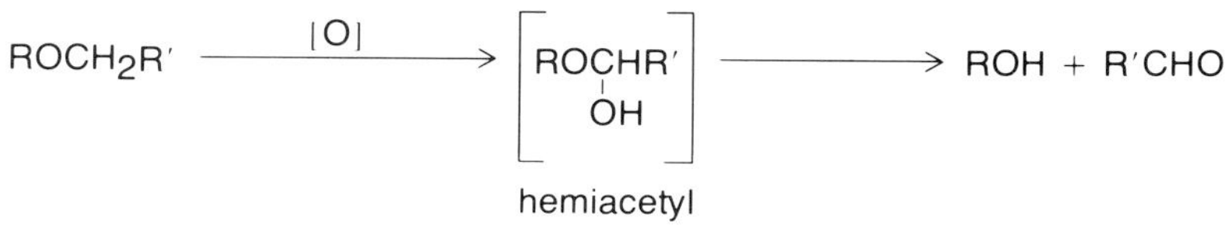

$$ROCH_2R' \xrightarrow{\;|O|\;} \left[\begin{array}{c} ROCHR' \\ | \\ OH \end{array} \right] \longrightarrow ROH + R'CHO$$

hemiacetyl

Dehalogenation. Dehalogenation is not the result of a direct attack on the carbon-halogen bond as previously had been thought. It is the result of oxidation of the halogen-containing carbon, producing a chemically unstable intermediate that decomposes to a carboxylic acid and liberates any halogens. Two halogens on the terminal carbon represent the optimal condition for dehalogenation, while a terminal carbon with three halogens is oxidized to a very limited degree.[11]

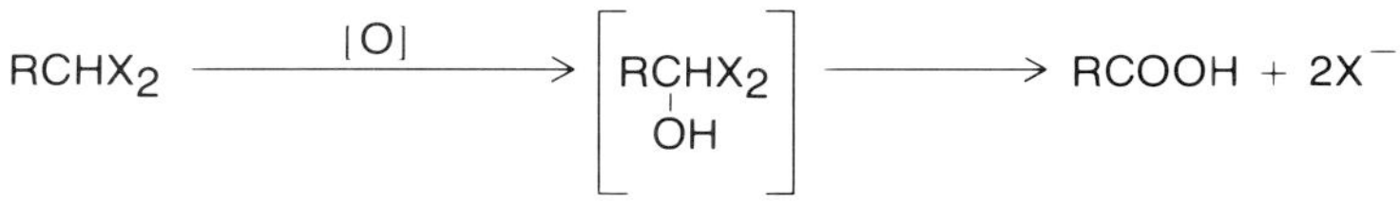

$$RCHX_2 \xrightarrow{\;|O|\;} \left[\begin{array}{c} RCHX_2 \\ | \\ OH \end{array} \right] \longrightarrow RCOOH + 2X^-$$

Epoxidation. An epoxide is formed when an oxygen atom is attached to two adjacent carbons of an olefin. Most epoxides are highly-strained molecules and extremely reactive because of the ease with which the ring can be opened. Some epoxides may be hydrated by the microsomal enzyme system epoxide hydrase.[12]

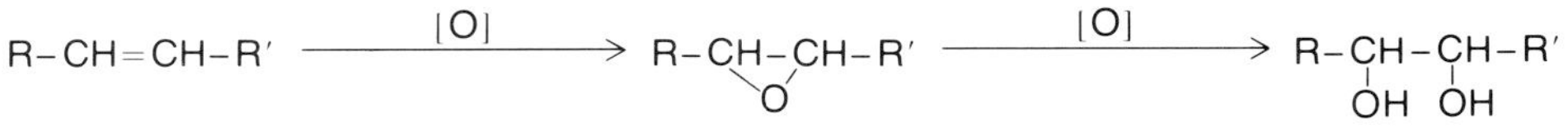

$$R-CH=CH-R' \xrightarrow{\;|O|\;} R-\underset{\underset{O}{\diagdown\diagup}}{CH}-CH-R' \xrightarrow{\;|O|\;} R-\underset{\underset{OH}{|}}{CH}-\underset{\underset{OH}{|}}{CH}-R'$$

Reduction. The mechanisms of reductive reactions catalyzed by the cytochrome P-450 enzyme system are very different from those of oxidative reactions. For reduction, it is thought that a substrate directly accepts electrons from cytochrome P-450 because oxygen inhibits the reaction. Reductions are most commonly associated with azocompounds and nitrocompounds but reductive metabolism involving cytochrome P-450 has also been confirmed for one anesthetic, halothane.[10]

$$CF_3CHBrCl \xrightarrow{\;e^-\;} [CF_3\dot{C}BrCl] \longrightarrow$$
$$CF_2=CBrCl + F^-$$

PHASE II REACTIONS

Phase II reactions may occur when the drug contains a group that is suitable for combination with an endogenous compound (i.e., glycine, sulfate, and glucuronic acid) to form readily excreted, polar, water soluble metaboliltes. A type of conjugation reaction is seen below.

$$UDPGA + ROH \xrightarrow{\text{glucuronyl transferase}} R-O-glucuronide + UDP$$

D-glucuronic acid can only be conjugated with a drug in its "active" form, uridine diphosphate glucuronic acid (UDPGA). UDPGA is condensed with a drug containing an appropriate chemical group, in this case a hydroxyl (–OH), catalyzed by glucuronyl transferase, an enzyme located in the rough endoplasmic reticulum of the liver. The resulting glucuronide is more water soluble because of the presence of a very polar sugar moiety. The free carboxyl ($-COO^-$) in the molecule further enhances water solubility because its pKa is usually lower than that of the drug-parent compound (substrate) and it is essentially completely ionized at body pH. The chemical groups on the drug molecule usually associated with conjugation reactions are: –OH, –COOH, –NH$_2$, and –SH. If the drug does not initially contain one or more of these groups it may attain one through a phase I reaction (i.e., by oxidation, reduction, or hydrolysis). One example of an anesthetic metabolite that results from multiple consecutive biotransformations is trichloroethanol, an end product of trichloroethylene[13, 14, 15] and possibly other anesthetics. It is only detected in the urine as its glucuronic acid conjugate, urochloralic acid.[16, 17]

ENZYME INDUCTION

Enzyme induction occurs when the number of molecules of a specific enzyme is increased due to accelerated synthesis or to decreased degradation. The mixed-function oxidase drug-metabolizing enzyme systems are generally inducible.[18] The phenomenon of enzyme induction is not common to all drugs. It appears to be independent of the chemical structure of the drug and unrelated to the nature of its pharmacologic or toxicologic activity. Furthermore, enzyme-inducing agents are highly lipophilic and are metabolized by the cytochrome P-450 enzyme system, which they induce. Induction is thought to be determined largely by the extent and duration of the interaction of the drug substrate (inducing agent) with the enzyme concerned.

Proliferation of the smooth endoplasmic reticulum, drug-metabolizing enzymes, as well as increased liver weight follow phenobarbital treatment.[19] NADPH-cytochrome P-450 reductase and cytochrome P-450 are preferentially increased. Available evidence indicates that enzyme induction of drug metabolizing enzymes results from both increased synthesis and decreased degradation of enzymes in liver cells of drug-treated animals. Large numbers of drugs and enzyme inducers may enhance the metabolism of other drugs as well as their own metabolism. In 1967, Conney[20] reported that over 200 drugs and chemicals were inducers of the hepatic mixed-function oxidase system in experimental animals. Since that time, several investigators have reported the nonspecific stimulation of drug-metabolizing enzymes by the inhaled anesthetics.[21, 22, 23]

Enzyme activity may also be increased without a change in the amount of enzyme present. An example of this phenomenon is substrate induction in chronic liver disease. Generally there is a decrease in the total number of liver cells. However, the amount of drug presented to any one cell is increased and thus the total amount of drug metabolized per cell is significantly increased. This phenomena, in part, may explain why fairly severe hepatic damage is measured before there is a noticeable alteration in drug metabolism.[24]

Several classes of drugs, including anticonvulsants, steroids, tranquilizers, sedatives, anesthetics, and insecticides, contain one or more members considered as enzyme inducers. With the prevalence of polypharmacy, enzyme induction may not be an uncommon phenomenon in patients undergoing surgery. Many case reports of drug toxicity have suggested enzyme induction as a causative factor; data, however, are often unconvincing. If a drug is toxic, its enhanced metabolism may decrease toxicity; however, if the metabolite is toxic, increased metabolism may increase toxicity. Enzyme induction does not necessarily result in the production of new or toxic metabolites or in the increased metabolism of all drugs. For example, metabolism of enflurane is not significantly increased in vivo following phenobarbital and phenytoin treatment in man[25] and animals[26,27] or in vitro in animals.[8,28] Likewise, even though several anesthetic metabolites are known to be toxic to man, a study of surgical patients whose enzymes were induced failed to show an increased incidence of toxic effects that could be attributed to enzyme induction.[29] The evidence in man is circumstantial at best, and animal studies of prolonged exposure have resulted in conflicting results. Regardless of the source of the enzyme-inducing agent, these compounds do have the potential to modify both the acute and chronic toxic effects of anesthetics.

ENZYME INHIBITION

Many compounds can inhibit the activity of the drug metabolizing enzyme system. The consequences of enzyme inhibition on pharmacologic activity and toxicity can be just as great as the effects seen with enzyme induction. Inhibition can result in an increased duration of pharmacologic or toxic effects, an accumulation of toxic compounds not normally achieved, or decreased pharmacologic or toxic effects.

Inhibitors can be of several types. One kind frequently encountered in clinical medicine is competitive inhibition resulting from two drug substrates competing for the same enzyme. Another type inhibitor is that which decreases the amount of cytochrome P-450 available to metabolize the drug. Two examples are inhibitors of protein synthesis (e.g., cyclohexamide) and chemicals that destroy cytochrome P-450 (e.g., methoxyflurane, enflurane, and halothane at mM concentrations).[30]

GENETIC-SPECIES VARIATION

Species variations in drug metabolism, both qualitative and quantitative, are the result of genetic differences. Differences may be observed in the metabolic pathways followed or in the ratios of metabolites from the same pathways. Qualitative differences generally result from the presence or absence of a specific enzyme in a particular species. Quantitative differences can result from variations in the amount and localization of enzyme, the presence of a natural inhibitor or competition of enzymes for substrate.

In man, genetic factors that are not readily evident under normal circumstances may play a significant role in the expression of a drug's therapeutic activity and toxicity. For example, physiological disposition of a drug may be unusual because of a structural variation in a serum protein responsible for binding drugs. This seemingly small alteration can affect chemical equilibrium and ultimately biological activity. Genetic factors appear to be more important than environmental factors (such as diet and pollution exposure) in determining the overall rate of drug metabolism and elimination, although enzyme induction and inhibition may account for some unusual drug responses seen in man. Studies of drug metabolism and elimination in twins have demonstrated far less variation in identical than in fraternal twins or in the normal population. This observation was consistent even when environmental factors (exposures) were quite dissimilar.[31]

METABOLISM OF SPECIFIC ANESTHETIC AGENTS

NONHALOGENATED INHALED ANESTHETICS

Diethyl Ether

$$CH_3-CH_2-O-CH_2-CH_3 \xrightarrow{|O|} |?| \longrightarrow CH_3-CHO + |?| + CH_3-CH_2OH$$

$$\longrightarrow CO_2 + \text{?-glucuronide}$$

Initial metabolism experiments by Haggard[32] demonstrated no in vivo biodegradation of diethyl ether. Subsequent studies with the radiolabeled compound, however, revealed biodegradation to $^{14}CO_2$ and nonvolatile urinary products.[33] The ether linkage is cleaved by enzymes of the hepatic mixed-function oxidase system producing products such as ethanol, acetic acid, and acetaldehyde, all of which are further oxidized to CO_2.[9, 34, 35] Diethyl ether has not been studied in vitro, but in vivo metabolism is enhanced following phenobarbital treatment. Chronic exposure of rats to subanesthetic concentrations of diethyl ether results in increased metabolism of several drugs,[22] elevated levels of hepatic microsomal enzymes,[23] and increased metabolism of diethyl ether and other inhaled anesthetics.[21]

Ethylene

$$H_2C=CH_2 \xrightarrow{|O|} |?| \longrightarrow CO_2 + |?|$$

Although initial experiments showed that ethylene was not metabolized, work by Van Dyke and Chenoweth[36] demonstrated $^{14}CO_2$ and labeled urinary products following the administration of ^{14}C-labeled ethylene.

Cyclopropane

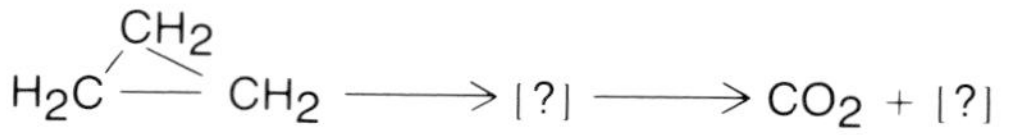

$$\overset{CH_2}{\underset{H_2C - CH_2}{\diagup \diagdown}} \longrightarrow |?| \longrightarrow CO_2 + |?|$$

Cyclopropane is the simplest cyclic compound that produces anesthesia. It is eliminated almost exclusively unchanged by the lungs. Van Dyke et al.[33] however, with the use of radiolabeled compounds, reported some conversion of cyclopropane to CO_2.

Nitrous Oxide

At present, there is no firm evidence that nitrous oxide is metabolized in vivo. However, nitrous oxide can produce enzyme induction in experimental animals following prolonged exposure.[9] A recent study of rats exposed to 20 percent nitrous oxide for 14 to 35 days resulted in inhibition of hepatic drug metabolism and induction of metabolism in the lung and testis.[37]

HALOGENATED INHALED ANESTHETICS

Chloroform

$$CHCl_3 \xrightarrow{|O|} CCl_3OH \longrightarrow COCl_2 + Cl^- \xrightarrow{|O|} |?| + CO_2 \longrightarrow Cl^- + |?|$$

Initial studies by Van Dyke et al.[33] showed metabolism of ^{36}Cl and ^{14}C chloroform. In vivo oxidative metabolism of chloroform results in the formation of trichloromethanol, which decomposes to phosgene[38] ($COCl_2$), which is in turn oxidatively dechlorinated or hydrolyzed to CO_2.[39,40] The metabolism of chloroform has been studied in two human volunteers.[41] Fifty percent of an administered $^{13}CHCl_3$ dosage was recovered as exhaled $^{13}CO_2$. Animal studies have shown that in the conversion of chloroform to CO_2 a reactive intermediate is formed that can bind with tissue macromolecules.[42,43,44] Metabolism and tissue binding can be induced by phenobarbital and inhibited by disulfiram.[43] Chronic exposure to chloroform results in the enhanced in vivo metabolism of hexobarbital and presumably other anesthetics.[22]

Trichloroethylene

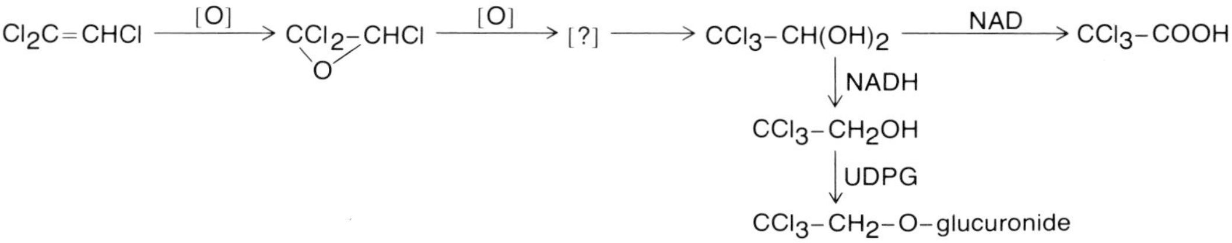

$$Cl_2C{=}CHCl \xrightarrow{\text{[O]}} \underset{\underset{O}{\diagup}}{CCl_2{-}CHCl} \xrightarrow{\text{[O]}} [?] \longrightarrow CCl_3{-}CH(OH)_2 \xrightarrow{\text{NAD}} CCl_3{-}COOH$$

$$CCl_3{-}CH(OH)_2 \xrightarrow{\text{NADH}} CCl_3{-}CH_2OH \xrightarrow{\text{UDPG}} CCl_3{-}CH_2{-}O{-}glucuronide$$

Trichlorethylene was the first inhaled anesthetic demonstrated to be metabolized.[45] In 1965, Byington and Leibman[13] demonstrated that metabolism occurred primarily by the hepatic mixed-function oxidases, via an epoxide and a rearrangement of chlorine atoms,[14] to chloral hydrate. This metabolite may be further transformed by oxidation to trichloroacetic acid by a soluble enzyme (requiring nicotinamide adenine dinucleotide [NAD]) or by reduction to trichloroethanol by alcohol dehydrogenase (requiring NADH, the reduced form of NAD).[15]

Trichloroacetic acid is excreted unchanged in the urine. Trichloroethanol is excreted in the urine as urochloralic acid, its glucuronic acid conjugate.[16,17] The in vitro metabolism of trichloroethylene to chloral hydrate is increased following phenobarbital pretreatment.[46]

Fluroxene

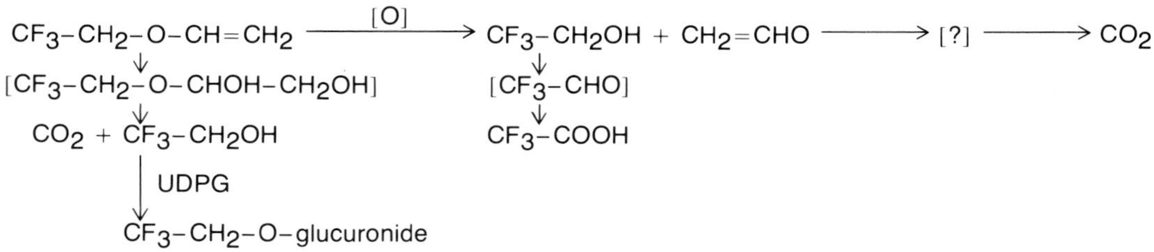

$$CF_3{-}CH_2{-}O{-}CH{=}CH_2 \xrightarrow{\text{[O]}} CF_3{-}CH_2OH + CH_2{=}CHO \longrightarrow [?] \longrightarrow CO_2$$

$$[CF_3{-}CH_2{-}O{-}CHOH{-}CH_2OH] \qquad [CF_3{-}CHO]$$

$$CO_2 + CF_3{-}CH_2OH \qquad CF_3{-}COOH$$

$$CF_3{-}CH_2OH \xrightarrow{\text{UDPG}} CF_3{-}CH_2{-}O{-}glucuronide$$

In man, fluroxene is metabolized in the liver primarily to trifluoroacetic acid. In mouse and dog the trifluoroethanol glucuronide has also been identified.[47] Fluroxene metabolism is increased by pretreatment with the enzyme inducers phenobarbital, 3-methylcholanthrene, and 3,4-benzpyrene.[48,49] In man, trifluoroethanol is produced in such small quantities that there appears to be little clinical risk from this metabolite.[50] Chronic exposure to fluroxene, like many other anes-

thetics, results in decreased hexobarbital sleeping time in rats.[22]

Halothane (Fluothane)

$$CF_3-CHClBr \xrightarrow{[O]} [CF_3-\overset{\bullet}{C}OCl] \xrightarrow{[HOH]} CF_3-COOH + Br^- + Cl^-$$

$$\downarrow e^-$$

$$[CF_3-\overset{\bullet}{C}HCl] \searrow CF_2=CBrCl + F^- \xrightarrow{[GSH?]} N-acetyl\ cysteine\ conjugate$$

$$\downarrow [?]$$

$$CF_3-CH_2Cl + Br^- \longrightarrow CF_2=CHCl + Br^- + F^-$$

Halothane was found to be significantly metabolized soon after its clinical introduction.[33,51,52] Its major metabolite in man and animals is trifluoroacetic acid, which is eliminated in the urine as the sodium salt.[34,51] Other urinary metabolites that occur in small amounts are Cl^-, Br^-, and F^-.[52] Although significant amounts of trifluoroethanol have been identified in urine of experimental animals, neither trifluoroethanol nor its glucuronide conjugates have been found in the urine of man. Likewise, trifluoroacetaldehyde has been proposed as a possible metabolite, but thus far has not been isolated. Recent studies by Sharp, et al.[53] have demonstrated the existence of several volatile metabolites as a result of reductive metabolism (requiring cytochrome P-450 in the absence of oxygen). Two direct reductive metabolites (di-

fluorochloroethylene and trifluorochloroethane) and a metabolite-decomposition product (difluorobromochloroethylene) were identified by gas chromatography–mass spectrometry in the exhaled gases of patients anesthetized with halothane. Induction of the hepatic drug-metabolizing enzyme system in experimental animals results in increased halothane metabolism and covalent binding of reactive intermediates to tissue macromolecules following administration of inducing agents such as phenobarbital[10,44,54,55] and Aroclor 1254.[56,57] Prolonged exposure to subanesthetic concentrations of halothane results in increased drug metabolism in experimental animals.[22,23]

Methoxyflurane (Penthrane)

$$CH_3-O-CF_2-CHCl_2 \xrightarrow{[O]} CH_3-O-CF_2-COOH + 2Cl^-$$

$$\downarrow [O] \qquad\qquad\qquad \downarrow$$

$$CH_2O + CF_2OH-CHCl_2 \qquad COOH-CF_2OH$$

$$\downarrow CO_2 \quad\downarrow HOH \qquad\qquad \downarrow$$

$$2F^- + COOH-CHCl_2 \qquad COOH-COOH + CH_2O + 2F^-$$

$$\downarrow [O]$$

$$2Cl^- + COOH-COOH$$

Metabolism of methoxyflurane has been studied extensively, both in vivo and in vitro. The molecule can be attacked at either the dichloromethyl group or at the ether linkage.[58,59] Major metabolites are F^-, dichloroacetic acid, and probably methoxydifluoroacetic acid although it has not yet been isolated.[9,58] This latter metabolite is acid labile and would be expected to break down in the environment of the kidneys and as a result release oxalic acid and more F^-. Loew et al.[11] had predicted from quantum mechanical calculations that the O-dealkylation of methoxyflurane would occur more rapidly than its dechlorination. This prediction was opposite that proposed by Holaday et al.[58]

and has now been seriously questioned by the experimental evidence of Ivanetich et al.[60] Metabolism of methoxyflurane is increased in vivo and in vitro following treatment with enzyme-inducing drugs such as phenobarbital[61,62] and phenytoin.[28] Its metabolism is subject to inhibition in vivo and in vitro by SKF-525A[60,61,63] and in vitro by metyrapone.[60] Prolonged exposure to methoxyflurane may result in the increased biotransformation of specific drugs by the decreased catabolism of NADPH-cytochrome P-450 reductase.

Enflurane (Ethrane)

$$CHF_2-O-CF_2-CHClF \xrightarrow{\ |O|\ } CHF_2-O-CF_2-COOH + Cl^- + F^-$$

$$\downarrow |O| \qquad\qquad\qquad\qquad \downarrow |O|$$

$$[CF_2O] + CF_2OH-CHClF \qquad\qquad [CF_2O] + COOH-CF_2OH$$

$$\downarrow HOH \qquad\qquad\qquad\qquad \downarrow HOH$$

$$2F^- + COOH-CHClF \qquad\qquad\qquad COOH-COOH + 2F^-$$

$$\downarrow |O|$$

$$Cl^- + F^- + COOH-COOH$$

Enflurane is slowly metabolized by the hepatic mixed-function oxidase system. The low rate of metabolism has made the study of its metabolism difficult. Even pretreatment with enzyme inducers such as phenobarbital[27,28] and phenytoin[28] only slightly increases enflurane metabolism. Metabolism under normal circumstance appears to occur only at the terminal fluoride containing carbon.[11] The metabolic pathway above seems most probable, although the difluoromethoxy-difluoroacetic acid has not been isolated.

Ivanetich et al.[60] have suggested from studies with the inducing agent, phenobarbital, and two enzyme inhibitors, SKF-525A and metyrapone, that only one form of cytochrome P-450 that is induced by phenobarbital is involved in the in vitro metabolism of enflurane. Two forms are responsible for metabolism of methoxyflurane. This would, in part, explain the differences observed in the degree of in vitro defluorination following phenobarbital pretreatment. Recently, Rice et al.[8] and Rice and Talcott[64] demonstrated significantly enhanced enflurane metabolism following treatment of rats with isoniazid. The reason for the fourfold enhancement of defluorination has not been fully explained, although there appears to be a shift in the type of cytochrome P-450 that is present in the microsomes isolated from isoniazid-treated rats. Similar to methoxyflurane, defluorination of enflurane is decreased following treatment with enzyme inhibitors SKF-525A[60,61,63] and metyrapone.[60] Exposure of rats to subanesthetic concentrations of enflurane significantly decreases hexobarbital sleeping time.[22]

Isoflurane

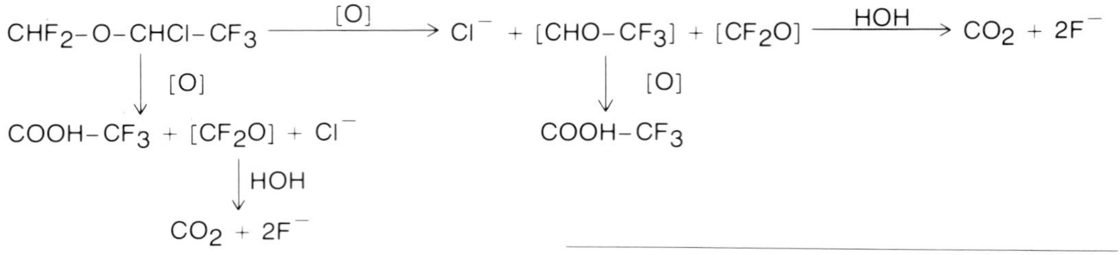

$$CHF_2-O-CHCl-CF_3 \xrightarrow{[O]} Cl^- + [CHO-CF_3] + [CF_2O] \xrightarrow{HOH} CO_2 + 2F^-$$

$$\downarrow [O]$$

$$COOH-CF_3 + [CF_2O] + Cl^- \qquad\qquad \downarrow [O]$$

$$\qquad\qquad\qquad COOH-CF_3$$

$$\downarrow HOH$$

$$CO_2 + 2F^-$$

The extremely low rate of metabolism appears to be due to the slow ether cleavage and release of $2F^-$ from the methyl group.[11,65] Work by Hitt et al.[66] has suggested the excretion of trifluoroacetic acid in the urine of rats and man. Trifluoroacetaldehyde and trifluoroacetylacylchloride, expected metabolic intermediates between isoflurane and trifluoroacetic acid, may also be produced. Although phenobarbital,[62,66] phenytoin,[28] and isoniazid[8,64] pretreatments increase the defluorination of isoflurane, enzyme induction does not seem to be of clinical significance. Isoflurane, like many ether anesthetics, enhances hexobarbital sleeping time following exposure of experimental animals to subanesthetic concentrations.[22]

Sevoflurane

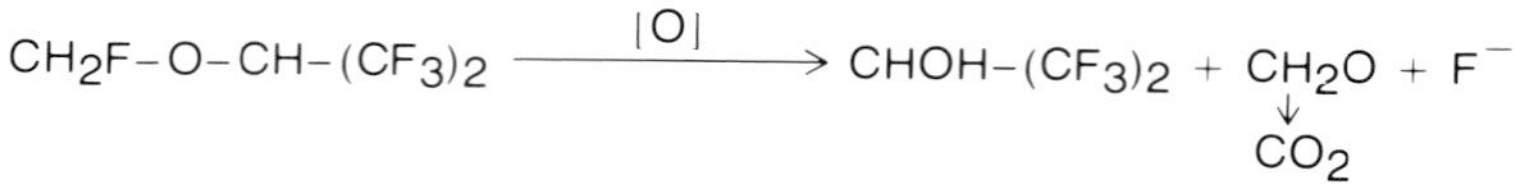

$$CH_2F-O-CH-(CF_3)_2 \xrightarrow{[O]} CHOH-(CF_3)_2 + CH_2O + F^-$$

$$\downarrow$$

$$CO_2$$

In vitro studies have shown that the rate of sevoflurane defluorination is approximately the same as that of methoxyflurane.[68,69] The trifluoromethyl group is not easily attacked enzymatically. Therefore it appears that the site of attack is at the ether linkage. The product, hexafluoroisopyropyl alcohol, would not be subject to further degradation although conjugation is a possibility. In vivo, there is far less serum F^- found with sevoflurane than with methoxyflurane.[68] This difference appears to be related to the differences in solubilities as well as to the fact that the sevoflurane metabolite is more stable. In vivo studies have shown increased sevoflurane defluorination following phenobarbital treatment.[69] In vitro, sevoflurane defluorination is increased by phenytoin[28] and isoniazid[8,64] as well as by phenobarbital.[69]

TOXICITY

MECHANISMS OF TOXICITY

The expression of drug toxicity is dependent upon various factors. This section discusses mechanisms of chemical toxicity that are considered applicable to the inhaled anesthetics. We have focused on mechanisms of tissue injury that are experimentally reproducible and consistent from one individual to another and not on toxic responses that are the result of a rare hereditary trait (i.e., inborn metabolic error). At present three general mechanisms of drug toxicity are applicable to tissue injury that is associated with the inhaled anesthetics. They are the intracellular accumulation of metabolites in toxic amounts, the formation of haptens that can initiate systemic hypersensitivity or immune responses, and the production of reactive intermediates that either adduct (form covalent bonds) to tissue macromolecules or initiate destructive chain reactions.

Each of the above mechanisms is dependent on the metabolism of the parent anesthetic compound. The first mechanism may result from the accumulation of high concentrations of a metabolite with a low toxic potency or the increased production (or decreased cellular secretion) of a highly toxic metabolite. The accumulation of metabolites in toxic quantities may intially occur as a result of other chemicals or pathologic states modifying drug metabolism. When the level of drug metabolites surpasses the intracellular "threshold" for toxicity, tissue injury may result from the direct or indirect actions of the metabolite. Toxicity may directly result from the actions of metabolites to inhibit or modify enzymatic and structural systems necessary for maintaining cellular integrity (e.g., membrane transport systems). Alternatively, metabolites may initiate unwanted pharmacologic actions that are indirectly toxic to the "target" cell. An example is the unwanted effect of a metabolite possessing vasoconstrictive properties; accumulation might initiate local tissue ischemia and thus promote cellular necrosis.

Probably the most important drug-mediated toxic mechanism is the production of reactive intermediates during drug metabolism. Intermediates are thought to initiate toxicity in two ways: they can form adducts (covalently bind) with macromolecules[70,71] or initiate aberrant free radical reactions.[72,73,74] Though few drugs are sufficiently reactive to form covalent bonds with cell constituents, covalent interactions between their reactive metabolites may occur with cell macromolecules (e.g., intracellular proteins, enzymes, nucleic acid). Bioactivation of chemically nonreactive compounds, such as the inhaled anesthetics,[75] may produce phase I metabolites that are capable of spontaneously forming covalent complexes with cell organelles and macromolecules.

One example of a potentially toxic covalent interaction is the binding of a reactive intermediate with tissue protein to produce a hapten-protein conjugate. Such a conjugate may in turn induce the synthesis of drug- or metabolite-specific antibodies and initiate hypersensitivity of immune responses.[76] The adduction of other reactive intermediates to tissue macromolecules might produce alterations in the normal operation of the cell by affecting organelles such as the endoplasmic reticulum, mitochondria, lysosomes, and the nucleus.[77] Other detrimental effects of covalent binding can result from the depletion of endogenous cellular compounds that are necessary for normal cell function.

One such compound necessary to cell homeostasis is glutathione. Intracellular glutathione and other sulfhydryl-containing compounds appear to function as natural cellular antioxidants.[74] When depleted of glutathione, the cell is susceptible to oxidant effects such as those produced by cytochrome P-450-mediated mono-oxygenases which continue to function in the absence of intracellular substrates by transfering electrons to cell lipids.[78] Under normal circumstances glutathione can terminate radical chain reactions by forming conjugates with radicals. In the absence of glutathione, however, destructive reactions continue and cell death can ensue.

Highly reactive metabolic intermediates such as arene oxides (a type of epoxide) may covalently bind to proteins, nucleic acids, and other cellular components.[79] Interaction between arene oxides and cellular components results in the formation of chemically stable, covalent drug-protein complexes, which subsequently may produce pathologic injuries such as hepatic necrosis,[74,80] mutagenesis, teratogenesis, and carcinogenesis.[12,81] Covalent binding of many classes of drug metabolites, in addition to the arene oxidases, may be responsible for initiation of organotropic and developmental carcinogenesis and teratogenesis[82] as well as drug allergies.[76] Many drugs, such as the inhaled anesthetics, are possible sources of free radical intermediates as a result of their phase I metabolism.

It has been proposed that the majority of drug effects, both therapeutic and toxic, occur through free radical mechanisms initiated by drug metabolism.[83] Most drugs are chemically stable. Drug metabolism may change this state by producing a single unpaired electron in an outer orbital shell. The result is a chemically reactive compound known as a free radical, which may be described as a molecule with one or more unpaired electrons. The activity of these short-lived, but highly reactive intermediates is extremely significant because they can initiate chain reactions and produce pathologic damage.[73, 84]

Free radical chain reactions consist of three phases. During the initiation phase, free radicals are generated by a single reaction or series of reactions. The propagation phase consists of a sequence of reactions that act to conserve or increase the numbers of free radicals. The termination phase is the destruction or inactivation of the generated free radicals. Once generated, radicals react with cellular components producing polymerization or cross-linking of enzymes and proteins,[85] auto-oxidation of lipids within the organelle membranes,[85] and damage to nucleic acids (e.g., main chain breaks in the nuclein acid strands or degradation of purine and pyrimidine rings).[86] Free radical reactions are generated during the normal course of cell metabolism.[78] Radical levels, however, are controlled in biologic tissues[87] such that they exist only in dilute concentrations (10^{-9}M).[84] It is only when aberrant radical reactions occur and endogenous antioxidants (e.g., glutathione) are depleted that tissue injury results.[73]

Generally, reactions of radical intermediates are assumed to be so rapid that none of them escape the tissue in which they are formed.[86] Since the inhaled anesthetics are strongly lipophilic, damage from their reactive intermediates can be expected to occur in lipid membranes. Several inhaled anesthetics have been implicated in the production of tissue injury via free radical initiated auto-oxidation of lipids (lipoperoxidation). Halothane and chloroform, at anesthetizing concentrations, stimulate lipoperoxidation in vivo in phenobarbital-pretreated rats.[88] Membrane lipids are especially rich in unsaturated fatty acids. These unsaturated compounds are highly susceptible to damage because the presence of a double bond weakens the carbon-hydrogen bond of the α-methylene carbon atom (i.e., the carbon atom adjacent to a carbon with an unsaturated bond). Free radicals initiate peroxidation by abstracting hydrogen from the α-methylene carbon.[73, 85] This results in a rearrangement of double bonds and a subsequent attack by oxygen resulting in cleavage of the radical. Unless terminated, the oxidative damage will be transferred to adjacent fatty acids.

The detrimental effects of covalent interaction on cell integrity may depend on the extent of covalent binding by free radicals and the cellular functions that are impaired. The exact way in which specific reactive intermediates (metabolites) initiate cellular injuries is not clear. For example, although the formation of free radicals and reactive intermediates is consistent with evidence showing that metabolites bind covalently to liver microsomes, there is no strict correlation between adduction and cell damage.[89] Determination of the first cellular function to be impaired is nearly impossible to prove experimentally because there may be stronger cellular adduction in nontarget cells and organs than in those suffering injury.

ACUTE TOXICITY

EFFECTS ON THE LIVER

Clinically, drug-mediated hepatotoxicity ranges in severity from a slight increase in serum liver enzymes to jaundice. The cause of this specific organ injury may be hepatocellular damage directly resulting from hepatotoxic agents or sensitizing agents, interference with bilirubin metabolism, or cholestasis. Direct hepatocellular injury, the first of these mechanisms, is probably responsible for the majority of anesthetic-mediated hepatotoxicity. Direct hepatotoxins cause dose-related and reproducible hepatic damage in man and animals. Two examples are carbon tetrachloride and chloroform. Sensitizing agents produce their toxic effects through hypersensitivity and immune reactions.

The extent of hepatotoxicity directly resulting from administration of inhaled anesthetics is difficult to determine. Several factors may predispose the liver to postoperative dysfunction and necrosis: chronic liver disease, viral infection (i.e., viral hepatitis and cytomegalovirus), septicemia, severe burns, pregnancy, nutritional deficiency, and previous or concommitant drug treatment. Many additional factors may be involved; for example, hypoxia, hypercarbia, and hypotension alone may cause liver damage. Strunin[90] suggests that most physiological alterations caused by hypoxia or hypercarbia are the result of changes in liver blood flow, rather than the result of direct anesthetic effects. Additionally, most surgical procedures, regardless of anesthetic technique (intravenous as well as inhalational), are probably followed by adverse changes in liver function. Usually these changes are minor and directly related to the surgical procedure.[91]

All anesthetic techniques reduce the liver blood flow to some degree.[92] Although studies in healthy volunteers have demonstrated no evidence of hypoxia or anaerobic metabolism, this may not be the case for patients with preexisting liver damage or other illnesses. In general, surgical manipulation, rather than the anesthetic agent, appears to be responsible for any decreases in liver blood flow.[93] Unfortunately, tests available to assess liver function are for the most part crude, inaccurate (i.e., not tissue specific), and only reflect abnormalities in the presence of severe disor-

ders. Traditional markers of liver function are serum protein, enzyme, and bilirubin concentrations. A change in serum enzymes may indicate leakage from damaged cells, failure of biliary secretion, or failure of synthesis. None of the enzymes routinely measured are entirely specific to the liver. Isoenzymes (subfractions of measurable enzymes) are occasionally used because they may be characteristic of a particular source, but only the aminotransferases and alkaline phosphatase have stood the test of time. Two aminotransferases (transaminases) routinely measured are aspartate aminotransferase (AST; formerly called glutamate-pyruvate transaminase [SGOT]) and alanine aminotransferase (serum glutamate-pyruvate transaminase [SGPT]). Aspartate aminotransferase is present in large amounts in the heart, liver, kidneys, and skeletal muscles. It is primarily a cytoplasmic enzyme and is commonly elevated following surgery, liver damage, or myocardial infarction. Although alanine aminotransferase is present in the liver in quantities less than that of AST, serum increases in this enzyme are considered more specific to the liver and significant elevations above normal levels are characteristic of hepatocellular damage.

Chloroform was discovered in 1831 and was first used in man in 1847.[94] The first two cases of jaundice and death were observed in the same year.[95] In 1912 it was suggested by the Committee on Anesthesia of the American Medical Association to cease chloroform use for minor and major operations because of occasional cardiovascular collapse following its administration.[96] Chloroform, however, was used until 1957.

Several investigators have observed the covalent binding of radiolabeled chloroform or its metabolites to hepatic tissues. Cohen and Hood[42] performed low-temperature whole body autoradiographic studies of $^{14}CHCl_3$ administered to mice by inhalation. Results indicate that nonvolatile radioactivity (i.e., metabolites) was primarily confined to the liver. Illett et al.[43] measured increased covalent binding of ^{14}C following the administration of $^{14}CHCl_3$ to mice pretreated with phenobarbital, an enzyme-inducing agent. When animals were pretreated with piperonyl butoxide, an enzyme-inhibiting agent, decreased covalent binding was measured. The extent of covalent binding closely paralleled the degree of hepatocellular damage. Brown[88] demonstrated increased lipoperoxidation in phenobarbital-pretreated rats. When chloroform metabolism was inhibited by SKF 525-A (2-diethylamino-2, 2-diphenylvalerate HC1) or DPPD (N,N'-diphenyl-p-phenylenediamine), lipoperoxidation was decreased. Enhanced covalent binding and lipoperoxidation in enzyme-induced animals presents a strong case for a reactive chloroform metabolite as the hepatotoxin.

In 1905, Bevan and Favill[97] concluded on the basis of four isolated case reports that diethyl ether was hepatotoxic. Later reviews of the cases, however, have pointed out that there was little solid evidence on which to base these conclusions. Studies in experimental animals have shown fatty changes and extensive degeneration in the liver, but not to the extent seen with the classic hepatotoxin chloroform.[98, 99]

To date there are no case reports of hepatic necrosis following nitrous oxide administration when hypoxia has been ruled out as a possible contributing factor.[72] Exposure of rats to 20 percent nitrous oxide for as long as 35 days resulted in no significant changes in liver serum enzymes or in glutathione content.[37] Nitrous oxide administered in combination with intravenous barbiturates, however, has been associated with several isolated reports of hepatic necrosis.[100, 101, 102, 103] No conclusions regarding the hepatotoxic potential of nitrous oxide can be drawn from the available evidence.

Cyclopropane was considered quite innocuous to the liver as regards toxicity[104] until 1964 when a report was published of three patients who developed hepatic dysfunction following its use with other anesthetics.[67]

Since then, various case reports have linked cyclopropane to hepatic damage.[101, 102, 103] The National Halothane Study reported that massive hepatic necrosis following cyclopropane administration occurred in an incidence of 1.70 in 10,000. However, in 24 of the 25 cases noted, the outcome of hepatic necrosis might have been due to the selection of cyclopropane for anesthetizing patients in shock. Liver injury in these cases might be explained on the basis that any anesthetic would produce splanchnic vasoconstriction in a shock patient.

Fluroxene was introduced in 1953[105] and was the first volatile fluorinated anesthetic used in man. Its hepatotoxic potential was first suggested in 1972 when Reynolds et al.[106] reported death following massive hepatic necrosis in a patient treated with phenobarbital and phenytoin and then anesthetized with fluroxene. Further evidence for the role of fluroxene in hepatic necrosis was reported by Harrison and Smith.[107] They observed that enzyme-induced cats exposed to fluroxene died of massive hepatic necrosis. They proposed that the necrosis after enzyme induction was due to damage initiated by the increased formation of free radicals or epoxidation of the vinyl radical. Postanesthetic deaths in dogs, cats, and rabbits after long and repeated exposure to trifluoroethanol, a metabolite of fluroxene, have implicated this compound in the genesis of liver damage.[108] Fluroxene has now been withdrawn from clinical use.

Halothane was prepared by Suckling in 1952[109] and was introduced into clinical practice in 1956.[110, 111] Several reports of postoperative jaundice and liver necrosis were published in 1963.[112, 113, 114] These case studies suggested that the clinical and pathologic findings resembled those classically ascribed to the hepatotoxin chloroform. These reports prompted a number of retrospective studies that in essence concluded that there was no evidence of an increased incidence in postoperative clinical hepatic damage as compared to other anesthetics. Because some fault could be found in all the retrospective studies (i.e., lack of proper control groups, inadequate numbers), the United States National Halothane Study was undertaken.[115,116] The incidence of fatal massive hepatic necrosis occurring in approximately 850,000 surgical patients was reviewed retrospectively. The committee came to the conclusion that "unexplained fever and jaundice in a specific patient following halothane might reasonably be considered a contraindication to subsequent use." However, Dykes and Bunker[117] observed that "there was not a single patient in the National Halothane Study who was jaundiced after administration of halothane, and died after a second administration, and who was found at necropsy to have suffered massive or intermediate hepatic necrosis." The true incidence of massive hepatic necrosis associated with halothane was 7 out of 250,000 halothane anesthetics or about 1 in 35,000, and not 1 in 10,000, as is sometimes reported.

In 1972 Strunin and Simpson[118] reviewed various reports and in conclusion suggested that the data could be arranged to support or deny almost any hypothesis linking halothane anesthesia to liver damage. Much of the pre-1970's data presented in support of the hypothesis of liver damage due to halothane appears not to have withstood critical examination. Although liver damage may rarely be associated with halothane anesthesia, the incidence, etiology, and interaction of other factors remains obscure.[119,120,121,122]

Determination of the exact mechanism of halothane-mediated hepatotoxicity has been seriously hampered because, until recently, investigators have been unable to produce hepatotoxicity in halothane-exposed experimental animals. Unlike chloroform and fluroxene, which produce fatty infiltration, centrilobular necrosis, and elevated transaminase values, prolonged exposure of animals to halothane produced no evidence of liver damage. Even phenobarbital treatment prior to halothane exposure did not result in consistent production of hepatotoxicity. Re-

cently, several animal models have been developed to define halothane-mediated hepatotoxicity. Centrilobular necrosis following halothane exposure occurs in rats pretreated with Aroclor 1254 (polychlorinated biphenyls)[56,57], isoniazid,[7] and triiodothyronine.[123] The Aroclor 1254 model has been abandoned because polychlorinated biphenyls themselves cause moderate alterations in liver ultrastructure and function. The mechanisms for halothane-induced hepatotoxicity in the isoniazid and triiodothyronine models have yet to be determined. In another model, the "halothane hypoxic model," phenobarbital pretreated rats are exposed to halothane under hypoxic conditions (FiO_2 = 7 to 14 percent).[124,125,126] This "hypoxic model" is based on the observation of reductive halothane metabolism under hypoxic conditions and the increased covalent binding of these reductive metabolites in vitro to liver protein and phospholipids.[10,55] The hepatic lesion in this model is of centrilobular origin, similar to that seen in man. This area has the lowest oxygen concentration and the highest metabolic rate and is thus most susceptible to hypoxic injury. Lesion intensity is dependent both on the degree of enzyme induction (the amounts of reactive intermediate formed) and the degree of hypoxia (the production of reductive metabolites). Although this model is reproducible and well defined, its clinical applicability is questionable because of the necessity of hypoxia for lesion production. The mechanism of halothane-induced hepatotoxicity remains obscure, although from the animal models it appears to depend upon the production of a reactive intermediate that either causes direct hepatocellular damage or initiates an immune-mediated response.

Methoxyflurane was first synthesized in the United States in 1958 and introduced clinically in 1960.[127] Although none of the metabolites of methoxyflurane are known to be hepatotoxic, there have been a number of reports of hepatic dysfunction and death from hepatic coma following methoxyflurane exposure. A review of 24 cases of methoxy-flurane-associated hepatitis by Joshi and Conn[128] presented evidence for a syndrome that is very similar to that described in 1976 by Walton et al.[122] for unexplained hepatitis following halothane administration. They concluded that a rare and indirect immunologic hepatic injury may occur which may have a direct effect on the liver by interfering with splanchnic circulation.[90,92,129] In man, the adverse minor changes in liver function,[130] as well as the changes seen in isolated liver preparations,[90] appear to be reversible and may be dose related. It is still unclear whether hepatic dysfunction, as measured by bromsulphalin (BSP) retention and hepatic enzyme elevation, is due to factors such as the depth and duration of the anesthetic exposure, the type of operation, and the extent of preexisting hepatic disease.

Enflurane was first used in North America in 1968.[131,132] There have been a few isolated case reports of liver damage associated with enflurance anesthesia.[133,134,135] However, over 10 million administrations of enflurane have been used without any syndrome similar to that of halothane hepatitis yet described.

Sevoflurane is an experimental drug. There have been several reports regarding its metabolism[68,69,136] and renal toxicity,[68,69] but only one study of hepatic function.[137] This study in untreated, phenobarbital- and Aroclor 1254–treated rats resulted in no significant changes in serum transaminases, liver triglycerides, or glutathione levels.[137] The possible hepatic toxicity of this drug in man can only be assessed in light of further clinical investigations.

EFFECTS ON THE KIDNEY

Inhaled anesthetics depress renal function during their administration. They decrease urine flow, glomerular filtration rate, renal blood flow, and electrolyte excretion. This depression, however, is secondary to effects on the cardiovascular, sympathetic, and endo-crine systems. Fortunately, changes in renal function almost always return to normal after anesthesia and surgery has terminated. If renal dysfunction persists into the postoperative period, the cause is often a combination of factors such as prior existence of renal or cardiovascular disease, severe fluid and electrolyte imbalance, and the administration of mismatched blood; the choice of anesthetic is usually unimportant.

More directly related to inhaled anesthesia is the toxic nephropathy that occasionally follows administration of fluorinated anesthetics. Methoxyflurane, which has the greatest nephrotoxic potential of any currently used anesthetic, provides a classic example of damage resulting from accumulation of a toxic metabolite.

Methoxyflurane

In 1966, vasopressin-resistant polyuric renal insufficiency was first reported in 13 of 41 patients receiving methoxyflurane anesthesia for abdominal surgery.[138] Subsequently, the causative agent was shown to be inorganic fluoride (F^-), an end-product of the biotransformation of methoxyflurane. The evidence is based on three observations. First, serum F^- levels following methoxyflurane administration in man are positively correlated with degree of renal dysfunction.[139] Second, F^- is a potent inhibitor of many enzyme systems including those thought to be involved with antidiuretic hormone.[140] Finally, vasopressin-resistant polyuric renal insufficiency similar to that seen in man and rats after prolonged methoxyflurane anesthesia, can be easily elicited in Fischer 344 rats injected with sodium fluoride.[141] Oxalic acid, another methoxyflurane metabolic end-product, is usually associated with classic anuric renal failure and not with the type of lesion seen following methoxyflurane.[142]

Fischer 344 rats provide a good animal model for methoxyflurane nephrotoxicity because they demonstrate renal changes following methoxyflurane that are similar to those seen in man. These changes include polyuria, hypernatremia, serum hyperosmolality, increased blood urea nitrogen (BUN) and creatinine, and decreased BUN and creatinine clearances. Furthermore, in this species as in man, the serum F^- threshold for renal dysfunction is about 50 μM.

The extent of nephrotoxicity in general surgical patients has now been correlated with methoxyflurane dosages (in MAC hours, i.e., the product of end-tidal concentration as a fraction of MAC and duration of anesthesia, in hours) and peak serum F^- levels.[143] The threshold of renal dysfunction occurs at dosages of about 2.5 MAC hours methoxyflurane, which corresponds to peak serum F^- levels of 50 to 60 μM. After 5 MAC hours methoxyflurane, serum F^- levels are 90 to 120 μM and patients have well-established but mild nephrotoxicity manifested by serum hyperosmolality, hypernatremia, polyuria, and low urinary osmolality. Seven to 9 MAC hours methoxyflurane lead to serum F^- levels up to 175 μM and marked nephrotoxicity.

Despite the overall correlation between nephrotoxicity and peak serum F^- levels, individual patients given the same methoxyflurane dosage vary in their nephrotoxic susceptibility. Genetic heterogeneity, drug interaction, preexistence of renal disease, and a host of other factors could account for the differences observed among patients. One example of a drug interaction is the additive nephrotoxic effect seen in a patient receiving both methoxyflurane and the aminoglycoside antibiotic gentamicin.[144] The same effect is seen in Fischer 344 rats in which concurrent administration of methoxyflurane and gentamicin produces greater nephrotoxicity than expected from either drug alone.[145]

Because methoxyflurane is a potent anesthetic and an excellent analgesic, many anesthesiologists still consider it a desirable drug. Its nephrotoxic potential, however, has severely limited its clinical usefulness. In an attempt to reduce methoxyflurane's biotransformation and the resultant production of F^-, deuterium has been substituted for hydrogen in the methoxyflurane molecule. The rationale for this substitution is that the C-D bond is less chemically reactive than the C-H bond. Thus, metabolism will be slowed when cleavage of the C-H bond is the rate-limiting step in a reaction. Data from both in vitro and in vivo studies indicate that when all four hydrogens are replaced by deuterium there is a modest decrease in F^- production.[146, 147] Furthermore, unlike ordinary methoxyflurane, the metabolism of completely deuterated methoxyflurane is not enhanced following enzyme induction with phenobarbital.[146] Unfortunately, the overall reduction in F^- production and the possible benefit to enzyme-induced patients are not sufficient to offer a significant clinical advantage.

Because it is difficult to regulate the exact alveolar concentration of methoxyflurane and thus remain below a nephrotoxic dose, Mazze[148] has suggested that the practicing anesthesiologist limit anesthetic duration. Two hours at a gradually decreasing inspired methoxyflurane concentration would appear to be safe for the majority of patients. However in patients on enzyme-inducing drugs the period of exposure to methoxyflurane should probably be reduced; in patients with preexisting renal impairment, methoxyflurane should be completely avoided.

Other Fluorinated Anesthetics

Because modern volatile inhalational anesthetics are fluorinated to reduce their flammability, they all theoretically possess nephrotoxic potential. Of the fluorinated anesthetics, halothane and enflurane are in widespread clinical use, whereas isoflurane and sevoflurane are in the developmental stage.

Halothane is not significantly defluorinated under normal clinical conditions and thus is not nephrotoxic.[143] Experimentally, halothane defluorination does occur in phenobarbital- or Aroclor 1254– pretreated rats under hypoxic conditions, but not to an extent associated with renal damage.[55] On the other hand, although defluorination for enflurane is much less than for methoxyflurane, evidence indicates that serum F^- levels may occasionally be high enough to produce mild renal impairment. In a study with Fischer 344 rats, 6 to 10 hours of 2.5 percent enflurane anesthesia produced mild vasopressin-resistant polyuric renal dysfunction.[26] Peak serum F^- levels were 40 to 57 μM, just reaching the threshold for renal toxicity; there was no increase in urinary oxalate excretion.

Surgical patients rarely show renal dysfunction following enflurane anesthesia.[149] Although serum F^- levels postanesthesia are significantly higher than background levels, they seldom reach the threshold for nephrotoxicity. In comparison with methoxyflurane, serum F^- levels following enflurane anesthesia peak earlier and fall more rapidly, emphasizing the important role that lipid solubility has in determining total F^- production (Fig. 14-3). In one study, peak serum F^- concentrations from nine surgical patients averaged 22.2 μM following enflurane exposures averaging 2.7 MAC hours.[149] The only controlled human study to show mild renal dysfunction following enflurane anesthesia involved 11 healthy volunteers.[150] After 9.6 MAC hours of enflurane, maximum urinary osmolality was reduced from approximately 1,050 to 800 mOsm/kg; mean serum F^- concentration was 33.6 μM. This mild impairment of renal concentrating ability, however, was not associated with hypernatremia, serum hyperosmolality, or increased serum creatinine or urea nitrogen and therefore was not regarded as clinically significant.

Based on the above data, enflurane appears to be safe but to have at least some potential for causing renal dysfunction. Whether this is clinically significant remains to be determined. In the meantime, it seems appropriate to avoid or limit the use of enflurane in patients with significant preexisting renal disease or in those undergoing renal transplantation.

Isoflurane, an isomer of enflurane, is defluorinated much less than enflurane. In nine surgical patients, mean peak serum F^- concentration measured 6 hours after anesthesia was only 4.4 μM.[65] Thus, isoflurane is not associated with F^- nephrotoxicity.

Sevoflurane is a new fluorinated ether anesthetic with a low blood-gas partition coefficient of approximately 0.6. Results of in vitro studies indicate that it is defluorinated more than enflurane but less than methoxyflurane. In a study using six healthy volunteers, serum F^- levels averaged 22 μM by the end of a 1 hour exposure to 3 percent sevoflurane, and had fallen to low levels by 24 hours after anesthesia.[136] Peak serum F^- levels, however, were not measured and anesthesia for longer than 1 hour was not performed. Thus, the clinical safety of this drug is yet to be established in more extensive human studies.

The Role of Enzyme Induction in Anesthetic Nephrotoxicity

Because anesthetics are defluorinated by the mixed-function oxidase system (cytochrome P-450), drugs that induce the enzymes of this system may lead to increased F^- production and nephrotoxicity. This effect has been clearly demonstrated with methoxyflurane; both Fischer 344 rats[151] and man[143] pretreated with the classic enzyme inducer, phenobarbital, show increased defluorination and nephrotoxicity. Another enzyme inducer, phenytoin, also increases methoxyflurane defluorination.[28]

The effects of phenobarbital and phenytoin on metabolism of other fluorinated anesthetics is less certain. Phenobarbital pretreatment increases in vitro and defluorination of sevoflurane,[69] while only slightly increasing that

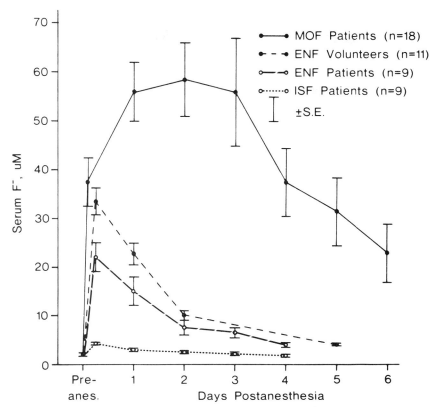

Fig. 14-3 Serum inorganic fluoride (F⁻) concentrations prior to and following enflurane, isoflurane, and methoxyflurane anesthesia. There was a significant increase in F⁻ concentrations immediately following enflurane anesthesia reaching a mean peak value of 22.2 ± 2.8 μM 4 hours after anesthesia was terminated; mean duration of anesthesia was 2.7 ± 0.3 MAC hours.[149] F⁻ levels in volunteers receiving enflurane anesthesia peaked at 33.6 ± 2.8 μM; mean duration of exposure was 9.6 ± 0.1 MAC hours.[150] Following 2 to 3 MAC hours of methoxyflurane,[143] mean peak serum F⁻ concentration was higher, 61 ± 8 μM, and declined more slowly than after enflurane. There was almost no increase in F⁻ following isoflurane administration.[65] (Cousins MJ, Greenstein LR, Hitt BA, et al: Metabolism and renal effects of enflurane in man. Anesthesiology 44:44, 1976)

of isoflurane.[27] Enflurane defluorination is not significantly increased.[27] The result with enflurane is surprising, but consistent with data obtained from a recent human study.[25] One hundred and two surgical patients were divided into the following four groups according to their drug intake histories: control (on no drug), 26 patients; chronic ethanol, 31 patients; chronic phenobarbital and/or phenytoin, 12 patients; and miscellaneous drugs, 33 patients. Regression lines of average peak serum F⁻ levels on enflurane dosage

were not significantly different among the groups. Thus, in this study, prior treatment of surgical patients with enzyme-inducing drugs did not increase serum F⁻ levels following enflurane anesthesia. Presumably, there is no increase in the rate of enflurane metabolism in vivo. In contrast with phenobarbital- or phenytoin-pretreated patients, there have been several cases observed in which patients pretreated with isoniazid demonstrate high serum F⁻ levels and transient urinary concentrating defect following enflurane anesthesia. Work in Fischer 344 rats has confirmed that unlike the classic enzyme inducers, phenobarbital and phenytoin, isoniazid increases enflurane defluorination.[7, 8, 149] Preliminary biochemical data also indicate that isoniazid may belong to a new class of enzyme inducers.[8] Such a chance finding reconfirms the necessity that anesthesiologists be constantly vigilant for dangerous interactions between anesthetic agents and other drugs.

EFFECTS ON THE GONADS

Evidence is gradually accumulating that inhaled anesthetics and their metabolites may be directly toxic to the testes. At present, the evidence is based on studies in experimental animals; human data is not yet available. Male LEW/f Mai rats exposed 8 hours daily to an atmosphere of 20 percent N_2O, 20 percent O_2 and 60 percent N_2 showed evidence of injury to seminiferous tubules after 2 days.[152] By 14 days, damage to spermatogenic cells was extensive. In another study, effects on spermatogonial cells of chronic exposure to a low dose N_2O-halothane mixture was assessed.[153] Exposure was either to air, 50 ppm $N_2O/1$ ppm halothane, or 500 ppm $N_2O/10$ ppm halothane and was for 7 hours/day, 5 days/week. Based on the data obtained, the invesigators concluded that chronic exposure to low dose N_2O-halothane causes dose-dependent chromosomal damage in spermatogonial cells. Finally, in a study that looked at mouse sperm morphology following exposure to anesthetics during early spermatogenesis, chloroform (0.08 percent and 0.04 percent), trichloroethylene (0.2 percent), and enflurane (1.2 percent) all increased the number of sperm abnormalities above background control; other inhaled anesthetics studied gave negative results.[154] However, because these data were collected in animals, the clinical relevance of these findings is difficult to assess.

CHRONIC TOXICITY

From the time chloroform hepatotoxicity was first recognized over 100 years ago, great emphasis has been placed on anesthetic-induced, acute organ toxicity. In recent years, proven methoxyflurane nephrotoxicity and suspicion that halothane may produce hepatotoxicity have enhanced interest in this topic. Historically, however, little thought has been given to possible long-term adverse effects on health from occupational exposure to trace concentrations of waste anesthetic gases.

Even if anesthetics have low potential for causing long-term toxicity, exposing a large population may represent a considerable public health hazard. In the United States, about 50,000 hospital operating room personnel, including anesthesiologists, nurse-anesthetists, and operating room nurses and technicians, are exposed daily to waste anesthetic gases.[155] Additionally, surgeons, dental personnel, veterinarians, and technical assistants have a variable but sometimes heavy exposure to anesthetics. For example, peak levels of at least 50 ppm halothane and 5,000 ppm nitrous oxide have occasionally been recorded in operating room and dental operatory atmospheres.[156, 157] The total number of exposed or potentially exposed personnel in the United States is about 225,000.[155]

Of particular concern are reports that inhaled anesthetics possess mutagenic, carcinogenic, and teratogenic potential. These topics are discussed in the following sections.

MUTAGENICITY

In recent years, investigators have become increasingly interested in mutagenic potential of inhaled anesthetics. There are several reasons. First, chemical mutagenicity and carcinogenicity are closely correlated. Thus, finding that a particular anesthetic is a mutagen also implies that it is a potential carcinogen and should be studied in an animal test system. Because in vitro assays for mutagenicity require much less time and expense than in vivo tests for carcinogenicity, they have become popular screening methods for detection of carcinogens. A second reason for identifying mutagens present in the environment is that they may pose a threat to the integrity of the human genome (the totality of genes and chromosomes) and thus to future generations of man.

To interpret results of in vitro mutagenicity tests with anesthetics, we must understand the mutation process. In a broad sense, mutation refers to heritable change in genetic information. Four types are generally recognized:

1. Base-pair mutation in which one of the four DNA bases (adenine, guanine, thymine, or cytosine) is replaced by one of the others.
2. Frame-shift mutation in which a base pair is added or deleted. In this case, all bases distal to the point of addition or deletion will be out of register, a potentially more serious mutation than the base-pair kind.
3. Large deletions or rearrangements of DNA segments.
4. Nondisjunction in which unequal partition of chromosomes occur between daughter cells.

It is not appropriate in this chapter to discuss every test system for chemical mutagenicity, because they include assays with bacteria, yeast, mammalian cells in culture, and intact mammals. Those that have been systematically applied to the inhaled anesthetics are the Ames *Salmonella*/mammalian microsome, the sister chromatid exchange, and the fibroblast/8-azaguanine resistance systems. The *Salmonella*/mammalian microsome system uses several strains of histidine dependent *S typhimurium*. Strains TA1535 and TA100 are most sensitive to base-pair

mutation, whereas strains TA1537 and TA98 are most sensitive to frame-shift mutation. Bacteria are plated on histidine-deficient culture medium together with the test chemical and a mammalian enzyme system (S-9 mix). The latter is a homogenate prepared most commonly from livers of mice or rats pretreated with enzyme inducers such as phenobarbital or Aroclor 1254. A NADPH-generating system is added to the homogenate. The S-9 mix is necessary because most chemicals are not directly mutagenic but require metabolic activation before becoming mutagens. They would therefore not normally be recognized in bacteria, which do not have the metabolic capability of mammalian cells. Under normal circumstances, only bacteria that spontaneously revert to their wild type (revertants), i.e., not requiring histidine, will grow. If a mutagen is present, the number of revertants increases and can be scored. All currently used and some previously used volatile and gaseous anesthetics have now been tested in this system.[158-161] Only divinyl ether and fluroxene gave unequivocally positive results.[159, 160] When tested at a 1 percent vapor concentration in desiccators, divinyl ether produced a dose-dependent increase in revertant colonies of strains TA1535 and TA100 in the absence of S-9 mix. The mutagenic response was enhanced when S-9 mix was included in the assay. In a liquid suspension assay, the mutagenic response occurred only in the presence of S-9 mix (Fig. 14-4). With fluroxene, a mutagenic response to strains TA1535 and TA100 occurred in liquid suspension at vapor concentrations between 3 percent and 30 percent only in the presence of S-9 mix[160] (Fig. 14-4). Mutagenic activity was not seen with strains TA1537 and TA98 nor with S-9 mix prepared from humans or uninduced rodents. Trichloroethylene was weakly mutagenic whereas other anesthetics, including nitrous oxide, halothane, enflurane, isoflurane, and methoxyflurane, were not mutagenic when tested in this system using a variety of bacterial strains, test con-

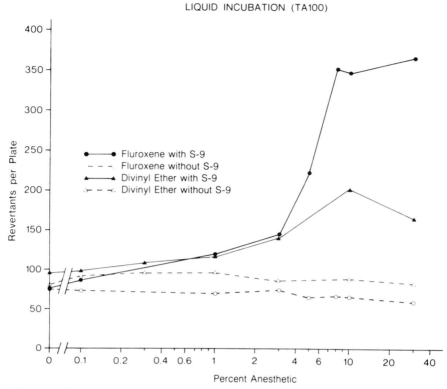

LIQUID INCUBATION (TA100)

Fig. 14-4 Number of revertant colonies per plate of S typhimurium, TA100, after liquid suspension with flueroxene or divinyl ether, with or without S-9. Both fluroxene and divinyl ether showed a dose-dependent mutagenic response at concentrations greater than 1 percent in the presence of S-9.[159, 160]

ditions, and multiple anesthetic concentrations.[158, 160, 161]

In addition to the anesthetics, several of their metabolites have been tested in the *Salmonella* system. Trifluoroacetic acid, trifluoroethanol, and trifluoroacetaldehyde hydrate were not mutagenic.[158, 162] A presumed halothane metabolite, 1,1-difluoro-2-bromo-2-chloroethylene (CF_2CBrCl), was not mutagenic in the standard *Salmonella* assay, but was weakly mutagenic when tested with exponentially growing bacteria.[163, 164, 165] Of two volatile halothane metabolites, 1,1,1-trifluoro-2-chloro-ethane (CF_3CH_2Cl) was not mutagenic, whereas 1,1-difluoro-2-chloroethylene (CF_2CHCl) was weakly mutagenic.[163, 165]

Finally, urine of anesthesiologists has been examined for mutagenic activity using the

Salmonella system. An early report indicated that 11 of 15 anesthesiologists, working in unscavenged operating rooms, had mutagens in their urine.[166] However, later studies in which more sensitive methods and larger numbers of operating room personnel were used did not confirm the earlier findings.[167]

In general, observations of sister chromatid exchanges (SCE) in Chinese hamster ovary cells have confirmed results from the bacterial assay.[168] SCE is a symmetrical exchange between a newly duplicated chromatid and its sister. Many chemicals that damage DNA also increase frequency of SCE. Following a 1 hour exposure of Chinese hamster ovary cells to 1 MAC divinyl ether, fluroxene, or ethyl vinyl ether, the SCE rate increased significantly above the background control level. The increase was greatest with ethyl vinyl

Table 14-1. Tests of Mutagenicity

Anesthetic	Positive	Negative
Halothane	D	A, 8-AzG, D, SCE
Nitrous oxide	D, T	A, 8-AzG, SCE
Chloroform	—	A, 8-AzG, SCE
Enflurane	—	A, 8-AzG, SCE
Methoxyflurane	—	A, SCE
Isoflurane	—	A, SCE
Cyclopropane	—	A
Diethyl ether	—	D, SCE
Trichloroethylene	A, M, S	A, SCE
Fluroxene	A, SCE	—
Divinyl ether	A, SCE	—

Abbreviations used: A = Ames *Salmonella* or *Escherichia*/mammalian microsome; 8-AzG = 8-azaguanine–Chinese hamster lung fibroblasts; D = *Drosophila;* M = Mouse spot test; S = Saccharomyces; SCE = Sister chromatid exchange–Chinese hamster ovary cells; T = Tradescantia.

ether and least with divinyl ether. Other anesthetics tested (Table 14-1) did not increase exchanges above control levels.[168]

Nitrous oxide, chloroform, halothane, and enflurane have been examined in the 8-azaguanine test system also.[169, 170] This mammalian cell assay utilizes Chinese hamster lung fibroblasts grown in culture. Normal cells contain an enzyme that allows 8-azaguanine (8-AzG), an analogue of guanine, to be incorporated into nucleic acids. However, when the normal cells incorporate 8-AzG instead of guanine into DNA, they fail to divide or thrive and soon die. On the other hand, mutant cells that do not contain the enzyme survive because 8-AzG is not incorporated into DNA. When normal cells were exposed to 75 percent nitrous oxide, 1 to 3 percent chloroform, 1 to 3 percent halothane, or 1.5 to 6.5 percent enflurane, no significant increase in numbers of mutations were observed.[169, 170]

From time to time, other test systems have been used to examine mutagenicity of anesthetics. In particular, trichloroethylene (TCE) has been extensively studied in a battery of tests because of its widespread commercial use other than as an anesthetic. Huge quantities are produced in the United States and other countries and it is now considered an important industrial pollutant present throughout many parts of the world. Mutagenicity tests with bacteria, yeast, and mice

show that TCE has weak to moderate genotoxicity (Table 14-1).

Several investigators have used the fruit fly, *Drosophila,* to examine the mutagenic potential of anesthetics. In a study performed in 1914, diethyl ether delivered by inhalation daily for about 11 days, did not produce mutations in *D empelophila.*[77] In another study, halothane administered three to four times a day for 12 days also had no mutagenic effect on mature sex cells of male *D melanogaster.*[171] In contrast, nitrous oxide increased the number of recessive sex-linked lethal mutations in *D melanogaster.*[172] Flies gassed in a 100 ml flask for 1 minute with 22 ml/min nitrous oxide, had a mutation rate of 2.82 ± 0.03, a value significantly higher than the air-treated controls. Halothane has been retested in *D melanogaster* using sex-linked recessive lethals as an indicator of genetic damage.[173] Adult males were exposed to halothane either for 14 days at 1,000 or 1,600 ppm (v/v) or for 1 or 2 days at 2,100 or 20,000 ppm. Results for experiments at high vapor concentrations, were uniformly negative. In several low concentration long-term experiments, a slight increase in mutation frequency was observed. Pooled data from these latter studies just reached significance at a 5 percent level. The investigators concluded that results were of borderline significance but indicated with a fair degree of probability

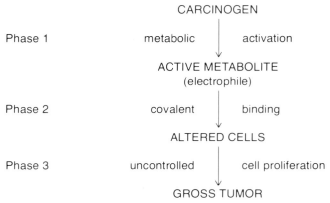

CARCINOGEN

Phase 1   metabolic | activation

ACTIVE METABOLITE
(electrophile)

Phase 2   covalent | binding

ALTERED CELLS

Phase 3   uncontrolled | cell proliferation

GROSS TUMOR

Fig. 14-5 Phases in chemical carcinogenesis.

that halothane was weakly mutagenic under the conditions used. It is clear that further studies with halothane, nitrous oxide, and other anesthetics using the same model system should be performed to assess the significance of these *Drosophila* experiments.

Finally, in two clones (02 and 4430) of *Tradescantia,* nitrous oxide increased the mutation rate of cells in petals and stamen hairs.[174] However, the maximum response rate was little more than twice the spontaneous rate and it was concluded that nitrous oxide was, at best, a weak mutagen.

Because of positive results obtained with nitrous oxide or halothane in the *Drosophila* or *Tradescantia* assays and the weakly positive results with some volatile halothane metabolites in the *Salmonella* assay, one cannot be dogmatic concerning the lack of mutagenicity of these anesthetics. Nonetheless, the *Salmonella*/mammalian microsome, the SCE, and the 8-azaguanine test systems are now considered well-validated methods for the detection of chemical mutagens/carcinogens. A summary of results obtained from studies that have used these assays and other test systems with inhaled anesthetics is shown in Table 14-1. Taken together, they provide reasonable evidence that under normal conditions, modern and many previously used inhaled anesthetics are not mutagens and, therefore, probably not carcinogens. On the other hand, the anesthetics that contain the vinyl moiety are mutagens and should be considered potential carcinogens.

CARCINOGENICITY

The development of chemically induced tumors (chemical carcinogenesis) has three broad phases (Fig. 14-5). The first involves metabolic activation of the administered chemical to a positively charged reactive intermediate or electrophile. The second is covalent binding of the electrophile to some critical tissue macromolecule. Although chemicals and metabolites bind to protein, RNA, and DNA, the latter is thought to be the target molecule for chemical carcinogenesis. After covalent binding has occurred, cells may be repaired, lay dormant, or progress to the third phase, which involves cellular proliferation and development of clinically apparent tumors. This phase is the least understood of the three because it occurs over a long time period and involves a multiplicity of mechanisms.

Covalent binding of reactive intermediates to tissue macromolecules is presumed to be necessary but not to be the only requirement for chemical carcinogenesis. As indicated in the section on specific organ toxicity, covalent binding of anesthetic metabolites has been recognized for many years. For example, low-temperature whole-body autoradiogra-

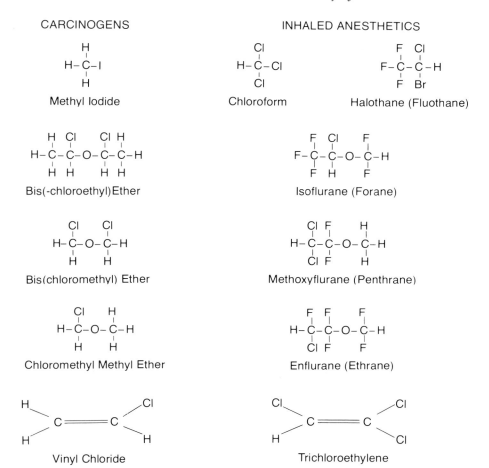

Fig. 14-6 Structural formulas of several known human carcinogens and the inhaled anesthetic agents.

phy has shown that in mice both chloroform and halothane fragments bind covalently to liver and other body tissues.[42, 175] Thus, some anesthetics satisfy at least one criterion for chemical carcinogenicity.

Other circumstantial evidence, often proposed as demonstrating an association between anesthetics and chemical carcinogens, is structural similarity (Fig. 14-6). For example, methoxyflurane, enflurane, and isoflurane are α haloethers as are the nonanesthetic but carcinogenic chemicals bis(chloromethyl) ether, chloromethyl methyl ether, and bis(α-chloroethyl) ether.[162, 176, 177] Halothane and chloroform are alkyl halides; methyl iodide, butyl bromide, and butyl chlo-

ride are from the same chemical group and are animal carcinogens.[178] Finally, the anesthetic agent and industrial solvent trichloroethylene is a halogenated alkene similar to the human[179] and animal carcinogen[180] vinyl chloride. Fluroxene and divinyl ether also contain the vinyl moiety. Although these observations on structure are suggestive, they are by no means proof that anesthetics have carcinogenic potential. Minor structural differences often impart major changes in function as has been clearly shown with aromatic hydrocarbons.[181] Epidemiologic surveys, animal studies, and in vitro carcinogenicity assays provide more definitive evidence.

Table 14-2. Epidemiologic Surveys of Cancer in Operating Room Personnel

Study	Year	Country	Results
Bruce et al.[182]	1968	USA	Neg.
Corbett et al.[183]	1973	USA	? Pos.—females
Bruce et al.[184]	1974	USA	Neg.
ASA Survey[185]	1974	USA	Pos.—females
			Neg.—males
Doll & Peto[186]	1977	UK	Neg.
Tomlin[187]	1979	UK	Neg.
Lew[188]	1979	USA	Neg.
Cohen et al.[189]	1979	USA	Neg.

At first sight, human epidemiologic studies would appear to provide the best method of establishing an occupational or treatment-related hazard. However, despite several studies concerning cancer among operating room personnel (Table 14-2), much controversy remains. In the largest study, the American Society of Anesthesiologists (ASA) surveyed retrospectively 49,595 United States operating room personnel.[185] A 1.3- to 2.0-fold increase in cancer rate was noted among female members of the ASA and the American Association of Nurse Anesthetists, compared to matched control groups. No increase in cancer rate was seen among surveyed males. However, some investigators have questioned the methods of data collection, statistical analysis, and conclusions of this study.[190] Interestingly though, in a recent large national survey of 60,000 female dental assistants and male dentists conducted in the United States, the female assistants working with inhaled anesthetics but not the male dentists working with these anesthetics were reported to have twice the incidence of cancer compared to those who did not work with these agents. The probability of obtaining such a result by chance was 0.06.[189] Nitrous oxide was used as the sole anesthetic in 81.3 percent of cases and in combination with potent agents, mainly halothane, in 18.7 percent of administrations. Consistent with these findings for female exposed personnel were results of an earlier study of 525 Michigan nurse-anesthetists.[183] When compared to the Connecticut Tumor Registry, the cancer in-

cidence for the year 1971 was well above expected. However, it is noteworthy that cancer incidences for all other years surveyed were not elevated, suggesting that the increase in 1971 was due to chance.

Not all investigators agree that the increased cancer incidences purported in these studies are real. Furthermore, no study has demonstrated the existence of a cause-and-effect relationship between anesthetics and cancer. Many other factors may account for the positive results seen. For example, after a careful review of epidemiologic data, several investigators have suggested that stress among operating room personnel was as likely a factor in occupational cancer as was contamination by trace concentrations of inhaled anesthetics.[191]

Other epidemiologic surveys that have examined cancer deaths rather than cancer incidence have been negative. In a retrospective survey in which 441 death certificates of ASA members, spanning the period from 1947 to 1966 were examined, there was no significant increase in deaths because of malignancies.[182] A prospective study of cause of death among 221 ASA members for the period 1967 to 1971 confirmed the earlier findings.[184] Both studies used age-corrected death rates among standard policy holders of the Metropolitan Life Insurance Company for comparison. In an English study, the death rate among 1,251 male, English anesthetists, over 35 years of age, who were followed prospectively for 20 years was compared with that of about 19,000 other physicians; the overall rate in both groups was 93 percent and the rate due to cancer was only 79 percent.[186] Finally, a joint study by the ASA and the American Cancer Society extended the earlier surveys of deaths among ASA members; the overall death rate for the period 1954 to 1976 was less than expected and the death rate due to cancer was the same as the estimated, contemperaneous death rates among all physicians.[188] In a brief critical review of most of the above studies, one author concluded there was little convincing evidence that cancer is an occupational hazard of working in the operating suite.[192] At present, there are no epidemiologic data concerning the cancer incidence among patients who have received one or more anesthetics.

The results of animal carcinogenicity experiments have been variable and their interpretation questionable.[193] When administered in extremely large dosages by oral gavage,[194] chloroform produced liver cancer in B6C3F1 mice and renal tumors in male or female Osborne-Mendel rats, whereas trichloroethylene[195] caused liver tumors in mice but not in rats. Fifty animals were used in both studies for each treatment and control group. Although oral gavage may be appropriate for studying dietary and therapeutic intake of chloroform or trichloroethylene, it is not clear if this route of administration is relevant to inhalational exposure of patients or operating room personnel. Indeed, it is well established that administering a drug by an unusual route often leads to confounding carcinogenicity data.[196] Furthermore, when trichloroethylene was studied, the agent tested contained 0.19 percent 1,2-epoxybutane and 0.09 percent epichlorohydrin, both known mutagens.[197, 198] Epichlorohydrin is also a rodent carcinogen.[199] The presence of these contaminants, though in trace amounts, casts doubt on the significance of data gathered on trichloroethylene carcinogenicity.

In the only positive study of an anesthetic administered via inhalation, the experimental anesthetic, isoflurane, showed an increased incidence of liver tumors in male, but not female, Swiss/ICR mice exposed in utero and for a short period postnatally.[200] Several factors, however, confound the interpretation of this study. For example, high levels of polybrominated biphenyls, which may have contributed to the increased liver tumor incidence, were present in livers of isoflurane-treated mice. In contrast, a more recent study did not demonstrate an increased incidence of liver or other tumors in Swiss/ICR mice exposed to either isoflurane, halothane, enflurane, methoxyflurane, or nitrous oxide.[201]

The exposure regimen was similar to that used in the previous study, although group sizes, about 200 animals, were much larger. Finally, two life-time carcinogenicity studies failed to demonstrate an increased incidence of benign or malignant tumors in experimental animals.[193, 202] The first used 161 Swiss/ICR mice to which a maximum tolerated dose of halothane was administered by inhalation.[193] Animals were exposed to 500 ppm for 2 hours/day, 3 days/week for 18 months and sacrificed after 20 months. The second study used groups of 50 Fischer 344 rats exposed for their life-time to several subanesthetic concentrations of a nitrous oxide–halothane mixture (50 ppm/1 ppm and 500 ppm/10 ppm).[202]

What can the practicing anesthesiologist conclude from these studies? Based on negative human epidemiologic and animal data we can say with some certainty that male operating room personnel do not have an abnormally increased rate of malignancy. There is much less certainty about cancer rate among females; although animal data have proved negative, epidemiologic data have shown a modest increase above expected levels.

TERATOGENICITY

Embryogenesis is an extremely complex process. It involves a number of interrelated events such as cell proliferation and death, differentiation, migration, and organization into organ systems. Disruption at any stage can have serious consequences for the developing embryo and fetus. Although the developmental process is remarkably consistent, embryogenesis is not always perfect; congenital malformations, both severe and trivial, are found in about 2 to 4 percent of all births in countries where records are kept.[203]

The term teratogenesis refers to adverse effects on developing biologic systems; namely, germ cells, embryos, fetuses, and immature postnatal individuals. The possible

Table 14-3. Teratogenic Mechanisms[206]

1. Mutation (four types—see text)
2. Interference with cell division
3. Alteration of nucleic acid function
4. Removal of cell precursor and substrates
5. Lack of energy sources
6. Enzyme inhibition
7. Change in cell membrane characteristics

mechanisms producing abnormal development (Table 14-3) are at present only partly understood. Mutations, especially those resulting in specific biochemical abnormalities and chromosomal nondisjunction, are well-established mechanisms of human congenital anomalies. Other mechanisms, such as interference with cell division and alterations of cell membrane, are less certain. These cellular effects, however, have been observed with inhaled anesthetics, at least at clinically used and higher concentrations.[204, 205] Although the cause of most defects remains unknown, chemical teratogenesis in man is well established (Table 14-4).

When discussing the possibility of anesthetic-produced carcinogenicity, we were most concerned about occupationally exposed personnel; a hazard to patients seemed much less likely in view of their short-term exposure. In contrast, patients administered anesthetics during pregnancy as well as operating room personnel exposed chronically to waste anesthetic gases may have an increased risk of spontaneous abortion or of bearing offspring with congenital defects. Thus, in the following sections we will consider the possible hazard to both groups.

The majority of surveys that have examined reproductive performance of operating room personnel are listed in Table 14-5.

Table 14-4. Known Human Chemical Teratogens*[206]

Androgenic hormones
Folic antagonists
Thalidomide
Organic mercury
Some hypoglycemics (?)
Some anticonvulsants (?)

* Account for only 2 to 3 percent of known causes of developmental defects in man.

Overall, the most consistent finding has been a higher than expected incidence of fetal wastage among female operating room personnel. For example, in a survey of 303 Russian anesthesiologists, 18 of 31 pregnancies ended in spontaneous abortion.[207] This study did not include a control population. In a later study of Danish anesthetists, approximately 20 percent of 392 pregnancies started after operating room employment, ended in spontaneous abortion compared with 10 percent of 212 pregnancies among the same group prior to employment.[208] Other studies from Finland, Britain, and the United States confirmed the higher incidence of spontaneous abortions. In the largest, about 50,000 operating room anesthesiologists, nurse-anesthetists, nurses, and technicians working in the United States and 24,000 unexposed physicians and nurses were surveyed.[185] The incidence of spontaneous abortion was 1.3 to 2 times higher among exposed than among unexposed females. Despite the existence of one negative survey,[209] collectively the above-mentioned studies provide reasonable evidence for an increased risk of spontaneous abortion among female operating room workers (Table 14-5). They do not necessarily prove that exposure to waste anesthetic gases is the cause.

Many studies have also assessed the incidence of both major and minor congenital malformations among the offspring of anesthetic-exposed females (Table 14-5). The findings have been less consistent than those for spontaneous abortion; negative or equivocal results have been generally obtained. Other hazards such as abortion among wives and malformation among offspring of exposed males have also been investigated (Table 14-5). Again, results have not been consistent among the studies and firm conclusions of possible hazards will have to await further investigation.

In 1961 the disastrous effects of thalidomide ingested during pregnancy were first recognized.[215] Since then, sophisticated animal studies have gradually been developed

Table 14-5. Epidemiologic Surveys of Adverse Reproductive Effects in Operating Room Personnel

			Results			
			Exposed Females		Wives of Exposed Males	
Authors	Year	Country	Spontaneous Abortion	Major Malformation	Spontaneous Abortion	Major Malformation
Vaisman[207]	1966	Russia	Pos.	Neg.	—	—
Askrog & Harvald[208]	1970	Denmark	Pos.	Neg.	Pos.	Neg.
Cohen et al.[210]	1971	USA	Pos.	—	—	—
Knill-Jones et al.[211]	1972	UK	Pos.	? Pos.	—	—
Rosenberg & Kirves[212]	1973	Finland	Pos.	Neg.	—	—
Corbett et al.[213]	1974	USA	—	Pos.	—	—
ASA survey[185]	1974	USA	Pos.	? Pos.	Neg.	? Pos.
Knill-Jones et al.[214]	1975	UK	Pos.	Neg.	Neg.	Neg.
Pharoah et al.[209]	1977	UK	Neg.	Pos.	—	—
Tomlin[187]	1979	UK	Pos.	Neg.	Neg.	Neg.

for examining potential teratogenicity of chemicals. Complete testing now involves assessing the effect of a chemical on many aspects of reproductive function, such as fertility, mating behavior, in utero embryonic and fetal wastage, congenital anomalies, and postnatal survival and behavior. Despite their apparent thoroughness, animal studies remain far from perfect. Apart from the difficulty extrapolating animal data to man, the number of animals exposed in any experiment is small compared with the number of humans exposed; thus, there is usually insufficient statistical power to evaluate the presence of a weak teratogen. Nonetheless, because direct human experimentation is obviously not possible, animal studies are still necessary and continue to provide useful information.

Effects of inhaled anesthetics on reproductive processes of experimental animals have been the subject of many reports. In some studies, to simulate occupational exposure, animals have received trace or subanesthetic concentrations of anesthetics by inhalation. The large number of such studies precludes a complete discussion in the present chapter. The interested reader is referred to two more-comprehensive reviews.[155,216] Several points are worth emphasizing, however. First, nitrous oxide and halothane have been the most commonly investigated agents, reflecting their widespread clinical use; other anesthetics have received less attention. Second,

many early investigators studied chick embryos, whereas today most prefer to use mammalian species because their reproductive physiology is closer to that of man. Third, few studies are complete by today's standards. For example, inadequate examination of maternal and fetal tissues is common, making it more difficult to be certain of negative results. Finally, the timing and method of anesthetic exposure and the dosages used vary considerably from study to study. Therefore, results obtained from different studies, even of the same agent, usually cannot be compared. Overall, the experimental evidence for adverse reproductive effects of anesthetic gases at concentrations found in the operating room is not strong. However, considerable doubt remains about the interpretation of these animal studies and their significance to occupational safety.

On the other hand, the detrimental effects of surgery and anesthesia on the pregnant patient is not in doubt. In the United States, at least 50,000 pregnant women (about 1.6 percent) undergo anesthesia and surgery during gestation for indications unrelated to pregnancy.[217] Operations for ovarian cysts, acute appendicitis, mammary tumors, and repair of incompetent cervix are most common. It is clear that the risk of unexpected abortion or premature labor is higher following an anesthetic. What is not immediately obvious is whether the patient's disease, surgery, anesthesia, or a combination of these is the precipitating cause. Another concern, though not yet substantiated, is that anesthesia during pregnancy leads to an increased incidence of congenital anomalies. We know that such an outcome is certainly not invariable and that pregnant patients who receive an anesthetic and do not abort usually deliver perfectly normal offspring. A case is reported of a woman who sustained severe head injury and received 17 general anesthetics during the course of her pregnancy; she was delivered by cesarean section of a normal male infant at 35 weeks gestation.[103] Follow-up at 6 months showed that the baby was normal and was reaching his milestones on schedule.

To assess the exact incidence of various anesthetic and surgery-related hazards occurring during pregnancy, at least two studies have been performed.[217,218] In the first, all obstetric records in the United States Naval Hospital in Portsmouth, Virginia were examined for the years 1957 to 1961.[218] During this period, 18,248 live births and 255 stillbirths were recorded; 67 patients had surgery during pregnancy, 24 having general and 43 having regional anesthesia. Nine stillbirths or abortions occurred after anesthesia, but no congenital anomalies were noted. Of the nine fetal losses, four were associated with appendiceal abscesses and four with Shirodkar procedures for incompetent cervical os. It was interesting that all nine cases resulting in fetal loss received spinal anesthesia, although the investigator attributed this to sampling bias. In the second and larger study, two sources of material were used.[217] The first was records of 9,073 obstetric patients delivered at the University of California Medical Center, San Francisco, between July 1959 and August 1964. The second source was records of 60,912 obstetric patients from 17 hospitals taking part in an Obstetrical Statistical Cooperative. Of the first group, 147 women (1.6 percent) had operations during their pregnancies. In the second group, 50 appendectomies and 17 Shirodkar procedures were recorded. Premature delivery after operation occurred in 8.8 percent; perinatal mortality

was 7.5 percent compared with 2 percent in the nonsurgical group. Based on a detailed analysis of data obtained from these records, the authors (Shnider and Webster) reached the following conclusions:

1. Premature labor after operation is mainly the result of the patient's surgical disease rather than the surgical or anesthetic technique, per se. In fact, no specific anesthetic technique, general or regional, had advantage in lowering the incidence of premature labor, perinatal mortality, or congenital anomalies.

2. There is a high incidence of premature labor and perinatal mortality associated with women undergoing operations for incompetent cervical os.

The authors also suggested that although the expected incidence of congenital anomalies was normal following operation, the number of cases was too small to give conclusive results. They therefore recommended that if possible, anesthesia not be administered during pregnancy or at least be delayed until after the period of maximum organogenesis (first trimester). Naturally, whether this advice can be heeded depends on the exact circumstances of each case. Although a number of uncertainties still remain, there has not been any recent evidence refuting or confirming the overall findings or recommendations of this important study.

Anesthetizing concentrations of inhaled anesthetics have been administered to pregnant experimental animals as a model for obstetric patients undergoing general anesthesia. In some cases, concentrations delivered and durations of exposure were even greater than those used clinically. If anything, results obtained at these higher concentrations are more difficult to interpret than at subanesthetic levels because the physiological effects expected at anesthetizing doses are not easily controlled. This is especially true for the most common type of study, which involves large numbers of small laboratory rodents. Since each animal cannot be monitored, the adverse effects of such factors as hypoxia, hypotension, hypothermia, and hyperthermia cannot be separated from the direct anesthetic effects.

Attention has recently focused upon another aspect of teratogenesis, effects of prenatal drug administration on postnatal behavior. The reason is the growing awareness that some teratogens may produce enduring behavioral deficits without any observable morphologic changes. Furthermore, while many organ systems are most sensitive to chemical teratogens during organogenesis in the first trimester, the central nervous system may be particularly vulnerable during myelination. In man, this period is probably from the seventh intrauterine month through the second postnatal month. Thus, a chemical may produce behavioral teratogenesis if administered late in gestation or even after birth.

Anesthetics have not escaped scrutiny as possible behavioral teratogens. In 1974, report of a rat study indicated that during development, exposure to as little as 10 ppm halothane caused lasting behavioral deficits and minor central nervous system damage.[219] Rats, 20 weeks old, exposed from conception to 60 days of age showed impairment of light-dark discrimination and food-motivated maze learning. Electron microscopy of cerebral cortex demonstrated neuronal degeneration and abnormal synapses. Because such a low halothane concentration is often found in the operating suite, the findings from the rat study caused great concern.

When performing studies in man, investigators have generally focused upon long-term behavioral effects of maternal obstetric medication, including epidural anesthesia. Claims have been made that if the mother is given medication at delivery, cognition, motor skills, and language ability of offspring are depressed for at least the first 7 years of life. These claims, however, remain extremely controversial. Behavioral abnormalities of offspring whose mothers received inhaled anesthetics have not been well studied. Furthermore, studies have not been done to assess neurobehavior in children of operating room personnel exposed to waste anesthetic gases. It is clear that considerable effort should be made in the coming years to determine whether inhaled anesthetics are behavioral teratogens in man.

REFERENCES

1. Daniels TC, Jorgensen EC: Physiochemical properties in relation to biologic action, Textbook of Organic Medicinal and Pharmaceutical Chemistry. 6th edition. Edited by Wilson, CO, Gisvold, O, Doerge, RF. Philadelphia, Lippincott, 1971, pp 5–67
2. Singer SJ: The molecular organization of biological membranes, Structure and Function of Biological Membranes. Edited by Rothfield L. New York, Academic Press, 1971, pp 146–222
3. Singer SJ, Nicolson GL: The fluid mosaic model of the structure of cell membranes. Science 175:720, 1972
4. DePierre JW, Dallner G: Structural aspects of the membrane of the endoplasmic reticulum. Biochim Biophys Acta 415:411, 1975
5. Omura T, Siekevitz P, Palade GE: Turnover of constituents of the endoplasmic reticulum membrane of rat hepatocytes. J Biol Chem 242:2389, 1967
6. Quinn GP, Azelrod J, Brodie BB: Species, strain and sex differences in metabolism of hexobarbitone, amidopyrine, antipyrine and aniline. Biochem Pharmacol 1:152, 1958
7. Rice SA, Maze M, Mazze RI, et al: Hepatotoxicity following halothane anesthesia in isoniazid treated rats. Fed Proc, 38:683, 1979
8. Rice SA, Sbordone L, Mazze RI: Metabolism by rat hepatic microsomes of fluorinated ether anesthetics following isoniazid administration. Anesthesiology 53:489, 1980
9. Van Dyke RA: Biotransformation; Handbook of Experimental Pharmacology. Edited by Chenoweth MB. New York, Springer-Verlag, 1972, p 345
10. Van Dyke RA, Gandolfi, AJ: Anaerobic release of fluoride from halothane. Relationship to the binding of halothane metabolites to hepatic cellular constituents. Drug Metab Dispos 4:40, 1976
11. Loew G, Motulsky H, Trudell J, et al: Quantum chemical studies of the metabolism of the

inhalation anesthetics methoxyflurane, enflurane, and isoflurane. Mol Pharmacol 10:406, 1974

12. Oesch F: Mammalian epoxide hydrases: Inducible enzymes catalyzing the inactivation of carcinogenic and cytotoxic metabolites derived from aromatic and olefinic compounds. Xenobiotica 3:305, 1973

13. Byington KH, Leibman KC: Metabolism of trichloroethylene in liver microsomes: II. Identification of the reaction product as chloral hydrate. Mol Pharmacol 1: 247, 1965

14. Daniel JW: The metabolism of ^{36}Cl-labeled trichloroethylene and tetrachloroethylene in the rat. Biochem Pharmacol 12:795, 1963

15. Leibman KC, McAllister WJ: Metabolism of trichloroethylene in liver microsomes: I. Characteristics of the reaction. Mol Pharmacol 1:239, 1965

16. Powell JF: Trichloroethylene: Absorption, elimination and metabolism. Br J Ind Med 2:142, 1945

17. Soucek B, Vlachova D: Excretion of trichloroethylene metabolites in human urine. Br J Med 17:60, 1960

18. Parke DV: Mechanisms and consequences of the induction of microsomal enzymes of mammalian liver. Biochem J, 130:53P, 1972

19. Remmer H, Merker HJ: Drug-induced changes in the liver endoplasmic reticulum. Association with drug-metabolizing enzymes. Science 142:1657, 1963

20. Conney AH: Pharmacological implications of microsomal enzyme induction. Pharmacol Rev 19:317, 1967

21. Brown BR Jr, Sagalyn AM: Hepatic microsomal enzyme induction by inhalation anesthetics: Mechanism in the rat. Anesthesiology 40:152, 1974

22. Linde HW, Berman ML: Non-specific stimulation of drug-metabolizing enzymes by inhalation anesthetic agents. Anesth Analg 50:656, 1971

23. Ross WT, Cardell RR: Proliferation of smooth endoplasmic reticulum and induction of microsomal drug-metabolizing enzymes after ether or halothane. Anesthesiology 8:325, 1978

24. Shideman FE, Kelly AR, Adams BJ: The role of the liver in the detoxification (Pentothal) and two other thiobarbiturates. J Pharmacol Exp Ther 91:331, 1947

25. Dooley JR, Mazze RI, Rice SA, et al: Is enflurane defluorination inducible in man? Anesthesiology 50:213, 1979

26. Barr GA, Cousins, MJ, Mazze RI, et al: A comparison of the renal effects and metabolism of enflurane and methoxyflurane in Fischer 344 rats. J Pharmacol Exp Ther 190:530, 1974

27. Hitt BA, Mazze RI: Effect of enzyme induction on nephrotoxicity of halothane related compounds. Environ Health Perspect 21:179, 1977

28. Caughey GH, Rice SA, Kosek JC, et al: Effect of phenytoin (DPH) treatment on methoxyflurane metabolism in rats. J Pharmacol Exp Ther 210:180, 1979

29. Greene NM: Halothane anesthesia and hepatitis in a high risk population. N Engl J Med, 289:304, 1973

30. Ivanetich KM, Lucas S, Marsh JA, et al: Organic compounds. Their interaction with and degradation of hepatic microsomal drug-metabolizing enzymes *in vitro*. Drug Metab Dispos 6:218, 1978

31. Cascorbi HF, Vessel ES, Blake DA: Genetic and environmental influence on halothane metabolism in twins. Clin Pharmacol Ther 12:50, 1971

32. Haggard HW: The absorption, distribution, and elimination of ethyl ether. J Biol Chem 59:737, 1924

33. Van Dyke RA, Chenoweth MB, Van Poznak A: Metabolism of volatile anesthetics. I. Conversion *in vivo* of several anesthetics to $^{14}CO_2$ and chloride. Biochem Pharmacol 13:1239, 1964

34. Cohen EN: Metabolism of the volatile anesthetics. Anesthesiology 35:193, 1971

35. Green K, Cohen EN: On the metabolism of ^{14}C-diethyl ether in the mouse. Biochem Pharmacol 20:393, 1971

36. Van Dyke RA, Chenoweth MB: Metabolism of volatile anesthetics. Anesthesiology 26:348, 1965

37. Rao GS, Meridian DJ, Tong YS, et al: Biochemical toxicology of chronic nitrous oxide exposures. Pharmacologist 21:216, 1979

38. Brown DM, Langley PF, Smith D, et al: Metabolism of chloroform. I. The metabolism of [^{14}C] chloroform by different species. Xenobiotica, 4:151, 1974

39. Paul BB, Rubinstein D: Metabolism of carbon tetrachloride and chloroform by the rat. J Pharmacol Exp Ther 141:414, 1963

40. Pohl LR, Martin JL, George JW: Mechanisms of $CHCl_3$ metabolism in rat liver microsomes. Pharmacologist 21:259, 1979

41. Charlesworth FA: Patterns of chloroform metabolism. Fed Cosmet Toxicol 14:59, 1976

42. Cohen EN, Hood N: Application of low-temperature autoradiography to studies of the uptake and metabolism of volatile anesthetics in the mouse. I. Chloroform. Anesthesiology 30:306, 1969

43. Illett KF, Reid WD, Sipes GI, et al: Chloroform toxicity in mice: Correlation of renal and hepatic necrosis with covalent binding of metabolites to tissue macromolecules. Exp Mol Path, 19:25, 1973

44. Scholler KL: Electron-microscopic and autoradiographic studies on the effect of halothane and chloroform on liver cells. Acta Anaesthesiol Scand (suppl) 32:5, 1968

45. Barrett HM, Johnston JH: The fate of trichloroethylene in the organism. J Biol Chem 127:765, 1939

46. Leibman KC, McAllister WJ: Metabolism of trichloroethylene in liver microsomes. III. Induction of the excretion of metabolites. J Pharmacol Exp Ther 157:574, 1967

47. Blake DA, Rozman RS, Cascorbi HF, et al: Anesthesia LXXIV: Biotransformation of fluroxene. I. Metabolism in mice and dogs *in vivo*. Biochem Pharmacol 16:1237, 1967

48. Ivanetich KM, Bradshaw JJ, Marsh JA, et al: The role of cytochrome P-450 in the toxicity of fluroxene (2,2,2-trifluoroethyl vinyl ether) anesthesia *in vivo*. Biochem Pharm 25:773, 1976

49. Ivanetich KM, Bradshaw JJ, Marsh JA, et al: The interaction of hepatic microsomal cytochrome P-450 with fluroxene (2,2,2-trifluoroethyl vinyl ether) *in vitro*. Biochem Pharm 25:779, 1976

50. Gion H, Yoshimura N, Holaday DA, et al: Biotransformation of fluroxene in man. Anesthesiology 40:553, 1974

51. Stier A: Trifluoroacetic acid as a metabolite of halothane. Biochem Pharmacol 12:544, 1964

52. Stier A, Alter H, Hessler O, et al: Urinary excretion of bromide in halothane anesthesia. Anesth Analg 43:723, 1964

53. Sharp JH, Trudell JR, Cohen EN: Volatile metabolites and decomposition products of halothane in man. Anesthesiology 50:2, 1979

54. Clauberg G: Untersuchungen uber den Einfluss von Inhalationsnarkose und Operation auf die Leberfunction unter besonderer Berucksichtigung des Halothans. Der Anaesthesist 19:324, 1970

55. Widger LA, Gandolfi AJ, Van Dyke RA: Hypoxia and halothane metabolism *in vivo;* release of inorganic fluoride and halothane metabolite binding to cellular constituents. Anesthesiology 44:197, 1976

56. Reynolds ES, Moslen MT: Halothane hepatotoxicity: Enhancement by polychlorinated biphenyl pretreatment. Anesthesiology 47:19, 1977

57. Sipes IG, Brown BR Jr: An animal model of hepatotoxicity associated with halothane anesthesia. Anesthesiology 45:622, 1976

58. Holaday DA, Rudofsky S, Treuhaft PS: Metabolic degradation of methoxyflurane in man. Anesthesiology 33:579, 1970

59. Van Dyke RA, Wood CL: Metabolism of methoxyflurane: Release of inorganic fluoride in human and rat hepatic microsomes. Anesthesiology 39:613, 1973

60. Ivanetich KM, Lucas SA, Marsh JA: Enflurane and methoxyflurane. Their interaction with hepatic cytochrome P-450 *in vitro*. Biochem Pharm, 28:785, 1979

61. Berman ML, Lowe HJ, Bochantin JS, et al: Uptake and elimination of methoxyflurane as influenced by enzyme induction in the rat. Anesthesiology 38:352, 1973

62. Mazze RI, Hitt BA, Cousins MJ: Effect of enzyme induction with phenobarbital on the *in vivo* and *in vitro* defluorination of isoflurane and methoxyflurane. J Pharmacol Exp Ther, 190:523, 1974

63. Fiserova-Bergerova V: Changes of fluoride content in bone: An index of drug defluorination in vivo. Anesthesiology 38:345, 1973

64. Rice SA, Talcott RE: Effects of isoniazid treatment on selected hepatic mixed function oxidases. Drug Metab Dispos 7:260, 1979

65. Mazze RI, Cousins MJ, Barr GA: Renal effects and metabolism of isoflurane in man. Anesthesiology 40:536, 1974

66. Hitt BA, Mazze RI, Cousins MJ: Metabolism of isoflurane in Fischer 344 rats and man. Anesthesiology 40:62, 1974

67. Bennike KW, Hagelsten JO: Cyclopropane hepatitis. A Danish disease? Lancet 2:255, 1964

68. Cook TL, Beppu WJ, Hitt BA, et al: Renal effects and metabolism of sevoflurane in Fischer 344 rats. An in vivo and in vitro com-

parison with methoxyflurane. Anesthesiology 43:70, 1975

69. Cook TL, Beppu WJ, Hitt BA, et al: A comparison of renal effects and metabolism of sevoflurane and methoxyflurane in enzyme induced rats. Anesth Analg 54:829, 1975

70. Miller EC, Miller JA: Mechanisms of chemical carcinogenesis: Nature of proximate carcinogens and interactions with macromolecules. Pharmacol Rev 18:805, 1966

71. Mitchell JR, Jollows DJ: Metabolic activation of drugs to toxic substances. Gastroenterology 68:392, 1975

72. Courville CB: Asphyxia as a consequence of nitrous oxide anesthesia. Medicine 15:129, 1936

73. Demopoulos HB: The basis of free radical pathology. Fed Proc 32:1859, 1973

74. DiLuzio NR: Antioxidants, lipid peroxidation and chemical-induced liver injury. Fed Proc 32:1875, 1973

75. Brown BR Jr, Sagalyn AM: Reactive intermediates of anesthetic biotransformation and hepatotoxicity, Molecular Mechanisms of Anesthesia. Edited by Fink BR. New York, Raven Press, 1975, pp 559–568

76. Levine BB: Immunochemical aspects of drug allergy. Br Rev Med 17:23, 1966

77. Morgan TH: The failure of ether to produce mutations in *Drosophila*. Am Nat 48:705, 1914

78. King MM, Lai EK, McCay PB: Singlet oxygen production associated with enzyme-catalyzed lipid peroxidation in liver microsomes. J Biol Chem 250:6496, 1975

79. Udenfriend S: Arene oxide intermediates in enzymatic hydroxylation and their significance with respect to drug toxicity, Drug Metabolism in Man. Edited by Vessell ES. Ann NY Acad Sci 179:295, 1971

80. Recknagel RO: Alterations produced in the endoplasmic reticulum by carbon tetrachloride. Minerva Med 69:455, 1978

81. Udenfriend S, Bartl P: Symposium on the Biochemistry and Metabolism of Arene Oxides. Nutley, NJ, Roche Institute of Molecular Biology, 1972

82. Druckrey H: Specific carcinogenic and teratogenic effects of "indirect" alkylating methyl and ethyl compounds and their dependency on stages of ontogenic development. Xenobiotica 3:271, 1973

83. Johnson MC, Swartz HM, Donati RM: Hematologic alterations produced by nitrous oxide. Anesthesiology 34:42, 1971

84. Pryor WA: Free radical reactions and their importance in biochemical systems. Fed Proc 32:1862, 1973

85. Tappel AL: Lipid peroxidation damage to cell components. Fed Proc, 32:1870, 1973

86. Myers LS Jr: Free radical damage of nucleic acids and their components by ionizing radiation. Fed Proc 32:1882, 1973

87. Demopoulos HB: Control of free radicals in biological systems. Fed Proc 32:1903, 1973

88. Brown BR Jr: Hepatic microsomal lipoperoxidation and inhalational anesthetics: A biochemical and morphologic study in the rat. Anesthesiology 36:458, 1972

89. Weinstein IB, Yamaguchi R, Gebert R, et al: Use of epithelial cell cultures for studies on the mechanism of transformation by chemical carcinogens. In Vitro 11:130, 1975

90. Strunin L: The liver and anaesthesia, Major Problems in Anaesthesia, Vol. 3. Edited by Mushin WW. London, W. B. Saunders Co Ltd, 1977, pp 144–146

91. Clarke RSJ, Doggart JR, Lavery T: Changes in liver function after different types of surgery. Br J Anaesth 48:119, 1976

92. Libonati M, Malsch E, Price HL, et al: Splanchnic circulation in man during methoxyflurane anesthesia. Anesthesiology 38:366, 1973

93. Gelman SI: Disturbances in hepatic blood flow during anaesthesia and surgery. Arch Surg 111:881, 1976

94. Simpson JY: On a new anaesthetic agent, more efficient than sulphuric ether. Lancet 2:549, 1847

95. Defalque RJ: The first delayed chloroform poisoning. Anesth Analg 47:374, 1968

96. Henderson Y, Cullen TS, Martin ED, et al: Report of the Committee on Anesthesia of the American Medical Association. JAMA 58:1908, 1912

97. Bevan AD, Favill HB: Acid intoxication, and late poisonous effects of anesthetics. Hepatic toxemia. Acute fatty degeneration of the liver following chloroform and ether anesthesia. JAMA 45:691, 754, 1905

98. Goldschmidt S, Ravdin IS, Lucke B: Anesthesia and liver damage. 1. The protective action of oxygen against the necrotizing effect of certain anesthetics on the liver. J Pharmacol Ex Ther, 59:1, 1937

99. Stephen CR, Margolis G, Fabian LW, et al: Laboratory observations with Fluothane. Anesthesiology 19:770, 1958

100. Caravati CM, Wootton P: Acute massive hepatic necrosis with fatal liver failure. South Med J 55:1268, 1962

101. Gingrich TF, Virtue RW: Postoperative liver damage. Is anesthesia involved? Surgery 57:241, 1965

102. Herber R, Specht, NW: Liver necrosis following anesthesia. Arch Intern Med 115:266, 1965

103. Slater EM, Gibson JM, Dykes MHM, et al: Postoperative hepatic necrosis. Its incidence and diagnostic value in association with the administration of halothane. N Engl J Med 270:983, 1964

104. Wylie WD, Churchill-Davidson HC: Anaesthesia and the liver, A Practice of Anaesthesia. London, Lloyd-Luke, 1962

105. Krantz JC, Carr CJ, Lu G, Bell FK: Anesthesia XL. The anesthesia action of trifluoroethyl vinyl ether. J Pharmacol Exp Ther 108:488, 1953

106. Reynolds ES, Brown BR Jr, Vandam LD: Massive hepatic necrosis after fluroxene anesthesia—a case of drug interaction. N Engl J Med 286:530, 1972

107. Harrison GG, Smith JS: Massive lethal hepatic necrosis in rats anesthetized with fluroxene after microsomal enzyme induction. Anesthesiology 39:619, 1973

108. Johnston RR, Cromwell TH, Eger EI II, et al: The toxicity of fluroxene in animals and man. Anesthesiology 38:313, 1973

109. Suckling CW: Some chemical and physical factors in the development of Fluothane. Br J Anaesth 29:466, 1957

110. Brennan RW, Hunter AR, Johnstone M: Halothane—a clinical assessment. Lancet 2:453, 1957

111. Johnstone M: The human cardiovascsular response to Fluothane anaesthesia. Br J Anaesth 28:392, 1956

112. Brody GL, Sweet RB: Halothane anesthesia as a possible cause of massive hepatic necrosis. Anesthesiology 24:29, 1963

113. Bunker JP, Blumenfeld CM: Liver necrosis after halothane anesthesia. Cause or coincidence? N Engl J Med 268:531, 1963

114. Lindenbaum J, Leifer E: Hepatic necrosis associated with halothane anesthesia. N Engl J Med 268:525, 1963

115. Bunker JP, Forrest WH, Mostseller F, et al: A Study of the Possible Association between Halothane Anesthesia and Postoperative Hepatic Necrosis. National Halothane Study. Washington, U.S. Government Printing Office, 1969

116. Subcommittee on the National Halothane Study of the Committee on Anesthesia, National Academy of Sciences-National Research Council. Summary of the National Halothane Study. Possible association between halothane anesthesia and postoperative necrosis. JAMA 197:775, 1966

117. Dykes MHM, Bunker JP: Hepatotoxicity and anesthetics. Pharmacol Physicians 4:15, 1970

118. Strunin L, Simpson BR: Halothane in Britain today. Br J Anaesth 44:919, 1972

119. Bottinger LE, Dalen E, Hallen B: Halothane-induced liver damage: An analysis of the material reported to the Swedish Adverse Drug Reaction Committee 1966–1973. Acta Anaesthesiol Scand 20:40, 1976

120. Inman WHW, Mushin WW: Jaundice after repeated exposure to halothane: An analysis of reports to the Committee on Safety of Medicines. Br Med J, 1:5, 1974

121. Moult PJA, Sherlock S: Halothane related hepatitis. A clinical study of twenty-six cases. Q J Med (New Series XLIV) 173:99, 1975

122. Walton B, Simpson BR, Strunin L, et al: Unexplained hepatitis following halothane. Br Med J 1:1171, 1976

123. Wood ML, Berman ML, Harbison RD, et al: Halothane-induced hepatic necrosis in triiodothyronine-pretreated rats. Anesthesiology 52:470, 1980

124. Jee R, Sipies IG, Gandolfi AJ, et al: Factors influencing halothane hepatoxicity in the rat hypoxic model. Toxicol Appl Pharmacol 52:267, 1980

125. McLain GE, Sipes IG, Brown BR Jr: An animal model of halothane hepatotoxicity. Anesthesiology 51:321, 1979

126. Ross WT Jr, Daggy BP, Cardell RR: Hepatic necrosis caused by halothane and hypoxia in phenobarbital-treated rats. Anesthesiology 51:327, 1979

127. Artusio JF Jr, Van Poznack A, Hunt RE, et al: A clinical evaluation of methoxyflurane in man. Anesthesiology 21:512, 1960

128. Joshi PH, Conn HO: The syndrome of methoxyflurane associated hepatitis. Ann Intern Med 80:395, 1974

129. Cale JO, Parks CR, Jenkins MT: Hepatic and renal effects of methoxyflurane in dogs. Anesthesiology 23:248, 1962

130. Dahlgren BE, Goodrich BH: Changes in

kidney and liver function after methoxyflurane (Penthrane) anesthesia. Br J Anaesth 48:145, 1976

131. Botty C, Brown B, Stanley V, et al: Clinical experiences with compound 347—a halogenated anesthetic. Anesth Analg 47:499, 1968

132. Dobkin HB, Heinrich, RG, Israel, JS, et al: Clinical and laboratory evaluation of a new inhalation agent: Compound 347 (CHF_2–O–CF_2–CHFCl). Anesthesiology 29:275, 1968

133. Deninger KJ, Lecky JH, Nahrwold ML: Hepatocellular dysfunction without jaundice after enflurane anesthesia. Anesthesiology 41:86, 1974

134. Sadove MS, Kim SI: Hepatitis after use of two different fluorinated anesthetic agents. Anesth Analg 53:336, 1974

135. Van der Reis L, Askin SH, Freckner GN, et al: Hepatic necrosis after enflurane anesthesia. JAMA 227:76, 1974

136. Holaday DA, Smith FR: Sevoflurane anesthesia and biotransformation in man. Anesthesiology 51:S27, 1979

137. Lynch S, Martis L, Woods E: Evaluation of hepatotoxic potential of sevoflurane in rats. Pharmacologist 21:221, 1979

138. Crandell WB, Pappas, SG, MacDonald A: Nephrotoxicity associated with methoxyflurane anesthesia. Anesthesiology 27:591, 1966

139. Mazze RI, Shue GL, Jackson SH: Renal dysfunction associated with methoxyflurane anesthesia. A randomized prospective clinical evaluation. JAMA 216:278, 1971

140. Smith FA (editor): Pharmacology of Fluorides. Vol. 20 of Handbook of Experimental Pharmacology. New York, Springer-Verlag, 1970

141. Mazze RI, Cousins MJ, Kosek JC: Dose-related methoxyflurane nephrotoxicity in rats: A biochemical and pathologic correlation. Anesthesiology 36:571, 1972

142. Jeghers H, Murphy R: Medical progress, practical aspects of oxalate metabolism. N Engl J Med 233:208, 1945

143. Cousins MJ, Mazze RI: Methoxyflurane nephrotoxicity: A study of dose response in man. JAMA 225:1611, 1973

144. Mazze RI, Cousins MJ: Combined nephrotoxicity of gentamycin and methoxyflurane anesthesia in man. A case report. Br J Anaesth 45: 394, 1973

145. Barr GA, Mazze RI, Cousins MJ, et al: An animal model for combined methoxyflurane and gentamicin nephrotoxicity. Br J Anaesth 45:306, 1973

146. Hitt BA, Mazze RI, Denson DD: Isotopic probe of the mechanisms of methoxyflurane defluorination. Drug Metab Dispos 7:218, 1978

147. McCarty LP, Malek RS, Larsen ER: The effects of deuteration on the metabolism of halogenated anesthetics in the rat. Anesthesiology 51:106, 1979

148. Mazze RI: The kidney: Anesthesia induced malfunction. 27th Annual Refresher Course Lectures of the American Society of Anesthesiologists, San Francisco, 1976, p 229

149. Cousins MJ, Greenstein LR, Hitt BA, et al: Metabolism and renal effects of enflurane in man. Anesthesiology 44:44, 1976

150. Mazze RI, Calverley RK, Smith NT: Inorganic fluoride nephrotoxicity: Prolonged enflurane and halothane anesthesia in volunteers. Anesthesiology 46:265, 1977

151. Cousins MJ, Mazze RI, Kosek JC, et al: The etiology of methoxyflurane nephrotoxicity. J Pharmacol Exp Ther 190:530, 1974

152. Kripke BJ, Kelman AD, Shah NK, et al: Testicular reaction to prolonged exposure to nitrous oxide. Anesthesiology 44:104, 1976

153. Coate WB, Kapp RW, Lewis TR: Chronic exposure to low concentrations of halothane-nitrous oxide: Reproductive and cytogenetic effects in the rat. Anesthesiology 50:310, 1979

154. Land PC, Owen EL, Linde HW: Mouse sperm morphology following exposure to anesthetics during early spermatogenesis. Anesthesiology, 51:S259, 1979

155. NIOSH: Criteria for a recommended standard . . . occupational exposure to waste anesthetic gases and vapors. DHEW (NIOSH), Publication No. 77–140, 1977

156. Millard RI, Corbett TH: Nitrous oxide concentration in the dental operatory. J Oral Surg 32:593, 1974

157. Pfaffli P, Nikki P, Ahlman K: Halothane and nitrous oxide in end-tidal air and venous blood of surgical personnel. Ann Clin Res 4:273, 1972

158. Baden JM, Brinkenhoff M, Wharton RS, et al: Mutagenicity of volatile anesthetics: Halothane. Anesthesiology 45:311, 1976

159. Baden JM, Kelley MJ, Mazze RI, et al: Mu-

tagenicity of inhalation anesthetics: Nitrous oxide, cyclopropane, trichloroethylene and divinyl ether. Br J Anaesth 51:417, 1979

160. Baden JM, Kelley MJ, Simmon VF, et al: Fluroxene mutagenicity. Mutat Res 58:183, 1978

161. Baden JM, Kelley MJ, Wharton RS, et al: Mutagenicity of halogenated ether anesthetics. Anesthesiology 46:346, 1977

162. Waskell L: Study of the mutagenicity of anesthetics and their metabolites. Mutat Res 57:141, 1978

163. Edmunds HN, Baden JM, Simmon VF: Mutagenicity studies with volatile metabolites of halothane. Anesthesiology 51:425, 1979

164. Garro AJ, Phillips RA: Mutagenicity of the halogenated olefin, 2-bromo-2-chloro-1, 1-difluoroethylene, a presumed metabolite of the inhalation anesthetic halothane. Environ Health Perspect 21:65, 1977

165. Waskell L: Lack of mutagenicity of two possible halothane metabolites. Anesthesiology 50:9, 1979

166. McCoy EC, Hankel R, Rosenkranz HS, et al: Detection of mutagenic activity in the urines of anesthesiologists: A preliminary report. Environ Health Perspect 21:221, 1977

167. Baden JM, Kelley MJ, Cheung A, et al: Lack of mutagens in urine of operating room personnel. Anesthesiology 53:195, 1980

168. White AE, Takehisa S, Eger EI II, et al: Sister chromatid exchanges induced by inhaled anesthetics. Anesthesiology 50:426, 1979

169. Sturrock JE: Lack of mutagenic effect of halothane or chloroform on cultured cells using the azaguanine test system. Br J Anaesth 49:207, 1977

170. Sturrock JR: No mutagenic effect of enflurane on cultured cells. Br J Anaesth 49:777, 1977

171. Krechkovsky EA, Shkvar LA: On the mutagenic effect of fluothane. Eksp Khir Anesteziol 18:72, 1973

172. Garrett S, Fuerst R: Sex-linked mutations in *Drosophila* after exposure to various mixtures of gas atmospheres. Environ Res 7:286, 1974

173. Kramers JC, Burm GL: Mutagenicity studies with halothane in *Drosophila melanogaster*. Anesthesiology 50:510, 1979

174. Sparrow AH, Schairer LA: Mutagenic response of *Tradescantia* to treatment with x-rays, EMS, DBE, ozone, SO_2, N_2O and several insecticides. Mutat Res 26:445, 1974

175. Cohen EN, Hood N: Application of low-temperature autoradiography to studies of the uptake and metabolism of volatile anesthetics in the mouse. III. Halothane. Anesthesiology 31:553, 1969

176. Leong BKJ, MacFarland HN, Reese WH: Induction of lung adenomas by chronic inhalation of bis (chloromethyl) ether. Arch Environ Health 22:663, 1976

177. Van Duuren BL, Goldschmidt BM, Katz C, et al: Alphaloethers: A new type of alkylating carcinogen. Arch Environ Health 16:472, 1968

178. Poirier LA, Stober GD, Shimkin MB: Bioassay of alkyl halides and nucleotide base analogs by pulmonary tumor response in strain A mice. Cancer Res 35:1411, 1975

179. Creech JL, Johnson MN: Angiosarcoma of the liver in the manufacture of polyvinyl-chloride. J Occup Med 16:150, 1974

180. Viola PL, Bigotti A, Caputo A: Oncogenic response of rat skin, lungs, and bone to vinyl chloride. Cancer Res 31:516, 1971

181. Cavalieri E, Calvin M: Molecular characteristics of some carcinogenic hydrocarbons. Proc Nat Acad Sci USA 68:1251, 1971

182. Bruce DL, Eide KA, Linde HW, et al: Causes of death among anesthesiologists: A 20-year survey. Anesthesiology 29:565, 1968

183. Corbett TH, Cornell RG, Lieding K, et al: Incidence of cancer among Michigan nurse anesthetists. Anesthesiology 38:260, 1973

184. Bruce DL, Eide KA, Smith NJ, et al: A prospective survey of anesthesiologist mortality, 1967–1971. Anesthesiology 41:71, 1974

185. American Society of Anesthesiologists: Report of an ad hoc committee on the effect of trace anesthetics on the health of operating room personnel. Occupational disease among operating room personnel: A national study. Anesthesiology 41:321, 1974

186. Doll R, Peto R: Mortality among doctors in different occupations. Br Med J 1:1433, 1977

187. Tomlin PJ: Health problems of anaesthetists and their families in the West Midlands. Br J Med 1:779, 1979

188. Lew EA: Mortality experience among anesthesiologists, 1954–1976. Anesthesiology 51:195, 1979

189. Cohen EN, Brown BW, Wu ML, et al: Occupational disease in dentistry and chronic

exposure to trace anesthetic gases. J Am Dent Assoc 101:21, 1980

190. Walts LF, Forsythe AB, Moore JG: Critique: Occupational disease among operating room personnel. Anesthesiology 42:608, 1975

191. Fink BR, Cullen BF: Anesthetic pollution: What is happening to us? Anesthesiology 45:79, 1976

192. Vessey MP: Epidemiological studies of the occupational hazards of anesthesia—a review. Anaesthesia 33:430, 1978

193. Baden JM, Mazze RI, Wharton RS, et al: Carcinogenicity of halothane in Swiss/ICR mice. Anesthesiology 51:20, 1979

194. Department of Health, Education and Welfare, FDA: Chloroform as an ingredient of human drug and cosmetic products. Fed Reg 14:15026, 1976

195. National Cancer Institute: Carcinogenesis technical report series, No. 2. Carcinogenesis bioassay of trichloroethylene. CAS No. 79-01-6, 1976

196. Oppenheimer BS, Oppenheimer ET, Danishefsky I, et al: Carcinogenic effect of metals in rodents. Cancer Res 16:439, 1956

197. Kucerova M, Zhurkov VS, Polivkova Z, et al: Mutagenic effect of epichlorohydrin, II. Analysis of chromosomal aberrations in lymphocytes of persons occupationally exposed to epichlorohydrin. Mutat Res 48:355, 1971

198. McCann J, Choi E, Yamasaki E, et al: The detection of carcinogens as mutagens in the *Salmonella*/microsome test: Assay of 300 chemicals, Part 1. Proc Natl Acad Sci USA 72:5135, 1975

199. Van Duuren BL, Goldschmidt BM, Katz C, et al: Carcinogenic activity of alkylating agents. J Natl Cancer Inst 53:695, 1974

200. Corbett TH: Cancer and congenital anomalies associated with anesthesia. Ann NY Acad Sci 271:58, 1976

201. Eger EI II, White AE, Brown CL, et al: A test of the carcinogenicity of enflurane, isoflurane, halothane, methoxyflurane and nitrous oxide in mice. Anesth Analg 57:678, 1978

202. Coate WB, Ulland BM, Lewis TR: Chronic exposure to low concentrations of halothane–nitrous oxide: Lack of carcinogenic effect in the rat. Anesthesiology 50:306, 1979

203. Klingberg MA, Weatherall JA (editors): Epidemiologic Methods for Detection of Teratogens. Basel, S. Karger, 1979

204. Sturrock JE, Nunn JF: Mitosis in mammalian cells during exposure to anesthetics. Anesthesiology 43:21, 1975

205. Trudell JR: A unitary theory of anesthesia based on lateral phase separations in nerve membranes. Anesthesiology 46:5, 1977

206. Wilson JE (editor): Environment and Birth Defects. New York, Academic Press, 1973

207. Vaisman AI: Working conditions in surgery and their effect on the health of anesthesiologists. Eksp Khir Anesteziol 3:44, 1967

208. Askrog V, Harvald B: Teratogen effect of inhalation anesthetics. Nord Med 83:498, 1970

209. Pharoah PO, Alberman E, Doyle P: Outcome of pregnancy among women in anaesthetic practice. Lancet 1:34, 1977

210. Cohen EN, Bellville JW, Brown BW: Anesthesia, pregnancy and miscarriage: A study of operating room nurses and anesthetists. Anesthesiology 35:343, 1971

211. Knill-Jones RP, Moir, DB, Rodrigues LV, et al: Anaesthetic practice and pregnancy: A controlled survey of women anesthetists in the United Kingdom. Lancet 1:1326, 1972

212. Rosenberg P, Kirves A: Miscarriages among operating theatre staff. Acta Anaesthesiol Scand 53:37, 1973

213. Corbett TH, Cornell RG, Endres JL, et al: Birth defects among children of nurse anesthetists. Anesthesiology 41:341, 1974

214. Knill-Jones RP, Newman BJ, Spence AA: Anaesthetic practice and pregnancy: A controlled survey of male anaesthetists in the United Kingdom. Lancet 2:807, 1975

215. McBride WG: Thalidomide and congenital anomalies. Lancet 2:1358, 1961

216. Ferstandig LL: Trace concentrations of anesthetic gases: A critical review of their disease potential. Anesth Analg 57:328, 1978

217. Shnider SM, Webster GM: Maternal and fetal hazards of surgery during pregnancy. Am J Obstet Gynecol 92:891, 1965

218. Smith BE: Fetal prognosis after anesthesia during gestation. Anesth Analg 42:521, 1963

219. Quimby KL, Katz J, Bowman RE: Behavioral consequences in rats from chronic exposure to 10 ppm halothane during early development. Anesth Analg 54:628, 1975

15

Pharmacology of Intravenous Narcotic Anesthetics

Theodore H. Stanley, M.D.

INTRODUCTION

Narcotics have been administered for hundreds of years to allay anxiety and pain associated with surgery.[1] Many of these compounds are now used not only as intravenous analgesic supplements but also as primary or sole intravenous anesthetics. Some investigators have recently suggested that with minor modifications, some new synthetic narcotics may qualify as the "ideal intravenous anesthetic."[2-6] In this chapter, I discuss the pharmacology and use of naturally occurring and synthetic intravenous narcotics in contemporary anesthetic practice.

HISTORY

An outline of the history of the use of narcotics in anesthesia is shown in Table 15-1. Opium was inhaled, ingested, and applied locally to wounds for its analgesic and hypnotic effects from biblical times until the 19th century. Unfortunately, these types of administration were fraught with difficulties, chief of which was variability in potency. As a result, either inadequate or no analgesia or overdose and death frequently occurred. The isolation by Serturner in 1809 of morphine as the most active of the more than 20 alkaloids

in opium and the invention of the syringe by Pravaz and the needle by Wood in 1853 finally allowed administration of narcotics in carefully measured doses.[1] Morphine then was frequently used intramuscularly for preoperative medication, as a supplement during ether or chloroform anesthesia, and postoperatively for analgesia. In the early 20th century, large amounts of morphine (1 mg/kg) plus scopolamine (1 to 3 mg/70 kg) were administered in divided doses intramus-

Table 15-1. A Brief History of the Use of Narcotics in Anesthesia

1. Opium—inhaled, ingested, applied topically from biblical times until the 19th century
2. Isolation of chemical structure of morphine—1809
3. Invention of syringe and hollow needle—1853
4. Morphine premedication—1870–1880
5. Morphine-scopolamine anesthesia—1880–1905
6. Morphine (narcotics) rarely used in the operating room—1905–1947
7. Neff introduces meperidine—N_2O anesthesia—1947
8. Narcotic-N_2O anesthesia gains popularity—1947–1969
9. Innovar-N_2O anesthesia—1963
10. Morphine-oxygen anesthesia (Lowenstein)—1969
11. Fentanyl-oxygen anesthesia (De Castro)—1970
12. Agonist-antagonist narcotics—1970's
13. Narcotics during inhalation of anesthesia—1970's
14. Newer narcotics as complete anesthetics—late 1970's

cularly as complete anesthesia.[7,8] Although initially popular, this technique rapidly fell into disfavor because of an alarming increase in operative mortality.[1,9] For the next 30 years, anesthesiologists rarely used narcotics intraoperatively.

Introduction of intravenously administered barbiturates, which are poor analgesics, led to renewed enthusiasm for the intraoperative use of narcotics. Two important events in this development were the synthesis of meperidine in 1939 and the advancement of a new anesthetic technique by Neff, Mayer, and de la Luz Perales in 1947.[10] Anesthesia was induced with nitrous oxide and maintained with both nitrous oxide and intermittent intravenous injections of meperidine. Many variations of the "nitrous oxide–narcotic" technique became popular. At first, thiopental (as an induction agent and/or as an additional supplement during maintenance), d-tubocurarine (for muscular relaxation), and a narcotic such as morphine, meperidine, or α-prodine were given. After the introduction of Innovar–nitrous oxide anesthesia[11] (Innovar consists of droperidol, a tranquilizer, and fentanyl, a short-acting narcotic), a variety of intravenous supplements were employed (including hypnotics, sedatives, tranquilizers, and additional analgesics) to be given in addition to the primary anesthetic which included a narcotic analgesic, nitrous oxide, thiopental, and a muscle relaxant.[12–16] These techniques were termed balanced anesthesia, presumably because each intravenous compound employed was selected and administered for a specific action, e.g., analgesia, sedation, amnesia, muscle relaxation. Lately, narcotics as well as other analgesics and hypnotics are being administered intravenously during anesthesia with potent inhaled anesthetics.[17] This practice is based on the belief that many of these drugs reduce the concentrations of inhaled anesthetics required for anesthesia and cause less depression of the cardiovascular system and other organ systems. Unfortunately, this last concept is not well documented.

More recently De Castro[18] and Lowenstein et al.[19] reintroduced the concept that high doses of narcotics could produce "complete" anesthesia. They administered fentanyl or morphine intravenously until consciousness was lost and then controlled ventilation with a high inspired concentration of oxygen. When morphine (0.5 to 1.0 mg/kg) was administered intravenously while patients breathed 100 percent oxygen, cardiovascular dynamics did not change in those patients without cardiac disease and frequently improved in those with significant valvular disease. These reports led to several additional studies evaluating morphine and other narcotics as the sole anesthetic for patients without cardiovascular reserve undergoing a major operative procedure.[20–23] Unfortunately, problems with incomplete amnesia,[24,25] histamine release,[25,26] prolonged postoperative respiratory depression,[27,28] increased blood volume requirements secondary to marked venovasodilation,[22] occasional severe hypotension,[24,25] and hypertension[21] have recently decreased the popularity of morphine as a "complete" anesthetic. In contrast, the new synthetic narcotic fentanyl has become popular not only as a component of balanced (nitrous oxide–narcotic) anesthesia[11,23] and as a supplement during inhalational anesthesia,[17] but also, in much larger (anesthetic) doses (50 to 100 μg/kg) as a primary or complete anesthetic.[2,3,25] Unfortunately, these large anesthetic doses of fentanyl also cause significant postoperative respiratory depression[2,3] and therefore are not frequently given to healthy patients undergoing routine operative procedures. However, like anesthetic doses of morphine, large intravenous doses of fentanyl produce complete anesthesia without depressing cardiovascular function and are therefore ideal for patients with little or no cardiovascular reserve. In addition, fentanyl-oxygen anesthesia apparently produces less prolonged postoperative respiratory depression, more cardiovascular stability, little or no histamine release, and no

Table 15-2. Classification of Narcotic Compounds

Occurring Naturally
   Morphine
   Codeine
   Papaverine

Semisynthetic
   Heroin
   Dilaudid

Synthetic
   Morphine derivatives (levorphanol)
   Methadone derivatives (methadone)
   Benzomorphan derivatives (pentazocine)
   Phenylpiperidine derivatives (meperidine and
     fentanyl)

venovasodilation when compared with morphine.[2,3,25–28]

Despite these problems, the use of narcotics as anesthetics probably will persist and possibly increase because of their minimal effect on most other organ systems when compared with inhaled anesthetics.[2–6]

CLASSIFICATION

Narcotics are usually classified as naturally occurring, semisynthetic, and synthetic (Table 15-2). Morphine, codeine, and papaverine, the only naturally occurring narcotics of clinical significance, are obtained from the poppy plant, *Papaver somniferum,* which is the source of the more than 20 pharmacologically active natural alkaloids that make up opium. These compounds can be divided into two chemical classes, the phenanthrenes (morphine and codeine) and the benzyliso-

quinoline derivatives (papaverine). Of the naturally occurring narcotics, only morphine is of importance as an intravenous anesthetic or analgesic.

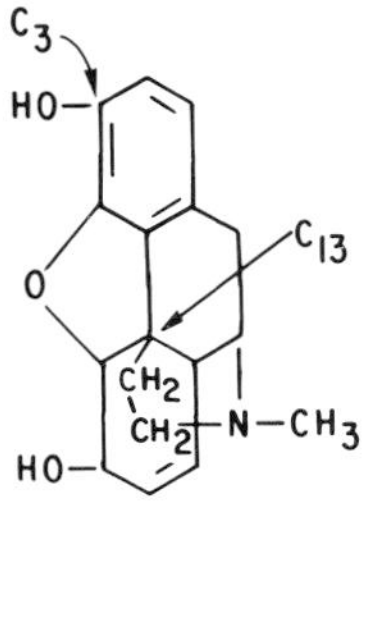

The semisynthetic narcotics are derivatives of morphine in which any one of several changes has been made, e.g., etherification of one hydroxyl group (codeine), esterification of both hydroxyl groups (heroin), oxidation of the alcoholic hydroxyl to a ketone, or saturation of a double bond on the benzene ring (hydromorphone hydrochloride [Dilaudid]).

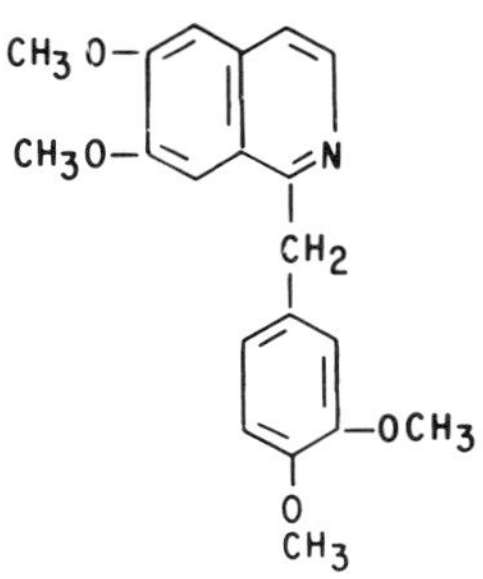

The synthetic compounds resemble morphine but are usually entirely synthesized. They are divided into four groups: the morphinan derivatives (levorphanol); the diphenyl or methadone derivatives (methadone, *d*-propoxyphene); the benzomorphans (phenazocine, pentazocine); and the phenylpiperidine derivatives (meperidine, fentanyl). Although many of these narcotics have been used intravenously for analgesia or anesthesia during surgery, only the phenylpiperidine derivatives currently play an important role in anesthesia.

MODE OF ACTION

The mode of action of narcotic compounds can be explained in terms of their structure and site of action and whether they interact with endogenous CNS peptides (Table 15-3).

STRUCTURE-ACTIVITY RELATIONSHIP

Structurally, narcotics are complex, three-dimensional compounds that usually exist as two optical isomers, i.e., molecules that are mirror images of each other and are identical in chemical composition but cannot be superimposed.[29] Usually only the *l*-rotatory isomer is able to produce analgesia.

A close relationship exists between the stereochemical structure of a narcotic compound and the presence or absence of analge-

MORPHINE

PAPAVERINE

**Table 15-3. Mode of Action of
Narcotic Compounds**

Structure-Activity
  Stereospecific
  Optical isomers (levo-active)
  Activity easily transformed
  Possess electron-rich carbon, basic nitrogen

Site of Action
  Specific periaqueductal gray area receptors
  Descending impulses from brain impair transfer of
    noxious impulses from periphery into spinal cord
  Spinal cord receptors (substantia gelatinosa)

Endogenous CNS (Opiate-like) Peptides
  Possess narcotic activity
  Enkephalins—pentapeptides
  Endorphins—larger peptides
  Produce analgesia in specific body areas as well as
    generally

sic activity.[30,31] Indeed, relatively minor changes in the conformation of the molecule, such as the degree of ionization produced by changing pH, may cause significant variation in pharmacologic activity of narcotic compounds.[31] Most narcotic compounds have a relatively rigid T-shaped structure.[29] They also usually possess an electron-rich hydroxyl or ketone group (carbon 3 in morphine) capable of hydrogen binding; a positively-charged basic nitrogen atom that can form an ionic bond; a quaternary carbon (carbon 13 in morphine) that is separated from the basic nitrogen by an ethane chain ($-CH_2-CH_2-$); and a flat benzene or 2-thienyl ring, which is a distance of 4.58 angstroms (from the center of the ring) from nitrogen.

SITE OF ACTION

Specific narcotic (opiate) receptors were assumed to exist in the CNS; however, they could not be identified because opiates bind to most biologic membranes. Recently techniques using highly specific radioactive opiates have enabled separation of binding sites, which allowed identification of these receptors.[32,33] Opiate receptors are concentrated in only a few areas of the brain and spinal cord.[33,34] For example, the periaqueductal gray matter of the brain stem, amygdala, cor-

pus striatum, and hypothalamus have very high concentrations of receptors that are involved with pain perception and integration and emotional responses to pain. The periaqueductal gray area is one of the few regions in which microinjections of morphine or direct electrical stimulation produce analgesia that can be blocked with naloxone.[32,34,35] According to Mayer et al.,[35] stimulation of periaqueductal gray receptors with morphine, electricity, or the endogenous opiate-like peptides creates a barrage of impulses that move down the central nervous system and inhibit the transmission of nociceptive information from peripheral nerves into the spinal cord. Apparently, the integrity of certain neurotransmitter systems connecting the pain-inhibiting system in the brain to the spinal cord is necessary for morphine to exert its analgesic action. Satoh and Takagi[36] found that morphine blockade of transmission of spinal cord potentials evoked by painful stimulation is inhibited by high spinal cord transsection.

Unfortunately, this theory of descending inhibition does not entirely explain morphine's analgesic action. The substantia gelatinosa of the spinal cord also possesses a dense collection of opiate receptors.[29,37,38] Direct application of narcotics to these receptors creates intense analgesia. Undoubtedly, narcotics produce analgesia by acting at receptors both in the spinal cord and in higher centers. Opiate receptors are also localized in the substantia gelatinosa of the caudal spinal trigeminal nucleus, the nucleus receiving pain fibers from the face and hands via branches of the 5th, 7th, 9th, and 10th cranial nerves.[32] Within the brain stem, opiate receptors are highly concentrated in the solitary nuclei that receive visceral sensory fibers from the ninth and tenth cranial nerves and the area postrema. Stimulation of the solitary nuclei depresses gastric secretion and the cough reflex and causes orthostatic hypotension. Stimulation of the area postrema with its chemoreceptor trigger zone results in nausea and vomiting.

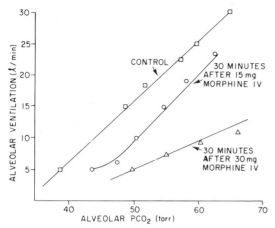

Fig 15-1. Effect of morphine (15 and 30 mg IV) on alveolar ventilation and alveolar PCO_2.

ENDOGENOUS CNS (OPIATE-LIKE) PEPTIDES

The specificity of CNS receptors for morphine and other narcotics led many investigators to believe that these receptors' normal function was to combine with an endogenous, narcotic-like compound probably involved in pain perception. In 1975, two pentapeptides that possessed significant opiate-like activity were found in the brain and were called enkephalins.[39] Although these pentapeptides were found throughout the brain and spinal cord, their highest density was in regions containing high concentrations of opiate receptors.[39,40] Outside the CNS, enkephalins

For many years morphine and most narcotics have been known to be effective in relieving dull, boring, poorly localized, visceral type pain but not nearly as effective in influencing highly localized somatotopic pain.[32] The lateral thalamic nuclei are involved with highly localized pain, whereas the medial thalamic nuclei mediate poorly localized and emotionally influenced pain. As might be expected, higher concentrations of opiate receptors recently have been found in medial than in lateral thalamic nuclei.

have only been found in the gastrointestinal tract.[34] The striking restriction of these compounds to these two areas suggests that they may act as neurohormones.

The enkephalins are not the only opiate-like peptides present in the central nervous system. Recently, larger peptides having different structures but possessing the whole sequence of amino acids found in the enkephalins have been detected in the pituitary gland.[41] These compounds, called endorphins, bind to opiate receptors and have marked narcotic activity. They were found to be part of an even larger pituitary extract, β lipotropin.

The exact relationship of enkephalins to endorphins and the purpose of both classes of peptides in the CNS are not completely understood. In synaptosomal opiate-binding assays, these peptides are indistinguishable from morphine in their activity.[41] The enkephalins and most of the endorphins are, on a molar basis, about as active as morphine.[41] In contrast, β endorphin is five to ten times more potent than morphine. Because enkephalins are degraded very rapidly when injected intravenously or even directly into cerebral ventricles, it is difficult to evaluate their analgesic actions in vivo. However, endorphins produce significant analgesia for 15 to 60 minutes. Remarkably, some endorphins appear to produce analgesia in specific body areas, i.e., α endorphin produces analgesia mostly of the face and neck, whereas β endorphin produces analgesia of the whole body. Endorphins also affect temperature, mood, and the secretion of other neurohormones.[41] The profound effects of each of the endorphins suggest that they may influence normal and abnormal behavior as well as drug addiction and withdrawal. Perhaps manipulation of the concentration of these peptides in the central nervous system, or administration of similar synthetic compounds, would produce desirable analgesic or anesthetic effects in patients undergoing operative procedures. Endorphins have been well reviewed by Guillemin.[42]

ANALGESIA-AMNESIA-ANESTHESIA

The reintroduction of morphine plus oxygen as an anesthetic technique in 1969 was based on the premise that large doses of morphine could produce anesthesia without significant changes in cardiovascular dynamics.[19] Unfortunately, doses of narcotics required to produce "complete" anesthesia may vary extensively from patient to patient.[28,43] The reasons for this variation are not understood and therefore prediction of narcotic anesthetic requirements is difficult. Generally, healthier patients (i.e., American Society of Anesthesiologists Class I or II) with normal or even high cardiac outputs prior to anesthesia require larger doses of narcotics for anesthesia than patients who have serious metabolic disease, cardiovascular limitations, or a reduced cardiac output.[2,3,28,43] Undoubtedly, differences in plasma protein binding, fat solubility, hepatic metabolism, renal excretion, and regional perfusion probably influence requirements for narcotics in a manner that has not been quantitated. Furthermore, when a narcotic is used either in large doses as a complete anesthetic or with supplements, such as nitrous oxide or other intravenous compounds, there are few reliable, measurable clinical indications that amnesia has been achieved. Profound analgesia and apnea can easily be achieved with narcotics without producing anesthesia.[22] While administration of supplements (nitrous oxide, diazepam, droperidol) or larger doses of narcotics will increase the likelihood of amnesia, undesirable effects are more likely to occur, e.g., prolonged postoperative respiratory depression after larger doses of some narcotics[27,28] and cardiovascular depression after administration of some supplements.[12,13]

The addition of supplements during narcotic anesthesia can provide certain advantages. Besides providing amnesia, addition of nitrous oxide,[44,45] diazepam,[2] and most other CNS depressants may decrease narcotic anesthetic requirements and the duration of post-

Table 15-4. Cardiovascular Actions of Narcotics

1. Large doses of some narcotics (morphine, fentanyl) have little influence on myocardial mechanics and cardiovascular dynamics.
2. Morphine can increase plasma catecholamines in man.
3. Anesthetic doses of fentanyl decrease plasma catecholamines in man.
4. Significant bradycardia, hypotension, hypertension, and tachycardia can occur during narcotic anesthesia.
5. Morphine but apparently not fentanyl, causes venodilation in a dose-dependent fashion.
6. Meperidine is a direct myocardial depressant.
7. Once produced, hypertension is difficult to treat during narcotic anesthesia.
8. Narcotic-induced bradycardia is usually due to central vagal nucleus stimulation.
9. Atropine premedication reduces but does not prevent narcotic-induced bradycardia.
10. Arrhythmias are less common during narcotic anesthesia than during potent inhalational anesthesia.
11. Morphine and perhaps other narcotics decrease pulmonary blood volume.

operative narcotic action. Supplementation with other drugs during narcotic anesthesia may also reduce an elevated arterial blood pressure and systemic vascular resistance (halothane),[46] decrease postoperative nausea and vomiting (intravenous droperidol),[47] and prevent cardiovascular stimulation (intravenous lidocaine) with intubation or surgery.[48]

CARDIOVASCULAR ACTIONS

This discussion of the cardiovascular effects (Table 15-4) of narcotics emphasizes morphine and to a lesser extent fentanyl (Sublimaze), meperidine (Demerol), and α-prodine (Nisentil). Although hypotension, hypertension, and cardiac arrhythmias have been described, morphine and fentanyl and some new narcotics, e.g., sulfentanil, usually produce minimal changes in cardiovascular dynamics.[2,19,49] For example, administration of morphine 1 mg/kg intravenously did not cause significant circulatory changes in patients without cardiac disease.[19] However, in patients with aortic valvular disease, stroke volume and cardiac output increased, proba-

Table 15-5. Blood Requirements During Operation and for the First Postoperative Day in 61 Patients Anesthetized with Morphine (1–4 mg/kg) plus Oxygen or Halothane (0.1–1.5%) plus 30% Nitrous Oxide and Oxygen and Undergoing Aortic Valve Replacement or Coronary Artery Bypass Operation

Pathology	Anesthetic	Mean Blood Requirements (ml) Intra-operative	Post-operative
Aortic valvular disease	Morphine	2822*	1091*
	Halothane	998	767
Coronary artery disease	Morphine	2763*	1418*
	Halothane	1726	708

* $P < .05$, Student's paired T-test when compared to halothane values.
(Stanley TH, Gray NH, Isern-Amaral JH, et al: Comparison of blood requirements during morphine and halothane anesthesia for open-heart surgery. Anesthesiology 41:34 1974.)

bly because myocardial depression does not occur after administration of morphine.[19, 50] In fact, Vasco and co-workers[51] found in dogs that morphine has a significant positive inotropic effect that was dependent on endogenous catecholamine release and was inhibited by β-adrenergic blocking agents or previous adrenalectomy. In a dose-dependent manner, morphine also increases the concentrations of catecholamines in both blood and urine of human subjects.[52–54] Although a similar effect has been described after administration of large doses (0.5 to 30 mg/kg) of fentanyl to dogs,[55] my co-workers and I recently found that anesthetic doses of fentanyl do not alter or may actually decrease plasma catecholamine concentrations in man.[56]

Despite these minimal cardiovascular effects, significant hypotension, hypertension, and cardiac arrhythmias have been seen after administration of morphine and other narcotics.[21, 24] Therefore, certain precautions should be observed during the induction and maintenance of anesthesia with morphine.

HYPOTENSION

Hypotension can occur during and following administration of even relatively small doses of morphine.[57] Due to arterial and venous dilation, increased vagal activity, and cardiac slowing, hypotension most often occurs in hypovolemic, hypertensive patients; in those having high vagal tone; or during rapid administration of morphine. Hypotension is less common (1) when morphine is given slowly (5 mg/min or slower); (2) when a rapid infusion of intravenous fluids is given concurrently; (3) in patients who are in a slight Trendelenburg (head down) position; and (4) in patients in congestive heart failure. These findings indicate that a large component of the hypotension from morphine is secondary to venodilation,[20, 22, 50, 58] which is probably due to a selective venous α-adrenergic blocking effect.[59] On the other hand, Zelis and co-workers[60, 61] found that morphine selectively impairs certain sympathetic reflexes involving peripheral veins, which they concluded was due to a CNS action of the drug. Apparently venoconstriction in response to tilting or inhalation of carbon dioxide is impaired by morphine, while venoconstriction caused by a single deep breath is not.[61] Whatever the mechanism, we found that in subjects given morphine, venodilation was dose-dependent and caused occasional hypotension during induction of anesthesia. When compared with patients anesthetized with halothane[62] (Table 15-5), these patients had increases in blood requirements during and after surgery. Venodilation and increased blood requirements apparently do not occur with lower doses of morphine (<0.5 mg/kg) plus N_2O.[63]

After administration of morphine, arterial vasodilation, in contrast to venodilation, lasts for only 15 to 30 minutes[64] and is probably related to histamine release[65] and the direct effects of morphine on vascular smooth muscle.[50] Although histamine release following morphine is variable, dose and rate of administration undoubtedly exert some influence. Hypotension secondary to histamine release can be corrected by vasopressors; however, administration of antihistamines either before or after morphine-induced hypotension is of no benefit.

Hypotension also occurs after the intravenous administration of meperidine.[66] Hypotension after meperidine is more frequent and more profound than after comparable doses of morphine. This is due to a significant negative inotropic effect of meperidine[66-68] as well as to a marked reduction in systemic vascular resistance. As a result, meperidine has had little value as a "complete" anesthetic, although it is still popular as a supplement in nitrous oxide–narcotic balanced anesthesia.[69] Meperidine, in contrast to morphine, rarely results in bradycardia but can cause tachycardia,[70] perhaps because of the structural similarity of meperidine to atropine.

Alpha-prodine, which is structurally similar to meperidine, has had limited use as an analgesic supplement in patients in the operating room and delivery suite. Unfortunately, while α-prodine is somewhat shorter-acting than meperidine, it possesses all of the latter's cardiovascular depressant qualities.[71]

MEPERIDINE   ALPHA-PRODINE

FENTANYL

Although fentanyl in large anesthetic doses (50 to 100 μg/kg in man) and in small analgesic doses (5 to 10 μg/kg) also reduces arterial blood pressure, it rarely reduces blood pressure below 90 torr systolic.[2,23] Hypotension, when it occurs after administration of fentanyl, is primarily due to bradycardia, and can be reversed with atropine, ephedrine, or even large doses of pancuronium.[72]

HYPERTENSION

Severe hypertension occasionally occurs during narcotic-oxygen or narcotic–nitrous oxide anesthesia,[21,24,73] usually in patients who have minimal impairment of cardiovascular reserve. Hypertension is less common in patients having valvular heart disease or in those who are severely ill.[74] The primary cause of hypertension during narcotic anesthesia may be incomplete amnesia and/or inadequate analgesia.[24,25] This possibility is supported by the occurrence of occasional intraoperative patient awareness when opioids are the major component of the anesthetic.[24] Also, hypertension is rare before endotracheal intubation or surgical stimulation,[73] which probably means that the sympathetic nervous stimulation and renin-angiotensin responses are not blocked by morphine in doses of 1 to 3 mg/kg.[53,75] However, larger doses of morphine (4 mg/kg or higher) block increases in circulating catecholamine levels in response to surgical stimulus.[52] Hypertension once it is produced during narcotic anesthesia is often difficult to treat. Higher doses of morphine, other narcotics, and even potent inhaled agents may not be effective in restoring blood pressure once noxious stimulation has elevated it. In these situations, vasodilators or adrenergic blockers may be required to treat hypertension. In addition, increased doses of morphine, a variety of intravenous hypnotics, or low concentrations of inhaled anesthetics may also be needed to avoid awareness.[24]

CARDIAC ARRHYTHMIAS

Bradycardia often occurs following the intravenous administration of some narcotics.[2, 76] This bradycardia, which is less frequent when induction of anesthesia is accompanied with nitrous oxide,[2, 76, 77] may be caused by stimulation of the sympathetic nervous system by nitrous oxide. Premedication with the belladonna drugs or glycopyrolate will attenuate or eliminate bradycardia after intravenous administration of morphine and fentanyl.[78] Although atropine (0.4 to 0.8 mg/70 kg intravenously) is usually effective in treating narcotic-induced bradycardia, occasionally these or even large doses (1 to 2 mg intravenously) are ineffective, and in such instances ephedrine (15 to 25 mg intravenously) is necessary.

Bradycardia from narcotics is relatively transient, usually lasting only 10 to 20 minutes and in the case of morphine is probably due to stimulation of the vagal nucleus in the medulla of the brain.[79] However, morphine may also have a direct effect on the sinoatrial (SA) node[80] and may depress atrioventricular conduction.[81] Although narcotics usually do not cause arrhythmias, large anesthetic doses of morphine (and probably other narcotics) can increase sinoatrial and atrioventricular block and decrease the duration of the refractory phase of atrial depolarization.[81] Although theoretically these effects could lead to the development of reentry-type arrhythmias, in practice this rarely occurs. Doses of epinephrine sufficient to induce arrhythmias in dogs recently were found to be no greater during narcotic–nitrous oxide anesthesia than during halothane, enflurane, or nitrous oxide anesthesia.[82] However, the incidence of malignant arrhythmias (ventricular tachycardia and ventricular fibrillation) was less with narcotics plus nitrous oxide than with most potent inhaled anesthetics.[82]

The most common arrhythmia, other than bradycardia, noted during narcotic anesthetic techniques is supraventricular tachycardia,[73] which usually occurs during or immediately following endotracheal intubation or surgical stimulation. Thus, inadequate anesthesia rather than a direct effect of the narcotic is probably responsible for the tachycardia. Some patients, however, experience supraventricular tachycardia during narcotic anesthetic induction without concurrent noxious stimulation, particularly following the use of large doses of meperidine and α-prodine, and occasionally morphine. While tachycardia following meperidine and α-prodine may be attributed to the structural similarity of these compounds to atropine, the tachycardia that occurs after morphine cannot. Such tachycardia is usually accompanied by facial and upper torso flushing. This suggests that increased blood concentrations of histamine and/or the catecholamines may be the explanation for this occasional finding.

PULMONARY VASCULATURE

The pulmonary vascular effects of only some narcotics have been studied. Morphine significantly increases pulmonary artery blood pressure and decreases pulmonary blood volume.[76, 83] Large doses of intravenous fentanyl occasionally increase pulmonary artery pressure in man.[84] The mechanism, or mechanisms, involved in producing these changes have not been elucidated. Other narcotics have not been well studied.

THE USE OF SUPPLEMENTS

During anesthesia, narcotics are frequently used with other drugs (supplements), of which nitrous oxide is the most common. While nitrous oxide alone has minimal effects on myocardial mechanics[85] and cardiovascular dynamics,[86] when combined with intravenously administered narcotics, myocardial depression frequently occurs.[20, 87, 88] (Table 15-6) After administration of morphine (2 mg/kg), McDermott and Stanley[87] found that nitrous oxide produced concentration-

Table 15-6. The Cardiovascular Effects of Supplements During Narcotic Anesthesia

1. Addition of N_2O to most narcotics produces cardiovascular depression.
2. Impairment of blood pressure during N_2O-narcotic anesthesia is usually much less than reduction of cardiac output.
3. Most supplements depress cardiac output when added during narcotic anesthesia.
4. Narcotics are added during potent inhalational anesthesia to decrease the concentration of the inhaled agent and to decrease cardiovascular depression.
5. Combinations of narcotics and inhaled compounds can result in severe cardiovascular depression.

dependent decreases in stroke volume, cardiac output, and arterial blood pressure and increases in systemic vascular resistances (Table 15-7). Impairment of cardiac output was always greater than the reduction in blood pressure because of an increase in peripheral vascular resistance. Heart rate was usually little changed by addition of nitrous oxide. Similar decreases in stroke volume and cardiac output and increases in peripheral vascular resistances have been found with lower doses of morphine,[73] other narcotics,[23, 69, 89] and Innovar[90] when combined with nitrous oxide. Surprisingly, cardiovascular depression during nitrous oxide–narcotic anesthesia appears not to be related to the plasma concentration of narcotic.[89]

When other intravenous supplements are combined with narcotics during anesthesia, cardiovascular depression can result. For example, when a barbiturate has been given for induction of anesthesia (thiamylal, 4 mg/kg intravenously), morphine (1 mg/kg intravenously) reduces cardiac output and stroke volume 30 to 40 percent and decreases arterial blood pressure 16 percent;[12] systemic vascular resistance is increased 35 percent. Similarly, intravenously administered diazepam (5 or 10 mg/70 kg), which has little cardiovascular effect when employed alone, markedly depresses cardiovascular function when given after morphine, fentanyl, and most narcotics.[2, 13] Of the intravenous compounds that have been studied, only scopolamine and droperidol appear *not* to produce significant cardiovascular depression when combined with intravenously administered narcotics.[13, 14]

Morphine, meperidine, and more recently fentanyl have also been combined with potent inhaled anesthetics.[17, 46] These techniques have varied from the addition of narcotics to patients who were primarily anesthetized with potent inhaled anesthetics[17] to the addition of inhaled anesthetics to narcotic-anesthetized patients.[46] These procedures have frequently included numerous other intravenous supplements as well. This approach is based on the unproven premise that narcotics will decrease the MAC and cardiovascular depression of the inhaled anesthetics, resulting in adequate anesthesia without marked cardiovascular depression.[17, 19, 45] However, low to moderate concentrations of halothane given after large doses of morphine produce marked cardiovascular depression.[46] Similar cardiovascular changes occur when fentanyl (200 μg intravenously) is given during enflurane–nitrous oxide anesthesia.[17] However, lower doses of fentanyl (50 to 100 μg) produced little change

Table 15-7. The Cardiovascular Effects of 0 to 50 Percent Nitrous Oxide During Morphine Anesthesia (Means)

Percent N_2O	0	10	20	30	40	50
Stroke volume (ml)	57	51*	50*	46*	42*	36*
Cardiac output (L/min)	5.2	4.6*	4.3*	4.0*	3.7*	2.9*
Systolic arterial blood pressure (torr)	124	119*	117*	109*	104*	94*
Peripheral resistance (PRU)	159	176*	183*	204*	259*	312*

* $P < .05$, Student's paired t-test when compared to control values.
(McDermott R, Stanley TH: The cardiovascular effects of low concentrations of nitrous oxide during anesthesia. Anesthesiology 41:89, 1974.)

Table 15-8. Respiratory Effects of Narcotics

1. Narcotics decrease the responsiveness of CNS respiratory centers to CO_2.
2. Narcotics impair respiratory reflexes and alter rhythmicity.
3. Respiratory rate is decreased before tidal volume.
4. Some narcotics (morphine, meperidine) can cause bronchoconstriction, and others can cause chest wall rigidity (fentanyl).
5. Large doses of narcotics impair ciliary motion.

in cardiovascular dynamics during enflurane–nitrous oxide anesthesia.

Narcotics decrease cerebral blood flow and intracranial pressure.[91–95] Thus, nitrous oxide–narcotic anesthesia with or without supplements is a popular technique for patients with increases in intracranial pressure (see Ch. 33). In dogs, some narcotics can transiently decrease cerebral oxygen consumption, but this decrease is usually less than the corresponding reduction in cerebral blood flow.[91,93,94] Whether narcotic anesthetic techniques should be used in patients with marginal cerebral circulation has not been resolved.

EFFECTS ON RESPIRATION

A summary of the respiratory effects of narcotics is shown in Table 15-8. All narcotics produce a dose-dependent depression of respiration,[96,97] primarily through a direct action on the brain stem respiratory centers. Narcotics markedly reduce the responsiveness of the brain respiratory centers to stimulation from carbon dioxide.[96] This is manifested by an increase in carbon dioxide threshold as well as a shift of the $PaCO_2$-alveolar ventilation response curve to the right[96] (Fig. 15-1). Narcotics also depress and interfere with pontine and medullary respiratory centers involved in respiratory rhythmicity and other respiratory reflexes. The latter effects tend to prolong respiration, increase the respiratory pauses, and delay expiration. Large doses of intravenous narcotics may also result in irregular respiratory rhythms and periodic breathing.

Small intravenous doses of morphine, meperidine, or fentanyl usually decrease respiratory rate without significantly changing tidal volume. Tidal volume may even be increased with therapeutic doses of morphine (10 mg or less intravenously) so that minute ventilation remains unchanged. In spite of normal tidal and minute volumes, $PaCO_2$ is usually elevated. Additional narcotic will decrease both respiratory rate and tidal volume. Anesthetic doses of pure agonist narcotics (as contrasted to agonist-antagonist narcotics) completely terminate involuntary breathing.[3,22] However, these patients may still be responsive to verbal command and may be able to initiate a normal tidal volume if requested to do so.

Morphine and meperidine can cause bronchoconstriction[98] that is probably due to a direct effect of morphine on bronchial smooth muscle and an indirect action of the compound through histamine release. When $PaCO_2$ is kept normal after administration of morphine, pulmonary dead space decreases. When $PaCO_2$ is allowed to rise, pulmonary dead space remains unchanged by morphine.[99] High doses of morphine (and probably many of the other narcotics) decreases bronchial ciliary motion.[100]

Many factors can change both the magnitude and duration of respiratory depression after narcotics (Table 15-9). Patients who are sleeping are usually more sensitive to the respiratory depressant effects of narcotics.[101] This can be of significance when patients who appear to be breathing adequately and sustaining a normal $PaCO_2$ after a narcotic anesthetic are allowed to fall asleep. Often, minute ventilation decreases and $PaCO_2$ increases. Perhaps even small doses of narcotics markedly potentiate the normal right shift of the $PaCO_2$-alveolar ventilation curve that occurs during natural sleep.[102] Another explanation might be that a secondary increase occurs in narcotic plasma concentrations due to sequestration of these compounds in the stomach and then reabsorption into plasma via the alkaline medium of the small intestine.[103,104] This mechanism, which occurs

Table 15-9. Factors which Influence Narcotic Respiratory Actions

1. Sleep
2. Age (higher plasma concentrations)
3. Urine output
4. Pain
5. Other drugs
6. Intestinal reabsorption
7. Diseases

after administration of both fentanyl and meperidine, may produce recurrent respiratory depression in some patients in the recovery room after apparent full recovery, even though additional narcotics had not been given.[104, 105]

Older patients are more sensitive to the respiratory depressant effects of narcotics than younger patients,[101] perhaps because older patients have higher plasma and probably brain narcotic concentrations than younger patients when these compounds are administered on a weight basis.[106] The respiratory depressant effects of narcotics are increased and often prolonged when administered with other CNS depressants, including the potent inhaled anesthetics,[97] alcohol,[101] barbiturates,[101] and most of the intravenous sedatives and hypnotics.

Pain, particularly surgically induced pain, counteracts the respiratory depressant effect of narcotic compounds.[97] Occasionally this pain can lead to postoperative problems in patients anesthetized with narcotics. Usually the sequence of events is as follows: a patient who was breathing adequately following surgery is then taken to the recovery room where it is noticed that respiratory rate is decreased or frank apnea has occurred. Although the main problem may be respiratory obstruction, a painful stimulus usually increases minute ventilation; however, when the stimulus is removed, inadequate respiration usually returns. The two choices of treatment would be (1) endotracheal intubation (if an endotracheal tube is not in place) and mechanical ventilation; or (2) administration of a narcotic antagonist.

Although almost all narcotics are metabo-

lized and little is excreted unchanged in urine (see section on pharmacodynamics), adequacy of renal function (urine output) may influence duration of narcotic activity.[28] After being anesthetized with large doses of morphine for open-heart surgery, patients having higher intraoperative and postoperative urine outputs excrete more morphine in their urine and are able to sustain adequate spontaneous ventilation sooner than are patients with lower urine outputs.[28] It is my clinical impression that patients anesthetized with other narcotics behave similarly.

Narcotic-induced respiratory depression can be antagonized by narcotic antagonists. Naloxone (Narcan) is the only narcotic antagonist currently available that does not have narcotic properties by itself. In my opinion, naloxone should be given only to antagonize a specific narcotic effect. Routine administration of naloxone following anesthesia in which narcotics were a primary component may incur complications, e.g., hypertension; tachycardia; acute, severe pain; and reappearance of narcotic effect some hours later, particularly after the use of large doses of narcotics. This reappearance of the narcotic effect is probably the most serious complication because it occurs reasonably rapidly in patients who minutes before were alert and therefore poorly monitored.

Interest in eliminating the addiction liability and the respiratory depressant effects of narcotics has in recent years led to the development of numerous synthetic compounds that have antagonistic as well as agonistic properties.[107–109] The first of these compounds, pentazocine, has as much respiratory depressant effect as equipotent analgesic doses of morphine.[108] Some of the new agonist-antagonist narcotics (butorphanol) supposedly produce only minimal respiratory depression irrespective of the dose.[109] Whether any of these newer narcotics will ultimately prove to have any significant advantage over the older compounds as intravenous analgesic supplements or anesthetics remains to be seen.

EFFECTS ON THE KIDNEY

The effects of morphine (10 to 30 mg/70 kg) on the kidney have been extensively studied in man and animals.[110,111] Most investigators agree that morphine can have significant antidiuretic properties, which may be due to a release of antidiuretic hormone (ADH).[110] However, in man this morphine-induced release does not occur except in unusual circumstances (i.e., when nausea and vomiting occur) or during surgical stimulation in lightly anesthetized patients.[110,112] Antidiuresis after morphine has, therefore, been related to a decrease in renal dynamics. Glomerular filtration rate decreases after morphine in man suggesting that this is the primary cause of reduced urine flow.[110,111] To compare anesthetics, we found that intraoperative and postoperative urine outputs of 61 patients undergoing similar open-heart operations with high dose morphine versus halothane anesthesia did not differ.[62]

My co-workers and I also studied the effects of morphine, 2 mg/kg intravenously, in volunteers whose ventilation was controlled to keep $PaCO_2$ within normal levels.[151] Morphine was given slowly with intravenous fluids in adequate amounts so that cardiovascular dynamics were unchanged. Under these conditions morphine had no effect on glomerular filtration rate, urine osmolarity, or urine output. However, addition of 60 percent nitrous oxide or a more rapid administration of morphine, so that arterial blood pressure and cardiac output were reduced, markedly diminished all of those tests of renal function. Recent work has confirmed that large doses of morphine and fentanyl probably do not stimulate ADH release in man.[3,11]

On the other hand, in supine, normovolemic, normocapnic dogs, morphine reduces urine output and increases urine osmolarity despite its minimal effects on cardiovascular dynamics.[113] These data suggest that morphine may increase blood levels of ADH in the dog.

In summary, morphine is not an antidiuretic in normovolemic, normocarbic supine man but is in the dog. In the absence of surgery, morphine does not stimulate release of ADH in man. If renal function does change during narcotic anesthesia and surgery, it is probably due to secondary changes in systemic and renal hemodynamics. Also, giving morphine to patients whose bladders are not catheterized may cause a decrease in urine output by an increase in detrusor and urethral shincter tone, resulting in retention of urine in the bladder.

EFFECTS ON THE GASTROINTESTINAL TRACT

Analgesic doses of many narcotics are significant emetics because they directly stimulate the emetic chemoreceptor trigger zone located in the area postrema of the medulla.[114] Another cause of vomiting after morphine is related to its ability to delay passage of gastrointestinal contents.[115] Morphine increases the tone of smooth muscles and tightens various sphincters such as the pyloric sphincter, the ileocecal valves, and Oddi's sphincter at the termination of the biliary tree.[115] Finally, vomiting after morphine can also be caused by an increased volume of secretions in the gastrointestinal tract.[116] That vomiting or nausea usually does not occur during induction of anesthesia with larger doses of narcotics suggests that narcotics may depress CNS emetic zones.

METABOLISM AND STRESS-FREE ANESTHESIA

The concept of stress-free anesthesia has recently been proposed.[117] Some neurolept anesthetic techniques (droperidol plus fentanyl and nitrous oxide), in contrast to most potent inhalational anesthetic techniques and even standard nitrous oxide–narcotic balanced anesthesia, tended to increase less, or not at all, the amount of stress-responding hormones produced during anesthesia and operation.[117] Specifically, stress-free anesthesia prevents increases in circulating catecholamines,[56] plasma glucocorticoids, and antidiuretic hormone.[3–5] Whether altering the stress response to surgery is advantageous or not is debatable.

EFFECTS ON NEUROMUSCULAR TRANSMISSION

In analgesic doses, narcotics have no demonstrable effect on neuromuscular transmission or the neuromuscular blocking drugs usually employed during anesthesia.[101] The influence of large anesthetic doses of narcotics on the neuromuscular junction and neuromuscular transmission has not been studied. Although muscle relaxants may not be required for surgery, they may still be necessary to relieve narcotic-induced muscle rigidity.[118–120] Muscle rigidity, which occurs primarily in the trunk muscles, usually occurs when intravenous narcotics are administered rapidly in high doses. All narcotics can produce rigidity, which may be enhanced by nitrous oxide.[118–120] In severe cases, ventilation may actually be impaired by rigidity of thoracic muscle, which is relieved by administering a depolarizing or nondepolarizing muscle relaxant. Muscle rigidity can also be minimized by a slow intravenous administration of narcotics, especially early in the anesthetic procedure.[3] In my experience, muscle rigidity rarely occurs after induction of anesthesia or during the operative procedure. It may be caused by the central action of narcotic anesthetics, since it is blocked by deep levels of anesthesia.[119]

PHARMACOKINETICS

Pharmacokinetics (Table 15-10) is the quantitative study of the disposition of drugs in the body and includes the processes of absorption, tissue distribution, biotransforma-

Table 15-10. Narcotic Pharmacokinetics

1. Most narcotics rapidly leave the blood stream.
2. Narcotics tend to accumulate in parenchymatous organs (lung, liver, kidney, spleen).
3. Chief metabolites of morphine and meperidine are the glucuronide conjugation products.
4. Only a small portion (< 1 percent) of any narcotic ever enters the brain.
5. Nonionized, nonprotein bound forms of narcotics penetrate into the central nervous system.
6. Very young and older animals and patients appear to require lower doses of narcotics.
7. Accumulation occurs with repeated doses of narcotics.
8. With anesthetic doses of narcotics, urine output appears to influence duration of narcotic action with morphine and perhaps other compounds as well.

tion, and removal of the drugs and their metabolites.

Because narcotics are usually given intravenously in anesthesia, absorption is a less significant factor in anesthesia than when these compounds are administered orally, intramuscularly, or subcutaneously.

DISPOSITION

Tissue uptake and disposition of narcotic compounds are governed by the same principles as apply to any other compound in the plasma. Rate of uptake is determined by delivery (blood flow) of the narcotic to a specific tissue, plasma concentrations of the narcotic at the tissue, and the capacity of the tissue to receive the drug (the mass of the tissue and the tissue plasma partition coefficient). Other important factors also influence the ability of narcotics and all intravenous compounds to penetrate tissues, e.g., the molecular size, ionization, lipid solubility, and protein binding of the compound. Because narcotics are generally small compounds, size is usually a minor factor in tissue permeability.

MORPHINE

When administered intravenously, morphine rapidly disappears from plasma. In man, IV administration of morphine, 10 mg,

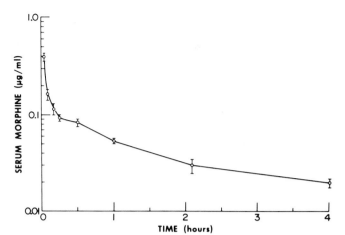

Fig. 15-2. Serum morphine concentrations in patients. Morphine was administered intravenously in a dose of 10 mg/70 kg. Results are the average values obtained from at least four patients per determination ± SE.

results in a serum morphine concentration of 0.5 µg/ml 2 minutes after injection. This concentration decreases to 0.1 and 0.08 µg/ml 5 and 30 minutes, respectively, after injection.[106] Thereafter, serum concentrations decrease much more slowly, reaching 0.06, 0.03, and 0.02 µg/ml 1, 2, and 3 hours, respectively, following administration (Fig. 15-2). From limited studies in man, anesthetic doses of morphine apparently produce only moderately higher blood concentrations than do analgesic doses.[121] Stanski and co-workers[121] found that intravenously administered morphine (1 mg/kg) resulted in initial (shortly after injection) plasma concentrations that varied between 0.85 and 2.5 µg/ml and fell to 0.4 to 0.6 µg/ml following redistribution in 1 hour and to 0.4 to 0.5 µg/ml by 2 hours following injection. The calculated elimination half-life was 137 minutes.

Lower total doses of morphine and fentanyl are required for complete anesthesia in patients having an impaired cardiovascular system.[2,3,22] No data are available to confirm whether this observation could be explained on a pharmacokinetic basis. However, Berkowitz et al.[106] found that patients 51 to 75 years of age averaged 70 percent higher (0.49 versus 0.29 µg/ml) serum morphine concentrations than patients 23 to 50 years of age following administration of 10 mg of morphine intravenously. Although cardiovascular dynamics were not measured in this study, cardiac output usually decreases with age.

Most of the small amount of injected morphine that gains access to the central nervous system appears in gray rather than white matter.[122] In rats, administration of morphine, 50 to 100 mg/kg intravenously, results in a peak brain concentration of only 3 to 26 µg/g of brain tissue.[122] Thus, in man, less than 0.1 percent of intravenously administered morphine probably enters CNS tissue at peak plasma concentrations.[122] The principal reasons for such poor penetration are that morphine is highly ionized (greater than 90 percent at physiological pH), protein bound (approximately 35 percent is bound to plasma proteins), and rapidly metabolized to morphine glucuronide. Since morphine has a pHa of 8.5, alkalinization of blood by administration of sodium bicarbonate should increase the concentration of nonionized morphine in plasma and secondarily increase concentrations in the CNS. Similar maneuvers performed during the postoperative period may impair movement of morphine out of CNS tissues and delay recovery. Recently Finck and co-workers[123] demonstrated that hypercarbia results in higher serum and brain concentrations than occur during normocarbia. One may assume that hypercarbia delays recovery from morphine anesthesia; however, no data exist to confirm this assumption. I

Table 15-11. Comparative Narcotic Potencies

Narcotic	Comparative Potency
Morphine	1
Meperidine	0.1
Fentanyl	150
Sulfentanil	1500
Dilaudid	5
Methadone	1.2
Nisentil	0.25
Heroin	2

believe postoperative recovery following narcotic administration is most rapid when $PaCO_2$ is within normal limits. Age also greatly influences CNS uptake of morphine in animals. Sixteen-day-old rats given intravenous morphine have brain levels of morphine that are approximately three times higher than those of 33-day-old injected animals.[124] Although the reason for this is unknown, perhaps newborn animals require less narcotics than do older animals for analgesia.

In contrast to the CNS tissues, tissues from other organs (particularly the kidney, lung, liver, and spleen, but also skeletal muscle) accumulate morphine rapidly.[124-126] The kidney has the greatest capacity to concentrate morphine.[124-126] Following a subcutaneous dose of morphine (5 mg/kg) in rats and dogs, levels of radioactive morphine in the kidney 60 minutes later are more than three times higher than that expected, assuming uniform distribution of the drug, and approximately 80 times greater than concentrations in the cerebrum. Most of the morphine found in renal tissue is located in the cortex and calices, suggesting highest concentration in those regions rich in glomeruli and tubules. Within the first 90 minutes, morphine found in the kidney and most other organs is both free (unbound to glucuronide) and bound. However, within 4 hours, approximately 75 percent of renal morphine is in the bound form.

In rats, uptake of morphine by the liver is markedly greater than by the brain (20 to 25 times higher) but less than by the kidney.[124-126] Although a more even distribution

of morphine occurs in the liver than in the kidney, areas of high concentration can be found in the portal areas. Free (unbound) morphine can be measured in the liver up to 90 minutes after administration of the compound, but within 4 hours all heptic morphine is in the glucuronide form.

MEPERIDINE

The pharmacokinetics of meperidine appear to be very similar to that of morphine. In human subjects, administration of meperidine, 50 mg intravenously, results in a serum concentration of 52 μg/ml in 1 minute, 24 μg/ml in 5 minutes, and 14 μg/ml in 30 minutes.[127, 128] Thereafter, meperidine serum concentrations decay slowly, reaching 10 μg/ml after 4 hours and 7 μg/ml after 8 hours. As with morphine, blood levels of meperidine

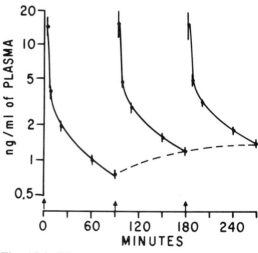

Fig. 15-3. Plasma concentrations of unchanged fentanyl following each of three doses (10μg/kg) administered intravenously at 90-minute intervals. Data points represent the means ± SEM for four dogs. The dotted line connects values for successive 90-minute intervals and indicates accumulation of fentanyl with repeated doses. (Murphy MR, Olson WA, Hug CC: Pharmacokinetics of ^{3}H-fentanyl in the dog anesthetized with enflurane. Anesthesiology 50:13, 1979.)

are directly related to the age of the patient.[127,129] Indeed, Chan et al.[129] reported that meperidine plasma concentrations following IV injection in patients over 70 years of age are about twice as large as those in patients under 30. In addition, more meperidine is bound to plasma proteins in older patients. These observations may partly explain why older persons seem to have greater and longer respiratory depression from meperidine. As with morphine, only a small amount of the administered meperidine passes into CNS tissues.[130,131] Burns et al.[130] demonstrated that 40 minutes after injection the highest concentration of meperidine (13 μg/g of tissue) appeared in the lung, and the lowest in fat. Also, patients with alcoholic cirrhosis have a greater volume of tissue distribution to which meperidine is distributed than nonalcoholic patients have and, as a result, lower plasma meperidine concentrations.[132] This may explain the increased tolerance of alcoholic subjects to meperidine and other narcotics.

FENTANYL

When administered in equipotent doses, fentanyl is more potent and has a shorter time of onset and duration of activity than either morphine or meperidine (Table 15-11). Following the IV administration of 0.1, 0.5, and 1.2 mg/m^2 (approximately 3, 15, and 30 μg/kg) of fentanyl in man, serum concentrations usually range from 30 to 40, 60 to 70, and 200 to 400 ng/ml, respectively, a few minutes after injection; but rapidly fall to approximately 20 percent of peak values in 5 minutes.[133] Thereafter, serum levels of fentanyl fall more slowly (average half-life is 10 to 20 minutes). Two hours after administration, serum fentanyl concentrations continue to decrease, but even more slowly than before (half-life of 1 to 4 hours). Subsequent injections of fentanyl produce higher and higher peak levels of fentanyl and slower serum

decay curves (Fig. 15-3). These findings indicate that fentanyl rapidly accumulates in tissues and is only slowly removed from these depots.[134]

When fentanyl was infused at a rate of 300 μg/min to produce anesthesia in patients with aortic valvular and coronary artery disease,[89] unconsciousness occurred when 18 μg/kg had been given. This dosage yields an average plasma concentration of 34 ng/ml at onset of unconsciousness. Infusion of additional fentanyl at the same rate produces average plasma concentrations of 48 and 54 ng/ml after 50 and 75 μg/kg. Fifteen and 45 minutes after infusion of fentanyl (75 μg/kg), plasma concentrations averaged 38 and 32 ng/ml, respectively. An hour later, plasma fentanyl concentration was still 29 ng/ml, and thereafter decayed slowly.

After a bolus IV injection of fentanyl, 20 μg/kg, in rabbits, brain concentrations reach 30 to 50 ng/g of wet tissue within 30 seconds. Brain concentrations of fentanyl decrease much more slowly than do its plasma concentrations.[135] Fentanyl brain levels are still approximately 50 percent of peak values 40 minutes after injection and only decrease to about 30 percent of peak values after 1 hour. The highest concentration of fentanyl within 30 seconds of an IV bolus injection of 20 μg/kg in rabbits occurred in the lungs, where levels of 1000 ng/g of tissue were measured.[135] Other tissues that concentrate fentanyl include the spleen and kidney (average tissue concentration = 300 to 400 ng/g of tissue after 30 seconds) and the heart (average tissue concentration = 100 to 150 ng/g of tissue after 30 seconds).[132] Decreases from peak concentrations in most of these organs also occur more slowly than do decreases in plasma concentrations. In contrast to the highly vascularized organs, which reach peak tissue levels 30 sec after intravenous administration of fentanyl, less highly perfused organs like skeletal muscle, intestinal wall, and liver reach maximum concentrations of fentanyl 5 minutes after injection. Fat slowly accumulates fentanyl, where the latter reaches maximal concentrations only 30 minutes after injection.

The rapid onset of fentanyl is undoubtedly related to its rapid appearance (within 30 seconds) in the brain. Fentanyl's ability to quickly gain access to most of the highly vascularized organs of the body suggests that perfusion is a dominant factor in its distribution. (In the rabbit, more than 90 percent of intravenously administered fentanyl [20 μg/kg] is gone from plasma within 5 minutes.) Another factor facilitating rapid distribution is the high solubility of fentanyl in lipids.[135] Although fentanyl is highly bound to plasma proteins (70 percent for fentanyl versus 35 percent for morphine), this does not appear to hinder its rapid appearance in CNS and other tissues.[135] One explanation is that almost 100 percent of the fentanyl bound to plasma protein is in a nonionized form that can readily penetrate the blood-brain barrier.

Thirty seconds after injection, approximately 25 percent of the fentanyl administered is in the lungs, and venous-arterial plasma differences are large.[135] Thereafter, these differences decrease, and within 5 to 10 minutes little or no difference exists. The short duration of action of fentanyl appears to be related to redistribution and rapid uptake by tissues other than the brain (particularly the lungs).

NALOXONE VERSUS MORPHINE

Naloxone (Narcan) is the drug of choice for treatment of narcotic overdose and postoperative respiratory depression induced by narcotics. It is a pure antagonist that has no apparent agonistic effects. Unfortunately, naloxone antagonizes the effects of morphine for only about 45 minutes. Ngai et al.[136] provided some interesting answers to this problem. In rats, equal IV doses of naloxone and morphine gave comparable peak serum drug concentrations and approximately the same

serum half-lives. These data do not seem to confirm the shorter duration of action of naloxone. However, naloxone leaves the brain at a much faster rate than does morphine.[136] Thus, a kinetic (brain) reason is probably the basis for this shorter duration of action. These data reinforce the advice that in cases of narcotic overdose or when large doses of narcotics have been given, the patient must be closely observed for possible recurrence of narcotic-induced depression after apparent naloxone-induced reversal.

BIOTRANSFORMATION (METABOLISM) AND EXCRETION

MORPHINE

The major metabolite of morphine is morphine-glucuronide, and the site of conjugation is at the 3-phenolic position.[124, 137, 138] Almost immediately after its intravenous administration, conjugation of morphine begins in the liver.[124, 137] Within 15 minutes of injection of morphine, 10 mg intravenously, Brunk and Delle[137] found high plasma concentrations of conjugated morphine (100 to 150 μg/ml). These concentrations peaked after 30 minutes and slowly declined over the next 24 hours. In human narcotic addicts, 60 to 80 percent of administered morphine is eventually conjugated to morphine 3-glucuronide and almost all of that is excreted in the urine.[138] In nonaddicted normal man, about 50 to 60 percent of intravenously administered morphine is conjugated with glucuronide and excreted in the urine.[124, 135, 139] Conjugated morphine accumulates in all tissues but especially in the kidney and gall bladder, the two organs principally involved in its excretion.[124, 126, 140] The percentage of bound morphine increases with time, especially in the kidney and liver. Six hours after IV administration of morphine, almost all renal and hepatic morphine is in the form of morphine 3-glucuronide. Similar changes probably occur in other organs, although few confirming data exist.

Formation of morphine glucuronide can be inhibited by some monoamine oxidase inhibitors, but not by aspirin or propranolol.[139, 141, 142] Phenobarbital and nalorphine increase the rate of morphine glucuronide formation but decrease the rate at which unconjugated morphine leaves the plasma.[140-144] Thus, some patients on chronic drug therapy may experience prolonged duration of drug activity after receiving standard morphine doses. In nonaddicted adult human subjects who received IV morphine (10 mg), approximately 8 to 10 percent of free morphine was excreted in the liver.[137] After the administration of anesthetic doses (1 to 3 mg/kg intravenously) in man, morphine is rapidly conjugated to morphine 3-glucuronide. During induction of anesthesia, 40 to 80 percent of excreted morphine is in the conjugated form.[28] This increases to 85 to 94 percent during the operative procedure and to greater than 95 percent during the first two postoperative hours. Only 8 to 12 percent of morphine administered in anesthetic doses is excreted in the urine unchanged.

Approximately 5 percent of morphine is n-demethylated, and almost all of this is excreted in the urine as normorphine.[137-142] Small amounts of morphine may be oxidized (dimerized) to form the dimer pseudomorphine, or methylated to form codeine.[124] Evidence that these metabolites are formed in any appreciable amounts in man is lacking.

Only about 5 to 10 percent of free morphine or its metabolites is excreted in feces, the only other significant excretory pathway for the alkaloid.[124, 145] Addicted dogs tolerant to morphine may excrete a greater proportion of morphine (15 to 26 percent), particularly in the conjugated form, in the feces than do nonaddicted dogs.[145] No such data are available for man. As mentioned previously, following anesthetic doses, excretion of morphine in man is directly related to urinary volume. Respiratory depression after morphine anesthesia and operation is probably inversely related to urine output and excretion of morphine. Thus, stimulating diuresis following morphine anesthesia may be an important clinical tool in promoting excretion of morphine and terminating its respiratory depressant effects. Lathrop and I found that patients with low urinary output had plasma concentrations of morphine-glucuronide that were 12 to 16 percent greater than those of patients with high urinary output.[28] Since little or no detectable free morphine was present in the plasma or urine postoperatively when patients were being evaluated postoperatively for adequacy of respiration, perhaps morphine 3-glucuronide has respiratory depressant actions of its own. Although morphine-glucuronide produces no effect on opiate receptors in the guinea-pig ileum,[146] the influence of morphine-glucuronide on respiratory rate, tidal volume, and ventilatory responses to increased inspired tensions of carbon dioxide, or any other determinant of medullary respiratory sensitivity, is not known.

MEPERIDINE

Meperidine is rapidly n-demethylated to normeperidine and hydrolyzed to meperidinic acid.[122, 127, 147] These reactions primarily take place in the liver. N-demethylation of meperidinic acid probably also takes place to reduce normeperidinic acid.[127, 147] All of these metabolites, as well as unaltered meperidine, are rapidly conjugated with glucuronide in the liver; thus, most of the meperidine found in urine is in the conjugated form.[147] Few data exist concerning the concentrations of the metabolites of meperidine within the central nervous system. This is unfortunate, since they may be involved in the total pharmacologic effect of meperidine. Only 2 to 6 percent of unchanged meperidine and 3 to 8 percent of bound or unbound normeperidine is excreted in the urine 48 hours after administration of meperidine.[127] Meperidinic and normeperidinic acid appear in minute amounts in urine; these amounts have not been carefully measured. Careful measurement of the fecal excretion of meperidine and its metabolites has also not been done.

FENTANYL

In rats, at least 80 to 90 percent of fentanyl is metabolized, probably in the liver, to 4-n-(N-propronyl-anilino)-piperidine.[148,149] Oxidative reactions also produce several metabolites in very small amounts.[149] Approximately 40 to 50 percent of administered fentanyl is excreted in the urine regardless of the dose, and about 10 percent of this is excreted as free fentanyl. Higher initial doses result in a greater percentage of free fentanyl in urine.[148] In rats, up to 30 percent of fentanyl in urine appears as free fentanyl following a subcutaneous administration of 3.0 mg/kg. In rats, approximately 40 percent of fentanyl, 320 μg/kg intravenously, is excreted in feces and 40 percent in urine. In the rabbit and rat, the greatest proportion of urinary fentanyl occurs during the first 8 hours after injection, and the greatest fecal concentration occurs in the next 16 hours.[149,150] In man, almost 70 percent of administered fentanyl is excreted in 4 days, the greatest amount appearing 8 to 24 hours after injection.[150] Comparison of rabbits and man suggests that metabolism of fentanyl is faster in rabbits. As mentioned above, early decreases in concentrations of fentanyl in plasma are primarily related to redistribution. After a few hours, however, excretion plays an increasingly important role.

REFERENCES

1. Foldes FF, Swerdlow M, Siker ES: Narcotics and Narcotic Antagonists. Springfield, IL, Charles C Thomas, 1964, pp 3–9
2. Stanley TH, Webster LR: Anesthetic requirements and cardiovascular effects of fentanyl-oxygen and fentanyl-diazepam-oxygen anesthesia in man. Anesth Analg 57:411, 1978
3. Stanley TH, Philbin DM, Coggins CH: Fentanyl-oxygen anesthesia for coronary artery surgery: Cardiovascular and antidiuretic hormone responses. Canad Anaesth Soc J 26:168, 1979
4. Hall GM: Analgesia and the metabolic response to surgery. Proc Roy Soc Med 3:19, 1978
5. Florence A: Attenuation of stress and haemodynamic stability. Proc Roy Soc Med 3:23, 1978
6. Hug CC, Murphy MR: Fentanyl disposition in cerebrospinal fluid and plasma and its relationship to ventilatory depression in the dog. Anesthesiology 50:342, 1979
7. Van Hoosen B: Scopolamine-Morphine Anaesthesia. Chicago, House of Manz, 1915
8. Smith RR: Scopolamine-morphine anesthesia, with report of two hundred and twenty-nine cases. Surg Gynecol Obstet 7:414, 1908
9. Sexton JC: Death following scopolamine-morphine injection. Lancet-Clinic 55:582, 1905
10. Neff W, Mayer EC, de la Luz Perales M: Nitrous oxide and oxygen anesthesia with curare relaxation. Calif Med 66:67, 1947
11. Holderness MC, Chase PE, Dripps RD: Use of a narcotic analgesic and a butyrophenone with nitrous oxide for general anesthesia. Anesthesiology 24:336, 1963
12. Stoelting RK: Influence of barbiturate anesthetic induction on circulatory responses to morphine. Anesth Analg 56:615, 1977
13. Stanley TH, Bennett GM, Loeser EA, et al: Cardiovascular effects of diazepam and droperidol during morphine anesthesia. Anesthesiology 44:255, 1976
14. Bennett GM, Loeser EA, Stanley TH: Cardiovascular effects of scopolamine during morphine-oxygen and morphine-nitrous oxide-oxygen anesthesia in man. Anesthesiology 46:225, 1977
15. Mannheimer WH: The use of morphine and intravenous alcohol in the anesthetic management of open heart surgery. South Med J 64:1125, 1971
16. Stanley TH: Blood pressure and pulse rate responses to ketamine during general anesthesia. Anesthesiology 39:648, 1973

17. Bennett GM, Stanley TH: Cardiovascular effects of fentanyl during enflurane anesthesia in man. Anesth Analg 58:179, 1979
18. De Castro J: Analgesic anesthesia based on the use of fentanyl in high doses. Anesthesia Vigile et Subvigile 1:87, 1970
19. Lowenstein E, Hallowell P, Levine FH, et al: Cardiovascular response to large doses of intravenous morphine in man. N Engl J Med 281:1389, 1969
20. Stoelting RK, Gibbs PS: Hemodynamic effects of morphine and morphine-nitrous oxide in valvular heart disease and coronary artery disease. Anesthesiology 38:42, 1973
21. Arens JF, Benbow BP, Ochsner JL: Morphine anesthesia for aorto-coronary bypass procedures. Anesth Analg 51:901, 1972
22. Stanley TH, Gray NH, Stamford W, et al: The effects of high-dose morphine on fluid and blood requirements in open-heart procedures. Anesthesiology 38:536, 1973
23. Stoelting RK, Gibbs PS, Creasser CW, et al: Hemodynamic and ventilatory responses to fentanyl, fentanyl-droperidol, and nitrous oxide in patients with acquired valvular heart disease. Anesthesiology 42:319, 1975
24. Lowenstein E: Morphine "anesthesia"—A Perspective. Anesthesiology 35:563, 1971
25. Hug CC: Pharmacology—anesthetic drugs, Cardiac Anesthesia. Edited by Kaplan JA. New York, Grune & Stratton, 1979, pp 3–37
26. Thompson WL, Walton RP: The elevation of plasma histamine levels on dogs following administration of muscle relaxants, opiates and macromolecular polymers. J Pharmacol Exp Ther 143:131, 1964
27. Bedford RF, Wollman H: Postoperative respiratory effects of morphine and halothane anesthesia: A study in patients undergoing cardiac surgery. Anesthesiology 43:1, 1975
28. Stanley TH, Lathrop GD: Urinary excretion of morphine during and after valvular and coronary-artery surgery. Anesthesiology 46:166, 1977
29. Snyder SH: Opiate receptors and internal opiates. Sci Am 236:44, 1977
30. Beckett AH, Casey AF: Synthetic analgesics, stereochemical considerations. J Pharm Pharmacol 6:986, 1954
31. Beckett AH: Analgesics and their antagonists: Some steric and chemical considerations. Part I. The dissociation constants of some tertiary amines and synthetic analgesics, the conformations of methadone-type compounds. J Pharm Pharmacol 8:848, 1956
32. Goldstein A: Opiate receptors. Life Sci 14:615, 1974
33. Pert CB, Kuhar MJ, Snyder SH: Opiate receptor autoradiographic localization in rat brain. Proc Natl Acad Sci USA 73:3729, 1976
34. Synder SH: Opiate receptors in the brain. New Engl J Med 296:266, 1977
35. Mayer DJ, Wolfe TL, Akil H, et al: Analgesia from electrical stimulation in the brainstem of the rat. Science 174:1351, 1971
36. Satoh M, Takagi H: Enhancement by morphine of the central descending inhibitory influence on spinal sensory transmission. Eur J Pharmacol 14:60, 1971
37. Yaksh TL, Rudy TA: Studies on the direct spinal action of narcotics in the production of anesthesia in the rat. J Pharmacol Exp Ther 202:411, 1977
38. Yaksh TL, Frederickson RCA, Huang SP, et al: In vivo comparison of the receptor populations acted upon in the spinal cord by morphine and pentopeptides in the production of analgesia. Brain Res 148:516, 1978
39. Hughes J, Smith TW, Kosterlitz HW, et al: Identification of two related pentapeptides from the brain with potent opiate agonist activity. Nature 258:577, 1975
40. Frederickson RCA: Enkephalin pentapeptides—A review of current evidence for a physiological role in vertebrate neurotransmission. Life Sci 21:23, 1977
41. Goldstein AL: Opioid peptides (endorphins) in pituitary and brain. Science 193:1081, 1976
42. Guillemin R: Endorphins, brain peptides that act like opiates. New Engl J Med 296:226, 1977
43. Stanley TH, Liu WS, Lathrop GD: The effects of morphine and halothane anaesthesia on urine norepinephrine during surgery for congenital heart disease. Canad Anaesth Soc J 23:58, 1976
44. Fraioli RL, Sheffer LA, Steffenson JL: The MAC equivalent of morphine, Abstracts of Scientific Papers. 1973 ASA Meeting, pp 253, 254
45. Eger EI II: Anesthetic Uptake and Action, Baltimore, Williams and Wilkins, 1974
46. Stoelting RK, Creasser CE, Gibbs PS, et al: Circulatory effects of halothane added to

morphine anesthesia in patients with coronary artery disease. Anesth Analg 53:449, 1974

47. Loeser EA: Unpublished data

48. Bidwai AV: Unpublished data

49. Van De Walle J, Lauwers P, Adriaensen H: Double blind comparison of fentanyl and sufentanil in anesthesia. Acta Anaesth Belg 27:129, 1976

50. Schmidt CF, Livingston AE: The action of morphine on the mammalian circulation. J Pharmacol Ex Ther 47:411, 1933

51. Vasco JS, Henney RP, Brawley RK, et al: Effects of morphine on ventricular function and myocardial contractile force. Am J Physiol 210:329, 1966

52. Stanley TH, Isern-Amaral J, Lathrop GD: The effects of morphine anesthesia on urine norepinephrine during and after coronary artery surgery. Can Anaesth Soc J 22:478, 1975

53. Stanley TH, Isern-Amaral J, Lathrop GD: Urine norepinephrine excretion in patients undergoing mitral or aortic valve replacement with morphine anesthesia. Anesth Analg 54:509, 1975

54. Balasaroswathi K, Glisson SN, El-Etr A, et al: Serum epinephrine and norepinephrine during valve replacement and aorto-coronary bypass. Canad Anaesth Soc J 25:198, 1978

55. Liu WS, Bidwai AV, Lunn JK, et al: Urine catecholamine excretion after large doses of fentanyl, diazepam and pancuronium. Canad Anaesth Soc J 24:371, 1977

56. Stanley TH, Berman L, Green O, et al: Fentanyl-oxygen anesthesia for coronary artery surgery: Plasma catecholamine and cortisol responses. Anesthesiology, 51:S139, 1979

57. Drew JH, Dripps RD, Conroe JH: Clinical studies on morphine II. Effects of morphine upon the circulation of man and upon the circulatory and respiratory responses to tilting. Anesthesiology 7:44, 1946

58. Henney RP, Vasko JS, Brawley RK, et al: The effects of morphine on the resistance and capacitance vessels of the peripheral circulation. Am Heart J 72:242, 1966

59. Ward JM, McGrath RL, Well JV: Effect of morphine on the peripheral vascular response to sympathetic stimulation. Am J Cardiol 29:659, 1972

60. Zelis R, Mansour EJ, Capone RJ, et al: The cardiovascular effects of morphine: The peripheral capacitance and resistance vessels in human subjects. J Clin Invest 54:1247, 1974

61. Zelis R, Flaim SF, Eisele JH: Effects of morphine on reflex arteriolar constriction induced in man by hypercapnia. Clin Pharmacol Ther 22:172, 1977

62. Stanley TH, Gray NH, Isern-Amaral JH, et al: Comparison of blood requirements during morphine and halothane anesthesia for open-heart surgery. Anesthesiology 41:34, 1974

63. Bedford F, Casey EJ: Unpublished data

64. Wong KC, Martin WE, Hornbein TF, et al: The cardiovascular effects of morphine sulfate with oxygen and with nitrous oxide in man. Anesthesiology 38:542, 1973

65. Thompson WL, Watton RP: The elevation of plasma histamine levels in dogs following administration of muscle relaxants, opiates and macromolecular polymers. J Pharmacol Exp Ther 143:131, 1964

66. Freye E: Cardiovascular effects of high doses of fentanyl, meperidine and naloxone in dogs. Anesth Analg 53:40, 1974

67. Strauer BE: Contractile responses to morphine, peritramide, meperidine and fentanyl: A comparative study of effects on isolated ventricular myocardium. Anesthesiology 37:304, 1972

68. Rees HA, Muir AL, MacDonald HR, et al: Circulatory effects of pethidine in patients with acute myocardial infarction. Lancet 2:863, 1967

69. Stanley TH, Liu WS: Cardiovascular effects of meperidine-N_2O anesthesia before and after pancuronium. Anesth Analg 56:669, 1977

70. King BD, Elder JD, Dripps RD: The effect of the intravenous administration of meperidine upon the circulation of man and upon the circulatory response to tilt. Surg Gynecol Obstet 94:591, 1952

71. Reddy P, Liu WS, Stanley TH, et al: Hemodynamic effects of anesthetic doses of alphaprodine and sufentanil in dogs. Anesthesiology 51:S102, 1979

72. Liu WS, Bidwai AV, Stanley TH, et al: The cardiovascular effects of diazepam and of diazepam and pancuronium during fentanyl and oxygen anesthesia. Canad Anaesth Soc J 23:395, 1976

73. Bennett GM, Stanley TH: Comparison of the cardiovascular effects of morphine-N_2O and fentanyl-N_2O balanced anesthesia in man. Anesthesiology 51:S102, 1979

74. Estafanous FG, Tarazi RC, Buckley S, et al: Arterial hypertension in immediate postoper-

ative period after valve replacement. Br Heart J 40:718, 1970

75. Bailey DR, Miller ED, Kaplan JA, et al: The renin-angiotensin-aldosterone system during cardiac surgery with morphine-nitrous oxide anesthesia. Anesthesiology 42:538, 1975

76. Lappas DG, Geha D, Fischer JE, et al: Filling pressures of the heart and pulmonary circulation of the patient with coronary artery disease after large intravenous doses of morphine. Anesthesiology 42:153, 1975

77. Stanley TH: Unpublished data

78. Liu WS, Bidwai AV, Stanley TH, et al: Cardiovascular dynamics after large doses of fentanyl and fentanyl plus N_2O in the dog. Anesth Analg 55:168, 1972

79. Robbins BH, Fitzhugh OG, Baxter JH Jr: The action of morphine in slowing the pulse. J Pharmacol Exp Ther 66:216, 1939

80. Kennedy BL, West TC: Effects of morphine on electrically-induced release of autonomic mediators in the rabbit sinoatrial mode. J Pharmacol Exp Ther 157:149, 1967

81. Eyster JAE, Meek WJ: Cardiac irregularities in morphine poisoning in the dog. Heart 4:542, 1952

82. Puerto BA, Wong KC, Puerto AX, et al: Epinephrine-induced dysrhythmias: Comparison during anesthesia with narcotics and with halogenated agents in dogs. Canad Anaesth Soc J 26:263, 1979

83. Roy SB, Singh I, Bhatia MH, et al: Effects of morphine on pulmonary blood volume in convalescents from high altitude pulmonary edema. Br Heart J 27:876, 1965

84. Hug C: Unpublished data

85. Goldberg AH, Sohn YZ, Phear WPC: Direct myocardial effects of nitrous oxide. Anesthesiology 43:61, 1975

86. Craythorne NWB, Darby TD: The cardiovascular effects of nitrous oxide in the dog. Br J Anaesth 37:560, 1965

87. McDermott R, Stanley TH: The cardiovascular effects of low concentrations of nitrous oxide during anesthesia. Anesthesiology 41:89, 1974

88. Lappas DG, Buckley MJ, Laver MB, et al: Left ventricular performance and pulmonary circulation following addition of nitrous oxide to morphine during coronary-artery surgery. Anesthesiology 43:61, 1975

89. Lunn JK, Stanley TH, Eisele J, et al: High dose fentanyl anesthesia for coronary artery surgery: Plasma fentanyl concentrations and influence of N_2O on cardiovascular responses. Anesth Analg 58:390, 1979

90. Dobkin AB, Pielock PA, Israel JS, et al: Circulatory and metabolic effects of Innovar-fentanyl-nitrous oxide anesthesia for major abdominal surgery in man. Anesth Analg 49:261, 1970

91. Michenfelder JD, Theye RA: Effects of fentanyl, droperidol and innovar on canine cerebral metabolism and blood flow. Br J Anaesth 43:630, 1971

92. Fitch W, Barker J, Jennett WB, et al: The influence of neuroleptanalgesic drugs on cerebral spinal fluid pressure. Br J Anaesth 41:800, 1969

93. Takeshita H, Michenfelder JD, Theye RA: The effects of morphine and N-allynormorphine on canine cerebral metabolism and circulation. Anesthesiology 37:605, 1972

94. Miller JD, Barker J: The effect of neuroleptic analgesic drugs on cerebral blood flow and metabolism. Br J Anaesth 41:554, 1969

95. Larson CP, Mazze RI, Cooperman LH, et al: Effects of anesthetics on cerebral, renal and splanchnic circulations: recent developments. Anesthesiology 41:169, 1974

96. Bellville JW, Seed JC: The effects of drugs on the respiratory response to carbon dioxide. Anesthesiology 21:727, 1960

97. Eckenhoff JE, Oechs R: The effects of narcotics and antagonists upon respiration and circulation in man. Clin Pharmacol Ther 1:483, 1960

98. Adriani J, Rovenstein EA: The effect of anesthetic drugs upon bronchi and bronchioles of excised lung tissue. Anesthesiology 4:253, 1943

99. Cooper DY, Lambertsen CJ: Effect of changes in tidal volume and alveolar carbon dioxide tension on physiological dead space. Anesthesiology 18:160, 1957

100. Van Dongen K, Leusing H: The action of opium-alkaloids and expectorants on the ciliary movements in the air passages. Arch Int Pharmacodyn 93:261, 1953

101. Foldes FF, Swerdlow M, Siker SS: Narcotics and Narcotic Antagonists. Springfield, IL, Charles C Thomas, 1964, pp 55, 56

102. Reed DJ, Kellog RH: Changes in respiratory response to CO_2 during natural sleep at sea level and at altitude. J Appl Physiol 13:325, 1958

103. Stoeckel H, Hengstmann JH, Schutter J: Pharmacokinetics of fentanyl as a possible explanation for recurrence of respiratory depression. Br J Anaesth 51:741, 1979

104. Trudnowski RJ, Gessner T: Gastric sequestration of meperidine following intravenous administration. Abstracts of Scientific Papers. 1975 ASA Meeting, pp 327–328

105. Becker LD, Paulson BA, Miller RD, et al: Biphasic respiratory depression after fentanyl-droperidol or fentanyl alone used to supplement nitrous oxide anesthesia. Anesthesiology 44:291, 1976

106. Berkowitz BA, Ngai SH, Yang JC, et al: The disposition of morphine in surgical patients. Clin Pharmacol Ther 17:629, 1975

107. Cass LJ, Frederick WS, Teodoro JV: Pentazocine as an analgesic. JAMA 188:112, 1964

108. Bellville JW: Pentazocine vs morphine. JAMA 189:332, 1964

109. Nagashima H, Karamanian A, Malovany R, et al: Respiratory and circulatory effects of intravenous butorphanol and morphine. Clin Pharmacol Ther 19:738, 1976

110. Papper S, Papper EM: The effects of pre-anesthetic, anesthetic and post-operative drugs on renal function. Clin Pharmacol Ther 5:205, 1964

111. Deutch S, Bastron RD, Pierce EC, et al: The effects of anesthesia with thiopentone, nitrous oxide, narcotics and neuromuscular blocking drugs on renal function in normal man. Br J Anaes 41:807, 1969

112. Philbin DM, Wilson NE, Sokoloshi I, et al: Radioimmunoassay of antidiuretic hormone during morphine anaesthesia. Canad Anaesth Soc J 23:290, 1976

113. Bidwai AV, Stanley TH, Bloomer HA: Effects of anesthetic doses of morphine on renal function in the dog. Anesth Analg 54:357, 1975

114. Wang SC, Glaviano VV: Locus of emetic action of morphine and hydregine in dogs. J Pharmacol Exp Ther 111:329, 1954

115. Chapman WP, Rowlands EN, Jones CM: Multi-balloon kymographic recording of the comparative action of demerol, morphine and placebo on the motility of the upper small intestine in man. N Engl J Med 243:171, 1950

116. Reynolds AK, Randall LO: Morphine and Allied Drugs. University of Toronto Press, Toronto, 1957

117. Reneman RS: Recent Experience with Fentanyl in Stress-Free Anesthesia. New York, Grune & Stratton, 1978

118. Freund FG, Martin WE, Wong KC, et al: Abdominal muscle rigidity induced by morphine and nitrous oxide. Anesthesiology 38:358, 1973

119. Gergis SD, Hoyt JL, Sokoll MD: Effects of Innovar and Innovar plus nitrous oxide on muscle tone and H-reflex. Anesth Analg 50:743, 1971

120. Sokoll MD, Hout JL, Gergis SD: Studies in muscle rigidity, nitrous oxide, and narcotic analgesic agents. Anesth Analg 51:16, 1972

121. Stanski DR, Greenblatt DJ, Lappas DG, et al: Kinetics of high dose intravenous morphine in cardiac surgery patients. Clin Pharmacol Ther 19:752, 1977

122. Mule SJ: Physiological dispositions of narcotic agonists and antagonists, Narcotic Drugs: Biochemical Pharmacology. Edited by Clouet DH. New York, Plenum Press, 1971,

123. Finck AD, Berkowitz BA, Hempstead J, et al: Pharmacokinetics of morphine: Effects of hypercarbia on serum and brain morphine concentrations in the dog. Anesthesiology 47:407, 1977

124. Way EL, Adler TK: The biological disposition of morphine and its surrogates. 1. Bull WHO 25:227, 1961

125. Wolff WA, Riegel C, Fry EG: The excretion of morphine by normal and tolerant dogs. J Pharmacol Exp Ther 47:391, 1933

126. Plant OH, Pierce IH: Studies of chronic morphine poisoning in dogs. V: Recovery of morphine from the tissues of tolerant and non-tolerant animals. J Pharmacol Exp Ther 58:437, 1936

127. Stambaugh JE, Warner IW, Sanstead JK, et al: The clinical pharmacology of meperidine—comparison of routes of administration. J Clin Pharmacol 16:245, 1976

128. Mather LE, Tucker GT, Pflug AE, et al: Meperidine kinetics in man: Intravenous injection in surgical patients and volunteers. Clin Pharmacol Ther 17:21, 1975

129. Chan K, Vaughan DP, Mitchard M: Plasma concentrations and urinary excretion of pethidine and metabolites, Abstracts of the Symposium on the Assessment of Drug Metabolism in Man—Methods and Clinical Applications. University of Dundee, 1974

130. Burns JJ, Bergen BL, Lief PA, et al: The physiological disposition and fate of meperidine (Demerol) in man and a method for its estimation in plasma. J Pharmacol Exp Ther 114:289, 1955

131. Plotkinoff NP, Elliot HW, Way EL: The metabolism of $N-C^{14}-H_3$ labeled meperidine. J Pharmacol Exp Ther 104:377, 1952

132. Koltz U, McHorse TS, Wilkinson GR, et al: The effects of cirrhosis on the disposition and elimination of meperidine in man. Clin Pharmacol Ther 16:667, 1974

133. Schleimer R, Benjamini E, Eisele H, et al: Pharmacokinetics of fentanyl as determined by radioimmunoassay. Clin Pharmacol Ther 23:188, 1978

134. Murphy MR, Olson WA, Hug CC: Pharmacokinetics of ^{3}H-fentanyl in the dog anesthetized with enflurane. Anesthesiology 50:13, 1979

135. Hess R, Herz A, Friedel K: Pharmacokinetics of fentanyl in rabbits in view of the importance of limiting the effect. J Pharmacol Exp Ther 179:474, 1971

136. Ngai SH, Berkowitz BA, Yan JC, et al: Pharmacokinetics of naloxone in rats and in man. Anesthesiology 44:398, 1976

137. Brunk SF, Delle M: Morphine metabolism in man. Clin Pharmacol Ther 16:51, 1974

138. Yeh SY: Urinary excretion of morphine and its metabolites in morphine-dependent subjects. J Pharmacol Exp Ther 192:201, 1975

139. Brunk SF, Dell M, Wilson WR: Morphine metabolism in man: Effect of aspirin. Clin Pharmacol Ther 15:283, 1974

140. Woods LA: Distribution and fate of morphine in non-tolerant and tolerant dogs and rats. J Pharmacol 112:156, 1954

141. Yeh SY, Mitchell CL: Effect of monoamine oxidase inhibitors on formation of morphine glucuronide. Biochem Pharm 21:571, 1972

142. Brunk SF, Dell M, Wilson WR: Effect of propranolol on morphine metabolism. Clin Pharmacol Ther 16:1038, 1974

143. Roerig DL, Hasegawa AT, Peterson RE, et al: Effect of chloroquine and phenobarbital on morphine glucuronidation and biliary excretion in the rat. Biochem Pharm 23:1331, 1974

144. Tampier L, Sanchez E, Mardones J: Effects of nalorphine on the in vitro morphine metabolism and on the p-nitrophenol conjugation in rat liver. Arch Int Pharmacodyn 188:290, 1970

145. Cochin J, Haggart J, Woods LA, et al: Plasma levels, urinary and fecal excretion of morphine in non-tolerant and tolerant dogs. J Pharmacol Exp Ther 111:74, 1954

146. Schulz R, Goldstein A: Inactivity of narcotic glucuronides as analgesics and on guinea-pig ileum. J Pharmacol Exp Ther 83:404, 1972

147. Way EL, Adler TK: The pharmacologic implications of the fate of morphine and its surrogates. Pharmacol Rev 12:382, 1960

148. Van Wijngaarden I, Soudijn W: The metabolism and excretion of the analgesic fentanyl (R 4263) by Wistar rats. Life Sci 7:1239, 1968

149. Maruyama Y, Hosoya E: Studies on the fate of fentanyl. Keio J Med 18:59, 1969

150. Hess R, Stiebler G, Herz A: Pharmacokinetics of fentanyl in man and the rabbit. Eur J Clin Pharmacol 4:137, 1972

151. Stanley TH, Gray NH, Bidwai AV, et al: The effects of high dose morphine and morphine plus nitrons oxide on urinary output in man. Can Anaesth Soc J 21:379, 1974

16

Pharmacology of Intravenous Non-Narcotic Anesthetics

Theodore H. Stanley, M.D.

INTRODUCTION

In contrast to anesthetic practice in Western Europe and in many other areas of the world, the use of intravenous, non-narcotic anesthesia in the United States is limited. One reason for this is the number of animal and human studies required by law and the consequent expense of getting a new drug (anesthetic) released in this country. Another, and perhaps more important, reason is the absence of new, *non-narcotic, intravenous anesthetics*. For, with the exception of ketamine and perhaps intravenous procaine, there are few *non-narcotic, intravenous anesthetics* available, only hypnotics, sedatives, and tranquilizers. Therefore, when one refers to intravenous anesthesia, one usually refers to the use of one or more hypnotics, sedatives, or tranquilizers in combination with a narcotic analgesic and with or without the addition of nitrous oxide. In the sense that most intravenous, non-narcotic anesthetics have little or no analgesic activity, this chapter discusses the pharmacology of a variety of compounds that are currently being used or are in the process of being developed as anesthetic induction agents or supplements.

THE BARBITURATES

The barbiturates were first synthesized in the late 19th century and introduced into medicine as hypnotics.[1] The parent molecule barbituric acid is a convulsant.[2] However, substitution on three key parts of the parent molecule (one or more organic radicals on carbon 5, an alkyl radical for the hydrogen atom attached to nitrogen 1, and a sulphur atom for the oxygen atom connected to carbon 2) results in compounds with a wide variety of actions.[2-5]

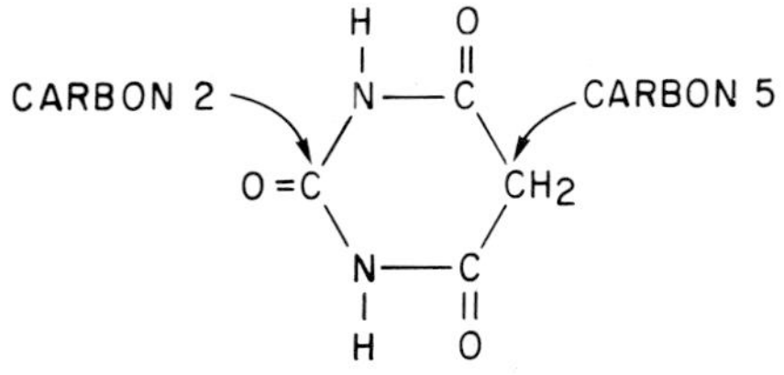

BARBITURIC ACID

Potency can be altered by many changes in the parent molecule; however, the most dynamic effects occur when the number of carbon atoms in the substituting group, or groups, on carbon 5 is increased (from 1 to 8

451

carbons) and further increased when these groups are branched or contain unsaturated carbon bonds. As potency increases so does toxicity and with substituting groups containing beyond seven or eight carbons, toxicity becomes very prominent.[2–5]

Substitution of certain groups on particular atoms of the parent compound produces effects that are radically different from each other. Therefore, while direct substitution with a phenyl group on carbon 5 results in an anticonvulsant, the presence of an alkyl group that contains an aromatic nucleus produces a convulsant compound. The two most important atoms with respect to the use of barbiturates in anesthesia are nitrogen 1 and carbon 2. Addition of a methyl group to nitrogen 1 results in a compound that is of short duration. Duration is also shortened by substitution of the oxygen attached to carbon 2 with sulphur (thiobarbiturate).

PHARMACOLOGIC ACTIONS

For matters of classification, the barbiturates are divided into four classes according to their duration of activity: long-acting, medium-acting, short-acting, and ultra-short-acting.[2] However, this classification is often altered depending on the route of administration (oral versus intravenous), dose, use of other compounds, and the species. Although only the ultra-short-acting barbiturates are commonly used in modern clinical anesthesia, all the nonconvulsive barbiturates depress the central nervous system. Their action is principally on the cerebral cortex and the reticular activating system but they also affect the cerebellar and vestibular systems and in high doses, the medullary, respiratory, and circulatory centers.[6–8] While the mechanisms by which they produce sedation and eventually unconsciousness is unknown, the barbiturates are said to "stabilize cerebral cellular membranes" and "elevate excitatory thresholds." Perhaps this occurs via their ability to inhibit oxidative phosphorylation.

Barbiturates do depress the oxidative uptake of phosphate and thus interfere with ATP foundation.[9, 10] They also inhibit the synthesis of acetylcholine and glutamine (probably via depression of ATP production).[11, 12] However, exactly how these changes result in hypnosis and eventually anesthesia is unknown.

HYPNOSIS, ANALGESIA, AND ANESTHESIA

Barbiturates produce hypnosis (sedation) with amnesia.[13] Larger doses generally produce greater effects until unconsciousness (anesthesia) occurs. When progressive deepening of hypnosis leads to unconsciousness, an excitatory period rarely intervenes.[13] In doses that are less than anesthetic, barbiturates do not produce analgesia,[14, 15] but, in fact, result in an increased sensitivity to somatic pain (antianalgesia).[16] Even in doses that produce light levels of anesthesia, barbiturates do not produce analgesia. With deeper anesthesia, analgesia, nonresponsiveness to surgical stimulation, does occur but at the expense of profound depression of the cardiovascular, respiratory, and renal organ systems. In addition, large, anesthetic doses of almost all barbiturates (including the ultra-short-acting compounds) produce prolonged periods of anesthesia and a long recovery period if used alone for surgical procedures lasting longer than 20 minutes.[8]

METABOLISM

Most barbiturates decrease total body and cerebral oxygen consumption.[8, 17, 18] Decreases in cerebral oxygen consumption occur without changes in blood glucose levels and appear to be greater than corresponding decreases in cerebral blood flow.[19] Such changes in cerebral metabolism may be protective to the poorly perfused or unperfused brain. This is discussed in further detail in Chapter 25. Barbiturates also result in vaso-dilation in skin and muscle vessels and via this mechanism cause an increase in skin blood flow and a decrease in body temperature.[20]

Absorption of most of the barbiturates can occur with oral or rectal administration (via the gastrointestinal tract), or intramuscular, subcutaneous, or intravenous injection.[8,21] Unfortunately, many intravenous solutions of the ultra-short-acting barbiturates can produce marked irritation and tissue necrosis when accidentally administered extravascularly.[8,21] This occurs becauses the solutions are alkaline (pH of sodium thiopental is 10.6 to 10.8).

ULTRA-SHORT-ACTING BARBITURATES—THIOPENTAL

In 1935 the work of Tabern and Volwiler[22] demonstrated that substitution of sulphur for oxygen at carbon 2 on the parent barbiturate compound significantly shortened the duration of barbiturate-induced narcosis. At the same time, Lundy[23] began clinical trials with the sulphur analogue of pentobarbital called thiopental (sodium ethyl [1-methyl butyl] thiobarbiturate). Thiopental (Pentothal) is a yellow powder with a bitter taste and slightly sulphurous smell.[8] It is a weak acid and is relatively insoluble in water or alcohol. The sodium salt of thiopental, made by adding 6 percent by weight sodium carbonate, is alkaline (pH 10.6 to 10.8), very soluble in water, and bacteriostatic.

SODIUM THIOPENTAL

PHARMACOKINETICS

Uptake, Redistribution, and Metabolism

Following intravenous administration, thiopental crosses the blood brain barrier and, if given in a sufficient dose, produces hypnosis in one circulation time.[2,5,8,23] Similar effects occur with other ultra-short-acting barbiturates, such as thiamylal and methohexital. With all these compounds, plasma to brain equilibrium occurs rapidly (in approximately 1 minute) because of high lipid solubility and lack of ionization and in spite of a high percentage of protein binding (65 to 75 percent).[5,8,24,25] Thiopental and the other ultra-short-acting barbiturates also rapidly diffuse into other highly vascularized tissues, such as the kidney, heart, and gastrointestinal tract.[24,25]

Thiopental rapidly diffuses out of the brain and other highly vascularized tissues and is redistributed to muscle, fat, and eventually all body tissues.[5,8,24–27] Redistribution to poorly vascularized tissues (fat) is a slow process taking minutes to hours but removal from brain usually occurs rapidly with brain levels down to half of peak levels after 5 minutes and to 10 percent of peak levels at 30 minutes.[28] It is because of this rapid removal from brain tissue that a single dose of thiopental is so short lasting.[24,25,28] The depth of anesthesia produced by thiopental depends upon its concentration in blood and brain tissue. However, the relationship is complex. When the initial dose is large, the brain concentration will be high as will the depth of anesthesia. However, the brain concentration when awaking occurs will be higher when a larger dose of thiopental had been given as compared to when a smaller dose had been given.[29] This phenomena is called acute tolerance and is important because higher subsequent doses are required for supplementation.

Metabolism following thiopental administration occurs much slower than redistribution and takes place primarily in the liver.[24, 26, 30] Less than 1 percent of an administered dose of thiopental is removed unmetabolized from the body via the kidney. Thiopental is metabolized at the rate of 16 to 24 percent an hour in man following a single dose.[30] The principal sites of metabolism are probably the substituents on carbon 5 (oxidation), carbon 2 (desulphurization), and the barbiturate ring (hydrolytic opening of the ring). A small amount of thiopental may also be metabolized in the kidney and brain. Significant depression of thiopental metabolism occurs in liver disease but this probably produces little clinical effect following a single injection of the compound.[5, 30] On the other hand, with prolonged administration of much larger doses of the drug, liver disease can greatly increase the duration of thiopental depression.[5] This occurs because redistribution occurs much more slowly, due to the fact that muscle and even fat stores have accumulated thiopental and therefore take it up slower. As a result, plasma and brain concentrations remain high and continue to do so until hepatic metabolism can remove a large percentage of the compound.

Circulatory Actions

In isolated mammalian hearts probably all barbiturates produce direct myocardial depression.[31-33] This occurs even at doses that do not change arterial blood pressure or result in apnea and is a dose-related phenomena, i.e., greater doses produce more myocardial depression. Thiopental produces little change or an increase in total peripheral resistance[34-36] but markedly increases venous vessel compliance with resultant venous pooling of blood and impaired venous return to the heart.[36, 37] Venous effects of thiopental are partly due to the actions of the drug on the central sympathetic apparatus in the medulla, as these effects appear to be much less evident or nonexistent after thiopental administration in sympathectomized animals.[38]

Thiopental results in dose-dependent decreases in arterial blood pressure, stroke volume, and cardiac output in unstimulated animals and man. Reductions in output vary from 10 to 25 percent with moderate doses of the compound (3 to 5 mg/kg) to 50 percent with larger doses (9 mg/kg).[20] Reflex tachycardia and, on occasion, compensatory increases in peripheral arterial resistance both before but especially after stimulation (e.g., tracheal intubation and surgical incision) may minimize decreases in cardiac output and blood pressure.[20, 39] Hypertensive and hypovolemic patients are more liable to sustain marked decreases in arterial blood pressure and cardiac output than normovolemic subjects. Similarly, rapid injections of thiopental produce much more marked derangements in cardiovascular dynamics than slower injections.[36] Indeed, injections of the compound at 50 mg/min in adults are often associated with no change in arterial blood pressure.[36, 40, 41]

Thiopental increases coronary artery blood flow but also increases heart rate and myocardial oxygen consumption.[39] Arrhythmias can occur following administration of thiopental and the other ultra-short-acting barbiturates particularly during spontaneous ventilation.[8, 32, 42] The most common of these are premature ventricular contractions. The incidence of arrhythmias varies from a few to as much as 20 percent.[42-44] The two most likely causes for these arrhythmias are myocardial sensitivity to a concurrent hypercania and increased cardiac vagal activity.

Respiratory Actions

Thiopental, as well as the other barbiturates, is a potent respiratory depressant.[8] Although the sequence of events following its administration varies with the patient, the dose, and the rate with which the compound is given, thiopental generally first produces an increase in tidal volume, for two or three breaths, and then apnea.[8, 45, 46] Apnea occurs when cerebral thiopental concentration is at peak level. Following apnea, respiration is resumed but at a much reduced rate and depth. The rate and depth of respiration depend on the absence or presence and degree of noxious (surgical) stimulation and the employment of other compounds, i.e., premedicants.[45,46] This is of particular importance when large, multiple doses of barbiturates have been used. In these situations patients may be breathing adequately when they leave the operating room but upon returning to the postanesthetic recovery area, where they are undisturbed, may experience severe respiratory depression.

As with most central depressants, thiopental interferes with the sensitivity of the medullary respiratory center to carbon dioxide.[46] In contrast to the narcotics, depth of respiration is generally decreased more than rate. Increases in arterial blood pressure, which generally occur with increases in $PaCO_2$, may be less marked or nonexistent because of the depressant effects of thiopental on the heart and peripheral vascular system.

Laryngeal reflexes are usually not depressed until large amounts of thiopental are administered and deep levels of narcosis are produced.[47,48] Stimulation of the tracheal bronchial tree during light levels of narcosis may result in laryngospasm or, worse yet, bronchospasm. The respiratory tract may be hypersensitive to stimuli during light thiopental anesthesia.[47,48]

Cerebral Actions

Cerebral metabolism and oxygen utilization are decreased after thiopental administration in proportion to the degree of cerebral depression.[17-19] Blood flow is also decreased but much less than oxygen consumption.[19] Theses changes are desirable because the ratio of cerebral perfusion to metabolism is increased. This can be used to advantage in patients with a marginally adequate cerebral circulation, i.e., patients with cerebral ischemia undergoing operation. The reduction in cerebral blood flow and increase in the cerebral perfusion/metabolism ratio also make

thiopental an ideal induction agent in patients with increased intracranial pressure (see Chs. 25 and 33).

Hepatic Function

While investigators initially suggested that thiopental may reduce hepatic blood flow[49,50] subsequent work demonstrated that these reductions were not due to thiopental but rather to hypocarbia, hypercarbia (with increased sympathetic activity), or the concomitant use of cyclopropane.[51,52] Thiopental probably reduces hepatic blood flow very little in healthy patients anesthetized with no other compound and maintained normocarbic.

In animals, prolonged thiopental administration decreases the ability of the liver to remove bromsulphthalein from the blood.[53] Thiopental, 20 mg/kg, given twice a day to dogs over a period of 2 to 3 weeks, increases prothrombin time and serum bilirubin levels for 4 days after termination of administration.[54] Yet with induction doses of thiopental (3 to 5 mg/kg) no change occurs in man in any postoperative index of liver function.[55] While larger doses of thiopental (average 15.5 to 18.5 mg/kg) for longer procedures do produce changes in a variety of hepatic function indices, the changes are not clinically significant and could, in fact, be related to operative procedure rather than thiopental.[55,56] The fact that there are case reports in which enormous doses of thiopental (25 to 34 g) have been given over a period of days without appreciable change in hepatic function suggests that if thiopental does produce hepatic toxicity, it must occur very rarely.[57]

Renal Function

In the absence of surgical stimulation, an induction dose of thiopental or light general anesthesia may not alter glomerular filtration rate but usually reduces renal blood flow.[58] Yet Habif et al.[49] found that thiopental reduced both glomerular filtration rate and renal blood flow during induction of anesthesia and that continued anesthesia and surgery produced little further change. Others have found little change in renal function during light levels of thiopental narcosis but significant depression during deep anesthesia.[58] Recovery in renal function occurs very rapidly after termination of thiopental-induced depression.[49] While the mechanism producing alteration of renal function during thiopental anesthesia has never been carefully studied, possibilities include increased secretion of antidiuretic hormone, direct vasoconstrictive action on the renal vasculature, and indirect effects, i.e., secondary to depression of arterial pressure and cardiac output. Prolonged oliguria, anuria, or histologic evidence of kidney pathology has never been reported after thiopental or any of the ultra-short-acting barbiturates.[8]

Other Organ Function

Thiopental and the barbiturates appear to have little effect on the gravid uterus[8] nor on the intensity or duration of action of the nondepolarizing relaxants.[8,59] Thiopental may protect against the pain and stiffness caused by succinylcholine.[60] Small doses or slow injection of larger doses of thiopental have little effect on the tone and motility of the stomach or gastrointestinal tract but rapid injection of large doses of thiopental (20 mg/kg) may cause complete cessation of the normal action of the pylorus, stomach, and small intestine.[61] Recovery of gastrointestinal function after thiopental is, however, rapid.

CLINICAL COMPLICATIONS

The highly alkaline (pH 10.6 to 10.8) sodium solutions of thiopental rarely produce pain on intravenous administration. In contrast, methohexital (sodium brevital), another popular ultra-short-acting barbiturate, does occasionally produce pain on intravenous injection.[62] High concentrations of either compound (5.0 percent thiopental; 2.0 percent methohexital) are not uncommonly followed by intravenous thrombosis. This complication rarely follows the use of lower concentrations (2.5 percent thiopental; 1.0 percent methohexital).[63]

Subcutaneous injection of thiopental, and to a lesser extent methohexital, results in local tissue irritation and if higher concentrations and sufficient volume are administered, tissue necrosis.[8] This appears to be less of a problem following intramuscular injections.[64,65]

Inadvertent intra-arterial injection of thiopental usually results in vascular spasm and intense pain.[8,65,66] Although a rare complication—estimated occurrence between 1 in 3,500 and 1 in 56,000 administrations—[8,67] intra-arterial injections can result in severe consequences. The intense arterial constriction that usually follows often results in the disappearance of distal arterial pulses and blanching of the limb followed soon after by severe cyanosis. Gangrene and permanent nerve damage have been reported after arterial injection of thiopental.[65] The mechanism, or mechanisms, producing these changes are not fully understood. Some have suggested that intra-arterial thiopental results in a release of norepinephrine.[68,69] Others have shown that crystals of insoluble thiopental form in the artery and either produce an intense vasospasm or are swept distally and occlude small arterioles.[70] Still other investigators have shown that hemolysis of erythrocytes and aggregation of platelets are induced by intra-arterial thiopental which may occlude distal vessels.[71] Methohexital can result in changes similar to those of thiopental. The damage is directly related to the dosage and concentration of the barbiturate injected. All vessels examined pathologically demonstrate a severe endoarteritis.[8,65] Treatment is immediate injection of a solution to dilute the concentration of the injected barbiturate (saline) or one that not only dilutes but also produces some degree of vasodilation (lidocaine or procaine). Heparin has also been injected into the artery.[63] Finally, sympathetic blockade of the extremity is employed by some.[65]

Excitatory Phenomena

Spontaneous tremor, muscle movement of hypertonus, occurs occasionally after intravenous injection of the ultra-short-acting barbiturates, particularly the methylated, carbon 2, compounds (e.g., methohexital).[72] Excitatory phenomena are more common after rapid injection. The exact cause of these phenomena are unknown.[72, 73]

Allergic and Unusual Reactions

In the over 40 years that the ultra-short-acting compounds have been used, few true allergies to them have been reported.[8, 65] In those few patients in whom barbiturate allergy has been detected, a previous strong allergic history has also been present.[65, 74] The allergy has usually manifested itself via skin rash and/or weals which, on occasion, have involved the larynx and glottis. Respiratory difficulty with bronchospasm, laryngospasm, and severe hypotension may occur.

More frequently ultra-short-acting barbiturates produce more dramatic than expected effects on the circulatory or cerebral systems. These so-called more susceptible people are usually elderly or possessed of low plasma proteins or significant liver dysfunction. In such individuals, usual dosage of thiopental or its conjoiners represent relative over-dosages and the prolonged effects they produce on the central nervous and cardiovascular systems are really not different than that which occurs following a large dose to a fit patient.

A potentially more serious reaction can occur following thiopental administration to patients with porphyria, a spectrum of diseases characterized by symptoms chiefly associated with the skin, nervous system, and alimentary tract. The porphyria diseases occur secondary to incomplete metabolism of porphyrin (also see Ch. 2).[75, 76] The most important of the porphyria diseases with regard to the anesthesiologist is acute, intermittent porphyria, which accounts for about 75 percent of the porphyrias seen in the United States.

The incidence of acute intermittent porphyria (AIP) is about 1 in 10,000. The active syndrome is characterized by abdominal pain, often described as colicky; tachycardia; hypertension; paresthesias, hypesthesias, or both; bulbar and/or peripheral nerve paralysis; and often psychotic behavior. A variety of normal physiological processes (pregnancy, short periods of minimal or absent food intake) and abnormal conditions (hepatic disease, anesthesia) can produce the active syndrome in patients with AIP in its latent phase.[75, 76] Anesthetic compounds that have been shown to trigger the syndrome include the barbiturates, the benzodiazepines, the ergot compounds, and some of the hydantoins.

The biochemical defect in AIP is an excess production of porphyrin precursors in the biosynthetic pathway to heme, which combines in hematopoietic tissue with globin to form hemoglobin. The rate-limiting enzyme in the sequence of reactions that ultimately forms heme is delta-aminolevulinic acid synthetase which is under feedback control by heme. In patients with AIP the controlling mechanism is defective and as a result many precursors of heme, particularly porphobilinogen and delta-aminolevulinic acid build up. Exactly how the buildup of these precursors, which are benign when given by themselves, produce the symptoms associated with the active AIP syndrome is unknown.

All patients with abdominal pain, especially of acute onset, may be in the early stages of an AIP attack. It is obvious that AIP should be ruled out, by analysis of urine and blood for porphyrins, before thiopental or any of the other triggering compounds that anesthesiologists may use are administered to these patients.

CURRENT CLINICAL USAGE

The ultra-short-acting barbiturates are almost exclusively used as intravenous induction agents or as supplements during anesthesia with nitrous oxide with or without other inhaled or intravenous compounds. On occasion, the ultra-short-acting barbiturates are used as complete anesthetics for extremely short, usually pain-free procedures, i.e., cardioversion or electroconvulsive procedures. In the latter case, one, two, or three intravenous boluses or a continuous, usually rapid infusion of the compounds are employed.

THE BENZODIAZEPINES

The benzodiazepines are classified as minor tranquilizers.[77] They produce, depending upon the dosage in which they are used, tranquility, sedation, drowsiness, or unconsciousness.[77,78] Interest in and development of these compounds originally arose out of the use of the phenothiazines for their soporific qualities in the 1950's.[79] The standard benzodiazepine with which all others are compared is diazepam (7-chloro-1,3-dihydro-1-methyl-5-phenyl-2*H*-1,4 benzodiazepin-2-one). Other benzodiazepines which have been used as intravenous sedatives, hypnotics and occasionally as anesthetics, include lorazepam, flunitrazepam, and most recently, midazolam.

Diazepam (Valium) is a crystalline, colorless, basic compound that is insoluble in water and has a molecular weight of 284.7.[79] Because of its aqueous insolubility, diazepam is dissolved in a vehicle composed of organic solvents. These consist of propylene glycol, ethyl-alcohol, and sodium benzoate in benzoic acid and make a slightly viscid solution with a pH of 6.6 to 6.9. This low pH is why this solution is painful on intravenous as well as intramuscular injection.[78] Commercial prep-

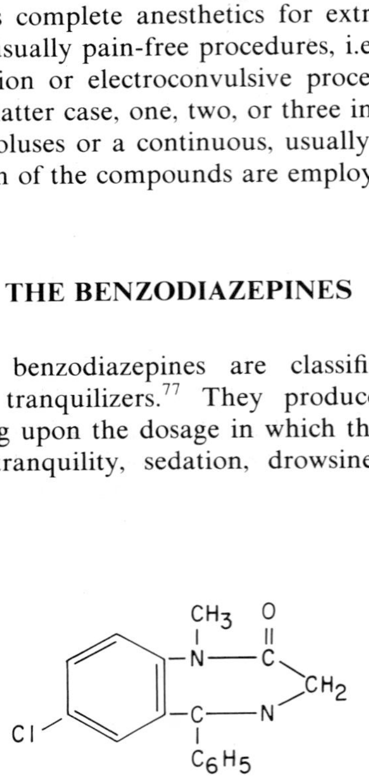

DIAZEPAM

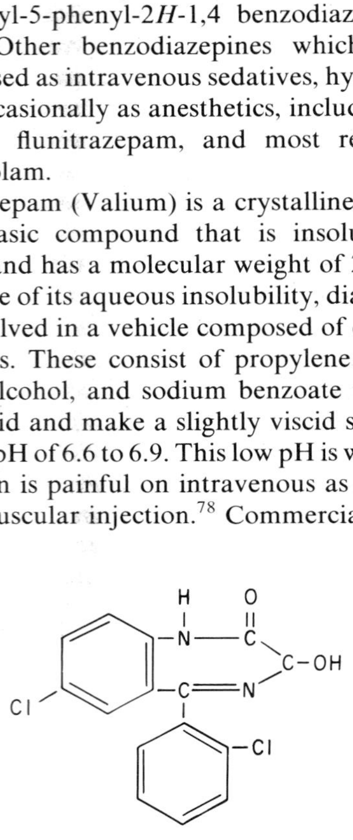

LORAZEPAM

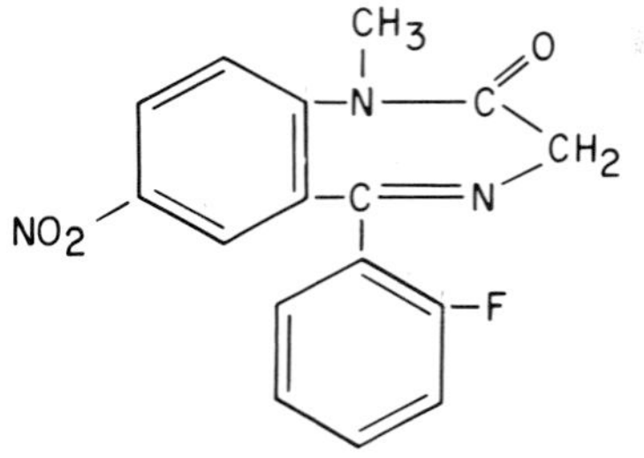

FLUNITRAZEPAM

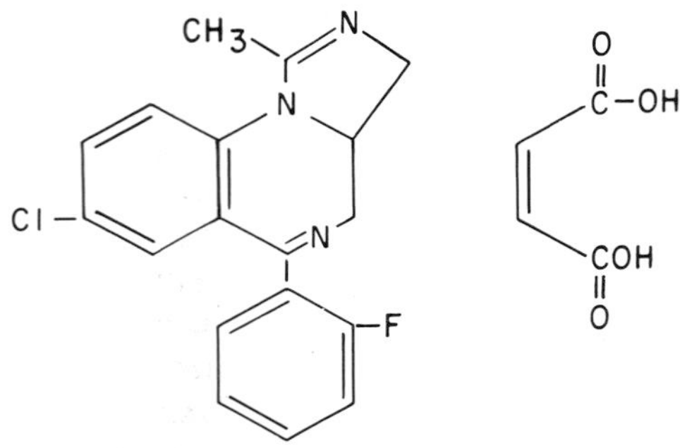

MIDAZOLAM

arations of both flunitrazepam and lorazepam also come in organic solvents, but they
are reported to be less irritating on injection
and followed by a lower incidence of venous
thrombosis.[79, 80] Midazolam, by contrast, is
water soluble and produces very little, if any,
pain on injection and a low incidence of venous thrombosis.[78, 81]

MECHANISM OF ACTION

Sedation following intravenous injection of
diazepam usually takes from 1 to 2 minutes.[79, 82, 83] This response is quite variable.
Indeed, in some patients as little as 5 mg/70
kg may produce unconsciousness and in
others as much as 1 mg/kg little more than
drowsiness. Narcotic compounds, given as
premedication or concurrently intravenously,
greatly potentiate the soporific effects of diazepam and all the benzodiazepines.[83] Although the reason for this is not entirely clear,
it may be related to the fact that both groups
are metabolically demethylated and may
compete for the same enzyme system in
vivo.[84]

The benzodiazepines interfere with interneuronal transmission at the level of the spinal cord. This probably accounts for their
muscle-relaxing action in spastic skeletal
muscular conditions.[79] Suprasinally, the
benzodiazepines interfere with the reticular
facilitatory system and depress the entire
limbic system, including the hypocampus, the
amygdala, the thalmus, the fornix, and the
angulate gyrus.[85, 86] Probably the action of the
benzodiazines on the limbic structures is most
responsible for their anticonvulsant effects,
however, a cortical depressant action cannot
be entirely ruled out.

Given alone, the benzodiazepines result in
little change in functions controlled by the
medulla (respiration and circulation). However, when combined with other intravenous
sedatives, hypnotics, or analgesics, severe
respiratory and circulatory depression can
occur.[83, 87, 88]

Diazepam, lorazepam, and probably most
of the benzodiazepines are good amne-
sics.[89–92] Retrograde amnesia does not follow
an induction of anesthesia with diazepam;
however, a number of investigators have
shown anterograde amnesia for periods of 30
minutes or more after 0.24 mg/kg of the
compound.[90] Anterograde amnesia may last
as long as 6 hours following lorazepam.[92] The
amnesic action of the benzodiazepines is most
marked when they are used to produce sedation, i.e., with regional anesthesia during operation. Patients may doze off to sleep but although they can be readily roused and can
answer questions rationally, they rarely remember these events postoperatively.

PHARMACOKINETICS

Following intravenous injections of 10 to
20 mg/70 kg given to adult volunteers, Baird
and Hailey found a rapid decline in plasma
levels of diazepam over a 10 to 20 minute period.[93] As has been found after oral administration, these investigators discovered a second peak in plasma diazepam concentrations
6 to 8 hours after injection. This delayed increase in plasma diazepam concentration
could account for the return of drowsiness
that has been reported by others and is
thought to occur secondary to enterohepatic
recirculation.[94]

The two most important metabolites of diazepam are desmethyldiazepam and hydro-
xydiazepam.[93] Desmethyldiazepam is only
slightly less potent than diazepam and its
plasma concentrations increase steadily over
approximately the first 24 hours after injection of diazepam. This metabolite undoubtedly also contributes to the return of drowsiness after apparent recovery following
diazepam administration.

Irrespective of its causation, return of
drowsiness after recovery from diazepam is of
profound clinical importance, especially
when the compound is used for outpatient
procedures. Patients should be cautioned

against driving or participating in any activity that requires a great deal of muscle coordination for at least 24 hours following any dosage of intravenous diazepam.

Diazepam is primarily metabolized in the liver.[95] Its half-life is prolonged in patients with hepatic cirrhosis[95] and those of advanced age.[96] On repeated administration diazepam and its metabolites accumulate, probably in adipose tissue, and result in prolonged somnolence.

Diazepam readily crosses the placenta and is found in fetal plasma in concentrations equal to and sometimes greater than those found in the maternal circulation.[97,98] The speed of diazepam's transfer into the fetus is probably related to its high solubility in lipids. Diazepam is also found in amniotic fluid although in lower concentrations than in fetal plasma.[99]

CARDIOVASCULAR ACTIONS

Intravenous injection of diazepam, even in large doses (0.5 to 1.5 mg/kg) produces only mild, if any, cardiovascular depression.[79] Animal work demonstrates that diazepam and the other benzodiazepines result in little change in ventricular contractility; heart rate; systemic, pulmonary artery, and atrial pressures; and the electrocardiogram.[100,101] Although diazepam, particularly large intravenous doses (1.0 mg/kg), does occasionally reduce arterial blood pressure, peripheral arterial resistance, and cardiac output, these changes are small, usually less than 20 percent, and not consistent, even in patients with severe cardiovascular disease.[102-105] Because of its benign actions on the cardiovascular system diazepam and, more recently, midazolam have become popular as induction agents and supplements in critically ill patients with cardiovascular disease.[104-106]

Diazepam is often used for intravenous sedation and amnesia in patients undergoing cardiac catheterization and electrical conversion.[78] Indeed, in these circumstances, increased coronary blood flow, increased myocardial function, and reduced myocardial oxygen consumption have all been described.[100,107]

The sites and mechanisms of action of diazepam and the other benzodiazepines on the heart and cardiovascular system have not been defined. Cardiovascular collapse and arrhythmias have occasionally been reported after the intravenous administration of diazepam.[108,109] Combinations of diazepam and narcotics, on the other hand, often produce severe cardiovascular depression.[87,88] The mechanism of this response is probably related to the sympatholytic effects of this combination of compounds.[110]

RESPIRATORY ACTIONS

Diazepam and the other benzodiazepines produce mild respiratory depression when injected intravenously.[101,104] Hypoventilation is primarily due to a decrease in tidal volume and occurs in spite of a small increase in respiratory rate.[104] Usually $PaCO_2$ is slightly elevated and PaO_2 slightly decreased, although this is certainly not always the case. Administration of diazepam, 10 mg intravenously, can occasionally produce apnea although $PaCO_2$ is often only marginally increased. Sadove et al.[111] found that diazepam did not change the respiratory response to increased inspired concentrations of carbon dioxide. However, as mentioned above, the response is usually quite different when diazepam or any of the other benzodiazepines are used together intravenously with narcotic compounds. In this situation profound and prolonged respiratory depression is usually produced.

NEUROMUSCULAR ACTIONS

The suggestion that the benzodiazepines might have an effect on the neuromuscular junction resulting in potentiation of the nondepolarizing muscle relaxants is controversial.[112,113] Still others have suggested that while the benzodiazepines result in little effect on neuromuscular function, the solvents in which they are commercially delivered may interfere with neuromuscular transmission.[114]

OTHER ORGAN SYSTEM EFFECTS

Diazepam has little, if any, effect on the vomiting centers nor on chemical-induced emesis (e.g. apomorphine).[79,112] There is one study that suggests that diazepine may protect against narcotic-induced vomiting.[83]

Although diazepam does not produce any change in any of the stress-responding hormones in man (the catecholamines, antidiuretic hormone, cortisol),[79] in dogs diazepam reduces narcotic-induced increases in plasma catecholamines.[110]

Diazepam and the benzodiazepines apparently result in little change in renal, hepatic, or biliary physiology and do not affect normal reproductive function in animals.[79] As mentioned previously, thrombosis and phlebitis have often been found after intravenous diazepam and less frequently after lorazepam and flunitrazepam. This complication occurs much more frequently when the drugs are injected into small veins and administered to the elderly.

MIDAZOLAM—THE NEW BENZODIAZEPINE

Midazolam (8-chloro-6-(2-flurophenyl-1-methyl)-4H-imidazo [1,5a] [1,4] benzodiazepine maleate), the new water soluble benzodiazepine currently undergoing clinical trials, has actions that are similar to diazepam.[78,81,106] However, midazolam is three times more potent than diazepam, has a shorter duration of activity and produces little, if any, venous sequelae on intravenous injection. In addition, Graham and co-workers[115] showed little placental transfer of midazolam. All of the above suggest that intravenous midazolam may be superior to diazepam as an anesthetic induction agent or hypnotic supplement.

CURRENT CLINICAL USES

The benzodiazepines are used intravenously as anesthetic induction agents, as hypnotic supplements during balanced anesthesia with other intravenous and/or inhalation compounds, as complete anesthetics in procedures for which little analgesia is required (e.g., cardioversion and electroconvulsive therapy), for sedation during regional anesthesia, and as anticonvulsants, especially after local anesthetic-induced convulsions. Their popularity in all these situations stems from their short onset of activity, which is only a little slower than intravenous thiopental in most cases, their amnesic qualities, and their relative lack of cardiorespiratory effects. Up until recently, the two most important problems in their intravenous use during anesthesia were thrombophlebitis and occasional prolonged duration of action. These problems may be less in frequency and intensity with midazolam. If so, the benzodiazepines will become even more important as intravenous anesthetics and anesthetic adjuvants.

BENZODIAZEPINE ANTAGONISM

Physostigmine, a tertiary amine capable of crossing the blood-brain barrier, has been shown to be effective in the antagonism of benzodiazepine-induced CNS depression as well as in CNS depression produced by a variety of sedatives and hypnotics.[116-118] Physostigmine's antagonistic actions may be due to an increase in brain acetylcholine secondary to inhibition of cholinesterase, but whether this is, in fact, the explanation is unknown. Alternatively, perhaps physostigmine's antagonistic action is nothing more than a generalized arousal effect. Disadvantages of physostigmine antagonism of benzodiazepine CNS depression include occasional nausea, vomiting, bradycardia, and in situations of benzodiazepine overdose, return of depression some hours later.[78, 116] All of the above reasons argue against physostigmine's routine use after employment of the benzodiazepines.

THE BUTYROPHENONES AND NEUROLEPTANALGESIA

The butyrophenones are classified as major tranquilizers.[119] The only one of clinical importance as an adjuvant intravenous anesthetic is droperidol, (dehydrobenzperidol). The butyrophenones induce a state of apathy and apparent mental detachment.[120] When combined with a narcotic they produce sedation and analgesia and if given in sufficient dosage, unconsciousness. The combination of a narcotic and a butyrophenone is called neuroleptanalgesia, a state of consciousness characterized by a trance-like demeanor in which immobility and analgesia exist.[120–122] Major surgical procedures can be performed with neuroleptanalgesia alone although nitrous oxide and when necessary a muscle relaxant are frequently added to the regimen, which is then called neuroleptanesthesia. The most popular of the neuroleptanalgesic combinations is Innovar, a mixture of droperidol (2.5 mg/ml) and fentanyl (0.05 mg/ml).[119]

DROPERIDOL

The concept of neuroleptanalgesia developed as the predecessor to the states of "artificial hibernation" produced by the French schools of anesthesia. These groups used "lytic cocktails"—mixtures of analgesics (most commonly meperidine) and tranquilizers (most commonly chlorpromazine or promethazine).[119] Neuroleptanalgesia was considered better than artificial hibernation because of greater cardiovascular stability and a more controllable duration of action. Unfortunately, neuroleptanalgesia, when used alone for major surgical procedures, can also result in cardiovascular instability (usually hypertension and/or tachycardia) and prolonged postoperative CNS depression (J. de Castro, personal communication). The latter occurs primarily due to the prolonged CNS depressant effects of the butyrophenones (e.g., droperidol). Because of this, most clinicians rarely employ pure neuroleptanalgesic techniques in the United States today. Rather, mixtures of other sedatives and hypnotics as well as droperidol, with a narcotic, a muscle relaxant, and nitrous oxide and/or a potent inhalation agent are the rule.[119, 123] These techniques are properly called balanced anesthesia. Rather than administer Innovar, some clinicians administer droperidol alone for its specific effects: sedation, hypnosis, amnesia, and a significant antiemetic action.[119, 123, 124]

MECHANISM OF ACTION

Droperidol interferes with CNS transmission at dopamine, noradrenaline, serotonin, and gamma-aminobutyric acid synaptic sites.[119, 125] The interference is probably due to competitive inhibition at the receptor. Inhibition at the dopaminergic site is the most likely cause for occasional extrapyramidal reactions (dyskinesia) and parkinsonian-like rigidity.[125, 126]

Droperidol has no analgesic effect by itself and when given alone appears to result in a patient who is placid, sleepy, and indifferent to his environment.[127, 128] However, when interviewed later, many patients given intramuscular or intravenous droperidol describe feelings of agitation and anxiety.[129] Droperidol does not potentiate the analgesic potency of narcotics given concurrently but may prolong their duration of activity.[127] The mechanism of this action is unknown.

Droperidol and other butyrophenones (e.g., haloperidol) inhibit the chemoreceptor trigger zone in the medulla and by this mechanism are effective postanesthetic antiemetics.[119,124] The butyrophenones appear, however, to have little effect on labyrinthine-induced vomiting.[78,79]

CARDIOVASCULAR, RESPIRATORY, AND OTHER ORGAN SYSTEM ACTIONS

With the exception of a small degree of hypotension, probably due to CNS and direct cardiac depression as well as to peripheral α-adrenergic blocking actions, droperidol produces little change in cardiovascular dynamics.[130–133] Generally, systemic and pulmonary vascular resistances are slightly decreased by droperidol; but these changes are usually transient, lasting only 15 to 20 minutes.[87,123,131] For unexplained reasons, droperidol occasionally may produce a dramatic decrease in peripheral arterial resistance and arterial blood pressure.[134] Droperidol appears to protect against catecholamine-induced cardiac arrhythmias.[135] Droperidol is also a cerebral vasoconstrictor, significantly decreasing cerebral blood flow,[136] but it does not seem to influence cerebral metabolic rate. While these latter actions may be used to benefit patients with increased intracranial pressure, they may be detrimental to those with cerebral ischemic disease although this latter fear has not been confirmed.

Droperidol does not effect respiratory or hepatic function and has little influence on secretions from the adrenal cortex but does decrease oxygen consumption and increase growth hormone and blood glucose levels.[137–141]

CURRENT CLINICAL USAGE

Droperidol, especially in small doses (10 mg), is still popular as an intravenous sedative and hypnotic supplement during nitrous oxide–narcotic anesthesia. It also has been advocated and is often used as a short-acting "afterload" reducer during anesthesia and in the postoperative period.[123] Finally, droperidol and haloperidol have experienced a reasonable popularity as antiemetics administered prophylactically during or at the end of surgery or after vomiting has occurred in the recovery room.[124]

THE EUGENOLS

Propanidid, a eugenol (a constituent of oil of cloves and cinnamon leaf oil), has achieved a reasonable degree of popularity as an intravenous hypnotic in Europe but has never been released in the United States. The reason for this is probably related to the high incidence of hypersensitivity reactions reported after its usage.[142,143]

Propanidid is 3-methoxy-4-(N,N diethyl-carbamoylmethoxy)-phenylacetic acid n-propylester.[142] It is a yellow oil with a pH of between 4 and 5 and is only slightly soluble in water. It is currently dissolved in a mixture of polyoxylated castor oil, sodium chloride, and water to form a 5 percent aqueous solution. Originally propanidid was dissolved in Cremophor EL, the solubilizing agent used with the steroid anesthetic, Althesin, which also has been reported to cause many allergic reactions.

PROPANIDID

MECHANISM OF ACTION

Propanidid is an ultra-short-acting hypnotic that produces, when injected in appropriate doses, amnesia and unconsciousness as fast as does thiopental (in one circulation time).[56] Propanidid, unfortunately, has no analgesic activity but also no antianalgesia action, in contrast to the barbiturates.[144, 145] Although the site of action of propanidid in the brain is unknown, EEG changes are similar to those found with the barbiturates.[142]

Excitatory muscle movements occur with propanidid in direct proportion to dosage.[142, 143, 146] Doses of 4 mg/kg result in abnormal muscle movements in approximately 10 percent of patients whereas doses of 14 mg/kg produce these effects in 70 percent of patients. Rapid injection of propanidid and the use of certain premedicants, i.e., the belladonnas and antihistamines, increase the incidence of excitatory muscle movements whereas other premedicants, the narcotics, decrease the incidence of these problems.[147]

CARDIOVASCULAR ACTIONS

Propanidid produces a decrease in arterial blood pressure in direct proportion to the dose administered.[144, 148] In doses of 4 mg/kg, half of the usual 7 mg/kg induction dose, propanidid results in less than a 10 percent reduction in arterial pressure. With an 8 mg/kg dose, however, decreases in arterial pressure of over 40 torr are common. Hypotension after propanidid is due to impaired myocardial contactile force and peripheral arterial vasodilation.[149, 150] Cardiac output usually falls during hypotension after propanidid but rapidly recovers to control values while blood pressure remains depressed. Heart rate is usually increased after propanidid.[151] This may explain why cardiac output returns to normal faster than arterial blood pressure. On the other hand, others have suggested that the initial depression of cardiac output and arterial blood pressure is due to the effects of propanidid and the more prolonged period of hypotension is secondary to a later release of histamine.[142]

Propanidid may result in transient A-V block in some patients but it also appears to have a quinidine-like action which has been suggested to be important to decreasing cardiac arrhythmias during laryngoscopy, tracheal intubation, and light inhalation anesthesia.[152]

RESPIRATORY AND OTHER EFFECTS

Propanidid results in an initial hyperventilation (which can be blocked via proper application of lidocaine to carotid chemoreceptors but not by vagotomy) and a secondary period of apnea.[153, 154] Narcotic premedication decreases respiratory stimulation and prolongs apnea.[155] In usual doses, propanidid, 6 to 8 mg/kg, results in cough, hiccup, and laryngospasm in less than 10 percent of patients.[146] This incidence rises with dosage, however. Propanidid prolongs the duration of succinylcholine-induced apnea.[156] It is felt that this occurs because both compounds are metabolized by pseudocholinesterase.[157] For unknown reasons propanidid also significantly decreases the incidence of muscle pains after succinylcholine.[156] Propanidid does not have an effect on indirect evoked muscle twitch in the cat.[158] However, Clarke et al.[156] found that *d*-tubocurarine requirements were increased in patients anesthetized with propanidid when compared to a similar series of patients anesthetized with thiopental.[156]

Propanidid has been shown to increase the incidence of nausea and vomiting when compared to other intravenous agents, especially when administered with nitrous oxide.[146, 159] The reason for this is unknown. Propanidid results in no change in liver, or hepatic, function when used in usual clinical doses, 6 to 8 mg/kg.[142, 147]

PHARMACOKINETICS

Following the rapid intravenous bolus administration of 7 mg/kg, plasma concentrations of propanidid reach 15 μg/ml in 1 minute but, because of rapid hydrolysis, they return to zero in 13 minutes.[157] Somewhat slower (over 20 seconds) injections of propanidid do not significantly change peak plasma concentrations of the compound but do increase the time that propanidid is measurable in the plasma.[160] When the same mg/kg dose is given, slower injections of propanidid produce EEG changes consistent with a depth of anesthesia that is less than that of bolus injections. However, recovery time is similar with the two methods of injection suggesting a phenomena of acute tolerance as can be observed after thiopental.[161]

Propanidid appears rapidly in all well-perfused tissues in the body, including the placenta and fetal circulation.[142, 143, 157] This occurs in spite of the fact that 40 percent of propanidid is bound to plasma proteins and is probably best explained by the compound's high solubility in lipids (heptane/water ratio 1.70 compared to 1.03 for thiopental). Anesthesia from propanidid is significantly prolonged and intensified by either a reduction in plasma protein concentration (secondary to more unbound, free propanidid) or a reduction of plasma pseudocholinesterase concentration (secondary to imparied propanidid metabolism).[142, 143, 157, 158, 162]

Plasma pseudocholinesterase is responsible for the rapid breakdown of propanidid.[142, 143, 157, 158, 162] Indeed, 98 percent of an administered dose of propanidid is metabolized at the ester linkage.[147] The remainder is destroyed by having the diethyl-amino group split off (see figure of propanidid). Destruction of propanidid can produce a transient decrease (as much as 20 percent following a bolus dosage of 7 mg/kg) in circulating pseudocholinesterase concentrations.[157] This explains the prolonged periods of apnea that follow the use of succinylcholine immediately after propanidid;[157, 158, 161] the duration of apnea from succinylcholine is increased by almost 4 minutes by propanidid.

Excretion of the metabolites of propanidid occurs rapidly. Ninety percent of the metabolites are excreted in the urine and up to 6 percent in the feces within 2 hours. The latter may help to explain why recovery following propanidid anesthesia is so rapid. Doenicke et al.[157] found entirely normal EEG patterns 30 minutes after IV administration of 500 to 1,000 mg doses of propanidid and absolutely no impairment of psychomotor performance 30 minutes later. Patients who receive 7 mg/kg of propanidid—with the exception of the old and critically ill, for whom dosage should probably be reduced anyway—have normal driving skills on a driving simulator 2 hours after intravenous injection.[143, 163] Rapid "clear-headed" recovery is one of the great advantages of propanidid and is the reason why it is so popular among its proponents, especially for outpatient surgery.[142, 143, 163]

HYPERSENSITIVITY

Although not reported in animals, hypersensitivity reactions secondary to propanidid have been reported in man.[142, 143, 164] The incidence of these reactions is difficult to estimate because their clinical appearance has been so varied. Everything from mild erythema, or skin rash, to urticaria, edema with or without severe hypotension, and bronchospasm have been reported after propanidid. Since hypotension is expected after propanidid in usual doses, it is not clear whether severe hypotension, as reported to be the only sign of hypersensitivity in some patients, was indeed that or simply a pharmacologic response to the drug. A further difficulty is that some degree of flushing occurs as a normal response to propanidid in many patients. Is this allergy or a normal pharmacologic response? Lorenz et al.[164] found that a fourfold increase in histamine (from a control value of 1 ng/ml to 4 ng/ml) is a normal response to propanidid. In some patients these authors found that histamine responses were more marked and the clinical reactions more severe, i.e., erythema more profound. In one patient plasma histamine increased to 100 ng/ml and a transient cardiac arrest occurred. These findings suggest that all patients sustain increases in circulating histamine after propanidid but that some patients respond with a greater outpouring of histamine than others. Unfortunately, the sophisticated immunologic studies that are required to determine whether the above responses are allergic or normal pharmacologic responses have not yet been performed. Considering the dwindling popularity of propanidid in Europe and the unlikelihood that it will ever be introduced into the United States, it is questionable whether these studies will ever be performed.

CURRENT CLINICAL USAGE

Propanidid's speedy onset and short duration of action make it ideal for outpatient surgery, for extractions in dental clinics, and as a supplement to narcotic analgesics or nitrous oxide and other inhalation agents in both short- and long-duration operative procedures.[142, 143] Propanidid's significant disadvantages, particularly cardiovascular depression, interaction with succinylcholine, and hypersensitivity-like responses, make it unlikely to ever achieve a great deal of popularity in Europe and will probably never allow it to be available for use in the United States.

THE STEROID ANESTHETICS

Although the hypnotic properties of the steroids have been known for many years,[165] only recently have any of these compounds come to a reasonable clinical trial.[143, 166] The reasons for this are complex and need not be discussed in this chapter except to note that onset of activity, venothrombosis, solubility in water, and the occurrence of unwanted re-

actions, particularly hypersensitive reactions, have been, and still are serious drawbacks of some of these compounds.[143, 166]

ALTHESIN

Althesin is currently the most popular steroid anesthetic. It is not, and probably never will be, available in the United States but it is often used in the British Isles. Althesin is a mixture of two steroids: alphaxalone (3α-hydroxy-5α-pregnane-11,20 dione) and alphadolone acetate (21-acetoxy-3α-hydroxy-5α-pregnane-11,20 dione), which are dissolved in Cremophor EL, a nonionic surface active solution of polyoxyethylated castor oil.[166] Alphaxalone is the most important of the two steroids and is employed in a ratio of 3:1 with respect to alphadolone. Indeed, the only real purpose for alphadalone is to increase solubility, as alphaxalone is not sufficiently soluble in Cremophor EL. However, alphadalone is about 50 percent as potent as alphaxalone and does, therefore, add somewhat to the hypnotic effect of the former.

CENTRAL NERVOUS SYSTEM EFFECTS

As with most of the intravenous anesthetics the mechanism by which Althesin produces anesthesia is unknown. However, doses of 1.8 mg/kg produce hypnosis in one circulation time.[167] Clinicians suggest that onset of sleep with Althesin appears to occur just a few seconds slower than thiopental;[143] perhaps this is because onset time is not as sudden with the former as it is with a bolus dosage of the latter. On the other hand, it is difficult to rapidly inject the more viscid Althesin solution and perhaps the difference is simply related to speed of injection of the two drugs. Althesin is not an analgesic.[142, 143]

Althesin produces EEG changes similar to those of thiopental, and they are, like those of thiopental, dose related and not restricted to any particular area of the brain.[168] Also as in thiopental use, cerebral blood flow, cerebral oxygen consumption, and intracranial pressure are significantly decreased by usually administered induction dosages (50 to 100 μg/kg) of Althesin.[169] Following administration of 50 μg/kg of Althesin, muscle tremors ocur in about 20 percent of patients. Muscle movements increase in frequence and severity as dosage and speed of injection are increased and, as with propanidid, may be further increased with scopolamine and reduced with narcotic premedication.

Duration of anesthesia following a single dose of Althesin (50 to 150 μg/kg) is 5 to 10 minutes longer than after a comparable dose of thiopental or methohexital.[163] Unlike propanidid, recovery from Althesin is often accompanied by disorientation, restlessness, confusion, and sometimes agitation.[163, 170] In simulated driving performances Kortilla et al.[163] found that impairment is still significant 6 hours following injection of a single dose of Althesin (85 μg/kg), whereas driving performance was always normal 4 hours after thiopental (4 mg/kg). This prolonged effect of Althesin on muscle coordination may be related to a pharmacologically active metabolite.

CARDIOVASCULAR ACTIONS

Althesin produces a little less cardiovascular depression than do similar doses of propanidid or thiopental.[171–174] Nonetheless, Althesin has significant negative inotropic effects on the myocardium.[172] Exactly what part Cremphor EL plays in this is not entirely clear. Some studies have shown that Cremphor EL does not alter the cardiovascular system when injected in doses that a patient might receive while being anesthetized with Althesin. Others have demonstrated significant increases in pulmonary vascular resistance, which may help explain the decrease in stroke volume and arterial blood pressure that usually accompany administration of Althesin.[175] Other changes associated with Althesin administration include a fall in central venous pressure and peripheral vascular

resistance and an increase in heart rate. With the exception of heart rate, the latter changes, as well as those of stroke volume and arterial blood pressure, are similar to those following comparable doses of thiopental.[173–175] Heart rate is increased much more after Althesin than after thiopental, and as a result cardiac output is rarely changed with Althesin whereas it usually is decreased with thiopental.[174]

RESPIRATORY ACTIONS

Althesin, like propanidid, often causes a short period of hyperventilation; however, this period only lasts for a few seconds.[146, 176–178] Apnea also occurs after Althesin.[176, 178] Fifty percent of patients receiving 100 μg/kg of Althesin and 33 percent of patients receiving 50 μg/kg are apneic at least for a short period of time.[178]

With doses of Althesin less than 100 μg/kg, coughing, hiccup, and laryngospasm occur in 5 to 15 percent of patients.[176–178] With higher doses of the drug the incidences of these problems increase significantly. Althesin does not interact with succinylcholine,[179] has little influence on respiratory or airway mechanics, and does not sensitize the chemoreceptors.[178] As with thiopental, laryngeal reflexes are usually completely suppressed with Althesin.[180]

OTHER ACTIONS

Althesin does not alter hepatic function in usual dosages and results in no greater incidence of venous thrombophlebitis than thiopental (2 to 3 percent).[181, 182] Some data suggest that nausea and vomiting following Althesin are not only significantly less than after propanidid but also less than after ketamine and the barbiturates as well.[183] This is, however, not confirmed in other studies.[184]

While Althesin in contrast to other intravenous anesthetics is highly toxic to fetal and neonatal mice,[185] it appears—at least in some studies—to be as good as thiopental as an induction agent for patients undergoing caesarean section.[186] Others have suggested that fetal acidosis occurs more frequently with Althesin than with thiopental as an induction agent.[187] Clearly, more human data is needed in this area.

METABOLISM

Peak plasma concentrations following doses of 50 to 200 μg/kg of Althesin range from 6.0 to 9.4 μg/ml.[188] At first recovery from anesthesia, Althesin blood levels range from 0.5 to 0.9 μg/ml.

Alphaxalone and alphadolone acetate are bound to a moderate extent by albumin and to a lesser extent by one of the globulin factors (total plasma protein binding = 35 to 50 percent).[189] Little of either steroid is redistributed to body fat, although uptake and then subsequent removal from the brain is rapid.[189, 190] Radiolabelled Althesin is concentrated in the liver and kidney, the two organs principally involved in its excretion.[190] Approximately 60 to 70 percent of radioactive Althesin winds up in the feces (via the biliary system) and 20 to 30 percent in the urine.[190] Urinary metabolites of Althesin are conjugated to glucuronide in man. No unmetabolized Althesin has been found in urine or feces in man.

The metabolites of Althesin have not been carefully studied as to their activity. Metabolism, at least in the rat, involves hydroxylation at the 2α and 16α positions in both molecules and perhaps an additional hydroxylation at the C_{21} position in alphadalone.

HYPERSENSITIVITY

There are numerous reports of hypersensitivity to Althesin.[143, 177, 191] Although many of these reports illustrate minor reactions to Althesin, others have been much more serious and include patient death. Some have estimated the frequency of hypersensitivity to Althesin at 1:900 to 1:1000. Because of this, it is doubtful that Althesin will ever be released in the United States.

MINAXOLONE

Minaxolone (28-ethoxy-3a-hydroxy-11a-dimethylamino-5a-pregnane-20-one) is a new water-soluble intravenous steroid anesthetic.[192] It is available as an aqueous water solution of sodium citrate and sodium chloride at a pH of 4 and a 5 mg/ml concentration of the steroid. Because of its water solubility there is hope that minaxolone may possess the desirable characteristics of Althesin—rapid anesthesia with minimal cardiovascular depression and little postoperative nausea and vomiting and thrombophlebitis—and not result in hypersensitivity.

So far, clinical investigation has demonstrated that minaxolone results in anesthesia in one circulation time, does not produce pain on injection, and has a recovery period similar to Althesin. Unfortunately a high "percentage"(65 to 75 percent) of patients demonstrate hypertonus and involuntary muscle movements, although these responses apparently do not interfere with operation (unparalyzed patients). Some hypotension (approximately 20 percent of patients sustain a decrease of arterial blood pressure of 20 torr or more) and apnea also occurs, although the duration and magnitude of respiratory depression is described as minimal.

At this time many more studies are needed with minaxolone before it can be ascertained what future, if any, the compound has as an intravenous anesthetic. There is some recent data (G. McDowell, personal communication) which indicate that minaxolone may be carcinogenic in animals. If that is documented, it will, unfortunately, end this potentially good anesthetic's clinical possibilities.

CURRENT CLINICAL USES

It is unlikely that Althesin, at least as currently used, i.e., dissolved in Cremphor EL, will ever be released in the United States because of the frequent and severe hypersensitivity reactions described with its use. This is unfortunate because the compound can be used as either a single dose induction agent or as a continuous infusion (with a narcotic analgesic) as a complete anesthetic technique with little alteration in cardiovascular dynamics, rapid recovery, and a low incidence of postoperative nausea and vomiting or venous sequelae. Whether minaxolone, a potential heir apparent as the best steroid anesthetic, will also possess these qualities and not be burdened with a high incidence of hypersensitivity reactions remains to be seen.

OTHER ANESTHETICS

ETOMIDATE

Etomidate (R-(+)-ethyl-1 (pentyethyl)-1H-imidazole-5-carboxylate sulfute) is a new carboxylated imidazole, which was first synthesized in 1965. In animals, etomidate is a potent hypnotic (25 times as potent as thiopental) with a wide margin of safety.[193, 194] Clinically, etomidate results in a rapid induction of anesthesia with minimal cardiovascular and respiratory changes.[195–199] The compound has been extensively studied in Europe and is undergoing clinical trial in the United States. Preparations are taking place to have the compound released into the United States as an intravenous induction

ETOMIDATE

agent and as a hypnotic supplement during intravenous and/or inhalation anesthesia.

CENTRAL NERVOUS SYSTEM ACTIONS

Etomidate does not produce analgesia but a number of experiments have presented evidence that the compound has a depressant action on the brain stem reticular formation.[193, 194, 200–202] Evans and Hill[201] showed in in vitro and in vivo experiments that etomidate produces a central depressant effect by a gamma-aminobutyric acid (GABA) mimetic action. They also showed that etomidate could be antagonized by GABA antagonists.[201] The influence and importance of GABA in central synaptic transmission is discussed elsewhere in this book. Briefly, GABA is an important central transmitter that may play an important role in awareness as well as muscle tone and control. Etomidate may also interact at GABA receptors in the cerebellar cortex and the basal ganglia.[202]

Etomidate decreases cerebral oxygen consumption, cerebral blood flow, and intracranial pressure.[203, 204] Preliminary work undertaken at Janssen Laboratories (A. Wauquien, unpublished data) suggest that etomidate protects transiently ischemic rat brains by prolonging the period of time circulation may be stopped before irreversible brain damage occurs and is an effective anticonvulsant. The latter findings have been confirmed in man (B. Cohn, personal communication).

Etomidate induces hypnosis a little slower than thiopental but within 1 minute all patients given 300 μg/kg are unconscious.[195–199, 205] The duration of the hypnotic effect of etomidate is dose dependent, the duration being doubled when the dose is doubled. Recovery following a single dose of etomidate is also rapid; approximately 2 to 3 minutes following induction of anesthesia with 300 μg/kg all patients are responsive. When compared to other intravenous anesthetics, recovery after etomidate appears to be slower than after propanidid but faster than that after thiopental.[195] However, like the duration of the hypnotic effect, recovery after etomidate is directly related to dosage.[193, 194, 205]

EEG changes after etomidate are similar to those after thiopental and, like those after thiopental, are dependent on the dose injection rate and the use of other compounds.[196, 197] While myoclomia and dyskinesia are sometimes seen after etomidate, they are not associated with epileptogenic or convulsant EEG changes. This suggests that etomidate's hypnotic effect is primarily related to depression of neocortical structures. Combinations of benzodiazepines or narcotics with etomidate suppress the motor phenomena sometimes seen after its administration but prolong the anesthesia and potentiate the EEG signs of depression[207] (H. Stoeckel, personal communication).

Etomidate (60 mg administered at a rate of 2 to 3 mg/min) decreases cerebral blood flow (mean decrease is 34 percent) and cerebral oxygen consumption (mean decrease 45 percent) in man.[203] These changes are similar to those found after comparable doses of thiopental and suggest that the compound may be useful in patients with increased intracranial pressure. A recent report demonstrates that etomidate significantly decreases intracranial pressure without changing cerebral perfusion pressure in patients with intracranial lesions.[204]

Cardiovascular Actions

In dogs, anesthetic doses of etomidate produce small decreases in aortic blood pressure and total peripheral vascular resistance.[194, 195, 205–207] Cardiac contractility is unchanged or slightly decreased and heart rate, cardiac output, and stroke volume are unchanged or somewhat increased by etomidate. Central venous pressure and myocardial oxygen uptake are unchanged following etomidate in dogs, while pulmonary artery and left ventricular end-diastolic pressures are transiently increased.

In patients without cardiopulmonary disease, etomidate (300 μg/kg) does not significantly change heart rate, stroke volume, or cardiac output but does decrease mean arterial blood pressure (15 percent), peripheral vascular resistance (17 percent), left ventricular max dp/dt, and calculated myocardial oxygen consumption (14 percent).[208] Similar findings have been reported following a similar dosage of etomidate in patients with significant cardiovascular disease.[197] These data suggest that etomidate may be of value as an induction agent in patients with little or no cardiac reserve. Cardiovascular changes associated with a continued etomidate infusion have not been adequately studied but are said to be similar to those following a single (bolus) injection[209] (P. Janssen, personal communication).

Respiratory Actions

Etomidate (0.3 mg/kg) decreases tidal volume (26 percent) and minute ventilation (21 percent) but increases respiratory rate (13 percent). On occasion, especially in the geriatric population, etomidate causes a transient (15 to 30 second) period of apnea.[210] The respiratory effects of a single dose of etomidate are transient, lasting 3 to 5 minutes, but usually result in a small, approximately 10 torr, decrease in PaO_2 in patients breathing room air.[210–212] The effects of a continuous infusion of etomidate on respiratory dynamics have not been carefully studied. However, Kalenda[213] suggests that when an induction dose of etomidate is given before fentanyl-N_2O anesthesia, postoperative respiratory depression can occasionally occur. This indicates that use of continuous etomidate infusions may also result in respiration depression when used in combination with narcotic supplements. Etomidate's influence on airway mechanics and ventilation/perfusion relations have not been evaluated following bolus doses or continuous infusions.

OTHER ACTIONS

Toxicology and teratology studies have demonstrated that etomidate produces little alteration of hepatic, renal, or hematologic function after daily administration of an anesthetic dose to dogs for 3 weeks.[205] Similar studies in man as well as etomidate's effects on the neuromuscular system have yet to be done.

Etomidate results in a high incidence of pain on injection (30 to 80 percent) and involuntary muscle movements (10 to 60 percent).[198,199,201] Nausea and vomiting can occur postoperatively after etomidate (as high as 30 percent in one study) and cough and hiccup on occasion (10 percent) during induction.[198] Preparation of etomidate in propylene glycol instead of an aqueous solution has reduced the incidence of pain on injection but not that of muscle movements.[207,209] Pain on injection can be further decreased by premedication or pretreatment of the vein with a narcotic (e.g., fentanyl 50 to 100 μg intravenously immediately before etomidate decreases the incidence of pain to 10 percent) or by selection of a large (ante cubital) vein.[209] Hypersensitivity to etomidate is rare.[205] Etomidate results in no detrimental effects when injected intra-arterially.[214]

PHARMACOKINETICS

Maximal blood levels of etomidate occur within 1 minute following injection of a bolus of the drug but decrease rapidly thereafter.[193,194,205,215,216] Uptake of the drug into the brain and other highly vascularized tissues (lung, kidney, muscle, heart, and spleen) occurs in spite of the fact that approximately 65 percent of etomidate is bound to plasma proteins. Because it is lipid soluble and soluble in the acid medium of the stomach, a slower uptake of etomidate occurs in fat and the stomach, with a maximal concentration in these organs occurring at 10 to 25 minutes after injection.

Etomidate is rapidly metabolized, mostly by hepatic cells, via hydrolysis of the ester group to the carboxylic acid of the drug. This metabolite is inactive. In man approximately 75 percent of administered etomidate is excreted in urine and 13 percent in feces in the first 24 hours after administration.

CURRENT CLINICAL USAGE

Etomidate has been used for a number of years in Europe as an induction agent because of its rapid onset of action, benign cardiovascular and respiratory actions, and short duration of action. More recently it is gaining popularity as the hypnotic component of a totally intravenous technique consisting of a continuous infusion of etomidate with intermittent injections of a short-acting narcotic (fentanyl and, most recently, afentanyl). Etomidate is particularly useful as a continuous infusion in elderly, sick patients and in outpatient surgery (A. Doenicke, personal communication). Discovery of etomidate's ability to decrease cerebral blood flow, cerebral metabolic rate, and intracranial pressure has indicated that the drug might be beneficial to neurosurgical patients and to those with potential or real brain injury. There are also reports (B. Cohn and B. S. Meldrum, personal communications) that etomidate is of value as an antiepileptic in status epilepticus. Unfortunately, pain on intravenous administration, which can be decreased but not eliminated with fentanyl pretreatment, and muscle movements occur with initial injection. It is said by European investigators (A. Doenicke and H. Stoeckel, personal communication) that these are not serious problems. Whether they will or will not prove to be serious problems in the United States remains to be seen. Attempts are being made to have etomidate available for use in the United States in the 1980's.

KETAMINE

Ketamine, 2-(O-chlorophenyl)-2-(methylamino)cyclohexanone HCl, was first synthesized by Stevens in 1963.[217] Ketamine has an asymmetric carbon (the hexamone carbon attached to nitrogen) and therefore exists as two isomers.[218,219] The dextrorotatory isomer is the more potent of the two isomers and produces less central nervous system and cardiovascular stimulation. Ketamine is a water soluble white crystal that, in an aqueous solution, has a pH between 3.5 to 5.5.[220]

KETAMINE

Central Nervous System Actions

Ketamine produces a state of unconsciousness described as dissociative anesthesia.[221] Patients appear cataleptic and have intense analgesia (which lasts into the postoperative period) and amnesia but appear to be only mildly sedated. Following intravenous administration of a usual anesthetic dose of ketamine, onset of unconsciousness takes from 20 to 60 seconds.[222] Defining onset time is often difficult, particularly after slow injection of ketamine, because the patients begin to gaze into space. Eyelash, corneal, and laryngeal reflexes are usually depressed and muscle tone is increased. Frequently, involuntary muscle movements and, occasionally, verbalization, all especially with surgical

stimulus, occur although patients are amnesic. In contrast to most of the intravenous anesthetics, premedication does not influence the magnitude of incidence of excitatory phenomena following ketamine.[220] Rarely do the excitatory phenomena present an anesthetic problem (i.e., result in respiratory obstruction) but when the problem does occur, surgery is often difficult.

In anesthetic doses, ketamine changes conscious alpha EEG rhythm to one composed primarily of theta waves and on occasion, bursts of delta activity.[223] Onset of delta activity coincides with loss of consciousness. Ketamine markedly alters visual and auditory evoked EEG responses.[217]

Detailed EEG studies suggest that ketamine produces a functional dissociation between the limbic and thalamoneocortical systems.[224] Corssen et al.[224] have demonstrated thalamoneocortical depression before limbic and reticular activating system depression. Whether any of the above EEG changes are the reason why ketamine often produces bizarre, frequently frightening dreams and visual disturbances is unclear. Pretreatment of patients with diazepam (0.2 mg/kg, IV) or treatment with 5 to 10 mg of diazepam just prior to termination of a ketamine anesthetic significantly decreases these psychic sequelae but does not eliminate them.[217,218]

Recovery from a single dose (2 mg/kg) of ketamine occurs in about 10 to 15 minutes.[220] Recovery after multiple injections is slower and following mixtures of ketamine and the benzodiazepines, butyrophenones, or other intravenous compounds is still slower.[217,225] Diplopia and other visual disturbances frequently persist or present for the first time on recovery and are disturbing. For this reason many clinicians advocate minimal vocal and visual contacts with patients during this interval.[220,222]

In contrast to the barbiturates, Althesin, and etomidate, ketamine (2 mg/kg) increases cerebral blood flow (80 percent), cerebral oxygen consumption (16 percent), and intracranial pressure (a variable amount depending on a variety of circumstances).[226] It is, therefore, potentially dangerous to use ketamine when patients have a raised intracranial pressure (see Ch. 33).

CARDIOVASCULAR ACTIONS

Ketamine, besides being a powerful analgesic, is the only intravenous anesthetic that routinely produces cardiovascular stimulation.[221] Heart rate, arterial blood pressure, and cardiac output are usually significantly increased.[217,220] The peak increases in these variables occur between 2 and 4 minutes after an intravenous injection and then slowly decline to normal over the next 10 to 20 minutes. The magnitude of tachycardia and hypertension are variable for reasons that are unknown. Other anesthetics may inhibit these responses.[227,228] Use of ketamine during potent inhalation anesthesia renders the compound a severe cardiovascular depressant. One reason for this may be that ketamine has a negative direct effect on the myocardium.[229,230] For cardiovascular stimulation to occur following ketamine, significant CNS depression must not already be present. Cardiovascular stimulation also is dependent on an intact, peripheral sympathetic nervous system.[231–233] This suggests that ketamine produces its cardiovascular stimulation via excitation of the central sympathetic apparatus. Evidence supporting ketamine's central sympathetic stimulating action includes the ability of halothane, high epidural anesthesia, hexamethonium, and phentolamine to prevent ketamine-induced hypertension and tachycardia.[227,228,231–233]

Increases in plasma epinephrine and norepinephrine occur, as early as two minutes, after intravenous ketamine[217] and return to control levels 15 minutes later. Perhaps ketamine has a cocaine-like action on adrenergic nerve terminals (that is, prevention of norepinephrine re-uptake).[235] Pretreatment with diazepam (0.2 mg/kg IV) immediately before ketamine prevents cardiovascular stimulation as well as increases in plasma catecholamines.[217] Indeed, arterial blood pressure, heart rate, and plasma catecholamines remain unchanged after injection of this combination. Similar protection against the cardiostimulatory effects of ketamine has been found by Bidwai (unpublished data), via prior or simultaneous administration of methohexital (1.0 to 1.5 mg/kg). The mechanism, or mechanisms, involved in the protective effects of these compounds is unknown but may be related to central sympathetic depression, as suggested above.

Dowdy and Daya[229] suggested a peripheral mechanism for the cardiovascular stimulation seen after ketamine. They showed that the drug desensitizes arterial baroreceptors. This reduces any negative feedback mechanisms on the vasomotor center and should promote hypertension and tachycardia. It is unclear whether baroreceptor desensitization or sympathetic stimulation is most responsible for the cardiovascular effects seen after ketamine.

Ketamine has been shown to have some antiarrhythmic properties, although it is rarely used for this purpose clinically.[229,230] Ketamine has been recommended as an anesthetic for patients with cardiac disease undergoing open heart surgery.[217,235,236] Some of these attempts have employed ketamine alone and others combinations of ketamine with diazepam. It appears clear to me that if ketamine can be administered in a way that prevents undue cardiovascular stimulation or depression, it may have great uses in these patients. On the other hand, the impressive cardiostimulatory effects of ketamine when used alone (which dramatically increase myocardial oxygen consumption) and occasional marked depression seen when the compound is used in combination with some central depressants, suggests caution. The same may not be so for patients in shock presenting for emergency surgery.[237] In this situation, ketamine's cardiostimulatory actions are generally of great advantage and because of this reason the compound has achieved a reasonable degree of popularity as an induction agent for patients in shock.

RESPIRATORY ACTIONS

In most patients ketamine slightly decreases respiratory rate for about 2 to 3 minutes.[220,238] On occasion, however, especially after narcotic premedication and/or rapid intravenous administration, ketamine can cause apnea.[238] Usually $PaCO_2$ is either unchanged or increased 2 or 3 torr after ketamine. Upper airway muscle tone is well maintained and upper airway reflexes are usually, but not always, active.[239] Because of the above, many clinicians have been tempted to use ketamine anesthesia without an endotracheal tube in spontaneously breathing patients who have a full stomach. A number of studies have shown that ketamine *does not* prevent aspiration in these situations.[239,240] Therefore, ketamine anesthesia clearly does not preclude use of an endotracheal tube in patients who may or do have a full stomach and a good chance of vomiting.

Small doses of diazepam (0.2 mg/kg) given before or during ketamine anesthesia have little effect on respiration. However, larger doses can produce profound and prolonged respiratory depression.[217,220] Ketamine dilates the bronchial tree and can antagonize the bronchoconstrictive actions of histamine, acetylcholine, and 5-hydroxytryptamine on the trachea and bronchi.[241] Ketamine has also been suggested as an ideal agent for patients with asthma.[242] Additional clinical work needs to be done before its use in this setting will be accepted.

OTHER EFFECTS

Ketamine produces little change in hepatic or renal function.[221,223] The duration of apnea and respiratory depression after suc-

cinylcholine (50 mg, IV) is significantly greater after ketamine than after thiopental[222] and may be secondary to the ability of ketamine to inhibit pseudocholinesterase activity.[243] There is one report that indicates that ketamine reduces requirements for *d*-tubocurarine.[244] This may be due to the reduced sensitivity of the postjunctional membrane to acetylcholine in the presence of ketamine.[245]

Ketamine does not increase plasma histamine concentrations and rarely causes a hypersensitivity response.[220] Some patients do sustain an erythematous rash early after its intravenous administration.

Following minor operations, ketamine may be associated with a somewhat increased incidence of nausea and vomiting than thiopental anesthesia.[246] In my experience, this also occurs when ketamine is used with nitrous oxide, diazepam, or narcotics for longer operations.

Ketamine crosses the placenta and can increase fetal muscle tone but it does not decrease uterine tone and has been found useful in low doses as an analgesic in caesarean section operations.[247]

METABOLISM

The metabolism of ketamine is complex. The drug is rapidly metabolized to norketamine (demethylated ketamine) in the liver via the hepatic P 450 microsomal system.[217] This compound can then undergo hydroxylation, dehydration, or both to form at least three other metabolites. Alternatively, ketamine may undergo direct hydroxylation of its cyclohexylamine ring in at least two sites. All of the metabolites are usually conjugated and most excreted in both urine and feces.

Ketamine reduces the MAC of halothane for several hours probably because of its high lipid solubility and conversion of ketamine to metabolite I, which possesses weak anesthetic properties.[248] Conversely, halothane prolongs the effect of ketamine by decreasing its uptake, distribution, redistribution, and metabolism.[248]

CURRENT CLINICAL USAGE

Ketamine has become extremely popular for burn patients, especially those requiring daily extensive dressing changes who have involvement of the face and hands such that airway manipulations and intravenous administrations of any compound is difficult.[220] In these situations ketamine can be administered intramuscularly (8 mg/kg) with an onset time only slightly higher than that following intravenous administration.[211, 220] Airway management is usually not a problem because essentially normal spontaneous respiration is maintained. While it is often difficult in these patients to monitor arterial blood pressure (a leg pressure cuff can be used), EKG and pulse can usually be obtained and are most often adequate monitors of the circulation because cardiovascular depression is quite rare.

As mentioned before, ketamine is also popular for induction of anesthesia in patients in shock and in poor risk geriatric patients because of its cardiostimulatory properties. Because of its rapid onset of action, ketamine is used as an intramuscular induction agent in children and in mentally retarded adult patients who may be difficult to manage.

Because of its high incidence of postoperative psychic phenomena, caution must be exercised in the use of ketamine for routine operative procedures where other anesthetic techniques may be equally as good.[220] However, if the uses of combinations of ketamine and diazepam or other compounds dramatically reduce the incidence of these problems, as the proponents of this technique suggest,[217] then this may no longer be an important problem.

Ketamine, alone, may be contraindicated in patients with severe hypertension, ischemic myocardial disease, and increased intracranial pressure. Ketamine should not be given when increases in heart rate, arterial blood pressure, cardiac output, intracranial pressure, cerebral blood flow, or cerebral metabolism are contraindicated. Ketamine, because it does not necessarily depress tracheal-laryngeal reflexes, is probably not a good agent to use in operations on the pharynx or larynx.

PROCAINE

Although extensively studied a number of years ago in the United States,[249–251] intravenous procaine has not achieved wide success as an anesthetic in the United States or Europe.[252] It has achieved wide success, however, in South America.[252] Advantages claimed for this technique include fast induction and recovery times, little influence on cardiorespiratory function, stability of cardiovascular dynamics during a variety of surgical stresses, residual postoperative analgesia, economy, easy supplementation with other agents, a paucity of nausea and vomiting, and absence of venous thrombotic effects.[252] Unfortunately, intravenous procaine must be used with other intravenous (e.g., thiopental and diazepam) and inhalation (e.g., nitrous oxide) anesthetics in order to insure surgical stability and hypnosis and avoid CNS excitatory actions (convulsions); its use must be avoided in patients with atrioventricular or intraventricular conduction defects or a history of epilepsy.[252]

The rationale that allows procaine to be used as an intravenous anesthetic is dependent on data indicating that the analgesic dose of the compound is one half of the convulsive dose and that when induction is carried out with thiopental (4 mg/kg, IV) the analgesic dose is one third of the convulsive dose. Induction is usually carried out in a standard fashion with conventional doses of diazepam or thiopental intravenously, followed by the intravenous administration of succinylcholine and endotracheal intubation.[252] Maintenance anesthesia is achieved with a 1 percent procaine infusion administered at a rate of 3 to 5 mg/kg/min supplemented with nitrous oxide (65 percent) in oxygen and often intermittent intravenous doses of meperidine and fentanyl. With signs of anesthetic lightness, the procaine infusion rate is increased. Usual doses of nondepolarizing muscle relaxants are required for muscle relaxation.

Although procaine does have good analgesic properties, the margin of safety in using the compound as the principal anesthetic is extremely narrow. When used as described above, there is little doubt that the need for narcotics and other supplements are significantly decreased. Thus, procaine may have use as a supplement during a variety of balanced anesthetic techniques. However, considering the serious problems that can and do occasionally arise (e.g., ventricular depression and convulsions) it is probably wisest to use procaine to supplement other analgesics (e.g., narcotics and nitrous oxide) rather than as the primary analgesic compound.

REFERENCES

1. Dundee JW, Wyant GM: Intravenous Anesthesia. Edinburgh, Churchill Livingstone, 1974, pp 1–5

2. Dundee JW, Wyant GM: Intravenous Anesthesia. Edinburgh, Churchill Livingstone, 1974, pp 23–63

3. Dundee JW, Barron DW: The barbiturates. Br J Anaesth 34:240, 1962

4. Dundee JW, Barron DW, King R: The effect of methylation on the anaesthetic action of ethyl-methyl-propyl-thiobarbiturate. Br J Anaesth 32:566, 1960

5. Dundee JW, Riding JE: A comparison of inactin and thiopentone as intravenous anaesthetics. Br J Anaesth 32:206, 1960

6. Maynert EW, Van Dyke HB: The absence of localization of barbital in divisions of the central nervous system. J Pharmacol Exp Ther 98:184, 1950

7. Donek, NS, Barlow CF, Roth LJ: An ontogenetic study of phenobarbital-C^{14} in cat brain. J Pharmacol Exp Ther 130:285, 1960

8. Dundee JW, Wyant GM: Intravenous Anesthesia. Edinburgh, Churchill Livingstone, 1974, pp 64–127

9. Aldridge WN: Action of barbiturates upon respiratory enzymes, Enzymes and Drug Action, Edited by Mongar JL, de Reuck AVS. Edinburgh, J & A Churchill, 1962, p 155

10. Brody TM, Bain JA: Effects of barbiturates on oxidative phosphorylation. Proc Soc Exp Biol Med 77:50, 1951

11. McLennan H, Elliott KAC: Effects of convulsant and narcotic drugs on acetylcholine synthesis. J Pharmacol Exp Ther 103:35, 1951

12. Kini MM, Quastel JH: Carbohydrate-amino acid interrelation in brain cortex in vitro. Nature (London) 184:252, 1959

13. Etsten B, Himwich HE: Stages and signs of pentothal anesthesia: Physiologic basis. Anesthesiology 7:536, 1946

14. Dundee JW: Alterations in response to somatic pain associated with anaesthesia. II: The effect of thiopentone and pentobarbitone. Br J Anaesth 32:407, 1960

15. Clutton-Brock J: Pain and the barbiturates. Anaesthesia 16:80, 1961

16. Robson JG, Davenport HT, Sugiyama R: Differentiation of two types of pain by anesthetics. Anesthesiology 26:31, 1965

17. Schmidt CF, Kety SS, Pennes HH: The gaseous metabolism of the brain and monkey. Am J Physiol 143:33, 1945

18. Pierce EC, Lambertsen CJ, Deutsch S, et al: Cerebral circulation and metabolism during thiopental anesthesia and hyperventilation in man. J Clin Invest 41:1664, 1962

19. Wechsler RL, Dripps RD, Kety SS: Blood flow and oxygen consumption of the human brain during anesthesia produced by thiopental. Anesthesiology 12:308, 1951

20. Conway CM, Ellis DB: The haemodynamic effects of short acting barbiturates. Br J Anaesth 41:534, 1969

21. Richards RK, Taylor JD: Some factors influencing distribution, metabolism and action of barbiturates: A review. Anesthesiology 17:414, 1956

22. Tabern DL, Volwiler EH: Sulfur-containing

barbiturate hypnotics. J Amer Chem Soc 57:1961, 1935

23. Lundy JS: Intravenous anesthesia: Preliminary report of the use of two new thiobarbiturates. Proc Mayo Clin 10:536, 1935

24. Brodie BB: Physiological disposition and chemical fate of thiobarbiturates in the body. Fed Proc 11:632, 1952

25. Goldbaum LR, Smith PK: The interaction of barbiturates with serum albumin and its possible relation to their disposition and pharmacological actions. J Pharmacol Exp Ther 111:197, 1954

26. Mark LC: Thiobarbiturates, Uptake and Distribution of Anesthetic Agents. Edited by Papper EM, Kitz RJ. New York, McGraw-Hill, 1963, pp 289–301

27. Price HL, Kovnat PJ, Safer JN, et al: The uptake of thiopental by body tissues and its relation to the duration of narcosis. Clin Pharmacol Ther 1:16, 1960

28. Price HL: A dynamic concept of the distribution of thiopental in the human body. Anesthesiology 21:40, 1960

29. Dundee JW, Price HL, Dripps RD: Acute tolerance to thiopental in man. Br J Anaesth 28:344, 1956

30. Mark LC, Brand L, Kamvyssi S, et al: Thiopental metabolism by human liver in vivo and in vitro. Nature 206:1117, 1965

31. Gruber CM, Baskett RF: The points of action of sodium phenobarbital and phenobarbital in lowering blood pressure. J Lab Clin Med 10:630, 1924

32. Gruber CM: The effect of anesthetic doses of sodium thiopental, sodium thio-ethamyl and pentothal sodium upon the respiratory system, the heart and blood pressure in experimental animals. J Pharmacol Exp Ther 60:143, 1937

33. Das SC: The influence of sodium evipan on the heart and circulation. Q J Exp Physiol 31:103, 1942

34. Fieldman EJ, Ridley RW, Wood EH: Hemodynamic studies during thiopental sodium and nitrous oxide anesthesia in humans. Anesthesiology 16:473, 1955

35. Johnson SR: The effect of some anaesthetic agents on the circulation in man. Acta Chir Scand 101 (suppl 158):501, 1951

36. Etsten B, Li TH: Hemodynamic changes during thiopental anesthesia in humans. Cardiac output, stroke volume, total peripheral resistance and intra-throracic blood volume. J Clin Invest 34:500, 1955

37. Eckstein JW, Hamilton WK, Mc Cammond JM: The effect of thiopental on peripheral venous tone. Anesthesiology 22:525, 1961

38. Skovsted P, Price ML, Price HL: The effect of short acting barbiturates on arterial pressure, preganglionic sympathetic activity and barostatic reflexes. Anesthesiology 33:10, 1970

39. Sonntag H, Hellberg K, Schenk H-D, et al: Effects of thiopental (Trapanal®) on coronary blood flow and myocardial metabolism in man. Acta Anaesthesiol Scand 19:69, 1975

40. Sankawa H: Cardiovascular effects of propanidid and methohexital sodium in dogs. Acta Anaesthesiol Scand (suppl) 17:55, 1965

41. Elder JD Jr, Nagano SM, Eastwood DW, et al: Circulatory changes associated with thiopental anesthesia in man. Anesthesiology 16:394, 1955

42. Irwin S, Stagg RD, Dunbar E, et al: Methitural a new intravenous anesthetic: Comparison with thiopental in the cat, dog, and monkey. J Pharmacol Exp Ther 116:317, 1956

43. Volpitto PP, Marangoni BA: Electrocardiographic studies during anesthesia with intravenous barbiturates. J Lab Clin Med 23:575, 1937

44. Woods LA, Wyngaarden JB, Rennick B, et al: Cardiovascular toxicity of thiobarbiturates: Comparison of thiopental and 5-allyl-5-(1 methyl)butyl-2-barbiturates (surital) in dogs. J Pharmacol Exp Ther 95:328, 1949

45. Eckenhoff JE, Helrich M: Study of narcotics and sedatives for use in preanesthetic medication. JAMA 167:415, 1958

46. Patrick RT, Faulconer AJ: Respiratory studies during anesthesia with ether and with pentothal sodium. Anesthesiology 13:252, 1952

47. Adriani J, Rovenstine EA: The effect of anesthetic drugs upon bronchi and bronchioles of excised lung tissue. Anesthesiology 4:253, 1943

48. Harrison GA: The influence of different anesthetic agents on the response to respiratory tract irritation. Br J Anaesth 34:804, 1962

49. Habif DV, Papper EM, Fitzpatrick HF, et al: The renal and hepatic blood flow, glomerular filtration rate, and urinary output of electrolytes during cyclopropane, ether and thio-

pental anesthesia, operation, and the immediate postoperative period. Surgery 30:241, 1951

50. Shackman R, Graber IG, Melrose DG: Liver blood flow and general anaesthesia. Clin Sci 12:307, 1953

51. Levy ML, Palazzi HM, Nardi GL, et al: Hepatic blood flow variations during surgical anesthesia in man measured by radioactive colloid. Surg Gyn Obst 112:289, 1961

52. Epstein RM, Wheeler HO, Frumin MJ, et al: The effect of hypercapnia on estimated hepatic blood flow, circulating splanchnic volume and hepatic sulfobromophithalein clearance during general anesthesia in man. J Clin Invest 40:592, 1961

53. Booker WM, Maloney AH, Tureman JR et al: Some metabolic factors influencing the course of thiopental anesthesia in dogs. Am J Physiol 170:168, 1952

54. Walton CH, Saldamando J, Egner WM: The effect of intravenous pentothal sodium with or without inhalation of oxygen on liver function. Anesthesiology 12:67, 1951

55. Dundee JW: Thiopentone as a factor in the production of liver dysfunction. Br J Anaesth 27:14, 1955

56. Clarke RSJ, Kirwan MJ, Dundee SW, et al: Clinical studies of induction agents. XIII: Liver function after propanidid and thiopentone anesthesia. Br J Anaesth 37:415, 1965

57. Dunkin LJ: Methohexitone in the management of a disturbed patient: A case report. Br J Anaesth 44:971, 1972

58. Maloney AH, Booker WM, Tureman JR, et al: Studies on renal function during various states of anesthesia produced by thiopental in dogs. Fed Proc 9:299, 1950

59. Secher O: Pilot investigation into the peripheral action of anaesthetics. Acta Pharmacol Toxicol 7:231, 1951

60. Craig HGL: The protective effect of thiopentone against muscular pain and stiffness which follows the use of suxamethonium chloride. Br J Anaesth 36:612, 1964

61. Gruber CM, Bruber Cm Jr: Effect of barbituric and thiobarbituric acid derivatives on pyloric sphincter and stomach in unanesthetized dogs. J Pharmacol Exp Ther 72:176, 1941

62. Taylor C, Stoelting VK: Methohexital sodium—A new ultra short-acting barbiturate. Anesthesiology 21:29, 1960

63. O'Donnell JF, Hewitt JC, Dundee JW: Clinical studies of induction agents. XXVIII: A further comparison of venous complications following thiopentone, methohexitone and propanidid. Br J Anaesth 41:681, 1969

64. Miller JR, Stoelting VK: A preliminary communication of the sleep producing effect of intramuscular methohexitone sodium in the pediatric patient. Br J Anaesth 35:48, 1963

65. Guerra F: Thiopental forever after, Trends in Intravenous Anesthesia. Edited by Aldrete JA, Stanley TH. Chicago, Year Book Medical Publishers, 1980, pp 143–150

66. Stone HH, Donnelly CC: The accidental intra-arterial injection of thiopental. Anesthesiology 22:995, 1961

67. Macintosh RR, Heyworth PSA, Elliot KAC: Intra-arterial injection of pentothal. Lancet 2:571, 1943

68. Burn JH, Hobbs R: Mechanism of arterial spasm following intra-arterial injection of thiopentone. Lancet 1, 1112, 1959

69. Burn JH: Why thiopoentone injected into an artery may cause gangrene. Br Med J 2:414, 1960

70. Waters DJ: Intra-arterial thiopentone (a physico-chemical phenomenon). Anaesthesia 21:346, 1966

71. Brown SS, Lyons SM, Dundee JW: Intra-arterial barbiturates: A study of some factors leading to intravascular thrombosis. Br J Anaesth 40:13, 1968

72. Dundee JW: Some effects of premedication on the induction characteristics of intravenous anaesthetics. Anaesthesia 20:299, 1965

73. Barron DW: Effect of rate of injection on incidence of side effects with thiopental and methohexital. Anesth Analg 47:171, 1968

74. Hayward JR, Kiester GL: Severe allergic reactions during thiopental sodium anaesthesia: Report of a case. J Oral Surg 15:61, 1957

75. Eales L, Dowdle EB: Clinical aspects of importance in the porphyrias. Br J Clin Pract 22:505, 1968

76. Eales L: Porphyria and thiopentone. Anesthesiology 27:703, 1966

77. Greenblatt DJ, Shader RI: Benzodiazepines. N Engl J Med 291:1011, 1239, 1974

78. Dundee JW: Benzodiazepines in anesthesia, Trends in Intravenous Anesthesia. Edited by

Aldrete JA, Stanley TH. Chicago, Year Book Medical Publishers, 1980, pp 219–234

79. Dundee JW: Wyant GM: Intravenous Anesthesia. Edinburgh, Churchill Livingstone, 1974, pp 249–273

80. Hegarty JE, Dundee JW: Sequelae after the intravenous injection of three benzodiazepines—diazepam, lorazepam and flunitrozepam. Br Med J 2:1384, 1977

81. Reves JG, Corssen G, Halcomb C: Comparison of two benzodiazepines for anesthetic induction: Midazolam and diazepam. Can Anaesth Soc J 25:211, 1978

82. Brown SS, Dundee JW: Clinical studies of induction agents. XXV: Diazepam. Br J Anaesth 40:108, 1968

83. Dundee JW, Haslett WHK, Keilty SR, et al: Studies of drugs given before anaesthesia. XX: Diazepam-containing mixtures. Br J Anaesth 42:143, 1970

84. Randall LO, Scheckel CL, Poole W: Pharmacology of medazepam and metabolites. Arch Int Pharmacodyn Ther 185:135, 1970

85. Ngai AH, Tseng DTC, Wang SC: Effect of diazepam and other central nervous system depressants on spinal reflexes in cats: A study of site of action. J Pharmacol Exp Ther 153:344, 1966

86. Himwich HE, Morillo A, Steiner WG: Drugs affecting rhinocephalic structures. J Neuropsych 4 (suppl 1): 15, 1962

87. Stanley TH, Bennett GM, Loeser EA, et al: Cardiovascular effects of diazepam and droperidol during morphine anesthesia. Anesthesiology 44:255, 1976

88. Stanley TH, Webster LR: Anesthetic requirements and cardiovascular effects of fentanyl-oxygen and fentanyl-diazepam-oxygen anesthesia in man. Anesth Analg 57:411, 1978

89. Brown PRH, Main DMG, Lawson JIM: Diazepam in dentistry. Report on 108 patients. Br Dent J 125:498, 1968

90. Pandit SK, Dundee JW: Preoperative amnesia: The incidence following the intramuscular injection of commonly used premedicants. Anaesthesia 25:493, 1970

91. Pandit SK: Antegrade amnesia effections of diazepam, hycosine, and pethidine. Postgrad Inst Med Ed & Res (Chandigarh) 4:151, 1970

92. George KA, Dundee JW: Relative amnesic actions of diazepam, flunitrazepam and lorazepam in man. Br J Clin Pharmacol 4:45, 1977

93. Baird ES, Hailey DM: Plasma levels of diazepam and its major metabolite following intramuscular administration. Br J Anaesth 45:546, 1973

94. Van der Klein E, Van Rossum JM, Muskens ETJM, et al: Pharmacokinetics of diazepam in dogs, mice and humans. Acta Pharmacol Toxicol 29 (suppl 3): 109, 1971

95. Andreasen PB, Hendel J, Greisen G, et al: Pharmacokinetics of diazepam in disordered liver function. Eur J Clin Pharmacol 10:115, 1976

96. Klotz U, Avant GR, Hoyumpa A, et al: The effects of age and liver disease on the disposition and elimination of diazepam in adult man. J Clin Invest 55:347, 1975

97. De Silva JAF, D'Aconte L, Kaplan L: The determination of blood levels and placental transfer of diazepam in humans. Curr Ther Res 6:115, 1964

98. Dawes GS: The distribution and action of drugs on the fetus in utero. Br J Anaesth 45:766, 1973

99. Idanpaan-Heikkila HJE, Jouppila PI, Puoluakka JO et al: Placental transfer and fetal metabolism of diazepam in early human pregnancy. Am J Obstet Gynecol 109:1011, 1971

100. Abel RM, Staroscik RN, Reis RL: The effects of diazepam (Valium) on left ventricular function and systemic vascular resistance. J Pharmacol Exp Ther 173:364, 1970

101. Rao S, Sherbaniuk RW, Prasad K, et al: Cardiopulmonary effects of diazepam. Clin Pharmacol Ther 14:182, 1973

102. Randall LO, Heise GA, Schallek W, et al: Pharmacological and clinical studies on Valium, a new psychotherapeutic agent of the benzodiazepine class. Curr Ther Res 3:405, 1961

103. Nutter DO, Massumi RA: Diazepam in cardioversion. N Engl J Med 273:650, 1965

104. Stovner J, Endresen R: Intravenous anaesthesia with diazepam. Proc 2nd Eur Cong Anesth. Acta Anaesthesiol Scand (suppl) 24:223, 1966

105. Knapp RB, Dubow H: Comparison of diazepam with thiopental as an induction agent in cardiopulmonary disease. Anesth Analg 49:722, 1970

106. Reves JG, Samuelson PN, Lunnan M: Effects of midazolam maleate in patients with elevated pulmonary artery occluded pressure, Trends in Intravenous Anesthesia. Edited by Aldrete JA, Stanley TH. Chicago, Year Book Medical Publishers, 1980, pp 253–257

107. Ikran H, Rubin AP, Jewkes RF: Effect of diazepam on myocardial blood flow of patients with and without coronary artery disease. Br Heart J 35:626, 1973

108. Rollason WN: Diazepam as an intravenous induction agent for general anesthesia, Diazepam In Anesthesia. Edited by Knight PF, Burgess CC. Bristol, Wright, 1968, pp 70–73

109. Barrett JS, Hey EB: Ventricular arrhythmias associated with the use of diazepam for cardioversion. JAMA 214:1323, 1970

110. Liu WS, Bidwai AV, Lunn JK, et al: Urine catecholamine excretion after large doses of fentanyl, fentanyl and diazepam and fentanyl, diazepam and pancuronium. Can Anaesth Soc J 24:371, 1977

111. Sadove MS, Balagot RC, McGrath JM: Effects of chlordiazepam and diazepam on the influence of meperidine on the respiratory response to carbon dioxide. J New Drugs 5:121, 1965

112. Stovner J, Endresen R: Diazepam in intravenous anaesthesia. Lancet 2:1298, 1965

113. Dretchen K, Ghoneim MM, Long JP: The interaction of diazepam with myoneural blocking agents. Anesthesiology 34:463, 1971

114. Webb SN, Bradshaw FG: An investigation, in cats, into the activity of diazepam at the neuromuscular junction. Br J Anaesth 45:313, 1973

115. Graham CW, Conklin KA, Katz RL, et al: A new psychotic agent for women during labor and delivery. Abstracts of Scientific Papers. 1977 ASA meeting, pp 97, 98

116. Bidwai AV, Stanley TH, Roberts C, et al: Reversal of diazepam induced post anesthetic somnolence with physostigmine. Anesthesiology 51:256, 1979

117. Hill GE, Stanley TH, Sentker CR: Physostigmine reversal of postoperative somnolence. Canad Anaesth Soc J 24:707, 1977

118. Holzgrafe RE, Vondrell JJ, Mintz SM: Reversal of postoperative reactions to scopolamine with physostigmine. Anesth Analg 52:921, 1973

119. Morrison JD: Neurolept techniques, Intravenous Anesthesia. Edited by Dundee JW, Wyant GM. Edinburgh, Churchill Livingstone, 1974, pp 207–218

120. De Castro G, Mundeleer P: Anesthesie sans sommeil, "Là neutoleptanalgesia." Acta Chir Belg 58:689, 1959

121. Nilsson E: Origin, rationale, and practical use of neuroleptanalgesia. Irish J Med Sci (series 8) 6:407, 1973

122. Nilsson E, Janssen P: Neuroleptanalgesia, an alternative to general anaesthesia. Acta Anaesthesiol Scand 5:73, 1961

123. Stanley TH: Cardiovascular effects of droperidol during enflurane and enflurane–nitrous oxide anesthesia in man. Can Anaesth Soc J 25:26, 1978

124. Loeser EA, Bennett G, Stanley TH, et al: Comparison of droperidol, haloperridol and prochlorperazine as postoperative anti-emetics. Can Anaesth Soc J 26:125, 1979

125. Janssen PAJ: The pharmacology of haloperidol. Int J Neuropsych 3 (suppl 1): 10, 1967.

126. Wiklund RA, Ngai SH: Rigidity and pulmonary edema after Innovar in a patient on levadopa therapy: Report of a case. Anesthesiology 35:545, 1971

127. Morrison JD, Load WB, Dundee JW: Controlled comparison of the efficacy of fourteen preparations in the relief of postoperative pain. Br Med J 3:287, 1971

128. Larson AG, Durh MB: A new technique for inducing controlled hypotension. Lancet 1:128, 1963

129. Clark MM: Droperidol in pre-operative anxiety. Anaesthesia 24:36, 1969

130. Puddy BR: Effects of droperidol on the vasoconstriction produced by noradrenaline, histamine, sympathetic nerve stimulation and potassium ions in the isolated rabbit auricular artery. Br J Anaesth 43:441, 1971

131. Whitwam JG, Rossel WJ: The acute cardiovascular changes and adrenergic blockade by droperidol in man. Br J Anaesth 43:581, 1971

132. Yelnosky J, Katz R, Dietrich EV: A study of some of the pharmacologic actions of droperidol. Toxicol Appl Pharmacol 6:37, 1964

133. Muldoon SM, Janssens WJ, Verbeuren TJ, et al: Alpha-adrenergic blocking properties of droperidol in isolated blood vessels of the dog. Br J Anaesth 49:211, 1977

134. Lawin P, Herden H, Badran H, et al: Drei Herstillstande bei Einleitung der Neurolept-

analgesia. Typ II Bei vorbehandelten Patienten mit vasodilatorischen Medikamenten. Anaesthetist 15:19, 1966

135. Long D, Dripps RD, Price HL: Measurement of antiarrhythmic potency of drugs in man: Effects of dehydrobenzperidol. Anesthesiology 28:318, 1967

136. Michenfelder JD, Theye RA: Effects of fentanyl, droperidol and Innovar on canine cerebral metabolism and blood flow. Br J Anaesth 43:630, 1971

137. Prys-Roberts C, Kelman GR: The influence of drugs used in neuroleptanalgesia on cardiovascular and ventilatory function. Br J Anaesth 39:134, 1967

138. Tornetta FJ, Boger WP: Liver function studies in droperidol-fentanyl anesthesia. Anesth Analg 43:544, 1964

139. MacDonald HR, Braid DP, Stead BR, et al: Clinical and circulatory effects of neuroleptanalgesia with dehydrobenzperidol and phenoperidine. Br Heart J 28:654, 1966

140. Oyama T, Takiguchi M: Effect of neuroleptanaesthesia on plasma levels of growth hormone and insulin. Br J Anaesth 42:1105, 1970

141. Oyama T, Takiguchi M: Effect of neuroleptanaesthesia on adrenocortical function in man. Br J Anaesth 42:425, 1971

142. Clarke RSJ: The eugenols, Intravenous Anesthesia. Edited by Dundee JW, Wyant GM. Edinburgh, Churchill Livingstone, 1974, pp 162–192

143. Kortilla K: Propanidid and althesin, Trends in Intravenous Anesthesia. Edited by Aldrete JA, Stanley TH, Chicago, Year Book Medical Publishers, 1980, pp 153–171

144. Wirth W, Hoffmeister F: Pharmakologische Untersuchungen mit Propanidid (3-Methoxy-4-(N,N-diathylcarbamoyl-methoxy)-phenylessigsaure-n-propylester), Die intravenose Kurznarkose mit dem neuen Phenoxyessigsaurederivat Propanidid (Epontol). Edited by Horatz K, Frey R, Zindler M. Berlin, Springer-Verlag, 1965, pp 17–47

145. Dundee JW, Clarke RSJ: Alterations in response to somatic pain associated with anesthesia, XVII: Propanidid (FBA. 1420) Br J Anaesth 37:121–125, 1965

146. Dundee JW, Clarke RSJ: Clinical studies of induction agents IX. A comparative study of a new eugenol derivative, FBA. 1420, with G.29.505 and standard barbiturates. Br J Anaesth 36:100–105, 1964.

147. Clarke RSJ, Dundee JW: Clinical studies of induction agents XII. The influence of some premedicants on the course and sequelae of propanidid anaesthesia. Br J Anaesth 37:51–56, 1965

148. Sankawa H: Cardiovascular effects of propanidid and methohexital sodium in dogs. Acta Anaesthesiol Scand (suppl) 17:55, 1965

149. Conway CM, Ellis DB, King NW: A comparison of the acute haemodynamic effects of thiopentone, methohexitone and propanidid in the dog. Br J Anaesth 40:736, 1968

150. Langrehr D: Endoanasthetische Wirkungen von Propanidid und ihre Bedeutung für das Verhalten von Kreislauf und Atmung, Die intravenose Kurznarkose mit dem neuen Phenoxyessigsaurederivat Propanidid (Epontol). Edited by Horatz K, Frey R, Zindler M. Berlin, Springer-Verlag, 1965, pp 239–247

151. Illes I: Cardiovascular effects of propanidid. Acta Anaesthesiol Scand (suppl) 17:45, 1965

152. Johnstone M, Barron PT: The cardiovascular effects of propanidid. A study in radiotelemetry. Anaesthesia 23:180, 1968

153. Howells TH, Radnay PA: Combination of propanidid with other anesthetics (inhalants). Acta Anaesthesiol Scand (suppl) 17:39, 1965

154. Gordh T: Analysis of hyperventilation in propanidid anaesthesia, Anaesthesiology und Wiederbelebung. Edited by Frey R, Kern F, Mayrhofer O. Berlin, Springer-Verlag, 1973, pp 131–136

155. Reichel Von G, Podlesch I, Ulmer WT, et al: Untersuchungen über die Wirkung des Kurznarkoticums Propanidid auf die Ventilation und den Gasstoffwechsel. Anaesthetist 14:184, 1965

156. Clarke RSJ, Dundee JW, Hamilton RC: Interactions between induction agents and muscle relaxants. Anaesthesia 22:235, 1967

157. Doenicke A, Krumey I, Kugler J, et al: Experimental studies of the breakdown of Epontol: Determination of propanidid in human serum. Br J Anaesth 40:415, 1968

158. Howells TH, Odell JR, Hawkins TJ, et al: An introduction to FBA. 1420: A new non-barbiturate intravenous anaesthetic. Br J Anaesth 36:295, 1964

159. Goldman V, Kennedy P: A non-barbiturate intravenous anaesthetic: Report of a pilot trial. Anaesthesia 19:424, 1964

160. Doenicke A, Kugler J, Kalmar L, et al: Klinische experimentelle Untersuchungen mit Propanidid. Anaesthesist 22:255, 1973

161. Scholtan VW, Lie SK: Kolloid-chenische Eigenschaften eines neuen Kurznarkoticums. Arzneim Forsch 16:679, 1966

162. Clarke RSJ, Dundee JW, Daw RH: Clinical studies of induction agents. XI. The influence of some intravenous anaesthetics on the respiratory effects and sequelae of suxamethonium. Br J Anaesth 36:307, 1969

163. Korttilla K, Linnoila M, Ertama P, et al: Recovery and simulated driving after intravenous anesthesia with thiopental methohexital, propanidid or alphadione. Anesthesiology 43:291, 1975

164. Lorenz W, Doenicke A, Meyer R, et al: Histamine release in man by propanidid and thiopentone: Pharmacological effects and clinical consequences. Br J Anaesth 44:355, 1972

165. Selye H: Anaesthetic effects of steroid hormones. Proc Soc Exp Biol Med 46:116, 1941

166. Dundee JW, Wyant GM: Intravenous Anesthesia. Edinburgh, Churchill Livingstone, 1974, pp 193–206

167. Clarke RSJ, Dundee JW, Carson IW: Some aspects of the clinical pharmacology of Althesin. Postgrad Med J 48 (suppl 2): 62, 1972

168. Scott DF, Virden S: Comparison of the effect of Althesin with other induction agents on electroencephalographic patterns. Postgrad Med J 48 (suppl 2): 93, 1972

169. Pickerodt VWA, McDowall DG, Coroneos NJ, et al: Effect of Althesin on cerebral perfusion, cerebral metabolism and intracranial pressure in the anaesthetized baboon. Br J Anaesth 44:751, 1972

170. Warren JB: Althesin in the dental chair. Postgrad Med J 48 (suppl 2): 130, 1972

171. Child KJ, Davis B, Dodds MG, et al: Anaesthetic, cardiovascular and respiratory effects of the new steroidal agent CT 1341: A comparison with other intravenous anaesthetic drugs in the unrestrained cat. Br J Pharmacol 46:189, 1972

172. Gordh T: The effect of Althesin on the heart in situ in the cat. Postgrad Med J 48 (suppl 2): 31, 1972

173. Savege TM, Foley EI, Coultos RJ, et al: CT 1341: Some effects in man. Anaesthesia 26:402, 1971

174. Savege TM, Foley EI, Ross L, et al: A comparison of the cardiorespiratory effects during induction of anaesthesia of Althesin with thiopentone and methohexitone. Postgrad Med J 48 (suppl 2):66, 1972

175. Prys-Roberts C, Föex P, Biro GP: Cardiovascular responses of hypertensive patients to induction of anaesthesia with Althesin. Postgrad Med J 48 (suppl 2): 80, 1972

176. Clarke RSJ, Dundee JW, Carson IW, et al: Clinical studies with induction agents. XL. Althesin with various premedicants. Br J Anaesth 44:845, 1972

177. Whitwam JG: Adverse reactions to IV induction agents. Br J Anaesth 50:677, 1978

178. Tomlin PJ: The respiratory effects of Althesin. Postgrad Med J 48 (suppl 2): 85, 1972

179. Foley EI, Walton B, Savage TM, et al: A comparison of recovery times between Althesin and methohexitone following anaesthesia for electro-convulsant therapy. Postgrad Med J 48 (suppl 2): 112, 1972

180. Carson IW, Moore J, Balmer JP, et al: Laryngeal competence with ketamine and other drugs. Anesthesiology 38:128, 1973

181. Clarke RSJ, Dundee JW, Doggart JR, et al: The effects of single and intermittent administrations of althesin and other intravenous anesthetics on liver function. Anesth Analg 53:461, 1974

182. Carson IW, Alexander JP, Hewitt JC, et al: Clinical studies of induction agents. XLI: Venous sequelae following the use of the steroid anaesthetic agent, althesin. Br J Anaesth 44:1311, 1972

183. Clarke RSJ, Montgomery SJ, Dundee JW, et al: Clinical studies of induction agents. XXXIX. CT1341, a new steroid anaesthetic. Br J Anaesth 43:947, 1971

184. Saarnivaara L: Comparison of thiopentone, althesin and ketamine in anaesthesia for otolaryngological surgery in children. Br J Anaesth 49:363, 1977

185. Gyermek LL: Increased toxicity of althesin in newborn animals. Br J Anaesth 46:704, 1974

186. Mahomedy MC, Downing JW, Mahomedy YH: Alfathesin for anaesthetic induction at caesarean section. S Afr Med J 49:1095, 1975

187. Clarke RSJ, Dundee JW, Carson IW: A new steroid anaesthetic: Althesin. Proc R Soc Med 66:1027, 1973

188. Kaplan SA, Jack ML, Alexander K, et al:

Pharmacokinetic profile of diazepam in man following single intravenous and oral and chronic oral administrations. J Pharm Sci 62:1789, 1973

189. Child KJ, Gibson W, Harnby G, et al: Metabolism and excretion of Althesin (CT 1341) in the rat. Postgrad Med J 48 (suppl 2):37, 1972

190. Card B, McCulloch RJ, Pratt DAH: Tissue distribution of CT 1341 (althesin) in the rat; an autoradiographic study. Postgrad Med J 48 (suppl 2):34, 1972

191. Watkins J, Ward AM: Adverse Response to Intravenous Drugs. London, Academic Press, 1978, pp 1–185

192. Dundee JW, Clarke RSJ, McNeill HG: Minoxolone: A preliminary communication, Trends in Intravenous Anesthesia. Edited by Aldrete JA, Stanley TH. Chicago, Year Book Medical Publishers, 1980, pp 259–263

193. Janssen PAJ, Niemegeers CJE, Schellekens KHL, et al: Etomidate, R-(+)-Ethyl-1-(α-methyl-benzl) imidazole-5-carboxylate (R 16659). Arzneim Forsch 21:1234, 1971

194. Janssen PAJ, Niemegeers CJE, Marsboom RPH: Etomidate, a potent non-barbiturate hypnotic. Intravenous etomidate in mice, rats, guinea-pigs, rabbits and dogs. Arch Int Pharmacol Ther 214:92, 1975

195. Doenicke A, Kugler J, Penzel G, et al: Hirnfunktion und Toleranzbreite nach Etomidate, einem neuen barbituratfreien applizierbaren Hypnoticum. Anaesthesist 22:357, 1973

196. Kugler J, Doenicke A, Laub M: The EEG after etomidate, Etomidate. Edited by Doenicke A. Berlin, Springer-Verlag, 1977, pp 31–48

197. Hempelman G, Oster W, Piepenbrock S, et al: Haemodynamic effects of etomidate—a new hypnotic—in patients with myocardial insufficiency, Etomidate, Edited by Doenicke A. Berlin, Springer-Verlag, 1977, pp 31–48

198. Holdcroft A, Morgan M, Whitwam JG, et al: Effect of dose and premedication on induction complications with etomidate. Br J Anaesth 48:199, 1976

199. Kay B: A clinical assessment of the use of etomidate in children. Br J Anaesth 48:207, 1976

200. Baiker-Hemerleın M, Kenins P, Kikiellus H, et al: Investigations on the site of the central nervous action of the short acting hypnotic R-(+)-ethyl-1-(α-methyl-benzl) imidazole-5-carboxylate (etomidate) in cats. Anaesthesist 28:78, 1979

201. Evans RH, Hill RG: GABA-mimetic action of etomidate. Experientia 34:1325, 1978

202. Hill RG, Taberner PV: Some neuropharmacological properties of the new non-barbiturate hypnotic etomidate (R-(+)-ethyl-1-(α-methyl-benzl) imidazole-5-carboxylate). Br J Pharm 54:241, 1975

203. Renou AM, Vernheit J, Macrez P, et al: Cerebral blood flow and metabolism during Etomidate Anaesthesia in man. Br J Anaesth 50:1047, 1978

204. Moss E, Powell D, Gibson RM, et al: Effect of Etomidate on intracranial pressure and cerebral perfusion pressure. Br J Anaesth 51:346, 1979

205. Reneman RS, Janssen PAJ: The experimental pharmacology of Etomidate, a new potent short-acting intravenous hypnotic, Etomidate. Edited by Doenicke A. Berlin, Springer-Verlag, 1977, pp 1–5

206. Zacharias M, Clarke RSJ, Dundee JW: Etomidate, Trends in Intravenous Anesthesia. Edited by Aldrete JA, Stanley, TH. Chicago, Year Book Medical Publishers, 1980, pp 173–187

207. Patschke D, Bruckner, JB, Gethmann JW, et al: A comparison of the acute effects of intravenous induction agents (thiopentone, methohexitone, propanidid, althesin, ketamine, piritramide and etomidate) on haemodynamics and myocardial oxygen consumption in dogs, Etomidate. Edited by Doenicke A. Berlin, Springer-Verlag, 1977, pp 49–71

208. Patschke D, Bruckner JB, Eberlein JH, et al: Effects of Althesin, Etomidate and Fentanyl on haemodynamics and myocardial oxygen consumption in man. Can Anaesth Soc J 24:57, 1977

209. Hempelmann G, Seitz W, Piepenbrock S: Kombination von Etomidate und Fentanyl. Anesthesist 26:231, 1977

210. Marquardt B, Waibel H, Bruckner JD: The influence of R 26 490 (etomidate sulfate) on ventilation and gas exchange, Etomidate. Edited Doenicke A. Berlin, Springer-Verlag, 1977, pp 113–118

211. Morgan M, Lumley J, Whitwam JG: Respiratory effects of etomidate. Br J Anaesth 49:233, 1977

212. Hempelmann W, Hempelmann G, Piepen-

broch S: A comparative study of blood gases and haemodynamics using the new hypnotic Etomidate, CT 1341, methohexitone, propanidid and thiopentone, Etomidate. Edited by Doenicke A. Berlin, Springer-Verlag, 1977, pp 119–129

213. Kalenda Z: The use of etomidate as an induction agent in Fentanyl anesthesia, Etomidate, Edited by Doenicke A. Berlin, Springer-Verlag, 1977, pp 130–139

214. Renemann RS, Verheyen F, Kruger R, et al: The effect of intra-arterial injection of etomidate and thiopental on the skeletal muscle and arterial wall-structures, Etomidate. Edited by Doenicke, A. Berlin, Springer-Verlag, 1977, pp 9–14

215. Heykants JJP, Meuldermans WEG, Michiels LJM, et al: Distribution, metabolism and excretion of etomidate, a short-acting hypnotic drug in the rat: Comparative study of (R)-(+) and (S)-(−)-etomidate. Arch Int Pharmacodyn Ther 216:113, 1975

216. Van Hamme MJ, Ghoneim MM, Ambre JJ: Pharmacokinetics of etomidate, a new intravenous anesthetic. Anesthesiology 49:274, 1978

217. Zsigmond EK, Domino EF: Clinical pharmacology and current uses of ketamine, Trends in Intravenous Anesthesia. Edited by Aldrete JA, Stanley TH. Chicago, Year Book Medical Publishers, 1980, pp 283–328

218. Marietta MP, Way WL, Castagnoli N Jr, et al: On the pharmacology of the ketamine en-antiomorphs in the rat. J Pharmacol Exp Ther 202:157, 1977

219. Ryder S, Way WL, Trevor AJ: Comparative pharmacology of the optical isomers of ketamine in mice. Eur J Pharmacol 49:15, 1978

220. Dundee JW, Wyant GM: Intravenous Anesthesia. Edinburgh, Churchill-Livingstone, 1974, pp 219–247

221. Corssen G, Domino FF: Dissociative anesthesia: Further pharmacologic studies and first clinical experience with the phencyclidine derivative CI-581. Anesth Analg 45:29, 1966

222. Bovill JG, Coppel DL, Dundee JW, et al: Current status of ketamine anaesthesia. Lancet 1:1285, 1971

223. Domino EF, Chodoff P, Corssen G: Pharmacologic effects of CI-581, a new dissociative anesthesia in man. Clin Pharmacol Ther 6:279, 1965

224. Corssen G, Miyasaka M, Domino EF: Changing concepts in pain control during surgery: Dissociative anesthesia, with CI-581: A progress report. Anesth Analg 47:746, 1968

225. Aldrete JA, McDonald JS: Low-dose ketamine-diazepam prevents adverse reactions, Trends in Intravenous Anesthesia. Edited by Aldrete JA, Stanley, TH. Chicago, Year Book Medical Publishers, 1980, pp 331–340

226. Dawson B, Michenfelder JD, Theye RA: Effects of ketamine on canine cerebral flow and metabolism: Modification by prior administration of thiopental. Anesth Analg 50:443, 1971

227. Stanley TH: Blood pressure and pulse-rate responses to ketamine during general anesthesia. Anesthesiology 39:648, 1973

228. Bidwai AV, Stanley TH, Graves C: The effects of ketamine on cardiovascular dynamics during halothane and ethrane anesthesia. Anesth Analg 54:588, 1975

229. Dowdy EG, Kaya K: Studies of the mechanism of cardiovascular responses to CI-581. Anesthesiology 29:931, 1968

230. Goldberg AH, Keane PW, Phear WPC: Effects of ketamine on contractile performance and excitability of isolated heart muscle. J Pharmacol Exp Ther 175:338, 1970

231. Traber DL, Wilson RD: Involvement of the sympathetic nervous system in the pressor response to ketamine. Anesth Analg 48:248, 1969

232. Traber DL, Wilson RD, Priano LL: Blockade of the hypertensive response to ketamine. Anesth Analg 49:420, 1970

233. Traber DL, Wilson RD, Priano LL: The effect of alpha-adrenergic blockade on the cardiopulmonary response to ketamine. Anesth Analg 50:737, 1971

234. Flacke JW, Flacke WE, Mehmed H, et al: A peripheral cocaine-like effect of ketamine. Abstracts of Scientific Papers, 1970 ASA meeting, pp 8–9

235. Corssen G, Allarde R, Brosch F, et al: Ketamine as the sole anesthetic in open heart surgery: A preliminary report. Anesth Analg 49:1025, 1970

236. Yoon M, Zsigmond EK, Kothary SP: A new anesthetic technique: Analgesia with diazepam-ketamine-pancuronium in cardiac surgical patients. Comm Anesth 5:10, 1975

237. Chaspakis G, Kekis N, Sakkalis C, et al: Use

of ketamine and pancuronium for anesthesia for patients in hemorrhagic shock. Anesth Analg 52:282, 1973

238. Podlesch I, Zindler M: Erste Erfahrungen mit dem Phencyclidinderivat Ketamine (CI-581) einen neuen intravenosen und intramuskularen Narkosemittel. Anaesthesist 16:299, 1967

239. Taylor PA, Towey RM: Depression of laryngeal reflexes during ketamine anaesthesia. Br Med J 2:688, 1971

240. Carson IW, Moore J, Balmer JP, et al: Laryngeal competence with ketamine and other drugs. Anesthesiology 38:128, 1973

241. El-Hawary MB, Mossad B, Abd El-Wahed S, et al: Effect of ketamine hydrochloride on the tracheobronchial tree. Mid East J Anaesthesiol 3:455, 1972

242. Corssen G, Gutierrez J, Reves JG, et al: Ketamine in anesthetic management of asthmatic patients. Anesth Analg 51:588, 1972

243. Kothary SP, Zsigmond EK: The effect of ketamine on human plasma cholinesterase in vitro and in vivo. Excerp Med Int Cong Ser 452:241, 1978

244. Johnston RR, Miller RD, Way WL: The interaction of ketamine with d-tubocurarine, pancuronium and succinylcholine in man. Anesth Analg 53:496, 1974

245. Cronnelly R, Dretchen KL, Sokoll MD, et al: Ketamine: myoneuronal activity and interaction with neuromuscular blocking agents. Eur J Pharmacol 22:17, 1973

246. Knox JWD, Bovill JG, Clarke RSJ, et al: Clinical studies of induction agents. XXXVI: Ketamine. Br J Anaesth 42:875, 1970

247. Peltz B, Sinclair DM: Induction agents for cesarean section: A comparison of thiopentone and ketamine. Anaesthesia 28:37, 1973

248. White PF, Marietta MP, Pudwill CR et al: Effects of halothane anesthesia on the biodisposition of ketamine in rats. J Pharmacol Exp Ther 196:545, 1976

249. Barbour CM, Tovell RM: Experiences with procaine administered intravenously. Anesthesiology 9:514, 1948

250. Fraser RJ, Kraft K: Pentothal-procaine analgesia. Anesth Analg 27:282, 1948

251. Birrtich NM, Powers WF: Intravenous procaine in thoracic surgery. Anesth Analg 27:181, 1948

252. Wikinski JA, de Wilcinski RLW, Ceraso O, et al: General anesthesia with intravenous procaine, Trends in Intravenous Anesthesia. Edited by Aldrete JA, Stanley TH. Chicago, Year Book Medical Publishers, 1980, pp 189–215

17

Pharmacology of Muscle Relaxants, Their Antagonists, and Monitoring of Neuromuscular Function

Ronald D. Miller, M.D.
John J. Savarese, M.D.

INTRODUCTION

In 1942 Griffith and Johnson[1] suggested that *d*-tubocurarine was a safe drug to use during surgery to help provide good skeletal muscle relaxation. One year later, Cullen[2] reported that *d*-tubocurarine had been given to 131 patients to produce additional skeletal muscle relaxation. In 1954 Beecher and Todd[3] published their famous report in which, by means of a multi-institutional survey, a sixfold increase in mortality rate was found for patients who received muscle relaxants versus those who did not receive muscle relaxants. This study had many faults in experimental design and thus did not deserve the publicity it received. In the subsequent years, the use of muscle relaxants has become a vitally important aspect of modern anesthesia practice.

Two philosophies govern the use of muscle relaxants. One end of the scale has been popularized by Gray and his co-workers in Liverpool, England: in this approach nitrous oxide, oxygen, and large doses of muscle relaxants constitute the sole anesthetic. With this type of anesthesia, patients will usually be amnesic. However, patients occasionally recall part or all of the conversations during surgery.[4] Awareness during surgery was vividly described in a recent editorial.[5] A trained medical person under general anesthesia described being completely awake during a cesarean section. She specifically stated that when she moved she was given more muscle relaxant (pancuronium) rather than more anesthesia. This inappropriate practice of giving muscle relaxants, instead of analgesics or hypnotics, when a patient moves in response to pain is unfortunately a prevalent practice. Often this practice is advocated in a patient who has an unstable circulatory status. In our opinion, muscle relaxants are often inappropriately given in this situation because concentrations or doses of analgesic or hypnotic drugs are poorly adjusted to the patient's physical state. As stated by Cullen and Larson[6] "It is, of course, true that muscle relaxants given inappropriately in these circumstances provide the surgeon with optimal conditions in a patient who does not move; unfortunately, ample evidence indicates that such misuse of muscle relaxants often means that a patient is paralyzed but not anesthetized—a state that may be satisfactory for the anesthetist and the surgeon but wholly unsatisfactory for the patient."

A further quote from Cullen and Larson[6]

emulates our own philosophy concerning muscle relaxant administration. "Relaxants used to cover-up deficiencies in total anesthetic management as in the prevention or treatment of laryngospasm, movement in response to pain and hypotension due to relative overdose of analgesic or hypnotic drugs (for a particular patient) represent an inefficient and inappropriate use of these valuable adjuncts to anesthesia." Muscle relaxants should be viewed as *adjuvants* not as substitutes for anesthesia. By giving them only in an anesthetized patient (i.e., no movement, hypertension, tachycardia, tearing, grimacing, etc.) and monitoring neuromuscular function, large doses of muscle relaxants can be avoided and this should decrease the incidence of prolonged paralysis and/or inadequate reversal.

In this chapter the clinical pharmacology and clinical use of muscle relaxants is discussed incorporating the overall philosophy that these drugs are adjuvants, not substitutes, for anesthesia. Lastly, diseases of the neuromuscular system, with which anesthesiologists are confronted, are discussed.

NORMAL NEUROMUSCULAR FUNCTION

Neuromuscular blockade and/or skeletal muscle relaxation can occur from interference with function at several sites: the central nervous system, the myelinated somatic nerve, unmyelinated motor nerve terminal, synthesis or hydrolysis of acetylcholine, cholinergic receptor and motor endplate, muscle membrane, and muscle contraction (excitation-contraction coupling). This subject has been reviewed recently by Waud and Waud,[7] Ali and Savarese,[8] and Feldman.[9]

The standard description of neuromuscular transmission is that upon arrival of an impulse at the motor nerve terminal, acetylcholine is released. Acetylcholine then diffuses across the synaptic cleft to the cholinergic receptor located on the motor endplate (Fig 17-1). When the receptor and acetylcholine combine, permeability of the membrane in the endplate region increases to sodium primarily, but also to potassium. Sodium moves from outside to inside the membrane, and the resting membrane potential changes from −90 mV to near zero. This change in mV is termed endplate potential. The magnitude of the endplate potential is directly related to the amount of acetylcholine released. If the potential is small (i.e., 60 mV or so), then permeability and therefore membrane potential return to normal without a propagated impulse. However, if the endplate potential is large, then the muscle membrane depolarizes, and the impulse will be propagated along the entire muscle fiber. Muscle contraction is then initiated by a process known as excitation-contraction coupling. The released acetylcholine is removed from the endplate region by diffusion and enzymatic destruction by acetylcholinesterase.

The above description of neuromuscular transmission, although accurate, is rather simplistic. Although it is beyond the scope of this chapter to provide a detailed description of neuromuscular transmission, some recent findings are outlined. From an anatomic view, the postsynaptic region is arranged in deep folds forming troughs at the mouths of which lie acetylcholine receptors. These folds appear to provide hydrolysis traps for acetylcholine, provide a channel for more rapid conduction of postsynaptic depolarization waves to trigger muscle action potentials, and provide more surface area for the passive spread of depolarization down the folds (Fig. 17-1).

Probably the major advance in neuromuscular function has been identification and isolation of the nicotinic acetylcholine receptor. The acetylcholine receptor is a macromolecule that, upon binding acetylcholine to a specific site, brings about translocation of cations across the postsynaptic membrane and thereby effects depolarization. The receptor is a glycoprotein of approximately 300,000 molecular weight and

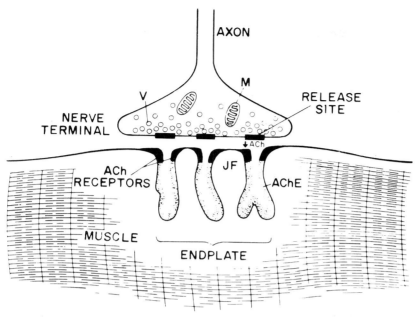

Fig. 17-1 Schematic representation of the neuromuscular junction (Reprinted by permission from Drachman DB: Myasthenia gravis. N Engl J Med 298:135, 1978.)

has a half-life of about a week. Each receptor molecule has one to two acetylcholine binding sites and a separate ion pore through which movement of sodium and potassium takes place.

Identification and isolation of the acetylcholine receptor has been made possible by the use of various snake venoms.[10] Three of these venoms, α bungarotoxin, α cobra, and β bungarotoxin, have been particularly useful. Alpha bungarotoxin binds *specifically* and *irreversibly* to the receptor. If bungarotoxin is labeled with radioactive iodine, the number and turn-over of receptors can be determined from the amount of bound radioactive isotope. Alpha cobra binds *reversibly* and therefore is useful for purification of the receptor. By binding the solubilized receptor to α cobra attached to sepharose beads, the specific receptor can be identified. Beta bungarotoxin probably does not affect the postsynaptic area but is a potent presynaptic blocker. It therefore is useful for examining presynaptic mechanisms of drugs.[11]

Although a clinician may be tempted to avoid reading any article of a study in which these snake venoms have been used, these venoms have already been used to solve some more practical problems:

1. The number of receptors increases or decreases in response to chronic neostigmine treatment. The number of receptors appears to change in the direction necessary to compensate for the change in acetylcholine concentration. This has implications concerning the massive hyperkalemic response to succinylcholine.

2. If 60 percent of the receptors are occupied by an α bungarotoxin, neuromuscular transmission in response to single pulses is not altered. However, if 80 percent of the receptors are blocked, neuromuscular transmission fails. This confirms the wide margin of safety of neuromuscular transmission and quantitatively the receptor occlusion studies of Waud and Waud.[12]

3. In myasthenia gravis the number of receptors is reduced, and the receptors are also more labile.

An explanation of why certain events, which are observed clinically (e.g. tetanic fade), occur is discussed in the section on monitoring neuromuscular blockade.

TYPES OF NEUROMUSCULAR BLOCKADE

Although neuromuscular blocking drugs probably act at several sites, their primary action is at the postsynaptic area. These drugs either cause a nondepolarizing, phase I (depolarizing) or phase II (dual, desensitization) block.

NONDEPOLARIZING

Classically, nondepolarizing neuromuscular blockers (*d*-tubocurarine, pancuronium, metocurine, gallamine, and ORG NC45—Norcuron) are thought to combine with the acetylcholine receptor, but not to activate them. If sufficient receptors are occupied by a muscle relaxant and are therefore unavailable to acetylcholine, neuromuscular transmission will fail. Because of a large margin of safety, 70 percent of the receptors can be blocked with no interference in the response to a single impulse. Specifically, Waud and Waud[12] found that the response to a single impulse (often called "twitch" response) does not decrease until 75 to 80 percent of the receptors are blocked. Neuromuscular transmission completely fails when 90 to 95 percent of the receptors are blocked. These concepts are responsible for our approach to monitoring neuromuscular function.

The preceding paragraph describes the classic mechanism of action of nondepolarizing muscle relaxants. Acetylcholine and the nondepolarizing muscle relaxants definitely have a presynaptic effect.[13, 14] The role of this presynaptic effect in producing neuromuscular blockade is controversial.[15] Presently most authors feel that the postsynaptic action is dominant and the presynaptic plays little role in producing a neuromuscular blockade.

By using a peripheral nerve stimulator, the following characteristics of a nondepolarizing block can be seen: (1) decreased contraction to a single impulse, (2) nonsustained response to a tetanic stimulus, (3) train-of-four ratio < 70 percent, (4) absence of muscle fasciculation prior to paralysis, (5) posttetanic facilitation, and (6) antagonism by acetylcholinesterase inhibitors.

PHASE I (DEPOLARIZING)

Although decamethonium is a depolarizing muscle relaxant, it is seldom administered to patients. Succinylcholine is the only one commonly used clinically. The neuromuscular effects of succinylcholine can conveniently be thought to be almost identical to those of acetylcholine except the former produces a longer effect. Succinylcholine reacts with the receptor to cause depolarization of the endplate that in turn spreads to and depolarizes adjacent membranes causing generalized disorganized contractions of muscle motor units. The latter is called succinylcholine-induced fasciculations by clinicians and can cause complications, which are discussed later. Because succinylcholine is not metabolized as rapidly as acetylcholine, the depolarized membranes remain depolarized and unresponsive to additional impulses. A neuromuscular block then results. As succinylcholine diffuses down a concentration gradient away from the endplate region, the membranes become repolarized and normal neuromuscular function results. Although the drug has presynaptic effects,[16] they are minor when compared to postsynaptic actions. A depolarizing neuromuscular blockade is therefore characterized by[8] (1) decreased response to a single impulse; (2) decreased amplitude, but sustained response to a tetanic stimulus; (3) if present, a train-of-four ratio > 70 percent; (4) muscle fasciculations prior to paralysis; (5) absence of posttetanic facilitation; and (6) augmentation of neuromuscular blockade by acetylcholinesterase inhibitors.

PHASE II (DUAL, DESENSITIZATION)

With prolonged or repeated exposure to succinylcholine, the initial depolarization decreases with time; in other words, the membrane becomes repolarized. Despite this repolarization, the membrane cannot be depolarized again by acetylcholine. The mechanism for the development of a phase II block is unknown. One hypothesis was that an inexcitable area develops on the investing membrane of the muscle immediately outside the endplate area which becomes repolarized shortly after the arrival of succinylcholine. This area presumably impedes centrifugal spread of an impulse initiated by acetylcholine's action on the receptor.[17] Because the endplate is partially repolarized and still does not respond to acetylcholine, the membrane is said to be desensitized to the affects of acetylcholine. Therefore Gissen et al.[18] proposed that the terms phase II and dual block be discontinued. They suggested that this block be called a "desensitization block." About ten years later, a group of experts met in London and concluded that this term inferred a rather simple explanation for a phase II block that had several exceptions. For example, a phase II block can often be antagonized by neostigmine or edrophonium.[19, 20] This group decided that it was preferable not to use the term "desensitization" and retain the term "Phase II," which does not imply a specific mechanism.[17]

The clinical characteristics of a phase II block are nearly identical to that of a nondepolarizing neuromuscular blockade—that is, a nonsustained response to a tetanic stimulus, the presence of posttetanic facilitation, and a train-of-four ratio < 50 percent. The transition from a phase I depolarizing neuromuscular block to a phase II block are described as follows:[8]

Stage 1—A typical depolarization block

Stage 2—Stage of tachyphylaxis: a diminished response following repeated doses

Stage 3—Stage of Wedensky inhibition: fade of successive EMG potentials in response to high-frequency (tetanic) stimulation. The response to slow rates of stimulation is sustained.

Stage 4—Stage of "fade and potentiation"; acetylcholinesterase inhibitors improve neuromuscular transmission

Stage 5—Nondepolarizing stage: all the signs of a nondepolarizing block are present. This block can be antagonized by acetylcholinesterase inhibitors.

There is a danger in labeling stage 5 the nondepolarizing stage. This infers that the mechanism of this blockade and a *d*-tubocurarine-induced neuromuscular blockade are exactly the same. Although the signs elicited by peripheral nerve stimulation are very similar, the mechanisms of blockade are probably different. This difference cannot be explained in detail because the mechanism by which succinylcholine causes a phase II block has not been fully elucidated.

MONITORING OF NEUROMUSCULAR FUNCTION

PERIPHERAL NERVE STIMULATION

Stimulating a peripheral nerve (usually the ulnar at the wrist or elbow) and visually observing contraction of the fingers (adductor pollicis and flexor digitorium muscles) is the most commonly advocated method of monitoring neuromuscular function clinically.[21, 22] This stimulation need not be restricted to the arm. Stimulating the facial or the motor nerves of a lower extremity, such as the peroneal nerve, and observing the magnitude of resultant muscular contraction can also be used for monitoring neuromuscular function.

This type of monitoring can be utilized to detect both magnitude and type of neuromuscular blockade. Quantitative conclusions must be guarded, however. Because of the wide margin of safety of neuromuscular function, a reduction in the contractile response to peripheral nerve stimulation is not quantitatively proportional to the action of

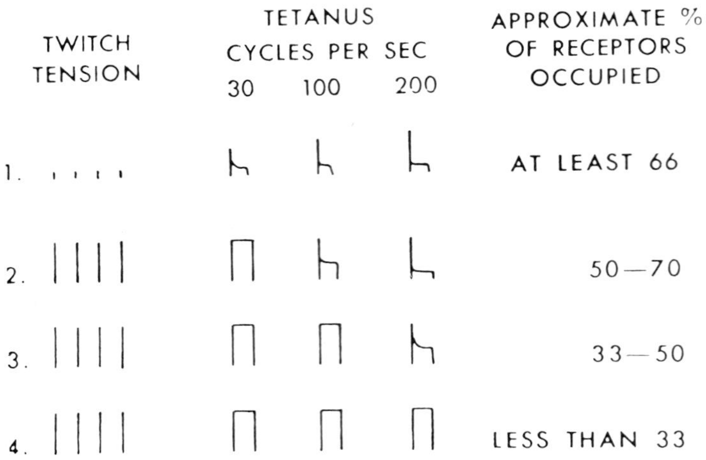

TWITCH TENSION	TETANUS CYCLES PER SEC			APPROXIMATE % OF RECEPTORS OCCUPIED
	30	100	200	
1. ˌ ˌ ˌ ˌ	⊓	⊓	⊔	AT LEAST 66
2. ‖‖‖	⊓	⊓	⊔	50 — 70
3. ‖‖‖	⊓	⊓	⊓	33 — 50
4. ‖‖‖	⊓	⊓	⊓	LESS THAN 33

Fig. 17-2 Correlation between twitch tension, response to tetanic stimuli of varying rates of stimulation, and the fraction of receptors occupied.[12]

relaxants at the receptor. For example, Waud and Waud[12] have demonstrated that the twitch response in the tibialis anterior muscle of the cat, analogous to the adductor response of the thumb, is not reduced unless more than 70 percent of the receptors are occupied by a nondepolarizing relaxant (Fig. 17-2). Twitch is completely eliminated when 90 percent of the receptors are occupied. In spite of this limitation, the twitch can be used as a quantitative monitor. DeJong[23] found that adjusting relaxant administration to maintain a faint but perceptible muscular contraction (twitch) in response to peripheral nerve stimulation assures adequate operating conditions while avoiding excessive relaxant administration. Even if the twitch has been abolished by inadvertant relaxant overdose, if one waits until the twitch reappears before administering subsequent relaxant, the incidence of failure of reversal can be attenuated.

Obviously, subtle degrees of neuromuscular blockade cannot be observed by monitoring the twitch. The neuromuscular junction must be stressed by a stimulus that is greater and longer in intensity than that used to elicit a single twitch. A sustained muscular contraction in response to a tetanic stimulus for 5 seconds is such a stimulus. Figure 17-2 correlates the fraction of receptors occupied with the ability to sustain contraction to varying degrees of tetanic stimuli. Unfortunately, tetanic stimuli are painful and are therefore of limited value in detecting subtle neuromuscular blockade in the unanesthetized patient (such as one in the recovery room).

Frequently, clinicians refer to partial reduction in twitch height in a manner that suggests that a muscle fiber can contract in a graded fashion. This simply is not true. Muscle contraction is an all-or-none phenomenon. Each fiber either contracts maximally or does not at all. Therefore when twitch height (adduction of thumb) is reduced, some fibers are contracting normally while others are still completely blocked. The stronger the response, the fewer fibers exist in a blocked state. Fade of muscular contraction in response to tetanic stimuli suggest that some fibers are more susceptible to being blocked by relaxants and need a greater release of acetylcholine to trigger their responses.[25]

MECHANICAL FORCE VERSUS ELECTROMYOGRAM

So far we have been discussing the observation or recording of mechanical force (i.e., adduction of the thumb). Epstein and Epstein[26] believe electromyography "simplifies routine clinical monitoring of curarization." Basically, with this technique the evoked action potential from several synchronously excited fibers (compound action potential) is recorded and displayed on an oscilloscope. The main difference is that the electromyogram has a rapid response, whereas mechanical force recordings have a slow response.

There are two advantages to having a rapid response. Rapid repetitive depolarization will appear as a single event in mechanical recordings, but can be separated by the electromyogram. For example, some stimulators deliver stimuli longer than the desired short one.[27] This may lead to paired muscle firing. While the electromyogram will separate these depolarizations, the response time of a mechanical recording is too slow and therefore they are viewed as a single depolarization. The second advantage is also based on the electromyogram's rapid response. As indicated previously, when determining whether contraction is sustained in response to a tetanic stimulus, the tetanic train usually must be maintained for about 5 seconds in order to be detected by the slow-responding mechanical recording. In contrast, the time required is much shorter with the rapid response of the electromyograph. This is a real advantage because the tetanic stimulus is so painful. Epstein and Epstein[28] have analyzed the electromyographic and mechanical response to tetanic stimuli. This analysis is recommended to those who seek more detailed information. Quantitation of neuromuscular block derived from electromyographic and mechanical recordings parallel each other.[28] Because instrumentation is usually not available clinically (oscilloscope or its equivalent[29]) for the electromyogram, recording of the mechanical force, in my opinion, is still preferred.

We believe, however, that the EMG is the monitor of the future and will be used routinely nearly as commonly as the electrocardiogram is presently used. We predict that nearly every anesthetic machine will have a neuromuscular monitor that will take less than 1 minute to set up. After application of two pasty electrodes to the ulnar nerve at the wrist and two additional electrodes over the adductor pollicis longus muscle, monitoring of neuromuscular function would be ready. The ulnar nerve would be stimulated, and the resultant EMG recorded, integrated, and displayed on a digital readout. The stimulator, integrator, and digital readout would be contained in one small unit mounted on an anesthetic machine. This approach has the advantage of not requiring observation of the hand. In other words, tucking the hand and arm in next to the patient to avoid interfering with the surgeon will not interfere with monitoring of neuromuscular function. Neuromuscular blockade will appear as a percent of control (e.g., 25 percent depression of the EMG twitch). Prototypes of this type of monitoring are already being tested clinically and appear to be quite promising (John Severinghaus, personal communication).

MECHANISM OF FADE AND POSTTETANIC FACILITATION

The hallmark of a nondepolarizing neuromuscular blockade is an inability to sustain contraction in response to a tetanic stimulus (usually 50 Hz for 5 seconds) and posttetanic facilitation (twitch after the response to tetanic stimuli is higher than the twitch immediately before tetanus). Before discussing the mechanism of these events, a discrepancy between pharmacologists and anesthesiologists should be explained. Pharmacologists frequently say that *d*-tubocurarine attenuates posttetanic facilitation, and yet anesthesiologists utilize its presence as an index of residual nondepolarizing block. This apparent discrepancy can be explained easily. Pharmacologists correctly state that the height of the posttetanic twitch is diminished by *d*-tubocurarine (Fig. 17-3). Anesthesiologists, however, utilize the ratio between the twitch height after and before the tetanic response. The ratio is increased during a partial nondepolarizing blockade in spite of the twitch after the tetanus being reduced in ac-

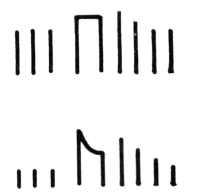

Fig. 17-3 Magnitude of posttetanic facilitation without and with a neuromuscular block from *d*-tubocurarine. Even though the magnitude of the posttetanic twitch is reduced, the ratio between the twitch after and before the tetanic stimulus is increased by *d*-tubocurarine. (Miller RD: Monitoring of neuromuscular blockade, Monitoring in Anesthesia. Edited by Saidman LJ, Smith NT. Reprinted by permission of John Wiley & Sons, Inc., New York, 1978.)

tual magnitude when compared with the control twitch height (Fig. 17-3).

The fade or unsustained contraction in response to a tetanic stimulus, which does not occur normally, does occur during a partial nondepolarizing block. After an initial burst, output of acetylcholine progressively decreases during tetanic stimulation. As pointed out by Waud and Waud,[12] the cholinergic receptor pool is so large (margin of safety of neuromuscular transmission is large) that a decrease in acetylcholine output does not result in transmission failure in the normal state. However with only 15 to 25 percent of the receptors free of relaxant, the decreased acetylcholine output is insufficient to maintain contraction and therefore "fade" occurs as acetylcholine diminishes during tetanic stimulation. During the interval between termination of the tetanic stimulus and the next single stimulus, acetylcholine mobilization and synthesis are still increased. This accounts for large posttetanic twitches (posttetanic facilitation) that rapidly return to the pretetanus height as acetylcholine

mobilization also returns to the pretetanus level.

TRAIN-OF-FOUR STIMULATION

Ali et al.[30] proposed train-of-four stimulation as the best choice for monitoring of neuromuscular function. Once again, the test that stresses the neuromuscular junction the most will be the most sensitive. The train-of-four simply uses a test of longer duration and greater intensity than the individual stimulus or twitch. Four supramaximal ulnar nerve stimuli at 2 Hz are delivered to the ulnar nerve,[30,31] and the ratio of the fourth to the first twitch amplitude is used as an index of nondepolarizing neuromuscular blockade (Fig. 17-4). This test does not require a control (prerelaxant) twitch and is not painful. However, 70 percent of the receptors can be occupied and still permit a normal train-of-four.[31] Thus, it is more sensitive than the single twitch, and of the same approximate sensitivity as tetanic stimulation at 50 Hz for 2.5 seconds. Furthermore, the train-of-four stimulation does not alter subsequent recovery from neuromuscular blockade as does tetanic stimulation.

We have found the train-of-four stimulation especially valuable in monitoring magnitude of neuromuscular blockade intraoperatively. Lee[32] observed that abolition of the fourth response of the train-of-four was associated with a 75 percent reduction in the standard twitch tension. Abolition of the third and second response of the train-of-four was correlated with 80 and 90 percent reductions of twitch tension respectively. When all four twitches in the train were absent, 100 percent or complete block was present. Thus, by counting the twitches in the train-of-four response, the magnitude of neuromuscular blockade can be clinically quantified. In an adequately anesthetized patient, we have found that adequate relaxation for abdominal surgery exists when two of the train-of-four responses are eliminated.

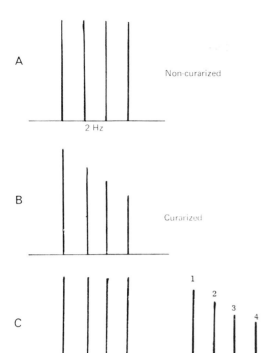

Fig. 17-4 Diagrammatic illustration of the evoked muscle twitch response to a train-of-four stimuli at 2 Hz in a noncurarized (A) and curarized (B) subject. The relationship between twitch one and twitch four reflects the extent of curarization. The greater the difference the greater the degree of curarization. (Ali HH: Quantitative assessment of residual antidepolarizing block (Part 1). Br J Anaesth 43:473, 1971.)

RECEPTOR OCCLUSION TECHNIQUES

Previously in this chapter, reference is made to the fraction of receptors that may be occupied during responses to various tests of neuromuscular function. Work on this subject has been performed primarily by Waud and Waud.[12,31] No one has the ability to count the number of receptors occupied by a relaxant. Rather, Waud and Waud estimated the fraction of receptors (without really knowing the absolute number of receptors) that must be unblocked by relaxant in order for tests of neuromuscular function to be normal. The technique estimates the fraction of receptors blocked by a nondepolarizing relaxant by determining a dose-response depolarization curve from various agonist doses (succinylcholine) in the absence and presence of the nondepolarizing blocker or antagonist (*d*-tubocurarine, pancuronium). The fraction of receptors unblocked by nondepolarizing relaxant or still available for neuromuscular transmission can be estimated from the dose ratio of the agonist and blocker. For example, in the presence of *d*-tubocurarine, 100 nmoles of succinylcholine might be required to produce the same degree of depolarization that 10 nmoles produced without *d*-tubocurarine. Since ten times more succinylcholine is required with *d*-tubocurarine, then 10 percent of the receptors are still free (or 90 percent of the receptors are blocked). All other tests used to measure neuromuscular function allow a normal response with a significant number of receptors still blocked, even at a tetanic stimulus of 200 Hz (Fig. 17-2). These results suggest that no test is available to determine whether all receptors are free of a relaxant.

RESPIRATION

Although we have just discussed the number of receptors occupied, the presence of posttetanic facilitation, and a sustained contraction in response to a tetanic stimulus, these factors are not really of prime importance. The presence of sustained adequate ventilation, particularly during stresses such as airway obstruction or vomiting, is what our main concern as anesthesiologists should be. In spite of the huge number of relaxant studies in the literature, there are few studies correlating tests of neuromuscular function with adequacy of ventilation and the conclusions are often incomplete. Walts et al.[33] concluded that sustained muscular contraction in response to tetanic stimulus (30 Hz) is a good test because it correlates with greater than 90 percent recovery of vital capacity and maximum voluntary ventilation in human volunteers. They concluded that the head-raising test is an unreliable index of recovery because it does not return to control when vital capacity and tetanic stimulation are within 90 percent of control. Perhaps the head-raising test is more sensitive. In fact, Johansen et al.[34] found head-lift and hand-grip strength to be 38 and 48 percent of control when both inspiratory and expiratory flow rates are greater than 90 percent of control. Furthermore, Ali et al.[30] found inspiratory force only 70 percent of control when vital capacity and expiratory flow rate are greater than 90 percent of control. Obviously, the most sensitive test stresses the neuromuscular junction the most. Sensitivity depends on both the intensity and duration of the stress applied. For example, a tetanic stimulus of 30 Hz for 10 seconds may be more stressful than one of 100 Hz for 1 second. A head-lift or hand-grip test may be insensitive when applied for 1 second or very sensitive when applied for 15 seconds. Obviously it becomes extremely important to define tests very carefully when making comparisons.[35, 36] In view of the scanty information available, we can only recommend that there are probably several sensitive tests available that can be used to stress the neuromuscular junction in a way that includes varying both the duration and intensity of stimulation.

patient is still under anesthesia, we frequently use a tetanic stimulus of 50 Hz or train-of-four, twitch height, tidal volume, and expiratory force to determine whether a neuromuscular blockade has been antagonized completely. Expiratory force can be determined by removing the rebreathing bag and occluding the outlet and observing the pressure on the circuit gauge (R. L. Katz, personal communication). The anesthesiologist should compare this pressure with expiratory force determined before relaxant administration. Of prime importance is using several tests and stressing the neuromuscular junction to detect possible subtle degrees of neuromuscular blockade.

Several authors recommend titrating the amount of acetylcholinesterase inhibitor to a specific end point, which is most frequently a tetanic stimulus of 30 to 50 Hz. Even though several tests may indicate normal neuromuscular function, we administer slightly more neostigmine or pyridostigmine than necessary to effect a sustained contraction in response to a tetanic stimulus of 30 to 50 Hz. For example, if 2.5 mg of neostigmine were sufficient to restore twitch height to control levels and sustain tetanus at 50 Hz, we would administer 3.0 mg of neostigmine in an effort to insure the availability of additional receptors needed to overcome airway obstruction. Later in this chapter antagonism of neuromuscular blockade is discussed in more detail.

CLINICAL CONCLUSION

In spite of the above considerations, we do not know what proportion of receptors must be available or how sensitive a test must be to insure adequate muscle strength to overcome airway obstruction and to permit coughing effectively. We have concluded that the anesthesiologist should not rely on one test, but should utilize as many tests as is practically possible (Table 17-1). For example, when the operative procedure is nearly finished and the

PHARMACOLOGY OF NONDEPOLARIZING MUSCLE RELAXANTS

Presently *d*-tubocurarine, pancuronium, metocurine (dimethyltubocurarine), and gallamine (Fig. 17-5) are the nondepolarizing muscle relaxants available for use in the United States. The doses under various clinical situations are listed in Table 17-2. These drugs are considered together in the subsections listed below.

Table 17-1. Suggested Comparison, Advantages, and Disadvantages of Tests of Neuromuscular Transmission

Test	Estimated Receptors Occupied (Percent)	Disadvantages
Tidal volume	80	Insensitive
Twitch height	75–80	Insensitive, uncomfortable, need to know twitch before relaxant administration
Sustained tetanus at 30 Hz	75–80	Insensitive, uncomfortable
Vital capacity	70–75	Insensitive, need patient cooperation
Train-of-four	70–75	Not very sensitive
Sustained tetanus at 100 Hz	50	Very painful
Inspiratory force	50	Sometimes difficult to perform without endotracheal intubation
Head lift and hand grip	33	Need patient cooperation

PHARMACOKINETICS AND PHARMACODYNAMICS

The rate of disappearance of muscle relaxant from blood is characterized by a rapid initial disappearance that is followed by a slower decay (Fig. 17-6). Distribution to tissues is the major cause of the initial decrease, whereas the slower decay is due to excretion. Because relaxants are highly ionized, they do not cross all membranes and have limited volume of distribution. The volume of distribution of relaxants[37] ranges from 80 to 140 ml/kg, which is not much larger than blood volume. If the volume of distribution is reduced, then the potency of muscle relaxant may be augmented. For example, if a disease state such as renal failure renders plasma proteins unable to bind *d*-tubocurarine, then the volume to which *d*-tubocurarine is distributed would be reduced making more available to the neuromuscular junction.[38] Reduced plasma protein binding would allow a more rapid excretion of *d*-tubocurarine by the kidney. The kidney eliminates *d*-tubocurarine by glomerular filtration. However,

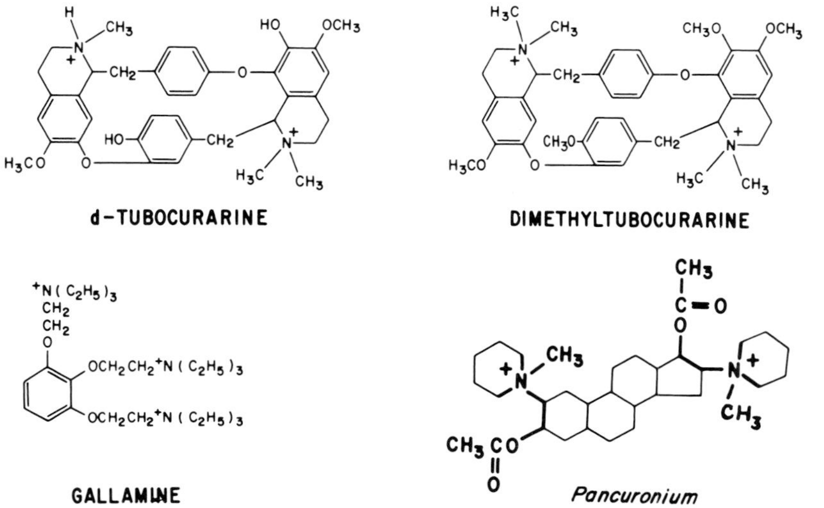

d–TUBOCURARINE

DIMETHYLTUBOCURARINE

GALLAMINE

Pancuronium

Fig. 17-5 Chemical formula of nondepolarizing neuromuscular blocking agents currently available in the United States.

Table 17-2. A Guide to Nondepolarizing Relaxant Dosage under Different Anesthetic Techniques*
(Dosages in mg/kg)

Drug	Potency Factor	Intubation	After Intubation		
			N₂O	Halothane (1 MAC)	Enflurane (1 MAC)
Pancuronium	1	0.06–0.08	0.04–0.06	0.03–0.04	0.02–0.03
Metocurine	4	0.3 –0.4	0.2 –0.25	0.1 –0.2	0.08–0.15
d-tubocurarine	7	0.5 –0.6	0.3 –0.4	0.2 –0.3	0.12–0.2
Gallamine	40	3.0 –4.0	2.0 –3.0	1.0 –2.0	0.8 –1.5
Approximate Fraction of "Intubing Dose"		1.0	0.7	0.5	0.3
Anesthetic Potency Factor			1.0	0.7	0.5

* Suggested dosages provide good intubating conditions under light anesthesia or satisfactory abdominal relaxation after intubation without a relaxant or with succinylcholine. Potency factors indicate the number of milligrams of other relaxants equal to 1 mg of pancuronium. Thus, pancuronium is 4, 7, and 40 times more potent than metocurine, d-tubocurarine, and gallamine. Fractions (bottom row) indicate amount of relaxant needed under indicated condition relative to dosage required for intubation. If the "potency factors" and the "intubating dose fractions" are known, then only the "intubating dose" for pancuronium need be remembered. The above table is intended as guide to dosage in general. Individual relaxant requirement should be confirmed with a peripheral nerve simulator. (Modified from Savarese JJ: Clinical use of muscle relaxants. Weekly Anesthesiology Update 2 (16):2, 1978.)

proteins are not filtered. So if *d*-tubocurarine is highly bound to protein, it will not be excreted readily by glomerular filtration. This would not be a factor with pancuronium, which probably is not bound to proteins to any extent.

The development of analytic techniques to measure muscle relaxant or antagonist concentrations in blood and other body tissues is of prime importance.[39–41] The plasma concentrations of neostigmine, pyridostigmine, edrophonium, pancuronium, and ORG NC 45 Norcuron (a new muscle relaxant) can now be measured by high pressure liquid chromatography, and the pharmacokinetics and pharmacodynamics of these drugs can now be studied. Why is this important clinically? Katz[42] and others have emphasized the variable response of patients to muscle relaxants. We believe this variability can, in large part, be explained by differences in pharmacokinetics and pharmacodynamics. For ex-

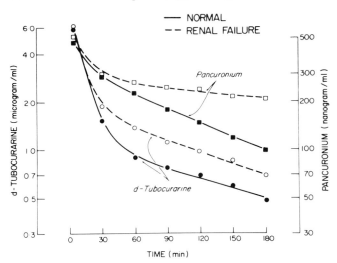

Fig. 17-6 Rates at which the plasma concentrations of *d*-tubocurarine and pancuronium decrease in patients with and without renal failure. Note that the decay rates are about the same in patients with normal renal function. However, the decay rate is much slower in patients with renal failure receiving pancuronium than those receiving *d*-tubocurarine. The data for pancuronium were obtained from McLeod, et al.[45] and for *d*-tubocurarine from Miller, et al.[37]

ample, What diseases and physiological changes alter the rate at which the relaxant leaves plasma and is eliminated (pharmacokinetics)? What diseases and physiological changes alter sensitivity of the neuromuscular junction to muscle relaxants (pharmacodynamics)? If the answers to these questions were available, anesthesiologists could be more selective in relaxant dose and avoid much of the "variability" described by Katz[26] and others.

Those pharmacokinetic factors that may alter muscle relaxant activity are (1) size of the initial dose, (2) renal failure, (3) biliary or liver disease, (4) anesthesia, (5) metabolism, (6) hypothermia, (7) age, (8) protein binding, (9) cerebrospinal fluid, and (10) metocurine. Although other factors undoubtedly exist, these are the ones that probably are the most important and that have been studied. Obviously, metocurine is not a factor. However, because metocurine's pharmacokinetics have not been emphasized previously, this drug is discussed separately.

SIZE OF INITIAL DOSE

Feldman[43] believes a strong affinity between muscle relaxant and receptor, rather than blood flow, produces the rate-limiting step in recovery from paralysis. Consequently, he argues that a single large bolus of relaxant given at the start of anesthesia will produce prolonged, adequate paralysis with a relatively low serum concentration of relaxant at the end of anesthesia. In contrast, he suggests that frequently repeated small doses of relaxant that are just sufficient to produce adequate paralysis will result in higher postoperative concentrations of relaxant. He believes that the latter approach is more likely to lead to residual postoperative paralysis with its attendant potential for respiratory complications.[43]

Certainly, initially administering large doses of muscle relaxant has its advantages. This technique will provide excellent surgical conditions and will mitigate the necessity of precisely regulating the anesthetic dose. However, the theory[27] that neuromuscular blockade may be easier to antagonize if a large (overdose) dose of muscle relaxant were given initially rather than small repetitive doses was recently tested. Ham et al.[44] found no difference in the pharmacokinetics and pharmacodynamics of *d*-tubocurarine when given by three dosage protocols: 20 mg/m^2 (about 34 mg/70 kg) as a single large bolus; repeated smaller doses of 5 mg/m^2 (about 8 mg/70 kg); or a continuous infusion titrated to maintain a constant 90 percent depression of twitch tension. Also, no difference in neostigmine antagonism between the three dosage schedules was found. These findings do not support Feldman's prediction of a lower serum muscle relaxant concentration with a large dose technique.[43]

Despite the lack of difference between the three dosage schedules in the Ham et al.[44] study, the use of small, frequent doses or continuous infusion of muscle relaxant while monitoring neuromuscular function with a peripheral nerve stimulator may have advantages over the large bolus technique. For example, the duration of neuromuscular blockade needed for a surgical procedure is not always predictable in advance; the large dose technique may result in 100 percent blockade, which cannot always be antagonized with anticholinesterase agents; with smaller doses or a continuous infusion the extent of neuromuscular blockade can be varied more readily with changing surgical needs.

RENAL FAILURE

Renal failure can profoundly affect the pharmacokinetics of relaxants. Gallamine, decamethonium, and probably metocurine are entirely dependent on renal excretion for their elimination. Recent studies in man indicate that pancuronium is more dependent on renal excretion than is *d*-tubocurarine

Table 17-3. Pharmacokinetics of Pancuronium in Patients with Normal Hepatic Function and Those with Cirrhosis[50]

Pharmacokinetic Variable	Normal Function (mean ± SE; N = 12)	Cirrhosis (mean ± SE; N = 14)
Distribution half life (min)	10.7 ± 1.3	23.7 ± 5
Elimination half life (min)	114 ± 10	208 ± 25
Clearance (ml/min/kg)	1.9 ± 0.1	1.5 ± 0.1
Volume of distribution (ml/kg)	279 ± 15	416 ± 58

(Fig. 17-6).[37,45,46] Even though the rate at which pancuronium and *d*-tubocurarine disappear from plasma is about the same with normal renal function, pancuronium disappears much slower during renal failure. However, Somogyi et al.[47] found the elimination half-life of pancuronium not to be prolonged by renal failure as much as that depicted in Figure 17-6. However, all investigators found much greater variability in patients with renal failure as compared to those with normal renal function. This probably reflects the varying associated problems (e.g., diabetes, anemia) in patients with renal disease. In any event, we still believe that *d*-tubocurarine probably is the preferred nondepolarizing relaxant for patients without renal function.[47]

Although the data in Figure 17-6 are convincing that *d*-tubocurarine is less dependent than is pancuronium on renal excretion for its elimination, this conclusion requires some caution. The immunoassay method measures only unchanged *d*-tubocurarine. The fluorimetric method does not distinguish between pancuronium and its metabolites. The slow rate at which pancuronium appears to leave the plasma (Figure 17-6) during renal failure may represent cumulation of relatively inactive metabolites. In spite of this analytic problem, we still believe that *d*-tubocurarine is less dependent on renal excretion for its elimination than is pancuronium. Metocurine has not been studied in patients with renal disease, but has been shown to be excreted nearly exclusively by the kidney in the dog. Furthermore, the occurrence of prolonged metocurine-induced paralysis, successfully treated by peritoneal dialysis or hemodialysis suggests that metocurine is also excreted entirely by the kidney in man.

BILIARY OR LIVER DISEASE

Several authors have suggested that relaxant requirement is increased[48] in patients with biliary or liver disease. Most of these opinions were based on rather scanty information. One might predict a prolonged neuromuscular blockade, since both *d*-tubocurarine and pancuronium are partly dependent on biliary excretion for their elimination. Somogyi et al.[49] found that the neuromuscular blockade and elimination half-life of pancuronium were prolonged in patients with extrahepatic biliary obstruction. Duvaldestin et al.[50] found that in patients with hepatic cirrhosis the volume of distribution is increased and the elimination half-life

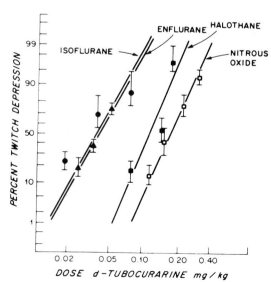

Fig. 17-7 The effect of anesthetics on a *d*-tubocurarine dose-response curve. (Ali HH, Savarese JJ: Monitoring of neuromuscular function. Anesthesiology 45:216, 1976.)

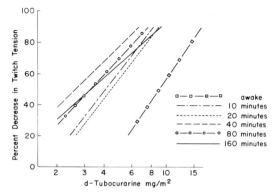

Fig. 17-8 The effect of duration of halothane anesthesia on a *d*-tubocurarine dose-response curve. (Miller RD, Criqui M, Eger EI II: The influence of duration of anesthesia on a *d*-tubocurarine neuromuscular blockade. Anesthesiology 44:207, 1976.)

of pancuronium is prolonged (Table 17-3). Because pancuronium is distributed to a larger volume in patients with cirrhosis, a larger dose of pancuronium may well be required to achieve a given neuromuscular blockade. However, once that neuromuscular blockade has been achieved, it should last longer because elimination is delayed. So, even though a larger dose of pancuronium may be required initially, subsequent doses can be smaller than normally expected.

ANESTHESIA

Inhaled anesthetics augment the neuromuscular block from nondepolarizing relaxants in a dose-dependent fashion (Fig. 17-7)[51] that surprisingly does not depend on the duration of anesthesia (for example, the case of halothane [Fig. 17-8]).[52] In contrast, enflurane's ability to enhance *d*-tubocurarine is time dependent and will be discussed later. Of those anesthetics studied, inhaled anesthetics augment the relaxants in decreasing order—isoflurane and enflurane > halothane > nitrous oxide–barbiturate–narcotic anesthesia (Figs. 17-7 and 17-9).[53–54] Several mechanisms have been proposed

by which inhaled anesthetics produce relaxation and augment the neuromuscular blockade from muscle relaxants. The mechanisms that are probably most important are those due to the ability of inhaled anesthetics to

(1) increase muscle blood flow—therefore, a greater fraction of the injected relaxant may reach the neuromuscular junction.[55] This probably is a factor only with isoflurane.

(2) induce relaxation at sites proximal to the neuromuscular junction, which obviously is the central nervous system.[56]

(3) not decrease release of acetylcholine from the motor nerve terminal.[57]

(4) have no demonstrable effect on the cholinergic receptor.[58,59]

(5) decrease the sensitivity of the postjunctional membrane to depolarization.[60,61]

(6) possibly act at a site distal to the cholinergic receptor and the postjunctional membrane, such as the muscle membrane.[58,59,61]

Conceptually, although most inhaled agents, such as halothane, do not decrease twitch tension, they reduce the margin of safety of neuromuscular transmission. Waud indicates that halothane acts at a site beyond the cholinergic receptor,[59,60] perhaps with either calcium conductance or release from depolarization, which may interfere with muscle contraction.[61] In an excellent review by Ngai,[61] it is emphasized that inhaled anesthetics are capable of producing relaxation through their action on the central nervous system with minimal neuromuscular blockade. So, adequate surgical conditions can exist without complete neuromuscular blockade,[61] when potent anesthetic vapors are given.

Despite changes in regional, renal, and hepatic blood flow, inhaled anesthetics have little or no effect on the pharmacokinetics of muscle relaxants in man.[67] The ability of inhaled anesthetics to augment a nondepolarizing neuromuscular blockade is a pharmacodynamic one—that is, the blood concentration of muscle relaxants required to

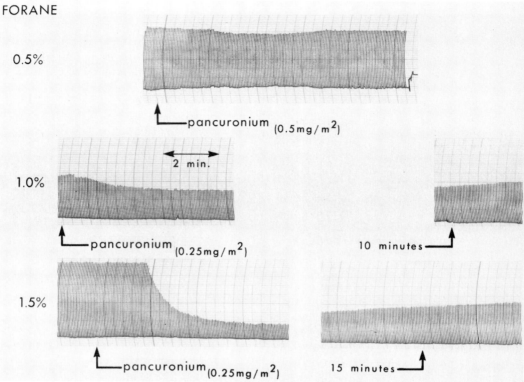

Fig. 17-9 The influence of anesthetic concentration on the magnitude of neuromuscular blockade from pancuronium. (Miller RD, Way WL, Dolan WM, et al: The dependence of pancuronium and *d*-tubocurarine induced neuromuscular blockades on alveolar concentrations of halothane and Forane. Anesthesiology 37:573, 1972.)

produce paralysis is decreased by inhaled anesthetics.

Unlike halothane, the ability of enflurane to enhance a *d*-tubocurarine neuromuscular blockade is time dependent. Stanski et al.[63] found that despite a constant blood level of *d*-tubocurarine, paralysis increased at a rate of 9 ± 4 percent/hr. This finding has been confirmed by Fahey et al. in an unpublished study. They have speculated that halothane achieves its maximal effect so rapidly because it acts on neural tissue (e.g., neuromuscular junction) where blood flow is high. Conversely they speculate that in addition to the neuromuscular junction, enflurane also acts on skeletal muscle where blood flow is less. Thus a longer time would be required for enflurane to achieve its maximal enhance-

ment of a nondepolarizing neuromuscular blockade.

METABOLISM

The only nondepolarizing muscle relaxant available in the United States that is metabolized is pancuronium. About 15 to 40 percent of an injected dose of pancuronium is deacetylated into 3-OH, 17-OH, or 3,17-OH pancuronium derivatives. (Fig. 17-10) The metabolites have been studied individually in anaesthetized patients.[64] The 3-OH metabolite is the most prominent in quantity and is the most potent; it is half as potent as pancuronium (Fig.17-11). Although the 3-OH metabolite has a duration of action similar to

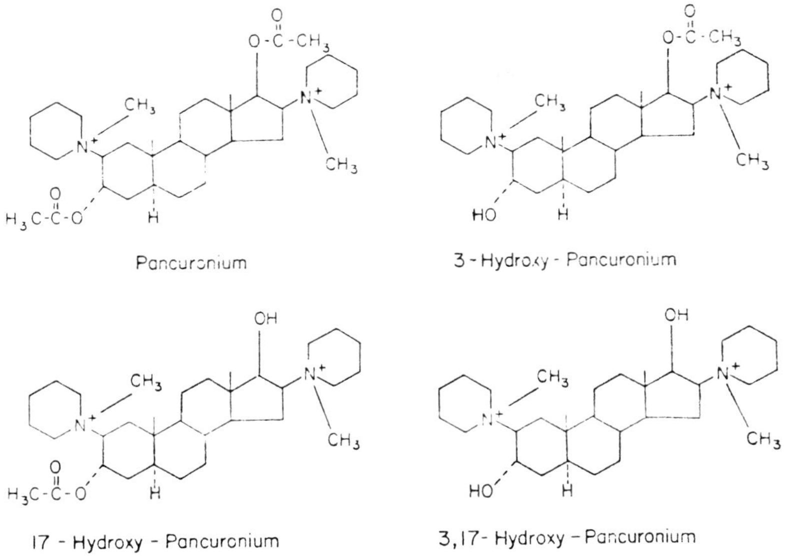

Fig. 17-10 Formula of pancuronium and its deacetylated metabolites.

Pancuronium

3 - Hydroxy - Pancuronium

17 - Hydroxy - Pancuronium

3,17- Hydroxy – Pancuronium

that of pancuronium and has similar pharmacokinetics, several questions remain. Is the block from the metabolite easily antagonized? Do the metabolites accumulate in patients with renal failure? Answers to these questions will soon appear. There is little doubt that the metabolism of pancuronium has clinical importance.

HYPOTHERMIA

Hypothermia prolongs a *d*-tubocurarine[65] and pancuronium[66] neuromuscular blockade. Blockades induced by both relaxants are prolonged because of delayed urinary and biliary excretion (Figure 17-12). With pancuronium, the block is also prolonged because of decreased metabolism into inactive metabolites.[66] Therefore hypothermia probably prolongs the block of pancuronium more than that of *d*-tubocurarine.

AGE

Several years ago, Stead[67] suggested that neonates were "miniature myasthenics." Certainly development of the neuromuscular junction is not complete at birth.[68] Premature infants are more susceptible to posttetanic exhaustion than term infants.[69] Goudsouzian[70] recently found that maturation of neuromuscular transmission occurs by the first 2 months of age. Despite the apparent immaturity of the neuromuscular junction at birth, investigators do not agree as to whether the newborn is more sensitive to nondepolarizing muscle relaxants.[67,71-77] The observed differences may be due to several factors including the type of anesthetic and different criteria used to determine dosages and/or levels of relaxation.

Only O'Keeffe et al.[78] have attempted to perform a pharmacokinetic and dynamic analysis of nondepolarizing muscle relaxants in children. With preliminary data they concluded that children (0 to 2 years old) are not more sensitive to *d*-tubocurarine than are adults. However, they did find that the elimination half-life ($t_{1/2\beta}$) was shorter and clearance from plasma quicker in children than in adults. Thus, given a sensitivity equivalent to adults, children may require repeated doses of *d*-tubocurarine at a greater frequency than adults.

Although there obviously is controversy regarding possible differences between neo-

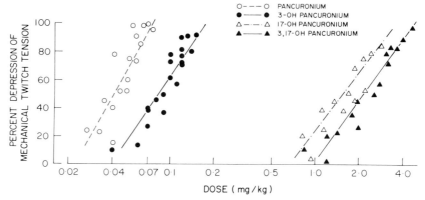

Fig. 17-11 Correlation between dose of muscle relaxant and depression of mechanical twitch tension. The lines represent analysis of linear regression. The correlation coefficients were 0.87, 0.92, 0.93, and 0.96 for pancuronium and its 3-OH, 17-OH, and 3,17-OH derivatives respectively. (Miller RD: Recent developments with muscle relaxants and their antagonists. Can Anaesth Soc J 26:83, 1979.)

nates and adults in their response to nondepolarizing muscle relaxants, this should be of little concern to the clinician. By gauging initial and repeated doses of nondepolarizing muscle relaxants according to objective criteria (e.g., stimulation of a peripheral nerve), overdoses and difficulties with antagonism of neuromuscular blockade can be avoided. Additional discussion of the use of muscle relaxants in children can be found in Chapter 36.

On the other end of the age scale, studies are now considering whether elderly patients (> 60 years) may respond differently than younger patients to nondepolarizing muscle relaxants. McLeod et al.[79] found that clearance of pancuronium was inversely related to age (Fig. 17-13). That is, patients in the third decade of life clear pancuronium from the plasma twice as fast as those in the ninth decade of life. Although neuromuscular function was not monitored, these authors predicted that the duration of neuromuscular blockade would be prolonged in the elderly. Also a

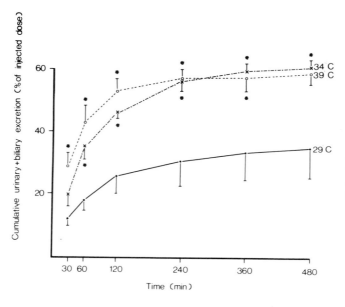

Fig. 17-12 Correlation between time after pancuronium 0.12 mg/kg and percentage of injected dose appearing in urine and bile. (Miller RD: Recent developments with muscle relaxants and their antagonists. Can Anaesth Soc J 26:83, 1979.)

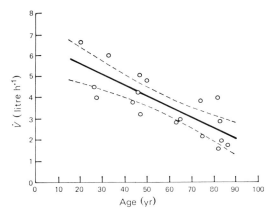

Fig. 17-13 Correlation between age (years) and pancuronium clearance from plasma ($\dot{V}$). (McLeod K, Hull CJ, Watson MJ: Effects of aging on the pharmacokinetics of pancuronium. Br J Anaesth 51:435, 1979.)

pharmacodynamic analysis (e.g., relationship between blood concentration of muscle relaxant and paralysis) has not been performed. With these limited data, we advise that elderly patients may require smaller doses of muscle relaxant and that the resultant neuromuscular blockade may be longer in duration. Thus the need for repetitive doses should be decreased in elderly patients.

PROTEIN BINDING

Sixteen percent of *d*-tubocurarine is bound to plasma albumen and 24 percent to gamma globulin.[80] While originally it was thought that pancuronium was not bound to plasma proteins, Thompson[81] recently demonstrated that 34 percent of pancuronium is bound to albumen and 53 percent to gamma globulin, and that 13 percent is unbound. Gallamine is bound to beta and gamma globulin, although the precise extent is unknown.[82] The clinical significance of protein binding is unclear. Theoretically, increasing binding would effectively increase the volume of distribution thus reducing free drug available at the site of action. Increased binding might also reduce renal elimination of the drug, since only free drug is filtered at the glomerulus. Finally the

possibility of another drug displacing the muscle relaxant from the protein and releasing it as active drug must be considered. However, Thompson has hypothesized that the number of binding sites may remain constant as plasma protein concentration increases if the proteins combine with their own binding sites.[81] Furthermore, binding of muscle relaxants with other sites such as cartilage and chondroitin sulfate may be qualitatively and quantitatively as important as plasma protein binding.[83] Therefore, it is difficult to predict the effect of alteration of protein binding on muscle relaxant pharmacokinetics. However, protein binding overall should not be of significant clinical concern. Even in patients with renal and hepatic disease, which are diseases well known to have altered protein binding to other drugs, the protein binding of *d*-tubocurarine is not altered.[84]

CEREBROSPINAL FLUID

Despite being ionized, intravenously administered nondepolarizing muscle relaxants do pass into the cerebrospinal fluid in amounts thought to be clinically significant.[85] However, neuromuscular blockade doses of gallamine given intravenously increase seizure threshold to lidocaine in dogs.[86] Forbes et al.[87] found that intravenously administered pancuronium reduced halothane anesthetic requirement (MAC) by 25 percent. Whether this was a central effect or was due to abolition of muscle spindle afferent input was not clarified. With these limited data, we conclude that small amounts of intravenously administered muscle relaxants do pass into the cerebrospinal fluid, but the clinical significance of this is unclear.

METOCURINE

Metocurine is being briefly considered separately to specifically discuss differences it may have from other nondepolarizing muscle

INHIBITION OF NEUROMUSCULAR AND AUTONOMIC FUNCTION BY d–TUBOCURARINE

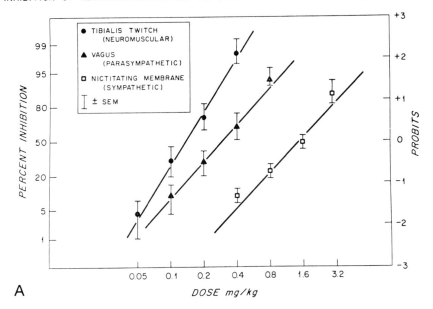

A

INHIBITION OF NEUROMUSCULAR AND AUTONOMIC FUNCTION BY PANCURONIUM

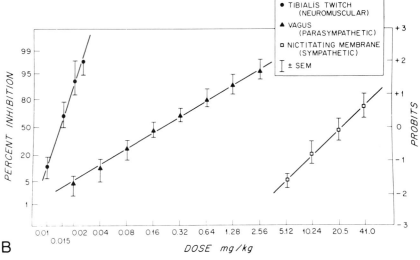

B

Fig. 17-14 (*A, B, & C*) Inhibition of neuromuscular and autonomic function by nondepolarizing relaxants in the cat. Note that autonomic and neuromuscular effects of *d*-tubocurarine occur within a narrow dose-range, whereas the side effects of metocurine are widely separated from its neuromuscular-blocking effect. The likelihood of hypotension during clinical use is, therefore, much less for metocurine than for *d*-tubocurarine. Pancuronium's principal autonomic effect, vagal blockade, becomes prominent as fully paralyzing doses are reached and exceeded. The vagolytic effect of gallamine (not shown) occurs within the same dose range as its neuromuscular blocking effect. Therefore, the likelihood of tachycardia during clinical use is greater for gallamine than for pancuronium.

INHIBITION OF NEUROMUSCULAR AND AUTONOMIC FUNCTION BY METOCURINE

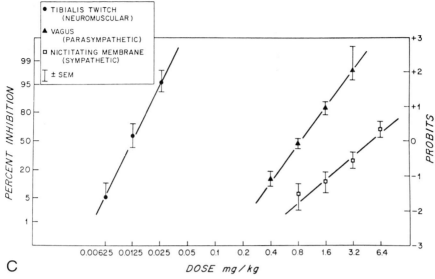

C

Fig. 17-14 (*continued*)

relaxants. Despite having the least cardiovascular effects of any nondepolarizing muscle relaxant in use in the United States, little has been published concerning its pharmacology. Savarese et al.[88] found metocurine approximately twice as potent as *d*-tubocurarine. However, the onset times and durations of action of *d*-tubocurarine and metocurine are similar. In a pharmacodynamic study correlating blood concentration with magnitude of neuromuscular blockade, Matteo and Khambatta[89] confirmed that metocurine is twice as potent as is *d*-tubocurarine.

The main difference is that *d*-tubocurarine is eliminated in the bile to a greater extent than is metocurine. Also, *d*-tubocurarine is less dependent on renal excretion for its elim-

ination, and probably is preferable to metocurine in patients with renal failure.[90]

CARDIOVASCULAR AND AUTONOMIC EFFECTS

All of the four nondepolarizing muscle relaxants produce cardiovascular effects. *d*-tubocurarine and, to a much lesser extent, metocurine produce hypotension. Pancuronium and gallamine produce tachycardia and, to a lesser extent, hypertension. Of these four muscle relaxants, metocurine produces the least cardiovascular change.[91,92] The autonomic effects of relaxants are summarized in Fig. 17-14*A*, *B*, and *C* and Table 17-4.

Table 17-4. Autonomic Effects of Neuromuscular Blocking Drugs

Drug	Autonomic Ganglia	Cardiac Muscarinic Receptors	Histamine Release
Succinylcholine	Stimulates	Stimulates	Slight
Decamethonium	None	None	None
d-tubocurarine	Blocks	None	Moderate
Metocurine	Blocks weakly	None	Slight
Gallamine	None	Blocks strongly	None
Pancuronium	None	Blocks weakly	None

HYPOTENSION

d-tubocurarine produces hypotension probably from liberation of histamine and in larger doses produces ganglionic blockade.[92,94] Dowdy et al.[95] proposed that hypotension was not from the *d*-tubocurarine itself but from the preservative in which it is stored. However within anesthetized patients, Stoelting[96] proved this theory not to be valid. Premedication with promethozine, an antihistamine drug, will attenuate *d*-tubocurarine–induced hypotension.[97] Hypotension is directly related to dose of *d*-tubocurarine and anesthetic depth,[94] especially if the anesthetic is a ganglionic blocker itself like halothane. With a light level of surgical anesthesia and the use of smaller doses of *d*-tubocurarine (15 mg/70 kg) the incidence of significant hypotension is markedly attenuated. Although hypotension can occur following administration of metocurine, the incidence and magnitude is much less than that associated with *d*-tubocurarine.

TACHYCARDIA

Pancuronium causes a moderate increase in heart rate and to a lessser extent cardiac output with little or no change in systemic vascular resistance.[98,99] Although this tachycardia has been attributed to a vagolytic action,[98] numerous investigators have implicated the sympathetic nervous system. Both indirect (release of norepinephrine from adrenergic nerve endings)[100,101] and direct (blockade of neuronal uptake of norepinephrine) mechanisms have been suggested.[101–103] Vercruysee et al.[104] suggested that both gallamine and pancuronium augment the release of norepinephrine in vascular tissues under vagal control. In studies in man, Roizen et al.[105] surprisingly found a decrease in plasma norepinephrine levels following administration of either pancuronium or atropine. They postulated that the increase in heart rate or rate-pressure product was be-cause pancuronium (or atropine) acts through baroreceptors to reduce sympathetic outflow. More specifically, pancuronium's vagolytic effect increases heart rate and hence blood pressure, which in turn influences the baroreceptors to decrease sympathetic tone. Support for this concept is provided by the fact that prior administration of atropine will attenuate or eliminate the cardiovascular effects of pancuronium.[98]

Gallamine increases heart rate by both vagolytic[106] and sympathetic stimulation.[107] Specifically, gallamine supposedly releases norepinephrine from adrenergic nerve endings in the heart by an unknown mechanism.[106] However, a positive chronotropic effect that places emphasis on the vagolytic mechanism has not been found in man.[108] It would not surprise us to ultimately find out that gallamine and pancuronium act by similar mechanisms.

ARRHYTHMIAS

Gallamine, *d*-tubocurarine, and succinylcholine actually reduce the incidence of epinephrine—induced arrhythmias.[109] Possibly because of enhanced atrioventricular conduction,[110] the incidence of arrhythmias from pancuronium appears to increase during halothane anesthesia.[98] Edwards et al.[111] observed a rapid tachycardia (> 150 beats/min) that progressed to atrioventricular dissociation in two patients anesthetized with halothane. The only common factor between these two patients was that they were both receiving tricyclic antidepressants. In further studies, Edwards et al.[111] found that the incidence of severe ventricular arrhythmia was common following pancuronium administration in dogs receiving halothane (but not enflurane) and chronically administered tricyclic antidepressants. We therefore conclude that the drug interaction between tricyclic antidepressants, halothane, and pancuronium must be avoided. Use of another muscle relaxant, such as *d*-tubocurarine, probably is the most convenient approach.

CLINICAL MANAGEMENT

We agree with Katz and Katz[112] who believe that muscle relaxants are widely abused but that little harm usually results because of the incredible safety of these drugs. However, to avoid prolonged paralysis and/or inadequate antagonism, using the lowest dose possible and yet providing adequate relaxation for surgery should be the main goal. Katz and Katz[112] recommend that the rational use of muscle relaxants can be achieved by the anesthesiologist who is familiar with the operative procedure and knows when muscle relaxants are required, has a method for assessing the magnitude and duration of action of the muscle relaxant, and understands the clinical pharmacology of the drug, including knowledge of side effects and complications of the relaxants.

The key factor is to avoid an overdose. In an adequately anesthetized patient, there is no reason to completely obliterate the twitch or train-of-four in response to peripheral nerve stimulation. In a patient who does not have a disease or is not receiving a drug that may influence the action of nondepolarizing muscle relaxants, we start with the intravenous administration of nondepolarizing relaxants, the dosage of which is dependent on the anesthetic being used as outlined in Table 17-2. Repetitive doses probably should be about $1/3$ to $1/5$ the initial dose and should not be given until some evidence of recovery from the previous dose is evident. Following these guidelines will help avoid an excessive neuromuscular blockade that cannot be antagonized.

PHARMACOLOGY OF DEPOLARIZING MUSCLE RELAXANTS

Although decamethonium is available, it is rarely used. Thus this entire section is devoted to the clinical pharmacology of succinylcholine (Fig. 17-15).

PHARMACOKINETICS AND PHARMACODYNAMICS

The extremely brief duration of action of succinylcholine is primarily due to its rapid hydrolysis by pseudocholinesterase, an enzyme of the liver and plasma. The initial metabolite, succinylmonocholine, is a much weaker neuromuscular blocker. It, in turn, is metabolized to succinic acid and choline. Pseudocholinesterase has an enormous capacity to hydrolyze succinylcholine at a very rapid rate such that a small fraction of the original intravenous dose actually reaches the neuromuscular junction. Since there is little or no pseudocholinesterase at the motor endplate, the neuromuscular blockade of succinylcholine is terminated by its diffusion away from the endplate into extracellular fluid. Pseudocholinesterase, therefore, influences the duration of action of succinylcholine by controlling the rate at which the latter is hydrolyzed before it reaches the endplate.

A succinylcholine neuromuscular blockade can be prolonged by a reduced quantity of normal enzyme or by an atypical form of pseudocholinesterase. Factors that have been described to lower pseudocholinesterase levels are (1) liver disease,[113] (2) pregnancy,[114] (3) phenelzine,[114] (4) echothiophate,[114] (5) cytotoxic drugs, (6) tetrahydroaminacrine,[115] (7) hexafluorenium,[114] (8) cancer,[116] and (9) acetylcholinesterase inhibitors.[117,118]

Despite all the publications and effort identifying those situations in which pseudocholinesterase levels may be low, this is of little concern. For example, Foldes et al.[113] found that when pseudocholinesterase was reduced to 20 percent of normal by severe liver disease, duration of apnea following succinylcholine administration was increased from a normal duration of 3 minutes to almost 9 minutes. Even when echothiophate eye treatment decreased pseudocholinesterase activity from 49 percent of control to no activity, the increase in deviation of neuromuscular blockade varied from 2 to 14 min-

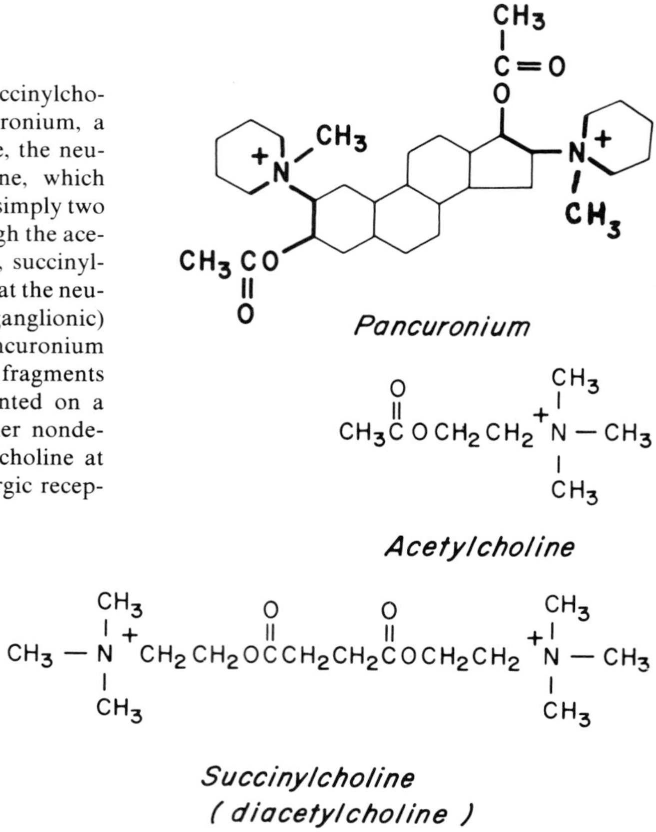

Fig. 17-15 Structural relationship of succinylcholine, a depolarizing agent, and pancuronium, a nondepolarizing agent, to acetylcholine, the neuromuscular transmitter. Succinylcholine, which was originally called diacetylcholine, is simply two molecules of acetylcholine linked through the acetate methyl groups. Like acetylcholine, succinylcholine stimulates cholinergic receptors at the neuromuscular junction and at nicotinic (ganglionic) and muscarinic autonomic sites. Pancuronium may be viewed as two acetylcholine-like fragments (outlined in dark print) properly oriented on a steroid nucleus. Pancuronium and other nondepolarizers inhibit the actions of acetylcholine at neuromuscular and autonomic cholinergic receptors.

Pancuronium

Acetylcholine

Succinylcholine
(diacetylcholine)

utes. In no patient did the total duration of neuromuscular blockade exceed 23 minutes.[114] In an extensive clinical study, Viby-Mogensen[119] confirmed these observations that duration of blockade from the usual clinical dose of succinylcholine is moderately increased by low pseudocholinesterase levels (Fig. 17-16).[119] Thus if repeated doses are given only when recovery from the previous dose of succinylcholine is evident, low pseudocholinesterase levels should slightly prolong a succinylcholine blockade and this should present no serious problem.

A succinylcholine neuromuscular blockade can be prolonged if the patient has an abnormal genetically derived variant of pseudocholinesterase. This variant was found by Kalow and Genest[120] to respond to dibucaine

differently than does normal pseudocholinesterase. Dibucaine inhibits normal pseudocholinesterase to a far greater extent than the abnormal enzyme. This observation led to the development of the "dibucaine number." Under standardized test conditions, dibucaine inhibits the normal enzyme about 80 percent and an abnormal enzyme about 20 percent (Table 17-5). Subsequently, many other genetic variants of pseudocholinesterase have been identified although the dibucaine-related variants are the most important. An excellent review by Pantuck and Pantuck[114] has a more detailed assessment of this topic.

The relationship between low dibucaine numbers and low pseudocholinesterase levels is often confusing. To repeat, a patient may

Table 17-5. Relationship between Dibucaine Number and Duration of Succinylcholine Neuromuscular Blockade

Type of Pseudocholinesterase	Frequency	Dibucaine Number*	Response to Succinylcholine
Homozygons typical	Normal	80	Normal
Heterozygons	1/480	50	Slightly prolonged
Homozygons atypical	1/3,200	20	Markedly prolonged

* The dibucaine number indicates the percentage of enzyme inhibited.

have a normal pseudocholinesterase level and yet with a low dibucaine number have a prolonged response to succinylcholine, indicating the presence of primarily atypical enzyme. Conversely the pseudocholinesterase level may be very low, and the patient may have a normal dibucaine number, but the response to succinylcholine may be slightly prolonged[119] because of the presence of only a small total quantity of enzyme, all of which is normal. In other words, the dibucaine number does not reflect the quantity of pseudocholinesterase present, but the quality of the enzyme, i.e., its ability to hydrolyze succinylcholine. Two other topics deserve mention in this section. Hexafluorenium is a nondepolarizing muscle relaxant that also inhibits pseudocholinesterase. Because of this later effect, it has been used to prolong the effect of succinylcholine so that the total dose of the latter can be reduced. Although some clinicians have successfully used this approach, it has not proven to be particularly advantageous and has not gained widespread popularity.

Lastly, the administration of blood or plasma has been recommended as therapy for a prolonged neuromuscular blockade in patients with low pseudocholinesterase levels.[121] Complete recovery from a pro-

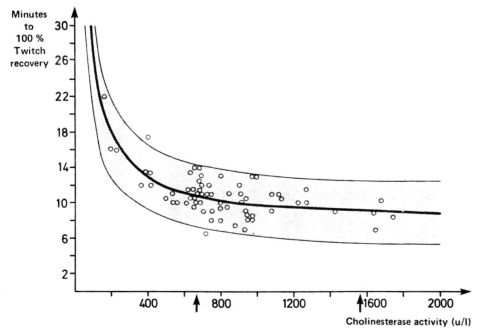

Fig. 17-16 Correlation between duration of succinylcholine neuromuscular blockade and pseudocholinesterase activity. (Viby-Mogensen J: Correlation of succinylcholine duration of action with plasma cholinesterase activity in subjects with the genotypically normal enzyme. Anesthesiology 53:517, 1980.)

longed response to succinylcholine can be achieved with controlled ventilation until the block spontaneously dissipates without significant morbidity or mortality. Considering the potential hazards of blood or plasma transfusion, this approach does not seem to be advisable.[122]

CARDIOVASCULAR EFFECTS

Succinylcholine-induced cardiac arrhythmias are many and varied. The drug stimulates all cholinergic autonomic receptors: nicotinic receptors in both sympathetic and parasympathetic ganglia[123] and muscarinic receptors in the sinus node of the heart. In low doses, both a negative inotropic and chronotropic response occurs that can be attenuated by prior administration of atropine. With large doses these effects may become positive.[124] One prominent clinical manifestation of this generalized autonomic stimulation is the development of cardiac arrhythmias. These are principally manifest as sinus bradycardia, junctional rhythms, and ventricular arrhythmias ranging from unifocal premature ventricular contractions to ventricular fibrillation in certain special circumstances (see below). Since many authors of clinical studies have noted these arrhythmias under various conditions in the presence of the intense autonomic stimulus of tracheal intubation, it is not entirely clear whether the cardiac irregularities are due to the action of succinylcholine alone or to the added presence of extraneous autonomic stimulation.

Sinus Bradycardia

The autonomic mechanism involved in sinus bradycardia is stimulatioin of cardiac muscarinic receptors in the sinus node, particularly in nonatropinized, relatively sympathotonic individuals, e.g., children.[125, 126] Sinus bradycardia has also been noted in adults[127] and appears more commonly after a second dose of the drug given approximately 5 minutes after the first. The bradycardia may be prevented by thiopental,[128] atropine, ganglion-blocking drugs, and nondepolarizing relaxants,[128, 129] the implication being that direct myocardial effects, increased muscarinic stimulation, and ganglionic stimulation may all be involved in the bradycardic response. The higher incidence of bradycardia after a second dose of succinylcholine[128] suggests that the hydrolysis products of succinylcholine (succinylmonocholine and choline) may "sensitize" the heart.

Nodal (Junctional) Rhythms

Nodal rhythms commonly occur as bradycardias that are slower than the sinus rate in existence before the administration of succinylcholine and intubation of the trachea. The mechanism probably involves relatively greater stimulation of cholinergic receptors in the sinus node, the result being suppression of the sinus mechanism and emergence of the atrioventricular node as the pacemaker. The incidence of junctional rhythm is higher after a second dose of succinylcholine[131] but is prevented by prior administration of *d*-tubocurarine.[127, 129]

Ventricular Arrhythmias

Succinylcholine, under stable anesthetic conditions, lowers the threshold of the ventricle to catecholamine-induced arrhythmias in the monkey and in the dog. Other autonomic stimuli, such as endotracheal intubation, hypoxia, hypercarbia, and operations, are probably additive to the effect of succinylcholine. To these stimuli must be added the possible influence of drugs such as digitalis, tricyclic antidepressants, monoamine oxidase inhibitors, exogenous catecholamines, and anesthetic drugs such as halothane and cyclopropane, all of which may lower the ventricular threshold for ectopic activity or increase the arrhythmogenic effect of the catecholamines. The influence of digitalis has been questioned, however.

Ventricular escape beats may also occur as a result of severe sinus and atrioventricular nodal slowing secondary to succinylcholine administration.

The occurrence of ventricular arrhythmias is further encouraged by the release of potassium from skeletal muscle as a consequence of the depolarizing action of the drug. Hyperkalemia from succinylcholine is discussed next.

COMPLICATIONS

HYPERKALEMIA

Clinical reports and experimental studies have clearly shown that patients with certain diseases or conditions may have an exaggerated release of potassium in response to succinylcholine, occasionally of such magnitude that cardiac arrest ensues. Conditions patients may have that are especially susceptible to a hyperkalemic response from succinylcholine are burns, trauma, nerve damage or neuromuscular disease, closed head injury, intra-abdominal infections, and renal failure.

Burns

Burn patients may have a significant increase in serum potassium following succinylcholine administration as high as 13mEq/L which has led to several cases of cardiac arrest. However, this susceptibility to hyperkalemia exists only between about 10 and 60 days postburn, is dose related, and varies directly with the extent of burn.[130] Pretreatment with nondepolarizing muscle relaxants is not effective. Despite this evidence our rule of thumb is that succinylcholine should not be given to a patient who has had the burn longer than a week. The 60-day

rule of thumb is only valid if the burn heals without infection. If infection is present, tissues are probably continuing to degenerate and therefore the 60-day rule during which time succinylcholine should not be given should be extended.

Trauma

Birch et al.[131] studying soldiers who had undergone trauma associated with the Vietnam War, found that a significant increase in serum potassium did not occur in 59 patients until about 1 week after injury, at which time a progressive increase in the serum potassium level occurred following infusion of succinylcholine. Three weeks after injury, three of these patients with especially severe injuries showed a marked hyperkalemia (increase greater than 3.6 mEq/L) which is sufficient to cause cardiac arrest. They found that administration of *d*-tubocurarine, 6mg, intravenously prevented the hyperkalemic response to succinylcholine. As with the burns, in the absence of infection or persistent degeneration of tissue, a patient is susceptible probably for 60 days following trauma or until adequate healing of damaged muscle has occurred.

Nerve Damage or Neuromuscular Disease

Cooperman[132] described 40 patients with neuromuscular disease, 15 of whom had an increase in serum potassium from 1 to 6 mEq/L after the intravenous administration of succinylcholine 1mg/kg. In another instance, Cooperman et al.[133] reported a hyperkalemic response, one of which was 9.05 mEq/L, in three patients with hemiplegia or paraplegia secondary to upper motor neuron lesions. Cooperman[132] concluded that the vulnerable period appears to be within the first 6 months after the acute onset of hemiplegia or paraplegia and within a longer period of time in patients with progressive disease such as muscular dystrophy. He speculated that in the latter instance, progressive muscle wasting or other structural change accounted for the prolonged susceptibility. He also found that the degree of hyperkalemia directly correlated with the degree and extent of muscle affected. The largest hyperkalemia was found in those patients with greater neurologic deficit and the involvement of more muscle mass. For a more intense clinical and pathophysiological discussion of this topic, the reader is referred to the excellent review of Gronert and Theye.[134]

Closed Head Injury

Stevenson and Birch[135] described a well-documented case in which a marked hyperkalemic response from succinylcholine occurred in a patient with a closed head injury without peripheral paralysis. One should be hesitant in concluding that succinylcholine should not be given to a patient with a closed head injury on the basis of this one case report. However, because this case was well documented, a high degree of suspicion should exist when giving succinylcholine to this group of patients.

Intra-abdominal Infections

Kohlschütter et al.[136] found that four of nine patients with severe abdominal infections had an increase in serum potassium (2.5 to 3.1 mEq/L) from succinylcholine. They concluded that if severe intra-abdominal infection has existed for longer than a week, a possible hyperkalemic response to succinylcholine should be considered.

Renal Failure

Several case reports suggest that patients with renal failure may be susceptible to a hyperkalemic response to succinylcholine.[137, 138]

However, in more controlled studies, patients were found not to be any more susceptible to an exaggerated response to succinylcholine than patients with normal renal function.[139-142] Korde and Waud[142] concluded that patients with a serum potassium above 5.5 mEq/L not only should not receive succinylcholine but also should not be anesthetized. However no data were presented to support this conclusion. In the senior author's experience in anesthetizing hundreds of patients with renal failure, succinylcholine often is the muscle relaxant of choice because of its lack of dependence on renal excretion for its elimination. One might postulate that if patients have uremic neuropathy, they may be susceptible to hyperkalemia from succinylcholine although the evidence supporting this view is scanty.[143, 144]

Increased Intraocular Pressure

Succinylcholine, when given by itself, usually causes an increase in intraocular pressure (IOP). The increased IOP is manifested 1 minute after injection, peaks between the second and fourth minute, and subsides by the sixth minute.[145] The mechanism by which succinylcholine increases IOP has not been clearly defined but involves contraction of tonic myofibrils or transient dilation of choroidal blood vessels. Despite this increase in IOP, use of succinylcholine for eye operations is not contraindicated unless the anterior chamber is open.

Numerous investigators have found that prior administration of a subparalyzing dose of nondepolarizing muscle relaxant (e.g., gallamine, 20 mg; d-tubocurarine, 3 mg; or pancuronium, 1 mg) will prevent the increase in IOP from succinylcholine.[146, 147] Yet Meyers et al.[148] were unable to confirm the efficacy of this approach. Despite this discrepancy, the senior author has successfully used this approach many times in providing anesthesia for patients with eye surgery. Also, the reader should consult Chapter 39. In the total picture, succinylcholine is only one of many factors, which includes endotracheal intubation and "bucking" on the tube, that may elevate IOP.[148] Of prime importance is insuring that the patient is well anesthetized and is not straining. There are several approaches to accomplish this goal.[146, 147, 149]

There probably are three situations in which succinylcholine should either be avoided or the above measures be taken to prevent its increasing IOP: if the patient is about to have repair of an ocular laceration, if the patient is about to have repair of a recent surgical incision that is coming apart, and if the patient's anesthesia lightens in the course of intraocular surgery. In the last case succinylcholine should not be given to quiet the patient, but the surgeon should be asked to pause while anesthesia is deepened without the use of muscle relaxants.[149]

INCREASED INTRAGASTRIC PRESSURE

Unlike the rather consistent increase in IOP, the increase in intragastric pressure (IGP) from succinylcholine is quite variable (Fig. 17-17). In fact, Miller and Way[150] found that 11 of 30 patients essentially had no increase in IGP. Yet 5 of 30 patients had an increase in IGP greater than 30 cm H_2O. The increase in IGP from succinylcholine appeared to be related to the intensity of fasciculations. Accordingly, when fasciculations were prevented by prior administration of gallamine, 20 mg, or *d*-tubocurarine, 3 mg, no increase in IGP was observed.

The increase in IGP from succinylcholine is presumed to be due to fasciculation of the abdominal skeletal muscle. This is not surprising, since more coordinated abdominal skeletal muscle activity (such as straight leg raising) may increase IGP to values as high as 120 cm H_2O. In addition to skeletal muscle fasciculations, the acetylcholine-like effect of succinylcholine may be partly responsible for the observed increases in IGP. Greenan[151] observed consistent increases in IGP of 4 to 7 cm H_2O with direct vagal stimulation. Therefore, prior administration of vagolytic

drugs may partly inhibit succinylcholine-induced increases in IGP. Thus, gallamine or pancuronium with their vagolytic actions should be more effective than *d*-tubocurarine in preventing the increase in IGP. This hypothesis, however, has not been tested.

Are the increases in IGP following succinylcholine administration enough to cause incompetence of the gastroesophageal junction? Generally IGP of greater than 28 cm H_2O is required to overcome the competence of the gastroesophageal junction. However, when the normal oblique angle of entry of the esophagus into the stomach is altered, as may occur with pregnancy, an abdomen distended by ascites or bowel obstruction, obesity, or a hiatus hernia, the IGP required to cause incompetence of the gastroesophageal junction is frequently less than 15 cm H_2O.[150] Under these circumstances, regurgitation of stomach contents following succinylcholine is a distinct possibility, and precautionary measures should be taken to prevent fasciculations.

Apparently succinylcholine does not appreciably increase IGP in infants and children.[152] This may be related to the minimal or absence of fasciculations from succinylcholine in these age groups.[152]

MUSCLE PAINS

The incidence of muscle pains following succinylcholine administration varies from 0.2 to 89 percent.[153] It occurs more frequently following minor surgery especially in women and in ambulatory rather than bedridden patients. Waters and Mapleson[154] postulated that the pain is secondary to damage produced in muscle by the unsynchronized contraction of adjacent muscle fibers just before the onset of paralysis. That damage to muscle may occur has been substantiated by finding myoglobinemia following succinylcholine.[155] If this hypothesis is valid, the prevention of fasciculations should eliminate muscle pain from succinylcholine. Prior administration of a subparalyzing dose of nondepolarizing muscle relaxant clearly prevents fascicula-

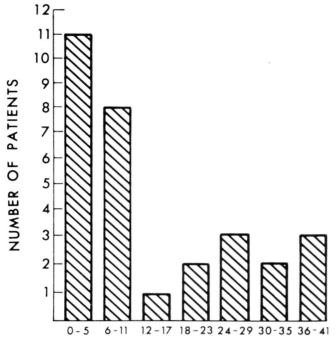

Fig. 17-17 Change in intragastric pressure from succinylcholine administration. Note that only a few patients had large increases in intragastric pressure. (Miller RD, Way WL: Inhibition of succinylcholine-induced increased intragastric pressure by nondepolarizing muscle relaxants and lidocaine. Anesthesiology 34:185, 1971.)

tions from succinylcholine.[156] Yet the efficacy of this approach in preventing muscle pains is questionable. Although some investigators claim that pretreatment with a subparalyzing dose of nondepolarizing muscle relaxant has no effect,[153] most feel that at least the pain from succinylcholine is attenuated.[154,156]

The senior author[157] believes the practice of preceding succinylcholine administration with a small dose of nondepolarizing muscle relaxant should be routine. The fasciculations certainly in no way are desirable. Furthermore, postoperative muscle pains and elevated IOP and IGP will be decreased or eliminated. Also succinylcholine-induced increases in serum creatinine phosphokinase and myoglobinuria may be attenuated. Although the succinylcholine dose should be increased by 30 to 50 percent, this appears to present no problems.[157] Occasionally patients may be very sensitive to these small doses of nondepolarizing muscle relaxants. Obviously, one

should not assume that these small doses of nondepolarizing muscle relaxants will never cause a clinically significant block. Therefore it almost goes without saying that these small, usually subparalyzing, doses of nondepolarizing muscle relaxants should not be administered in the absence of equipment for resuscitation.[158]

INTERACTION WITH
NONDEPOLARIZING MUSCLE
RELAXANTS, NEOSTIGMINE, AND
PYRIDOSTIGMINE

Nondepolarizing (*d*-tubocurarine, pancuronium, and gallamine) and depolarizing (succinylcholine and decamethonium) muscle relaxants are antagonistic[159,160] or additive[161] depending upon the experimental design. Both types of relaxants are administered concomitantly in three possible situations:

Table 17-6. Clinical Characteristics of a Phase I and Phase II Neuromuscular Blockade from Succinylcholine

Characteristic	Phase I	Transition	Phase II
Tetanic stimulation	No face	Slight fade	Fade
Posttetanic facilitation	None	Slight	Yes
Train-of-four	Slight fade	Moderate fade	Marked fade
Train-of-four ratio	> 0.7	0.4–0.7	< 0.4
Edrophonium	Augment	Little effect	Antagonize
Recovery	Rapid	Rapid	Increasingly prolonged
Dose requirements (mg/kg)	2–3	4–5	6 or more

(Adapted from Lee C, Katz RL: Neuromuscular pharmacology. Br J Anaesth 52:73,1980.)

1. Succinylcholine is commonly given to facilitate intubation of the trachea, and then a longer-acting nondepolarizing relaxant such as *d*-tubocurarine or pancuronium is administered. Presumably the block from a nondepolarizing relaxant will not be altered if given after the block from succinylcholine has dissipated; however, Katz[161] reported that prior administration of succinylcholine nearly doubled the depression of twitch height from the same dose of pancuronium. A comparable increase in duration of block occurred. Although succinylcholine and *d*-tubocurarine are supposedly antagonistic,[162] Katz et al.[161] have speculated that perhaps the endplate is still desensitized from the first dose of succinylcholine. If so, this may account for the unexpected increase in duration of nondepolarizing block when preceded by succinylcholine.

2. A small dose of a nondepolarizing agent is commonly given prior to giving succinylcholine to prevent some of the adverse effects of the latter. This approach is discussed above in the section under muscle pains.

3. *d*-tubocurarine can be injected for prolonged relaxation, and then the shorter-acting succinylcholine can be given to facilitate closure of the peritoneum. The amount of succinylcholine required for adequate relaxation is directly dependent on the amount of residual *d*-tubocurarine effect present.[159] Despite the questionable pharmacologic reasoning, concomitant administration of an antagonist and agonist in appropriate doses appears to be effective.[157] Whether it is the best way to solve the problem is the subject of much debate. Many prefer to give an additional dose of nondepolarizer that can be easily an-

tagonized at the end of the operation or to deepen anesthesia. The latter approach is our preference.

Another interaction with succinylcholine involves neostigmine or pyridostigmine. For example, after *d*-tubocurarine has been used for an intra-abdominal surgery of long duration and the neuromuscular blockade reversed by neostigmine, the surgeon announces that he needs another 15 minutes to retrieve a remaining sponge. Should succinylcholine be given? Our experience is that succinylcholine, 100 mg/70 kg, given intravenously, produces a neuromuscular blockade that normally lasts 5 to 10 minutes but will last up to 60 minutes when given soon after administration of neostigmine. Sunew and Hicks[163] found that the effect of succinylcholine, 1mg/kg, was prolonged from 11 to 35 minutes when given 5 minutes after administration of neostigmine, 5 mg. This can partly be explained by inhibition of pseudocholinesterase by neostigmine and to a lesser extent by pyridostigmine.

CLINICAL MANAGEMENT

The changing characteristics of a succinylcholine neuromuscular blockade from a clinical point of view have been nicely reviewed by Lee and Katz[164] (Table 17-6).

Although the response to tetanic stimuli can be used, train-of-four stimulation has proven to be a very useful guide in detecting the transition from a phase I to a phase II block (Table 17-6). Clearly both the dose and the time of administration of succinylcholine are important variables, although the relative contribution of each has not been established. Practically, if the use of the drug is terminated shortly after train-of-four fade is clearly evident, rapid return of normal neuromuscular function will ensue. Also whether antagonism of a phase II block should be attempted has always been controversial. However, it is now clear that if the train-of-four ratio is less than 0.4, administration of edrophonium or neostigmine results in prompt antagonism. Ramsey et al.[165] recommend that antagonism of a succinylcholine-induced phase II block with edrophonium or neostigmine should be attempted after spontaneous recovery of the twitch has been observed for a period of 20 to 30 minutes and has reached a plateau phase with further recovery proceeding slowly. They state that in this situation, edrophonium and neostigmine invariably produce "dramatic" acceleration of the return of train-of-four toward normal. Ramsey et al.[165] state that the dosage guideline in Table 17-6 apply to only halothane or enflurane anesthesia. With nitrous oxide intravenous anesthesia, the dosage guidelines are more variable. The increased variability of muscle relaxant response during nitrous oxide intravenous anesthesia is also true with nondepolarizing muscle relaxants.[62] in any event, monitoring neuromuscular function via peripheral nerve stimulation, such as the train-of-four, will help avoid succinylcholine overdose, detect development of a phase II block, follow its rate of recovery, and assess the effect of edrophonium or neostigmine on the recovery from a phase II block.

ANTAGONISM OF A NONDEPOLARIZING NEUROMUSCULAR BLOCKADE

The criteria for determining whether a block has been antagonized have been described in the section on monitoring of neuromuscular function. Neostigmine and pyridostigmine antagonize a nondepolarizing neuromuscular blockade by increasing the availability of acetylcholine at the muscle endplate mainly by inhibition of acetylcholinesterase and to a much lesser extent by increased release of transmitter from the motor nerve terminals.[166] For more detailed information concerning the chemistry of acetylcholinesterase inhibition by edrophonium, neostigmine, or pyridostigmine, the reader is referred to the excellent work of Kitz.[167, 168]

FACTORS THAT MAY INTERFERE WITH ANTAGONISM

Our approach is not to give more antagonist if neostigmine (2.5 to 5.0 mg/70 kg) or pyridostigmine (10 to 20 mg/70 kg) fail to antagonize the block. These doses maximally inhibit acetylcholinesterase and larger doses may cause a block themselves.[169] If these doses fail to antagonize the block, the cause for the inadequate antagonism should be sought. Some of these causes are listed below.

INTENSITY OF NEUROMUSCULAR BLOCKADE

The degree of neuromuscular blockade at the time when neostigmine is administered determines the speed and extent of antagonistic action by neostigmine. When twitch height is more than 20 percent of control, time from neostigmine administration (2.5 mg) to attainment of control twitch height is 3 to 14 minutes. When twitch heights are less than 20 percent of control, recovery takes 8 to 29 minutes (Fig. 17-18).[170] Our observations indicate that most attempts to antagonize the block occur when a 90 to 100 percent depression of twitch tension exists. It should not be surprising if 30 to 45 minutes are required for twitch height to return to control levels or even longer for a sustained contraction in response to a tetanic stimulus of 50 Hz.

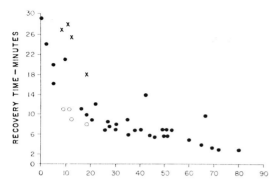

Fig. 17-18 Correlation between twitch height when a bolus of neostigmine, 2.5 mg, was given IV and time it took for twitch height to return to its control height. (Katz RL: Clinical neuromuscular pharmacology of pancuronium. Anesthesiology 34:550, 1971.)

RELAXANT BEING ANTAGONIZED

The neuromuscular blockade from gallamine resists reversal by neostigmine more than do those from *d*-tubocurarine and pancuronium. Monks[171] found that neostigmine-induced recovery from a *d*-tubocurarine or pancuronium block was faster than recovery from a gallamine block. He concluded that a *d*-tubocurarine or pancuronium block is "more easily reversed" than a gallamine block. Although these studies infer that gallamine—which required more neostigmine for reversal—is less desirable, all the gallamine blocks in our study[172] were completely antagonized by neostigmine. Monks[171] did not follow the twitch response until complete recovery occurred. Does the fact that gallamine requires more neostigmine for antagonism represent an undesirable clinical effect? We suspect not.

ACID-BASE STATE

Respiratory acidosis may augment a nondepolarizing neuromuscular blockade but, more importantly, limits and prevents its antagonism (Fig. 17-19).[173, 174] In other words, it is impossible to antagonize a nondepolarizing neuromuscular blockade in the presence of significant respiratory acidosis ($PaCO_2$ >50 torr). This has many clinical ramifications. For example, if a patient hypoventilates in the recovery room, attempts to antagonize a residual *d*-tubocurarine block may fail. Administration of narcotics to relieve pain may increase the likelihood of this untoward event. Such a sequence contains an element of potential positive feedback in which respiratory depression produces more acidosis and relaxant effect and, hence, more respiratory depression.

Although metabolic acidosis might also be predicted to prevent antagonism by neostigmine, this has not been substantiated.[173, 174] To our surprise, metabolic alkalosis, but not metabolic acidosis, prevented neostigmine antagonism of *d*-tubocurarine and pancuronium (Fig. 17-19).[173, 174] These results suggest that extracellular hydrogen ion concentration (pH) per se may not be as important as changes in electrolytes and intracellular pH. Metabolic alkalosis produced by infusion of sodium bicarbonate will also decrease extracellular potassium and calcium levels. We found recently that if calcium and potassium levels are not allowed to decrease, metabolic alkalosis does nothing to a pancuronium neuromuscular blockade or its antagonism by neostigmine. These findings suggest that looking at extracellular (pH) alone is insufficient to predict the effect of acid-base changes on neostigmine antagonism of nondepolarizing relaxants. Frequently, a bolus of bicarbonate will transiently increase twitch tension. It is then concluded that metabolic alkalosis antagonizes a nondepolarizing block. We submit that this type of study has little or no relation to the clinical situation in which metabolic alkalosis has existed for several hours or days with associated electrolyte abnormalities. What does the clinician do with such confusing information concerning metabolic acid-base changes? Because so many factors are involved, the simplest and most obvious advice is to maintain a normal acid-base state.

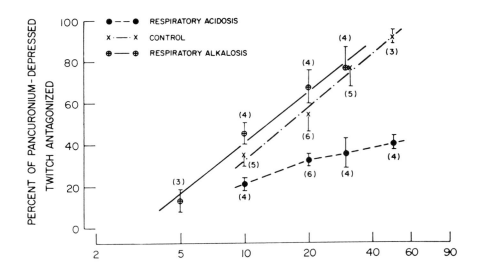

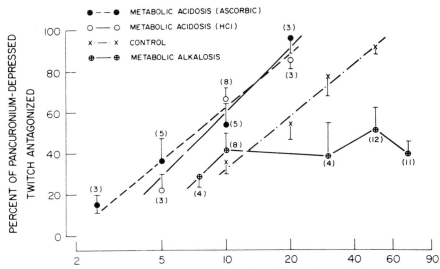

Fig. 17-19 Influence of changes in acid-base status on the ability of neostigmine to antagonize a pancuronium neuromuscular blockade. Note that with respiratory acidosis and metabolic alkalosis, neostigmine, even in large doses, does not antagonize the blood. (Miller RD, Roderick L: The influence of acid-base changes on neostigmine antagonism of a pancuronium neuromuscular blockade. Br J Anaesth 50:317, 1978.)

ELECTROLYTE IMBALANCE

Although the subject of several review articles,[175, 176] little data are available on the effect of electrolyte imbalance on a nondepolarizing neuromuscular blockade and its antagonism by neostigmine. Low extracellular concentrations of potassium apparently enhance the block from nondepolarizing relaxants and diminish the ability of neostigmine to antagonize the block. This prediction is based on the increase in endplate transmembrane potential that results from a higher ratio of intracellular to extracellular potassium. Thus a decrease in extracellular potassium causes hyperpolarization and in-

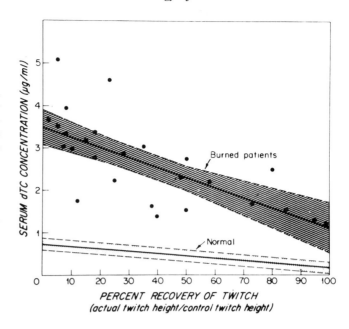

Fig. 17-20 Correlation between serum concentration of *d*-tubocurarine (dTC) and percent depression of twitch height in patients with and without burns. Note that the burned patients appear to be relatively resistant to *d*-tubocurarine. (Martin JAJ, Szyfelbein SK, Ali HH, et al: Increased *d*-tubocurarine requirement following major thermal surgery. Anesthesiology 52:352, 1980.)

creases resistance to depolarization. However, the endplate is only one part of the contractile mechanism, the remainder of which may be affected in a contrary fashion. For example, a low extracellular potassium level also should increase the transmembrane potential of the motor nerve terminal. Although the threshold for depolarization is increased once depolarization occurs, the nerve action potential will be larger, and this should augment acetylcholine release and postjunctional depolarization. Which of the opposing prejunctional and postjunctional changes from hypokalemia are dominant is difficult to ascertain. Furthermore, patients with an imbalance in potassium may have other diseases or injuries that alter their response to muscle relaxants (e.g., patients with burns; see Fig. 17-20 and p. 528).

Cohen[176] and Feldman[175] speculate that, in chronic diseases, both intracellular and extracellular potassium decrease without affecting transmembrane potential. Therefore, the response to muscle relaxants and their antagonists should be normal. However, the muscle transmembrane potentials are changed in patients who are severely ill or even bedridden for a few days.[177] Also, severe dehydration should concentrate the relaxant present in plasma, thereby increasing muscle relaxant activity.

As with acid-base studies, a common error with some studies, in our opinion, is to administer a bolus of some electrolyte such as potassium and to assume that the result resembles the clinical problem of chronic hyperkalemia, which may be present in a patient for hours or days. Studies in these types of patients are difficult because many factors exist that may alter muscle relaxant action. We attempted to develop an animal model that would simulate the type of chronic hypokalemia anesthesiologists may observe in patients. Cats were given a diuretic without potassium supplement for 15 days. We found that less pancuronium was required for neuromuscular blockade and more neostigmine was required for antagonism.[178] Even though the differences were small, we were always able to antagonize the block completely. Assuming this animal model approximates the clinical situation, changes in potassium appear to be of minor consequence.

SUMMARY

In view of these factors and the pharmacokinetic ones presented in the section on the pharmacology of nondepolarizing muscle relaxants, more than 5 mg/70 kg of neostigmine or 20 mg/70 kg of pyridostigmine should not be given unless certain questions have been answered. These questions are as follows:

1. Has enough time been allowed for the neostigmine or pyridostigmine to antagonize the block, i.e., at least 15 to 30 minutes?
2. Is the neuromuscular blockade too intense to be antagonized?
3. What is the acid-base and electrolyte status?
4. What is the temperature?
5. Is the patient receiving any drugs that may make antagonism difficult?
6. Has excretion of the relaxant been reduced?

Quite often answers to these questions will provide the reason for failure of neostigmine or pyridostigmine to antagonize the nondepolarizing neuromuscular blockade.

CARDIOVASCULAR EFFECTS OF ANTAGONISM

Because only the nicotinic effects of neostigmine and pyridostigmine are desired, the muscarinic effects must be blocked by atropine or glycopyrrolate. It is our practice to administer atropine (1.0 to 1.5 mg/70 kg) with neostigmine (2.5 to 5.0 mg/70 kg) or pyridostigmine (10 to 15 mg/kg). Although a controversial question, we believe the amount of atropine required to prevent undesirable muscarinic effects is the same whether pryidostigmine or neostigmine is used.[178]

Although many clinicians advise establishing a vagolytic effect from atropine before administering neostigmine, this is unnecessary because the vagolytic effects precede the cardiac muscarinic effects of neostigmine by 1 to 2 minutes. We administer neostigmine or pyridostigmine and atropine concomitantly. Other muscarinic effects of neostigmine and pyridostigmine have not been studied comparatively. Other than a slightly longer duration of action, pyridostigmine appears to offer no advantage over neostigmine.

Although the mixture of neostigmine or pyridostigmine with atropine in the above dose ratios usually produces no significant cardiovascular problems, atrioventricular block, atrioventricular conduction disturbances, bradycardia, and even cardiac arrest can occur.[179] These problems seem to be more likely in elderly patients or in those receiving various drugs with cardiovascular effects, such as tricyclic antidepressants.[180] Because of its longer duration of action, glycopyrrolate has been shown to provide prolonged cardiac protection against the muscarinic effects of neostigmine or pyridostigmine.[181] The onset of its cardiac antimuscarinic effect is slower than that of atropine and comparable to the onset of the muscarinic-stimulating effect of neostigmine. As a result, the net effect on heart rate when neostigmine and glycopyrrolate are given simultaneously is minimal. It does not penetrate the blood brain barrier as well as atropine. The dose of glycopyrrolate is about 0.2 mg for each 1.0 mg of neostigmine injected.

PHARMACOKINETICS OF NEOSTIGMINE, PYRIDOSTIGMINE, AND EDROPHONIUM

Even though the anticholinesterases—neostigmine, pyridostigmine, and edrophonium—have been used for many years to antagonize a nondepolarizing neuromuscular blockade, until recently nothing was known about their pharmacokinetics and dynamics in anesthetized patients. This deficiency was

Table 17-7. The Pharmacokinetics of Neostigmine (N), Pyridostigmine (P), and Edrophonium (E) in Patients Without and With Renal Failure.[182-184]

Measure	Without Renal Failure		
	N	P	E
Distribution half-life (min)	3.4	6.7	7.2
Elimination half-life (min)	77	113	110
Volume of central compartment (L/kg)	0.2	0.3	0.3
Total serum clearance (ml/kg/min)	9.1	8.6	9.5

Measure	With Renal Failure		
	N	P	E
Distribution half-life (min)	2.5	3.9	7.0
Elimination half-life (min)	181	379	304
Volume of central compartment (L/kg)	0.3	0.4	0.3
Total serum clearance (ml/kg/min)	4.8	3.1	3.9

largely due to lack of a suitable analytic technique to measure the concentration of these drugs in body fluids, most importantly serum. Recently we developed a high pressure liquid chromatography method by which the serum concentrations of neostigmine, pyridostigmine, edrophonium, and their metabolites can be measured.

The kinetics of these three drugs in patients with and without renal failure are summarized in Table 17-7.[182-184]

Several important clinical conclusions can be derived from these data:

1. The longer duration of action of pyridostigmine probably has a pharmacokinetic basis in view of the longer elimination half-life.[182, 183]

2. By comparing elimination half-lives in patients with and without renal failure, we conclude that renal excretion accounts for about 50 percent of neostigmine's excretion and about 75 percent of that of pyridostigmine and edrophonium. Of prime importance clinically is that renal failure delays plasma clearance of neostigmine, pyridostigmine, and edrophonium as much if not more than that of pancuronium and *d*-tubocurarine. Therefore if proper doses of anticholinesterase drugs are given and overdoses of muscle relaxants are avoided, renal failure should not be associated with "recurarization."[182, 183]

3. Edrophonium has long been thought not to be a suitable antagonist because its duration of action is too short. However, when larger doses (i.e., 0.5 to 1.0 mg/kg) are used, sustained antagonism of a nondepolarizing neuromuscular blockade results.[185, 186] In fact, the elimination half-life of edrophonium is similar to that of neostigmine or pyridostigmine[184] (Table 17-7). That edrophonium has a quicker onset of action and probably fewer muscarinic side effects, may justify more frequent use of this drug when antagonizing a nondepolarizing neuromuscular blockade.

DRUG INTERACTIONS

There are so many drugs that have been shown to interact with neuromuscular blockers and/or their antagonists in animals that it is beyond the scope of this chapter to review them all. The reader is referred to excellent reviews on drug interactions for more detailed information.[8, 187-189]

ANTIBIOTICS

More than 140 reports concerning enhancement of neuromuscular blockade from muscle relaxants by antibiotics have ap-

Table 17-8. The Interaction Between Antibiotics, Muscle Relaxants, Neostigmine, and Calcium

Antibiotic	Increase in Neuromuscular Block		Neuromuscular Block from Antibiotic-*d*Tc Antagonized by:	
	*d*Tc*	Sch*	Neostigmine	Calcium
Neomycin	Yes	Yes	Usually	Usually
Streptomycin	Yes	Yes	Usually	Usually
Gentamicin	Yes	†	Sometimes	Usually
Kanamycin	Yes	Yes	Sometimes	Sometimes
Paromomycin	Yes	†	Yes	Yes
Viomycin	Yes	†	Yes	Yes
Polymyxin A	Yes	†	No	No
Polymyxin B	Yes	Yes	No‡	No
Colistin	Yes	Yes	No	Sometimes
Tetracycline	Yes	No	Partially	Partially
Lincomycin	Yes	†	Paritally	Partially
Clindamycin	Yes	†	Partially	Partially

* *d*TC is *d*-tubocurarine-like drugs, which include other nondepolarizing muscle relaxants. Sch is succinylcholine.

† Not studied.

‡ Block is augmented by neostigmine.

peared in the literature.[36] Many of the antibiotics have been shown to have a magnesium-like depression of the evoked release of acetylcholine (prejunctional). Yet these same antibiotics have postjunctional activity.[190–192] Many investigators have attempted to classify antibiotics according to whether the prejunctional or postjunctional activity is dominant. The search for a common mechanism of antibiotic-induced neuromuscular blockade probably is futile because of several possible mechanisms inherent in the variety of antibiotics that can cause blockade. In other words, the mechanisms of neuromuscular blockade are probably different for the various antibiotics, which may account for some of the conflicting suggestions for effective remedies in the case reports (Table 17-8). Despite the intensive and excellent work of Singh et al.[191–192] attempting to elucidate the mechanisms of action of several antibiotics, they can only conclude in one of their publications[192] that

> Our present results confirm that the aminoglycoside streptomycin acts primarily by a calcium-reversible prejunctional mechanism, whereas the other antibiotics tested act by different mechanisms. As the nature of the components of mixed pre- and post-

junctional block produced by polymyxin B, lincomycin and clindamycin are yet unknown, reversibility of these antibiotics by standard reversal agents remains difficult to predict and in the clinical situation it may be preferable to continue artifical ventilation until the return of spontaneous respiration.

Clinical experience with the antibiotics is summarized in Table 17-8. However, our approach to a prolonged neuromuscular blockade involving antibiotics is really quite straightforward.[193] We arbitrarily administer neostigmine up to 5 mg/70 kg; more neostigmine may augment the block. When this is ineffective, ventilation should be controlled until the neuromuscular blockade terminates spontaneously. We no longer recommend the use of calcium for two reasons. First, the antagonism calcium produces usually is not sustained. Second, calcium may antagonize the antibacterial effect of the antibiotics.

MAGNESIUM AND CALCIUM

The effects of magnesium- and calcium-induced alterations of neuromuscular blockade have been studied in animals and in man. Magnesium sulfate, given for treatment of preeclampsia and eclamptic toxemia, enhances the neuromuscular blocking properties of both *d*-tubocurarine and succinylcholine.[194, 195] Magnesium decreases the amount of acetylcholine released from the motor nerve terminal, the depolarizing action of acetylcholine on the postjunctional membrane and the excitability of the muscle fiber itself, and the amplitude of the endplate potential.[196] Thus, magnesium enhances *d*-tubocurarine–induced blockade by reducing acetylcholine output from the motor nerve terminal and by reducing sensitivity of the postjunctional membrane. We cannot explain why the action of succinylcholine is enhanced, unless a desensitization block rapidly occurs with high plasma magnesium levels.

Although calcium enhances the release of acetylcholine from the motor nerve terminal and enhances excitation-contraction coupling in muscle,[197] it also stabilizes the postjunctional membrane. This stabilization may explain why calcium only partially antagonizes magnesium–*d*-tubocurarine–induced blockade.[195] Calcium is less effective in antagonizing magnesium-succinylcholine-induced blockade and will augment a desensitization block from succinylcholine. Again, this is probably explained by membrane stabilization.[198] A prolonged block should be anticipated when a magnesium-relaxant combination is used, since neostigmine and calcium are only partially effective antagonists.

LOCAL ANESTHETICS AND ANTIARRHYTHMICS

In large doses, most local anesthetics block neuromuscular transmission; and in smaller doses, they enhance the neuromuscular block from both nondepolarizing and depolarizing muscle relaxants.[199, 200] Telivuo and Katz[199] found an additional decrease in twitch height and tidal volume from lidocaine, mepivacaine, prilocaine, and bupivacaine in patients partially paralyzed with nortoxiferine. Thus

local anesthetics given as antiarrhythmic agents intraoperatively or postoperatively may augment a residual neuromuscular block. The ability of neostigmine to antagonize a combined local anesthetic-relaxant neuromuscular blockade has not been studied.

In low doses, local anesthetics depress posttetanic potentiation, and this is thought to be a neural, prejunctional effect.[201] With higher doses, local anesthetics block acetylcholine-induced muscular contractions, and this suggests that local anesthetics have a stabilizing effect on the postjunctional membrane.[202] Also, local anesthetics have a direct effect on the muscle membrane by decreasing the strength of contraction of a curarized or denervated muscle in response to a single shock.[203] Procaine has been shown to displace calcium from the sacrolemma and thus inhibit caffeine-induced contraction of skeletal muscle.[204] Most of these mechanisms of action probably apply to all the local anesthetics. In addition, procaine inhibits plasma cholinesterase and may augment the effects of succinylcholine. In essence, local anesthetics have actions on the presynaptic, postjunctional, and muscle membranes.

Several drugs used for the treatment of arrhythmias also augment the block from muscle relaxants, particularly that of *d*-tubocurarine.[205] For example, patients have become "recurarized" after receiving quinidine in the recovery room. These cases may represent unrecognized residual curarization that was augmented by the administration of quinidine. Quinidine potentiates the neuromuscular block from both nondepolarizing and depolarizing muscle relaxants;[206] edrophonium was ineffective in antagonizing a nondepolarizing blockade after quinidine. In these clinical doses, quinidine appears to act at the prejunctional membrane as judged by its lack of effect on acetylcholine-evoked twitch. However, large, nonclinical doses of quinidine given intra-arterially produce a neuromuscular blockade of the depolarizing type which is augmented by edrophonium.[207]

HYPOTENSIVE DRUGS

Both hexamethonium and trimethaphan produce neuromuscular blockade alone and enhance the blockade produced by *d*-tubocurarine.[208] However, these studies were performed in the rat diaphragm preparation with large doses of hypotensive drugs. Despite occasional clinical reports,[209] we believe trimethaphan rarely interacts with muscle relaxants in a clinically important manner.

Nitroglycerine has been found to prolong a pancuronium neuromuscular blockade but not that from any other neuromuscular blocker.[210,211] The mechanisms for this selective action of nitroglycerin have not been elucidated.

DIURETICS

In patients undergoing renal transplantation, the intensity and duration of *d*-tubocurarine neuromuscular blockade was increased following a dose of furosemide 1 mg/kg IV.[212] This has been investigated further with the rat diaphragm and cat soleus preparations (work in progress). In the rat diaphragm, the concentration of *d*-tubocurarine required for neuromuscular blockade is markedly reduced at clinically relevant doses of furosemide. This diuretic has an effect on the nerve terminal (presynaptic) probably relating to the cyclic nucleotide system. Furosemide appears to inhibit the cyclic AMP system and reduce the output of transmitter which results in enhancement of *d*-tubocurarine blockade. Clinically this effect is documented and significant.[212]

In contrast, mannitol appears to have no effect on a nondepolarizing neuromuscular blockade. Furthermore, increasing urine output by administration of mannitol has no effect on the rate at which *d*-tubocurarine, and presumably other muscle relaxants, are eliminated in the urine.[213] However, this lack of effect on the excretion of *d*-tubocurarine should not be surprising. Urinary excretion of *d*-tubocurarine depends on glomerular filtration. Mannitol is an osmotic diuretic and exerts its effect by altering the osmotic gradient within the proximal tubules so that water is retained within the tubules. Thus, an increase in urine volume in patients with adequate glomerular filtration would not be expected to increase excretion.

DISEASES THAT MAY ALTER MUSCLE RELAXANT ACTION

The following diseases are complex in their pathology and physiology. Only that aspect directly relating to the use of muscle relaxants is discussed.

MYASTHENIA GRAVIS

The pathology and therapy are superficially reviewed earlier in this chapter and in Chapter 2. Also, other authors have presented excellent reviews of this topic.[214–216] As far as muscle relaxants are concerned, myasthenic patients respond as if already partially curarized. Therefore, they are very sensitive to nondepolarizing and somewhat resistant to depolarizing muscle relaxants, although the latter has not been well documented.

When presented with the problem of anesthetizing one of these patients, avoidance of all muscle relaxants would be preferred. Usually an inhaled anesthetic by itself will provide sufficient relaxation of skeletal muscle including that necessary for endotracheal intubation.

Before giving muscle relaxants, the anesthesiologist should be sure that a profound neuromuscular blockade does not already exist; there may be other reasons for inadequate surgical exposure. The status of neuromuscular blockade should be evaluated by use of a peripheral nerve stimulator. If the twitch or train-of-four is already markedly depressed, administration of additional muscle relaxant may induce a block that is difficult to antagonize, particularly in a patient with myasthenia gravis. If additional relaxation is required, we prefer deepening anesthesia. For example, the enflurane concentration could be increased, or administration of a small dose of thiopental may be adequate. If a muscle relaxant is needed, then a small dose (e.g., *d*-tubocurarine, 1 to 3 mg/70 kg, or pancuronium, 0.5 to 1 mg/70 kg) can be given, but prolonged weakness should be anticipated.

Feldman[216] recommends that because of an unpredictable drug response it is probably safer to ventilate these patients electively during the postoperative period than to resort to giving large doses of anticholinesterase drugs. This recommendation is consistent with our experience and that often described in the literature[217] that surgery and anesthesia often completely alter the states of myasthenia gravis in an unpredictable manner. Even if a patient is well-controlled preoperatively, the doses of anticholinesterase drugs required may radically change postoperatively. For that reason a recommended approach is to withhold all anticholinesterase medication for 12 to 24 hours preoperatively. Postoperatively, anticholinesterase and steroid therapy is initiated with extreme caution because the sensitivity of the patient to these drugs may have changed.

MYASTHENIC SYNDROME (EATON-LAMBERT SYNDROME)

This syndrome is an association between carcinomatous conditions (especially oat-cell carcinoma of the bronchus) and motor neuropathy and resembles myasthenia gravis. These patients are unusually sensitive to both nondepolarizing and depolarizing muscle relaxants.

MYOTONIA

The myotonic syndromes include myotonia congenita, myotonia dystrophica, and paramyotinia congenita. With the latter condition, myotonia appears only upon exposure to cold.

Myotonic dystrophy (atrophica), which is the most common of the three, is an inherited, autosomal dominant disease. Clinical features include weakness and wasting of the facial, cervical, and proximal limb muscles; frontal baldness; cataracts; gonadal atrophy; thyroid nodules; endocrine failure; and voluntary and percussion myotonia. Continuous, low-voltage activity with high-voltage, fibrillation-like potential bursts will be evident on the electromyogram. A mechanical stimulus will evoke a burst of rhythmic activity of 90 to 100/sec, which eventually slows to low-voltage activity, the so-called dive-bomber effect. Cardiac conduction defects as well as myocardial failure are commonly present. Respiratory involvement is also common, secondary to weakness of skeletal muscles. While the carbon dioxide response curves are normal, mechanical ability is impaired, as reflected by a diminished vital capacity, forced vital capacity in 1 second, and maximum expiratory force. In addition, some patients have weakness of pharyngeal muscles with recurrent aspiration pneumonitis. The onset of the disease is most common in the second to fourth decade and progresses to atrophy in later years.

Anesthetic and operative mortality is increased for several reasons. The most common complication is respiratory failure postoperatively due to decreased mechanical ability, which interferes with deep breathing and coughing. Intraoperatively, cardiac conduction abnormalities may cause hemodynamic instability. Generalized myotonia may follow administration of succinylcholine in some patients. In some cases the severity of the myotonic response has precluded attempts to control ventilation. Although it is difficult to collect a large clinical experience[218] Mitchell et al.[219] thoroughly evaluated three patients with myotonia dystrophica and their response to muscle relaxants and concluded that (1) the response to nondepolarizing muscle relaxants is normal; (2) patients with myotonia are more likely than normal patients to develop apnea after administration of sedative or anesthetic drugs; and (3) the use of depolarizing muscle relaxants is hazardous because marked generalized contracture of skeletal muscle may develop, preventing adequate airway maintenance and ventilation.

Also, the use of anticholinesterases may exacerbate myotonia, although this is not well documented and was not confirmed by Mitchell et al.[219] Should myotonia develop intraoperatively, muscular blockers will not attenuate myotonia because it is primarily a muscle membrane disease.

Myotonia may also develop in response to percussion or to shivering postoperatively. Local infiltration of the involved muscles with local anesthetics may attenuate percussion myotonia. Quinine and procainamide have been used for generalized myotonia. Although several anesthetic approaches probably are satisfactory, we have used small doses of thiopental and volatile anesthetic agents, avoiding all muscle relaxants. We believe the trachea should remain intubated until the patient has demonstrated adequate mechanical ventilatory ability postoperatively. Regional anesthesia may be used but will not block the myotonic response. Intravenous regional anesthesia might be useful in appropriate cases and offers the advantage of attenuating the myotonic response. A clinical series, however, has not been reported utilizing this technique.

FAMILIAL PERIODIC PARALYSIS

This disease is associated with hyperkalemia, hypokalemia, or normokalemia characterized by intermittant attacks of skeletal-muscle weakness and flaccid paralysis, which usually spare the bulbar musculature. With the hypokalemic type, intravenous fluids should avoid a large carbohydrate or salt load and hypokalemia. Postoperatively, if such a patient is weak, it usually is secondary to hypokalemia. In general, muscle relaxants should be avoided although Siler and Discavage[220] noted a normal response to succinylcholine. In contrast, the hyperkalemic patients should have their carbohydrate stores maintained with dextrose-rich, potassium-free intravenous solutions. Muscle relaxants, especially succinylcholine, probably should be avoided. Succinylcholine can cause myotonia in these patients.[221]

UPPER AND LOWER MOTOR NEURON DISEASE

The potential hazards in giving succinylcholine to patients with upper or motor neuron disease is described earlier in this chapter. Their response to nondepolarizing muscle relaxants is probably greater than normal. This was well documented by Rosenbaum et al.[222] who found that *d*-tubocurarine, 1.5 mg, given over a 30 minute period to a man with amyotrophic lateral sclerosis caused difficulty with speech and swallowing.

By administering small doses of nondepolarizing muscle relaxants plus monitoring with a peripheral nerve stimulator, the anesthesiologist should be able to avoid significant problems in these patients. However, monitoring with a peripheral nerve stimulator may not be reliable in patients with an upper motor neuron lesion.[223] Monitoring of the unaffected limb or other confirmatory measures of neuromuscular blockade should be used in these patients.

BURNS

The problems with burns and succinylcholine are well documented. Recently, Martin et al.[224] found that following burns of more than 25 percent of body surface area, both the total doses of *d*-tubocurarine and serum concentration necessary to attain a given twitch depression are greatly increased (Fig. 17-20, on p. 521). The mechanism of this increased *d*-tubocurarine requirement was not elucidated.

NEW DRUGS

Several groups are seeking a short-acting nondepolarizing muscle relaxant with no cardiovascular effects. Durant et al.[225] found that ORG NC45 (Norcuron) indeed seemed to meet these requirements. Since then, from initial clinical trials, we believe ORG NC45 has[226] a duration of action ⅓ to ½ that of pancuronium, little or no cumulative effect, easy reversibility with neostigmine, and no cardiovascular effects. In unpublished studies from the senior author's laboratory, Fahey, Morris, and Cronnelly found ORG NC45 to have a much shorter elimination half-life than that of other nondepolarizing muscle relaxants. In animal studies, over half of an injected dose of ORG NC45 was eliminated in the bile. Because ORG NC45 is not heavily dependent on the kidney for its elimination, it appears to be an ideal muscle relaxant to use in patients with impaired renal function.

Atracurium is another nondepolarizing muscle relaxant that is undergoing clinical trials.[227] It has many of the same characteristics of Norcuron, but its metabolism has not been studied extensively. However, it may undergo *Hoffman elimination,* a form of spontaneous breakdown of the quaternary group dependent on alkaline pH. If these routes of metabolism are proven for atracurium, then it might be inferred that the drug does not depend on renal or hepatic mechanisms for its elimination. A nondepolarizing relaxant that has an extremely short duration of action (10 to 15 minutes) because of rapid hydrolysis by pseudocholinesterase has recently undergone clinical trial.[228] This agent (BW785U), however, has a prominent histamine-releasing property that may prevent its clinical acceptance. Another ester material, BW444U, is more slowly hydrolyzed by pseudocholinesterase, but lacks significant side effects and is expected to have a duration of action ⅓ that

of pancuronium and *d*-tubocurarine. It is likely that it will not depend greatly on the liver or kidney for its elimination. In summary, we believe the day will come when there is a muscle relaxant with all the advantages of succinylcholine but none of the disadvantages.

In the area of new antagonists, studies in animals indicate that 4-aminopyridine has several advantages over neostigmine and pyridostigmine, including longer duration of action, antagonism of antibiotic neuromuscular blockades when neostigmine often fails, and no muscarinic stimulation so that no atropine is required. In spite of these advantages, 4-aminopyridine alone probably will not be useful clinically because the doses required for complete antagonism ($> 1 \text{ mg/kg}^{-1}$) also stimulate the central nervous system and cause postoperative restlessness and confusion (S. Agoston, unpublished data). Obviously what is needed is a 4-aminopyridine that does not cross the blood brain barrier.

Although 4-aminopyridine appears not to be useful alone as an antagonist, it may offer a significant advantage when combined with neostigmine. Four-aminopyridine markedly potentiates the antagonist activity of both neostigmine and pyridostigmine.[229] For example, 4-aminopyridine, 20 mg/70 kg, does nothing by itself. Yet it reduces the amount of neostigmine or pyridostigmine required by 60 to 70 percent.[230] The combination of neostigmine or pyridostigmine with 4-aminopyridine may diminish or eliminate the disadvantages that these drugs have when given individually. The amount of atropine required is reduced by 60 to 70 percent. Also, possibly a predictable antagonism of an antibiotic neuromuscular blockade may exist. These potential advantages are sufficient to warrant further studies with the combination of 4-aminopyridine with neostigmine or pyridostigmine.

Four-aminopyridine is an interesting compound, which may have other applications. It has been used to prevent ketamine-induced dreams[231] and to treat myasthenia gravis.[232]

Thus, the full potential of this drug may not as yet have been identified.

REFERENCES

1. Griffith HR, Johnson GE: The use of curare in general anesthesia. Anesthesiology 3:418, 1942

2. Cullen, SC: The use of curare for improvement of abdominal relaxation during inhalation anesthesia—report on 131 cases. Surgery 14:261, 1943

3. Beecher HK, Todd DP: A study of deaths with anesthesia and surgery. Am Surg 140:2, 1954

4. Cormack, RS: Awareness during surgery—a new approach. Br J Anaesth 51:711, 1979

5. Editorial (no author): On being aware. Br J Anaesth 51:711, 1979

6. Cullen SC, Larson CP, Jr: Essentials of Anesthetic Practice. Chicago, Year Book Medical Publishers, 1974

7. Waud BE, Waud DR: Physiology and pharmacology of neuromuscular blocking agents, *Muscle Relaxants.* Edited by Katz RL. Amsterdam, Excerpta Medica, 1975, pp 1–58

8. Ali HH, Savarese JJ: Monitoring of neuromuscular function. Anesthesiology 45:216, 1976

9. Feldman SA: Muscle Relaxants. Philadelphia, WB Saunders, 1979, pp 11–34

10. Chang CC: Use of alpha- and beta- bungarotoxins for the study of neuromuscular transmission. Anesthesiology 48:309, 1978

11. Lee C, Yang E, Katz, RC: Interactions of neuromuscular effects of edrophonium, alpha-bungarotoxin and beta-bungarotoxin. Anesthesiology 48:311, 1978

12. Waud BE, Waud DR: The relation between tetanic fade and receptor occlusion in the presence of competitive neuromuscular block. Anesthesiology 35:456, 1971

13. Hubbard JI, Wilson DF, Miyamoto M: Reduction of transmitter release by d-tubocurarine. Nature 223:531, 1969

14. Galindo A: Prejunctional effect of curare: Its relative importance. J Neurophysiol 34:289, 1971

15. Averbach A, Betz W: Does curare affect transmitter release? J Physiol (Lond) 213:691, 1971

16. Standaert FG, Adams JE: The actions of succinylcholine on the mammalian motor nerve terminal. J Pharmacol Exp Ther 149:113, 1965

17. Hunter AR, Feldman SA: Muscle Relaxants. Br J Anaesth 48:277, 1976

18. Gissen AJ, Katz RL, Karis JH et al: Neuromuscular block in man during prolonged arterial infusion with succinylcholine. Anesthesiology 27:242, 1966

19. Crul JF, Long GJ, Brunner EA et al: The changing pattern of neuromuscular blockade caused by succinylcholine in man. Anesthesiology 27:729, 1966

20. Miller RD, Stevens WC: Antagonism of succinylcholine paralysis in a patient with atypical pseudocholinesterase. Anesthesiology 36:511, 1972

21. Katz RL, Katz GJ: Clinical considerations in the use of muscle relaxants, Muscle Relaxants. Edited by Katz RL. Amsterdam, Excerpta Medica, 1975, pp 313–334

22. Churchill-Davidson HC: A portable peripheral nerve stimulator. Anesthesiology 26:224, 1965

23. DeJong RH: Controlled relaxation. JAMA 197:393, 1966

24. Ngai SH, Hanks EC, Farhie SE: Effects of anesthetics on neuromuscular transmission and somatic reflexes. Anesthesiology 26:162, 1965

25. Feldman SA: Measurement of neuromuscular block, Measurement in Anesthesia. Edited by Feldman SA, Leigh JM, Spierdijk J. Netherlands, Leiden University Press, 1974, pp 39–47

26. Epstein RM, Epstein RA: Electromyograph in evaluation of the response to muscle relaxants, Muscle Relaxants. Edited by Katz RL. Amsterdam, Excerpta Medica, 1975, pp 299–312

27. Epstein RA, Wyte SR, Jackson SH, et al: The electromechanical response to stimulation by the block-aid monitor. Anesthesiology 30:43, 1969

28. Epstein RA, Epstein RM: The electromyogram and the mechanical response of indirectly stimulated muscle in anesthetized man following curarization. Anesthesiology 18:212, 1973.

29. Epstein RM, Epstein RA, Lee ASJ: A recording system for continuous evoked electromyography. Anesthesiology 38:287, 1973

30. Ali HH, Wilson RS, Savarese JJ, et al: The effect of tubocurarine on indirectly ilicited train-of-four muscle responses and respiratory measurements in humans. Br J Anaesth 47:570, 1975

31. Waud BE, Waud DR: The relation between the response to "train-of-four" stimulation and receptor occlusion during competitive neuromuscular block. Anesthesiology 37:413, 1972

32. Lee C: Train-of-four quantitation of competitive neuromuscular block. Anesth Analg 54:649, 1975

33. Walts LF, Levin N, Dillon JB: Assessment of recovery from curare. JAMA 213:1894, 1970

34. Johansen SH, Jorgensen M, Molbeck S: Effect of tubocurarine on respiratory and nonrespiratory muscle power in man. J Appl Physiol 19:990, 1964

35. Miller RD: Factors affecting the action of muscle relaxants, Muscle Relaxants. Edited by Katz RL. Amsterdam, Excerpta Medica, 1975, pp 163–191

36. Miller RD: Antagonism of neuromuscular blockade. Anesthesiology 44:293, 1976

37. Miller RD, Matteo R, Benet LZ, et al: Influence of renal failure on the pharmacokinetics of *d*-tubocurarine in man. J Pharmacol Exp Ther 202:1, 1977

38. Miller RD, Eger EI II: Early and late relative potencies of pancuronium and *d*-tubocurarine in man. Anesthesiology 44:297, 1976

39. Horowitz PE, Spector S: Determination of serum *d*-tubocurarine concentration by radioimmunoassay. J Pharmacol Exp Ther 185:94, 1973

40. Cronnelly R, Stanski DR, Miller RD, et al: Renal function and the pharmacokinetics of neostigmine in anesthetized man. Anesthesiology 51:222, 1979

41. Kersten VW, Meijer DKF, Agoston S: Fluorimetric and chromatographic determination of pancuronium bromide and its metabolites in biological materials. Clin Chem Acta 44:59, 1973

42. Katz RL: Neuromuscular effects of *d*-tubocurarine, edrophonium and neostigmine in man. Anesthesiology 28:327, 1967

43. Feldman SA: The rational use of muscle relaxants, Muscle Relaxants. London, WB Saunders, 1973, pp 149–155

44. Ham J, Miller RD, Sheiner LB, et al: Dosage-schedule independence of *d*-tubocurarine pharmacokinetics and pharmaco-dynamics and recovery of neuromuscular function. Anesthesiology 50:528, 1979

45. McLeod K, Watson MJ, Rawlings MD: Pharmacokinetics of pancuronium in patients with normal and impaired renal function. Br J Anaesth 48:341, 1976

46. Buzello W, Agoston S: Kinetics of intercompartmental disposition and excretion of tubocurarine, gallamine, alcuronium and pancuronium in patients with normal and impaired renal function. Anesthetist 27:319, 1978

47. Somogyi AA, Shanks CA, Triggs EJ: The effect of renal failure on the disposition and neuromuscular blocking action of pancuronium bromide. Eur J Clin Pharmacol 12:23, 1977

48. Cohen EN: Patients with altered sensitivity. Clin Anesth 2:76, 1966

49. Somogyi AA, Shanks CA, Triggs EJ: Disposition kinetics of pancuronium bromide in patients with total biliary obstruction. Br J Anaesth 49:1103, 1977

50. Duvaldestin P, Agoston S, Henzel E, et al: Pancuronium pharmacokinetics in patients with liver cirrhosis. Br J Anaesth 50:1131, 1978

51. Miller RD, Way WL, Dolan WM, et al: The dependence of pancuronium and *d*-tubocurarine induced neuromuscular blockades on alveolar concentrations of halothane and Forane. Anesthesiology 37:573, 1972

52. Miller RD, Criqui M, Eger EI II: The influence of duration of anesthesia on a *d*-tubocurarine neuromuscular blockade. Anesthesiology 44:207, 1976

53. Miller RD, Way WL, Dolan WM, et al: Comparative neuromuscular effects of pancuronium, gallamine, and succinylcholine during Forane and halothane anesthesia in man. Anesthesiology 35:509, 1971

54. Fogdall RP, Miller RD: Neuromuscular effects of enflurane alone and in combination with *d*-tubocurarine, pancuronium, and succinylcholine in man. Anesthesiology 42:173, 1975

55. Vitez TS, Miller RD, Eger EI II: An in vitro comparison of halothane and isoflurane potentiation of neuromuscular blockade. Anesthesiology 41:53, 1974

56. Gergis SD, Dretchen KL, Sokoll MD, et al: Effect of anesthetics on acetylcholine release from the myoneural junction. Proc Soc Exp Biol Med 141:629, 1972

57. Waud BE, Waud DR: The effects of diethyl ether, enflurane, and isoflurane at the neuromuscular junction. Anesthesiology 42:275, 1975

58. Waud BE, Waud DR: Comparison of drug-receptor dissociation constants at the mammalian neuromuscular junction in the presence and absence of halothane. J Pharmacol Exp Ther 187:40, 1973

59. Karis JH, Gissen AJ, Nastuk WL: Mode of action of diethyl ether in blocking neuromuscular transmission. Anesthesiology 27:42, 1966

60. Gissen AJ, Karis JH, Nastuk WL: Effect of halothane on neuromuscular transmission. JAMA 197:770, 1966

61. Ngai SH: Action of general anesthetics in producing muscle relaxation: Interaction of anesthetics with relaxants, Muscle Relaxants. Edited by Katz RL. Amsterdam, Excerpta Medica, 1975, pp 279–297

62. Stanski DR, Ham J, Miller RD, et al: Pharmacokinetics and pharmacodynamics of *d*-tubocurarine under nitrous oxide–narcotic and halothane anesthesia. Anesthesiology 51:235, 1979

63. Stanski DR, Ham J, Miller RD, et al: Time dependent increase in sensitivity to dTC during enflurane anesthesia. Anesthesiology 51:S269, 1979

64. Miller RD, Agoston S, Booij LDHJ, et al: The comparative potency and pharmacokinetics of pancuronium and its metabolites in anesthetized man. Anesthesiology 207:539, 1978

65. Ham GC, Miller RD, Benet LZ, et al: The pharmacokinetics and pharmacodynamics of *d*-tubocurarine during hypothermia in the cat. Anesthesiology 49:324, 1978

66. Miller RD, Agoston S, Van der Pol F, et al: Hypothermia and pharmacokinetics and pharmacodynamics of pancuronium in the cat. J Pharmacol Exp Ther 207:532, 1978

67. Stead AL: The response of newborn infants to muscle relaxants. Br J Anaesth 27:124, 1955

68. Kelly SS, Roberts DV: The effect of age on the safety factor in neuromuscular transmission in the isolated rat. Br J Anaesth 149:217, 1977

69. Kolnigsberger MR, Patten B, Lovelace RE: Studies of neuromuscular function in the newborn—a comparison of myoneural function in the full term and premature infant. Neuropediatric 4:350, 1973

70. Goudsouzian NG: Maturation of neuromuscular transmission in the infant. Br J Anaesth 52:205, 1980

71. Bennet EJ, Ignacio A, Patel K et al: Tubocurarine and the neonate. Br J Anaesth 48:687, 1976

72. Bush GH, Stead AL: The use of *d*-tubocurarine in neonatal anesthesia. Br J Anaesth 34:721, 1962

73. Churchill-Davidson HC, Wise RP: The response of the newborn infant to muscle relaxants. Can Anaesth Soc J 11:1, 1964

74. Long G, Bachman L: Neuromuscular blockade by *d*-tubocurarine in children. Anesthesiology 28:723, 1967

75. Goudsouzian NG, Ryan JF, Savarese JJ: The neuromuscular effects of pancuronium in infants and children. Anesthesiology 41:95, 1974

76. Goudsouzian NG, Donlon JV, Savarese JJ, et al: Re-evaluation of dosage and duration of action of *d*-tubocurarine in the pediatric age group. Anesthesiology 43:416, 1975

77. Goudsouzian NG, Liu L, and Savarese JJ: Metocurine in infants and children. Anesthesiology 49:266, 1978

78. O'Keeffe C, Gregory GA, Stanski DR et al: *d*-tubocurarine: pharmacodynamics and kinetics in children. Anesthesiology 51:S270, 1979

79. McLeod K, Hull CJ, Watson MJ: Effects of aging on the pharmacokinetics of pancuronium. Br J Anaesth 51:435, 1979

80. Ghoneim MM, Pandya H: Binding of tubocurarine to specific serum protein fractions. Br J Anaesth 47:853, 1975

81. Thompson JM: Pancuronium binding by serum proteins. Anaesthesia 31:219, 1976

82. Skivington MA: Protein binding of three tritiated muscle relaxants. Br J Anaesth 44:1030, 1972

83. Olsen GD, Chan EM, Riker WK: Binding or *d*-tubocurarine, di(methyl[14]C) ether iodine and other amines to cartilage, chondroitin sulfate and human plasma proteins. J Pharmacol Exp Ther 195:242, 1975

84. Ghoneim MM, Kramer SE, Bannow R, et al: Binding of *d*-tubocurarine to plasma protein in normal man and in patients with hepatic or renal disease. Anesthesiology 39:410, 1973

85. Matteo RS, Pua EK, Khambatta HJ, et al:

Cerebrospinal fluid levels of *d*-tubocurarine in man. Anesthesiology 46:396, 1977

86. Munson ES, Wagman IH: Elevation of lidocaine seizure threshold by gallamine. Arch Neurol 28:329, 1973

87. Forbes AR, Cohen NH, Eger EI II: Pancuronium reduces halothane requirement in man. Anesth Analg 58:497, 1979

88. Savarese JJ, Ali HH, Antonio RP: The clinical pharmacology of metacurine. Anesthesiology 47:277, 1977

89. Matteo RS, Khambatta HJ: Relation of serum metocurine concentration to neuromuscular blockade in man (abstr). Anesthesiology 51:S287, 1979

90. Meijer DKF, Weitering JG, Vermeer GA, et al: Comparative pharmacokinetics of *d*-tubocurarine and metocurine in man. Anesthesiology 51:402, 1979

91. Basta JW, Lichtiger M: Comparison of metocurine and pancuronium-myocardial tension-time index during endotracheal intubation. Anesthesiology 46:366, 1977

92. Savarese JJ: The autonomic margins of safety of metocurine and *d*-tubocurarine in the cat. Anesthesiology 50:40, 1979

93. McCullough LS, Reier CE, Delauaois AL, et al: The effects of *d*-tubocurarine on spontaneous postganglionic sympathetic activity and histamine release. Anesthesiology 33:328, 1970

94. Munger ML, Miller RD, Stevens WC: The dependence of *d*-tubocurarine induced hypotension on the alveolar concentration of halothane and the presence of nitrous oxide. Anesthesiology 40:442, 1974

95. Dowdy EG, Holland WC, Yamaka I: Cardioactive properties of *d*-tubocurarine with and without preservatives. Anesthesiology 34:256, 1971

96. Stoelting RK: Blood-pressure responses to *d*-tubocurarine and its preservatives in anesthetized patients. Anesthesiology 35:315, 1971

97. Stoelting RK, Longnecker DE: Effects of promethazine on hypotension following *d*-tubocurarine use in anesthetized patients. Anesth Analg 51:509, 1972

98. Miller RD, Eger EI II, Stevens WC: Pancuronium induced tachycardia in relation to alveolar halothane, dose of pancuronium, and prior atropine. Anesthesiology 42:352, 1975

99. Stoelting RK: The hemodynamic effects of pancuronium and *d*-tubocurarine in anesthetized patients. Anesthesiology 36:612, 1972

100. Domenech JS, Garcia RC, Sasiain JMR, et al: Pancuronium bromide: An indirect sympathomimetic agent. Br J Anaesth 48:1143, 1976

101. Docherty JR, McGrath JC: Sympathomimetic effects of pancuronium bromide on the cardiovascular system of the pithed rat. Br J Pharmocol 64:589, 1978

102. Quintana A: Effect of pancuronium bromide on the adrenergic reactivity of the isolated rat vas deferens. Eur J Pharmacol 46:275, 1977

103. Ivankovich AD, Miletich DJ, Albrecht RF, et al: The effect of pancuronium on myocardial contraction and catecholamine metabolism. J Pharm Pharmacol 27:837, 1975

104. Vercruysse P, Bossuyt P, Hanegreefs G, et al: Gallamine and pancuronium inhibit pre- and post-junctional muscarinic receptors in canine saphenous veins. J Pharmacol Exp Ther 209:225, 1979

105. Roizen MF, Forbes AR, Miller RD, et al: Similarity between effects of pancuronium and atropine on plasma norepinephrine levels in man. J Pharmacol Exp Ther 211:419, 1979

106. Eisele JH, Marta JA, Davis HL: Quantitative aspects of the chronotropic and neuromuscular effects of gallamine in anesthetized man. Anesthesiology 35:630, 1971

107. Brown BB Jr, Crout JR: The sympathomimetic effect of gallamine on the heart. J Pharmacol Exp Ther 172:266, 1970

108. Reitan JA, Fraser AI, Eisele JH: Lack of cardiac inotropic effects of gallamine in anesthetized man. Anesth Analg 52:974, 1973

109. Wong KC, Wyte SR, Martin WE, et al: Antiarrhythmic effects of skeletal muscle relaxants. Anesthesiology 34:458, 1971

110. Geha DG, Cozelle BC, Raessler KL, et al: Pancuronium bromide enhances atrioventricular conduction in halothane-anesthetized dogs. Anesthesiology 46:342, 1977

111. Edwards R, Miller RD, Roizen MF, et al: Cardiac effects of imipramine and pancuronium during halothane and enflurane anesthesia. Anesthesiology 50:42, 1979

112. Katz RL, Katz GJ: Clinical considerations in the use of muscle relaxants, Muscle Relaxants. Edited by Katz RL. Amsterdam, Excerpta Medica, 1975, pp 313

113. Foldes FF, Rendell-Baker L, Birch JH: Causes and prevention of prolonged apnea with succinylcholine. Anesth Analg 35:609, 1956

114. Pantuck EJ, Pantuck CB: Cholinesterases and anticholinesterases, Muscle Relaxants. Edited by Katz RL. Amsterdam, Excerpta Medica, 1975, pp 143

115. Lindsay PA, Tumley J: Suxamethonium apnoea mask by tetrahydroaminacrine. Anaesthesia 33:620, 1978

116. Kaniaris P, Fassoulaki A, Tiarmakopoulou K, et al: Serum cholinesterase levels in patients with cancer. Anesth Analg 58:82, 1979

117. Kopman AF, Strachovsky G, Lichtenstein L: Prolonged response to succinylcholine following physostigmine. Anesthesiology 49:142, 1978

118. Bentz EW, Stoelting RK: Prolonged response to succinylcholine following pancuronium reversal with pyridostigmine. Anesthesiology 44:258, 1976

119. Viby-Mogensen J: Correlation of succinylcholine duration of action with plasma cholinesterase activity in subjects with the genotypically normal enzyme. Anesthesiology 53:517, 1980

120. Kalow W, Genest K: A method for the detection of atypical forms of human serum cholinesterase. Determination of dibucaine numbers. Can J Biochem 35:339, 1957

121. Epstein HM, Jarzensky D, Zuckerman L, et al: Plasma cholinesterase activity in bank blood. Anesth Analg 59:211, 1980

122. Schuh FT: Pseudocholinesterase activity of human whole blood, bank blood, and blood protein solutions. Anaesthetist 24:103, 1975

123. Galindo AHF, Davis TB: Succinylcholine and cardiac excitability. Anesthesiology 23:32, 1962

124. Goat VA, Feldman SA: The dual action of suxamethonium on the isolated rabbit heart. Anaesthesia 27:149, 1972

125. Craythorne NWB, Turndorf H, Dipps RD: Changes in pulse rate and rhythm associated with the use of succinylcholine in anesthetized patients. Anesthesiology 21:465, 1960

126. Leigh MD, McCoy DD, Belton KM, et al: Bradycardia following intravenous administration of succinylcholine chloride to infants and children. Anesthesiology 18:698, 1957

127. Stoelting RK, Peterson C: Heart-rate slowing and junctional rhythm following intravenous succinylcholine with and without intramuscular atropine preanesthetic medication. Anesth Analg 54:705, 1975

128. Schoenstadt DA, Whitcher CE: Observations on the mechanism of succinylcholine-induced cardiac arrhythmias. Anesthesiology 24:358, 1963

129. Mathias JA, Evans-Prosser CDG, Churchill-Davidson HC: The role of nondepolarizing drugs in the prevention of suxamethonium bradycardia. Br J Anaesth 42:609, 1970

130. Schaner PJ, Brown RL, Kirksey TD, et al: Succinylcholine-induced hyperkalemia in burned patients. Anesth Analg 48:764, 1969

131. Burch AA, Mitchell GD, Playford GA, et al: Changes in serum potassium response to succinylcholine following trauma. JAMA 210:490, 1969

132. Cooperman LH: Succinylcholine-induced hyperkalemia in neuromuscular disease. JAMA 213:1867, 1970

133. Cooperman LH, Strobel GE Jr, Kennell EM: Massive hyperkalemia after administration of succinylcholine. Anesthesiology 32:161, 1970

134. Gronert GA, Theye RA: Pathophysiology of hyperkalemia induced by succinylcholine. Anesthesiology 43:89, 1975

135. Stevenson PH, Brich AA: Succinylcholine-induced hyperkalemia in a patient with a closed head injury. Anesthesiology 51:89, 1979

136. Kohlschütter B, Baur H, Roth F: Suxamethonium-induced hyperkalaemia in patients with severe intra-abdominal infections. Br J Anaesth 48:557, 1976

137. Roth F, Wuthrich H: The clinical importance of hyperkalemia following suxamethonium administration. Br J Anaesth 41:311, 1969

138. Powell JN: Suxamethonium-induced hyperkalaemia in a uraemic patient. Br J Anaesth 42:806, 1970

139. Walton JD, Farman JV: Suxamethonium, potassium and renal failure. Anaesthesia 28:626, 1973

140. Miller RD, Way WL, Hamilton WK, et al: Succinylcholine-induced hyperkalemia in patients with renal failure? Anesthesiology 36:138, 1972

141. Powell R, Miller RD: The effect of repeated

doses of succinylcholine on serum potassium in patients with renal failure. Anesth Analg 54:746, 1976

142. Korde M, Waud BE: Serum potassium concentrations after succinylcholine in patients with renal failure. Anesthesiology 36:142, 1972

143. Walton JD, Farman JV: Suxamethonium hyperkalemia in uremic neuropathy. Anaesthesia 28:666, 1973

144. Powell JN, Golby M: The pattern of potassium liberation following a single dose of suxamethonium in normal and uraemic rats. Br J Anaesth 43:662, 1971

145. Pandey K, Badola RP, Kumar S: Time course of intraocular hypertension produced by suxamethonium. Br J Anaesth 44:191, 172

146. Konchigeri HN, Lee YE, Venugopal K: Effect of pancuronium on intraocular pressure changes induced by succinylcholine. Can Anaesth Soc J 26:479, 1979

147. Miller RD, Way WL, Hickey RF: Inhibition of succinylcholine-induced increased intraocular pressure by nondepolarizing muscle relaxants. Anesthesiology 29:123, 1968

148. Meyers EF, Krupin T, Johnson M, et al: Failure of nondepolarizing neuromuscular blockers to inhibit succinylcholine-induced increased intraocular pressure, a controlled study. Anesthesiology 48:149, 1978

149. Chandrashekhar J, Bruce DL: Thiopental and succinylcholine: Action on intraocular pressure. Anesth Analg 54:471, 1975

150. Miller RD, Way WL: Inhibition of succinylcholine-induced increased intragastric pressure by nondepolarizing muscle relaxants and lidocaine. Anesthesiology 34:185, 1971

151. Greenan J: The cardio-oesophageal junction. Br J Anaesth 33:432, 1961

152. Salem MR, Wong AY, Lin YH: The effect of suxamethonium on the intragastric pressure in infants and children. Br J Anaesth 44:166, 1972

153. Brodsky JB, Brock-Utne JG, Samuels SI: Pancuronium pretreatment and post-succinylcholine myalgias. Anesthesiology 51:259, 1979

154. Waters DJ, Mapleson WW: Suxamethonium pains: Hypothesis and observation. Anaesthesia 26:127, 1971

155. Ryan JF, Kagen LJ, Hyman AI: Myoglobinemia after a single dose of succinylcholine. N Engl J Med 285:824, 1971

156. Jansen EC, Hansen PH: Objective measurement of succinylcholine-induced fasciculations and the effect of pretreatment with pancuronium of gallamine. Anesthesiology 51:159, 1979

157. Miller RD: The advantages of giving *d*-tubocurarine before succinylcholine. Anesthesiology 37:568, 1972

158. Rogoff RC, Lippman M, Walts LF: An unusual sensitivity to *d*-tubocurarine. Anesthesiology 41:397, 1974

159. Walts LF, Dillon JB: Clinical studies of the interaction between *d*-tubocurarine and succinylcholine. Anesthesiology 31:39, 1969

160. Sugai N, Hughes R, Payne JP: The effect of suxamethonium alone and its interaction with gallamine on the indirectly elicited tetanic and single twitch contractions of skeletal muscle in man during anaesthesia. Br J Clin Pharmacol 2:391, 1975

161. Katz RL: Modification of the action of pancuronium by succinylcholine and halothane. Anesthesiology 35:602, 1971

162. Jenkinson DH: The antagonism between *d*-tubocurarine and substances which depolarize the motor end-plate. J Physiol 152:309, 1960

163. Sunew KY, Hicks RG: Effects of neostigmine and pyridostigmine on duration of succinylcholine action and pseudocholinesterase activity. Anesthesiology 49:188, 1978

164. Lee C, Katz RL: Neuromuscular pharmacology. Br J Anaesth 52:73, 1980

165. Ramsey FM, Lebowitz PW, Savarese JJ, et al: Clinical characteristics of long term succinylcholine neuromuscular blockade during balanced anesthesia. Anesth Analg 59:110, 1980

166. Riker WF, Standaert FG: The action of facilitatory drugs and acetylcholine on neuromuscular transmission. Ann NY Acad Sci 135:163, 1966

167. Kitz RJ: The chemistry of anticholinesterase activity. Acta Anaesthesiol Scand 8:197, 1964

168. Kitz RJ: Molecular pharmacology of acetylcholinesterases, A Guide to Molecular Phar-

macology and Toxicology. Edited by Featherstone RM. New York, Marcel Dekker, 1977, pp 333–374

169. Payne JP, Hughes R, Azawi SA: Neuromuscular blockade by neostigmine in anaesthetized man. Br J Anaesth 52:69, 1980

170. Katz RL: Clinical neuromuscular pharmacology of pancuronium. Anesthesiology 34:550, 1971

171. Monks S: The reversal of nondepolarizing relaxants. Anesthesia 27:313, 1972

172. Miller RD, Larson CP Jr, Way WL: Comparative antagonism of *d*-tubocurarine-, gallamine-, and pancuronium-induced neuromuscular blockades by neostigmine. Anesthesiology 36:503, 1972

173. Miller RD, Van Nyhuis LS, Eger EI II, et al: The effect of acid-base balance on neostigmine antagonism of *d*-tubocurarine-induced neuromuscular blockade. Anesthesiology 42:377, 1975

174. Miller RD, Roderick L: The influence of acid-base changes on neostigmine antagonism of a pancuronium neuromuscular blockade. Br J Anaesth 50:317, 1978

175. Feldman SA: Effect of changes in electrolytes, hydration, and pH upon the reactions to muscle relaxants. Br J Anaesth 35:546, 1963

176. Cohen EN: Patients with altered sensitivity. Clin Anesth 2:76, 1966

177. Cunningham JN Jr, Carter NW, Rector FC Jr, et al: Resting transmembrane potential difference of skeletal muscle in normal subjects and severely ill patients. J Clin Invest 50:49–59, 1971

178. Fogdall RP, Miller RD: Antagonism of *d*-tubocurarine- and pancuronium-induced neuromuscular blockades by pyridostigmine in man. Anesthesiology 39:504, 1973

179. Tan CK, Balasaraswathi K, El-Etr AA: Neostigmine induced Wencheback phenomena. Anesthesiology Rev 7:28, 1980

180. Glisson S, Fajardo L, El-Etr AA: Amitriptyline therapy increases electrocardiographic changes during reversal of neuromuscular blockade. Anesth Analg 57:77, 1978

181. Ramamurthy S, Shaker MH, Winnie AP: Glycopyrrolate as a substitute for atropine in neostigmine reversal of muscle relaxants. Can Anaesth Soc J 19:4, 1972

182. Cronnelly R, Stanski DR, Miller RD, et al:

Renal function and the pharmacokinetics of neostigmine in anesthetized patients. Anesthesiology 51:222, 1979

183. Cronnelly R, Stanski DR, Miller RD, et al: Pyridostigmine kinetics with and without renal function. Clin Pharmacol Ther 28:78, 1980

184. Morris R, Fahey R, Miller RD, et al: Pharmacokinetics of edrophonium in anesthetized man. Anesthesiology (In press)

185. Kopman AF: Edrophonium antagonism of pancuronium-induced neuromuscular blockade in man. Anesthesiology 51:139, 1979

186. Bevan DR: Reversal of pancuronium with edrophonium. Anaesthesia 34:614, 1979

187. Emery ERJ: The influence of drugs used in therapeutics on the action of muscle relaxants. Br J Anaesth 35:565, 1963

188. Argov Z, Mastaglia FL: Disorders of neuromuscular transmission caused by drugs. N Engl J Med 301:409, 1979

189. Miller RD: Factors affecting the action of muscle relaxants, Muscle Relaxants. Edited by Katz RL. Amsterdam, Excerpta Medica, 1975, pp 165–193

190. Lee C, de Silva AJC: Acute and subchronic neuromuscular blocking characteristics of streptomycin: A comparison with neomycin. Br J Anaesth 51:431, 1979

191. Singh YN, Harvey AL, Marshall IG: Antibiotic-induced paralysis of the mouse phrenic nerve-hemidiaphragm preparation, and reversibility by calcium and by neostigmine. Anesthesiology 48:418, 1978

192. Singh YN, Marshall IG, Harvey AL: Depression of transmitter release and postjunctional sensitivity during neuromuscular block produced by antibiotics. Br J Anaesth 51:1027, 1979

193. Miller RD: The reversal of neuromuscular blockade. Regional Refresher Courses in Anesthesiology 5:134, 1977

194. Giesecke AH, Morris RE, Dalton MD, et al: Of magnesium, muscle relaxants, toxemic parturients, and cats. Anesth Analg 47:689, 1968

195. Ghoneim MM, Long JP: The interaction between magnesium and other neuromuscular blocking agents. Anesthesiology 32:23, 1970

196. del Castillo J, Engbaek L: The nature of the

neuromuscular block produced by magnesium. J Physiol 124:370, 1954

197. Manthey AA: The effect of calcium on the desensitization of membrane receptors at the neuromuscular junction. J Gen Physiol 49:963, 1966

198. Badola RP, Chatterji S, Pandey K, et al: Effects of calcium on neuromuscular block by suxamethonium in dogs. Br J Anaesth 43:1027, 1971

199. Telivuo L, Katz RL: The effects of modern intravenous local analgesics on respiration during partial neuromuscular block in man. Anaesthesia 25:30, 1970

200. Usubiaga JE, Wikinski JA, Morales RL, Usubiaga LE: Interaction of intravenously administered procaine, lidocaine and succinylcholine in anesthetized subjects. Anesth Analg 46:39, 1967

201. Usubiaga JE, Standaert F: The effects of local anesthetics on motor nerve terminals. J Pharmacol Exp Ther 159:353, 1968

202. Kordas M: The effect of procaine on neuromuscular transmission. J Physiol 209:689, 1970

203. Gelser RM, Matsuba M: Neuromuscular blocking actions of local anesthetics. J Pharmacol Exp Ther 103:314, 1951

204. Thorpe WR, Seeman P: The site of action of caffeine and procaine in skeletal muscle. J Pharmacol Exp Ther 179:324, 1971

205. Harrah MD, Way WL, Katzung BG: The interaction of d-tubocurarine with antiarrythmic drugs. Anesthesiology 33:406, 1970

206. Miller RD, Way WL, Katzung BG: The potentiation of neuromuscular blocking agents by quinidine. Anesthesiology 28:1036, 1967

207. Miller RD, Way WL, Katzung BG: The neuromuscular effects of quinidine. Proc Soc Exp Biol Med 129:215, 1968

208. Deacock AR, Hargrove RL: The influence of certain ganglionic blocking agents on neuromuscular transmission. Br J Anaesth 34:357, 1962

209. Wilson SL, Miller RN, Wright C, et al: Prolonged neuromuscular blockade associated with triméthaphan. Anesth Analg 55:353, 1976

210. Glisson SN, El-Etr AA, Lim R: Prolongation of pancuronium-induced neuromuscular blockade by intravenous infusion of nitroglycerine. Anesthesiology 51:47, 1979

211. Glisson SN, Sanchez MM, El-Etr AA, et al: Nitroglycerin and the neuromuscular blockade produced by gallamine, succinylcholine, d-tubocurarine and pancuronium. Anesth Analg 59:117, 1980

212. Miller RD, Sohn YJ, Matteo RS: Enhancement of d-tubocurarine neuromuscular blockade by diuretics in man. Anesthesiology 45:442, 1976.

213. Matteo RS, Nishitateno K, Pua EK, et al: Pharmacokinetics of d-tubocurarine in man: Effect of an osmotic diuretic on urinary excretion. Anesthesiology 52:335, 1980

214. Grob D, Namba T: Characteristics and mechanisms of neuromuscular block in myasthenia gravis. Ann NY Acad Sci 274:143, 1976

215. Engel WK: Myasthenia gravis, corticosteroids, anticholinesterase. Ann NY Acad Sci 274:623, 1976

216. Feldman SA: Muscle relaxants in pathologic states, Muscle Relaxants. Philadelphia, WB Saunders, 1979, pp 108–116

217. Hedley-Whyte J, Burgess GE III, Feeley TW, et al: Respiratory management of peripheral neurologic disease, Applied Physiology of Respiratory Care. Boston, Little, Brown, 1976, pp 245–256

218. Hook R, Anderson EF, Noto P: Anesthetic management of a paturient with myotonia atrophica. Anesthesiology 43:689, 1975

219. Mitchell MM, Ali HH, Sauarese JJ: Myotonia and neuromuscular blocking agents. Anesthesiology 49:44, 1978

220. Siler JN, Discavage WJ: Anesthetic Management of hypokalemic periodic paralysis. Anesthesiology 43:489, 1975

221. Flewellen EH, Bodensteiner JB: Anesthetic experience in a patient with hyperkalemic periodic paralysis. Anesth Rev 7:44, 1980

222. Rosenbaum KJ, Neigh JL, Strobel GE: Sensitivity to nondepolarizing muscle relaxants in amyotrophic lateral sclerosis: Report of two cases. Anesthesiology 35:638, 1971

223. Graham DH: Monitoring neuromuscular block may be unreliable in patients with upper-motor-neuron lesions. Anesthesiology 52:74, 1980

224. Martin JAJ, Szyfelbein SK, Ali HH, et al: Increased d-tubocurarine requirement fol-

lowing major thermal injury. Anesthesiology 52:352, 1980

225. Durant NN, Marshall IG, Savage DS, et al: The neuromuscular and autonomic blocking activities of pancuronium, Org NC 45, and other pancuronium analogues, in the cat. J Pharm Pharmacol 31:831, 1979

226. Fahey M, Morris R, Miller RD, et al: Clinical pharmacology of ORG NC45 (Norcuron™). Anesthesiology (in press)

227. Hunt TM, Hughes R, Payne JP: Preliminary studies with atracurium in anesthetized man. Br J Anaesth 52:238, 1980

228. Savarese JJ: Personal communication

229. Miller RD, Dennissen PAF, van der Pol F, et al: Potentiation of neostigmine and pyridostigmine by 4-aminopyridine in the rat. J Pharm Pharmacol 30:699, 1978

230. Miller RD, Booij LDHJ, Agoston S, et al: 4-Aminopyridine potentiates neostigmine and pyridostigmine in man. Anesthesiology 50:416–420, 1979

231. Agoston S, Salt PJ, Erdmann W, et al: Antagonism of ketamine-diazepam anesthesia by 4-aminopyridine in human volunteers. Br J Anaesth 52:367, 1980

232. Lundh H, Milsson O, Rosen I: Effects of 4-aminopyridine in myasthenia gravis. J Neuro, Neurosurg, Psychiatr 42:171, 1979

18

Pharmacology of the Autonomic Nervous System

Ronald D. Miller, M.D.
Robert K. Stoelting, M.D.

ANATOMY

The autonomic nervous system is subdivided into two major divisions, the sympathetic and parasympathetic. This applies only to the efferent components of the autonomic nervous system. The same division cannot be made for the afferent fibers because they usually serve the somatic as well as the autonomic nervous system. The anatomy of the autonomic efferent fibers is illustrated in Figure 18-1. The cell of origin lies in the central nervous system. The ganglion consists of a number of cell bodies and is the site of synapse between preganglionic and postganglionic fibers. The preganglionic fibers are myelinated and the postganglionic fibers are not. A more detailed description of the anatomy of the autonomic nervous system can be found in Bhugat[1] and Mayer.[2]

From an anatomic point of view, several differences exist between the sympathetic and parasympathetic nervous systems. The sympathetic nervous system is distributed throughout the body whereas the parasympathetic fibers are more limited. As illustrated in Figure 18-1, the parasympathetic nervous system has its terminal ganglia very near to the organs innervated and thus is more lim-

ited and discrete in its discharge of impulses than is the sympathetic nervous system.

TRANSMISSION

Transmission of impulses involves release of a neurotransmitter. Those fibers that release acetylcholine are called cholinergic and those that release norepinephrine are called adrenergic (Fig. 18-1). Cholinergic fibers include preganglionic fibers to all ganglia, postganglionic parasympathetic fibers to smooth muscle, heart, and glands, and postganglionic sympathetic fibers to sweat glands. Adrenergic fibers include postganglionic sympathetic fibers to smooth muscle, heart, and glands.

RECEPTORS

ADRENERGIC

Traditionally, there are two types of adrenergic receptors. Alpha receptors, when stimulated, cause excitatory responses. Beta receptors, when stimulated, cause inhibitory responses. Dopamine, which can activate

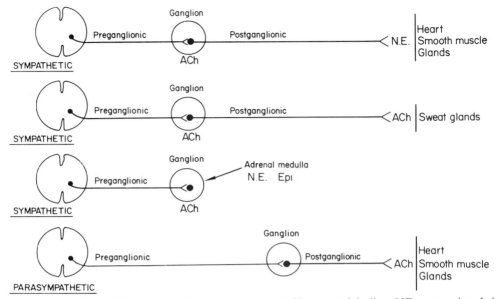

Fig. 18-1 Classification of the antonomic nervous system. ACh = acetylcholine, NE = norepinephrine, and Epi = epinephrine.

both α and β receptors, also acts on specific dopamine receptors that are located in the coronary, renal, cerebral, and mesenteric vessels. When these receptors are stimulated, vasodilation of those vessels occurs. This vasodilation is antagonized by haloperidol but not by a β-blocking drug, propranolol.

Alpha receptors can be subdivided into α_1 and α_2 receptors. Alpha$_1$ receptors are postsynaptic and mediate typical α-adrenergic effects, primarily smooth-muscle contraction (Table 18-1). Conversely, α_2 receptors are primarily presynaptic. Because discovery of the α_2 receptor is fairly recent, its function will be described. A detailed discussion of α-adrenergic receptor subtypes has been provided by Hoffman and Lefkowitz.[3] The function of an α_2 receptor is illustrated in Figure 18-2. Basically, stimulation of the presynaptic α_2 receptor inhibits norepinephrine release from the nerve terminal, whereas drugs that block α_2 receptors enhance norepinephrine release. Since some drugs appear to have selective α_1 or α_2 effects, this subdivision of α receptors is potentially clinically impor-

tant. For example, phentolamine is an equipotent α_1 and α_2 blocker. Although useful in treatment of patients with pheochromocytoma, phentolamine because it produces tachycardia is not helpful in treating primary systemic hypertension. The tachycardia probably occurs because blockade of α_2 presynaptic receptors in the heart leads to increased release of norepinephrine into the synaptic cleft through blockade on the α_2 receptor-mediated autoinhibitory effect of endogenous norepinephrine. This increased concentration of norepinephrine would then cause enhanced stimulation of β-adrenergic receptors in the heart, resulting in positive inotropic and chronotropic effects. Obviously, a drug that only blocks α_1 receptors (e.g., prazosin) would be preferable.

In 1967, β receptors were divided into β_1 and β_2 receptors.[4] Beta$_1$ receptors, such as those that mediate the effects of catecholamines in the heart, are those at which norepinephrine and epinephrine are approximately equipotent. Beta$_2$ receptors are those at which epinephrine is much more potent

Table 18-1. Classification of Responses of Various Organs to Autonomic Stimulation

Organ	Receptor	Response Adrenergic	Response Cholinergic
Heart			
S-A node	β_1	Tachycardia	Bradycardia
Atria	β_1	Increased automaticity	Decreased contractility
A-V node and conduction	β_1	Increased conduction rate	Decreased conduction rate
Ventricle	β_1	Increased contractility and conduction velocity	Slight decrease in contractility
Blood Vessels			
Skin and mucosa	α	Constriction	Dilation
Skeletal muscle	α & β_2	Constriction > dilation	Dilation
Coronary	α & β_2	Construction and dilation	Dilation
Gastrointestinal Tract			
Motility and tone	$\alpha_2 \beta_2$	Decrease	Increase
Sphincters	α	Contraction	Relaxation
Urinary Bladder			
Detrusor	β	Relaxation	Contraction
Sphincter	α	Contraction	Relaxation
Eye			
Radial muscle, iris	α	Contraction	No effect
Ciliary muscle	β	Relaxation for far vision	Contraction for near vision
Skin			
Pilomotor	α	Contraction	No effect
Sweat glands	α	Localized secretion	Generalized secretion

than norepinephrine. Receptors that mediate smooth-muscle relaxation in bronchial smooth muscle are good examples of β_2 receptors.

The location and function of these receptors are listed in Table 18-1.

CHOLINERGIC

Cholinergic receptors are subdivided into muscarinic and nicotinic receptors because muscarine and nicotine were found to stimulate these receptors. The muscarinic receptors

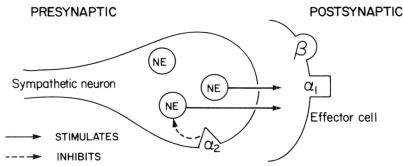

Fig. 18-2 Schematic representation of the synapse of the sympathetic neuron and effector cell, showing presynaptic and postsynaptic receptors. Stimulation of α_2 receptors inhibits norepinephrine (NE) release. (Modified and reproduced with permission from Ram CVS, Kaplan NM: Alpha- and beta-receptor blocking drugs in the treatment of hypertension, Current Problems in Cardiology. Edited by Harvey WP, et al. Copyright © 1979 by Year Book Medical Publishers, Inc. Chicago.)

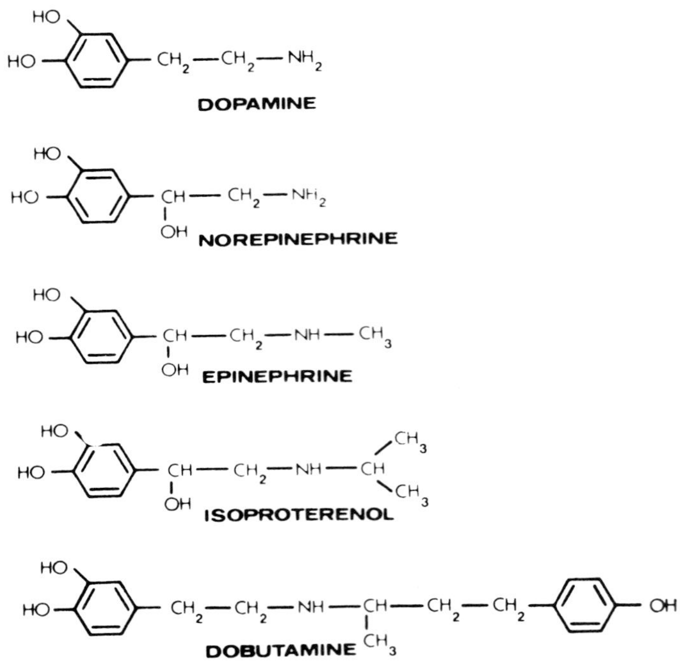

Fig. 18-3 Chemical structure of the endogenous and synthetic catecholamines. Any compound with hydroxyl groups on the 3 and 4 positions in the benzene ring of phenythylamine is a catecholamine. The first endogenous catecholamine, dopamine, is 3,4-dihydroxyphenylethylamine. Hydroxylation of the beta carbon of dopamine results in norepinephrine. Methylation of the terminal amine of norepinephrine results in epinephrine. Adding an isopropyl rather than a methyl group produces isoproterenol. Dobutamine is a combination of dopamine and isoproterenol. (Reprinted by permission. From Sonnenblick EH, Frishman WH, Le Jemtel TH: Dobutamine: A new synthetic cardioactive sympathetic amine. The New England Journal of Medicine 300:17, 1979.)

are blocked by atropine. The nicotinic receptors are classically further divided into ganglionic receptors, which are blocked by hexamethonium, and skeletal muscle receptors, which are blocked by *d*-tubocurarine. Atropine, hexamethonium, and *d*-tubocurarine compete with acetylcholine for binding sites on the receptors. For example, if atropine sufficiently blocks the muscarinic receptors, then acetylcholine will be unable to stimulate these receptors. See Table 18-1 for location and function of these receptors.

CATECHOLAMINES

Catecholamines are compounds with hydroxyl groups on the 3 and 4 positions in the benzene ring of phenylethylamine (Fig. 18-3). Endogenous catecholamines are dopamine, norepinephrine, and epinephrine. Dopamine serves as a precursor of norepinephrine and is a neurotransmitter in the brain. Norepinephrine is present in postganglionic sympathetic nerve endings and acts locally on

receptors (effector cells) as the neurotransmitter for the peripheral sympathetic nervous system. Epinephrine is produced in the adrenal medulla and acts on distant target organs. Catecholamines that do not occur endogenously are isoproterenol and dobutamine.

BIOSYNTHESIS

Synthesis of catecholamines involves a series of enzyme-controlled steps that begin with the active transport of tyrosine from the circulation into the postganglionic sympathetic nerve ending (Fig. 18-4).[5] The enzyme tyrosine hydroxylase converts tyrosine to dihydroxyphenylalanine (DOPA). This is a rate-limiting step in which catecholamine synthesis can be inhibited by either increased circulating norepinephrine or by drugs that are specific tyrosine hydroxylase inhibitors. DOPA is decarboxylated to dopamine, which is then transported from the cytoplasm of the nerve ending into the storage vesicle. Here

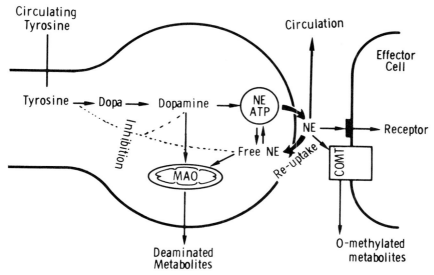

Fig. 18-4 Schematic representation of adrenergic nerve endings and how norepinephrine is produced and terminated. MAO = monoamine oxidase, NE = norepinephrine, ATP = adenosine triphosphate, and COMT = catechol-*O*-methyl transferase. (Bhagat BD: Mode of Action of Autonomic Drugs. Graceway Publishers, New York, 1979.)

dopamine is converted to norepinephrine by dopamine β oxidase. An additional enzyme, phenylethanolamine N-methyltransferase, present only in chromaffin cells, methylates approximately 85 percent of the norepinephrine formed in the adrenal medulla to epinephrine. Glucocorticoids from the adrenal cortex pass through the adrenal medulla and are capable of activating this enzyme, so that in stress states there is increased epinephrine production.

Although their function and location are described in Table 18-1, adrenergic receptors have not been isolated chemically; however, it is likely that the enzyme adenylate cyclase (AC), located in the cell membrane, is part of the receptor mechanism. Conceptually, this enzyme has two components (Fig. 18-5).[2] The site facing the cell exterior recognizes the specific neurotransmitter or hormone. This recognition activates the site facing the interior of the membrane. Activation of this latter site catalyzes the conversion of adenosine triphosphate (ATP) to cyclic 3', 5'-adenosine monophosphate (cAMP). The subsequent

increase of intracellular cAMP is thought to be responsible for the β effects of catecholamines. The biologic role of another cyclic nucleotide, 3', 5'-guanosine monophosphate (cGMP) is less well understood. Nevertheless, cGMP is thought to mediate the cellular effects of acetylcholine and possibly the α effects of catecholamines. cAMP and cGMP may be referred to as "second messengers," emphasizing their role in activating other enzymes (protein kinases) necessary for responses to neurotransmitters, hormones, and drugs. Enzymatic hydrolysis of cAMP by phosphodiesterase (PDE) is the main physiologic mechanism for terminating the action of cAMP.

In addition to activating AC, catecholamines regulate the responsiveness of the receptor. This is reflected by decreased responsiveness (refractoriness) to catecholamines with chronic exposure. For example, asthmatics treated chronically with a β agonist manifest decreased bronchodilatation in response to catecholamines. Refractoriness is most likely due to a decreased number of β

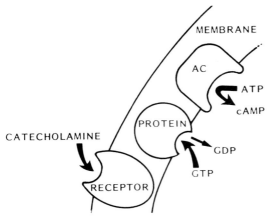

Fig. 18-5 Catecholamines are speculated to attach to receptors (adenylate cyclase, AC) on cell membranes ultimately producing increased intracellular cyclic 3′,5′-adenosine monophosphate (cAMP) and the characteristic beta response. ATP = adenosine triphosphate, GDP = guanosine diphosphate, GTP = guanosine triphosphate.

receptors that occur with chronic catecholamine stimulation.[6]

INACTIVATION OF NOREPINEPHRINE

Termination of norepinephrine activity at the receptor is due almost entirely to reuptake of this neurotransmitter from the receptor and synaptic cleft back into the sympathetic nerve ending (Fig. 18-4). Following reuptake, a small amount of norepinephrine is deaminated in the cytoplasm by monamine oxidase (MAO). The remaining norepinephrine is transported into the storage vesicle for reuse. This reuptake plus continued biosynthesis provides a large norepinephrine reserve and explains the difficulty in producing neurotransmitter depletion with drugs.

The process for norepinephrine reuptake into the postganglionic sympathetic nerve endings and storage vesicles is not specific for norepinephrine. Structurally similar compounds (guanethidine, metaraminol) may enter the nerve ending and storage vesicle by the same mechanism and result in depletion of the neurotransmitter. In contrast, drugs (ephedrine, cocaine, tricyclic antidepressants) may interfere with the reuptake mechanism resulting in an enhanced response to catecholamines—i.e., more norepinephrine is available to receptors.

A small amount of norepinephrine escapes reuptake into the nerve ending and enters the circulation. This norepinephrine is metabolized by both MAO and catechol-*O*-methyl transferase (COMT) primarily in the liver and kidney. Epinephrine released by the adrenal medulla is inactivated by the same enzymes. The final metabolic product is vanillyl-mandelic acid (VMA), while homovanillic acid is the major metabolite of dopamine. Less than 5 percent of the norepinephrine released from the nerve ending escapes reuptake and metabolism to appear unchanged in the urine. This emphasizes the difficulty in judging sympathetic nervous system activity at the receptor by measuring serum or urinary norepinephrine concentrations. Furthermore, serum norepinephrine concentrations may be influenced by events other than release from the nerve ending, such as altered reuptake or changes in MAO and/or COMT activity. Despite these limitations, measurement of norepinephrine concentrations in blood and urine remains the most useful method of appraising sympathetic nervous system activity.

Subtle changes in neurotransmitter release (as may be produced by anesthetic drugs) are best determined by measuring norepinephrine concentrations. In contrast, total norepinephrine production (as with pheochromocytoma) is best reflected by VMA concentrations, since this represents both intraneuronal breakdown (but never released) and the metabolized norepinephrine escaping reuptake. Dopamine β oxidase is simultaneously released from the nerve ending with norepinephrine. Therefore, measurement of serum dopamine β oxidase concentrations may also serve as an index of sympathetic nervous system activity.

PHARMACOLOGY OF SPECIFIC CATECHOLAMINES AND OTHER SYMPATHOMIMETIC DRUGS

A summary of the relative potency of these drugs on adrenergic receptors is presented in Table 18-2. A comparison of the cardiovascular effects of these drugs is summarized in Table 18-3.

NOREPINEPHRINE

As the neurotransmitter released from postganglionic sympathetic nerve endings, nonepinephrine is responsible for maintaining blood pressure by appropriate adjustments in peripheral vascular resistance. Norepinephrine-induced vasoconstriction increases systolic, diastolic, and mean arterial pressures. $Beta_1$ effects on the heart are overshadowed by the α_1 effects of this catecholamine on the peripheral vasculature. Cardiac output may be reduced, despite the increased blood pressure reflecting the effect of increased ventricular afterload and baroreceptor-mediated reflex bradycardia. Prevention of bradycardia with atropine unmasks the positive chronotropic and inotropic effects of norepinephrine. $Beta_2$ effects of norepinephrine are minimal. The cardiovascular effects of norepinephrine are summarized in Figure 18-6.

Table 18-2. Relative Adrenergic-Receptor Activity of Sympathomimetic Amines

Drug	Alpha	$Beta_1$	$Beta_2$
Norepinephrine	+++	++	−
Epinephrine	+	++	++
Isoproterenol	−	+++	+++
Dopamine*	++	++	+
Dobutamine	+	++	+
Phenylephrine	+++	−	−
Methoxamine	+++	−	−
Metaraminol	++	+	+
Ephedrine	++	+	+

Codes used: − = no change, + = slight stimulation, ++ = moderate stimulation, +++ = marked stimulation.
* Causes renal and mesenteric dilation by stimulating dopaminergic receptors.

Table 18-3. Relative Potencies of Sympathomimetic Drugs

Drug	MAP	HR	CO	TPR	RBF
Norepinephrine	↑↑↑	↓*	↓*	↑↑↑	↓↓↓
Epinephrine	↑↑	↑↑	↑↑	↑↑	↓↓
Isoproterenol	↓	↑↑↑	↑↑↑	↓↓	↑
Dopamine	↑	↑↑	↑↑↑	↑	↑↑↑
Dobutamine	↑	↑	↑↑↑	↑ or ↓	↑ or ↓
Phenylephrine	↑↑↑	↓*	↓*	↑↑↑	↓↓↓
Methoxamine	↑↑↑	↓*	↓*	↑↑↑	↓↓↓
Metaraminol	↑↑	↑	↑ or ↓*	↑↑	↓↓
Ephedrine	↑↑	↑	↑	↑↑	↓↓

Abbreviations used: MAP = mean arterial blood pressure, HR = heart rate, CO = cardiac output, TPR = total peripheral resistance, RBF = renal blood flow; ↑ = slight, ↑↑ = moderate, ↑↑↑ = marked increase.
* Decreases in heart rate are not a direct effect, but are due to reflex bradycardia.

EPINEPHRINE

Clinically, the catecholamine epinephrine may be used to (1) treat congestive heart failure, (2) relieve bronchospasm (see Ch. 22), (3) provide local hemostasis, (4) limit systemic absorption of local anesthetics (see Ch. 19), and (5) produce vigorous ventricular fibrillation during cardiopulmonary resuscitation (see Ch. 46).

Epinephrine stimulates α_1, β_1, and β_2 receptors. Low doses stimulate α_1 receptors in the skin, mucosa, and hepatorenal vasculature while β_2 stimulation predominates in skeletal muscle. The net effect is a preferential distribution of cardiac output to skeletal muscle and a decreased systemic vascular resistance. Renal blood flow is greatly reduced even with an unchanged blood pressure. Stimulation of β_1 receptors increases heart rate and contractility, producing an increased cardiac output. Since the blood pressure is not greatly elevated, compensatory baroreceptor reflexes do not prevent the increased cardiac output produced by epinephrine. $Beta_1$ stimulation also increases automaticity and contributes to ventricular irritability. The cardiovascular effects of epinephrine are summarized in Figure 18-7.

Epinephrine has the most significant effects of all the catecholamines on metabo-

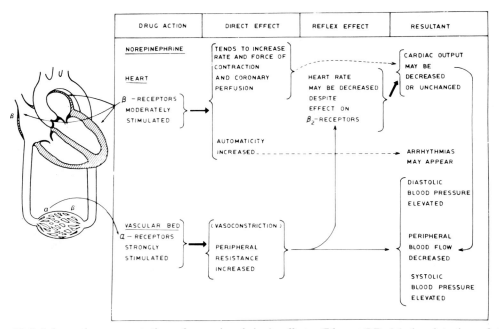

Fig. 18-6 Schematic representation of norepinephrine's effects. (Bhagat BD: Mode of Action of Autonomic Drugs. Graceway Publishers, New York, 1979.)

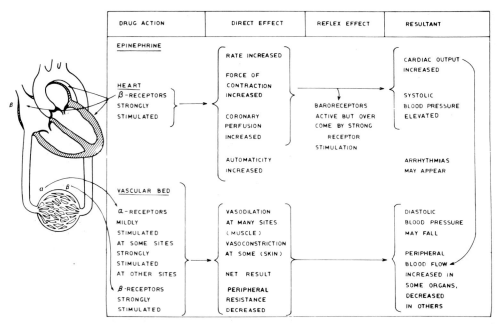

Fig. 18-7 Schematic representation of epinephrine's effects. (Bhagat BD: Mode of Action of Autonomic Drugs. Graceway Publishers, New York, 1979.)

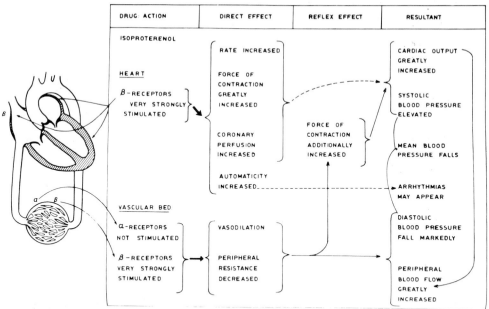

Fig. 18-8 Schematic representation of isoproterenol's effects. (Bhagat BD: Mode of Action of Autonomic Drugs. Graceway Publishers, New York, 1979.)

lism. Beta$_1$ stimulation from epinephrine increases liver glycogenolysis and adipose tissue lipolysis while α_1 stimulation inhibits insulin release. Epinephrine release during anesthesia and operation (or any form of trauma) is the most plausible explanation for the characteristic hyperglycemia of the perioperative period.

ISOPROTERENOL

Isoproterenol, a synthetic catecholamine, is a potent stimulant of β_1 and β_2 receptors with no significant effect on α_1 receptors. Myocardial contractility, heart rate, systolic blood pressure, and automaticity increase while systemic vascular resistance (muscle, renal, and pulmonary) and diastolic blood pressure decrease. (Fig. 18-8). The net effect is an increase in cardiac output and occasionally a reduction in mean arterial pressure. Bron-

chodilatation is accompanied by significant cardiovascular effects, since isoproterenol does not discriminate between β_1 and β_2 receptors. In contrast, specific β_2 agonists (terbutaline) produce a much smaller cAMP increase in myocardial cells.

Excessive tachycardia and simultaneous diastolic hypotension may reduce coronary blood flow at the same time myocardial oxygen requirements are increased by tachycardia. The above events, combined with a high incidence of ventricular dysrhythmias and diversion of blood flow to skeletal muscle, detract from the value of this catecholamine, particularly in patients with coronary artery disease. The major application of isoproterenol (0.05 to 0.1 μg/kg/min) is for patients with valvular heart disease (right ventricular dysfunction and pulmonary hypertension) who may benefit from a more rapid heart rate plus decreased systemic and pulmonary vascular resistance.

DOPAMINE

The catecholamine dopamine has replaced other preparations for use in clinical situations characterized by decreased cardiac output and increased left ventricular end-diastolic pressure. Depending on the dose, dopamine directly stimulates postsynaptic dopaminergic, β, and α receptors. Dopamine is unique among the catecholamines in its ability to stimulate dopaminergic receptors (3 to 10 μg/kg/min) and redistribute blood flow to the kidneys. In addition, β stimulation increases cardiac output with only a slight increase in heart rate or systemic vascular resistance. Dopamine also exerts part of its inotropic effect by releasing endogenous norepinephrine, which may predispose to ventricular dysrhythmias. Furthermore, this indirect stimulation may be an unreliable mechanism when cardiac catecholamine stores are depleted as with chronic congestive heart failure. Alpha effects of dopamine predominate with doses above 20 μg/kg/min.

Several investigators have observed increased pulmonary artery occluded pressure (PAOP) during dopamine administration particularly when infusion rates exceed 5 μg/kg/min.[7, 8] This shift of the left ventricular function curve towards greater filling pressures may produce an increased myocardial wall tension and oxygen demand. The ability of dopamine to exert inotropic effects and to increase PAOP concomitantly is not shared by other catecholamines. The speculated mechanism for this increased preload is dopamine-induced redistribution of blood volume from the periphery to the central circulation due to venous constriction. In addition, dopamine may reduce left ventricular compliance.

Hess et al.[8] recently demonstrated that the simultaneous administration of intravenous nitroglycerin (0.5 μg/kg/min) during dopamine infusion (8 μg/kg/min) prevented the increase in PAOP without offsetting the desirable effects on cardiac output. The beneficial effects of adding nitroglycerin to dopamine may be especially helpful for patients with congestive heart failure or pulmonary hypertension who need inotropic support with dopamine.

DOBUTAMINE

Dobutamine, a recently introduced synthetic catecholamine, has structural characteristics of both dopamine and isoproterenol.[9] Removal of the side-chain hydroxyl groups from the isoproterenol portion decreases arrhythmogenicity but retains the inotropic properties. Dobutamine acts selectively on β_1 receptors without significant effects on β_2 or α_1 receptors. Unlike dopamine, this catecholamine does not act indirectly by stimulating endogenous norepinephrine release nor does it stimulate dopaminergic receptors to increase renal blood flow.

The most prominent effect during dobutamine infusion (2 to 20 μg/kg/min) is a dose-dependent increase in cardiac output without marked changes in heart rate. Systemic and pulmonary vascular resistances may decrease. This ability to increase contractility with minimal chronotropic or α_1 stimulation is unique to dobutamine. In contrast to dopamine, the left ventricular filling pressure tends to decrease during dobutamine infusion. The cardiovascular effects make dobutamine useful for treating acute cardiac failure characterized by low cardiac output and elevated diastolic filling pressures. Dobutamine may be ineffective for those patients who also need increased systemic vascular resistance to elevate blood pressure.

PHENYLEPHRINE AND METHOXAMINE

Phenylephrine and methoxamine are essentially pure α receptor stimulators, causing vasoconstriction with no stimulatory effects on the heart or central nervous system. The cardiovascular effects of phenylephrine are summarized in Figure 18-9. Because of

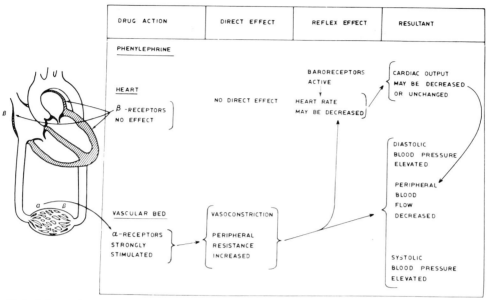

DRUG ACTION	DIRECT EFFECT	REFLEX EFFECT	RESULTANT

PHENYLEPHRINE

HEART

β -RECEPTORS
NO EFFECT

NO DIRECT EFFECT

BARORECEPTORS
ACTIVE

HEART RATE
MAY BE DECREASED

CARDIAC OUTPUT
MAY BE DECREASED
OR UNCHANGED

DIASTOLIC
BLOOD PRESSURE
ELEVATED

PERIPHERAL
BLOOD
FLOW
DECREASED

VASCULAR BED

α-RECEPTORS
STRONGLY
STIMULATED

VASOCONSTRICTION

PERIPHERAL
RESISTANCE
INCREASED

SYSTOLIC
BLOOD PRESSURE
ELEVATED

Fig. 18-9 Schematic representation of phenylephrine's effects. (Bhagat BD: Mode of Action of Autonomic Drugs. Graceway Publishers, New York, 1979.)

marked α receptor stimulatory effects, an increase in both systolic and diastolic pressures occur. This hypertensive response evokes a reflex bradycardia as outlined in Figure 18-10.

EPHEDRINE

Ephedrine has both indirect and direct effects. It causes an increase in mean arterial blood pressure due to release of norepinephrine from its storage sites (Table 18-3). This is called an *indirect* effect because ephedrine itself does not cause the increase in blood pressure. Conversely, ephedrine does not depend on release of norepinephrine to stimulate the heart (a *direct* effect).

Ephedrine is widely used in anesthesia for treatment of hypotension in obstetrics and during spinal or epidural anesthesia. When ephedrine is given repeatedly (e.g., > 75 mg/70 kg), tachyphylaxis often occurs.

METARAMINOL

Metaraminol, like ephedrine, has both indirect and direct effects. However, the peripheral vascular effects appear to be more dominant than those that occur with ephedrine. Because of α receptor stimulation, metaraminol increases total peripheral resistance and therefore blood pressure (Table 18-3). However, metaraminol does have a direct stimulatory effect on the heart, although certainly less than that of ephedrine.

Metaraminol depletes and replaces norepinephrine from its storage site and then acts as a false transmitter. The false transmitter is then released in response to adrenergic nerve stimulation and is about one tenth as potent as norepinephrine. As a result, vascular tone is reduced resulting in a fall in arterial blood pressure. Thus with administration of metaraminol for longer than 2 to 3 hours, hypotension may develop.

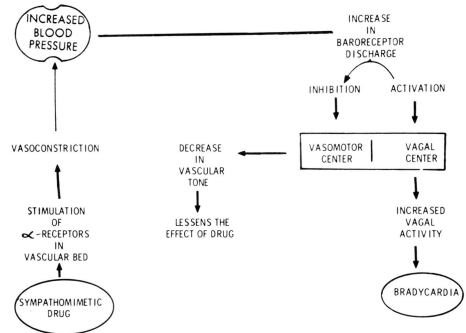

Fig. 18-10 Schematic representation of the reflex response evoked by a sympathomimetic drug such as phenylephrine. (Bhagat BD: Mode of Action of Autonomic Drugs. Graceway Publishers, New York, 1979.)

PHARMACOLOGY OF ANTIHYPERTENSIVE DRUGS

The pharmacology of the various antihypertensive drugs are briefly discussed in this section. However, the preoperative evaluation of a patient who is hypertensive and may be taking these drugs is discussed in Chapter 2. The antihypertensive drugs can be classified according to their main mechanisms of action (Table 18-4).

CENTRAL SYMPATHOLYTIC DRUGS

RESERPINE (SERPASIL)

Reserpine prevents norepinephrine accumulation in the storage vesicles but not in the nerve ending, so that the neurotransmitter is vulnerable to oxidation by the enzyme monoamine oxidase (Fig. 18-4). The net effect is gradual depletion of norepinephrine as the storage granules deplete their contents spontaneously or in response to nerve stimulation. Also, reserpine depletes the adrenal medulla of catecholamines. This results in a dose-dependent impairment of sympathetic nervous system function. However, complete depletion of norepinephrine seems unlikely in humans, as reserpine's toxicity limits the total adult reserpine dose to about 0.5 mg/70kg/day.

Reserpine readily crosses the blood-brain barrier and can cause sedation, tranquilization, mental depression, decreased anesthetic requirement, and occasional parkinsonian-like rigidity. Most of these effects probably reflect depletion of central nervous system norepinephrine or dopamine. In higher doses, reserpine increases gastric acid secretion, thereby increasing the incidence of peptic ulcer disease.

Table 18-4. Classification of Antihypertensive Drugs

Central sympatholytic drugs
   Reserpine
   Alpha-methyldopa
   Clonidine

Peripheral sympatholytic drugs
   Guanethidine

Beta-adrenergic blocking drugs
   Propranolol
   Metoprolol

Alpha-adrenergic blocking drugs
   Phenoxybenzamine
   Phentolamine
   Prazosin

Ganglionic blocking drugs
   Pentolinium
   Trimethaphan

Dilators of vascular smooth muscle
   Hydralazine
   Minoxidil
   Diazoxide
   Sodium nitroprusside
   Nitroglycerin

ALPHA-METHYLDOPA (METHYLDOPA, ALDOMET)

Methyldopa is also a centrally acting anti-hypertensive agent whose mechanism of action is incompletely understood. Present evidence indicates that the drug has to be metabolized to α-methylnorepinephrine in the brain to be effective.[10] In turn, α-methyl-norepinephrine interacts with central α-adrenergic receptors to decrease sympathetic outflow.[11] Methyldopa decreases blood pressure by reducing both the cardiac output and peripheral resistance.[12] The plasma half-life of the drug is only 1 to 2 hours, but its hypotensive effect can last as long as 24 hours, probably because the active metabolite α-methylnorepinephrine has a long half-life in the brain.[13]

A major side effect involves depression of the central nervous system, including drowsiness, decreased intellectual drive, and forgetfulness. Impotence and dryness of the mouth also are seen with the chronic use of methyldopa.

A positive direct Coombs' test will develop in about 25 percent of persons on long-term methyldopa therapy, which in itself is harmless, except for difficulty in crossmatching blood for tranfusions.[14] However, in 1 to 5 percent of patients with a positive Coombs' test secondary to methyldopa, hemolytic anemia will develop, which will necessitate the cessation of the drug. In addition to hemolysis, use of methyldopa has been associated with fever and hepatic dysfunction that can resemble either acute hepatitis or chronic active hepatitis.[15] The hematologic and hepatic effects may complicate the postoperative evaluation of a jaundiced patient especially when halothane has been used (see Ch. 14).

Patients receiving methyldopa may manifest a hypertensive response when also receiving propranolol.[16] Propranolol probably blocks the usual vasodilating effects of α-methylnorepinephrine so that only the potent α-stimulating effects of the methyldopa metabolite are apparent. Thus, the anesthesiologist should consider this hazard when contemplating the intraoperative administration of propranolol to a patient receiving methyldopa.

Dementia has been observed in patients first treated with methyldopa and subsequently with the butyrophenone haloperidol.[17] This dementia may be caused by the ability of both drugs to prevent dopamine from reaching the central nervous system receptor. Thus, if a patient is taking methyldopa, perhaps Innovar should not be used because it contains another butyrophenone, droperidol.

CLONIDINE (CATAPRES)

Clonidine is a central-acting antihypertensive drug that has α-adrenergic agonist properties. When given acutely, clonidine produces α-adrenergically mediated vasoconstriction. However, clonidine also inhibits sympathetic outflow from the central nervous system and increases the depressor effects of baroreceptor stimulation.[18, 19] This biphasic effect of the drug is frequently best seen in patients receiving large doses (> 1.0 mg/70kg/day) wherein the initial response is hypertension followed by a more prolonged hypotension due to inhibition of sympathetic outflow from the central nervous system.[20]

Because of the reduced sympathetic activity, clonidine lowers blood pressure by decreasing both cardiac output and peripheral resistance. The pharmacokinetics of clonidine indicate that the drug has a half-life of about 12 hours and its duration of action is also about 12 hours, although the range for both variables can span from 6 to 24 hours.[19]

The main problems with clonidine are the disturbing side effects to the central nervous system that include sedation and inability to concentrate. Dryness of the mouth secondary to decreased saliva flow is very common. The drug ordinarily does not cause orthostatic hypotension, but orthostatic hypotension can occur if the patient is dehydrated intravascularly.

Among the most serious side effects described for clonidine are rebound hypertension and signs of sympathetic overactivity 8 to 36 hours following sudden withdrawal of the drug. Elevated serum and urinary levels of catecholamines also have been noted in clonidine withdrawal.[21, 22] If use of clonidine must be discontinued, a regimen involving tapering the drug dosage over several days to a week is desirable. If rebound hypertension occurs, it can be treated by reinstituting clonidine. Obviously, the night before surgery is not the time to consider withdrawing clonidine. Such a decision could lead to hypertensive problems in the perioperative period.

PERIPHERAL SYMPATHOLYTIC DRUGS

Guanethidine

Because of its basic guanidine group, guanethidine does not enter the brain and, consequently, lacks any significant effect on the central nervous system.[23] The drug, transported into presynaptic sympathetic neurovesicles by the norepinephrine pump, depletes and inhibits the release of the norepinephrine, resulting in a functional sympathetic denervation.[24] The pharmacokinetics of the drug is complicated and includes an elimination half-life of about 5 days.

Because guanethidine has to enter the adrenergic neuron to be active, any drug that interferes with the norepinephrine pump will inhibit its hypotensive effect. The tricyclic antidepressant drugs are potent in this respect and can totally reverse guanethidine's hypotensive effect.[25] In addition, phenothiazines, ephedrine, amphetamines, and cocaine can block uptake of guanethidine into nerve endings.[26] Guanethidine lowers blood pressure mainly by decreasing cardiac output through a reduction in venous return, an effect that is exaggerated when the patient is in an upright position. The side effects of the drug are secondary to unwanted aspects of adrenergic blockade.

BETA-ADRENERGIC BLOCKING DRUGS

Propranolol (Inderal)

Propranolol blocks both the β_1 (cardiac) and β_2 (vascular, bronchial) adrenergic receptors. Propranolol also has a membrane-stabilizing or "quinidine-like" effect, which probably accounts for its effectiveness in treating digitalis intoxication.

One of propranolol's most common indications is for the treatment of hypertension. Because selective β_2 antagonism has not been shown to lower blood pressure, it appears that inhibition of the β_1-adrenergic receptor is responsible for the lowering of blood pressure. Although propranolol may lower blood pressure because it decreases plasma renin activity, there is substantial evidence against that being the only explanation for its hypotensive action.[27] Propranolol, when given chronically, lowers renin activity after the first dose, but the hypotension may not occur for as long as a week after the initiation of therapy.[28] Propranolol, when given intravenously, lowers renin activity immediately but the blood pressure does not decrease as rapidly.[29]

Propranolol probably decreases blood pressure by decreasing cardiac output. The physiological sequences after administration of propranolol are as follows: there is an immediate decrease in cardiac output but an increase in peripheral vascular resistance such that blood pressure does not change; the change in peripheral vascular resistance over several weeks readjusts close to baseline so that the chronic decrease in cardiac output results in arterial hypotension. Because not all people respond to β-blocking doses of propranolol in the treatment of hypertension, no single mechanism explains propranolol's ability to decrease blood pressure.

Ischemic heart disease is also a common indication for the use of propranolol. The drug is very effective in increasing exercise tolerance in angina pectoris; helping to salvage ischemic myocardium in the presence of acute myocardial infarction; and alleviating life-threatening arrhythmias, especially tachyarrhythmias. About 40 to 70 percent of the drug is extracted by the liver before systemic availability; thus, there is a large variation among patients in the drug levels after a standard dose.[30] Because measurements of its presence in the blood are not readily available, looking at decrements in tachycardia in response to exercise may be a reasonable way to evaluate the extent of β blockade. The half-life of the drug is usually 4 to 6 hours, but its hypotensive effect can last much longer. Side effects of propranolol include heart failure, atrioventricular block, hypoglycemia, asthma, central nervous system disturbances, and peripheral vascular compromise. In addition, propranolol blocks some of the warning signs and symptoms of hypoglycemia; therefore, its use may be contraindicated in insulin-dependent diabetic patients.

If an overdose of propranolol has been given, a specific pharmacologic β agonist, isoproterenol, may be able to antagonize both the negative chronotropic and inotropic effects of propranolol. However, huge doses of isoproterenol may be required. Calcium chloride, up to 7 mg/kg by intravenous bolus, may be a better choice. If readily available, cardiac pacing may be equally effective.

METOPROLOL (LOPRESSOR)

Metoprolol is a selective β_1-adrenergic blocker. Thus, like propranolol, metoprolol effectively inhibits the inotropic and chronotropic effects of isoproterenol. Conversely, metoprolol does not inhibit the vasodilator effects of isoproterenol. This relative β_1 selectivity of metoprolol is the basis for its potential therapeutic advantage over less selective drugs.

ALPHA-ADRENERGIC BLOCKING DRUGS

PHENOXYBENZAMINE (DIBENZYLINE) AND PHENTOLAMINE (REGITINE)

Phenoxybenzamine and phentolamine have little clinical value in treatment of ambulatory essential hypertension. Both drugs act as competitive blockers by occupying the α-receptors and by preventing the usual neurotransmitter-receptor interactions. The major disadvantage of α-adrenergic blockers is impairment of compensatory vasoconstriction, and this could lead to subsequent orthostatic hypotension. Marked decreases in blood pressure may occur with blood loss and conceivably in response to sudden position changes or positive intrathoracic pressure. Furthermore, increased myocardial oxygen requirements may result from lack of β-receptor blockade, subsequent reflex tachycardia, and increased myocardial contractility. Prevention or treatment of hypertensive responses to endogenous (pheochromocytoma) or exogenous catecholamines is the most frequent indication for α-adrenergic blockade.

Prazosin (Minipress)

This drug was initially marketed as a peripheral vasodilator because of its ability to inhibit phosphodiesterase, but it is also a potent postsynaptic α-adrenergic inhibitor. Because the in vitro concentration necessary to inhibit phosphodiesterase is almost 1,000 times that required to inhibit α-adrenergic receptors, prazosin probably works through its α-adrenergic-blocking properties.[31] Prazosin, like other α-adrenergic blocking agents, can cause orthostatic hypotension. This effect is especially prominent during the first few doses and seems to lessen with continued use of the drug. Unlike other peripheral vasodilators, prazosin does not stimulate the release of renin or cause reflex tachycardia in the face of low blood pressure.[32, 33] That prazosin is a selective α_1-adrenergic blocker probably explains the lack of renin release or reflex tachycardia (Fig. 18-2).[3] The absence of high potency at α_2 receptors goes along with a norepinephrine release that would not be enhanced. Other drugs that enhance norepinephrine overflow would tend to enhance renin release directly. This effect does not occur with prazosin. Conversely, a drug such as phentolamine is not as effective as an antihypertensive agent probably because blockade of α_2-adrenergic receptors causes a loss of feedback inhibition of norepinephrine release. This would tend to counteract α_1-receptor blockade.

GANGLIONIC BLOCKING DRUGS

Pentolinium (Ansolysen) and Trimethaphan (Arfonad)

Pentolinium and trimethaphan produce ganglionic blockade by occupying receptor sites and stabilizing the postsynaptic membranes against the actions of acetylcholine liberated from presynaptic nerve endings. Thus they lower blood pressure by lowering vascular resistance. In addition, trimethaphan also has a direct smooth muscle relaxing effect and releases histamine. With the advent of selective sympathetic nervous system inhibitors, ganglionic blockers are seldom employed for control of blood pressure in ambulatory patients.

DILATORS OF VASCULAR SMOOTH MUSCLE

Hydralazine (Apresoline)

Hydralazine probably interferes with calcium transport in arterial vascular smooth muscle and lowers blood pressure by vasodilation. Since baroreceptors remain intact, increased sympathetic outflow to the myocardium and peripheral vasculature in response to lowered blood pressure may offset the desired antihypertensive effect. This reflex stimulation is prevented by combining this drug with other antihypertensives, such as guanethidine or propranolol. In contrast, orthostatic hypotension is not a problem because cardiovascular reflexes and sympathetic nervous system function are not altered.

The side effects of hydralazine are mainly related to the reflex sympathetic changes it produces. Palpitations and tremors can be reasonably controlled with β-adrenergic receptor antagonists. The drug should not be used in patients with angina because it can precipitate myocardial infarction.

Minoxidil (Loniten)

Minoxidil is a drug whose mechanism of action is very similar to hydralazine except that it is more effective.[34] The plama half-life is approximately 4 hours. The net effect can last as long as 24 hours, probably because the drug accumulates in vascular tissues, the site of its pharmacologic effect. As with any peripheral vasodilator, the use of minoxidil is associated with reflex tachycardia and salt and water retention;[35] thus, this drug is most effective when used with a diuretic and a β-adrenergic blocking agent. Pulmonary hypertension has been described with the use of minoxidil, but in these cases the elevated cardiac output, fluid overload, and left ventricular failure contributed more to the pulmonary hypertension than did an elevated pulmonary vascular resistance due to minoxidil.

The major problems associated with the drug have been avid salt and water retention and unwanted hair growth. Salt and water retention can usually be controlled by the use of potent loop diuretics, but patients with moderate renal failure occasionally escape the effects of the diuretics. Unwanted hair growth is especially unesthetic for women, but aside from cosmetic consequences, it has no harmful effect.

DIAZOXIDE (HYPERSTAT)

Diazoxide is a nondiuretic thiazide derivative that has been used for the management of postoperative hypertension. This drug reduces systolic and diastolic blood pressures by a direct relaxant action on arteriolar smooth muscle. It has no significant effect on sympathetic reflexes, so that the decrease in peripheral vascular resistance is accompanied by a reflex increase in heart rate and cardiac output. A single intravenous injection of diazoxide of 2.5 to 5.0 mg/kg over 10 to 20 seconds rapidly lowers blood pressure to an acceptable level in 2 to 5 minutes. Blood pressure gradually returns to control levels over the next 12 hours. The absence of a sedative effect allows the physician to evaluate the patient's mental status. Although excessive hypotension is unlikely, a disadvantage compared with nitroprusside is the inability to adjust the dose of diazoxide in accordance with the patient's response. It must be remembered that the response to diazoxide is accentuated in patients who are given drugs such as propranolol or guanethidine, since

the reflex-sympathetic responses to decreased blood pressure are blocked. When used in patients with eclampsia, diazoxide acts as a powerful uterine relaxant, but contractions may be reestablished with oxytocin.

NITROPRUSSIDE (NIPRIDE) AND NITROGLYCERIN (NITROL)

Sodium nitroprusside is a very potent intravenous antihypertensive agent that has acquired popularity in the past 5 years. The molecular structure of the drug has a ferrous center surrounded by five cyanide groups and a nitrosyl group. It is the nitrosyl group that is responsible for the drug effect on vascular smooth muscle. Unlike the other peripheral vasodilators (diazoxide, hydralazine, minoxidil), nitroprusside has a significant dilatory effect on both the venules and arterioles, thus both preload and afterload are affected. Also, unlike the other vasodilators, the use of nitroprusside is not associated with a significant reflex increase in cardiac output. The advantage of nitroprusside is its very rapid action, which allows for fine adjustment of blood pressure by titrating the infusion rate. The disadvantage of the drug is the close nursing supervision that is required because accidental speeding up of the intravenous infusion will result in severe hypotension. The drug is unstable when exposed to light; therefore, the infusion bottle should be wrapped in aluminum foil and a fresh solution should be prepared every 4 hours.

The use of nitroprusside during anesthesia to deliberately produce hypotension is discussed in Chapter 33. Briefly, an infusion rate of 0.5 to 5.0 μg/kg/min is usually adequate with the lowest doses required in the presence of potent inhaled anesthetics. Since nitroprusside has no effect on the myocardium or the autonomic nervous system, the cardiac output is usually unchanged or even increased when the blood pressure is lowered. Cyanide toxicity should be suspected in any patient who is resistant (who requires greater than 10 μg/kg/min) or who develops tachyphylaxis or metabolic acidosis. Nitroprusside should be immediately discontinued in such patients and appropriate cyanide antagonists employed if hypotension or metabolic acidosis persists (see Ch. 33). The pharmacology and toxicology of nitroprusside have been well reviewed by Tinker and Michenfelder,[36] Rauscher et al.,[37] and Cohen and Burke.[38]

Fahmy[39] proposed that nitroglycerin may be preferred to nitroprusside as a drug to produce deliberate hypotension. Traditionally, nitroglycerin has been used to decrease peripheral vascular resistance in patients with heart failure after acute myocardial infarction and to decrease hypertension during coronary artery surgery. In a study in which 44 patients received nitroglycerin and 47 received nitroprusside, Fahmy[39] concluded that nitroglycerin was an effective drug to use for deliberate hypotension. He further postulated that nitroglycerin may be superior to nitroprusside because the former drug decreases diastolic blood pressure more than does nitroprusside. Because coronary perfusion is indirectly dependent on arterial diastolic pressure, preservation of adequate myocardial perfusion during hypotension may be more likely with nitroglycerin than with nitroprusside. This hypothesis is attractive but unproven.

PHARMACOLOGY OF CHOLINERGIC AND ANTICHOLINERGIC DRUGS

As described in the section under cholinergic receptors, these drugs can be pharmacologically subdivided into nicotinic and muscarinic drugs. The nicotinic system involves ganglionic and neuromuscular transmission. Ganglionic blockers are discussed in the section on "antihypertensives." Neuromuscular transmission is discussed in Chapter 17. Therefore only muscarinic drugs will be discussed in this section.

MUSCARINIC DRUGS

The classic muscarinic agonist is acetylcholine. The muscarinic effects of acetylcholine are summarized in Figure 18-11. Although acetylcholine is a tremendously important endogenous transmitter, it is not used clinically probably because of its rapid hydrolysis by acetylcholinesterase. Methacholine, carbachol, and bethanechol are less rapidly hydrolyzed and therefore their effects are longer acting. Still, their importance and use is limited.

Of more importance are drugs that inhibit acetylcholinesterase and thereby indirectly cause muscarinic stimulation. From the anesthesiologist's point of view, reversal of neuromuscular blockade is an example in which the anticholinesterase drugs are commonly used. In this situation, the anesthesiologist desires only the nicotinic and not the muscarinic effects of the anticholinesterases. Therefore a muscarinic blocker, such as atropine or glycopyrrolate, is also given. Those anticholinesterase drugs, such as neostigmine, pyridostigmine, and edrophonium, used for antagonism of a nondepolarizing neuromuscular blockade are reversible inhibitors of acetylcholinesterase. Physostigmine is also a reversible inhibitor of acetylcholinesterase, but it is not used to reverse neuromuscular blockade. Physostigmine is used to treat the so-called central anticholinergic syndrome, which is discussed later.

Irreversible inhibitors of acetylcholinesterase include organophosphorous compounds, which form a virtually irreversible combination with cholinesterase. They are used primarily as insecticides and potentially as warfare agents. The only drugs of this group used medically are the eye drops echothiophate and isoflurophate. Those compounds that are used as insecticides are a frequent cause of poisoning among agricultural workers. These insecticides are very potent and are absorbed rapidly through unbroken skin. Because the insecticides cause

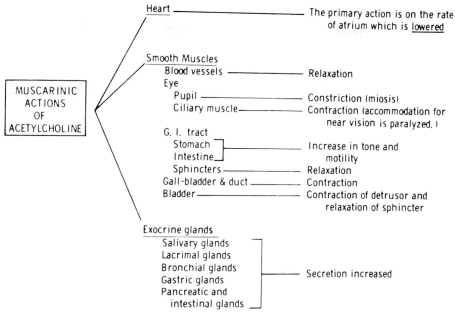

Fig. 18-11 Summary of the muscarinic effects of acetylcholine. (Bhagat BD: Mode of Action of Autonomic Drugs. Graceway Publishers, New York, 1979.)

an accumulation of acetylcholine at all cholinergic sites, the signs and symptoms are those of excess acetylcholine. The muscarinic signs and symptoms are listed in Figure 18-11. Nicotinic manifestations may include muscular fasciculation, cramps, and weakness. It is beyond the scope of this chapter to discuss the treatment of insecticide intoxication in detail, but the drug pralidoxime is a specific antidote. This drug, sometimes referred to as 2-PAM, reverses the effects of acetylcholinesterase inhibitors including skeletal muscle and, to a lesser extent, muscarinic effects.

MUSCARINIC BLOCKING DRUGS

Atropine is the classic muscarinic blocking drug, although scopolamine and glycopyrrolate (Robinul) are also commonly used in anesthesia. Classically, these drugs are viewed

as competitive antagonists of acetylcholine on tissues innervated by postganglionic cholinergic nerves and on smooth muscles that respond to acetylcholine. These sites and effects are summarized in Table 18-1 and Figure 18-11.

This simple view of atropine's effects explain most of the drug's action. However, Flacke and Flacke[40] emphasize that these muscarinic blocking drugs are not pure antagonists. Atropine and scopolamine, in small doses, cause bradycardia, which was originally thought to be a central vagal stimulatory effect. However, because atropine can cause bradycardia, even in the presence of bilateral vagotomy, this finding dictates a conclusion that these drugs must have a peripheral site of action. The only conclusion that can be reached is that atropine must have a weak peripheral agonist effect.

To further complicate the mechanism of action of atropine, Flacke and Flacke[40] have summarized the work of other investigators and concluded that atropine also has an indirect effect resulting from a block of the inhibition or attenuation of the release of the sympathetic transmitter norepinephrine in organs with dual, antagonistic innervation. This effect of atropine on the release of norepinephrine during simultaneous stimulation of sympathetic and vagal nerves may explain the so-called sympathomimetic effect of atropine.

There are marked variations in sensitivity of different effector organs to antimuscarinic drugs, and differences between different drugs in relative potency.[41] For example atropine is a more potent blocker of cardiac vagal effects than scopolamine, whereas scopolamine is more potent as an antisialogogue.

Atropine and scopolamine are nonpolar tertiary amines and therefore easily penetrate lipid membranes, such as the blood-brain barrier. In contrast glycopyrrolate (Robinul) is a polar quaternary amine; and because this limits its passage across the blood-brain barrier, this drug should have fewer central effects.[42] Numerous investigators[43-45] feel that glycopyrrolate is superior to atropine or scopolamine because of increased antisialogogue activity and less tachycardia and central nervous system effects. The reader is referred to the excellent review of Flacke and Flacke[40] and Chapter 3 for a more detailed evaluation of glycopyrrolate.

CENTRAL ANTICHOLINERGIC SYNDROME (ATROPINE PSYCHOSIS)

Atropine and scopolamine, as well as plant extracts containing belladonna alkaloids, can cause the "central anticholinergic syndrome." Symptoms range from sedation and stupor to anxiety, restlessness, hyperactivity, disorientation, and hallucinations. Because there are numerous muscarinic receptors in the brain, muscarinic blockers, which cross the blood-brain barrier, can cause this syndrome.

The central anticholinergic syndrome is not limited to atropine-like drugs, but can be caused by hundreds of drugs[40] that contain central anticholinergic activity. These range from tricyclic antidepressants to antihistamines. Physostigmine, a tertiary acetylcholinesterase inhibitor, is a specific antidote producing almost immediate reversal of the signs and symptoms. Drugs like neostigmine and pyridostigmine are not effective antidotes. This is because they are quaternary actylcholinesterase inhibitors and therefore do not cross the blood-brain barrier.

Lastly, physostigmine has been used to treat central nervous system depression from drugs with no known anticholinergic activity, such as diazepam. Perhaps physostigmine is a nonspecific central nervous system stimulant or analeptic, independent of its anticholinergic action. Flacke and Flacke[40] emphasize that an acetylcholinesterase inhibitor facilitates cholinergic transmission even if no receptor antagonist is present. Therefore, physostigmine may be effective indirectly in treating central nervous system anticholinergic activity.

REFERENCES

1. Bhagat BD: Mode of Action of Autonomic Drugs. Graceway Publishers, Flushing, New York, 1979
2. Mayer SE: Neurohumoral transmission and the autonomic nervous system, The Pharmacological Basis of Therapeutics. 6th edition. Edited by Gilman AG, Goodman LS, Gilman A. New York, MacMillan, 1980
3. Hoffman BB, Lefkowitz RJ: Alpha-adrenergic receptor subtypes. N Engl J Med 302:1390, 1980
4. Lands AM, Arnold A, McAuliff JP, et al: Differentiation of receptor systems activated by sympathomimetic amines. Nature 214:597, 1967
5. Axelrod J, Weinshilboum R: Catecholamines. N Engl J Med 287:237, 1972
6. Galant J, Duriseti L, Underwood S, et al: Decreased beta-adrenergic receptors on poly-

morphonuclear leukocytes after adrenergic therapy. N Engl J Med 299:933, 1978

7. Leier C, Heban P, Huss P, et al: Comparative systemic and regional haemodynamic effects of dopamine and dobutamine in patients with cardiomyopathic heart failure. Circulation 58:466, 1978

8. Hess W, Klein W, Mueller-Busch C, et al: Haemodynamic effects of dopamine and dopamine combined with nitroglycerin in patients subjected to coronary bypass surgery. Br J Anaesth 51:1063, 1979

9. Sonnenblick EH, Frishman WH, LeJemtel TH: Dobutamine: A new synthetic cardioactive sympathetic amine. N Engl J Med 300:17, 1979

10. Henring M, Rubenson A: Evidence that the hypotensive action of α methyl-DOPA is mediated by central actions of methylnoradrenaline, J Pharm Pharmacol 23:407, 1971

11. Heise A, Kroneberg G: Alpha-sympathetic receptor stimulation in the brain and hypotensive action of α-methyl DOPA. Eur J Pharmacol 17:315, 1972

12. Lund-Johansen P: Alpha-methyldopa and beta blockers in hypertension—A comparison of their hemodynamic effects. Clin Exp Pharmacol Physiol (suppl) 4:23, 1978

13. Freed CR, Quintero E, Murphy RC: Hypotension and hypothalamic amine metabolism after long-term α methyldopa infusion. Life Sci 23:313, 1978

14. Carstairs KC, Breckenridge A, Dollery CT, et al: Incidence of positive direct Coombs' test in patients on alpha methyldopa. Lancet 2:133, 1966

15. Rodman JS, Deutch DJ, Gutman SI: Methyldopa hepatitis. Am J Med 60:941, 1976

16. Nies AS, Shand DG: Hypertensive response to propranolol in a patient treated with methyldopa—a proposed mechanism. Clin Pharmacol Ther 14:823, 1973

17. Thornton WE: Dementia induced by methyldopa with haloperidol. N Engl J Med 294:1122, 1976

18. Reid JL, Wing LMH, Mathias CJ, et al: The central hypotensive effect of clonidine—Studies in tetraplegic subjects. Clin Pharmacol Ther 21:375, 1977

19. Pettinger WA: Clonidine, a new antihypertensive drug. N Engl J Med 293:1179, 1975

20. Hunyor SN, Bradstock K, Somerville PJ, et al: Clonidine overdose. Br Med J 4:23, 1975

21. Hansson L, Hunyor JN, Julius S, et al: Blood pressure crises following withdrawal of clonidine, with special reference to arterial and urinary catecholamine levels, and suggestions for acute management. Am Heart J 85:605, 1973

22. Reid JL, Dargie HJ, Davies DS, et al: Clonidine withdrawal in hypertension—Changes in blood pressure and plasma and urinary noradrenaline. Lancet 1:1171, 1977

23. Chang CC, Costa E, Brodie BB: Interaction of guanethidine with adrenergic neurons. J Pharmacol Exp Ther 147:303, 1965

24. Oates JA, Mitchell JR, Feagin OT, et al: Distribution of guanidium antihypertensives—Mechanism of their selective action. Ann NY Acad Sci 179:302, 1971

25. Mitchell JR, Cavanaugh JH, Arias L, et al: Guanethidine and related agents—III. Antagonism by drugs which inhibit the norepinephrine pump in man. J Clin Invest 49:1596, 1970

26. Woosley RA, Walter I, Oates JA, et al: Antagonism of antihypertensive and sympathoplagic effects of guanethidine by ephedrine in man. Clin Res 24:259, 1976

27. Buhler FR, Laragh JH, Baer L, et al: Propranolol inhibition of renin secretion. N Engl J Med 287:1209, 1972

28. Tarazi RC, Dustan HP: Beta adrenergic blockade in hypertension. Am J Cardiol 29:633, 1972

29. Julius S, Esler M: Autonomic nervous cardiovascular regulation in borderline hypertension. Am J Cardiol 36:685, 1975

30. Shand DG: Drug therapy—Propranolol. N Engl J Med 293:280, 1975

31. Cambridge D, Davey MJ, Messingham R: Prazosin, a selective antagonist of post synaptic α adreno receptors. Br J Pharmacol 59:5144, 1977

32. Wood AJ, Bolli P, Simpson FO: Prazosin in normal subjects: Plasma levels, blood pressure and heart rate. Br J Clin Pharmacol 3:199, 1976

33. Bolli P, Wood AJ, Simpson FO: Effects of prazosin in patients with hypertension. Clin Pharmacol Ther 20:138, 1976

34. Gottlieb TB, Katz FH, Chidsey CA: Combined therapy with vasodilator drugs and beta adrenergic blockade—A comparative study of minoxidil and hydralazine. Circulation 45:571, 1972

35. Dormois JC, Young JL, Nies AS: Minoxidil in severe hypertension: Value when conven-

tional drugs have failed. Am Heart J 90:360, 1975

36. Tinker JH, Michenfelder JD: Sodium nitroprusside. Anesthesiology 45:340, 1976

37. Rauscher LA, Jurst JM, Collins GM: Nitroprusside toxicity in a renal transplant patient. Anesthesiology 49:428, 1978

38. Cohen JN, Burke LP: Nitroprusside. Ann Intern Med 91:752, 1979

39. Fahmy NR: Nitroglycerin as a hypotensive drug during general anesthesia. Anesthesiology 49:17, 1978

40. Flacke JW, Flacke W: Cholinergic and anticholinergic drugs, Drug Interactions in Anesthesia. Edited by Smith NT, Miller RD, Corbascio AN. Philadelphia, Lea & Febiger, 1981, pp. 113–128

41. Eger EI II: Atropine, scopolamine and related compounds. Anesthesiology 23:365, 1962

42. Proakis AG, Harris GB: Comparative penetration of glycopyrrolate and atropine across the blood-brain and placental barriers in anesthetized dogs. Anesthesiology 48:339, 1978

43. Ostheimer GW: A comparison of glycopyrrolate and atropine during reversal of nondepolarizing neuromuscular blockade with neostigmine. Anesth Analg 51:468, 1972

44. Oduro KA: Glycopyrrolate methobromide. 2. Comparison with atropine sulfate in anesthesia. Can Anaesth Soc J 22:466, 1975

45. Winnie AP: Anticholinergic agent and anesthesia: Antiarrhythmic or arrhythmogenic? Anesthesiol Rev 6:11, 1979

Section I

Preparation of the Patient/Use of Anesthetic Agents:
   Regional Anesthesia

19

Pharmacology of Local Anesthetic Drugs

John J. Savarese, M.D.
Benjamin G. Covino, Ph.D., M.D.

INTRODUCTION

Local anesthesia may be produced by many tertiary bases and certain alcohols. However, all clinically useful materials are either aminoesters or aminoamides. These materials, when applied in sufficient concentration at the site of action, prevent conduction of electrical impulses by the membranes of nerve and muscle. When local anesthetic agents are given systemically, the functions of cardiac, skeletal, and smooth muscle as well as the transmission of impulses in the peripheral and central nervous systems and within the specialized conducting system of the heart may all be altered. Local anesthetics may provide analgesia of various parts of the body by topical application, by injection in the vicinity of peripheral nerve endings and major nerve trunks, or by instillation within the epidural or subarachnoid spaces. Specific clinical applications of local anesthetics will be considered in other chapters, especially 20 and 21. In this chapter the basic and clinical pharmacology of local anesthetics is presented.

BASIC PHARMACOLOGY

CHEMISTRY

THE LOCAL ANESTHETIC MOLECULE

The typical local anesthetic molecule, exemplified by lidocaine (Fig. 19-1), is a tertiary amine separated at a distance of 6 to 9 angstroms from an unsaturated (aromatic) ring system (usually a benzene ring) by an intermediate chain. The tertiary amine is a base (proton acceptor). The intermediate chain contains either an ester (–CO–) or amide (–CNH–) linkage; local anesthetics may therefore be classified as ester or amide compounds. The amide or ester linkage contributes to anesthetic potency, since its removal results in a decrease in activity. The aromatic ring system gives a lipophilic character to its

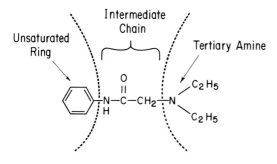

LIDOCAINE

Fig. 19-1 The chemical formula of lidocaine, showing the three essential portions of a local anesthetic molecule.

Table 19-1. Representative Local Anesthetic Agents in Common Clinical Use

Generic* and Common Proprietary Name	Chemical Structure	Approximate Year of Initial Clinical Use	Main Anesthetic Utility	Representative Commercial Preparation	Maximum Dose (mg)
Cocaine	$CH_2-CH-CHCOOCH_3$ / $NCH_3-CHOOC_6H_5$ / $CH_2-CH-CH_2$	1884	Topical	Bulk powder	200
Benzocaine Americaine	H_2N—(ring)—$\overset{O}{C}-OC_2H_5$	1900	Topical Topical	20% ointment 20% aerosol	—
Procaine Novocain	H_2N—(ring)—$COOCH_2CH_2N(C_2H_5)(C_2H_5)$	1905	Infiltration Spinal	10 & 20 mg/ml solutions 100 mg/ml solution	1000
Dibucaine Nupercaine	quinoline, OC_4H_9, $CONHCH_2N(C_2H_5)_2$	1929	Spinal	0.667, 2.5, & 5 mg/ml solutions	100
Tetracaine Pontocaine	$H_9C_4-N(H)$—(ring)—$COOCH_2N(CH_3)(CH_3)$	1930	Spinal Spinal	Niphanoid crystals—20 mg/ml 10 mg/ml solutions	200
Lidocaine Xylocaine	(ring with CH_3, CH_3)$NHCOCH_2N(C_2H_5)(C_2H_5)$	1944	Infiltration Peripheral nerve blocks Epidural Spinal Topical Topical	5 & 10 mg/ml solutions 10, 15, & 20 mg/ml solutions 10, 15, & 20 mg/ml solutions 50 mg/ml solution 2.0% jelly, viscous 2.5%, 5.0% ointment	500

Generic/Trade name	Structure	Year	Route	Concentration	Maximum dose (mg)
Chloroprocaine Nesacaine		1955	Infiltration Peripheral nerve blockade Epidural	10 mg/ml solution 10 & 20 mg/ml solutions 20 & 30 mg/ml solutions	1000
Mepivacaine Carbocaine		1957	Infiltration Peripheral nerve blockade Epidural	10 mg/ml solution 10 & 20 mg/ml solutions 10, 15, & 20 mg/ml solutions	500
Prilocaine Citanest		1960	Infiltration Peripheral nerve blockade Epidural	10 & 20 mg/ml solutions 10, 20, & 30 mg/ml solutions 10, 20, & 30 mg/ml solutions	900
Bupivacaine Marcaine		1963	Infiltration Peripheral nerve blockade Epidural	2.5 mg/ml solutions 2.5 & 5 mg/ml solutions 2.5, 5, & 7.5 mg/ml solutions	200
Etidocaine Duranest		1972	Infiltration Peripheral nerve blockade Epidural	2.5 & 5 mg/ml solutions 5 & 10 mg/ml solutions 5 & 10 mg/ml solutions	300

* USP nomenclature
(Modified from Covino BG, Vassallo HG: Local Anesthetics: Mechanisms of Action and Clinical Use. New York, Grune & Stratton, 1976, by permission.)

Table 19-2. Relative in Vitro Conduction Blocking and Physicochemical Properties of Various Agents

Agent	Relative Conduction Blocking Properties*			Physicochemical Properties		
	Potency	Onset	Duration	pKa	Lipid Solubility	Protein Binding
Low potency						
Procaine	1	1	1	8.9	0.6	5.8
Intermediate Potency						
Mepivacaine	2	1	1.5	7.6	1.0	77
Prilocaine	3	1	1.5	7.7	0.8	55
Chloroprocaine	4	0.8	0.75	8.7	—	—
Lidocaine	4	0.8	1.5	7.7	2.9	64
High Potency						
Tetracaine	16	2	8	8.5	80	76
Bupivacaine	16	0.6	8	8.1	28	95
Etidocaine	16	0.4	8	7.7	141	94

* Data derived from isolated frog sciatic nerve.
(Covino BG, Vasallo HG: Local Anesthetics: Mechanism of Action and Clinical Use. New York, Grune & Stratton, 1976, by permission.)

portion of the molecule, whereas the tertiary amine end is relatively hydrophilic, particularly since it is partially protonated and bears a positive charge in the physiological pH range. Lidocaine, for example, is 65 percent protonated at pH 7.4. The chemical formulae of commonly administered local anesthetic drugs are given in Table 19-1.

STRUCTURE-ACTIVITY RELATIONS AND PHYSICOCHEMICAL PROPERTIES

The intrinsic potency and duration of action of local anesthetics may be modified by certain changes within the molecule.

Lipophilic-Hydrophilic Balance

The lipophilic versus hydrophilic character of the local anesthetic molecule may be affected by altering the size of alkyl substitution in the vicinity of either the tertiary amine or the aromatic ring. Materials of more lipophilic nature are obtained by increasing the size of alkyl substitution. These agents are more potent and longer lasting than their more hydrophilic congeners. For example,

etidocaine, which has three more carbon atoms in the amine end of the molecule, is four times more potent and five times longer lasting than its chemical relative lidocaine when these materials are compared in the isolated frog sciatic nerve. Two other examples of increased potency and duration of action in the more lipophilic members of related pairs of compounds are mepivacaine and bupivacaine and procaine and tetracaine (Table 19-2); in the case of these pairs, a butyl group is added to the aromatic portion (tetracaine) or to the tertiary amine area (bupivacaine) of the molecule (see also Table 19-1).

Hydrogen Ion Concentration

Local anesthetics in solution exist in a chemical equilibrium between the basic uncharged form (B) and the charged cationic form (BH^+). At a certain hydrogen ion concentration (pH) specific for each drug, the concentration of local anesthetic base is equal to the concentration of charged cation. This hydrogen ion concentration is called the pKa. The relationship may be expressed as follows:

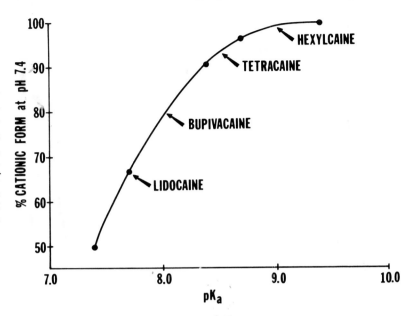

Fig. 19-2 The relationship of pKa to the percentage of local anesthetic cation present at pH 7.4. (Covino BG, Vassallo HG: Local Anesthetics: Mechanisms of Action and Clinical Use. New York, Grune & Stratton, 1976, by permission.)

$$pH = pKa - \log (BH^+ - B)$$

The pKa values for standard local anesthetic agents are listed in Table 19-2.

The pH of the surrounding medium into which the local anesthetic is injected influences drug activity by altering the relative percentage of agent present in the basic or protonated forms. The relationship between pKa and the percentage of local anesthetic present in the cationic form is shown in Fig. 19-2. The reasons for this pH effect on local anesthetic behavior are discussed in the section on mechanism of action.

Protein Binding

A direct correlation exists between local anesthetic potency, lipophilic character, and duration of action versus protein binding (Table 19-2). In general, the potent, long acting, highly lipophilic agents such as tetracaine, etidocaine, and bupivacaine are far more highly protein-bound than their more hydrophilic counterparts (procaine, lidocaine, and mepivacaine).

NERVE STRUCTURE AND FUNCTION

ANATOMY OF THE PERIPHERAL NERVE

Each peripheral nerve axon possesses its own cell membrane, the axolemma, within which is contained the axoplasm. Nonmyelinated nerves, such as autonomic postganglionic fibers, are also encased in a Schwann-cell sheath. Most motor and sensory fibers are also wrapped in several layers of myelin, a lipoid-insulating membrane that separates the axon itself from the Schwann-cell sheath. Myelin greatly increases the speed of nerve conduction by producing saltatory conduction via the nodes of Ranvier, which are periodic interruptions in the myelin sheath. A classification of peripheral nerves according to fiber size and physiological properties is presented in Table 19-3.

A typical peripheral nerve consists of several groups of axons, or fascicles. Each ax̲ has its own connective tissue coverin̲ endoneurium. Each group of axons i̲ by a second connective tissu̲ perineurium. The entire nerv̲

Table 19-3. Classification of Peripheral Nerves According to Fiber Size and Physiological Properties

Fiber Class	Subclass	Myelin	Diameter (μ)	Conduction Velocity (M/sec)	Location	Function
A	α	+	6–22	30–120	Afferent to and efferent from muscles and joints	Motor, proprioception
	β	+	6–22	30–120	Afferent to and efferent from muscles and joints	Motor, proprioception
	γ	+	3–6	15–35	Efferent to muscle spindles	Muscle tone
	δ	+	1–4	5–25	Afferent sensory nerves	Pain, temperature, touch
B		+	< 3	3–15	Preganglionic sympathetic	Various autonomic functions
C	sC	−	0.3–1.3	0.7–1.3	Postganglionic sympathetic	Various autonomic functions
	dγC	−	0.4–1.2	0.1–2.0	Afferent sensory nerves	Pain, temperature, touch

(Bonica JJ: Principles and Practice of Obstetric Analgesia and Anesthesia. Philadelphia, FA Davis, 1967.)

an outer sheath called the epineurium (Fig. 19-3). In order to reach its site of action (the nerve axon), therefore, a local anesthetic molecule must traverse four or five (in the case of a myelinated nerve) connective tissues and/or lipid membranous barriers.

STRUCTURE OF THE AXONAL MEMBRANE

Early proposals by Danielli and Davson[1] and by Robertson[2] have led to the concept that biologic membranes consist of a bimolecular lipid layer, sandwiched between nonlipid proteinaceous monolayers (Fig. 19-4). Probably the most widely accepted current membrane model is that of Singer and Nicholson[3] ("fluid mosaic model"—Fig. 19-5). This model envisions a membrane consisting of a lipid matrix, bimolecular in nature, composed of long-chain fatty acids with polar heads (phosphatidyl choline, phosphatidyl inositol), the long lipid chains being oriented towards the middle of the bilipid layer. The polar heads of these molecules border on two separated aqueous environments: the extracellular fluid space exteriorly and the cell cytoplasm interiorly. Imbedded within the lipid matrix are several types of globular protein structures, some located exteriorly, some on the interior aspect, and some passing through the membrane. As in the case of the lipids, the ore hydrophilic, charge-bearing portions of proteins are considered to be oriented towards the water phase, especially on the extracellular fluid side of the cell membrane. The more hydrophobic areas of these proteins probably interact with the lipids of the membrane in the interior of the bilipid layer.

The general membrane concept of Singer and Nicholson[3] is adaptable to conducting membranes. The membrane proteins may form the framework for "channels" responsible for the transmembrane conductance of sodium and potassium ions necessary to generate the changes in membrane potential responsible for the propagation of nerve impulses. Specific local anesthetic receptors may exist in these channels. The concept is a dynamic one, involving much interaction between membrane lipids and proteins.

PHYSIOLOGY OF NERVE CONDUCTION

The neural membrane is able to maintain a voltage difference of 60 to 90 mV between its inner and outer aspects because it is relatively impermeable to sodium ions. An active, energy-dependent mechanism, the sodium-potassium pump, maintains this potential difference by constant extrusion of sodium from within the cell (Fig. 19-6). Although the membrane is freely permeable to potassium ions, an intracellular to extracellular potassium ratio of 150 mEq to 5 mEq per liter or 30:1, is maintained because of the active exchange of intracellular sodium for extracellular potassium and because of the retentive

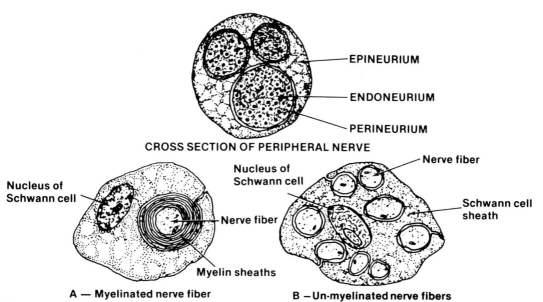

Fig. 19-3 Diagrammatic cross-sections through a peripheral nerve (top) and myelinated and unmyelinated fibers (bottom). Note organization of peripheral nerve into bundles, or fascicles. (Covino BG: Mechanism of action of local anesthetic agents, Topical Reviews in Anesthesia. Vol 1. Edited by Norman J, Whitwam JG. Bristol, Wright, 1980, pp 85–134.)

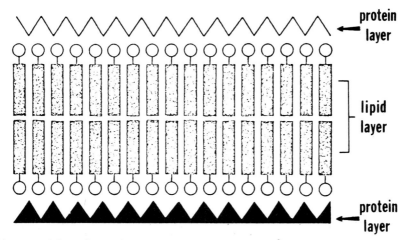

Fig. 19-4 Diagram of the unit membrane suggested by Robertson.[2] Two layers of long-chain fatty acids with polar heads (circles) oriented toward the water phases of extracellular and intracellular fluid and lipid chains (rectangles) oriented toward the center of the membrane were conceptualized as sandwiched between layers of protein. (Covino BG, Vassallo HG: Local Anesthetics: Mechanisms of Action and Clinical Use. New York, Grune & Stratton, 1976 by permission.)

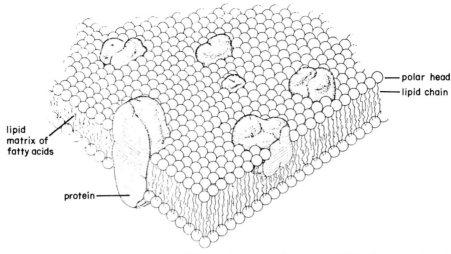

polar head
lipid chain

lipid
matrix of
fatty acids

protein

Fig. 19-5 The Singer-Nicholson model, which envisions a relatively fluid lipid bilayer in which proteinaceous structures are imbedded. Some of the proteins which project all the way through the membrane may constitute the essential portions of ionic channels responsible for transmembrane sodium and potassium conductance. (Singer SJ, Nicolson GL: The fluid mosaic model of the structure of cell membranes. Science 175:720–731, 1972. Copyright 1972 by the American Association for the Advancement of Science.)

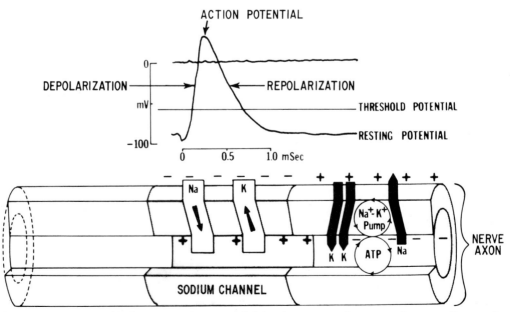

ACTION POTENTIAL

DEPOLARIZATION — REPOLARIZATION

THRESHOLD POTENTIAL

RESTING POTENTIAL

Na   K   Na⁺-K⁺ Pump   ATP

SODIUM CHANNEL

NERVE AXON

Fig. 19-6 The relationship between action potential development and transmembrane sodium and potassium conductance changes in peripheral nerve membrane. An energy-dependent mechanism, the sodium-potassium pump, normally maintains an intracellular to extracellular potassium ratio of 30:1 by constant extrusion of sodium. A voltage differential of approximately −90 mV is thereby maintained between the interior and exterior aspects of the membrane. (Covino BG, Vassallo HG: Local Anesthetics: Mechanisms of Action and Clinical Use. New York, Grune & Stratton, 1976, by permission.)

effect of negatively charged intracellular proteins on intracellular potassium.

The nerve at rest behaves as a potassium electrode according to the Nernst equation:

$$E = \frac{-RT}{nF} \ln \frac{(K^+) i}{(K^+) o}$$

where E = membrane potential; R = gas constant (8.315 joules); T = temperature (celsius); n = ionic valence (1 in the case of potassium); F = Faraday's constant (96,500 coulombs); ln = natural logarithm; and (K^+) = Potassium concentration inside (i) and outside (o) the cell.

For potassium, therefore:

$$E = -58 \log 30, \text{ or } -85.7 \text{ mV}$$

During normal excitation (depolarization) of a nerve, the permeability to sodium increases rapidly, altering the resting membrane potential from approximately -90 mV to -50mV. At this critical threshold potential, a dramatic sudden maximal increase in sodium permeability occurs. The resultant sudden inward rush of sodium ions rapidly reverses membrane potential to the $+30$ to $+40$ mV range. This process takes only 0.1 to 0.2 msec. During the next 0.4 to 0.6 msec, sodium permeability rapidly diminishes and potassium permeability increases markedly, until the resting membrane potential is reestablished. Finally the transmembrane ionic gradients for sodium and potassium are reestablished by the active pumping mechanism. The time course of these conductance changes is shown in Fig. 19-7. The ionic fluxes that occur during depolarization and repolarization are passive phenomena, since each ion is moving down its concentration gradient.[4]

If the critical threshold potential is achieved during local depolarization of a conducting membrane, then propagation of the depolarization will proceed along the entire length of the membrane. The conduction of an impulse is an all-or-none phenomenon in that if the critical threshold is not reached

during a local depolarization, then conduction of the impulse will not occur.[4]

MECHANISM OF ACTION OF LOCAL ANESTHETIC DRUGS (PHARMACODYNAMICS)

Active Form

Local anesthetic bases are poorly soluble in water but are soluble in relatively hydrophobic organic solvents. Therefore, as a matter of convenience, most of these drugs are marketed as the hydrochloride salts, which are soluble in water but insoluble in organic solvents. The pKa of the drug and the tissue pH will determine the amount of drug that exists as free base or as positively charged cation when injected into living tissue.

A lengthy debate has taken place over the issue of which form of the local anesthetic is actually responsible for prevention of impulse propagation. Early observations that alkaline solutions of local anesthetics more effectively blocked nerve conduction[5] led to the belief that the tertiary base is the so-called active form. Subsequently, the investigations of Ritchie, et al.[6,7] showed that in the isolated rabbit vagus nerve containing an intact sheath, the rate of onset of conduction block increased as the bathing medium was made more alkaline. On the other hand, in the desheathed isolated frog sciatic nerve, the onset of block was more rapid under more acidic conditions. These contrasting observations led to the postulation that the uncharged base traverses the lipophilic nerve sheath more easily, but once this passage has occurred, the positively charged cation binds to the axonal membrane to block conduction. These investigators concluded that both forms of local anesthetic must be present for greatest effectiveness. Further evidence that the cation is the active form of local anesthetics was presented by Narahashi, et al.[8-10] who perfused squid giant axons with quaternary derivatives of lidocaine and found that these materials,

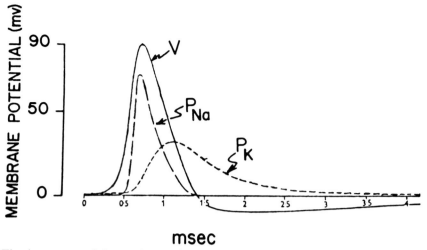

msec

Fig. 19-7 The time course of changes in membrane potential (V) and sodium and postassium permeability (P_NA and P_K) during action potential development in squid axon. (Modified by Strichartz[15] from Hodgkin AL, Huxley AF: A quantitative description of membrane current and its application to conduction and excitation in nerve. J Physiol (Lond) 117:500, 1952.)

which bear a permanent positive charge, are just as effective in preventing the excitation process in nerve as their tertiary amine analogues when they both are placed on the interior aspect of the axonal membrane.

These observations, however, do not explain the moderately high local anesthetic activity of materials such as benzocaine, which exist only in an uncharged form.

THE ELECTROPHYSIOLOGICAL EFFECT OF LOCAL ANESTHETICS

The resting membrane potential of nerve is not affected by various concentrations of local anesthetics.[11] As the concentration of local anesthetic applied to the nerve is increased, a decrease in the rate and degree of depolarization is produced. Inhibition of depolarization increases with time as the concentration of drug is maintained. Since both the rate of repolarization and the conduction velocity are diminished and the refractory period is prolonged, the number of action potentials that a nerve is capable of transmitting per unit of time decreases as the drug concentration increases, until complete block is

achieved when the nerve is unable to depolarize to the threshold potential.[12] The most important of the above mechanisms is reduction of the rate of depolarization during action potential development.

The above electrophysiological effects of local anesthetics are a direct consequence of inhibition of membrane conductance of sodium and potassium ions, especially sodium. Tetrodotoxin, a substance secreted by the Japanese puffer fish, produces conduction blockade in peripheral nerves by completely inhibiting sodium conductance without affecting potassium conductance.[13] On the other hand, tetraethylammonium, which inhibits potassium conductance, does not affect action potential development and nerve conduction.[14]

MEMBRANE SITE OF ACTION OF LOCAL ANESTHETICS

Local Anesthetic Receptors

As mentioned earlier, changes in membrane potential in nerves are most likely due to the transmembrane passage (conductance) of sodium and potassium ions through specialized proteinaceous "channels." Recent evidence suggests that local anesthetics inhibit sodium flux by acting on specific receptors that control gate mechanisms responsible for conductance changes in sodium channels.[11, 15, 16]

The exact site of conduction block by local anesthetics within the sodium channel has been a subject of much investigation. Two receptor sites are recognized, located on the external and internal aspects of the sodium channel.[15, 16]

The external receptor site is blocked by the two biotoxins, tetrodotoxin and saxitoxin.[17] Both of these substances are positively charged.

The internal receptor site, on the other hand, is blocked by clinically useful local anesthetics in their charged forms and also by their quaternary (charged) derivatives when the latter substances are placed on the internal surfaces of nerve axons.[8, 9, 16, 18, 19] In actual clinical practice the uncharged form (tertiary base) is placed in the vicinity of the external surface of the neural membrane and must traverse it to reach the interior aspect of the sodium channel, where it acquires its positive charge and interacts with the internal receptor site.

An alternative receptor theory is that of Hille, in which he postulates a single local anesthetic receptor located on the inner aspect of the sodium channel.[16] This structure may interact with neutral or charged local anesthetics. The pathway of arrival of anesthetic at this receptor site, however, is considered to differ depending on the type of anesthetic in question. Hille theorizes that the sodium channel may exist in any of three states (resting, open, or inactivated), which may undergo transition from one form to another (Fig. 19-8). Following nerve stimulation, the closed channels open to allow passage of sodium ions. The charged quaternary forms of local anesthetics as well as the positively charged biotoxins, being hydrophilic, must use this pathway to reach the internal receptor site, since they are unable to traverse the lipid portions of the membrane. Neutral relatively lipophilic drugs such as benzocaine do not require the presence of open sodium channels but may reach the internal receptor by penetration of the lipid portions of the membrane. Clinically used local anesthetics such as lidocaine may reach the internal receptor by either pathway: via membrane lipid as the uncharged base or via open sodium channels as the charged protonated form. To quote Hille, "To the old question of inside vs outside action, the answer is within the membrane, and to the old question of cation vs free base the answer is both, but with different pathways and hence with different phenomenology."[16] Hille's single receptor theory assumes that the charged biotoxins, saxitoxin and tetrodotoxin, must reach this receptor via the external opening of the sodium channel, since they do not block conduction when placed on the internal aspect of axonal membranes. Hille's concept is consistent with the observation that neutral local anesthetics such as benzocaine do not show stimulus frequency-dependent blocking characteristics whereas clinically used agents, which may exist in the charged form, do show such behavior. The reason, according to Hille, would be that the higher the frequency of stimulation, the greater the number of open gates might exist in sodium channels per unit of time and, therefore, the greater the opportunity for charged local anesthetic molecules to traverse open sodium channels to reach internal receptor sites.

The Surface Charge Theory

This hypothesis proposes that the lipophilic portion of the local anesthetic molecule binds to nonspecific ubiquitous sites within axonal membrane lipids, leaving the protonated positively charged amine terminal of the molecule on the external surface of the membrane.[20]

An accumulation of sufficient positive charges would tend to neutralize the relative electronegativity of the external membrane

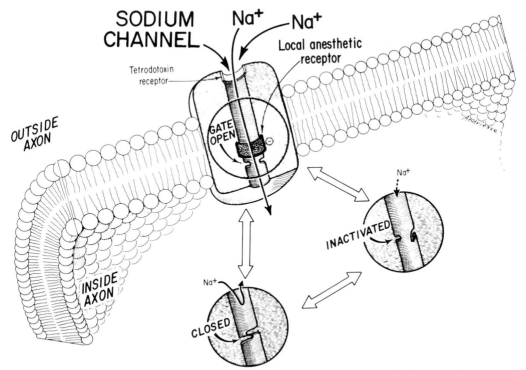

Fig. 19-8 The sodium channel in nerve depicted according to the Singer-Nicholson membrane model.[3] The channel probably traverses a protein structure which spans the entire thickness of the axonal membrane. According to Hille,[16] a gating mechanism located on the internal aspect of the sodium channel controls the inward transit of sodium ions. In the resting axon the gate is closed and does not allow passage of sodium ions. During action potential development, the gate opens to allow the inward rush of sodium responsible for initial axonal depolarization. The gating mechanism may be inactivated by local anesthetics which bind to specific receptors in the sodium channel. According to Hille,[16] a single receptor on the inner aspect of the channel binds all types of local anesthetics, though the route of arrival of the various types of local anesthetic molecules to the receptor may differ. A second receptor may exist to which the biotoxins tetrodotoxin and saxitoxin may bind. This receptor is probably located at the external opening of the sodium channel.

surface, resulting in an increase in the transmembrane potential, without altering the intracellular resting potential.[21] A sufficient increase in the transmembrane potential would inhibit the ability of an electrotonic current from a nearby unanesthetized portion of nerve membrane to depolarize the treated area to its threshold for firing. Conduction blockade would then result.

The surface charge theory requires that the charged form of local anesthetics be the active form. This has been demonstrated by Ritchie et al.,[6] Narahashi et al.,[8–10] and Strichartz.[19] It explains the apparent antagonism

between calcium and local anesthetics and the positive correlation of local anesthetic potency with lipid solubility but does not account for the activity of neutral drugs, such as benzocaine, that do not exist in a charged form.[12]

The Membrane Expansion Theory

This theory proposes that the interaction of relatively hydrophobic local anesthetic molecules with membrane lipids causes a conformational change in the organization of membrane lipids, resulting in membrane expansion. This is essentially an extension of the Meyer-Overton theory for general anesthetics, and assumes an intramembrane site of action for local anesthetics. Expansion of conducting membranes should theoretically reduce the size of sodium channels, thereby preventing sodium conductance changes and inhibiting depolarization. Reversal of the local anesthetic action of uncharged local anesthetic molecules by high ambient pressures ("pressure reversal") has been demonstrated by some investigators to occur, as in the case of general anesthetics. Charged local anesthetics, however, such as tetrodotoxin and QX572, the quaternary derivative of lidocaine, are resistant to pressure reversal.[22] "Pressure reversal" of the actions of uncharged local anesthetics is still open to question, since other investigators have been unable to demonstrate it.[23]

The membrane expansion concept is readily applicable to the action of neutral substances such as benzocaine but does not explain the local anesthetic activity of charged molecules.

Cm: Minimum Anesthetic Concentration

The minimum concentration of local anesthetic necessary to block impulse conduction along a given nerve fiber within a reasonable standard period of time is termed the Cm, or minimum anesthetic concentration. Concentrations lower than the Cm will not inhibit conduction at all. The study of a series of local anesthetics under standard conditions of nerve fiber size and timing generates a series of Cm values that reflect the relative potencies of the various drugs. In addition, variation of the experimental conditions for a single anesthetic, such as changes in electrolyte concentrations and acid-base status, may affect the Cm. Information obtained in such studies is often clinically pertinent. The Cm is, therefore, a standard of local anesthetic

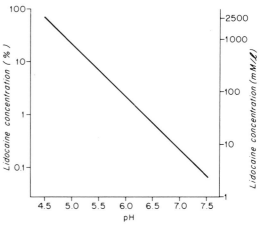

Fig. 19-9 The minimum concentration of lidocaine necessary to block nerve conduction (Cm) expressed as a function of ambient pH. Note that a 100 times greater concentration of lidocaine is necessary to block conduction at pH 5.0 than at pH 7.0. See text for further details. (Modified from deJong RH: Physiology and Pharmacology of Local Anesthesia. 1970. Courtesy of Charles C Thomas, Publisher, Springfield, Illinois.)

potency, analogous to the minimum alveolar concentration (MAC) for inhaled anesthetics.[24] A variety of factors may affect Cm. Some of these are:

Fiber Size. Larger nerve fibers require higher concentrations of local anesthetic for inhibition of impulse conduction. Their Cm values will be relatively high.

pH. The Cm of a given anesthetic is less at a high pH than at a low pH. Thus, in a sheathed nerve the Cm for lidocaine is 100 times less at a pH of 7.0 than at a pH of 5.0 (Fig. 19-9).

Calcium Concentration. Local anesthetic potency correlates directly with inhibition of calcium binding by phospholipids. The local anesthetic effect of most drugs is inversely proportional to the calcium concentration of the test medium.

Nerve Stimulation Rate. Individual anesthetic potency in vitro is directly proportional to the rate of nerve stimulation, a greater apparent potency being noted at high stimulation rates.

Classification of Local Anesthetics According to Site of Action

Takman[25] has classified local anesthetics according to their various proposed sites and mechanisms of action as follows:

Class A. Substances acting only at specific receptors on the external surface of the sodium channel (e.g., the charged biotoxins tetrodotoxin and saxitoxin).

Class B. Substances acting mainly at receptors on the internal (axoplasmic) side of the sodium channel (e.g., quaternary derivatives of lidocaine).

Class C. Substances acting nonspecifically within the lipids of nerve membrane to cause membrane expansion (benzocaine, n-butanol, and other neutral uncharged substances).

Class D. Agents acting both at the axoplasmic (internal) end of the sodium channel on specific receptors and within membrane lipids by physicochemical mechanisms, i.e., membrane expansion. Most clinically used local anesthetics fit into this class, since they exist both as the uncharged tertiary base and charged protonated form. The cationic form would, therefore, be expected to act specifically on internal receptors, while the uncharged base should interact with membrane lipids to cause expansion).

Summary: Mechanism of Action of Local Anesthetics

The sequence whereby clinically used local anesthetics produce inhibition of axonal conduction has been summarized by Covino[12] as follows:

1. Clinically used local anesthetics exist in solution as both charged and uncharged forms, the relative proportions depending on the pH of the solution, the pH at the site of injection, and the pKa of each drug.

2. The charged lipophilic tertiary base form diffuses more readily across neural sheaths and the axonal membrane to reach the inter-nal aspect of the sodium channel. The base is protonated within the axoplasm and binds as the charged cation to a specific receptor within the internal opening of the sodium channel, thereby inhibiting sodium conductance. This loss of membrane permeability to sodium prevents cell membrane depolarization and the propagation of action potentials.

3. The clinically used local anesthetics act primarily upon specific receptors located at the internal opening of sodium channels. Other possible sites of action include nonspecific absorption within cell membrane lipids, resulting in "membrane expansion" and sodium channel narrowing, and diffusion of the uncharged base via hydrophobic pathways through membrane lipids to reach the specific receptor site where protonation and binding occur within the internal opening of the sodium channel.

4. The biotoxins saxitoxin and tetrodotoxin interact with a different specific receptor located on the external aspect of the sodium channel. Alternatively, according to Hille,[16] they may reach a single common receptor site located on the internal aspect of the internal sodium channel gate by traversing the channel via the external opening.

5. An older mechanism, the surface charge theory,[20] is still favored by some investigators. This mechanism assumes penetration of the axonal membrane by the lipophilic portion of local anesthetic molecules and neutralization of axolemmal surface negative charges by the positively charged terminal amino group of the molecule. This mechanism obviates the necessity for a specific local anesthetic receptor.

CLINICAL PHARMACOLOGY

CHOICE OF LOCAL ANESTHETIC

A list of local anesthetic agents available for clinical use together with the type of regional anesthetic for which each drug is commonly administered, is given in Table 19-1.

The choice of local anesthetic drug involves an assessment of the following general factors: the operative site and the nature and duration of the surgical procedure; the type of regional anesthesia to be performed; the patient's size and shape and general state of health, including any significant metabolic disorders or major ongoing organ system impairment; and the intrinsic durations of action of the drugs themselves.

Only general considerations are treated in this section. Further details may be obtained by consulting the chapters on spinal and epidural anesthesia (Ch. 21) and nerve blocks (Ch. 20).

OPERATIVE SITE AND DURATION OF OPERATION

One of the primary factors governing the choice of drug and the type of regional anesthesia to be administered is the nature and duration of the procedure. In anticipating the duration of surgery, one must consider the procedure itself and the experience and ability of the surgeon. Before administering any regional anesthetic, it is useful to have a realistic estimate of the surgeon's anticipated operative time. The local anesthetic administered should provide at least a 50 to 100 percent longer duration of analgesia than this estimate to account for surgical preparation time and for any unanticipated difficulty during the case and possibly to provide a brief period of analgesia in the recovery room. Of course, these problems can be minimized by the use of a continuous technique.

TYPE OF REGIONAL ANESTHESIA

The duration of action of a single local anesthetic varies with the site of injection. Table 19-4 compares the durations of action of lidocaine and bupivacaine at various sites. In

general, the duration is shortest with each agent where central neural block (spinal anesthesia) is performed, and longest when major peripheral nerves are blocked, e.g., brachial plexus block. Kinetic factors underlying these differences are discussed in the next section.

PATIENT SIZE AND METABOLIC-PHYSIOLOGICAL STATUS

Patient size indirectly affects local anesthetic choice, since not all local anesthetics are available for all types of regional anesthesia (e.g., spinal anesthesia—see Table 19-1). The patient's own anatomy is a major governing factor regarding such dilemmas as spinal versus epidural anesthesia or brachial plexus block via the supraclavicular, interscalene, or axillary routes. In a markedly obese subject, for example, spinal anesthesia with tetracaine might be considered more convenient and more likely to succeed than epidural anesthesia with bupivacaine or etidocaine. Similarly, in a bull-necked individual, brachial plexus block via the axillary route might prove more technically facile than via the interscalene or supraclavicular routes because the landmarks might be easier to define. Patient disease factors may markedly affect the disposition of local anesthetics by the body. Their clinical durations of action may be prolonged especially by liver disease in the case of the amide-type local anesthetics and by atypical pseudocholinesterase or deficiency in the typical form of that enzyme in the case of the ester-type drugs.

DURATION OF ACTION OF THE DRUG

Each local anesthetic has been noted to provide analgesia over a range of time. Table 19-4 contrasts the durations of action of lidocaine, an intermediate-duration agent, and bupivacaine, a long-acting drug. Procaine and chloroprocaine are generally classified as

Table 19-4. Onset and Duration of Action of Lidocaine and Bupivacaine Following Various Forms of Regional Anesthesia*

Anesthetic Procedure	Lidocaine			Bupivacaine		
	Solution	Sensory Onset (Min)	Sensory Duration (Min)	Solution	Sensory Onset (Min)	Sensory Duration (Min)
Infiltration						
a. Extravascular	1% w/epi 1:200,000	—	416.2 ± 25.8	0.25% w/epi 1:200,000	—	428.6 ± 39.9
b. Intravenous Regional	0.5%	—	111.0 ± 26.6	0.25%	—	344.0 ± 27.7
Peripheral Nerve Blockade						
a. Ulnar Nerve Block	1% w/epi 1:200,000	3.00 ± 0.5	178.0 ± 17	0.25% w/epi 1:200,000	16.00 ± 4.7	395.0 ± 22
b. Brachial Plexus Block	1% w/epi 1:200,000	14.04 ± 3.83	195.0 ± 26.3	0.25% w/epi 1:200,000	23.26 ± 7.93	613.0 ± 126
Central Neural Blockade						
a. Epidural	2% w/epi 1:200,000	5.07 ± 0.58	156.6 ± 15	0.5% w/epi 1:200,000	6.27 ± 1.19	228.6 ± 23
b. Subarachnoid	5%	4.30 ± 1.5	94.0 ± 28	1%	30–90 sec	128.0 ± 19

(Covino BG, Vassallo HG: Local Anesthetics: Mechanisms of Action and Clinical Use. New York, Grune & Stratton, 1976, by permission.)
* All values ± standard error.
Epi = epinephrine.

short-acting local anesthetics; lidocaine, mepivacaine, and prilocaine are considered to have intermediate durations of action; and tetracaine, bupivacaine, and etidocaine are long-acting drugs.

The duration of local anesthetic effect may be lengthened by increased dosage (either by increasing the volume or concentration of drug)[26] or by addition of a vasoconstricting substance, e.g., epinephrine or phenylephrine. The vasoconstrictor decreases the rate of venous removal of drug from the site of injection, thereby prolonging the block. The effect is most notable during spinal anesthesia and peripheral nerve block, where the sites of injection are relatively avascular. The duration of block by drugs such as bupivacaine and etidocaine, which are highly lipid-soluble and relatively potent vasodilators, is least affected by epinephrine, particularly when injection is performed into a relatively adipose but well-perfused area such as the epidural space.[27]

The onset of local anesthetic block is accelerated by the use of carbonated solutions of local anesthetics.[28,29] The improved local anesthetic effect probably is due to greater availability of free base.

DEVELOPMENT OF TACHYPHYLAXIS

The development of decreased local anesthetic effect following repetitive dosage during continuous regional anesthetic techniques is termed tachyphylaxis. The process has been carefully studied during epidural anesthesia by Bromage et al.[30] and Cohen et al.[31]

The mechanism for the development of tachyphylaxis appears to involve local pH changes occurring in the immediate vicinity of the nerves. Local anesthetic solutions, which are commonly marketed as the hydrochloride salts, are mildly acidic (pH 4 to 6). On injection into tissue, the salts are buffered to physiological pH, thereby providing sufficient quantities of the base for diffusion through axonal membranes. Repeated injections consume locally available buffering capacity such that a buildup of the charged form develops, leaving inadequate concen-

Table 19-5. Various Preparations Intended for Topical Anesthesia

Anesthetic Ingredient	Concentration (%)	Pharmaceutical Application Form	Intended Area of Use
Benzocaine	1–5	Cream	Skin and mucous membrane
	20	Ointment	Skin and mucous membrane
	20	Aerosol	Skin and mucous membrane
Cocaine	4	Solution	Ear, nose, throat
Dibucaine	0.25–1	Cream	Skin
	0.25–1	Ointment	Skin
	0.25–1	Aerosol	Skin
	0.25	Solution	Ear
	2.5	Suppositories	Rectum
Cyclonine	0.5–1	Solution	Skin, oropharynx, tracheobronchial tree, urethra, rectum
Lidocaine	2–4	Solution	Oropharynx, tracheobronchial tree, nose
	2	Jelly	Urethra
	2.5–4	Ointment	Skin, mucous membrane, rectum
	2	Viscous	Oropharynx
	10	Suppositories	Rectum
	10	Aerosol	Gingival mucosa
Tetracaine	0.5–1	Ointment	Skin, rectum, mucous membrane
	0.5–1	Cream	Skin, rectum, mucous membrane
	0.25–1	Solution	Nose, tracheobronchial tree

(Covino BG, Vassallo HG: Local Anesthetics: Mechanisms of Action and Clinical Use. New York, Grune & Stratton, 1976, by permission.)

trations of base available for axonal diffusion. The clinical result is apparent tolerance to the anesthetic effect, most noticeable in areas of the body with limited buffer reserve, such as cerebrospinal fluid (continuous spinal anesthesia).[31] The probability of occurrence of tachyphylaxis with local anesthetics is directly proportional to the pKa. Drugs such as mepivacaine having pKa values closest to 7.4 (Table 19-2) are most likely to show tachyphylaxis.

TOPICAL ANESTHESIA

Some of the local anesthetics are effective when applied topically in sufficient concentration. Table 19-5 summarizes commonly available topical anesthetic preparations and their clinical applications. Topical use of local anesthetics is generally safe; however, since high concentrations of drugs are employed and are readily absorbed via mucous

membranes, the toxic properties of local anesthetics may become manifest, especially when excessively large volumes of topical preparations are spread over broad areas of mucous membrane. The work of Adriani and Campbell[32] illustrates this rather well (Fig. 19-10).

KINETICS OF NERVE BLOCK

In major peripheral nerve trunks, axonal bundles, or fasciculi, that are situated close to the surface of the nerve trunk are called mantle bundles. Those located in the interior are termed core bundles. In the extremities, proximal sensory distribution is supplied by the mantle bundles, whereas peripheral innervation arises from core bundles. During performance of major nerve blocks in the extremities, analgesia first develops proximally and then spreads distally (Fig. 19-11). This clinical observation is consistent with the

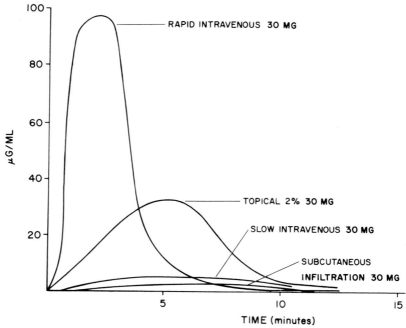

Fig. 19-10 Comparative speed of uptake and peak serum level attained when 30 mg lidocaine is administered by various routes. (Modified from Adriani J, Campbell B: Fatalities following topical application of local anesthetics to mucous membranes. JAMA 162:1527, 1956. Copyright 1956, American Medical Association.)

above described anatomic location of the nerve supplies to the various parts of the extremity. The local anesthetic must diffuse across greater distances and through more membranous barriers to reach core bundles.[24,33]

During major peripheral nerve block, e.g., brachial plexus block, it has been observed that motor blockade frequently develops prior to sensory block because, as described by Winnie et al.,[33] the distribution of motor fibers in core bundles is peripheral to the distribution of sensory axons. The local anesthetic reaches the motor fibers of core bundles first, thus explaining the observation that 1 percent solutions of lidocaine, mepivacaine, and prilocaine often produce motor block in advance of anesthesia of the fingers.[33] These solutions contain sufficient concentrations of local anesthetic to easily produce conduction block in the larger motor A fibers (see Table

19-3). Winnie et al.[33] also noted that during the use of a local anesthetic solution such as 0.25 percent bupivacaine, which contains barely enough local anesthetic concentration to produce any motor block at all, sensory block does precede motor block.

The clinical kinetics of nerve block described above differ from classical neurophysiological studies; in the latter, the speed of onset of conduction block is always inversely proportional to fiber size, the smaller sensory and autonomic fibers being blocked first, followed by larger motor and proprioceptive axons.[34] This difference is explained by the fact that these neurophysiological studies were performed on single nerve fibers, where diffusion distance and fiber location do not come into play. In contrast, during clinical block of major nerve trunks in situ, fiber location and tissue barriers are important factors.[33]

HYPERSENSITIVITY

Ester derivatives of para-aminobenzoic acid, such as procaine and tetracaine, have been responsible for most reports of hypersensitivity to local anesthetics, while true allergy to the amide-type drugs is undoubtedly extremely rare.[35] Patients subjected to skin testing for possible allergy to local anesthetics responded only to the ester-type compounds, whereas no skin reaction at all was noted after intracutaneously administered amide local anesthetics.[36] Forty-two percent of 60 nonallergic individuals skin tested by Aldrete and Johnson[36] developed a wheal and flare from subcutaneously administered ester-type compounds, whereas 72 percent (8 or 11) subjects who had previous histories of "allergic" reactions to local anesthetics showed such a positive response to the esters but not to the amides.

It is generally assumed on the basis of the Aldrete and Johnson study[36] that individuals suspected of allergy who undergo skin testing and show negative reactions to local anesthetics may safely receive drugs that produce no response. There is undoubtedly a high percentage of false positive results in this type of screening procedure.

True hypersensitive responses to local anesthetics, when they do occur, may manifest themselves as generalized erythema, edema, respiratory wheezing and/or dyspnea, hypotension, tachycardia, headache, or loss of consciousness (all symptoms of histamine release and all occurring within only a few minutes of local anesthetic administration). Treatment is supportive and therapeutic: maintenance of the airway with administration of oxygen by assisted or controlled ventilation; circulatory support by proper positioning, fluids, and possibly vasopressors; and administration of antihistamines and corticosteroids to control the physiological effects of systemic histamine release.

While hypersensitivity reactions to local anesthetics are rare, toxic responses to absolute or relative local anesthetic overdosage, to

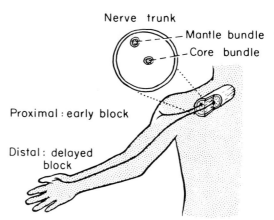

Fig. 19-11 The relative locations of mantle and core bundles in a nerve trunk. Proximal areas of the extremity are innervated by mantle bundles, while distal areas are served by core bundles. Within each bundle, motor fibers are distributed exterior to sensory fibers. Thus, sensory block proceeds from proximal to distal regions, and motor block may become apparent before distal sensory block.[33] See text for further details. (Modified from deJong RH: Physiology and Pharmacology of Local Anesthesia. 1970. Courtesy of Charles C Thomas, Publisher, Springfield, Illinois.)

inadvertent intravascular injection, or to very rapidly absorbed ordinary doses, are undoubtedly much more common and are in fact an important consideration during the performance of every regional anesthetic technique. This is particularly true when relatively large drug dosage is necessary to provide the desired type of anesthesia and when an injection is made into a highly vascular area where rapid absorption may occur, such as during caudal or paracervical[37] anesthesia.

SYSTEMIC EFFECTS OF LOCAL ANESTHETICS (LOCAL ANESTHETIC TOXICITY)

Local anesthetics, when given directly intravenously in large doses or when rapidly absorbed from peripheral sites, may achieve

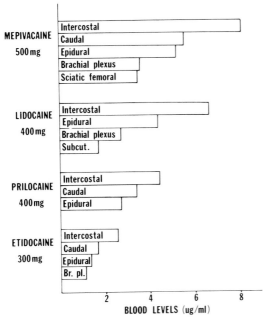

Fig. 19-12 Peak serum levels of local anesthetics attained during the performance of various types of regional anesthetic procedures. (Covino BG, Vassallo HG: Local Anesthetics: Mechanisms of Action and Clinical Use. New York, Grune & Stratton, 1976, by permission.)

high enough blood concentrations to affect the physiology of several organ systems, principally the heart and peripheral circulation and the central nervous system. These systemic effects may be considered therapeutic in some cases (e.g., the intravenous administration of lidocaine for control of ventricular extrasystoles) or as side effects or toxic effects in other cases, depending on the severity of patient response. A continuum of effect probably exists dependent on the serum concentration, with mild side effects occurring at lower serum concentrations and becoming more striking as serum levels increase. Threshold dosages producing early symptoms and signs of CNS toxicity in man are listed in Table 19-6. These dosages may be considered as maximum recommended

quantities, particularly during intercostal, caudal, or paracervical block (vascular areas). Approximate serum levels resulting during the use of various local anesthetics for several types of regional anesthesia are shown in Fig. 19-12.

CENTRAL NERVOUS SYSTEM

Increasing the local anesthetic dosage, resulting in rising serum levels, produces a consistent pattern of CNS symptomatology in man due to easy passage of local anesthetics from the bloodstream into the brain. At recommended clinical dosage for regional anesthesia, serum levels usually remain well below recognized toxic concentrations unless rapid absorption occurs due to inadvertent intravascular injection or due to injection into a highly vascular locale. Early symptoms and signs of toxicity include tinnitus, light-headedness, visual and auditory disturbances, restlessness, garrulousness, slurred speech, nystagmus, shivering, and muscular tremors. The EEG pattern during early toxicity is not diagnostic.[4,24]

Progression of dosage and serum level beyond these early stages of toxicity results in the development of EEG seizure activity with tonic-clonic convulsions followed by CNS depression. The convulsive stage may not be manifest, with toxicity initially becoming apparent as CNS depression, particularly during the administration of lidocaine and procaine.[38]

Mechanism of CNS Toxicity of Local Anesthetics

The general pattern of local anesthetic effect on all excitable membranes is depression of conduction due to inhibition of sodium conductance. Toxic levels of local anesthetics probably initially lead to depression of cortical inhibitory pathways,[39,40] thereby allowing unopposed activity of an excitatory nature. This transitional stage of unbalanced excitatory and inhibitory activity is followed by generalized CNS depression if higher serum levels are reached.[41]

CARDIOVASCULAR SYSTEM

The cardiovascular effects of local anesthetics occur either indirectly because of inhibition of autonomic pathways during regional anesthesia, e.g., during high spinal or epidural anesthesia, or because of a direct depressant action on cardiac or vascular smooth muscle or on the myocardial conducting system. The blockade of sympathetic efferent fibers that occurs during central neural blockade is really a therapeutic effect and is not considered further in this section.

The mechanism of direct cardiovascular depression by local anesthetics again involves effects on ionic conductance in myocardial and smooth muscular conducting membranes and in the myocardial conducting system.

During phase 4 diastolic depolarization of myocardial cells, a gradual decrease of potassium permeability normally occurs. This effect, particularly in ventricular muscle, is diminished or abolished by antiarrhythmic doses of lidocaine and results in a prolongation or abolition of phase 4.[42] Higher doses of lidocaine result in a slowing of phase 0 depolarization (the rapid spike phase). This effect is presumably due to inhibition of sodium conductance, as during conduction blockade in peripheral nerves.

The normal electrocardiogram is little affected by ordinary antiarrhythmic doses of lidocaine. Toxic doses, however, slow conduction in the heart, the ECG manifestation being an increased PR interval and QRS duration and sinus bradycardia, all of which reflect a decrease in automaticity.[4] Other local anesthetics have been shown to possess antiarrhythmic effects but have not been as extensively studied as lidocaine.

INTRA-ARTERIAL INJECTION OF LOCAL ANESTHETICS

A most interesting explanation for the occasional occurrence of syncope and/or apparent local anesthetic toxicity after relatively small doses of local anesthetics may be inadvertent intra-arterial injection under high pressure with consequent brief reverse arterial blood flow resulting in the direct delivery of high concentrations of drug to the brain or heart or both.[44,45] Aldrete et al.[44] have shown that injection of as little as 3 mg/kg lidocaine into the lingual artery in baboons resulted in internal carotid arterial lidocaine concentrations of 30 μg/ml, a level far above that previously reported by Munson et al.[46] to be the threshold for convulsive activity in monkeys. Injections into the brachial artery of 7 mg/kg lidocaine in the Aldrete study produced lidocaine concentrations greater than 100 μg/ml in the internal carotid artery, showing that moderate intra-arterial doses of local anesthetics, when injected under pressure even at considerable distance from cerebral vessels, may easily produce toxic responses. Clearly not only the anatomic site of injection but also the speed of and force behind the injection must be considered as factors influencing local anesthetic toxicity. Certainly the maximum safe dosage of local anesthetic varies according to the conditions under which the anesthetic is administered.

INHIBITION OF CATECHOLAMINE UPTAKE BY COCAINE

The reuptake of epinephrine and norepinephrine by adrenergic nerve endings is a principal mechanism of their bioinactivation. Cocaine markedly inhibits this process,[47] thereby potentiating responses to exogenous or endogenously released catecholamines. The result may be marked pressor responses and/or ventricular arrhythmias. Probably the most likely cause of death under general anesthesia in patients who have received cocaine (e.g., for topical anesthesia of the airway) is ventricular fibrillation. Certainly topical anesthesia with cocaine should not be used in arrhythmia-prone patients, in subjects in whom halothane or cyclopropane anesthesia is planned (because these general anesthetics increase myocardial sensitization to catecholamine-induced arrhythmias), or in patients receiving infusions of catecholamines for circulatory support.

METHEMOGLOBINEMIA

The administration of large doses (greater than 10 mg/kg) of prilocaine during regional anesthetic procedures may lead to the accumulation of a metabolite (o-toluidine), which is an oxidizing agent capable of converting hemoglobin (Hb^{++}) to methemoglobin (Hb^{+++}). When sufficient methemoglobinemia is present (3 to 5 g/100 ml) the subject may appear cyanotic and the blood may acquire a brownish discoloration. Such levels of methemoglobinemia are safe in healthy individuals but any such slight impairment of oxygen transport in subjects with cardiac or pulmonary disease or in infants (whose erythrocytes are relatively deficient in methemoglobin reductase) may warrant immediate treatment.

Reducing agents such as methylene blue (1 to 5 mg/kg) or, less satisfactorily, ascorbic acid (2 mg/kg) may be given intravenously to rapidly convert methemoglobin to hemoglobin.[48]

LOCAL TISSUE TOXICITY

Neither local anesthetics themselves nor commonly included antibacterial preservatives such as methylparaben have been shown to produce any neurotoxic effect when administered at recommended clinical concentrations. An inadvertent injection of relatively large volumes of 2 or 3 percent chloroprocaine into the subarachnoid space during the intended performance of epidural block has recently been reported to result in sensory and motor deficits persisting for several weeks (after the initial total spinal anesthesia had subsided).[49-51] The reported sequelae were most probably due to the low pH (3.12 to 3.16) of these solutions of 2-chloroprocaine hydrochloride, rather than to any effect of the drug itself. The poor buffering capacity of CSF may also have contributed to the above complication, since this factor must have prolonged the exposure of the fibers within the subarachnoid space to this rather acidic medium.[51]

TREATMENT OF TOXIC RESPONSE TO LOCAL ANESTHETICS

Supportive therapy (airway management, circulatory maintenance) of systemic toxic responses to local anesthetic overdosage is similar to measures outlined in the section on hypersensitivity. In addition, if marked CNS excitation or frank convulsive manifestations are present, they may be terminated with small intravenous doses of a short-acting barbiturate, e.g., thiopental 1 to 2 mg/kg, or muscular manifestations may be treated with a short-acting neuromuscular blocking agent, e.g., succinylcholine 0.5 to 1.0 mg/kg, particularly if airway management is jeopardized by repeated convulsions. In the latter case, intubation of the trachea under succinylcholine-induced paralysis will not only facilitate airway management but also prevent pulmonary aspiration of gastric secretions in the presence of continued CNS depression.

Avoidance of local anesthetic toxicity by limiting dosage to the smallest amounts necessary for performance of any regional anesthetic procedure is really the first step in management of local anesthetic toxicity. Premedication with a benzodiazepine, such as diazepam 0.1 to 0.2 mg/kg, probably

Table 19-6. Threshold for Production of CNS Toxicity by Local Anesthetics in Man and Monkey

Agent	Threshold Dose (mg/kg) Producing CNS Symptoms in Man	Approximate Serum Level (μg/ml) Producing Convulsive Activity in the Monkey
Procaine	19.2	—
Chloroprocaine	22.8	—
Lidocaine	6.4	18–26
Mepivacaine	9.8	22
Prilocaine	>6.0	20
Bupivacaine	1.6	4.5–5.5
Etidocaine	3.4	4.3
Tetracaine	2.5	—

(Adapted from Covino BG, Vassallo HG: Local Anesthetics: Mechanisms of Action and Clinical Use. New York, Grune & Stratton, 1976, by permission.)

Code used: — = not known.

provides significant prophylaxis against the CNS toxic effects of local anesthetics and is a second important step.[52, 53]

PHARMACOKINETICS

The absorption, distribution, and excretion of local anesthetics may be considered from two points of view. First, under the most common clinical conditions, the drugs are injected into an area that is relatively sequestered from the circulation (a depot site) for the production of regional anesthesia. Second, the drugs, particularly lidocaine, may be given directly intravenously for control of ventricular arrhythmias, as cough suppressants or as adjuncts to general anesthesia. Under either condition of clinical administration, the general pattern of distribution, metabolism, and elimination (distribution kinetics) of local anesthetics is similar, although the actual rates of handling of various drugs by the body are different and are markedly influenced by the chemical and physicochemical properties of the drugs. Rates of absorption into the central compartment (absorption kinetics) during the two methods of administration are obviously different: uptake from depot sites during regional anesthesia is relatively slow and dependent upon the degree of perfusion of each site, with peak serum levels being reached within 15 to 30 minutes.[54] On the other hand, peak levels are reached immediately after intravenous injection.

ABSORPTION KINETICS FROM DEPOT SITES

Systemic absorption of local anesthetic from the site of a regional anesthetic is modified by the following factors: dosage; site of injection, particularly with respect to local perfusion and drug-tissue binding; addition of vasoconstricting substances; physicochemical properties of the drugs; and pharmacologic properties of the drugs.[4, 54] Peak serum levels of various local anesthetics resulting after dosage usually employed for brachial plexus or peridural anesthesia are given in Table 19-7 and may be compared with minimum dosages noted to cause threshold CNS symptoms in man (Table 19-6). It is evident from Tables 19-6 and 19-7 that the relatively large doses of local anesthetic given for regional anesthesia in man produce serum levels that may approach concentrations resulting in convulsant activity in monkeys and by inference in man as well. Figure 19-13 illustrates the continuum of local anesthetic blood levels associated with therapeutic and toxic effects in man.

Table 19-7. Usual Peak Serum Levels of Local Anesthetics in Man after Peridural Anesthesia or Brachial Plexus Block

Drug	Dose (mg)	Serum Concentration (μg/ml)
Lidocaine	400–600	2–7
Prilocaine	400–600	2–5
Mepivacaine	400–600	2–6
Bupivacaine	150–400	1.5–2.5
Etidocaine	150–300	1.0–2.5

(Tucker GT, Mather LE: Clinical pharmacokinetics of local anesthetics. Clin Pharmacokinet 4:241, 1979.)

Dosage

Peak local anesthetic blood levels are directly related to dosage, regardless of the injection site or the volume of solution employed.[4, 12]

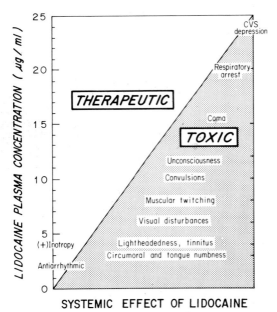

SYSTEMIC EFFECT OF LIDOCAINE

Fig. 19-13 The continuum of therapeutic and toxic effects of systemically-absorbed local anesthetics (lidocaine is used as an example). As serum levels increase, desirable antiarrhythmic properties yield to more serious undesirable actions upon the central nervous and circulatory systems. (Modified from Mather LE, Cousins MJ: Local anesthetics and their current clinical use. Drugs 18:185, 1979.)

Site of Injection

Irrespective of the local anesthetic agent employed, regional anesthetics performed at various anatomic sites produce peak blood levels of drug that as a rule vary directly with the local vascularity of the site. Systemic absorption of local anesthetic, as reflected in maximum blood level of drug, generally occurs in the following decreasing order according to the site of injection for regional anesthesia: intercostal > caudal > epidural > brachial plexus > sciatic-femoral block (Fig. 19-12).

Vasoconstrictor Substances

Vasoconstrictors such as epinephrine reduce systemic absorption of local anesthetics from depot sites by decreasing regional perfusion in these areas. This is true especially for intermediate- and short-duration drugs such as procaine, lidocaine, and mepivacaine, with the exception of prilocaine. Neuronal uptake (binding) of drug is presumably enhanced by this mechanism, and the potential systemic toxic effects of the drugs are reduced, since blood levels are lowered by approximately 33 percent. The combination of reduced systemic absorption and enhanced uptake by nerve is responsible for extension of the local anesthetic effect by roughly 50 percent.[4, 54, 55]

Vasoconstrictors are less effective in prolonging the anesthetic properties of the more lipid-soluble long-acting drugs bupivacaine and etidocaine, possibly because these materials are highly tissue bound in the first place (because of their lipid solubility) and because their relatively potent vasodilating properties may counteract the epinephrine effect.[4]

Physicochemical Properties

The net systemic absorption of the highly lipophilic agents bupivacaine and etidocaine is comparatively less than the net uptake of

Table 19-8. Disposition Kinetics of Amide Local Anesthetics

Pharmacokinetic Parameter	Lidocaine	Mepivacaine	Bupivacaine	Etidocaine
Vd_{ss} (L)	91 ± 15	84 ± 35	73 ± 26	133 ± 75
$t\frac{1}{2}\ \alpha_1$ (h)	0.16 ± 0.003	0.012 ± 0.007	0.045 ± 0.03	0.036 ± 0.01
$t\frac{1}{2}\ \alpha_2$ (h)	0.16 ± 0.03	0.12 ± 0.04	0.48 ± 0.19	0.31 ± 0.09
$t\frac{1}{2}\ \beta$ (h)	1.6 ± 0.3	1.9 ± 0.8	2.7 ± 1.3	2.7 ± 1.1
Cl (L/min)	0.95 ± 0.21	0.78 ± 0.25	0.58 ± 0.23	1.11 ± 0.34

Abbreviations used: Vd_{ss} = volume of distribution (steady state); $t\frac{1}{2}\ \alpha_1$ = rapid distribution half-life; $t\frac{1}{2}\ \alpha_2$ = intermediate distribution half-life; $t\frac{1}{2}\ \beta$ = elimination half-life; Cl = clearance values.

(Adapted from Tucker GT, Mather LE: Clinical pharmacokinetics of local anesthetics. Clin Pharmacokinet 4:241, 1979.)

lidocaine or mepivacaine, probably because of greater tissue binding at the site of injection.[4, 54] Since a relatively smaller fraction of the more lipid-soluble agents is taken up into the central compartment, the safety margin for avoidance of toxicity is greater for the long-acting drugs.[54] This factor is especially important in obstetrics, where local anesthetic-induced fetal depression is directly related to the maternal blood level.[48]

Pharmacologic Properties

The lipid soluble materials etidocaine and bupivacaine have a more pronounced vasodilator property than lidocaine and mepivacaine. The prominence of this effect in bupivacaine and etidocaine minimizes vasoconstrictor-modulated increased duration of nerve block in the case of these drugs and tends to oppose the effect of tissue binding in limiting blood levels achieved.[4]

DISTRIBUTION KINETICS

Kinetic studies after intravenous slow-bolus infusions of amide-type local anesthetics into human volunteers have been carried out by Tucker and Mather.[54] Serial plasma levels obtained over 3 to 6 hours yielded curves best expressed mathematically as triexponential functions corresponding with an assumed three-compartment distribution model in man.

Pharmacokinetic data (Table 19-8) indicate that the amide local anesthetics are widely distributed after intravenous bolus administration, with a suggestion of sequestration in certain storage sites, possibly fatty areas (steady-state volumes of distribution are greater than total body water volumes). An initial rapid distribution phase ($t_{1/2}\ \alpha_1$) probably indicates uptake into highly perfused organs (brain, liver, kidney, heart) with a slower distribution phase ($t_{1/2}\ \alpha_2$) corresponding with uptake by intermediately-perfused tissues (muscle, gut). Clearance values (Cl) and elimination half-lives ($t_{1/2}\ \beta$) for amide local anesthetics probably represent mainly hepatic metabolism, since renal excretion of unchanged drug accounts for less than 5 percent of dosage.[54]

Pharmacokinetic studies of ester-type agents are not available, principally because plasma half-lives in vitro are extremely short (less than 1 minute for procaine and 2-chloroprocaine) due to rapid hydrolysis by plasma cholinesterase.[56]

METABOLISM AND EXCRETION

The detoxification and elimination of local anesthetics follows the general pattern of drug metabolism: that is, the drugs are converted either in the liver or the plasma to

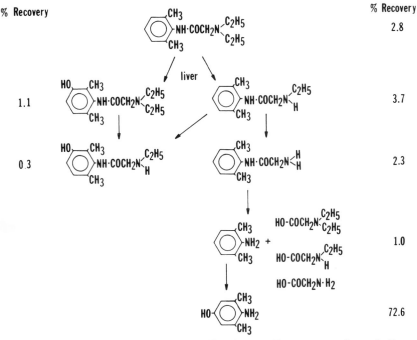

% Recovery

2.8

1.1

liver

3.7

0.3

2.3

1.0

72.6

Fig. 19-14 Suggested pathways of lidocaine metabolism in man. Percentages of metabolites recovered in urine are given at left and right. The major pathway involves N-dealkylation, hydrolysis of the amide linkage, and ring hydroxylation. See text for details. (Covino BG, Vassallo HG: Local Anesthetics: Mechanisms of Action and Clinical Use. New York, Grune & Stratton, 1976, by permission.)

more water-soluble metabolites for excretion in the urine. Since local anesthetic bases (the uncharged form) are relatively insoluble in water, little or no urinary excretion (less than 5 percent of an injected dose) of this form occurs.[54] Acidification of urine, however, will promote ionization of the tertiary base to the more water-soluble quaternary form, which is more readily excreted and not so easily reabsorbed by the renal tubules. Eriksson[57] for example has shown that urinary excretion of prilocaine may be increased to as much as 20 percent of an injected dose by urinary acidification.

Amide Agents

The amide linkage is hydrolyzed by liver microsomal enzymes. This initial step converts the amide base to an -amino carboxylic acid and a cyclic aniline derivative. Complete metabolism usually involves several further steps such as ring hydroxylation (of the aniline moiety) and N-dealkylation (of the aminocarboxylic acid). The suggested pathway for lidocaine in man is shown in Fig. 19-14. There is considerable variation in the rate of liver metabolism of individual amide compounds, the approximate order being prilocaine > etidocaine > lidocaine > mepivacaine > bupivacaine.[4]

The metabolism of amide local anesthetic drugs is clinically relevant in two areas: first, prilocaine metabolism results in the production of o-toluidine (the aniline derivative), which can oxidize hemoglobin to the ferric form possibly resulting in clinically significant methemoglobinemia (see local anesthetic toxicity). Second, decreased metabolism of amide local anesthetics in patients with liver disease may lead to relatively higher plasma levels of these materials, thereby increasing the possibility of systemic toxic manifestations.[58,59]

Ester Agents

The ester local anesthetics are hydrolyzed at varying rates by plasma cholinesterase into relatively water-soluble amino alcohols and carboxyloic acids. The breakdown products are pharmacologically inactive, although the para-aminobenzoic acid moieties of procaine, tetracaine, and chloroprocaine have been implicated as antigens in true hypersensitivity reactions. Rates of hydrolysis in the following order have been reported by Foldes et al.:[56] 2-chloroprocaine > procaine > tetracaine. Individuals who are homozygotic for the atypical form of plasma cholinesterase will metabolize ester local anesthetics much more slowly than normal individuals and are consequently at greater risk for toxic responses to this class of compounds, since higher serum levels are more easily achieved.[60]

REFERENCES

1. Danielli JF, Davson HA: A contribution to the theory of permeability of thin fibers. J Cell Comp Physiol 9:89, 1936
2. Robertson JD: The ultrastructure of cell membranes and their derivatives. Biochem Soc Symp 16:3, 1959
3. Singer SJ, Nicholson GL: The fluid mosaic model of the structure of cell membranes. Science 175:720, 1972
4. Covino BG, Vassallo HG: Local Anesthetics: Mechanisms of Action and Clinical Use. New York, Grune & Stratton, 1976
5. Shanes AM: Electrochemical aspects of physiological and pharmacological action in excitable cells. II. The action potential and excitation. Pharmacol Rev 10:165, 1958
6. Ritchie JM, Ritchie B, Greengard P: The active structure of local anesthetics. J Pharmacol Exp Ther 150:152, 1965
7. Ritchie JM, Ritchie B, Greengard P: The effect of the nerve sheath on the action of local anesthetics. J Pharmacol Exp Ther 150:160, 1965
8. Narahashi T, Frazier DT, Yamada M: The site of action and active form of local anesthetics. I. Theory and pH experiments with tertiary compounds. J Pharmacol Exp Ther 171:32, 1970
9. Frazier DT, Narahashi T, Yamada M: The site of action and active form of local anesthetics. II. Experiments with quaternary compounds. J Pharmacol Exp Ther 171:45, 1970
10. Narahashi T, Yamada M, Frazier DT: Cationic forms of local anesthetics block action potentials from inside the nerve membrane. Nature 223:748, 1969
11. Shanes AM, Freygang WH, Grundfest H, et al: Anesthetic and calcium action in the voltage-clamped squid giant axon. J Gen Physiol 42:793, 1959
12. Covino BG: Mechanism of action of local anesthetic agents. Topical Rev Anesth 1:85, 1980
13. Hille B: The common mode of action of three agents that decrease the transient change in sodium permeability in nerves. Nature (London) 210:1220, 1966
14. Hille B: The selective inhibition of delayed potassium currents in nerve by tetraethylammonium ion. J Gen Physiol 50:1287, 1967
15. Strichartz G: Molecular mechanisms of nerve block by local anesthetics. Anesthesiology 45:421, 1976
16. Hille B: Local Anesthetics: Hydrophilic and hydrophobic pathways for the drug-receptor reaction. J Gen Physiol 69:497, 1977
17. Narahashi T, Anderson NC, Moore JW: Comparison of tetrodotoxin and procaine in internally perfused squid giant axons. J Gen Physiol 50:1413, 1967
18. Hille B: The pH-dependent rate of action of local anesthetics on the node of Ranvier. J Gen Physiol 69:475, 1977
19. Strichartz GR: The inhibition of sodium currents in myelinated nerve by quaternary derivatives of lidocaine. J Gen Physiol 62:37, 1973
20. Skou JC: Local anaesthetics. VI. Relation between blocking potency and penetration of a monomolecular layer of lipoids from nerves. Acta Pharmacol Toxicol 10:325, 1954
21. Singer MA: Interaction of local anesthetics and salicylate with phospholipid membrane. Can J Physiol Pharmacol 51:785, 1973
22. Kendig JJ, Cohen EN: Pressure antagonism to

nerve conduction block by anesthetic agents. Anesthesiology 47:6, 1977

23. Roth SA, Smith RA, Paton WDM: Pressure antagonism of anesthesia-induced conduction failure in frog peripheral nerve. Br J Anaesth 48:621, 1976

24. deJong RH: Physiology and Pharmacology of Local Anesthesia. Springfield, Illinois, Charles C Thomas, 1970

25. Takman BH: The chemistry of local anesthetic agents: Classification of blocking agents. Br J Anaesth (suppl) 47:183, 1975

26. Crawford OB: Comparative evaluation in peridural anesthesia of lidocaine, mepivacaine and L-67, a new local anesthetic agent. Anesthesiology 25:321, 1964

27. Blair MR: Cardiovascular pharmacology of local anaesthetics. Br J Anaesth (suppl) 47:247, 1975

28. Bromage PR: A comparison of the hydrochloride and carbon dioxide salts of lidocaine and prilocaine in local anaesthesia. Acta Anaesthesiol Scand (suppl) 16:55, 1965

29. Bromage PR, Burfoot MF, Crowell DE, et al: Quality of epidural blockade. III. Carbonated local anaesthetic solutions. Br J Anaesth 39:197, 1967

30. Bromage PR, Pettigrew RT, Crowell DE: Tachyphylaxis in epidural analgesia: I. Augmentation and decay of local anesthesia. J Clin Pharmacol 9:30, 1969

31. Cohen EN, Levine DA, Colliss JE, et al: The role of pH in the development of tachyphylaxis to local anesthetic agents. Anesthesiology 29:994, 1968

32. Adriani J, Campbell B: Fatalities following topical application of local anesthetics to mucous membranes. JAMA 162:1527, 1956

33. Winnie AP, LaValley DA, DeSosa B, et al: Clinical pharmacokinetics of local anesthetics. Can Anaesth Soc J 24:252, 1977

34. Gasser HS, Erlanger J: The role of fiber size in the establishment of a nerve block by pressure or cocaine. Am J Physiol 88:58, 1929

35. Aldrete JA, Johnson DA: Allergy to local anesthetics. JAMA 207:356, 1969

36. Aldrete JA, Johnson DA: Evaluation of intracutaneous testing for investigation of allergy to local anesthetic agents. Anesth Analg 49:173, 1970

37. Gordon HR: Fetal bradycardia after paracervical block: Correlation with fetal and maternal blood levels of local anesthetic (mepivacaine). N Engl J Med 279:910, 1968

38. Usubiaga JE, Wikinski J, Ferrero R, et al: Local anesthetic-induced convulsions in man—an electroencephalographic study. Anesth Analg 45:611, 1966

39. deJong RH, Robbes R, Corbin RW: Central actions of lidocaine upon synaptic transmission. Anesthesiology 30:19, 1969

40. Warnick JE, Kee RD, Yim GKW: The effects of lidocaine on inhibition in the cerebral cortex. Anesthesiology 34:327, 1971

41. Wagman IH, deJong RH, Prince DA: Effects of lidocaine on the central nervous system. Anesthesiology 28:155, 1967

42. Kabela E: The effects of lidocaine on potassium efflux from various tissues of dog heart. J Pharmacol Exp Ther 184:611, 1973

43. Dunbar RW, Boettner RB, Gatz RN, et al: The effects of mepivacaine, bupivacaine, and lidocaine on digitalis-induced ventricular arrhythmias. Anesth Analg 49:761, 1970

44. Aldrete JA, Romo-Salas F, Arora S, et al: Reverse arterial blood flow as a pathway for central nervous system toxic responses following injection of local anesthetics. Anesth Analg 57:428, 1978

45. Covino BG: Systemic toxicity of local anesthetic agents (editorial). Anesth Analg 57:387, 1978

46. Munson ES, Tucker WK, Ausinsch B, et al: Etidocaine, bupivacaine and lidocaine seizure thresholds in monkeys. Anesthesiology 42:471, 1975

47. MacMillan WH: Hypothesis concerning the effect of cocaine on the action of sympathomimetic amines. Br J Pharmacol 14:385, 1978

48. Ralston DH, Shnider SM: The fetal and neonatal effects of regional anesthesia in obstetrics. Anesthesiology 48:38, 1978

49. Ravindran R, Bond VR, Tasch MD, et al: Prolonged neural blockade following regional analgesia with 2-chloroprocaine. Anesth Analg 59:447, 1980

50. Reisner LS, Hochman BN, Plumer MH: Persistent neurologic deficit and adhesive arachnoiditis following intrathecal 2-chloroprocaine injection. Anesth Analg 59:452, 1980

51. Covino BG, Marx GF, Finster M, et al: Prolonged sensory/motor deficits following inadvertent spinal anesthesia (editorial). Anesth Analg 59:399, 1980

52. Munson ES, Wagman IH: Diazepam treatment of local anesthetic-induced seizures. Anesthesiology 37:523, 1972

53. deJong RH, Heavner JE: Diazepam prevents local anesthetic seizures. Anesthesiology 34:523, 1971

54. Tucker GT, Mather LE: Clinical pharmacokinetics of local anesthetics. Clin Pharmacokinet 4:241, 1979

55. Mather LE, Cousins MJ: Local anesthetics and their current clinical use. Drugs 18:185, 1979

56. Foldes FF, Davidson GM, Duncalf D, et al: The intravenous toxicity of local anesthetic agents in man. Clin Pharm Ther 6:328, 1965

57. Eriksson F: Prilocaine: An experimental study in man of a new local anesthetic with special regards to efficacy, toxicity, and excretion. Acta Chir Scand (suppl) 358:1, 1966

58. Selden R, Sasahara AA: Central nervous system toxicity induced by lidocaine. Report of a case in a patient with liver disease: JAMA 202:908, 1967

59. Aldrete JA, Homatas J, Boyes RN, et al: Effects of hepatectomy on the disappearance rate of lidocaine from blood in man and dog. Anesth Analg 49:687, 1970

60. Foldes FF, Foldes VM, Smith JC, et al: The relation between plasma cholinesterase and prolonged apnea. Anesthesiology 24:208, 1963

20

Nerve Blocks

Terence M. Murphy, M.B., Ch.B.

INTRODUCTION

Regional anesthesia can provide almost ideal conditions for surgery and postoperative pain relief. Optimal surgical conditions including relaxation of skeletal musculature are provided with lack of reflex response. Regional anesthesia usually is stable to the cardiovascular and respiratory systems, and often enables surgical maneuvers without compromising the protection of the airway in an individual with a full stomach.

There are, however, disadvantages to the technique. The most significant, perhaps, being its incidence of failure. For unlike general anesthesia, which can permit successful completion of the surgery virtually 100 percent of the time, regional anesthesia is associated with an incidence of failure that varies depending upon the skill and expertise of the anesthesiologist. Also, the needles that are used to produce the block can traumatize the target nerves and also other important structures, such as pleura and blood vessels, causing pneumothorax, intravascular injections with possible toxic overdoses of local anesthetic, and/or bleeding and hematoma.

Success with regional anesthesia depends on placing the needle near the target nerve and keeping it there during injection of local anesthetic. This requires intimate knowledge of the surface landmarks and overall anatomy of the area. This anatomic knowledge

will facilitate positioning of the needle and also enable avoidance of important structures. Knowledge of peripheral neural anatomy will permit interpretation of the defects in a partially failed block and enable such to be "rescued" by supplemental nerve block analgesia.

In addition to anatomic expertise in positioning the needle, it is important to appreciate the pharmacology of the agents used along with their pharmacokinetics (see Ch. 19).[1]

The successful practice of regional anesthesia also depends significantly on the anesthesiologist having a good rapport with the patient and the ability to psychologically manage a patient during what is often a stressful period (i.e., immediately preoperatively). With the judicious use of analgesic supplements, such as infiltration of local anesthetic agents and administration of oral and injectable analgesics and/or sedative hypnotics, the skilled anesthesiologist can ensure that the administration of regional analgesia is not an unpleasant experience for the patient.

A frequent criticism of regional anesthesia is the extra time it takes to do it compared with that of induction of general anesthesia. This can be a legitimate complaint, although if the patient's welfare is improved by taking extra time such delays are justified. However, to optimally utilize regional anesthesia in a clinical setting, appropriate space and staff should be used to enable the patients to be prepared ahead of time. It is unsatisfactory to attempt to perform detailed and prolonged nerve block procedures in a hurried fashion with an impatient surgical audience. The establishment of nerve block ahead of the required hour is ideal and this involves judicious use of induction rooms and support personnel.

CLINICAL MANAGEMENT

For optimal use of regional anesthesia for surgery, appropriate patient selection and preparation is critical. Trying to coerce a reluctant patient (or surgeon or both) to consider regional anesthesia, not only raises ethical questions but usually ends in an unsatisfactory situation for all concerned, not the least of whom is the anesthesiologist.

Patients who have had previous unpleasant experiences with regional anesthesia are probably the most difficult to prepare for further regional anesthesia. For that reason, it is vitally important that if regional anesthesia is inadequate or insufficient, patients be adequately covered with other forms of analgesia, either intravenous narcotics or inhaled agents, such that they do not have unpleasant recollections of the event; unpleasant memories may jeopardize their acceptance of regional anesthesia on a later occasion when it may be the anesthetic of choice.

PREOPERATIVE VISIT

Patients should be put at ease with regard to regional anesthesia early in the preoperative visit. It is the rare patient who wishes to, or should, be kept wide awake during the operative procedure. The vast majority of patients, particularly for elective surgery, are more comfortable and better served if the regional anesthetic procedure is accompanied by a light sleep or certainly amnesic tranquilization. Therefore the patient should be reassured during the opening conversation at the preoperative visit with such phrases as "before you go to sleep, we suggest . . . ," following which the clinician should then go on to describe the induction of regional anesthesia. The reassurance that they will be asleep and oblivious of the surgical environment is usually sufficient to obtain the cooperation of most patients. The vast majority of patients are not so much concerned with the induction of the regional anesthetic as the prospect of being wide awake during operations. This latter prospect precipitates fear, apprehension, and often refusal of regional anesthesia.

In addition to a standard preoperative evaluation, an examination of the landmarks needed for the particular regional technique is necessary; this is to confirm that there are no cutaneous infections or other impediments, such as old operative scars and osseous fusions, which could mitigate against the performance of the anesthetic. A full explanation of the preoperative sequence including premedication, transport to the operating room, positioning for block, and intravenous and other needle placement, will help reassure the patient at this stage; particularly, reassurance of the use of local anesthetic infiltration of superficial and deep tissues will help to allay the patient's concerns about the needle insertion. If a stimulating needle is to be used, the patient can at this stage be advised about the possibility of muscle contractions during the block. Also confirmation of a normal clotting mechanism should be attained. If abnormal, this would obviously bias against the use of regional anesthesia, certainly around the neuraxis or major blood vessels.

PREOPERATIVE PREPARATION IN OPERATING SUITE

The induction of regional anesthesia should take place ideally in an induction area separate from the noise and clatter of the operating room. Induction rooms can be as grand as facilities permit or may be a spare operating room or a corner of the recovery area. Ideally, they should provide enough space for appropriate positioning of the patient and ready access to facilities needed for inducing positive pressure respiration and rapid endotracheal intubation. The need for resuscitation and intubation may arise during the induction sequence because of the development of unexpected collapse due to drug overdose, total spinal anesthesia, allergic reactions, etc.

Upon greeting the patient, the clinician can evaluate the efficacy of the preoperative medication. If this medication is found wanting, supplemental analgesics and/or sedative hypnotics can be administered through an intravenous catheter placed in a site that will not interfere with the planned surgery. Drugs such as diazepam 2 to 5 mg/70 kg are often very useful for allaying apprehension at this stage. Some patients seem to need an inordinate amount of diazepam to become sedated and tranquil in this stressful situation. In such patients, a small dose of 25 to 50 mg of sodium thiopental is often all that is needed to reinforce the effect of small doses of diazepam. If cooperation of the patient is required for positioning, or reporting of paresthesias, or both, during the regional anesthetic procedure, then it is important not to excessively premedicate the patient, because he will be unable to cooperate. However, if a regional procedure (e.g., intercostal block) does not require cooperation, then the anesthesiologist can be more generous with sedation. Adequate monitoring of airway and cardiovascular functions are as essential during regional anesthesia as during other phases of anesthesiology during which the patient's protective reflexes may be compromised by excessive sedation. Do not underestimate the power of the spoken word in reassuring patients. Many anesthesiologists use hypnosis both knowingly and unknowingly in reassuring and acquiring the cooperation of patients during this stressful preoperative period. Appropriate preparation at the preoperative visit the evening before helps the clinician to induce a hypnotic trance during the preoperative pe-

riod and thus preclude the use of pharmacologic sedation.

Because there is a significant failure rate in regional anesthesia, even in experienced hands, it is always important to advise the patient that an additional local anesthetic injection may be necessary, even when it appears that the procedure has been completed with the first attempt. It is detrimental to the patient/physician relationship to assure the patient that the block is "all completed" and then some time later have to inform the patient that the block has not worked and a repeat attempt is needed. Therefore, such phrases as "I have injected an appropriate dose of anesthetic for your size and weight. It is sometimes necessary to inject more but we will wait and see if the first injection is adequate" or some personal variation of this theme is appropriate.

Since regional anesthesia is unfortunately but practically often induced in a situation where the operating team is waiting and ready to begin, it is sometimes necessary for the anesthesiologist to commit himself to starting the operation when the block appears to be effective even if he is not 100 percent certain of this. On such occasions, it is vitally important to have all the equipment ready for a rapid induction of an alternative, i.e., general anesthesia if this should be necessary.

If the block does not take effect, it is an entirely unsatisfactory situation for all concerned to have the surgical incision commence when the patient has intact sensation. Because of the concept of differential block,[2] many patients will have analgesia but will still have intact proprioception at the time of skin incision. This may be alarming to them. Depending on the patient, an explanation may be all that is required or a small bolus of rapidly acting intravenous anesthetic, such as thiopental 25 to 75 mg, may be appropriate to sufficiently depress consciousness so that the proprioceptive stimuli from the scalpal blade does not produce patient anxiety and/or withdrawal responses. This small bolus of thiopental can be a very useful prerequisite to skin incisions in regional anesthesia. In the event that the block is inadequate, the anesthesiologist will be able to detect this by such reflex responses as tachycardia or hypertension or even by facial grimaces (screwing up of eyes) or frank movement of the head and/or limbs. With an appropriate bolus of drug, the patient will probably not have recall of this unpleasant event. The skilled anesthesiologist will be able to expeditiously induce general anesthesia with a rapid injection of a larger dose of thiopental or similar drug and then proceed to alternative anesthetic strategies, such as inhaled agents, narcotics, and even muscle relaxants. Therefore, prior to skin incision, always confirm the availability of a functioning anesthesia machine and that the induction drugs and endotracheal intubation equipment are *immediately* at hand. Of course, much of this equipment should already be available when performing the regional block in case a toxic reaction occurs in response to the local anesthetic (see Ch. 19).

The experienced anesthesiologist can "rescue" a failed block to the extent that the failure of the block and the subsequent rescue do not interfere with the surgery. A successful rescue prevents the patient and surgeon from forming adverse opinions about the disadvantages of regional anesthesia and does not prejudice them against using this technique on a subsequent occasion when the regional anesthetic may be essential for the patient's welfare. If general anesthesia is contraindicated and the regional anesthetic effect is essential, then it is vitally important to ascertain that the block is, in fact, effective prior to attempting the commencement of surgery.

INTRAOPERATIVE MANAGEMENT

It is tempting with a satisfactory regional anesthetic to assume that the patient may need less attentive monitoring than with a general anesthetic. This is not true. In the patient who is awake, continual attention will be necessary to assure his comforts with regard to the position of unblocked parts of his body. In the patient who is asleep, vigilance will be necessary to prevent reflex or spontaneous uncooperative movements of the patient that could interfere with the progress of surgery. The vast majority of patients are better off sedated and at least amnesic if not actually sleeping during this procedure, and there are many effective ways of producing this sedation during regional anesthesia.

If an adequate premedication has been administered, this will often ensure patient sleep and comfort during the procedure. However, supplemental sedatives and/or narcotics may be needed from time to time. Diazepam is appropriate as are some of the longer acting barbiturates (e.g., pentobarbital) for longer cases. Thiopental is often abused when sedating these patients. Thiopental has a very brief action and can be a potent depressant of respiratory and cardiovascular reflexes. Therefore it must be used judiciously and certainly not in large amounts to cover up inadequate regional anesthesia.

There are several different and satisfactory ways of assuring patient sedation, sleep, or both during regional anesthesia. Continuous intravenous drip administration of short-acting barbiturates, such as methohexital (Brevital), can provide sedation and suppress reflex responses to painful regional anesthetic induction, such as intercostal blocks and epidural insertion of needles. This is also a possible option for continued sedation during surgery. The supplementation of 50 to 75 percent nitrous oxide in oxygen is another ideal analgesic and sedative technique. This is stable with regard to cardiovascular and respiratory variables and readily reversible at the end of the procedure.

POSTOPERATIVE PATIENT MANAGEMENT

Regional anesthesia may have its major benefits in the postoperative recovery period. Here analgesia continues and depending on whether a continuous technique has been used, reinjections can continue this analgesia well into the postoperative phase.

Patients should remain in the recovery room until stable cardiovascular and respiratory variables have been monitored for at least one hour. This is particularly so if such techniques as high epidural or spinal blocks have been used, but is perhaps less necessary if a peripheral nerve block was utlized. In the latter case, the patient can often return to the ward provided protection for the anesthetized part is insured with splints, dressings, paddings, and instructions to the patient and the nursing staff.

Physicians and nurses familiar with recovery rooms are readily appreciative of the postoperative tranquility and comfort of the patient with a satisfactory regional block as opposed to the often stormy early postoperative situation of patients recovering from general anesthesia.

PREMEDICATION

Patient personalities will run the whole gamut from the phlegmatic individual whose stoical and cooperative acceptance are extensive to the somatically sensitive patients who must be rendered virtually anesthetic prior to the introduction of skin wheals. Usually preparation for regional anesthetic blocks that demand or require patient feedback with regard to paresthesias and other problems precludes premedication that is too heavy. For most patients, a narcotic or a sedative hypnotic or both suffice. Morphine 10 to 15 mg/70 kg or diazepam 10 mg/70 kg is usually sufficient. If the patient is unduly apprehensive upon arrival in the operating suite, additional diazepam can be titrated intravenously. Diazepam also is a very useful premedicant for those blocks in which large doses of local anesthetic agents are infiltrated, because by raising the convulsive threshold to these drugs it provides protection against toxicity from an overdose of these agents.[3]

The combination of the synthetic narcotic fentanyl and the buterophenone droperidol

(Innovar) 1 to 2 ml has proved popular with many regional anesthesiologists. This produces a very tranquil and cooperative patient who can often give rational feedback with regard to paresthesias but does not experience the emotional reactions and reflexes.

For those procedures that do not require patient cooperation to report paresthesias, it is permissible to use heavier premedications. Such procedures would be intercostal or paravertebral blocks and those techniques requiring use of a nerve stimulator during which patient cooperation is less necessary. For example, the combination of a barbiturate with a narcotic (for example, nembutal 100 mg with morphine 10 mg) can be used. However, it is by no means essential to use heavy premedication. The anesthesiologist skilled in these regional anesthetic techniques should be able to perform them using appropriate reassurance and adequate infiltration of local anesthetic with minimal discomfort to the patient. By employing adequate preparation at the time of the preoperative visit the evening before and gentle and expert technique, the anesthesiologist should be able to utilize regional anesthesia without resorting to heavy premedication.

The routine use of atropine and scopolamine, which is practiced for general anesthesia in many centers, probably should be avoided for routine use in regional anesthesia. These drying agents frequently leave the patient with an uncomfortable and dry mouth, which can often be a source of great concern and discomfort in an otherwise satisfactory regional anesthetic experience. However, atropine is often used to treat the bradycardia occasionally accompanying those regional techniques that result in high spinal anesthesia.

EQUIPMENT

Although many regional anesthesia practitioners use disposable equipment, usually nondisposable, good quality equipment will facilitate the vast majority of regional anes-

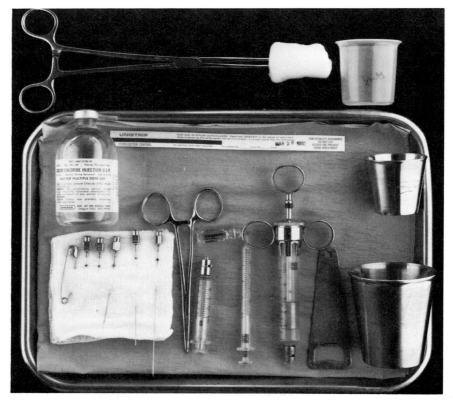

Fig. 20-1 A suitable tray for use in regional anesthetic blocks. Note the selection of different lengths of 22 gauge stainless steel, nondisposable needles with security bead; the control syringe; the selection of beakers for drugs and solution for skin preparation; the small tuberculin syringe for accurate transfer of epinephrine to drug solution; and the bottle of normal sodium chloride for dilution of drug as needed for the different concentrations that are required for skin wheals, infiltration, and conduction nerve anesthesia.

thetic techniques. The use of flimsy, ill-fitting disposable equipment can jeopardize chances of success. Figure 20–1 shows a suitable tray for use in regional block anesthesia.

NEEDLES

Needles should be of good quality stainless steel, with Luer-Lok and a security bead. Needles of 22-gauge will prove satisfactory for the vast majority of regional techniques; a relatively blunt point rather than a long sharp taper is best. Long thin-tapered needles have a tendency to pierce nerves, whereas blunter needles will tend to push the nerve ahead of them and thus reduce the risk of neural damage[4]. An integral part of many regional anesthetic techniques involves appreciating both the resistance of tissues the needle is passing through and the changes of resistance that occur in certain specific blocks when the needle passes through tissue of different density (such as axillary sheath or psoas fascia). This sensation of resistance, or lack of same, will be more effectively transmitted to the operator's hand when a blunter rather than a sharp point is used. In the latter case, the needle tends to part the tissues and this detracts from transmission of sensation from needle point to operator (Fig. 20-2).

Handling of needles is most important. In

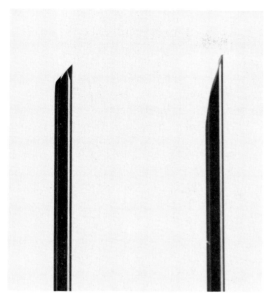

Fig. 20-2 Note the shallow bevel of the needle on the left, which is the optimal type of point for regional anesthesia because it is less likely to traumatize nerves than the sharper needle shown on the right. Also, the losses of resistance, which are an important feedback technique for identifying needle position, are more easily obtained with a blunter rather than a sharper needle. Twenty-two–gauge needles are optimal for the vast majority of regional anesthesia.

cific depth (for example, in paravertebral blocks, where the transverse process is located, then the needle realigned and advanced an additional 1.5 cm), the middle or ring finger may be used as a marker. The rubber stopper from the local anesthetic bottle may also be used as a marker on the needle.

SYRINGES

The use of a control syringe is highly desirable for the majority of regional anesthetic procedures. A control syringe with ring holders permits one-handed aspiration during the block. This is important for ascertaining that the needle point has not entered a vascular conduit or the subarachnoid space (blood or cerebrospinal fluid will be aspirated). By permitting one-handed operation of the syringe and drug administration, the operator's other hand is free to stabilize the relationship of the needle to the patient. In many anesthetic blocks, the needle is initially correctly located only to be misplaced by aberrant movements of the patient, the needle, the operator, or all three. By stabiliz-

all regional anesthesia the main goal is to transmit what is happening at the needle point to the sensory cortex of the operator. For this reason, it is best to hold the needle as a pen is held: the needle is held by muscles of the hand, which serve as appropriately sensitive transducers because they have a relatively large cortical representation; the needle should not be locked in a fixed hand with the coarser muscular movements of the elbow, shoulder, and trunk muscles being used, since these muscles have relatively parsimonious cortical representation.

The needle, therefore, should be held by the hub between the thumb, index, and middle fingers, using the ring and middle finger as needed for stability (Fig. 20-3). In certain blocks where the needle is related to specific bony landmarks and then advanced to a spe-

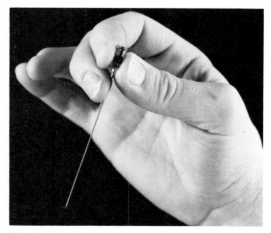

Fig. 20-3 For regional anesthetic blocks, the needle is held firmly with the thumb, index, and middle fingers and positioned utilizing the small muscles of the hand for more accurate placement.

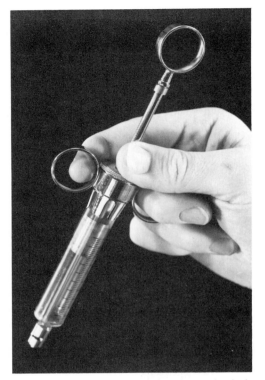

Fig. 20-4 To grip the control syringe, the index and middle fingers hold the syringe barrel via control rings; the thumb can be used to secure the metal piston and prevent drug leaking from syringe during transfer. During injection, the thumb is inserted in the ring on the piston and pressure on this ring enables detection of "losses of resistance" to injection as the syringe and needle are advanced.

ing the needle in relationship to the patient so that they move as one, the needle is more likely to remain in close approximation to the nerve target. A glass-barrelled metal piston control syringe is optimal because the supporting thumb does not contaminate the fluid path as it does with an all-glass syringe (Fig. 20-4). These syringes demand more maintenance for they must be disassembled after each use for thorough cleaning. However, they are much more satisfactory and effective to use than other syringes, especially the poor quality disposable kind. Their free-running piston-like barrel gives much more appropriate feedback for losses of resistance than the rubberized plungers of plastic syringes, which do not run so freely and can give false information on resistance of tissues. The high quality glass and metal control syringes are much more effective "transducers."

Facility with using the Luer-Lok syringe requires that prior to locking the needle on the syringe, the hand is pronated and applied to the needle. Then the act of supination brings the needle and syringe into locked unison.

SAFETY PRECAUTIONS

Whenever large doses of local anesthetic are administered or smaller doses administered close to the neuraxis (for example, stellate ganglion and interscalene paravertebral blocks) certain safety precautions should be taken and certain resuscitation equipment must be available.

An intravenous portal, usually in the form of a continuous intravenous drip, is a necessary safeguard. This is essential for administering both fluid volume and drugs such as vasopressors should this be necessary to support a hypotensive situation. It may also serve as an emergency route for the administration of such drugs as diazepam or short-acting barbiturates in the event of local anesthetic toxic convulsions or the need for supplemental sedation.

The equipment necessary for emergency endotracheal intubation must be readily available in these circumstances. This, of course, includes a functioning laryngoscope, a selection of endotracheal tubes with intact cuffs, and a means of delivering oxygen via positive pressure. An Ambu bag would be regarded as the bare minimum for this, and an anesthesia machine should usually be available.

During the injection of local anesthetic drugs, aspiration tests are mandatory. Since needles can move unknowingly, it is always important to aspirate at the beginning, during, and end of injections to ensure that the needle remains in the same anatomic location and does not trespass into adjoining blood vessels, subarachnoid spaces or other areas.

To ascertain that the drug is being placed in the correct location, a test dose of local anesthetic should first be administered. Usually a dose of 3 to 5 ml is appropriate. The volume of the test dose will vary as to its anatomic site. For instance, when concerned about the possibility of an intravascular injection while performing, for example, a stellate ganglion block, a much smaller test dose is required because a dose as small as 0.25 ml of 1 percent lidocaine solution when injected into the vertebral artery can produce quite profound sequela of transient CNS convulsions. On the other hand, if one is administering a test dose for, perhaps, an epidural anesthetic, then it is necessary to use up to 100 mg of lidocaine to ensure detection of accidental intrathecal placement of the needle or catheter. It is also essential to administer test doses that contain 1:200,000 solution of epinephrine, as this concentration of epinephrine will produce a transient tachycardia if the drug is accidentally injected into a blood vessel.

GENERAL TECHNIQUE

POSITIONING OF THE NEEDLE

In seeking to approximate the needle point to the nerve in question, there are several techniques that can be used. These are as follows.

ELICITATION OF PARESTHESIA

The needle is inserted according to surface landmarks and advanced in the direction of the nerve until the needle locates the nerve and the patient states that a paresthesia oc-

curred in the peripheral distribution of that nerve. Although this remains one of the standard techniques of needle positioning, it has disadvantages. It is uncomfortable. Because of the distractions of the discomfort of the needle, some patients cannot or will not cooperate to yield objective information with regard to paresthesia. In brief, the elicitation of paresthesia is more successful in the phlegmatic, cooperative, somewhat stoical individual than it is in the anxious and hypersensitive type. Paresthesias have been shown to be associated with an increase in postblock nerve lesions in axillary blocks.[5]

APPROXIMATION TO BONY LANDMARKS

The firm sensation of underlying bone enables the operator to ascertain the position of same and when particular nerves bear a constant relationship to a bony prominence, this can facilitate approximating needle to nerve. For example, the paravertebral nerves lie caudad and deep to the vertebral transverse processes and thus the needle has only to be maneuvered at the appropriate depth caudad to this process to produce blockade.

LOSS OF RESISTANCE

In other nerve blocks (for example, axillary approaches to the brachial plexus) the nerves lie in a compartment that is surrounded by a resilient sheath of fibrous tissue, i.e., the axillary sheath. In these instances, the loss of resistance as the needle first meets the sheath, presses against it, and then passes through as the sheath suddenly gives way, is confirmatory evidence of placement in the correct anatomic compartment. Other examples of loss of resistance are the "popping" through the prevertebral fascia in approaches to the brachial plexus between the scalene muscles in the neck and classically, of course, traversing the ligamentum flavum in epidural anesthesia.

APPROXIMATION TO ARTERIES

In certain positions, the nerves run in conjunction with arteries and the transmission of arterial pulsation to the needle as occurs in, for example, the transmitted aortic pulsations in a celiac block or the brachial artery pulsations in an axillary block will confirm that the needle is in close position to the artery and therefore the nerve target.

One method of ensuring approximation of needle to nerve occurs in axillary block of the brachial plexus when the anesthesiologist attempts to anesthetize the posterior cord. It is feasible to enter the brachial artery as confirmed by aspiration tests of blood and then to advance the needle through the posterior wall of the artery until aspiration of blood is no longer possible. The needle is then deemed to be lying in close approximation to the posterior cord; a bolus of local anesthetic here will block that cord and its radial nerve derivative.

USE OF STIMULATING NEEDLES

Apart from the elicitation of sensory paresthesia, all of the above attempts to localize the needle are indirect methods. Probably the most direct method and the one that has considerable success is to use a "stimulating needle." Most of the arrangements for making these needles are custom-made by individual anesthesiologists. Basically what is needed is a relatively low frequency pulse-generated electric current that can be transmitted via the exploring needle.[6,7] A ground connection to the patient at a distal site is required. Nerve stimulators used for monitoring neuromuscular blockade can be easily modified for this purpose.[8]

By using a current of 2 to 20 volts of brief duration and a repetition rate of 2 to 3 pulses per second, the motor components of the nerve that are to be blocked can be stimulated. This procedure provides objective evidence of the proximity of needle to nerve. It also permits adequate and even heavy sedation with preoperative analgesics so that the patient is unaware of the discomforts of the needling procedure; thus, it has greater patient acceptance. Such an arrangement has been used in my practice for the past 10 years and has proved eminently satisfactory.

NERVE BLOCKS OF THE UPPER EXTREMITY

To successfully achieve regional analgesia of the upper extremity, knowledge of the anatomy of the brachial plexus and of the anatomic distribution of its principal branches is needed. Knowing the branches is necessary to individually block these nerves when selective and discrete analgesia of part of the upper extremity is needed or when a supplement to a brachial plexus block that is deficient in one or more of its major components is needed.

APPLIED ANATOMY OF THE BRACHIAL PLEXUS

The brachial plexus is derived from the anterior primary rami of C5, C6, C7, C8 and T1. These nerves emerge in the paravertebral gutter of the appropriate vertebra and at this site they lie sandwiched between the anterior and middle scalene muscles that arise from the anterior and posterior tubercles, respectively, of the cervical vertebra. These scalene muscles pass downwards and laterally from the cervical vertebrae; the anterior being inserted into the scalene tubercle of the first rib and the scalenus medius being inserted into a quadrangular area between the neck and the subclavian groove of the first rib. Across these two muscles is stretched the prevertebral fascia. As the brachial plexus and subclavian artery emerge between the muscles, they produce a "tenting" effect in the fascia; a tube (sheath) of prevertebral fascia then surrounds the artery and plexus and continues distally and is then called the axillary sheath. This sheath then extends into the middle and distal thirds of the arm. The brachial plexus and its terminal branches are contained within this sheath, distributed around the artery. The plexus may be effectively blocked with single injections into the sheath either in the paravertebral region, between the scalene muscles, as it passes over the first rib, or in the axilla (Fig. 20-5).

The brachial plexus, therefore, is composed of roots that lie between the scalene muscles. The trunks of the brachial plexus lie in the posterior triangle of the neck. The divisions of the plexus surround the artery behind the clavicle. At the outer border of the first rib, the cords of the plexus are formed that pass into the axilla where the branches arise.

In the formation of the plexus, the nerve roots of C5 and C6 unite to form the upper trunk. C7 continues undivided as the middle trunk and C8 and T1 unite to form the lower trunk. These three trunks are stacked vertically between the scalene muscles and in the posterior triangle of the neck above the subclavian artery. Each of these trunks divides into an anterior and posterior division behind the clavicle and these divisions give rise to the cords that surround the subclavian vessel. The two superior anterior divisions form the lateral cord (which will eventually give rise to the median nerve) and this lies to the lateral side of the artery. All three posterior divisions form the posterior cord, which will give rise eventually to the radial nerve, and this lies posterior to the artery. The inferior anterior division continues as the medial cord on the medial side of the artery and this will eventually give rise to the ulnar nerve.

The branches of the brachial plexus are primarily from the roots and from the cords. There are in essence no branches from the trunks or the divisions.

BRANCHES FROM THE ROOTS

The branches from the roots are all motor and supply the rhomboid muscles (C5) the subclavian muscle (C5–C6), and the serratus anterior muscle (the larger branch from C5, C6, and C7). These branches are usually only anesthetized in the interscalene approach to the brachial plexus.

The suprascapular nerve arises from the junction of C5 and C6. This supplies the muscles of the dorsal aspect of the scapula (supraspinatus and infraspinatus) after the nerve passes through the suprascapular foramen on the superior border of the scapula. The suprascapular nerve also gives a significant contribution to the sensory supply of the shoulder joint. This nerve is often irritated during the performance of an interscalene approach to the brachial plexus; this irritation manifests as a dull paresthesia referred to the scapula and/or shoulder joint.

BRANCHES FROM THE LATERAL CORD

The main branch of the lateral cord is the lateral head of the median nerve, which together with the medial head (from the medial cord) forms the median nerve lying on the lateral side of the artery in the distal axilla. In the axillary approach to the brachial plexus when the needle is positioned lateral to the brachial artery a paresthesia of the median nerve distribution to the thumb, index, and middle fingers is to be expected.

The other clinically important branch of the lateral cord is the musculocutaneous nerve. This arises from the plexus, leaves the axillary sheath high in the axilla, and enters into the substance of the coracobrachialis muscle. Therefore, in the axillary approach to brachial plexus blocks, unless the anesthetic is deposited sufficiently proximal in the sheath, this nerve will be spared and the block will be unsatisfactory. (The musculocutaneous nerve is "musculo" to the flexor muscle of the arm—biceps and brachialis—and "cu-

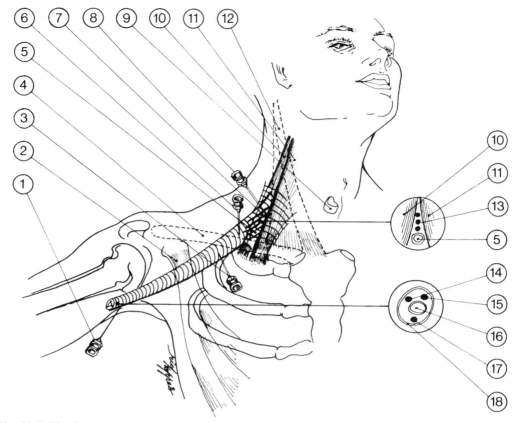

Fig. 20-5 The four approaches for blocking the brachial plexus and the relations of this plexus as it emerges from between the two scalene muscles, acquires its tubular sheath of prevertebral fascia, and passes into the axilla in close relationship to the axillary artery.

Axillary approach (1). Note the relationships of the main nerves to the artery in this axillary approach as shown in the insert diagram. The lateral cord (15) is lateral to the axillary artery (16). The medial cord (17) is medial and below the vessel, and the posterior cord (14) is posterior to the vessel. The vessel and these three nerves are all contained within the tubular prolongation of the prevertebral fascia, and the axillary sheath (18). Injections are made into this fascial and sheath envelope to block the three main nerves.

Infraclavicular approach (3). The needle is inserted 2.5 cm below the midpoint of the clavicle (4) and medial to the coracoid process of the scapula (2). This block also endeavors to deposit anesthetic within the axillary sheath and at this level the musculocutaneous nerve is usually still contained within the sheath.

Supraclavicular block (6). The needle is inserted 2 cm above the midpoint of the clavicle (4) and drug is deposited around the trunks of the brachial plexus as they cross the first rib enclosed within the fascial sheath along with the subclavian artery (5).

Interscalene approach (8). The needle is inserted posterior to the sternomastoid muscle (12) between the anterior (11) and middle scalene muscles (10) to block the brachial plexus components (7) at the level of the cricoid cartilage (9). This block is shown in the insert in more detail where the brachial plexus components (13) are stacked vertically above the subclavian artery (5) between the anterior (11) and middle (10) scalene muscles.

taneous" to the lateral border of the forearm.)

The remaining branch of the lateral cord is the lateral pectoral nerve, which is primarily a motor nerve to the pectoralis major muscle, and it is usually not clinically important in brachial plexus blocks.

BRANCHES FROM THE MEDIAL CORD

The important branches of the medial cord are the medial head of the median nerve, which crosses the axillary artery anteriorly, and the ulnar nerve. The ulnar nerve is the largest branch of this cord. It pursues a posteromedial course in relation to the artery in the axilla. The other important cutaneous branches of the medial cord are the medial cutaneous nerves of the arm and forearm, respectively. The medial cutaneous nerve of the arm runs on the medial side of the axillary vein and supplies skin over the front and medial aspect of the arm from axilla to elbow. The medial cutaneous nerve of the forearm runs distally between artery and vein, pierces the deep fascia of the arm just above the elbow, and supplies skin on the front and medial aspect of the forearm. The medial pectoral nerve is the remaining branch. This supplies both pectoral muscles.

BRANCHES FROM THE POSTERIOR CORD

Of the five branches, the radial is the continuation of the posterior cord. It leaves the axilla through the triangular space between the triceps, teres major, and humerus. The other large branch is the axillary nerve, which exits through the posterior wall of the axilla giving branches to the shoulder joint, the deltoid, and teres minor muscles prior to terminating in a cutaneous branch; the latter supplies an area of skin over the lateral upper third of the arm. The remaining branches of the posterior cord compose the large branch to the latissmus dorsi muscle and the upper

and lower subscapular nerves, which supply the muscles of the ventral aspect of the scapula (i.e., subscapularis and teres major).

TECHNIQUES OF BRACHIAL PLEXUS BLOCK

INTERSCALENE APPROACH

In the interscalene approach, the object is to deposit the local anesthetic at the roots of the brachial plexus as they lie between the anterior and middle scalene muscles.[9] This block is carried out at the C6 vertebral level. This is found by identifying the cricoid cartilage; a perpendicular line is drawn posterior from this cartilage to intersect the posterior border of the sternomastoid muscle at or close to the interscalene groove. The external jugular vein is a fairly constant landmark as it often crosses the sternomastoid muscle at the same site as the interscalene groove. The deep structures lying in the posterior triangle at this point are palpated with the exploring forefinger, which is moved in a horizontal back and forth direction at right angles to the interscalene groove to identify this hiatus between the two scalene muscles. By having the patient take slow, deep breaths at this stage, the scalene muscles will often be more easily palpated.[10]

When the groove is identified, the needle is inserted at right angles to the skin in a caudad and medial direction. The structures lying between the skin and the brachial plexus are primarily the platysma muscle and the prevertebral fascia and various amounts of subcutaneous fat depending on the morphology of the patient. In slim individuals, the needle need only be inserted about 1 cm and paresthesias of the C5 and C6 dermatomes to the radial border of forearm, thumb, or index finger are often obtained at shallower depths than this. The important maneuver is to ensure that the needle is positioned deep to the prevertebral fascia in the interscalene groove. A stimulating needle will give good objective

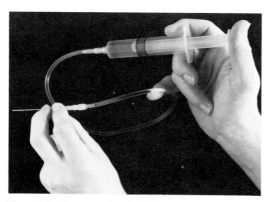

Fig. 20-6 The use of a flexible extension tube between the injecting needle and the injecting syringe prevents the transference of aberrant movements of the syringe to the needle and therefore reduces the chances of the needle moving away from the target. This particular arrangement (the "immobile needle") is used in those relatively superficial blocks where the depth of needle insertion is so shallow that is does not afford any stability to the needle. This occurs in axillary blocks, interscalene blocks, and femoral sheath blocks. The needle is stabilized by forming a "bridge" with the anesthesiologist's hand between the needle hub and the patient. The injecting syringe can then be moved with relative impunity without fear of dislodging the needle.

confirmation by stimulating the C5 and C6 myotomes (biceps and brachialis contractions). Any of these above confirmatory signs are good evidence that the needle is in close proximity to the upper roots of the brachial plexus and an indication to proceed with the injection. Stabilization of the needle is of critical importance in this as it is in many other blocks; in addition, the use of a flexible extension tube from needle to a syringe reservoir is a distinct advantage in this particular block,[11] as is the cooperation of an assistant to manipulate the injection syringe while the anesthesiologist stablizes the needle in relation to the plexus (Fig. 20-6).

After aspiration tests are satisfactory, 30 to 40 ml of local anesthetic are injected and should be contained deep to the prevertebral fascia. Any "ballooning" of subcutaneous tissues in the neck is an indication that the an-

esthetic is probably being deposited superior to the fascia, and this will prove an unsatisfactory block. The complete volume of anesthetic is injected at this site, and no further attempts need be made to elicit paresthesia of deeper components of the plexus (C7 and C8 or T1). In contrast to more peripheral blocks of the plexus, the onset of the block follows a dermatomal and myotomal pattern, as occurs with epidural blockade—i.e., the anesthetic spreads from C5 distally down to T1, with the progress of anesthesia down the preaxial border to the thumb and forefingers, spreading across the fingers medially to the small digit, and then ascending up the postaxial border of the limb to the axilla. The myotomes are also sequentially anesthetized in this same fashion of C5 through T1. Therefore the first muscle group to be effectively anesthetized is usually the biceps and brachialis, the flexors of the elbow; this is in contrast to the axillary block, where this is usually the last muscle group to be anesthetized because of the difficulty of ensuring anesthesia of the musculocutaneous nerve in an axillary approach. The last myotome to be anesthetized in an interscalene block is that of T1, which involves the small muscles of the hands. Therefore, when patients can no longer adduct and abduct their fingers, the interscalene block can be deemed to be complete.

This block has obvious advantages over more peripheral blocks for operations around the shoulder and arm. It is eminently suitable for surgical procedures on the acromioclavicular joint and the clavicle and for reducing dislocated shoulders. With effective cranial spread of anesthetic to involve cervical plexus, and adequate caudad spread to anesthetize all of the brachial plexus, it can be used for operations on the shoulder joint itself. It is usual for this block to anesthetize the deep cervical plexus, C2, C3, and C4 by craniad spread in the paravertebral spaces. This is more likely to happen if the patient is lying flat and no pressure is applied above the injection site. However, if the surgery is on the distal parts of the upper extremity, particularly if it involves the postaxial border, caudad spread is more important than craniad. Therefore, the patient is positioned sitting at an angle of 45 degrees, and pressure is applied over the superior part of the interscalene groove during the injection in an attempt to encourage the spread of the local anesthetic to the more caudal elements of the brachial plexus.[12] One of the limitations of this block is the fact that such caudad spread cannot be consistently produced, and for surgical procedures that involve the postaxial border of the upper extremity, the onset of anesthesia in this area is often prolonged. However, for procedures on the preaxial border, the onset is more rapid than other brachial plexus blocks.

Complications of the interscalene block involve accidentally placing the needle in the vertebral artery that is very close to the nerves, passing between the foramina transversaria, anterior to the anterior primary rami. Even small quantities of local anesthetic injected into this vessel produce large concentration in the cerebral circulation with convulsions.[13] Therefore, aspiration tests are always mandatory. If the needle is used as described with a caudad direction, the obliquity of the articulation of the cervical vertebrae should prevent the needle entering the neuraxis. However, if the needle is used in a horizontal or cephalad direction, the risk of the needle passing between the vertebrae or through a paravertebral foramen into the epidural and/or spinal compartment and/or neuraxis is a potential danger. Epidural spread of anesthetic[14] and total spinal[15] anesthetic have been reported with this technique. Therefore, the needle should always be directed caudad. If the above-described technique is followed, the needle should be well above the apical pleura. Pneumothorax is a potential risk here with deeper needling, although the incidence of pneumothorax with interscalene block should be less than with the conventional supraclavicular approach.

SUPRACLAVICULAR APPROACH

The classic supraclavicular approach attempts to block the trunks of the brachial plexus as they cross the first rib in the posterior triangle of the neck.[16] The landmarks for this are 1 to 2 cm above the midpoint of the clavicle. Palpation of the subclavian artery is possible in slim individuals, and the nerve trunks are posterosuperior to the vessel at this point. Traditionally, the needle is inserted at right angles to the skin in all planes and advanced until either a paresthesia is obtained in the upper extremity or the first rib is contacted as an endpoint. The needle is then "walked" along the first rib in anteroposterior directions until paresthesias are obtained. At this site the brachial plexus is at its most compact (i.e., it is reduced to three elements, the upper, middle, and lower trunks). Local anesthetic deposited here will provide effective and complete anesthesia of the upper extremity, with the exception of the intercostobrachial nerve component. Because the trunks are probably the bulkiest components of the brachial plexus, the onset of anesthesia tends to be slower here than it would be for, as an example, an interscalene block. A significant complication with this block is the incidence of pneumothorax, which even in good hands occurs 1 percent of the time[17] and probably occurs subclinically much more often, maybe even 20 percent.[18]

AXILLARY APPROACH

The axillary approach has proved an effective and safe means of regionally anesthetizing the upper extremity.[18] It is the preferred technique for procedures distal to the elbow. Its main drawbacks are the difficulty in ensuring anesthesia of the musculocutaneous nerve and that it is not suitable for surgical procedures of the proximal arm or shoulder.

The arm is abducted to an angle of 90 degrees, and if the upper extremity is sufficiently mobile an even greater angle is optimal by having the patient place his hand behind his head. This gives excellent exposure to the axilla, which may be shaved at the anesthesiologist's discretion. The landmark here is the axillary artery whose pulsations are palpated in the anterior interval between the deltoid and latissimus dorsi muscles high in the axilla. A skin wheal of local anesthetic is placed over the artery, and the needle is inserted until it pops through the axillary sheath. At this stage it is feasible to inject the total (40 ml) volume in the axillary sheath and await the onset of block. If paresthesia is required for confirmation of needle position, then after entering the axillary sheath the needle is positioned first on the superolateral aspect of the axillary artery, where a median nerve paresthesia is sought and elicited when referred paresthesia to the thumb or preaxial fingers is identified by the patient. A bolus of 10 ml of local anesthetic is deposited at this site, and the exploring needle then positioned on the medial aspect of the artery at a posterior plane; ulnar paresthesias to the fifth digit are sought and when obtained a bolus of 10 ml of anesthetic is inserted at this point. Options for anesthetizing the radial component of the brachial plexus are to position the needle posterior to the vessel either by transfixing the vessel or by approaching it from the posterior medial aspect; a further 10 ml are deposited if and when a radial paresthesia is obtained. In practice it is usually satisfactory to deposit anesthesia when there are two paresthesias on the median and ulnar side of the artery. The application of distal pressure to the axillary sheath either with a tourniquet or the anesthesiologist's hand is recommended in an attempt to ensure that the anesthetic moves proximally to the place in the sheath where the musculocutaneous nerve exits.[12] A cuff of anesthesia over the proximal medial aspect of the axilla is recommended to anesthetize the intercostobrachial nerve. This is the lateral branch of the T2 intercostal nerve, which innervates skin for a variable extent in the axilla and medial border of the

arm. Usually an adequate skin wheal over the axillary artery is sufficient to anesthetize this nerve. If it is not anesthetized, it can cause discomfort usually in relation to the tourniquet pressure.

INFRACLAVICULAR APPROACH

As an alternative approach to the brachial plexus block, Raj[19] described a method—the infraclavicular approach—whereby the needle is inserted 2 cm below the midpoint of the inferior border of the clavicle and the anesthesiologist using a modified nerve stimulator locates the brachial plexus with a laterally directed needle from this insertion point. Advantages of this approach would be in those situations where the axillary approach or approaches to plexus in the posterior triangle were contraindicated for one reason or another (e.g., patient positioning difficulties, fractures, and infections). It would have an advantage over the axillary approach of introducing the anesthetic more cephalad in the axillary sheath and thereby would assure block of the musculocutaneous nerve. No significant side effects have been reported with this technique as yet, although if the needle was directed medially in error, pneumothorax would certainly be a risk. This technique has been modified by Sims[19a] whereby the needle puncture is made at a more lateral site in the interval between the coracoid process of the scapula and the inferior border of the clavicle. Again, a nerve stimulator is used and contact with the plexus is reached at a distance of 2 to 3 cm from the skin wheal. Thirty-five ml of local anesthetic injected at this site yeild satisfactory analgesia.

BLOCKS OF PERIPHERAL NERVES

Specific nerves can be blocked alone for limited surgery over their distribution. More frequently, peripheral block is required to

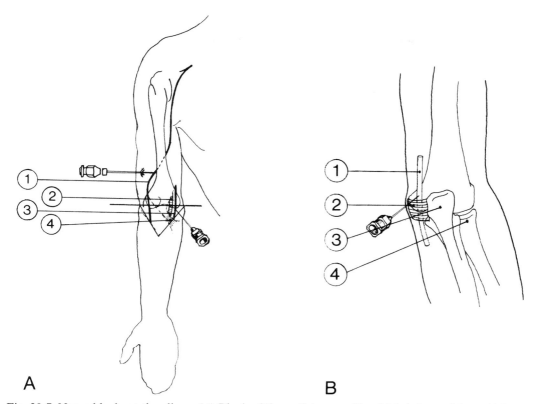

Fig. 20-7 Nerve blocks at the elbow. (*A*) Block of the radial nerve (1), which is located 8 cm (4 finger-breadths) above the lateral epicondyle as it curves from the posterior to the lateral aspect of the humerus. The median nerve (3) is blocked at the level of the humeral epicondyles in the medial angle of the antecubital fossa medial to the pulsations of the brachial artery (2) and the biceps tendon aponeurosis (4). (*B*) Block of the ulnar nerve at the elbow. The ulnar nerve (1) is blocked on the posteromedial aspect of the elbow joint. The nerve is readily palpated between the olecranon process of the ulnar (3) and the medial epicondyle of the humerus (2). It is usually blocked above the level of the elbow joint where the nerve is more mobile and less likely to be traumatized by the needle. Number 4 is the head of the radius.

supplement an unsatisfactory brachial plexus block in which component nerves have been spared.

RADIAL NERVE BLOCK

The radial nerve can be blocked both in the arm and at the wrist. The landmarks for block in the arm are on the lateral border at the junction of the middle and lower thirds. This site is found by measuring 4 fingerbreadths above the lateral epicondyle of the humerus; the nerve can be palpated at this site in some

individuals where it emerges from its course in the spiral groove of the humerus. The block is shown in Figure 20-7*A*. After appropriate skin wheals, a needle is inserted down to the humerus and local anesthetic is deposited in a fan-like fashion along the lateral border of the humerus at the junction of its middle and lower third. A radial nerve paresthesia to the dorsum of thumb or first fingers is confirmatory evidence of correct position. A total of 5 to 10 ml of drug is usually needed.

At the wrist, the radial nerve is found at the level of the proximal flexor crease on the radial side of the radial artery (Fig. 20-8). The artery is palpated and a bolus of 3 ml of a local anesthetic is inserted lateral to it; a subcutaneous cuff of anesthesia is deposited on the lateral and dorsal aspects of the radial side of the wrist at this level to anesthetize those branches of the radial nerve that have left the parent trunk in the lower third of the forearm.

MEDIAN NERVE BLOCK

The median nerve can be blocked conveniently at the level of the elbow or at the wrist. At the elbow, the median nerve is the most medial content of the antecubital fossa and the landmark for localization is the brachial artery. The brachial artery is found immediately medial to the biceps tendon at the level of the flexion crease of the elbow, and medial to it is the median nerve (Fig. 20-7*A*). A bolus of 5 ml of local anesthetic injected at this site will effect analgesia of the peripheral distribution of the median nerve, i.e., the palmar aspects of the thumb, index, and middle fingers, and half the ring finger and the corresponding nailbeds of the same digits. Median nerve block at this site will also produce motor blockade of those median-innervated wrist flexor muscles of the forearm and thenar muscles.

At the wrist, the median nerve is located at the level of the proximal flexion crease between the palmaris longus and the flexor carpi radialis tendons (Fig. 20-8). The main body of the nerve passes deep to the flexor retinaculum. However, a superficial palmar branch arises from the nerve proximal to the flexor retinaculum and passes superficial to this retinaculum subcutaneously to supply an area of skin over the lateral aspect of the thenar eminence and adjacent palm. This superficial palmar branch is blocked by subcutaneous infiltration between skin and flexor retinaculum at the puncture site for the median nerve block. For anesthesia of the parent nerve, the needle is advanced through

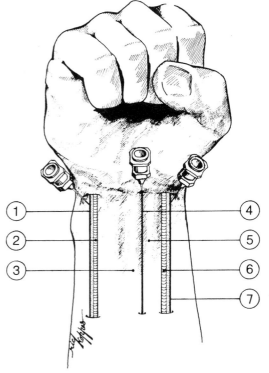

Fig. 20-8 Various blocks at the wrist. The ulnar nerve (1) is blocked medial to the ulnar artery (2). The median nerve (4) is blocked between the tendons of palmaris longus (3) and flexor carpi radialis (5). The radial nerve (7) is blocked lateral to the radial artery (6). It is often necessary to put a cuff of local anesthetic over the lateral and dorsal aspects of the wrist to block those terminal divisions of the radial nerve that have branched proximal to blocking the main branch.

the flexor retinaculum until a loss of resistance is appreciated and then a bolus of 3 ml of local anesthetic will affect anesthesia of the median nerve. Because the nerve is confined in the carpal tunnel at this stage, it is not advisable to actively seek paresthesia lest the nerve be traumatized. This compact carpel fascial compartment acts as a reservoir to keep the anesthetic in close approximation to the nerve. Successful block of the median nerve of the wrist will result in analgesia of the lateral three and a half fingers and the corresponding nailbeds on the dorsal surface and of motor block of the muscles of the thenar eminence and the lumbrical muscles of the first and second fingers.

ULNAR NERVE BLOCK

The ulnar nerve can be blocked at the elbow and wrist. This nerve is identified at the elbow where it runs posteriorly to the medial epicondyle of the humerus where it is subcutaneous and readily palpable. It is suggested that analgesia be produced by infiltration proximal to the medial epicondyle, as the nerve is more mobile at this site and less likely to be traumatized by the needle (Fig. 20-7*B*). Five to 10 ml of anesthetic is required.

At the wrist, the ulnar nerve lies on the medial (or ulnar side) of the ulnar artery and is blocked in this situation at the level of the proximal flexor crease (Fig. 20-8). Three ml of local anesthetic is injected at this site medial to the ulnar artery. Block results in analgesia of the palmar and dorsal surfaces of the lateral one and a half digits and all of the small muscles of the hand except those of the thenar eminence and the first and second lumbrical muscles.

NERVE BLOCKS OF THE LOWER EXTREMITY

In contrast to the upper extremity where the brachial plexus is a relatively compact neural bundle contained in its own fascial sheath and therefore eminently suitable to single needle techniques, the nerve supply to the lower extremity is widely separated. The embryologic nerve supply to the lower extremity is the sciatic nerve but because the lower extremity has "borrowed" considerable skin and musculature from the trunk, this borrowed tissue maintains its original nerve supply from the lumbar plexus with its femoral, obturator, and lateral femoral cutaneous components. Therefore, the lower extremity is supplied by four principal nerves, which

are widely separated from each other as they enter the thigh, and as such, require needling procedures in different locations to produce nerve block of the lower limb. Appreciation, however, of the formation of the lumbar plexus does permit needling in the paraspinal areas where the plexus is formed and enables analgesia of the derivatives of the lumbar plexus to be achieved with just a one-needle technique in the so-called psoas compartment block. A separate needling technique, however, is required for the sciatic nerve and this is traditionally achieved by a posterior approach in the buttock. It is also appropriate to appreciate the peripheral anatomy of the derivatives of the lumbar and sciatic plexus so that more discrete nerve blocks can be produced for limited procedures.

APPLIED ANATOMY OF THE LUMBAR PLEXUS

The lumbar plexus is formed from the anterior primary rami of the paravertebral nerves T12 to L4. The upper two components—T12 and L1—are concerned with the nerve supply of the anterior abdominal wall. The lower components—L2, L3, and L4—are primarily destined for the skin and musculature of the anterior and medial components of the thigh. Enroute to this final destination, they supply psoas major and quadratus lumborum muscles on the posterior abdominal wall. After supplying these muscles, they divide into anterior and posterior divisions within the substance of the psoas major muscle. The anterior divisions form the obturator nerve and the posterior divisions form the femoral nerve. These nerves emerge from the posterior aspect of the psoas major muscle where they lie between it and the quadratus lumborum in the so-called psoas compartment. This appears to be an anatomic compartment that can be filled with an injection of local anesthetic to anesthetize these derivatives of the lumbar plexus.

OBTURATOR NERVE

The anterior divisions of L2, L3, and L4 form the obturator nerve, which then emerges from the medial border of the psoas major muscle. It crosses the alar of the sacrum and leaves the pelvis via the anteromedial aspect of the obturator foramen. It supplies the parietal peritoneum on the sidewalls of the pelvis and having left the obturator canal, it divides into anterior and posterior divisions. These are primarily motor nerves of supply to the adductor compartment of the thigh. The posterior division is primarily distributed to the deeper adductor muscles with a terminal twig that accompanies the femoral artery and eventually provides sensation to part of the knee joint. The anterior division on entering the thigh supplies a branch to the hip joint, branches to the adductor muscles, and a final cutaneous branch that supplies a variable area of skin over the lower third of the medial border of the thigh.

FEMORAL NERVE

The femoral nerve is the other main component of the lumbar plexus and is formed within the substance of psoas major muscle by the posterior divisions of L2, L3, and L4. It emerges from the lateral border of the psoas major muscle in the iliac fossa, running down in the groove between psoas and iliacus deep to the iliac fascia, and enters the thigh by passing beneath the inguinal ligament to the lateral side of the femoral artery. It is the nerve of supply to the muscles in the anterior compartment of the thigh (quadriceps, sartorius, etc.) and supplies the skin over the anterior aspect of the thigh from just below the inguinal ligament to the knee. The terminal branch of the femoral nerve is the saphenous nerve, which passes through the canal under the sartorius muscle to reach the medial aspect of the knee. The saphenous nerve pursues a course posterior to the long saphenous vein and usually divides into two nerves, which accompany the vein on either side and pass anterior to the medial malleolus and sometimes extend as far forward as the proximal phalanx of the great toe. Thus the saphenous nerve supplies a strip of skin down the medial side of the leg from knee to great toe.

LATERAL FEMORAL CUTANEOUS NERVE

This nerve is formed from the posterior divisions of L2 and L3 within the psoas major muscle. It emerges from the lateral border of this muscle and crosses the iliac fossa deep to the dense fascia covering the iliacus muscle. It enters the thigh by piercing the inguinal ligament 1 to 2 cm from the anterior superior iliac spine. It supplies part of the parietal perineum of the iliac fossa and, after entering the thigh, divides into anterior and posterior branches about 2 cm below the inguinal ligament. These branches pierce the deep fascia lata of the thigh and then supply cutaneous sensation to the lateral aspect of the thigh down to the knee.

TECHNIQUES OF LUMBAR PLEXUS BLOCK

As with the brachial plexus, the lumbar plexus component nerves can be anesthetized at different sites along their course—from the plexus origins in the paravertebral gutter through its formation in the psoas compartment where the nerves are deep to the psoas major muscle and iliacus fascia. Alternatively, they can be blocked as the individual nerve branches enter the thigh.

PARAVERTEBRAL BLOCK

The intent with the paravertebral block is to deposit the local anesthetic at the paravertebral foramen with paravertebral blocks at

L2, L3, and L4. Because of the continuity of the paravertebral space, it is feasible by depositing a large quantity, e.g., 15 ml of local anesthetic at the L3 space, for it to diffuse craniad and caudad to block all three nerves. This is not as predictable as doing three separate paravertebral nerve blocks. The needles are inserted 2.5 cm lateral to the cephalic end of the lumbar vertebra spine, after appropriate skin wheals, to a depth of approximately 3 to 4 cm where the marble-like periosteum of the transverse process is located. The needle is then "walked" posteriorly until it slips off the transverse process. It is advanced another 1 to 2 cm and paresthesias may be sought at this depth between the transverse processes above and below this space. Here a stimulating attachment on the needle is a distinct advantage for obtaining objective information with regard to its placement. The nerve block is accomplished by injecting 5 ml at each site.

BLOCK IN THE "PSOAS COMPARTMENT"

As the lumbar plexus forms within and emerges from the psoas major muscle, it lies wedged between this muscle anteromedially and quadratus lumborum and iliacus muscles posteriorly and laterally. All these muscles lie deep to the dense fascia over the posterior abdominal and pelvic walls, and local anesthetic injected into this fascial compartment between the two muscle masses of psoas major anteriorly and quadratus lumborum and iliacus posteriorly will distribute itself around the lumbar plexus and provide the appropriate block.[20] There are two main routes of approach to this compartment.

Posterior Approach

In this approach, a needle is introduced paravertebrally 3 cm caudad to the intercristal plane 5 cm from the midline (Fig. 20-9). The intent is for the 15 cm needle to be ad-

vanced anteriorly cephalad and lateral to the transverse processes of L5. If it contacts same, it is walked laterally off this process cephalad to the pelvic brim. It traverses the quadratus lumborum muscle and a loss of resistance can be felt by the educated hand as the needle emerges from the anterior border of quadratus lumborum at a depth of about 12 cm. The intent is to place the lumen of the needle where the lumbar plexus is situated: deep to the posterior abdominal wall fascia, anterior to quadratus lumborum and posterior to the psoas major muscle (Figs. 20-10 and 20-11). Different techniques have been described for effecting the block, including distending the space with 20 cc of air prior to injecting the local anesthetic.[20] The use of the stimulating needle is an excellent way of obtaining objective evidence that the needle is in close proximity to the lumbar plexus. It will be necessary to ascertain movements of the vasti and adductor muscles of the thigh to confirm this and not to be confused by direct stimulation of psoas major muscle; the latter can produce flexion of the hip and mislead the operator into thinking that he is stimulating lumbar plexus when he is actually producing a direct effect on the muscle belly of psoas major. Thirty ml injected into this compartment will produce an effective block of the lumbar plexus.

Perivascular or Inguinal Approach

The femoral nerve, lateral femoral cutaneous nerve, and the obturator nerve are formed deep to the deep fascia on the posterior pelvic walls. Local anesthetic injected from below the inguinal ligament under pressure will track up into this compartment between psoas major and iliacus muscles and spread to involve these three major nerve derivatives of the lumbar plexus.[21]

The technique for this is to introduce the needle below the inguinal ligament lateral to the pulsations of the femoral artery, to direct the needle cephalad, and to inject (after ap-

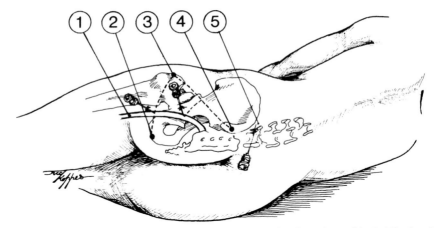

Fig. 20-9 The posterior approach to both the sciatic nerve and lumbar plexus block. The landmarks for the sciatic nerve block are the posterior superior iliac spine (4) and the greater trochanter (3). The sciatic nerve is located 4 to 5 cm caudad to the midpoint of this line at which site it can often be located on deep palpation in slim individuals. A needle is inserted at this site and paresthesia to the leg or foot confirms correct placement. Alternatively the sciatic nerve (1) can be located just medial to the midpoint of a line joining the greater trochanter (3) to the ischial tuberosity (2). For lumbar plexus block from this posterior approach, the needle is inserted to a depth of approximately 12 cm at point (5), which is 3 cm caudad from the intercristal plane, 5 cm from the midline, and lateral to the L5 vertebral spine.

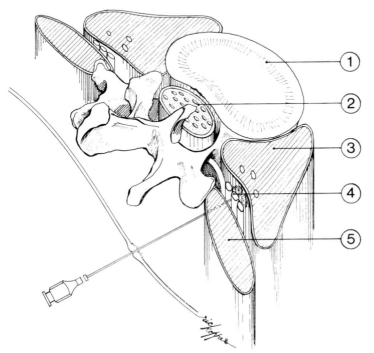

Fig. 20-10 The relationships of the lumbar plexus in the psoas compartment block, when the needle is inserted lateral to the L5 vetebra (1). The lumbar plexus nerves (4) lie between the psoas major muscle (3) anterior and the quadratus lumborum muscle (5) posterior. The landmarks for the needle insertion are shown in Figures 20-9 and 20-14; the needle is inserted through the paraspinal muscle mass until loss of resistance and/or paresthesia is obtained, as the needle passes anterior to the quadratus lumborum muscle.

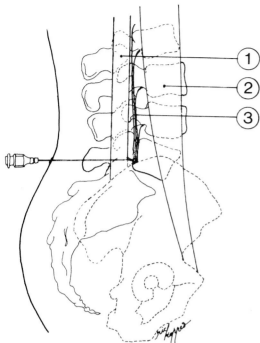

①
②
③

Fig. 20-11 A view of the psoas compartment block, showing the needle inserted at the level of L5 and advanced to a depth of approximately 12 cm where it contacts the branches of the lumbar plexus (3) as they lie between the quadratus lumborum muscle (1) and the psoas major muscle (2).

propriate aspiration tests) 20 to 30 ml of local anesthetic. With 20 ml this technique produces predictable anesthesia of the femoral and lateral femoral cutaneous components, but to ensure obturator nerve involvement, larger volumes (e.g., 30 ml) appear to be needed.

BLOCKS OF PERIPHERAL NERVES

FEMORAL NERVE BLOCK

The femoral nerve passes under the inguinal ligament lateral to the femoral artery at approximately the midinguinal point (i.e., half-way between the pubic tubercle and an-terior superior iliac spine) and divides into its leash of terminal branches immediately below the inguinal ligament. These branches are deep to the deep fascia (fascia lata) of the thigh.

The needle is introduced lateral to the artery just below the midpoint of the inguinal ligament (Fig. 20-12). A loss of resistance is obtained as it "pops" through the fascia lata; a paresthesia may be sought, although injection of a bolus of 10 to 15 ml of local anesthetic at this site is usually effective in blocking the femoral nerve. This will anesthetize the anterior compartment of the thigh and the distribution of the saphenous nerve on the medial aspect of the leg. Because the main trunk of the femoral nerve has divided into its many terminal branches just below the inguinal ligament, a convincing paresthesia is sometime difficult to elicit, probably because the small nerve branches tend to move away from the advancing needle. Therefore, again a stimulating attachment to the needle will help. In combination with the obturator, lateral femoral cutaneous, and sciatic nerves, this block is essential for effective analgesia of the lower extremity. The Femoral nerve block is also useful alone or in combination with the lateral femoral cutaneous nerve block for isolated surgical procedures, such as skin graft from the anterior and lateral surfaces of the thigh.

LATERAL FEMORAL CUTANEOUS NERVE BLOCK

The lateral femoral cutaneous nerve is blocked either above or below its site of emergence through the inguinal ligament 1 to 2 cm medial to the anterior superior iliac spine (Fig. 20-12). Because the nerve lies in the fascial gutter of the reflection of the inguinal ligament, it is readily blocked at this site by injecting 5 ml of local anesthetic. The classic landmarks are 2 cm medial and 2 cm below the anterior superior iliac spine. Infiltration with 5 to 8 ml of local anesthetic is

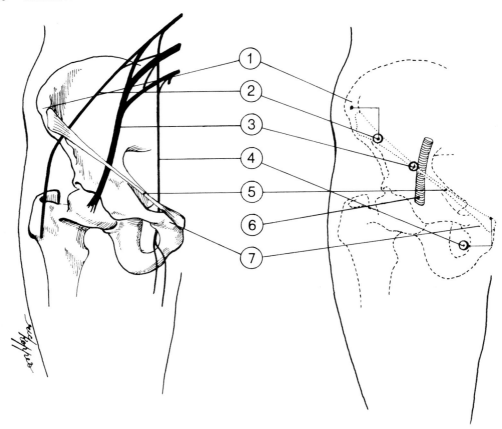

Fig. 20-12 Block of the lateral femoral cutaneous, femoral, and obturator nerves. Landmarks for this block are the anterior, superior iliac spine (1) and the pubic tubercle (7). These two points are joined by the inguinal ligament (5). The lateral femoral cutaneous nerve (2) is blocked 2 cm mediad and caudad to the anterior superior iliac spine. The femoral nerve (3) is blocked just below the midpoint of the inguinal ligament where the former is located lateral to the pulsations of the femoral artery (6). The obturator nerve (4) is blocked as it emerges from the obturator foramen 2 cm lateral and caudad to the pubic tubercles.

usually sufficient to block this nerve. Paresthesia may be obtained. This is entirely a sensory nerve and there is no advantage to be gained from using a stimulating needle.

OBTURATOR NERVE BLOCK

The obturator nerve is situated much deeper than the femoral and lateral femoral cutaneous nerves, as it enters the thigh through the obturator foramen. The landmarks for this block are 2 cm medial and 2 cm caudad to the pubic tubercle (Fig. 20-12). A 10 cm needle will suffice in all but the most obese patients. It is introduced at right angles to the skin at this above site and advanced until it locates the inferior pubic ramus. It is then "walked" medially and cephalad until it slips off the bone and lies at the obturator foramen. A paresthesia may be sought by adjusting the needle position at this site for confirmation of placement. This is a difficult block for the operator and an uncomfortable one for the patient. It can be more expeditiously performed by using a nerve stimulator attachment to the needle, and the objective contractions of the adductor muscles on the medial side of the thigh are confirmatory evidence of needle placement.

Shortly after leaving the obturator foramen, the obturator nerve divides into anterior and posterior divisions that descend in the thigh, separated from each other by the adductor brevis muscle. It is feasible when using a nerve stimulator to just locate the posterior division; if the local anesthetic is only injected here, it will produce motor paralysis of adductor magnus and the genicular branch of the obturator to the knee joint but will not produce block of the anterior division, which supplies the adductor brevis, gracilis, and cutaneous supply over the medial aspect of the thigh. Therefore, it is important to attempt to block the nerve as close to its emergence from the obturator foramen as possible. Although the obturator nerve characteristically has a dermal distribution over the lower third of the medial side of the thigh, branches from the anterior division often supply more cephalad areas of the medial aspect of the thigh. Parks[22a] has modified this approach with success.

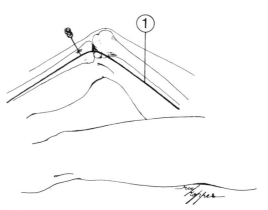

Fig. 20-13 The saphenous nerve (1) leaves the thigh on the medial aspect of the knee and is blocked by infiltrating a cuff of anesthesia over the medial side of the head of the tibia below the knee joint.

phenous nerve block can enable the commencement of surgery on the foot while the analgesia of the main femoral nerve is developing to cover subsequent tourniquet discomfort (Fig 20-13).

SAPHENOUS NERVE BLOCK

The saphenous nerve is the only part of the femoral nerve that supplies the lower extremity below the level of the knee. Therefore, in surgical procedures on this part of the lower extremity, it is sufficient to block the saphenous nerve and not necessary to produce complete femoral nerve analgesia unless a tourniquet is used. It is anesthetized by placing a cuff of anesthetic over the medial aspect of the proximal end of the tibia just below the knee. It accompanies the long saphenous vein and if that vein can be identified, infiltration on both sides of the vein will effect analgesia. This nerve block is sometimes useful for "rescuing" a sciatic femoral block for surgery of the foot or leg when the femoral component is either failed or is slow in onset. A sa-

SCIATIC NERVE BLOCK

The sciatic nerve is the largest peripheral nerve in the body and it is feasible to block this from posterior,[16] anterior,[22] or lateral[23] approaches at the hip. The most popular method is the posterior approach in the buttock.

The landmarks for blocking the sciatic nerve in the buttock are the posterior superior iliac spine and the greater trochanter. A line joining these two bony prominences is bisected. At a point 5 cm caudad on this line, a skin wheal is made for the puncture site for the nerve block (Figs. 20-9 and 20-14). The mass of the buttock determines the appropriate length of needle to use. This may be a 6 cm needle in a slim individual or a 10 cm needle in a more steatopygous type. As the needle is inserted and moved in a fan-like direction at right angles to the course of the sciatic nerve, the first paresthesia obtained is

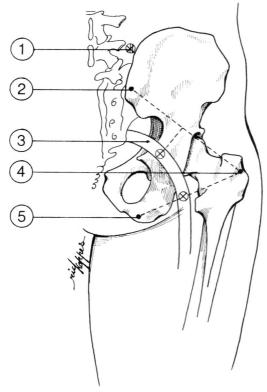

Fig. 20-14 The sciatic nerve (3) emerges from the greater sciatic notch and proceeds with a convex course in the buttocks to enter the thigh between the ischial tuberosity and the head of the femur. It can be blocked in the buttocks 4 to 5 cm caudad to the midpoint of a line joining the posterior superior iliac spine (2) to the greater trochanter (4). An alternative site for block in this region is at approximately the halfway point on a line joining the ischial tuberosity (5) to the greater trochanter (4). Sometimes the sciatic nerve lies medial to this midpoint. This figure also shows the site of entrance for the psoas compartment block. The needle is inserted at position 1, which is between the iliac crest and the L5 vertebra 3 cm caudad to the intercristal plane and 5 cm from the midline.

usually down the posterior aspect of the thigh due to the needle contacting the posterior cutaneous nerve of the thigh, which lies superficial to the sciatic in the buttock. This may be taken as a good indication that the needle is in

close proximity to the sciatic; 25 ml of local anesthetic is injected at this site or ideally a little deeper when a paresthesia to the foot confirms placement. Because of its large size and compact nature, care should be exercised not to repeatedly needle the nerve and an initial "gentle" paresthesia to the leg or foot should be sought.

An alternative approach for the sciatic nerve in this region is to block it as it leaves the buttock. This site is located at or medial to the midpoint of a line joining the greater trochanter to the ischial tuberosity. A similar paresthesia of the posterior cutaneous nerve of the thigh is usually first met with although if the sciatic nerve itself is contacted, then the paresthesia usually radiates to the foot.

The patient is usually positioned prone for a sciatic nerve block, although it is feasible to perform the posterior approach with the patient in the lateral decubitus position or even with the patient supine and the thigh flexed at the hip.[24] In this latter situation, an assistant is needed to hold the leg in position.

NERVE BLOCKS AT THE ANKLE

For surgical procedures on the foot that do not require a thigh or leg tourniquet it is feasible to anesthetize the nerves supplying the foot as they cross the ankle joint. Because the nerve supply to the foot involves several branches, the local anesthetic must be deposited in several sites to produce an effective block.

APPLIED ANATOMY OF THE ANKLE AND FOOT

The nerve supply of the foot is primarily from derivatives of the sciatic nerve, namely, its tibial, sural and, peroneal branches. As mentioned above the saphenous terminal branch of the femoral nerve also contributes to the innervation of the foot. The posterior tibial nerve enters the foot on the medial aspect with the posterior tibial artery. It divides at the level of the medial malleolus into medial and lateral plantar nerves that are distributed in the sole in a comparable pattern to the median and ulnar nerves in the hand, i.e., the medial plantar nerve supplies the skin of the preaxial three and a half digits and the lateral plantar supplies the skin of the postaxial one and a half digits (the fifth and half of the fourth toe). The sural nerve enters the foot laterally behind the lateral malleolus and supplies skin on the posterolateral aspect of the heel and the lateral aspect of the foot as far forward as the base of the small toe.

The peroneal nerves both superficial and deep supply the dorsal aspects of the foot. The superficial peroneal nerve supplies all of the dorsal aspects of the foot and the medial side of the great toe except the interdigital cleft between the great and second toe, which is supplied by the terminal branch of the deep peroneal nerve.

The saphenous nerve distribution and block is discussed in the section on the femoral nerve.

TECHNIQUES

The posterior tibial nerve is located on the medial aspect of the ankle posterior to the medial malleolus. It is located by palpating the pulsations of the adjacent posterior tibial artery, which lies usually anterior to the nerve. Infiltration of 5 ml of local anesthetic injected posterolateral to the artery at the level of the medial malleolus will produce anesthesia of the medial and lateral plantar nerves, that is, anesthesia of the sole and also the nail beds of the distal phallanges. A 4 to 6 centimeter needle is usually appropriate. Paresthesias may be elicited, but usually 5 ml of anesthetic solution is injected between skin and tibia, posterior to the pulsations of the artery about one fingerbreadth behind the medial malleolus (Fig. 20-15*A*).

SURAL NERVE BLOCK

The sural nerve, a superficial nerve, is blocked by a subcutaneous infiltration of local anesthetic on the lateral aspect of the ankle. This cuff of anesthesia is infiltrated from the lateral malleous to the Achilles tendon at the level of the ankle joint, usually using a total of 5 to 10 ml of local anesthetic (e.g., 1 percent lidocaine) (Fig. 20-15*A*).

SAPHENOUS AND PERONEAL NERVE BLOCKS

The saphenous and peroneal nerves supply the dorsal aspect of the foot. The saphenous nerve is situated anterior to the medial malleous running in company with the long saphenous vein. The superficial peroneal branches run subcutaneously over the lateral part of the line joining the medial and lateral malleoli across the dorsum of the foot. Therefore a subcutaneous cuff of anesthesia infiltrated from medial to lateral malleoli with the main amounts being deposited in the medial and lateral thirds of this line will yield analgesia of the skin of the dorsum of the foot (Fig. 20-15*B*).

The only remaining part of the foot that will have skin sensation at this stage is the interdigitial cleft between the great and second toe. If this must be anesthetized for the required surgery, the deep peroneal (anterior tibial) nerve is blocked at the level of the malleoli by identifying the tibialis anterior tendon by having the patient dorsiflex his foot. Palpation lateral to this tendon at the level of the malleoli will locate the pulsation of the anterior tibial artery. The nerve lies lateral to this artery, between the vessel and the extensor hallucis longus tendon deep to the extensor retinaculum. Therefore, a 5 cm needle is inserted at this point. A loss of resistance is detected as the needle passes through the flexor retinaculum, and although paresthesias are sometimes obtained to the

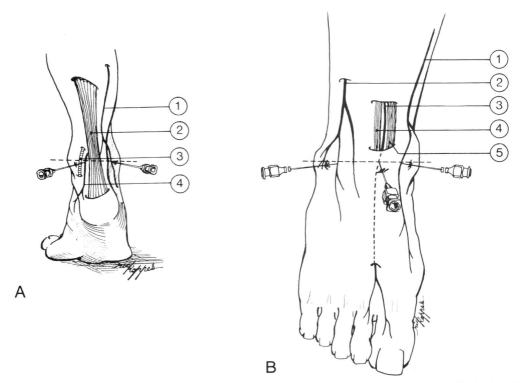

Fig. 20-15 Nerve blocks at the ankle. (*A*) Both the posterior tibial and the sural nerves are blocked at the level of the malleoli. The posterior tibial nerve (4) is located between the medial malleolus and the Achilles tendon (2). It lies posterior to the posterior tibial artery (3) at this level. The branches of the sural nerve (1) are anesthetized by infiltrating a cuff of anesthesia from the lateral malleolus to the Achilles tendon. (*B*) Nerve block of the dorsum of the foot involves the block of three nerves. The terminal branch of the saphenous nerve (1) is blocked by an infiltration cuff of anesthesia over the medial malleolus. The terminal branches of the superficial peroneal nerve (2) are anesthetized by a similar cuff of anesthesia over the lateral third of the dotted line joining the two malleoli. The deep peroneal (anterior tibial nerve) (3) is located at a deeper level on this same line between the tibialis anterior tendon (5) on its medial side and the extensor hallucis longus tendon (4) laterally. The tibialis anterior artery can sometimes be palpated at this level medial to the nerve.

first interdigital cleft, usually infiltration deep to the extensor retinaculum at this point will produce satisfactory analgesia of the deep peroneal nerve (Fig. 20-15*B*).

Use of this technique does not preclude a tourniquet; an Esmarch bandage can be applied to the foot from toes to the malleoli and the bandage then released distally leaving the proximal bandage in situ as a tourniquet.[25] Like most other forms of regional anesthesia this affords excellent pain relief, and because no major muscle groups in the lower extrem-ity are compromised for the procedure, early ambulation is feasible.

NERVE BLOCKS
IN THE HEAD AND NECK

Regional anesthesia of the head and neck was extensively used in days before general endotracheal anesthesia. It is used less often now but is still useful in individual clinical situations, especially for postoperative pain re-

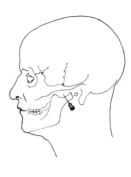

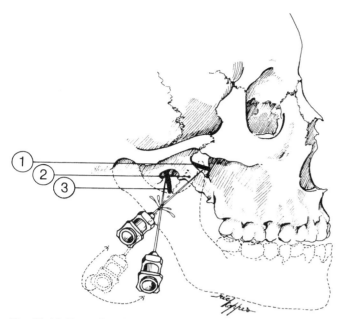

Fig. 20-16 Second and third division trigeminal nerve blocks. The needle is introduced (as shown in the smaller drawing) through the coronoid notch of the mandible, which is located under the midpoint of the zygoma and palpated by opening and closing the jaw. The needle is advanced to the lateral pterygoid plate (2) and for the second division block it is walked anteriorly into the pterygomaxillary fissure where the second division maxillary nerve (1) is located. To block the third division mandibular nerve (3), the needle is walked posteriorly off this lateral pterygoid plate until a paresthesia is obtained into the lower jaw.

lief and for the relief of chronic pain problems in the head and neck.

The important sensory nerves in this area are the trigeminal, glossopharyngeal, vagus, and cervical plexus.

TRIGEMINAL NERVE BLOCK

The trigeminal nerve divides into its three main branches in the middle cranial fossa. The first division passes through the superior orbital fissure, crosses the orbit, and is distributed to the forehead, nose, and upper eyelid. The second division leaves the middle cranial fossa through the foramen rotundum and is distributed to the derivatives of the upper jaw. Its cutaneous distribution is primarily to the cheek, upper lip, and zygoma regions. The third division exits from the skull

through the foramen ovale to enter the infratemporal fossa where it divides into its terminal divisions; the latter supply the muscles of mastication and sensation to the derivatives of the lower jaw, including the skin over the lower jaw, the temporal region, and even the vertex. It also supplies the skin of the upper two-thirds of the anterior surface of the ear. It is the nerve of supply to the mucous membrane over the anterior two-thirds of the tongue and the floor of the mouth.

With the advent of alternative techniques for the treatment of trigeminal neuralgia, there is now less need for Gasserian ganglion nerve block (Ch. 38). There is, however, still need for the second and third division blocks of the trigeminal nerve for various pain states and operative and postoperative analgesia. For discrete surgical procedures on the face under local anesthesia, block of the peripheral branches of the trigeminal nerve are sometimes indicated.

MAXILLARY AND MANDIBULAR NERVE BLOCK

The maxillary and mandibular nerves—two main branches of the trigeminal cranial nerve—can be blocked after they leave the foramina in the middle cranial fossa.

The maxillary division may be anesthetized as it exits from the skull through the foramen rotundum in the anterior wall of the middle cranial fossa and comes to lie in the pterygopalatine fossa between the skull and the upper jaw. The nerve can be blocked at this site via an approach across the infratemporal fossa as described below. The mandibular nerve, which is the nerve of supply to the derivatives of the lower jaw, leaves the skull through the foramen ovale in the floor of the middle cranial fossa; at this exit point it is situated immediately posterior to the lateral pterygoid plate of the sphenoid bone, which serves as a landmark.

For both these blocks, the needle is introduced through the coronoid notch of the mandible, which is below the midpoint of the zygoma (Fig. 20-16). The needle is advanced across the infratemporal fossa until it strikes the lateral pterygoid plate, which is on the medial wall of this anatomic compartment. To produce a second division (maxillary nerve block) the needle is walked anteriorly along the lateral pterygoid plate until it advances deeper into the pterygopalatine fossa. It is advanced a further centimeter and a bolus of 3 ml of local anesthetic is injected at this site. This will produce analgesia of the second division of the trigeminal nerve—an area that includes the upper jaw and its derivatives including the skin over the cheek, upper lip, and lower eye lid. For the third division mandibular nerve block, the needle is walked posteriorly off the lateral pterygoid plate and a bolus of 3 ml of local anesthetic is injected at the posterior limit of this plate; this

injection often creates a mandibular nerve paresthesia to the ipsilateral lower jaw and/or lower lip.

Complications of the second division block are that of puncture of one of the terminal branches of the maxillary artery or its venae comitantes with possible retro-orbital hematoma. It is also possible if the needle is inserted too deeply, to transgress on retro-orbital structures with spread of local anesthetic to optic nerve, resulting in temporary blindness. Therefore, small, discrete quantities of anesthetic should be used and the needle should not be angled cephalad in this approach. If the needle is introduced through the coronoid notch, it is difficult, if not impossible, for the needle to be manipulated into the retro-orbital area.

Complications of the third division block can result if the needle, inserted too deeply beyond the posterior limits of the lateral pterygoid plate, punctures the superior constrictor muscle of the pharynx; the needle point will then lie within the pharynx, which is a potentially infected area, and be withdrawn through the infratemporal fossa and possibly seed bacteria. This, however, appears to be more a theoretic than real problem.

BLOCK OF OTHER PERIPHERAL BRANCHES OF THE TRIGEMINAL NERVE

The terminal branches of the trigeminal nerve supply the skin of the face. The first division branches supply the brow, upper eyelid, and nose. The second division branches supply the skin of the cheek, lower eyelid, and zygoma region. The third division terminal branches supply the skin of the lower jaw, the temporal region, and the upper two-thirds of the anterior surface of the ear. Block of the second (maxillary) and third (mandibular) divisions are described above.

The terminal nerves of these three divisions emerge onto the face through foramina that lie in the same vertical plane as the pupil when the eye is looking directly forward.

The supraorbital branches of the first division can be blocked above the eyebrow in this plane. In practice, a cuff of anesthesia is infiltrated over the medial half of the forehead above the eyebrow; this infiltration of local anesthetic will anesthetize the supraorbital and supratrochlear terminal branches of the first division (ophthalmic) of the trigeminal nerve and thus anesthetize the forehead. Surgical procedures limited to this area can then be performed. The skin of the nose is supplied by the infratrochlear nerve superiorly and the external nasal nerve over the lower part of the nose and tip. The infratrochlear nerve is anesthetized by infiltrating the local anesthetic at the junction of the nasal bones and cartilage. This block can be used to anesthetize the tip of the nose for surgical procedures in that area.

The infraorbital or terminal branch of the second division (maxillary nerve) of the trigeminal nerve can be blocked one fingerbreadth below the orbital margin in the vertical line of the pupil. Infiltrations at this point can be made either extraorally or intraorally and will provide anesthesia over the cheek and upper lip.

The mental nerve is the terminal branch of the third division; this nerve emerges through the mental foramen and varies in position from inferior to superior border of the mandible from infancy to old age. This foramen is also situated in the same vertical plane as the pupil when the eye is looking directly forward, and the nerve can be blocked either extraorally or intraorally at this site. Analgesia of the ipsilateral lower lip will result.

GLOSSOPHARYNGEAL NERVE BLOCK

The glossopharyngeal nerve exits from the skull through the jugular foramen along with the internal jugular vein, the vagus, and the accessory nerves. It sweeps forward, closely related to the styloid process of the sphenoid bone and the large vessels of the internal carotid and internal jugular vein. Its sensory supply is to the posterior one-third of the tongue, the pharnyx, and the superior surface of the epiglottis; its motor supply is to the muscles of deglutition. Blocking this nerve is necessary in certain terminal cancer conditions and as a diagnostic maneuver in the rare phenomenon of glossopharyngeal tic pain, which is a similar problem to trigeminal neuralgia but occurs in the distribution of the glossopharyngeal nerve. Because of its close proximity to the vagus and accessory nerves after it leaves the skull through the jugular foramen, it is best to try and block the nerve at a more distal site as it sweeps around the styloid process of the temporal bone. This site is located by finding the midpoint of the line joining the angle of the mandible to the mastoid process. It is sometimes possible on deep pressure to palpate the styloid process at this site. A 6 cm needle is inserted to a depth of approximately 3 to 4 cm and contact is sought with the styloid process. If a glossopharyngeal paresthesia to the pharynx or posterior tongue is obtained, then this is taken as confirmatory evidence of correct needle placement. In the event that no paresthesia is obtained, the needle is aligned posterior to the styloid process and 3 to 5 ml of local anesthetic is injected. It is still possible that spread will occur to involve the vagus nerve and maybe the accessory nerve with resultant laryngeal anesthesia and weakness of the sternomastoid and trapezius muscles respectively. Because of the proximity of the large vessels, aspiration tests with a small 0.25 ml test dose are mandatory.

Successful block will result in analgesia of the ipsilateral posterior one-third of the tongue, the tonsillar area, and the pharynx. This block is useful for patients who have carcinoma in these areas. Since such patients have often had a radical neck resection and the stermomastoid muscle has been removed, identification of the styloid process and, therefore, glossopharyngeal block is much easier.

VAGUS NERVE BLOCK

The vagus nerve is widely distributed. Its important branches for regional anesthesia are those sensory branches to the larynx and trachea. It is useful to block these for intubation procedures and also to treat chronic pain due to cancer of the larynx or trachea.

The sensory and motor supply of the larynx and trachea are the superior and recurrent laryngeal branches of the vagus. The superior laryngeal branches leave the vagus high in the neck and sweep forward below the greater cornu of the hyoid bone; here the nerve divides into an internal laryngeal branch that pierces the thyroid membrane and supplies the laryngeal inlet down to the level of the vocal cords. An external branch passes down external to the larynx to provide motor supply to the cricothyroid muscle.

The recurrent laryngeal nerve follows different courses on the right and left sides of the neck. On the right side of the neck, the nerve arises from the vagus low in the neck, passes around the subclavian artery and runs up to the larynx in the groove between trachea and esophagus. On the left side, the nerve arises from the vagus in the thorax and loops around the arch of the aorta (more specifically the ductus arteriosis) and again passes to the larynx in the groove between esophagus and trachea. The recurrent laryngeal nerve is the nerve of supply to all the muscles of the larynx except the cricothyroid muscle mentioned above, which is innervated by the superior laryngeal nerve. The recurrent laryngeal nerve also supplies sensation to the larynx below the vocal cords and to the trachea.

The superior laryngeal nerve is readily and easily blocked as it passes below the greater cornu of the hyoid bone. Although the recurrent laryngeal nerve can be blocked in the groove between trachea and esophagus (and frequently is as a complication of stellate ganglion block), the most effective way to block this distribution is usually by means of a transtracheal or peroral spray of the area.

CERVICAL PLEXUS BLOCKS

The cervical plexus is derived from the C1, C2, C3, and C4 spinal nerves. C1 is primarily involved in motor supply to the muscles of the suboccipital triangle. Cervical nerves 2, 3, and 4 contribute to the deep and superficial cervical plexus, which supply the musculature of the neck in a segmental fashion and form the dermatomal supply to the skin of the neck from the trigeminally innervated face down to the axial lines of the upper extremity; at the latter, C4 innervated skin meets the T2 dermatomes of the trunk.

The deep cervical plexus forms in the paravertebral region of the second, third, and fourth cervical vertebrae. The nerves arise between the scalene muscles in craniad continuity with the nerves that form the brachial plexus. Therefore, block of the brachial plexus via the interscalene approach will frequently involve cephalad spread that anesthetizes the deep cervical plexus producing dermatomal and myotomal anesthesia of the neck.

The deep cervical plexus is electively blocked for such neck surgery as thyroidectomies and tracheostomies. Traditionally it was produced by inserting three needles, one each at C2, C3, and C4, posterior to a line joining the mastoid process to Chassiagnac's turbercle of the sixth cervical vertebra. The C4 level is located at the intersection of this line with a horizontal line drawn through the lower border of the ramus of the mandible. In fact, a single needle technique and injection of 10 ml or so of anesthetic at this single level (C4) will usually produce a satisfactory cervical plexus block. More recently, Winnie[26] has suggested producing such a block by introducing the needle higher in the interscalene groove than that for brachial plexus block and by using digital pressure caudad to the injection site to direct the anesthetic to the cervical plexus. Both these above methods afford satisfactory deep cervical plexus block anesthesia of the deep muscle and the skin of the neck. This block will not, of course, anesthetize the vagally innervated viscera of the larynx and trachea. If such a bilateral cervical plexus block is used for tracheostomy, either local spray or laryngeal nerve analgesia will be required to supplement the block.

If only cutaneous analgesia is needed in the neck, then a superficial cervical plexus block will suffice. These nerves are located at or about the midpoint of the posterior border of the sternomastoid muscle. From this point, they radiate like the spokes of a wheel anteriorly (anterior cervical nerves), inferiorly (supraclavicular nerves), and superiorly and posteriorly (great auricular nerve). They can be anesthetized by the infiltration of local anesthetic over the posterior border of the sternomastoid muscle in its middle third. Ten to 15 ml of local anesthetic injected at this site will produce analgesia over the C2, C3, and C4 dermatomes. If the infiltration is carried out deep to the deep fascia over the posterior triangle of the neck in this site and motor blocking concentrations of drug are used, then the accessory nerve may also be involved in this block; the patient should thus be warned that for the duration of the block he may develop a drop shoulder due to trapezius muscle paralysis.

Complications of cervical plexus block are primarily those of accidental injection or spread of the local anesthetic into the vertebral artery (producing systemic toxic convulsion reactions) or accidental injection into the cervical epidural or subarachnoid space (producing high or total spinal anesthesia). To prevent intravascular injection, aspiration tests are, of course, mandatory. In an attempt to prevent accidental subarachnoid injection into dural sleeves of the subarachnoid space and/or accidental injection through the paravertebral foramina, caudad direction of the needle and aspiration tests for cerebrospinal fluid must be made. However, a negative aspiration test does not necessarily mean that the needle point has not been situated in a dural sleeve of the subarachnoid space. Therefore, a small test dose of 2 ml is appropriate. If motor-blocking concentrations of drug are used, deep cervical plexus block will usually produce phrenic nerve palsy. Because the diaphragm is innervated only in its central part by the phrenic nerve and laterally by the lower intercostal nerves, phrenic nerve block does not necessarily overly compromise respiration at rest. However, in patients, such as paraplegics or quadraplegics, who have a paralyzed chest wall, a motor block of the phrenic nerve can cause considerable if not complete respiratory embarrassment; this block is best avoided in those with high level spinal cord injuries.

INTERCOSTAL NERVE BLOCKS

Intercostal nerve blocks are very useful for surgical anesthesia and for the control of postoperative and other acute pain states such as that resulting from broken ribs.[27]

APPLIED ANATOMY

Intercostal nerves T1 through T12 are the anterior primary rami of the segmental nerves of supply to the body wall of the thorax and abdomen. They pursue a circumferential course around the trunk, supplying intercostal and abdominal wall muscles and skin on the anterior and lateral walls of the trunk. In the thorax their course is under the inferior margin of the rib of the same segmental level. A neurovascular bundle of vein, artery, and nerve run together deep to the intercostal muscles in the intercostal space.

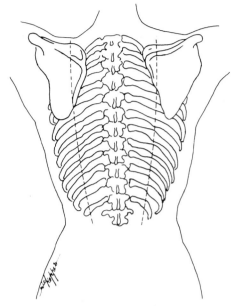

Fig. 20-17 Dorsal view of the patient's position for intercostal nerve block. The intercostal blocks are performed along the dotted lines shown in the diagram, which is the site in which the ribs first become palpable and is approximately 8 to 10 cm from the midline (about one handwidth). Note that the upper extremities are swung upwards rotating the scapula away from the midline and permitting access to the sixth, fifth, and sometimes even fourth intercostal space.

TECHNIQUE

Depending on the extent of the analgesia required, the intercostal nerve can be blocked at any stage in its course. To effectively pro-duce analgesia of the anterior and lateral thoracic and abdominal walls, it needs to be blocked before the lateral cutaneous branches arise at the midaxillary line. Therefore, it is usually blocked 8 cm from the midline posteriorly, where the rib can be palpated. Because of the angle of the rib as it arises from the vertebra, the rib is not palpable in the immediate paravertebral region and only becomes subcutaneous approximately 8 cm from the midline (Fig. 20-17). The ribs are identified at this site; the arms are abducted and placed alongside the head. This assures rotation of the scapula and enables ribs 6 through 4 to be palpated and the appropriate intercostal nerve blocked if this is required. When the arms are by the side, the ribs are covered by scapula and therefore cannot be palpated.

A skin wheal is made over the intercostal space and then the skin wheal is pulled cephalad so that it rests over the rib above the nerve to be blocked (Fig. 20-18). A short bevel 4 to 5 cm needle is inserted through the skin as the wheal is held over the rib, and the periosteum of the rib is used as the end point for needle advancement. A little local infiltration of this periosteum makes the procedure more comfortable for the patient. The needle is now walked off the inferior border of the rib by withdrawing the needle to subcutaneous tissue and permitting the skin to retract caudally as the needle is walked along the rib. As the needle slips off the lower border of the rib it will pop through the intercostal muscle and a loss of resistance will be

Fig. 20-18 Intercostal nerve block. (*A*) The intercostal space is identified by the index and middle fingers ▶ of the anesthesiologist's nondominant hand. Numbers point to rib (1); intercostal neurovascular bundle containing intercostal vein, artery and nerve from within out (2); intercostal muscles both internal and external (3); lung (4); and visceral and parietal pleural layers (5).

(*B*) The anesthesiologist's fingers move the skin wheal cephalad over the rib above the intercostal space. The needle is now inserted at this site so that the rib acts as a bony end point to prevent accidental excessive advancement with possible pleural puncture.

(*C*) The needle is walked caudally as the skin wheal is allowed to retract in a similar direction. As the needle slips off the lower end of the rib it pierces the intercostal muscles and enters the potential space between these muscles and the parietal pleura. A subtle loss of resistance is often appreciated at this stage and an injection is made into this space without any active attempts to seek paresthesia.

appreciated. The patient is told to hold his breath to reduce movement and possible needle displacement. The needle is then "locked" at this site, aspiration tests performed, and 5 ml of local anesthetic injected. A series of intercostal blocks from T4 through T12 will produce effective and profound analgesia of the anterior abdominal wall and along with a celiac plexus block (see Ch. 38) will permit extensive intra-abdominal surgery. Individual blocks on combinations of intercostal nerves can be used to produce more focal analgesia as may be required for cholecystectomy or thoracotomy, postoperative pain control, or for pain relief for broken ribs.

PARAVERTEBRAL NERVE BLOCKS

The paravertebral segmental nerves can be blocked in the paravertebral space from C1 to L5. The technique in all cases is a modification of a similar approach of locating the bony landmark, usually the transverse process or the lamina of the appropriate vertebra, and then walking the needle off the transverse process or lamina into the paravertebral space. This space readily communicates with adjacent paravertebral spaces, and if a large volume of local anesthetic is injected into one space, it will spread to anesthetize adjacent nerves. This block is used primarily for diagnostic work, although it is quite feasible to produce operative anesthesia by a combination of paravertebral nerve blocks. This technique might be considered for operative use in those patients in whom there is some contraindication to blocks that are closer to the neuraxis, such as spinal or epidural blocks. Such contraindications might occur in those with clotting defects or congenital or postoperative bony impediments that preclude spinal or epidural anesthesia.

LUMBAR PARAVERTEBRAL BLOCK

The technique for this paravertebral block is as follows. A skin wheal is raised 2.5 cm lateral to the rostral end of the spine of the lumbar vertebra of the level to be blocked. An 8 cm needle is introduced through this wheal and advanced until contact with the transverse process is obtained. The needle is now walked posteriorly off the transverse process and advanced an additional 1.0 to 2.0 cm so that it lies in the paravertebral space; if this space is flooded with 5 ml local anesthetic, analgesia of the nerve should occur. If paresthesias are required, the needle is walked the length of the paravertebral space to the transverse process below until the paresthesia is obtained. A stimulat-

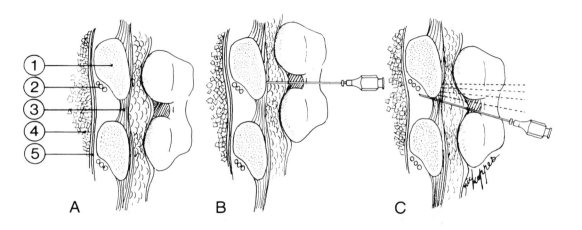

1
2
3
4
5

A   B   C

ing needle is of great assistance in such procedures.

THORACIC PARAVERTEBRAL BLOCK

The principle of the thoracic paravertebral block is the same as with the block in the lumbar region, although here the landmarks are less clear. The reason for this is that the obliquity of angle of the thoracic vertebral spines are such that in the midthoracic region the spines may overlap the vertebral level two spinal segments below. Therefore, it is not clinically feasible to predictably and specifically block a particular thoracic paravertebral nerve without the use of roentgenographic confirmation. Because of the risk of pneumothorax with this block, the strategy is to insert the needle 1 cm paravertebrally and using the lamina as an end point walk the needle laterally into the paravertebral space in the hope that with this approach there will be less likelihood of contacting parietal pleura. This approach is useful for postthoracotomy pain relief, when usually the existence of chest drains and the like preclude the concerns about pneumothorax. Because of the location of the scapula, intercostal block for the first three or four intercostal nerves is usually not feasible, and to produce analgesia of these to treat, for example, a fractured rib, paravertebral blocks would need to be done.

SACRAL NERVE BLOCK

Transsacral block of sacral nerves 1 through 4 is, in essence, a paravertebral block and the nerves are approached through the posterior sacral foramina. These blocks are used usually diagnostically and therapeutically for urologic problems of bladder spasm in patients with spinal cord damage. They can also be used diagnostically and therapeutically in certain pain states, but they have limited application for surgery because there are simpler ways of effecting analgesia in these dermatomes (by either caudal or sciatic nerve anesthesia).

ANATOMY

The posterior sacral foramina lie in a paramedian position on the dorsal aspect of the sacrum. The landmarks for identifying these foramina are shown in Figure 20-19*A*. The S1 posterior foramina is located 1 cm medial and superior to the posterior superior iliac spine. A mark made at this site is joined to a point 1 cm lateral and cephalad to the ipsilateral sacral cornu and the remaining sacral foramina of S2, S3, and S4 are found at equidistant intervals on this line.

TECHNIQUE

It is important to appreciate the dorsal convexity of the sacrum and to note that the sacral foramina are not parallel to each other but related to each other more like radii of the same circle. Therefore, needles successfully positioned in the sacral foramina will diverge from each other and not be parallel (Fig. 20-19*B*). This convexity of the sacrum is more marked in the female pelvis than male. This can be an uncomfortable block because of the frequent contact with periosteum that is sometimes necessary before successfully walking the needle into the foramina. Therefore, generous subcutaneous and periosteal infiltrations of local anesthetics should be made. The needles, once they enter the foramina, are advanced for 1 to 2 cm or until a paresthesia of the ventral sacral root is obtained.

Complications of this procedure are that of occasional epidural or even subarachnoid spread, especially from the upper S1 and S2 nerves. Another complication can result from too deep an advancement of the needle so that it exits from the anterior sacral foramen into the pelvis, where the rectum is a close

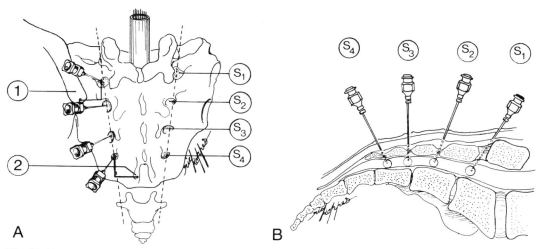

Fig. 20-19 (*A & B*) Transsacral block. The sacral nerves are blocked via the posterior sacral foramina S1, S2, S3, and S4. S1 is located 1 cm medial and cephalad from the posterior superior iliac spine (1). S4 sacral foramina is located 1 cm lateral and cephalad from the sacral cornu (2). S3 and S2 are at approximate equidistant intervals along this line. Note the dorsal convexity of the sacrum. Because of this, the posterior sacral foramina are not parallel to each other and therefore when correctly positioned, the needles are not parallel.

relation; if this occurs the needle could theoretically be inserted into a highly infected area and then subsequently withdrawn, seeding pathogenic bacteria in the sacral canal. This however appears to be of more theoretic than practical concern.

INTRAVENOUS REGIONAL ANESTHESIA

Intravenous regional anesthesia, first described by Bier[28] at the turn of the century, has proven a very useful and safe block for extremity analgesia. It is ideally suited for surgical procedures on the hand or forearm and lends itself well to the emergency situation when skilled anesthetic help is not at hand. Its safety has permitted its use by many nonanesthetic personnel and the morbidity and mortality from its widespread use is minimal.[29–32]

The principle employed is that of isolating the vascular supply to the distal extremity by a proximally placed tourniquet on the arm or thigh. The limb is ideally exsanguinated prior to inflating the tourniquet and then the isolated vascular segment is injected with a weak local anesthetic solution (e.g., 0.5 percent lidocaine or 0.25 percent bupivacaine) that will produce a rapid onset analgesia which will last until the tourniquet is deflated.[33]

TECHNIQUE

Because the tourniquet produces pain after 30 to 40 minutes, a double tourniquet system is used as follows.

An intravenous portal is established distally in the limb to be blocked; this opening should be as close to the operative site as convenience permits. The intravenous cannula is attached via an extension tube to a reservoir syringe of local anesthetic. The double tourniquet is applied proximally to the limb (either arm or thigh) and the limb is then elevated above the level of the trunk. If the clinical conditions permit, an Esmarch bandage is applied to the limb from the distal aspects of the digits to tourniquet. The proximal tourniquet is now inflated to 50 cm above systolic blood pressure and the Esmarch bandage removed. The local anesthetic is injected (50 ml for an upper extremity, 100 ml for a lower extremity) and a cadaveric mottling is noticed in the skin as the remaining blood is displaced from the vascular system. The onset of anesthesia is rapid, usually within 5 to 10 minutes, and surgery can proceed.

It is customary to remove the intravenous cannula prior to the onset of surgery, although this is by no means essential; if an extended surgical procedure is envisaged, it is as well to leave the portal in situ so that if it is necessary to release the tourniquet from time to time, the limb can be reinjected after reinflation. After the initial injection, analgesia is produced up to, but not including, the limb under the proximal tourniquet. Most patients will tolerate this tourniquet discomfort for a 20 to 40 minute interval depending on the nature of the patient. When the patient complains of tourniquet discomfort, then the distal tourniquet is inflated over what will be analgesic skin. When tests have confirmed the efficacy of this distal tourniquet, then the proximal tourniquet is deflated, usually with much relief to the patient. The patient will now remain comfortable for an additional 15 to 30 minutes before the distal tourniquet starts to produce discomfort. All in all, one can anticipate probably 45 to 60 minutes of maximum satisfactory analgesia with this above technique. If the surgery is going to be longer than this, then deflation of the tourniquet with subsequent reexsanguination and reinjection will probably be necessary or selection of an alternative anesthetic technique will be needed. Usually with deflation of the tourniquet, sensation returns rapidly to the limb. If bupivacaine is used, however, there is often a 10 minute or so "grace" period when analgesia remains, and this permits those surgeons who require it to test for hemostasis prior to placing the last skin sutures.[34]

With deflation of the tourniquet, local anesthetic is flushed out into the system and theoretically poses a potential for toxic reactions. In actual fact, these are a rare event with this technique. Although the venous blood draining the limb often has quite high concentrations of local anesthetic, by the time this venous blood from the limb has passed through the lungs and becomes mixed with the rest of the venous return, the systemic arterial levels are usually much lower.[35] Vigilant monitoring will detect cardiovascular depression at this time, usually manifested by bradycardia of about 10 beats a minute, but this is usually not significant clinically.[36] There have also been reports of an isolated transient asystole.[37] By and large, however, this intravenous technique is very safe and lends itself well to the ambulant outpatient or emergency patient who needs such procedures as a Colley's fracture reduction and repairs of lacerations. Phlebitis has been reported as a sequel to this anesthetic procedure when chloroprocaine was used and for this reason, it is probably best to avoid using this agent with this technique.[37a]

COMPLICATIONS OF REGIONAL NERVE BLOCKS

SYSTEMIC LOCAL ANESTHETIC TOXICITY

Whenever large quantities of local anesthetic are administered or smaller quantities injected near blood vessels, the risk of intravascular accidental injection is ever present and systemic toxic reactions can result. For the most part, these crises are best prevented by frequent aspiration tests to ascertain that the needle has not entered the lumen of a blood vessel and by strict observance of safe limits of injection dose. Diazepam (0.15 mg/kg) raises the convulsion threshold to local anesthetics by about 50 percent[3] and, therefore, as mentioned above is a useful premedication. In the event that convulsions occur, the danger is of hypoxic insult to the central nervous system and oxygenation is critical. One hundred percent oxygen by mask, with positive pressure if need be, must be administered and the airway protected by intubation if necessary. Small titrated doses of a CNS depressant, diazepam 1 to 5 mg/70 kg or thiopental 25 to 50 mg/70 kg, will usually abort the attack and neither positive pressure nor intubation are required unless frank convulsions uncontrolled by the above simple method occur.

Injections of local anesthetic drugs around the neuraxis, even in small quantities, can result in epidural or even subarachnoid spread via inadvertently placing the needle through the paravertebral foramen or injection into dural sleeves that extend distal to this foramen. The management of total spinal and high epidural blocks is discussed in Chapter 21.

LOCAL TISSUE TOXICITY

When used in conventional concentrations, local anesthetics have not been shown to produce localized nerve damage, and in preparations *in vitro* irreversible nerve block is only produced by concentrations in excess of those used clinically.[38] The addition of epinephrine to local anesthetic solutions is frequently used to prolong the block and reduce the uptake of local anesthetic from the site of injection. Provided an optimal concentration is used, i.e., 1/200,000, there does not appear to be any complication associated with its use.[39] Epinephrine should not be added to the local anesthetic solution for ring blocks of the digits and penis because tissue ischemia may result. Selander[40] has recently shown, in studies with animals, an increased incidence of axonal degeneration with epinephrine containing bupivacaine.

PROLONGED BLOCK

There is considerable individual variation in the duration of action of local anesthetic agents in different patients. In the event that an unduly prolonged block persists beyond the expected recovery time, the priorities are to ensure that the anesthetized area is protected with splints, padding, and support to prevent trauma to the part. A comprehensive neurologic evaluation is necessary to ascertain the status of the defect. It is often appropriate at this stage to enlist the second opinion of neurologists and physiatrists to document the sensory and motor defects and maybe by the use of electromyography, to ascertain the site of any lesion.[41] In the event that permanent block results, a comprehensive evaluation by these specialists is in order and their contact with the patient must be maintained.

DIFFERENTIAL DIAGNOSIS OF NERVE DAMAGE

It is important when evaluating nerve damage that has occurred following the regional anesthetic technique to ascertain the neurologic characteristics of the defect and to see if it correlates with the peripheral distribution of the alleged nerve that was damaged.

There are many instances of nerve damage being due to other problems than the anesthetic when there is faulty positioning of patients during surgery and pressure produces paresis of the nerve involved. Such examples are either the saphenous or lateral popliteal nerve being compressed against lithotomy stirrups. Also, the sciatic nerve has been injured in thin individuals by the pressure of lying on an operating table for prolonged periods, and the sciatic nerve is also at risk in the immediate postoperative period from intragluteal injections. The femoral nerve can be damaged by use of self-retaining retractors in lower abdominal procedures and the prolonged and inappropriate use of a tourniquet can result in nerve damage.[42]

It is vitally important to ascertain if some of the above factors are responsible for the defects often ascribed to the local anesthetic technique.

INFECTION

Infection is rarely seen if conventional techniques of sterilization of equipment and aseptic procedures are used. Local anesthetics appear to have antimicrobial activity, being bacteriostatic and possibly bacteriocidal.[43] Severe and fulminating infections due to bowel organisms have been described from time to time, usually when injections have occurred in contaminated areas, such as in the perineum at the time of giving birth.[44]

HEMATOMAS

Hematoma formation following nerve block procedures can cause permanent nerve damage.[45] To reduce the incidence, it is important, if at all possible, to avoid using regional anesthesia in those patients on anticoagulation therapy. Sometimes it is a difficult decision to deny the patient the benefits of a regional nerve block when general anesthesia is perhaps contraindicated, and some of these difficult decisions can only be applied on an individual basis at this moment in time because of a lack of sufficient data on this subject. It is usually wise to avoid needling procedures in anticoagulated patients.

PNEUMOTHORAX

Pneumothorax is a risk in any nerve block that involves insertion of the needle in relationship to the thoracic cage, such as intercostal blocks, brachial plexus blocks, and thoracic paravertebral blocks. As skill is gained in accomplishing these blocks the incidence of pneumothorax is less, but even in expert hands these sequelae occur from time to time.[17]

Pneumothorax should be suspected in any patient complaining of breathlessness after a nerve block procedure in the region of the thoracic cage. Physical examination of the chest may reveal the presence of pneumothorax, which can be confirmed with a chest radiograph. If pneumothorax is less than 20 percent, symptomatic therapy, bedrest and observation are usually all that is required until spontaneous recovery occurs. However, if greater than this, close observation is necessary, and should the lung fail to reexpand in 24 hours, active decompression is probably indicated. This is accomplished by insertion of a chest tube with an underwater seal through the second intercostal space in the midclavicular line. If after a nerve block procedure the anesthesiologist is concerned that the needle may have punctured the pleura, it is advisable to have the patient remain at quiet bed rest under supervision for the next 24 hours because clinically significant pneumothorax can develop later than the immediate postblock period.

Although it is possible to practice anesthesia using general inhalational techniques alone, those anesthesiologists with skill in regional nerve blocks will be able to offer their patients and surgical colleagues an alternative and, many times, an improved service, not only at the time of operation, but also for pain relief in the postoperative period. It does require greater preparation at the time of the preoperative visit and also in the immediate presurgical induction period. However, the anesthesiologist who acquires the technical and nontechnical skills of handling patients under regional anesthesia will find much personal satisfaction in this extension of his repertoire.

REFERENCES

1. Winnie AP: Clinical pharmacokinetics of local anesthetics. Can Anesth Soc J 5: 24, 1971
2. De Jong RH: Physiology and Pharmacology of Local Anesthesia. Springfield, IL, Charles C Thomas, 1970
3. De Jong RH; Heavner JE: Local anesthetic seizure prevention: Diazepam versus Pentothal. Anesthesiology 36: 449, 1972
4. Selander D, Dhuner KG, Lundborg G: Peripheral nerve injury due to injection needles

used for regional anesthesia. Acta Anaesthesiol Scand 21: 182, 1977

5. Selander I, Edshage S, Wolff T: Paresthesia or no paresthesia? Nerve lesions after axillary blocks. Acta Anaesthesiol Scand 23: 27, 1979

6. Greenblatt GM, Denson JS: Needle nerve stimulator-locator nerve blocks with new instrument for locating nerves. Anesth Analg 41:599, 1962

7. Montgomery SJ, Raj PP, Nettles D, et al: The use of nerve stimulator with standard unsheathed needles in nerve blockade. Anesth Analg 52: 827, 1973

8. Wright BD: A new use for the block-aid monitor and plastic intravenous cannulas for nerve blocks. Anesthesiology 31:290, 1969

9. Winnie AP: Interscalene brachial plexus block. Anesth Analg 49: 455, 1970

10. Sharrock NE, Bruce G: An improved technique for locating the interscalene groove. Anesthesiology 44: 431, 1976

11. Winnie AP: An immobile needle for nerve blocks. Anesthesiology 31: 577, 1969

12. Winnie AP, Rodonjic R, Akkineni SR, et al: Factors influencing distribution of local anesthetic injected into the brachial plexus sheath. Anesth Analg 48: 225, 1979

13. Korevaar WC, Burney RG, Moore PA: Convulsions during stellate ganglion block. A case report. Anesth Analg 58: 329, 1979

14. Kumar A, Battit GE, Froese AB, et al: Bilateral cervical and thoracic epidural blockade complicating interscalene brachial plexus block: A report of two cases. Anesthesiology 35: 650, 1971

15. Ross S, Scarborough CD: Total spinal anesthesia following brachial plexus block. Anesthesiology 39: 458, 1973

16. Moore DC: Regional Block. 4th edition. Springfield, IL, Charles C Thomas, 1965

17. Moore DC: Complications of Regional Anesthesia. Springfield, IL, Charles C Thomas, 1955

18. De Jong RH: Axillary block of brachial plexus. Anesthesiology 22: 215, 1961

19. Raj PP, Montgomery SJ, Nettles D, et al: Infraclavicular brachiah plexus block. A new approach. Anesth Analg 52: 897, 1973

19a. Sim JK: A modification of landmarks for infraclavicular approach to brachial plexus block. Anesth Analg 56:554, 1977

20. Chayden D, Nathan H, Chayden M: The psoas compartment block. Anesthesiology 45: 95, 1976

21. Winnie AP, Ramamurthy S, Durran Z: The inguinal perivascular technic of lumbar plexus anesthesia: The 3 in 1 block. Anesth Analg 52: 989, 1973

22. Beck GP: Anterior approach to sciatic nerve. Anesthesiology 24: 222, 1963

22a. Parks CR, Kennedy WF: Obturator nerve block: A simplified approach. Anesthesiology 28:775, 1967

23. Ichiyanagi K: Sciatic nerve block: Lateral approach with the patient supine. Anesthesiology 20: 601, 1969

24. Raj PP, Parks RI, Watson TD, et al: A new single position supine approach to sciatic femoral block. Anesth Analg 54: 489, 1975

25. Schurman DJ: Ankle block for foot surgery. Anesthesiology 44: 348, 1976

26. Winnie AP, Ramamurthy S, Durrani Z, et al: Cervical plexus block simplified: A single injection technique. Anesth Analg 54: 370, 1975

27. Moore DC, Bridenbaugh LD: Intercostal block in 4333 patients: Indications, technique and complications. Anesth Analg 41: 1, 1962

28. Bier A: Versuche über Cocainisirung des Rückenmarkes. Dtsch A Chir 51: 361, 1899

29. Holmes CM: Intravenous regional analgesia. A useful method of producing analgesia of the limbs. Lancet 1: 245, 1963

30. Kennedy BR, Duthie AM, Parbrook GD, et al: Intravenous regional analgesia: An appraisal. Br Med J 5440: 954, 1965

31. Erickson E: Illustrated Handbook in Local Anaesthesia. Copenhagen, Munksgaard, 1969

32. Ericksen E, Person A, Ortengren B: Intravenous anaesthesia. An attempt to determine the safety of the method and a comparison between prilocaine and lidocaine. Acta Chir Scand (suppl.) 358: 47, 1966

33. Raj PP, Garcia CE, Burleson JW, et al: The site of action of intravenous regional anesthesia. Anesth Analg 51: 776, 1972

34. Evans CJ, Dewar JA, Boyes RW, et al: Residual nerve block following intravenous regional anaesthesia. Br J Anaesth 46: 668, 1974

35. Tucker GT, Boas RA: Pharmacokinetic aspects of intravenous regional anesthesia. Anesthesiology 34: 538, 1971

36. Kew MC, Lowe JP: The cardiovascular complications of intravenous regional anesthesia. Br J Surg 58: 179, 1971

37. Thorn-Alquist AM: Intravenous regional anesthesia. A 7-year survey. Acta Anaesthesiol Scand 15: 23, 1971

37a. Harris WH: Choice of anaesthetic agents for intravenous anaesthesia. Acta Anaesthesiol Scand (suppl.) 36:47, 1969

38. Skou JC: Toxicity of local anesthetics. Acta Pharmacol Toxicol 10: 292, 1954

39. Dhuner KG: Frequency of general side reactions after regional anesthesia with mepivacaine with and without vasoconstrictors. Acta Anaesthesiol Scand (suppl.) 48: 23, 1972

40. Selander D, Brattsand R, Lundborg G, et al: Local anesthetics: Importance of mode of application, concentration and adrenalin for the appearance of nerve lesions. Acta Anaesthesiol Scand 23: 127, 1979

41. Jebsen RH: Electrodiagnosis in nerve root syndromes. Northwest Med 65: 107, 1966

42. Moldaver J: Tourniquet paralysis syndrome. Arch Surg 68: 136, 1954

43. Schmidt RM, Rosenkranz HS: Antimicrobial activity of local anesthetics: Lidocaine and procaine. J Infect Dis 121: 597, 1970

44. Hibbard LT, Synder EN, McVann RN: Subgluteal and retropsoal infection in obstetric practice. Obstet Gynecol 39: 137, 1972

45. Wooley BJ, Vandam LD: Neurological sequelae of brachial plexus nerve block. Ann Surg 149: 53, 1959

21

Spinal, Epidural, and Caudal Anesthesia

Terence M. Murphy, M.B., Ch.B

SPINAL AND EPIDURAL ANESTHESIA

HISTORY

Corning[1] probably first attempted to administer medication into the subarachnoid and epidural spaces. By producing spinal anesthesia with cocaine in dogs, he suggested that this may have some potential for surgery.

Administration of spinal and epidural anesthesia in humans was introduced at the turn of the century. Bier[2] performed spinal anesthesia in 1899 and Siccard[3] and Cathelin[4] introduced epidural analgesia 3 years later in 1901. Because of the efficacy of these forms of anesthesia in contrast to the general anesthetic techniques used at that time, spinal and epidural anesthesia achieved wide popularity and were extensively used until the discovery of the anesthetic potential of the muscle relaxants in clinical surgery in 1946. Then followed a decline in the utilization of regional anesthesia, and a generation of physicians grew up to regard such procedures as historic techniques—although a few enthusiasts maintained their skills, largely because of individual effort and dedication.

With the "rediscovery" of regional anesthesia in recent decades, its success (particularly that of continual epidural anesthesia in obstetrics) has fired the enthusiasm of many anesthesiologists to extend its scope back into the operating room. Thus, spinal and epidural anesthesia, along with other forms of regional anesthesia, are finding a renewed application in pain relief for patients during and after surgery, for obstetric patients, and for patients with chronic pain.

FUNDAMENTAL CONSIDERATIONS

Both epidural and spinal anesthesia can produce profound anesthesia over large areas by anesthetizing nerve pathways to, from, and maybe even within the neuraxis. Both techniques usually produce satisfactory muscle relaxation, which is quite profound with spinal anesthesia and with the more concentrated anesthetic solutions introduced into the epidural space. The gastrointestinal tract is usually contracted, and this facilitates surgical exploration of the abdomen and especially closure of abdominal wounds. With both techniques, selective anesthesia of the operative site can be produced, which enables patients to undergo extensive abdominal, pelvic, obstetric, and lower extremity surgery with minimal impairment of cardiovascular or respiratory stability. The patient may even be wide awake if desired, although most patients prefer sedation or sleep. Both of these techniques may even be used for upper abdominal and thoracic surgery, although they are usually used in combination with light general anesthesia and an endoctracheal tube to protect the airway and facilitate controlled ventilation.

These versatile techniques of spinal and epidural anesthesia do, however, have their limitations. They probably have a higher degree of failure than general anesthetic techniques; therefore, patients or surgeons who have experienced this disadvantage, often have prejudices against spinal and epidural anesthesia. Because both spinal and epidural anesthetics can interrupt the thoracolumbar sympathetic outflow, profound vasodilation and hypotension may occur. Another limiting feature of these forms of anesthesia is their finite duration: analgesia from a local anesthetic drug deposited around the neuraxis will wear off in time. If surgical analgesia should be required in excess of this, then supplemental anesthesia must be given. This objection is circumvented by the introduction of continuous techniques whereby catheters can be inserted into the epidural space. Reinjection of anesthetic can be administered throughout the perioperative period. It is also feasible to produce segmental anesthesia—particularly with epidural techniques—wherein selective dermatomes and myotomes are anesthetized for both intraoperative anesthesia and especially for postoperative analgesia. In certain types of upper abdominal surgery such as cholecystectomies or gastric bypass procedures where the surgical incision is limited to just a few dermatomes, a very small dose of local anesthetic administered via a thoracic epidural technique can give very satisfactory postoperative anesthesia.[5,6] Looking to the future, the technology used in the placement of epidural catheters may also have considerable application for the administration of narcotic analgesics in the epidural and/or spinal area for prolonged analgesia. Pure analgesia can be provided by administering such drugs as morphine into the epidural space; this type of analgesia unlike that of the local anesthetic drugs is unassociated with the concomitant sympathetic and motor blockades that produce hypotension and muscle weakness.[7–10]

APPLIED ANATOMY

As with other forms of regional anesthesia, an understanding of the anatomy of the area involved is very important. For spinal and epidural anesthesia, the applied anatomy of the spinal canal and its contents, namely the spinal cord and the meninges, is important to understand. The topographical arrangements of the spinal levels of sensory, motor, and autonomic components in the spinal cord should also be understood.

The Spinal Canal

This bony canal extends from the foramen magnum to the sacral hiatus and is formed anteriorly by the bodies of the vertebra, laterally by the pedicles, and posteriorly by the lamina. Between the bony vertebra, the intervertebral discs and the ligaments joining the lamina and spines comprise additional boundaries; the only openings in the canal are the intervertebral foramina, which permit the passage of the segmental nerves and blood vessels. Contained within the canal is the spinal cord surrounded by its three membranes, which from within to the periphery are the pia mater, arachnoid mater, and dura mater.

The spinal dura mater, also called the theca, is a direct continuation of the fibrous layer of the dura mater from the skull and extends from the foramen magnum to the second sacral segment. Although firmly attached in the skull, it is free of bony attachments in the spinal canal. Immediately within the dura mater and separated from it only by a thin film of lymph is the spinal arachnoid mater. The pia mater surrounds the spinal cord; the former's lateral extensions, the ligamentum denticulatum, stretch laterally from the spinal cord on each side and attach the cord to the dura-arachnoid at the intervals between the intervertebral foramina through which the spinal nerves exit.

The spinal cord is an elongated cylinder that lies in the spinal canal. It extends the length of the spinal canal in fetal life, but because of differential growth of the spinal canal, the lower end of the cord at birth is at the L3 level and its tapered caudal limit, the conus medullaris, assumes its adult position at the L1-L2 junction at the end of the second decade of life.

The dura mater maintains its embryologic attachments at the S2 level; thus below the conus medullaris is a relatively large subarachnoid compartment stretching from L1 to S2 that contains the cauda equina—those spinal nerve roots that are bathed in cerebrospinal fluid and destined for body levels below L1.

It is in this area of the spinal canal, between the level of the conus medullaris (i.e., the upper border of the L2) and the upper border of the sacrum (the L5-S1 interspace), that subarachnoid and epidural punctures are classically and most frequently performed. When undertaken at these levels, the spinal cord is not in danger of needle trauma. Both subarachnoid and epidural puncture can be performed at other levels of the spinal canal, although to prevent damage to the spinal cord greater technical expertise is demanded when these needling procedures are undertaken above L2. Because of the continuous dorsal plate of the sacrum, the only practical approach for introducing local anesthetic agents into the sacral part of the spinal canal is via the sacral hiatus.

The subarachnoid space surrounds the spinal cord between the pia and the arachnoid membranes. Its lower limit is the termination of the dural sac at the second sacral vertebral level and superiorly it communicates with the cerebrospinal fluid in the cranial and ventricular cavities. Spinal or subarachnoid anesthesia involves the introduction of local anesthetic agents into this compartment. Although it is possible to introduce local anesthetic agents at any spinal level, it is usually performed below the termination of the spinal cord at L2, where the subarachnoid space contains the cauda equina. The spinal puncture is usually performed at the L3-L4 or L4-L5 intervertebral space.

The epidural space is that compartment between the dura mater and the bony and ligamentous walls of the spinal canal. It is a potential space. In life it is filled with extradural fat and the internal vertebral plexus of veins, which are arranged in two paramedian channels extending the length of the epidural space from cranium to sacrum. These veins drain the blood from the meninges and the vertebral bodies to the segmental veins via the intervertebral foramina. The segmental nerves, as they leave the dura mater, cross this epidural space before exiting from the spinal canal through the intervertebral foramina. Epidural anesthesia is usually performed at similar lumbar levels to spinal anesthesia, but can be used in thoracic and sacral areas for specific indications.

In summary, subarachnoid, or spinal, puncture is theoretically and technically feasible anywhere from the foramen magnum to the lower limits of the dura mater at S2. Epidural puncture is possible throughout the length of the spinal canal—from the upper cervical regions to the sacral hiatus. In the vast majority of these regional anesthetic techniques, subarachnoid anesthesia and peridural anesthesia are administered via the L3-L4 or the L4-L5 interspaces. Epidural anesthesia is also frequently used via the sacral hiatus and is sometimes used in the thoracic area to produce segmental anesthesia for both intraoperative and postoperative pain control. When used in this latter situation, the epidural anesthesia is usually performed in the midthoracic level (i.e., T4 to T8), because in this area the spinal cord is thinnest between the enlargements for the two major limb plexuses—brachial and lumbosacral; therefore there is theoretically more room and presumably a greater margin of safety between the borders of the spinal canal and the outer surface of the spinal cord to permit the placement of needles, catheters, and anesthetic drugs.

IDENTIFICATION OF SPINAL VERTEBRAL LEVEL

The spinous processes of L2 through L5 are more or less horizontal in direction and therefore are good landmarks for the bodies of the same vertebrae. With the exception of the T1 and T2 vertebrae, all the other spinous processes have a distinct caudad direction; in the middle thoracic area, the spinous processes may well overlap vertebral bodies two segments lower in the column. The only vertebra that can be identified with any certainty on clinical examination is the vertebra prominens, C7, which is the vertebra first palpated at the caudal limit of the ligamentum nuchae at the base of the neck. The line joining the iliac crests passes through the L4 vertebra or the L4-L5 space and thus permits identification of these two lower vertebrae with a degree of certainty. With the arms by the sides the horizontal line joining the lower parts of both scapulae passes usually through the T7 vertebral spine. Any other vertebrae are usually found clinically by counting from these known levels, but the further one gets from C7 and L4, the less reliable the clinical identification is and radiographs are then necessary.

THE DERMATOMES

An intimate knowledge of the sensory, motor, and autonomic distribution of the different spinal nerves is very important for the correct conduct of spinal and epidural anesthesia and particularly for the interpretation of its effects and complications. This then requires knowledge of the dermatomes and myotomes of the body. The peripheral distribution of the autonomic nervous system is much less precisely understood and probably subject to greater variation than the sensory

and motor systems. Those topics are covered well in most basic anatomy text books. Last[11] provides an excellent and concise account of this topic and a summary is given below.

A dermatome is that area of skin supplied by a single spinal nerve. The face is supplied by trigeminal dermatomes and the rest of the body skin is supplied in sequence by dermatomes C2 through S5. Adjacent dermatomes overlap considerably except across axial lines. Axial lines are defined as those lines separating discontinuous dermatomes; such lines are found on limbs and on the trunk adjacent to limbs. As the developing limb bud grows out from the axial skeleton it carries with it the dermatomes destined for that limb, and thus a "dermatomal gap" is produced on the trunk, examples being where the C4 dermatome of the neck lies adjacent to the T2 dermatome of the upper thorax. The dermatomes in between, i.e., C5 through T1, have migrated out onto the developing limb. The dermatome distribution is as shown in Figure 21-1. Limb dermatomes are distributed in an orderly sequence along the preaxial and postaxial borders of the limb. The dermatome arrangement of the lower extremity is more complex than the orderly arrangement seen in the upper extremity because of the adduction and medial rotation of the mature lower limb from its embryonal position.

There is an orderly distribution of these limb dermatomes, which follows a set pattern: both the upper and lower extremity are supplied by five spinal nerves, the central nerve being distributed most distally in the limb and the two craniad and caudad nerves being distributed symmetrically on the preaxial and postaxial borders. The lower extremity has "borrowed" considerable skin and musculature from the trunk to form the flexor compartment of the thigh; this skin and musculature is innervated by lumbar plexus L1, L2, and L3, which is developmentally trunk skin and muscle and not embryologically part of the main nerve supply of the lower extremity.

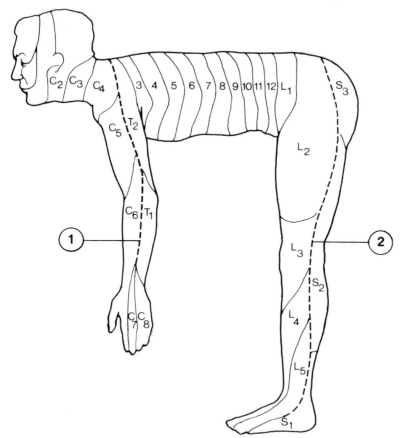

Fig. 21-1 The dermatomes of the body show an orderly craniad to caudal sequence. By positioning the body as shown, the complex arrangement of dermatomes on the limbs is more readily understood. On the upper extremity, the limb dermatomes are distributed symmetrically about the axial line (1). Note that dermatomes C5 and C6 are distributed on the preaxial border of the limb and the postaxial dermatomes, C8, T1, and T2, are distributed on the postaxial part of the limb. C7, which is the central dermatome of the limb, is distributed more distally, that is, over the middle finger. There is an orderly sequence on the trunk from T3 to L1.

The dermatome distribution of the lower extremity is also arranged around the axial line (2). Large areas of skin, i.e., L2 and L3, have been borrowed from the trunk to supplement the true leg dermatomes of L4 through S3. Note as in the upper extremity, the craniad dermatomes, L4 and L5, are distributed on the preaxial border of the limb and the caudad dermatomes, S2 and S3, are distributed on the postaxial border of the limb. The central dermatome S1 is distributed over the lateral aspect of the plantar surface and lateral border of the foot. (After Foerster I: Brain 56:1, 1933. By permission of Oxford University Press.)

THE MYOTOMES

Like skin, muscles are supplied by segmental nerves. Last[11] has simplified the bewildering complexity of muscle innervation, especially that of the limbs, by pointing out that there appear to be spinal centers for joint movements and that these spinal centers tend to occupy four continuous segments in the cord.

The two craniad segments innervate one movement of the joint and the two lower

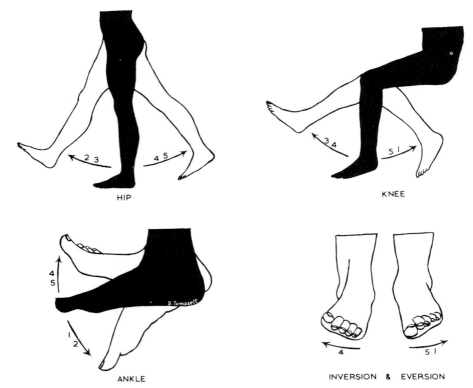

Fig. 21-2 Spinal segmental innervation (myotomes) of the lower extremity. (Last RJ: Anatomy, Regional and Applied. 6th edition. Edinburgh, Churchill Livingstone, 1978.)

segments innervate the opposite movement. For example, the elbow joint is supplied by C5, C6, C7, and C8. C5 and C6 supply the flexors (biceps and brachialis) and C7 and C8 supply the extensors of this joint (triceps). In contrast to the dermatomal distribution, the myotomal arrangement in the lower extremity is simpler than the upper extremity. It is as follows:

The center for the hip joint is L2, L3, L4, and L5. The knee joint is also supplied by four adjacent levels, but one level lower (L3, L4, L5, and S1). Similarly, the ankle joint is more distally supplied by L4, L5, S1, and S2. The arrangement is as shown in the following outline and in Figure 21-2, both from Last.[11]

The upper extremity is a little more complicated because some of the fine delicate control movements of the hand and shoulder are controlled by single spinal segments (for

Hip	Knee	Ankle
L2 L3 } Flex		
	L3 L4 } Extend	
		L4 L5 } Dorsi-flex
L4 L5 } Extend		
	L5 S1 } Flex	
		S1 S2 } Plantar-flex

(Modified from Last RJ: Anatomy, Regional and Applied. 6th edition. Edinburgh, Churchill Livingstone, 1978.)

example, the small muscles of the hand are all controlled by the T1 segment). However, there is still a progression from craniad to caudad of spinal segments as each joint is considered from proximal to distal limb. Therefore, the shoulder joint is controlled by C5, C6, C7, and C8 with adduction being primarily C5, and abduction C6, C7, and C8. The elbow joint, as mentioned, is C5, C6, C7,

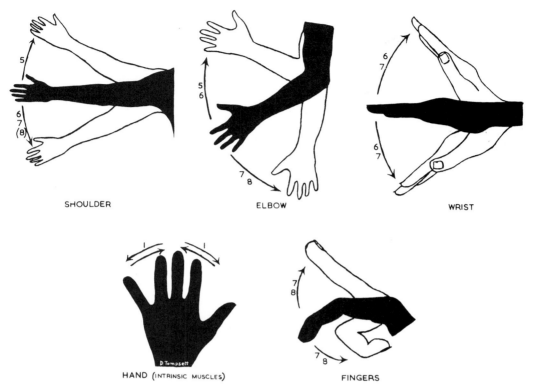

SHOULDER   ELBOW   WRIST

HAND (INTRINSIC MUSCLES)   FINGERS

Fig. 21-3 Spinal segmental innervation (myotomes) of the upper extremity. (Last RJ: Anatomy, Regional and Applied. 6th edition. Edinburgh, Churchill Livingstone, 1978.)

and C8. The wrist joint is C6 and C7 for both flexion and extension of the wrist, and flexion and extension of the metacarpals are controlled by the C7 and C8 spinal segments. T1 controls the small muscle movements of the hand, i.e., abduction and adduction of the digits (Fig. 21-3).

THE SYMPATHETIC NERVOUS SYSTEM

The spinal connector cell bodies for the sympathetic nervous system lie in the spinal cord from the C8 to L2 segments. Their efferents exit in the anterior roots of spinal nerves T1 through L2. Distal to the junction of ante-

Shoulder	Elbow	Wrist	Digits	
C5 } Flex	C5 C6 } Flex	C6 C7 } Flex & Extend	C7 C8 } Flex & Extend	
C6 C7 C8 } Extend	C7 C8 } Extend		T1 } Adduction & Abduction	

rior and posterior primary rami, the sympathetic efferent fibers leave the somatic segmental nerve in the white (medullated) ramus communicans to enter the sympathetic trunk. The sympathetic trunk extends along the

vertebral bodies from the base of the skull to the coccyx. The trunk is irregularly ganglionated. There are usually 3 cervical ganglia, 11 thoracic, 4 lumbar, and 4 sacral. Only the ganglia in the T1 to L2 levels receive white

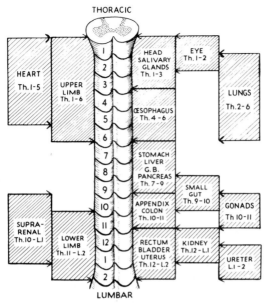

THORACIC

Fig. 21-4 Spinal levels of sympathetic connector cells. (Last RJ: Anatomy, Regional and Applied. 6th edition. Edinburgh, Churchill Livingstone, 1978.)

rami. The cervical, lower lumbar, and sacral parts of the trunk obtain their efferent fibers as a continuation of the thoracolumbar outflow.

The sympathetic trunk has both somatic and visceral branches. The somatic branches leave the ganglia as gray rami communicans, and enter the segmental somatic nerves. The sympathetic nerves are thus distributed to the somatic nerves, which convey the sympathetic vasoconstrictor, sudomotor, and pilomotor fibers to the area of distribution of the nerve.

Visceral branches from the sympathetic trunk leave the trunk and form plexuses for the various visceral destinations, for example, cardiac, pulmonary, celiac, superior, and inferior hypogastric. The cardiac, esophageal, pulmonary, and celiac plexuses receive a parasympathetic supply from the vagus, whereas the inferior hypogastric and pelvic plexuses receive their parasympathetic efferents from the pelvic parasympathetic outflow from levels S2, S3, and S4.

The sympathetic nervous system also contains many afferent sensory fibers from the viscera. These travel by the sympathetic nerves, the appropriate visceral plexus, and then via the sympathetic trunk and white rami back to the neuraxis. The somatic afferent fibers usually travel along blood vessels and somatic spinal nerves.

There appear to be spinal levels for these different sympathetic innervations (Fig. 21-4). Although knowledge is limited about the specific levels, they act as a very useful guide when determining the appropriate levels of analgesia needed for surgery on particular viscera. For example, as can be seen in Figure 21-4 although the surgical skin incision for operation on the testes might involve a dermatomal level of T12, it is necessary to have at least a T10 block to assure visceral analgesia. Similarly, surgery may be performed on the foot with a spinal block that extends no higher than L3. But if a thigh tourniquet is used, the discomfort generated from this tourniquet may well travel along sympathetic afferents that are entering the spinal cord at higher levels than L3; therefore, for satisfactory analgesia, a block usually to T10 or above is needed. It is conceivable that some of the sympathetic afferents may well enter the spinal cord at levels higher than those traditionally claimed. This provides a working hypothesis for some of the enigmatic pain complaints that are occasionally observed under what appear to be satisfactory levels of spinal and epidural anesthesia. Also, because of the concept of differential nerve blockade (i.e., local anesthetic drugs more easily and freely diffuse into and block sympathetic nerves more rapidly than the larger and more heavily myelinated sensory and motor nerves) it is conceivable that the anesthetic can be removed from the smaller nerves more easily and the sympathetic nerves may easily recover in advance of their somatic counterparts. Thus one may still have what appears to be adequate skin anesthesia when the visceral afferents for these spinal levels have recovered.[12] This could be an explanation for some of the enigmatic phenomena seen when patients complain of pain during visceral manipulations in what appears to be a satisfactory somatic block.[13]

CLINICAL ASPECTS

PREOPERATIVE EVALUATION PERIOD

The preoperative evaluation and approach for spinal and epidural anesthesia is very similar to the comments outlined in Chapter 20.

With the popularity of peridural techniques for obstetric anesthesia, many patients are aware of and receptive to the advantages of peridural anesthesia. The term spinal anesthesia still has fearful implications for many patients who have often heard of unsubstantiated tales of paralysis. Sometimes a simple explanation of the facts is sufficient to reassure most patients. However, patients who have personally, or whose close friends or relatives have, suffered unpleasant experiences during the induction or maintenance of regional anesthesia are often very difficult to convince. This is one reason why in the event of a partial or complete failure of a regional anesthetic technique, efforts should always be made so that the patient is not inconvenienced, or worse still, made to suffer discomfort to prove the inadequacy of the block. With spinal and epidural anesthesia, heavier preoperative sedation can be used than in those regional anesthetic techniques for which patient cooperation is required. Thus, generous doses of narcotics, sedative hypnotics, or both will protect the patient from the discomfort of the passage of the relatively large needles required for epidural techniques and also provide some protection from anxiety from a failed block; such doses will also prepare the way for the expeditious induction of general anesthesia if this becomes necessary.

PREMEDICATION

Many of the comments in Chapter 20 about premedication of the patient for a regional anesthetic are appropriate here. It is important to explain to the patient ahead of time the sequence of events and reassure him as to the advisability of the spinal or epidural anesthetic. Because neither spinal nor epidural anesthesia relies on patient cooperation and feedback to any great extent, moderately heavy premedication can be given. If, however, it is necessary to perform the procedure in the sitting position, a heavily premedicated patient may not be able to cooperate.

Usually premedication will include a narcotic (morphine 0.2 mg/kg IM or meperidine 1.5 mg/kg IM 1 hour before the procedure). The narcotic can often be combined with a barbiturate (pentobarbital 2 to 3 mg/kg) or diazepam 0.1 mg/kg. Antisialogogues are usually not required or desirable—the patient may have a satisfactory block for the surgery and keep complaining of a dry mouth.

POSITIONING OF THE PATIENT FOR THE PUNCTURE

The Sitting Position

The patient is positioned sitting on the operating table at approximately its midpoint. The knees are bent and the feet rest on a stool adjusted to an appropriate height; the patient is instructed to fold his arms and usually rest them on a suitable stand or lean on an assistant at this stage. This puts the patient's spine in an optimal position for performing a lumbar puncture, either via the midline or paramedian approach. This position is ideally suited to puncture at any level.

It is probably the optimal position for a spinal puncture and should be used if the patient can conveniently assume this position. It is particularly effective when the hyperbaric spinal techniques are used for perineal lower extremity or obstetric procedures. The anesthesiologist sits or stands on the opposite side of the operating table. The vertebrae are usually centrally positioned in the midline in this situation; and this position greatly facilitates lumbar and thoracic peridural anesthesia in the obese, in whom the identification of vertebrae and midline is often quite difficult in the lateral decubitus position. When spinal puncture and injection have been produced, the patient may remain in the sitting position if perineal anesthesia is all that is required. If a higher block is needed, then with the help of assistants after the patient's legs are swung up onto the table, the patient is placed in the supine position.

The Lateral Decubitus Position

The lateral decubitus position is probably the most common position for spinal and epidural anesthesia in surgical and obstetric practice. Here the patient lies on his or her side and if a hyperbaric technique is to be used, the side for surgical exploration is the dependent one. Optimal positioning is essential to facilitate satisfactory completion of the lumbar puncture. The patient's back should be parallel to the edge of the table, and ideally the shoulders and iliac crest should be vertical. The thighs should be flexed on the trunk and the head and neck flexed on the thorax. This produces maximal curvature of the lumbar spines with separation of their spinous processes, which facilitates midline and paramedian approaches. The anesthesiologist usually will find this block accomplished more conveniently if he sits facing the patient's back and the table is adjusted to a convenient working height. The spinal tray and its equipment should be positioned on the side of the anesthesiologist's dominant hand. The anesthesiologist should be able to perform satisfactory lumbar puncture with the patient lying on either side, although the right-handed anesthesiologist will usually find this procedure easier if the patient lies on his left side and the left-handed anesthesiologist will usually find it easier with the patient lying on his right side.

The Prone Position

For hypobaric techniques in the perineal area (as used for drainage of pilonidal cysts, rectal, and other perineal surgery) the patient is often placed in a so-called jackknife position. This position lends itself well to hypobaric spinal anesthesia, and lumbar puncture is usually accomplished in what will be the position for operation. Here the anesthesiologist usually stands to one or the other side. The lumbar puncture is accomplished via either a midline or paramedian approach. If narrow gauge needles (i.e., number 25) are used, it is sometimes necessary to actively aspirate cerebrospinal fluid by attaching a syringe to the needle to confirm that the needle is in the subarachnoid space. This method is used because the low CSF pressure at this level in this position may hamper the freeflow of CSF up the needle. A distinct advantage of this position is that the patient does not need to be moved into a different position for the surgery.

APPROACHES TO THE EPIDURAL AND SPINAL CANALS

These canals are usually approached from a posterior aspect via a midline or paramedian approach. Each of these approaches has its merits and should be included in the anesthesiologist's repertoire. It also is theoretically possible to perform epidural and subarachnoid placement of local anesthetic agents through the paravertebral foramen and even via an anterior intraoperative approach through the intervertebral disc.

The Midline Approach

The needle is introduced into the vertebral canal via an approach in the midline between adjacent vertebral spines; the angle of this approach will vary depending upon the vertebral level at which puncture is performed. In the lumbar region, the needle will be entering almost in a perpendicular fashion; whereas the angle will become more acute in the thoracic area.

In a typical lumbar puncture, the interspinous ligament is located by selecting appropriate adjacent spines and palpating the space between them. Having raised a skin wheal at this site, the anesthesiologist inserts the needle between the spines; a slight cephalad inclination is used when inserting the needle. Having pierced the surpraspinous ligaments, the needle will then enter the interspinous ligament and if kept in a perpendicular plane will traverse this ligament down to the base of the spine; at the latter point, it will engage the ligamentum flavum in the midline. Further advancement will result in the needle entering the epidural space and subsequently the subarachnoid space.

The main advantage of this technique is its simplicity. It is atraumatic and extensive infiltrations with local anesthetics are usually not required. Also, because the epidural veins tend to be situated laterally, the central area is relatively avascular. Thus perhaps there is less risk of intravascular injection and toxic side effects.

Young individuals usually have mobile spines. Because they can assume a cooperative curved posture, the midline approach works admirably. The disadvantages of the midline approach are primarily encountered in the more difficult cases. In those individuals who because of age, infirmity, or inability

to cooperate cannot assume the flexed posture, adjacent vertebral spines can be in apposition making it very difficult to insert a needle between them. With thoracic spinal and epidural puncture, a correct placement of the needle in the midline becomes more difficult with the marked overhang of thoracic spinous processes. In these difficult situations, the paramedian approach can prove indispensable to a successful block.

The Paramedian Approach

In the paramedian approach, the needle is introduced to one or the other side of the midline. The exact distance from the midline is not critical, but most authors recommend a distance of 1 to 2 cm. For a straight-forward puncture in the lumbar areas, this is done lateral to the interspinous gap. The needle is then advanced in this paramedian location alongside but lateral to the interspinous ligament. The needle then transverses the paraspinal dorsal muscle mass. At the appropriate depth, the needle will engage the ligamentum flavum in its lateral intralamina fibers; further advancement is marked by first an increase in resistance followed by a loss of resistance as the epidural space is entered. Further advancement will place the needle in the subarachnoid space.

An additional refinement of the paramedian technique is to introduce the needle lateral to the spine itself and to advance it parallel to the spine until the bony end point of the lamina is reached. This provides an indication of the correct depth of the ligamentum flavum. By "walking" the needle along the lamina, usually in a cephalad fashion, the ligamentum flavum at the cephalic end of the lamina will be located. There is a marked change in consistency as the needle is slipped off the marble-like bone onto the ligamentum flavum, which has the consistency of leather. Further advancement of the needle through the ligamentum flavum will result in it entering the epidural space and with further advancement it enters the subarachnoid space.

The paramedian approach can be used anywhere from the lumbosacral hiatus to the foramen magnum. It is a predictable and consistent method for affecting either epidural or subdural needle placement; in addition, it somewhat frees the anesthesiologist from his dependency upon whether the patient can cooperate by appropriately flexing his spine because it is impossible for the patient, even in full extension, to occlude this route to the epidural or subarachnoid space. It is also very useful in obese patients because the appropriate depth of needle insertion can be determined by first locating the recognizable end point of vertebral lamina and then walking the needle to the ligamentum flavum.

The Lumbosacral Puncture—
The Taylor Approach

The lumbosacral puncture is a very useful approach described by Taylor in 1942[14] and is a variation of the conventional paramedian approach. The Taylor approach is used at the L5-S1 interspace, the largest interspace in the vertebral column, offering a larger target to the spinal needle than does the conventional paramedian or the midline approach. The needle is introduced through a skin wheal 1 cm medial and 1 cm cephalad to the posterior superior iliac spine. The needle is directed

cephalad and medially; if the dorsal surface of the sacrum is contacted, the needle is walked cephalad until it slips off the surface of the sacrum and pierces the ligamentum flavum and then the dura mater[14] (Fig. 21-5).

EQUIPMENT

Although disposable equipment is less satisfactory than quality reusable material, an exception may be made in the case of the disposable spinal anesthetic trays. These tend to be quite satisfactory for routine clinical use. This is so because the straightforward end point of spinal needle placement, i.e., the definitive objective sign of CSF fluid aspiration, requires only modest kinesthetic expertise and the disposable needles and syringes provided in such trays are suitable for the purpose.

For epidural trays, however, I prefer reusable sets of high quality epidural needles and glass syringes (provided detergents are avoided in the cleaning of such equipment). These trays can be reused extensively without any significant problem as long as they are steam autoclaved at 225° to 260° F at 18 to 20 lbs. pressure for 30 minutes and then vacuum dried. The use of sterilizer indicators, both inside and outside the tray, confirm the efficacy of the autoclaving process. Trays should be resterilized if not used for about 2 weeks. (See Fig 20-1.) The needles used are described in the following sections.

Fig. 21-5 The dorsal view of the fourth and fifth lumbar vertebrae, their relationship to the sacrum and ▶ iliac bones, and the most frequently used approaches for needle puncture in subarachnoid and lumbar peridural techniques. Numerals represent the following: (1) the cauda equina; (2) the dura mater; (3) the ligamentum flavum at the L3-L4 interspace; (4) the midline approach for spinal and epidural techniques where the needle is introduced between the spines of L3 and L4 vertebrae, traversing the supraspinous and interspinous ligaments before piercing the ligamentum flavum; (5) the paramedian approach at this level where the needle puncture site is 1 to 2 cm lateral to the above midline approach; if the initial approach results in contacting the lamina of the vertebrae as shown in the dotted needle silhouette, then the needle is walked cephalad and medially until it slips off the lamina and contacts ligamentum flavum as shown; (6) the large interspace between S5 and L1, which is situated 2 cm medial and cephalad from (7) the posterior superior iliac spine; (8) the needle can be introduced at this site in the "Taylor" approach for either subarachnoid or epidural puncture.

SPINAL ANESTHESIA (SUBARACHNOID BLOCK)

Although spinal anesthesia has provoked controversy throughout its 80-year history and its popularity has waxed and waned, it has nevertheless stood the test of time. An understanding of its physiological effects and the use of both improved equipment and sterilizing techniques have rendered it an eminently safe form of anesthesia for appropriate selected patients. Unfortunately, because of a few well-publicized cases of permanent neurologic damage during an era when modern sterilizing and autoclaving techniques were not used, spinal anesthesia still has a poor reputation. Thus there are still many patients who have fears of the technique and require often considerable education, explanations, and reassurance at the preoperative visit. Several large scale studies have, however, attested to its safety.[15-18] Its increasing popularity and use are entirely justified because few anesthetic techniques offer such excellent operating conditions, proven patient safety, and economy of anesthetic effort and resources.

NEEDLES FOR SUBARACHNOID PUNCTURE

The majority of spinal punctures are performed with either 25 or 22 gauge needles. A 3½-inch length is sufficient to reach the subarachnoid space in all but massively obese

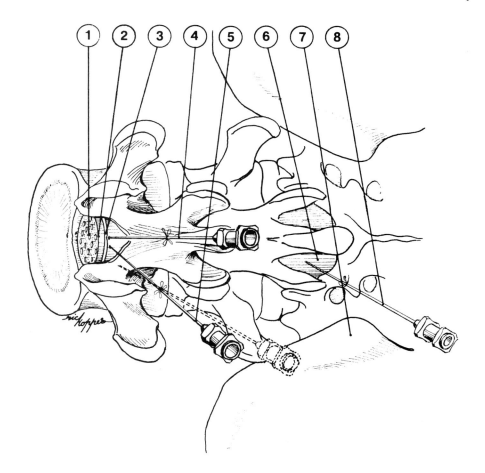

patients, for whom a 5-inch needle is sometimes required.

The advantage of a 22 gauge needle is primarily that of facility of puncture. This more rigid needle gives better feedback and proprioceptive information from the needle tip to the operator with regard to the tissue structures through which it passes. Because it is more rigid than the pliable 25 gauge needle, the 22 gauge needle can be more easily directed. The only disadvantage of the 22 gauge needle is the increased incidence of postspinal headache when this size needle is used in younger patients.

The use of 25 gauge needles reduces the incidence of postspinal headache to as low as 1 percent.[19] The main disadvantage of the 25 gauge needle is that it is relatively easily distorted and bent with inappropriate usage. It is optimally used with an introducer, and usually a thin-walled 18 gauge 1½-inch needle is sufficient for this purpose. If the initial needle path is incorrect, it can be corrected by withdrawing the needle tip into the introducer and then realigning the more rigid introducer to the angle desired before reinserting the 25 gauge spinal needle through the introducer at the new angle. The thin 25 gauge needle gives less effective proprioceptive feedback (than 22 gauge) when passing through the various tissue planes such as ligamentum flavum and dura, but the educated hand soon comes to recognize these losses of resistance. Another relative disadvantage of the smaller gauge needles is the longer time it takes for CSF fluid to track back through the needle. Therefore appropriate time should be taken before acknowledging the fact that the needle is not in the subarachnoid space. The presence of CSF can be ascertained more rapidly by using an aspirating syringe on the needle. This delay in the spontaneous appearance of CSF through these needles is more pronounced when the needle is used in the prone jackknife position where gravity mitigates against CSF rising in the needle.

Needle Bevels

As with other forms of regional anesthesia, a somewhat shorter bevel needle is desirable for subarachnoid block. Not only will this give a better feel for resistance changes as the needle passes through ligamentum flavum and dura, but it will usually prove more satisfactory upon injecting solutions into the subarachnoid space. A disadvantage of needles with long bevels is that even with an incomplete puncture of the dura, it is feasible to aspirate cerebrospinal fluid, even though only part of the bevel may be sitting in the subarachnoid space. A subsequent injection of drug in this position can deposit part of the anesthetic in the extradural space and thus give inadequate spinal anesthesia.

The types of bevels that have been produced for spinal anesthesia basically fall into two types: those with a cutting bevel, such as a Pitkin needle, or those with a noncutting pencil type point, such as the Green or Whittaker needles. The rationale behind using the noncutting type of bevel is that it parts rather than cuts longitudinal fibers of the dura. Thus when the noncutting needle is removed, the defect in the dura would be more likely to seal than if a cutting needle had been used. Although there is no definitive information on the relative merits of these cutting points, Phillips[19] claims a reduced incidence of headache using Green-type needles rather than those with a cutting edge. However his results may be explained by the smaller size of the pencil point needle.

The currently available 25 gauge needles usually are suitable for most spinal anesthetics. For those patients who have increased risk of postdural puncture headache, use of a 26 gauge needle should be considered. In most older patients, a 22 gauge needle can be used without the likelihood of producing a headache.

26 Gauge Needle

The incidence of postspinal headache probably can be reduced still further by the use of even finer needles.[20] A 26 gauge needle is available and the usual practice is to insert it through a 21 gauge introducer. This 3½-inch introducer is inserted via midline or paramedian approaches to the epidural space and then the 26 gauge needle is passed through it and used to complete the subarachnoid puncture leaving only a very small hole in the dura. This technique would be indicated in those patients who are at maximal risk for a postspinal headache, i.e., individuals who have suffered from this complication in the past, parturients, and those, such as outpatients, who are likely to be ambulatory shortly after their spinal puncture.

A 32 gauge needle technique has been described[21] but has not found wide use, presumably because of the practical details of the use and maintenance of these needles plus the difficulty of aspirating through them.

Handling Needles for Subarachnoid Puncture

As described in Chapter 20, on regional nerve blocks, the main goal in using any percutaneous technique is to ascertain what is happening at the pointed end of the needle and to obtain maximal proprioception feedback as to the placement of this point in relation to tissue planes, losses of resistance, etc. It is best to use the fine transducers of the small muscles of the hand and thenar eminence rather than to lock the wrist and elbow in a fixed position and use the coarser muscles of the shoulder girdle with their relatively parsimonious cortical representation. I prefer to hold needles much as a pen is held, so as to better appreciate their placement.

Another approach is to insert the spinal needle by gripping it with both hands and resting the wrist and forearm on the back of the patient. Winged needle adaptations have been constructed to facilitate such an approach. The thesis behind this approach is that there is greater control over the needle and thus movements of the patient are less likely to result in inappropriate advancement of the needle and a possible trauma to the nerves in the subarachnoid space. There is no doubt that this technique works well and is probably the most universally taught method for subarachnoid puncture.

SUBARACHNOID PUNCTURE

The subarachnoid space is reached by either midline or lateral paramedian approaches as described above (Fig. 21-5). When the needle has passed through the dura, the stylet is withdrawn and free flow of cerebrospinal fluid is proof that it is in the correct compartment. The needle should now be rotated through four quadrants and the CSF flow should continue either spontaneously or by aspiration in each quadrant to ascertain that the lumen of the needle is positioned within the subarachnoid space. After locking the needle with the nondominant hand and stabilizing it in relation to the patient's back, the anesthesiologist attaches the syringe containing the spinal anesthetic solution. A further brief aspiration test confirms that the lumen is still within the subarachnoid space and has not been dislodged by the act of attaching the syringe, and the drug is then injected. A further brief aspiration test when 50 percent of the solution has been injected confirms the position of the needle, and a repeat aspiration test when all the solution has been injected will offer further confirmation that the solution has been injected into the correct subarachnoid compartment. The delicate 25 gauge needles can be dislodged from their original subarachnoid position as syringes are attached to the needle.

There are different ways of stabilizing the spinal needle once it is in situ. A favorite and extensively used technique is to place the dorsum of the nondominant hand on the adjacent part of the patient's back and form a tripod with the thumb, index, and forefinger by grasping the needle hub; this forms a stable base for securing the needle position during the attachment and removal of syringe or syringes.

The rate of injection of the solution is important in determining the ultimate height of the block.[22] Rapidly injected solutions tend to produce turbulence and therefore a higher block, whereas more slowly injected solutions will assume more discrete positions depending on their hypobaricity or hyperbaricity. Use is sometimes made of these phenomena by employing barbotage techniques when a high block is needed. In this technique, the local anesthetic solution is partially injected and then by aspirating quantities of CSF into the syringe, reinjection is undertaken, this procedure can be repeated several times during the injection to fairly efficiently distribute the local anesthetic over a wider area in the subarachnoid space.

"Bloody Tap"

Occasionally after puncture of the dura and removal of the stylet from the needle, blood will flow through the needle. The blood should be allowed to continue to drip, and usually if it is in the subarachnoid space, the solution will clear after several drops. Clear CSF can then be aspirated and the injection may proceed. If, however, blood continues to flow from the needle, then the needle is probably in the lumen of a blood vessel. The needle probably should be repositioned until clear cerebrospinal fluid is aspirated.

Difficult Spinal Taps

Despite following traditional techniques, it is often very difficult to successfully position the needle in the subarachnoid space. On such occasions, the patient's position should be checked because this may have altered during the course of attempted puncture, particularly in the lateral position. The patient may have been appropriately flexed initially, but in response to discomfort, a more extended spinal position may have developed making midline puncture much more difficult. To prevent this from occurring, the help and encouragement of an assistant to maintain the patient in a flexed position with the knees up to the chest and the head bent down with the chin on the chest is invaluable. Should, however, the patient's cooperation be less than ideal, this would be an indication to consider a paramedian approach, which is much less dependent upon the patient being in an optimally flexed position. If failure persists, do not hesitate to return to basics and plot out landmarks again. If the patient is heavily draped, it is quite feasible for the patient to have moved without the operator detecting this. By relocating the appropriate spines, iliac crests, etc., a fresh approach will often lead to a successful puncture.

Once facility has been acquired in the different approaches to the subarachnoid space, the anesthesiologist usually can successfully complete successful subarachnoid puncture. However, with less experience, there will be patients in whom, despite repeated attempts and what seems like appropriate techniques, failure results. Unless a spinal anesthesia is absolutely essential, the operator should certainly consider alternative methods, even general anesthesia rather than persist in inconveniencing the patient and the operating room team by prolonged and fruitless attempts at block. Such an event is a demoralizing experience for all concerned—the patient, the anesthesiologist, and the often impatient surgical team. However, if the spi-

Table 21-1. Doses of Drugs (in mg) Commonly Used in Hyperbaric Subarachnoid Blocks*

Drug	Low block to L1	Midblock to T10	High block to T6
Procaine	50	75	100
Lidocaine	25	50	75
Tetracaine	7	10	12

* These mg doses are a guide and apply to solutions mixed in 2 ml of 10 percent dextrose.

nal anesthesia is essential for the patient's welfare, then even prolonged time taken to insure success is justified.

DRUGS USED IN SPINAL ANESTHESIA

The local anesthetics used today appear to be quite safe for subarachnoid administration, and in clinically used dosages, do not appear to be neurotoxic[19] (Table 21-1). The drugs are selected primarily with regard to their duration of action and therefore can be classified into short-, intermediate-, and long-acting. The duration of these drugs can be enhanced by utilizing the vasoconstrictive properties of added epinephrine, and thus a spectrum of preparations of various durations can be selected depending upon the clinical need. One of the limitations of spinal anesthesia is the fact that it does have finite duration: if the surgical procedure is unexpectedly prolonged, such that the spinal anesthetic dissipates before the completion of surgery, alternative techniques have to be used. In practice, however, it is usually feasible to coordinate the duration of the spinal anesthetic with the surgery. Continuous spinal techniques have been described whereby a catheter is placed in the subarachnoid space. Although this is technically feasible and may well be an underutilized technique, it does not appear to have found widespread use, presumably because of the potential for increased incidence of postspinal headaches.

Procaine in doses of 50 to 100 mg can give spinal anesthesia from the groin to the costal margin respectively when administered in the lumbosacral area. The duration of procaine is approximately 30 to 60 minutes and with the addition of epinephrine 0.2 mg, this can be extended by about 50 percent. Procaine is used primarily for short surgical procedures and does require the cooperation of a well-coordinated surgical team to enable the completion of the procedure prior to the block wearing off. Lidocaine in approximately half the procaine doses will yield twice the anesthesia time and doses of 25 to 50 mg of lidocaine in 2 ml of hyperbaric solution will provide a low or high spinal anesthetic as needed. Mepivacaine is very similar in its properties to lidocaine with regard to both dosage and extent of anesthesia, but it tends to last a little longer. Tetracaine is probably the most widely used agent for spinal anesthesia and has a long and proven track record. Tetracaine produces predictable and satisfactory sensory and motor blockade that lasts from approximately 90 to 120 minutes; this time can be increased by the addition of epinephrine. Doses of from 5 to 12 mg will provide a low to high spinal anesthesia as required. Dibucaine in doses from 2.5 to 5 mg can provide longer anesthesia of 2 to 3 hours duration.

Bupivacaine, when used in the subarachnoid space, appears to produce block characteristics very similar to tetracaine. Surprisingly, it does not seem to produce a longer duration of analgesia and the motor blockade is significantly greater with tetracaine than with bupivacaine.[23] See Chapter 19 for more details concerning the pharmacology of local anesthetics.

Addition of Vasoconstrictors

The duration of spinal anesthesia can be increased by approximately 50 percent if epinephrine is added to the solution injected. A dose of 0.2 mg (i.e., 0.2 ml of the standard 1:1,000 solution ampule) appears to be the optimal amount. This does not produce any systemic affects in contrast to the epinephrine added to the large volumes of epidural anesthetic solution. The epinephrine is usually added to the local anesthetic solution immediately prior to injection. This is preferable to using the premixed solutions, which require a buffered pH value that impairs the quality of the local anesthetic blockade.[24]

Phenylephrine (Neo-Synephrine) has been used in dosages of 2 to 5 mg as an additive to prolong the duration of spinal anesthesia. It does this most effectively because it is a potent vasoconstrictor, and it can almost double the duration of the spinal anesthetic. The addition of phenylephrine should obviously be considered for use in prolonged surgical situations.[24]

Baricity of Solution

Spinal anesthetic solutions can be either hyperbaric, hypobaric, or isobaric. In the hyperbaric technique, which is the technique most frequently used, the drugs are usually mixed with 10 percent dextrose solution. Being heavier than spinal fluid, this solution will settle to the most dependent aspect of the subarachnoid fluid column, which will depend on the position of the patient. For perineal or lower extremity surgical procedures, the patient can be placed in a sitting position. The hyperbaric solutions will bathe the lower sacral roots and produce a solid perineal and lower extremity anesthesia. For unilateral surgical procedures, such as on one lower extremity, the patient may be positioned with that side lowermost and the hyperbaric solution permitted to preferentially bathe those roots prior to positioning the patient for the subsequent surgery. Attempts to produce strictly unilateral spinal anesthesia do not succeed even when the patient is left undisturbed in that lateral position for several minutes. This is because after surgical positioning, the solution inevitably spreads to the opposite side; the more profound block, however, will be found on the originally dependent side. When the patient is turned supine, the curves of the lumbar spine with its maximal convexity at the L3 level will determine the flow of the hyperbaric solution (i.e., if the solutions are injected below L3, they will tend to gravitate caudad; whereas if injected above L3, they will flow cephalad and therefore produce a higher block). Also, by appropriately positioning the patient in either Trendelenburg or anti-Trendelenburg position, the hyperbaricity of the solution can be utilized to permit the spread of the spinal anesthetic up or down. Most hyperbaric solutions will have "fixed" by about 20 minutes after injection. The ultimate spinal anesthetic level will be decided by then although there are many reported examples of spinal anesthetic levels changing after this interval of time, a fact that further emphasizes the need for constant monitoring of these patients.

Hypobaric spinal anesthesia is a less frequently but probably under utilized technique. In this method, the drug is usually mixed with sterile water or saline. Because there is an enhanced local anesthetic effect with hypobaric solutions, less milligram dosage is required although the drug is usually mixed in an increased volume to produce a similar block to those doses and volumes used with hyperbaric techniques. Hypobaric spinal anesthesia is especially good for perineal and rectal procedures, such as sigmoidoscopy and hemorrhoidectomy, where the surgical approach requires the patient to be in the Buie or jackknife prone position. With the patient flexed in this position, the highest part of the spinal canal is the sacral area; hypobaric solutions introduced in the lumbosacral area will float to the caudal end of the subarachnoid space and produce effective analgesia of the sacral dermatomes. This particular approach has the added advantage that the position for the spinal puncture and the surgery are the same and the patient does not need to be moved between block and surgery. Hypobaric techniques are useful for those surgical procedures in which the patient remains in the lateral position with the surgical site uppermost, such as for a total hip arthroplasty. Here the hypobaric injection of 4 to 6 ml of water containing 4 to 6 mg of tetracaine will produce an effective anesthesia. With these hypobaric techniques, it is, of course, important to maintain the head at a lower level than the lumbosacral area to prevent the hypobaric solution rising and producing a higher block than required.

Isobaric techniques are not widely used but may be indicated when anesthesia is required at a specific level. Usually the spinal puncture is made and a quantity of spinal fluid withdrawn and this is used as the diluent for mixing the local anesthetic, e.g. tetracaine crystals. When reinjected back into the spinal canal, this solution tends to remain in the injected area, irrespective of the positioning of the patient. This is occasionally useful in those procedures (such as extensive lower extremity surgery or hip fracture) in which it is often humane to anesthetize the patient in his own bed prior to undergoing the extensive and elaborate positioning that is often necessary prior to commencing such surgical procedures. If hyperbaric or hypobaric techniques are used in such a situation, the often vigorous and extensive movement of the patient can produce unplanned spread of the local anesthetic agent.

A further use of agents of different baricity in spinal anesthesia is for diagnostic and therapeutic nerve blocks, wherein small aliquots of hypobaric or hyperbaric local anesthetic or neurolytic agents can be injected at any spinal level to produce either temporary or permanent nerve block (Fig. 21-6). Spinal puncture can be made at any level from the foramen magnum to the lumbosacral junction and individual spinal nerves can be selectively blocked by appropriate patient positioning.[25]

For example, with carcinoma of the breast with infiltration of the chest wall restricted to one side, the patient can be positioned with that side uppermost. By arranging the patient on a flexed table, the appropriate dermatomes can be positioned at a higher level than the head or lower body. A spinal puncture done at this level can then permit the "floating" of hypobaric solutions of local anesthetics for diagnostic purposes. Using this same technique, absolute alcohol can be used for therapeutic neurolysis in volumes of 0.25 to 0.5 ml at the appropriate dermatomes; tests for sensation changes should be conducted prior to proceeding with larger volumes. Traditionally, the patient in this situation is also positioned with the uppermost side of the body angled forward so that this hypobaric solution would preferentially perfuse the posterior rather than the anterior roots to produce a sensory rather than motor block (Fig. 21-6). The involvement of motor block is not so crucial in such areas as the midthorax where only intercostal muscle action would be compromised. Motor sparing is usually stressed for the more important limb muscles, although a sensory deafferented limb is not a functional extremity.

If hyperbaric selective spinal root block is required with the use of, for example, phenol solutions, then the positioning requirements are the reverse of that described above for the hypobaric techniques (i.e., the effected dermatomes are positioned lowermost with the patients head and lower body arranged above the level of the block). The spinal puncture is performed at the appropriate level and small doses (i.e., 0.5 ml) of 10 percent phenol in glycerine are usually used. Phenol is a much less painful injection than alcohol. The relative merits of the neurolytic effects of these drugs are still a matter of controversy and individual preference.[25-27]

TOTAL SPINAL ANESTHESIA

This technique was used in the early days following the introduction of spinal anesthesia by Bier[2] and was enthusiastically proposed by Jonnesco[28] who used combinations of stovaine and strychnine for high spinal anesthesia, even in pediatric neurosurgical cases. More recently, total spinal anesthesia

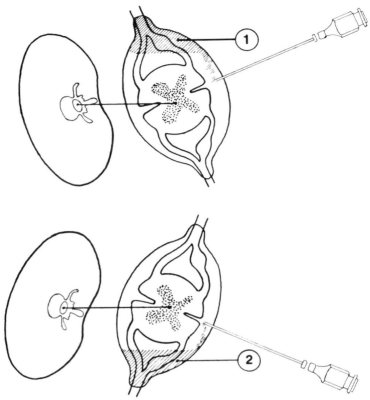

Fig. 21-6 The hypobaric and hyperbaric techniques in subarachnoid puncture. The upper diagram is a transverse section of the patient positioned for hypobaric techniques with either local anesthetic or neurolytic substances; the needle is introduced into the subarachnoid space and the nerves to be blocked are positioned uppermost. By slowly injecting the hypobaric agent, it will rise to float on top of the CSF in the subarachnoid space and selectively anesthetize the posterior root ganglion (1). To maximize this, the patient is rotated forwards so that the hypobaric solution will preferentially perfuse the ganglion on the dorsal root. In the lower diagram, the patient's position is altered for hyperbaric techniques; the patient is positioned with his uppermost side rotated posteriorly to improve perfusion of the posterior root ganglion with the hyperbaric anesthetic or neurolytic agent (2).

has been found to provide excellent operating conditions for abdominal surgery. However, with the large doses of local anesthetic, i.e., 30 to 40 ml of 1 percent lidocaine or mepivicaine, motor paralysis of the legs persisted for 4 hours or more postoperatively. The greatest disadvantage of the technique was the finite duration of the anesthesia lasting anywhere from 90 to 150 minutes, and the patients frequently required supplemental general anesthesia as visceral sensation returned prior to the completion of the surgery. The other disadvantage was that in those patients on whom

the surgery finished before the total spinal anesthesia had receded, artificial respiration was required in the recovery room.

EFFECTS OF SPINAL ANESTHESIA

A differential nerve blockade can exist because weaker solutions are required to block the smaller autonomic C fibers than the larger sensory or motor fibers. Thus a differential zone of anesthesia exists at the upper end of a spinal block. Greene[29] has shown that the level of autonomic sympathetic block is usually two or more segments higher than the sensory block, which in turn is higher than the level of motor block. The significant effect is that the autonomic paralysis is always about two segments higher than the spinal level as determined by pinprick. The higher this sensory block ascends in the thoracic region, the greater is the sympathetic denervation. If the sensory level of spinal block is in the T4 to T3 region, then a complete sympathetic paralysis with profound hypotension may occur.

Effects on Cardiovascular Performance

Because of the sympathetic blockade, spinal anesthesia is usually associated with a fall in arterial blood pressure. This could theoretically compromise coronary perfusion, but because of the decreased afterload, the oxygen requirements for the myocardium are less and usually the coronary perfusion is adequate.[30] Because of these reasons it is not necessary to maintain a "normal" blood pressure. Because the cause of hypotension is usually due to a decreased venous return, a head-down tilt and administration of crystalloids intravenously is usually effective therapy. The patient does not usually need α-stimulating drugs to produce vasoconstriction because this can increase the afterload and the oxygen requirements at a time when the oxygen supply may be diminished because of reduced coronary perfusion. If excessive fluids are given intravenously in this situation, hemodilution with a decrease in the oxygen-carrying power may result.

Effects on Respiratory Function

Respiratory function is usually unimpaired with low spinal anesthetics. But as the height of the spinal anesthetic increases to include thoracic myotomes there is an ascending intercostal muscle paralysis. This, however, has

little, if any, effect on respiratory efficiency in the supine resting surgical patient.[31] Even with total intercostal muscle paralysis, the phrenic drive to the diaphragm is sufficient to maintain respiratory homeostasis. Even with profound blockade up to high thoracic or low cervical areas, arterial blood gas values are usually normal except in the grossly obese patients. These latter individuals will usually need respiratory assistance in the form of endotracheal intubation with positive pressure respiration. Patients with such high blocks cannot, however, cough effectively because of abdominal and thoracic wall muscle paralysis. Therefore any clinical situation that demands the patient clear his airway could compromise ventilation.

Usually when respiration fails in conjunction with a high spinal anesthetic, it is most likely to be due to the hypotension with its resultant ischemia of the respiratory centers in the medulla. The treatment for spinal anesthesia–induced hypotension is outlined under complications.

Effects on Brain-Blood Flow

Cerebral blood flow is unaffected during spinal anesthesia unless profound hypotension occurs as a complication. Autoregulation maintains cerebral perfusion, although Kleinerman et al.[32] showed that hypertensive patients may experience decreases in cerebral blood flow associated with spinal anesthesia–induced hypotension.

COMPLICATIONS OF SPINAL
ANESTHESIA

Hypotension

Hypotension is one of the more common accompaniments of spinal anesthesia. It is usually a reflection of the discrepancy between the capacity of the vascular system and the volume of blood available to fill it. Spinal anesthesia that extends into thoracic levels and above, reduces sympathetic tone and therefore causes peripheral vasodilatation. Blood pools in the periphery and if the venous return is not assisted by gravity (head-down position), then a reduction in cardiac output will result in a fall in arterial blood pressure. This fall in blood pressure is accentuated with increasing elevation of the upper body.

If the patient is kept in a head-down position and any preexisting hypovolemia is corrected by adequate fluid replacement, then usually the cardiac output is maintained and the systemic blood pressure will drop a modest 10 to 15 percent; the latter is usually a reflection of the decreased peripheral vascular resistance.

With head-down tilt, healthy patients tolerate this reduced blood pressure well. Although this hypotension could theoretically compromise coronary perfusion, the decreased afterload that is present with systemic vasodilation reduces the oxygen requirements for the myocardium and coronary perfusion is usually adequate. The vast majority of hypotensive episodes witnessed with developing spinal anesthesia can be treated by intravenous crystalloid administration and the Trendelenburg position.

With ascending sympathetic blockade, the cardiac accelerator fibers that emerge in the upper four thoracic spinal nerves are blocked. Thus the resultant unopposed vagal tone may produce bradycardia, which can result in a reduced cardiac output and contribute to hypotension. Bradycardia may also be produced by decreased stimulation of stretch receptors on the right side of the heart.[19] This bradycardia component of the hypotension may be expeditiously treated with the administration of atropine 0.5 to 1 mg administered intravenously.[33]

Treatment of Hypotension. The slight drop in blood pressure that occurs with most spinal anesthetics probably does not need any specific treatment. A greater fall in blood pressure can be treated by administration of fluids intravenously and the Trendelenburg position. Atropine, 0.3 to 0.6 mg/70 kg, can be given should bradycardia occur.

If the hypotension does not respond to these methods, then vasoconstrictors can be given. Pure α-stimulating vasoconstrictors are less desirable because although they will often increase the blood pressure, they do so at the expense of increasing afterload and thereby increasing myocardial oxygen demand at a time when this may be compromised. Use of the combined α- and β-stimulating drugs (such as ephedrine in doses of 10 to 50 mg IV) is preferred, because this not only produces the desired peripheral vasoconstriction but also promotes central cardiac stimulation.[34]

The above therapeutic approaches apply only to the patient who is normovolemic. With considerable hemorrhage as may occur in trauma or obstetrics, hemostasis is often maintained by intense vasoconstriction. To produce extensive sympathetic blockade in such individuals by means of a spinal anesthetic can result in a precipitous and life-threatening hypotension. For this reason, spinal anesthesia is not indicated in patients who have recently undergone massive hemorrhage unless the intravascular volume has been adequately replaced.

Postspinal Headache

Headache is a frequent sequela to anesthesia and surgery. True spinal headache is due to a persistent CSF leak through the needle hole in the dura mater. This headache is characterized by its dependence on posture. Any attempt to assume the upright position elicits a severe occipital and often circumferential headache, which is relieved by resuming the supine position. In its milder forms, the headache will often spontaneously resolve during the first postoperative days and should be treated conservatively with supine bed rest and copious administration of oral and/or intravenous fluids along with appropriate systemic analgesics. However, for those refractory headaches that are incapacitating and/or for those that do not respond to conservative measures in the first day or so, an epidural blood patch should be considered.[35-37] By administering 5 to 10 ml of the patient's own (aseptically drawn) blood, into the epidural space at the site of the previous lumbar puncture, prompt and efficient relief of pain usually results. It can be repeated in those small percentage of patients who do not get long relief from the first injection. This type of procedure is usually utilized for those cases of inadvertent dural puncture that occur during attempted epidural anesthesia using large bore 18 gauge needles. Should this occur, it is justifiable to place a prophylactic blood patch via the needle or catheter once it is positioned in the epidural space.

Nausea and Vomiting

Nausea and vomiting occurs often during the early induction phases of a high subarachnoid block when hypotension occurs. It is usually effectively treated by restoring the blood pressure with fluid, or vasopressors, or both. It is often self-limiting and the administration of oxygen by mask can be beneficial. The administration of atropine in the presence of bradycardia will also often help.[33]

Urinary Retention

Urinary retention is frequently seen in the postoperative period and is often due to persistent blockade of the nerve supply to the bladder. If large amounts of intravenous fluid had been administered, one should be alert for bladder distension because this may require catheter drainage.

Backache

The ubiquitous complaint of backache is no more common after atraumatic spinal anesthesia than it is after general anesthesia,[38]

and symptomatic treatment is all that is required.

Neurologic Sequelae

Reports of neurologic damage following spinal anesthesia are exceedingly rare. Reviewing the experience in excess of half a million spinal anesthetics, Lund[16] could not find one case of permanent motor paralysis. In another long-term follow-up study of 10,000 cases of spinal anesthesia, Dripps and Vandam[15] found only a single incident of neurologic complication, which may well have been due to a coincident meningioma in that patient. In a series in excess of 3,000 patients, Nolte[17] described one patient with a peripheral neuropathy that could have been caused by the spinal anesthetic.

Evaluation and treatment of neurologic deficits after spinal anesthesia are the same as those described in Chapter 20 for nerve block anesthesia.

CONTRAINDICATIONS TO SPINAL ANESTHESIA

There are relatively few absolute contraindications to spinal anesthesia. Obviously patient refusal or an utterly uncooperative patient who cannot or is not able to keep still during the needling procedure would be obvious examples. To prevent transmission of infected organisms into the subarachnoid space, infection in the injection sites, such as cutaneous pustules and bed sores, would prohibit needling in the area. Raised intercranial pressure is an absolute contraindication to spinal anesthesia as it is to lumbar puncture techniques in general because of the danger of producing herniation of the conus medullaris through the foramen magnum. Because of the risk of uncontrolled bleeding in the spinal canal with its subsequent pressure injury to vital nerve elements, spinal anesthesia is probably contraindicated in patients with any clotting defects or in those who are receiving anticoagulant therapy. The place of spinal anesthesia in those patients receiving "mini-dose" heparin prophylaxis treatments is still controversial. There does not appear to be any evidence to suggest that there is an increased risk of spinal hemorrhage in such situations, but the medicolegal climate suggests caution with needling procedures within the neuraxis during any heparin therapy.

SPINAL NEUROLYTIC BLOCK

Patients with an ongoing cancer frequently have pain due to afferent nociceptive input from this disease. Although selective peripheral nerve blocks are sometimes indicated, the extent of the disease, or its potential spread, or both may require neurolytic block at a relatively central location at spinal nerve roots. The introduction of small amounts of neurolytic agents (alcohol or phenol), into the subarachnoid space, can denervate large parts of the body. By utilizing the hyperbaric and hypobaric nature of these agents (compared with CSF) and appropriate patient positioning, selective denervation can frequently be obtained. These neurolytic blocks usually involve destruction of the posterior root ganglion and, as such, produce a denervation that does not cause the post neurolytic neuralgia that often accompanies neurolysis performed peripherally.[26] The optimal site for spinal and neurolytic block is where the afferent nociceptive pathway is remote from the limb plexuses and nerve pathways concerned with sphincter control (e.g., unilateral cancer in the chest wall and breast). It is theoretically possible to produce selective sensory block and to spare other modalities (motor power and sphincter control). However, because of a high complication rate that varies with the site of the block, the patient must be advised of the risks of the procedure. Often the patient's deteriorating clinical condition is such that the patient and the physician are prepared to accept some of the risks

of the spread of neurolytic agents to nerve pathways other than those conducting the pain.[25, 26]

The following neurolytic agents are those most frequently used in the spinal canal.

Ethyl Alcohol

Ethyl alcohol is usually used in absolute concentrations for subarachnoid neurolytic block. It is readily available in 2 ml ampules and is conveniently titrated during the block using a 1 ml tuberculin syringe. Weaker solutions of alcohol have been suggested in an attempt to perhaps produce selective destruction of smaller sensory fibers and in the hope of preserving larger motor fibers. There is little information to suggest that this is possible or effective.

Phenol

Phenol is a popular neurolytic agent. It is not commercially available for medical use and needs to usually be specially prepared by the hospital pharmacy services. It is used in strengths up to 10 percent and is classically mixed in glycerine to produce a hyperbaric solution.

Because of its poor solubility in water, phenol is usually dissolved in warm glycerine; it is usually convenient to make a 10 percent solution, which can then be diluted if weaker concentrations are needed. Phenol solutions tend to discolor on exposure to light and therefore should be kept in a dark place. Usually such solutions are stable for approximately 12 months. It is convenient to have the pharmacy make up sterile supplies of 1 g of phenol crystals, which can then be dissolved in the appropriate amount of warmed sterile glycerine just prior to use. Ten percent phenol solutions are usually predictably neurolytic, whereas with the 5 percent solution it is often difficult to obtain any objective neurolysis.

Technique of Neurolytic Subarachnoid Block

The patient position will vary depending on whether a hyperbaric (phenol) or a hypobaric (alcohol) neurolytic agent is used.

With alcohol, the spinal segments to be blocked are positioned uppermost and the remaining nerves are positioned at a lower level, usually by flexing the table with the head and pelvis at a lower position than the area to be blocked; this is done to attempt to prevent the spread of neurolytic agent to the limb plexuses, cranial nerves, and autonomic nerve components controlling sphincters. If hyperbaric phenol is used, then the positions are reversed, i.e., the area to be blocked is positioned at the lowest level and the operating room table is adjusted so that the head and lower spinal areas are at a higher position.

In an attempt to preferentially perfuse the posterior roots and the sensory ganglion, the body should be rotated as shown in Figure 21-6.

The safest approach is to use very small aliquots of neurolytic agent, i.e., 0.25 to 0.5 ml, and to note the effect of each bolus prior to proceeding with further injections. Thus, neurolysis can be controlled and too extensive a spread prevented. Because the extent of neurolysis should be tested frequently during the procedure, there is a practical advantage to using hypobaric solutions such as alcohol: the upper side of the patient is much more accessible for testing with pin prick then the under side of the patient particularly when the patient is surrounded by pillows, sandbags, and other support aids.

When terminal sacral neurolysis is required of the lower sacral nerve roots, the prone flexed jackknife position is good for the use of alcohol, as the sacral areas are readily available for testing with pin prick in this situation. When hyperbaric techniques are used, the patient is positioned sitting and this often precludes access to the perineal area for adequate testing during the procedure.

Comparison Between Alcohol and Phenol

Controversy exists concerning the relative merits of these two agents. This probably stems from the fact that the extent and duration of neurolytic blocks with both agents are exceedingly variable. Although analgesia for several months is desired, frequently pain relief is much shorter. Alcohol is more convenient to obtain, being commercially available in 2 ml ampules. It also tends to give a more rapid onset and enables the operator to see the effect at the time of the procedure, whereas the effect of phenol may alter over the 24 hours following the block. The disadvantage of alcohol is that it is an exceedingly painful injection, although this discomfort is very short-lived and usually tolerated satisfactorily by most patients.

Epidural Neurolytic Injections

In an attempt to control chronic pain states, neurolytic agents have occasionally been injected into the epidural space. Phenol (in doses of 5 to 10 percent concentrations, usually in aqueous solution) has been used most widely for this effect.[25] There is limited evidence from which to draw specific conclusions about the merits of neurolytic epidural blocks.[27] Characteristically the somatic evidence for blockade (i.e., dermal analgesia) dissipates very rapidly; with the weaker 5 percent solutions, it is often difficult to detect—even on the day following the blockade. However, patients have reported prolonged pain relief, even with the persistence of dermal sensation. With the concentrations used above, motor blockade has not been a significant long-term complication, and therefore epidural neurolysis may have some application when chemically neurodestructive procedures are needed in an area where motor blockade must be spared, e.g., in the area of the limb plexuses. Of course, whenever neurolytic agents are injected around the neuraxis, there is always cause for considerable concern, particularly that of the possibility of accidental subdural puncture with large doses of neurolytic drugs, which could prove catastrophic.

EPIDURAL ANESTHESIA

Epidural anesthesia, like spinal anesthesia, attempts to produce regional nerve block. There are, however, salient differences in the nature of the block produced and the physiological responses to it. In general, epidural anesthesia tends to produce a less "solid" block than spinal anesthesia. The disparity between motor and sensory levels is usually more marked with epidural anesthesia than with spinal anesthesia. Although the mechanisms for epidural block is still a matter of debate,[39] it probably produces a maximal initial effect on the nerves as they traverse the epidural space. Selective segmental blockade can more easily be achieved, and this will leave sensation intact above and below the blocked segments. At the same sensory level, the physiological responses to epidural and spinal anesthesia are often quite different. The onset of sympathetic blockade is usually slower with epidural anesthesia and thus permits adequate compensatory vasoconstriction in the unblocked parts of the body. This difference is probably most marked in the older, less vasoreactive age groups.

Another salient difference between the two techniques is that much larger doses of local anesthetic agent are injected into the epidural space. These drugs can produce a systemic effect after uptake from the injection site in contrast to the much smaller doses used in spinal anesthesia, which have little or no systemic effects. Although mean arterial blood pressure changes are often similar with subarachnoid and epidural blocks, there are often significant cardiovascular differences when epinephrine is added to the epidural solutions. Epinephrine can produce a marked rise in cardiac output due to the β-stimulating effect of the low circulating levels of epineph-

rine that are absorbed from the epidural space.

The injection of local anesthetic drugs in the epidural space requires different needles than for spinal anesthesia and also requires catheters to enable reinjection to take place.

The different sites of needle insertion for spinal and epidural puncture, are shown in Figure 21-7.

There are several varieties of epidural needles available, and individual enthusiasts have modified both ends of the needle for specific purposes.

Epidural needles basically come in two types. Those in which the orifice is at the distal end of the needle (Crawford)[40] and those in which the blunt leading edge of the needle has a lateral opening at the tip (Tuohy). The reason for this latter construction is an effort to reduce the incidence of dural puncture: it is postulated that the blunt leading end of the Tuohy-type needle will be less likely to puncture the dura as it enters the epidural space. In the open-ended needles such as the Crawford, this risk of dural puncture is reduced by the injection of a bolus of saline or air as the epidural space is entered; this bolus is intended to push the dura away from the advancing needle. Both needles have their advocates, and if used appropriately, both seem to have a low incidence (0.5 percent) of dural puncture.[26, 39]

The hub end of the needle has been modified, usually by the attachment of "wings" or large spool-type hubs to ostensibly facilitate handling of the needle. These refinements have individual enthusiastic support but are not essential for satisfactory performance of epidural anesthesia.

These needles are usually available in an 18 gauge thin-wall model whose internal diameters will permit the passage of the epidural catheters commercially available. They should be inserted with the stylet in situ down to ligamentum flavum to prevent depositing

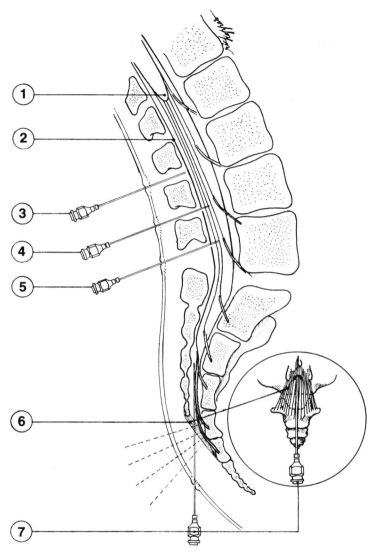

Fig. 21-7 Subarachnoid and peridural approaches. A longitudinal section through the lumbar and sacral areas show the positions and relationships of subarachnoid and epidural needle placements in these sites. Numerals represent as follows: (1) the conus medullaris of the distal cord at the level of L2 (below this point, the spinal canal contains the cauda equina); (2) the dura mater; (3) a lumbar epidural needle placement at the L3-L4 interspace with the needle point situated in the epidural space; (4) s subarachnoid needle placement at the L4-L5 interspace with the needle situated in the subarachnoid compartment containing the cauda equina; (5) a needle position in the subarachnoid space at the L5-S1 interspace (Taylor approach); and (6) the sacrococcygeal ligament, which is the site of puncture for caudal epidural anesthesia. The dotted lines in the sacrococcygeal ligament show the needle approach, whereby the needle is first introduced at a steep angle to effect puncture of the sacrococcygeal ligament; having pierced the ligament, the needle contacts the bony endpoint of the dorsal aspect of the ventral plate of the sacrum and then by a series of needle readjustments, a more acute angle is adopted and the needle threaded into the sacral canal as shown in the inset (7). The latter shows the dorsal view of the needle in situ piercing the sacrococcygeal ligament, which is shown stretching from the sacral cornu above to the coccyx below.

an epidermal plug of tissue into the neuraxis.[41]

TECHNIQUE OF EPIDURAL ANESTHESIA

Probably the most commonly used technique for inserting the needle in the epidural space is determining the loss of resistance to injection as the needle passes from the dense ligamentum flavum into the epidural space where there is free flow to injection. With the Tuohy- and Crawford-type needles, the needle is inserted with the stylet in situ down into the area of the ligamentum flavum. The stylet is then removed and the resistance to injection is checked either intermittently or continuously as the needle is slowly advanced through the ligamentum flavum. As the needle passes ventral to the ligamentum flavum there is little, if any, resistance to injected air or fluid and a negative aspiration test suggests that the needle lumen is now in the epidural space.

The midline technique is preferred by many anesthesiologists because it is easy to identify in most patients and is less vascular as the needle passes through ligamentous structures throughout its course, i.e., supraspinous, interspinous, and ligamentum flavum. The epidural space also is less vascular in the midline, since the epidural venous plexuses tend to be distributed in bilateral paramedian channels. One of the disadvantages of the midline technique is the lack of feedback as to the exact depth of the ligamentum flavum. Therefore continued testing of resistance to injection is necessary once an appropriate depth of needle insertion has been reached.

With paramedian techniques and using usually the Crawford tip (although the Tuohy may be used in this situation), the needle is inserted lateral to the spinous process below the space selected for puncture. The needle is inserted parallel to the line of the vertebral spine and adjacent to it, and it is usual to locate the lamina of the vertebra at a depth of 4 to 7 cm. This then is very useful feedback as to the depth of the ligamentum flavum, and by walking the epidural needle in a cephalad and medial direction off the lamina, the sensation transmitted along the needle will change from that of hard marble-like bone to a more resilient leather-like ligamentum. The stylet is now withdrawn from the needle and a syringe of either air or saline is attached. The needle is now moved through the ligamentum flavum very slowly and constant pressure is applied to the attached syringe barrel so that as the needle lumen enters the epidural space a bolus of air or saline will be flushed out of the syringe; the latter is to detect the loss of resistance identifying the epidural space and also hopefully to push the dura away from the advancing needle point.

It is of paramount importance that the needle traverse the ligamentum flavum in a controlled fashion. The usual way to do this is to apply resistance to its advancing motion with the anesthesiologist's nondominant hand. The dominant hand will be applied to the syringe testing the resistance of the barrel throughout the movement. There is individual preference as to the best ways to achieve this. I prefer to place the dorsum of the nondominant hand adjacent to the needle as it is embedded in the ligamentum flavum and using a tripod consisting of thumb, forefinger, and middle finger of this hand to secure the hub of the advancing needle and thus provide resistance to the advancing force that is applied by the dominant hand. In this way the needle advanced through ligamentum flavum is under control, and as the loss of resistance sensation is appreciated, the needle does not move forward in an uncontrolled fashion.

An alternative technique that is often used with the Tuohy needle in the midline approach is to advance the needle 1 mm at a time as it crosses the ligamentum flavum, testing each time for loss of resistance with either air or fluid. Both techniques work well as experience is gained and individual preference is the determining factor.

A drop of saline placed on the open hub of such needles will be "sucked in" as the needle enters the epidural space with its subatmospheric pressure, and this has been used as an indicator in the "hanging drop" method of Gutierrez as described in a book on epidural anesthesia by Bromage.[39]

EPIDURAL CATHETERS

By placement of a malleable epidural catheter through the needle, this form of anesthesia has the main advantage over spinal anesthetics in that it can provide continuous reinjection opportunities. Most of the modern catheters are nylon or Teflon and perform well. The ideal catheter should have an external diameter that passes through the standard epidural 18 gauge thin-wall needles and have walls thick enough so that kinking does not occur during taping and patient positioning. They should be biologically inert and have some distance markers to ascertain how far the catheters have been threaded through the needle. Ideally they should be radiopaque so that their position can be checked by radiographs if necessary. Most cannulas come with a metal stylet to provide rigidity for threading in the epidural space. Because the stylet could theoretically make the catheter so rigid that it might puncture the dura, the stylet should be withdrawn 1 or 2 cm from the tip of the catheter so that the leading edge of the catheter presents a soft and pliable front as it is advanced in the epidural space; this hopefully will reduce the incidence of both dural and/or epidural vein puncture.

Despite these techniques, catheters from time to time will find their way into epidural veins or subarachnoid spaces either at the time of insertion or hours or days later. This fact reaffirms the mandatory requirement of test doses whenever epidural catheters are either injected for the first time or the tenth time! Because of the pulsating nature of the spinal cord and its surrounding membranes, it is not surprising that over the course of time

catheters can erode their way into a subdural setting. Once threaded through the introducing needle (either Tuohy or Crawford), the catheter should never be withdrawn through the needle as this can transect the catheter. If the catheter needs to be withdrawn, the needle and catheter must be removed simultaneously.

MECHANICAL AND OTHER AIDS TO DETERMINE EPIDURAL NEEDLE PLACEMENT

The ingenuity of individual anesthesiologists has been exercised in attempts to produce mechanical and other indicators for correct placement of the needle in the epidural space. Most of these are devices to detect the subatmospheric pressure that exists in this space and usually use capillary attachments with fluid indicators (Odom) or inflated balloons (MacIntosh) that deflate upon entering the epidural space. Other springload devices have been used to facilitate the loss of resistance phenomena as the epidural needle passes from dense ligamentum flavum into the lower resistance of the epidural space. However, most of these devices tend to be more trouble than they are worth and in my opinion the physician's own kinesthetic sense is probably the best transducer and indicator.

THORACIC EPIDURAL ANESTHESIA

One of the disadvantages of lumbar or caudal epidural anesthesia is the fact that very large volumes of drug often need to be used if analgesia is needed in the high abdominal or thoracic area. For such procedures as thoracotomy or cholecystectomy, this results in excessive blockade in the pelvic and lower extremity regions, which is not necessary for this surgery. Consequently postoperatively, analgesia recedes from the operative site at an early stage and yet the lower extremities are still blocked for a considerable time. By depositing the local anesthetic in the thoracic epidural space, segmental analgesia can be achieved in the required thoracic dermatomes with much smaller quantities of drug. This leaves the pelvic and lower extremity dermatomes and myotomes unblocked, which permits the patient to move the lower extremities postoperatively. One option for producing thoracic epidural blockade is to thread a catheter into the thoracic area from below. Attempts to predictably thread catheters any distance in the lumbar epidural space are fraught with failure. For example, knots can form in a catheter or the catheter can be diverted out of a paravertebral foramen and produce a unilateral paravertebral block. For this reason, thoracic placement of the epidural needle and catheter has been undertaken by many authors and has proven an eminently safe form of anesthesia.[6, 42] Small doses of local anesthetic of as little as 0.5 ml per thoracic spinal segment will give satisfactory anesthesia for operative and especially postoperative analgesia.

The main deterrent to thoracic epidural anesthesia is the theoretic possibility of producing trauma to the spinal cord by the epidural needle. Although theoretically this is a possibility, neurologic deficits following this procedure are rare. The reasons for this may be that thoracic epidural techniques are usually performed by individuals who already have considerable expertise in the conventional lumbar approaches. Also anatomically, there is an additional safety factor if the blocks are restricted to the midthoracic area because in this part of the spinal canal, the spinal cord is at its thinnest between the two enlargements of the brachial and lumbosacral plexuses. Therefore there is a greater distance from ligamentum flavum to the dorsum of the cord in the midthoracic than in the lower or upper thoracic areas. However, it should be borne in mind that there is the potential for catastrophic trauma to the spinal cord with the epidural needle, and therefore this technique should be reserved for those with proven manual dexterity in the other epidural approaches. The technique is appropriate for operative anesthesia in the thoracic and upper abdominal areas and is enjoying a renewed utilization with the increased incidence of gastric bypass techniques for surgery in grossly obese patients;[6] in these patients (who are at increased risk for postoperative pulmonary and other complications) it can provide not only satisfactory analgesia during the procedure, but with very small doses administered either intermittently or by continuous perfusion in the postoperative period, permit early activity and even ambulation. (Fig. 21-8).

DRUGS USED IN EPIDURAL
ANESTHESIA (SEE TABLE 21-2)

Lidocaine

Lidocaine is an excellent drug for epidural anesthesia. It is usually used in 1 percent solutions for analgesia and 2 percent solutions for intraoperative anesthesia. It is characterized by a relatively rapid onset, and the doses needed vary from a maximum of 1.6 ml of 2 percent lidocaine per segment for young adults to half that amount for the elderly. Unless combined with epinephrine, caudal anesthesia is often unsatisfactory when administered via the lumbar approach. This is probably because of the fact that the drug, although it spreads caudally, is not maintained in contact with the nerves long enough to produce a solid block. Motor blockade with 2 percent lidocaine is often limited to the myotomes adjacent to the site of injection. The further the myotomes are from this site, the less satisfactory the motor block; thus, for lumbar epidural anesthesia, there is often profound motor blockade of the hip flexors, but the patient often can still quite actively produce plantar flexion of the feet, even when there is satisfactory abdominal surgical anesthesia. Mepivacaine is very similar to lidocaine but lasts a little longer.

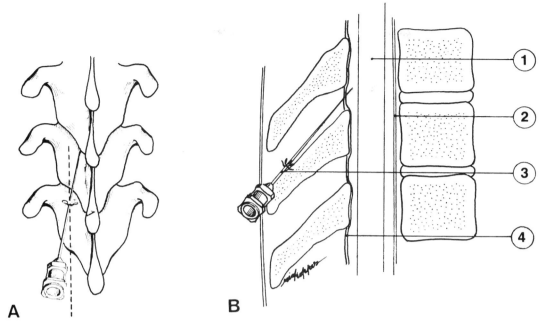

Fig. 21-8 Thoracic epidural puncture. (*A*) The paramedian approach to the epidural space in the thoracic region wherein the initial track of the needle as shown by the dotted line contacts the bony endpoint of the lamina of the thoracic vertebrae; the needle is then repositioned by walking along this lamina in a cephalad and medial fashioin until it locates the ligamentum flavum between the overlapping lamina. The angle of introduction of the needle is much steeper here than in the lumbar region. This is necessary because of this oblique overhang of the vertebral lamina. (*B*) The acute angle of approach of the needle as seen in a sagittal section. Numerals represent (1) the thoracic spinal cord surrounded by dura mater; (2) the anterior longitudinal ligament; (3) the needle piercing the ligamentum flavum with its tip in the epidural space; and (4) the ligamentum flavum.

Bupivacaine

The long-acting amide anesthetic bupivacaine is another very satisfactory drug to use in epidural anesthesia. A solution of 0.5 percent will produce good analgesia and usually 0.75 percent is used to produce operative anesthesia. Bupivacaine is characterized by a relatively slower onset than lidocaine. It tends to spread equally as well in the epidural space, producing operative anesthesia for a period in excess of that produced by lidocaine. Bupivacaine is, however, characterized by producing much longer anesthesia than lidocaine in the dermatomes and myotomes adjacent to the injected site in the epidural space. Thus, although the anesthesia at the upper limits of the block may recede early, anesthesia persists for a considerably longer time than lidocaine at the level of the block. Thus for postoperative pain relief, it would be ideal to have the catheter positioned at those dermatome levels that correspond to the site of maximal discomfort. With this set-up, relatively small doses of bupivacaine can give prolonged analgesia. When administered in the lumbar epidural space, there appears to be relatively poor caudal spread with bupivacaine as there is with lidocaine. Often the bupivacaine does not penetrate the large S1 and L5 segmental nerves to their central core, and this frequently results in a sparing of sensation in the distal distribution of these nerves over the foot.[43-45] Motor block with bupivacaine, 0.75 percent, tends to be more profound and of longer duration than that of lidocaine, lasting approximately 2 to 3 hours.[45]

Etidocaine

Etidocaine closely parallels bupivacaine in its characteristics[45] with regard to sensory blockade, although it has a much faster onset degree and duration of motor block than does bupivacaine. Studies in patients as well as in human volunteers have attested to the similarities in the sensory block characteristics of these agents.[13] But when used clinically, a higher degree of unsatisfactory analgesia with etidocaine with regard to both intraoperative and postoperative analgesia is more evident.[13] There is not as yet a satisfactory explanation for this, although there is some evidence to suggest that etidocaine is less efficient in producing small fiber blockade; the latter is indicated by evidence that suggests bupivacaine is more efficient at providing both more effective and lengthier sympathetic block than etidocaine.[45]

Tetracaine

Tetracaine has been used infrequently for epidural anesthesia. In a 0.5 percent solution it does produce satisfactory sensory and motor blockade; however, it appears to spread poorly in the peridural space and has not found widespread use.

Chloroprocaine

The short duration of chloroprocaine has prevented its widespread use for surgical anesthesia. However, because of low systemic toxicity and relatively rapid onset, it has recently become popular for obstetric anesthesia. Combining it with bupivacaine to provide a rapid onset and long-acting drug combina-tion has been attempted, but the combination has not proved to be an arithmetic sum of the different characteristics of the individual components.[46]

Adhesive arachnoiditis and associated sensory and motor deficits have followed the inadvertent subarachnoid injection of large doses of chloroprocaine; the low pH of the solution has been indicted as a possible cause of these complications. Thus, if using this solution for epidural anesthesia and should an inadvertent subarachnoid injection occur, the chloroprocaine should be flushed with isotonic saline out of the subarachnoid space as soon as possible.[46a]

Block Characteristics of Commonly Used Agents

The characteristics of onset of epidural anesthesia are similar for both the shorter-acting lidocaine and the longer-acting bupivacaine and etidocaine. Onset of anesthesia occurs first at the site of injection and then spreads cephalad at a faster rate than caudally. This is probably because the size of the upper lumbar and thoracic nerves is smaller, which permits more rapid penetration of the drug than does the larger size of the lower lumbar and upper sacral nerves. Maximal spread is achieved in approximately 20 to 30 minutes. The resultant level is usually maintained for a period of approximately 1 to 1½ hours with lidocaine and 2 to 3 hours with initial doses of either bupivacaine or etidocaine. The block with lidocaine regresses quite rapidly, usually over a 15 to 30 minute period. Analgesia usually persists longest in those segments first blocked, where presumably the maximal concentration of drug is placed. With the longer-acting agents bupivacaine and etidocaine, however, there is often a persistent "tail" of anesthesia that is maintained in the segments adjacent to the injection site. Thus although "operative anesthesia" (i.e., analgesia of the abdominal wall and contents) dissipates after 2 to 3 hours,

**Table 21-2. Dose, Latency, and Duration of
Local Anesthetic–Induced Epidural Anesthesia***

Drug	Concentration (%)	Dose (mg)/ Segment	Latency (min)	Duration (min)	Quality
Chloroprocaine	3	45	12	60	Good
Procaine	5	60	20	60	Poor
Tetracaine	0.5	7	18	145	Poor
Dibucaine	0.33	45	40	200	Poor
Lidocaine	2	31	16	46	Good
Mepivacaine	2	31	17	60	Good
Bupivacaine	0.75	9	16	210	Good
Etidocaine	1	15	10	170	Good
Bupivacaine	0.5	7	18	120	Poor

* These doses are for young adults and should be decreased according to increasing age.[68, 69, 70] These data are for local anesthetics without epinephrine, which will increase the shorter acting drugs by 50 percent (see text).

there is often a tail of anesthesia that persists in those dermatomes adjacent to the injection site, i.e., over the groin and thigh areas (see Fig. 21-9).

A unilateral epidural block usually can not be achieved even with appropriate positioning. However, such aberrations do occur spontaneously from time to time.[47] Possible explanations are meningeal septa or more likely that the epidural catheter has threaded out of a paravertebral foramen.

Anesthetic Sparing of Lower Lumbar and Sacral Segments

With the use of the long-acting agents bupivacaine and etidocaine in lumbar epidural anesthesia, many patients have inadequate analgesia in the lower leg and foot areas.[43] This phenomena is almost certainly due to lack of penetration of the drug into the larger L5-S1 nerve roots. The drug obviously spreads down into the sacral areas, because analgesia of more distal nerves is frequently present (Fig. 21-9). This lack of penetration is less evident with lidocaine. However, if epinephrine is not included in the lidocaine solutions injected into the lumbar area, then satisfactory caudal analgesia frequently does not result.[12]

If block is required in these L5 and S1 dermatomes, then a low lumbar approach

should be used and the catheter directed caudally, or alternatively caudal epidural anesthesia should be performed allowing the local anesthetic to be deposited at the nerve roots.

PHYSIOLOGICAL EFFECTS OF
EPIDURAL ANESTHESIA

Effects on Cardiovascular Performance

Effects of Epidural Anesthesia. Early authors assumed that hypotension produced by epidural anesthesia was explained entirely by sympathetic blockade but that the hypotension was less in both frequency and magnitude than that encountered with spinal anesthesia. However, the degree of hypotension was later observed to be similar to that of spinal anesthesia, but the onset was significantly slower. Studies by Ward[48] in human volunteers receiving both spinal and epidural anesthesia showed that marked cardiovascular changes were associated with the epinephrine-containing solutions that were used in the epidural blocks.

That high epidural block is associated with hypotension has been known for many years, and it was ascribed originally to dilatation of both resistance and capacitance vessels. Defalque[49] demonstrated that the degree of hy-

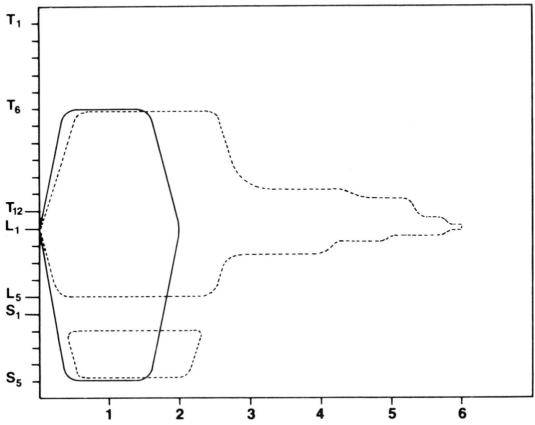

Fig. 21-9 Shown are the block spreading characteristics of lidocaine and bupivacaine injected into the epidural space via catheter at L1. The vertical axis represents the spinal segment levels from T1 through S5 and the horizontal axis is time in hours. Lidocaine anesthesia is shown by the area within the solid line and bupivacaine by the areas within the dotted lines.

Anesthesia commences and last longest at the site of the injection (L1) for both agents. Cephalad spread is usually more rapid in onset than caudad spread for both drugs and the sacral sparing effect that is seen with bupivacaine, whereby the L5 and S1 dermatomes may remain unblocked, is shown. Various degrees of this sparing can occur from complete absence of block, as shown, through to a late onset and early regression in these dermatomes. The operative analgesia of the abdominal wall lasts longer with bupivacaine than lidocaine and the cessation of anesthesia in lidocaine is much more precipitous; when lidocaine starts to wear off, it rapidly dissipates, whereas with bupivacaine—although there is a fairly steep curve as the block wears off from above downwards—the segments adjacent to the injection site are persistently blocked, often for a period of another 2 to 3 hours after the regression of anesthesia over the abdominal wall segment.

potension bore a linear relationship to the height of the block. Bonica et al.[50] found that normovolemic human volunteers were well able to compensate for this vasodilation with blocks as high as the fifth thoracic dermatome. However, anesthesia above this level also blocks the cardioaccelerator fibers with appreciable decreases in blood pressure, heart rate, and cardiac output.[51]

Effects of the Local Anesthetic Agent. When large doses of local anesthetics are injected into the epidural space, significant systemic blood levels of these agents occur, particularly over time with reinjections. It has been assumed that the systemic effects of these agents would increase any hypotension that occurs as a result of the vasomotor block of epidural anesthesia. However, cardiovascular stimulatory effects have been implicated, particularly from lidocaine. Two possible mechanisms for this are that of a centrally mediated effect relying on the integrity of central and peripheral nervous pathways and of a peripheral effect similar to the potentiation of endogenous catecholamines by cocaine.[52]

Effects of Added Vasoconstrictor. Epinephrine produces both an α effect characterized by vasoconstriction of resistance and capacitance vessels and a β effect that produces increases in heart rate, stroke volume, and cardiac output, which are accompanied by a vasodilation and a fall in peripheral resistance. This β effect is noted with the low circulating levels of epinephrine in epidural anesthesia. In contrast, phenylephrine when used with epidural anesthetic agents produces a decrease in cardiac output and an increase in mean arterial pressure and total peripheral resistance.[44]

Effects on Organ Blood Flow

Hepatic blood flow decreases during peridural anesthesia with lidocaine alone, probably because there is an increased splanchnic vascular resistance and a slight decrease in arterial pressure. This is in contrast to what is seen with high spinal anesthesia, in which the decrease in hepatic blood flow is due to the decrease in arterial pressure because the vascular resistance is not significantly elevated.[53, 54] The differences are presumably due to the sympathetic blockade plus the elevated blood lidocaine levels, since they persist beyond the effect of the circulating epinephrine (i.e., when the cardiac output and splanchnic vascular resistance return to normal after 30 minutes, the hepatic blood

flow decreased the same degree as peridural anesthesia with lidocaine alone).[54] Spinal and epidural anesthesia produces a less profound reduction in splanchnic blood flow than the general anesthetic agents except halothane.[39]

Epidural anesthesia produces a decrease in glomerular filtration rate and renal plasma flow, which reflects the reduction in arterial pressure produced by both plain and epinephrine-containing local anesthetic solutions.[53]

Effects on Respiration

Deafferentation of the abdomen and chest wall leads to reduction of sensory input to the respiratory motor nuclei and a subsequent reduced but adequate motor output carried by the phrenic nerves. Spontaneous respiration with high epidural blockade, even with light general anesthesia, usually maintains satisfactory respiratory exchange,[31] even with upper abdominal surgery. The arterial blood gas values remain in a normal acceptable range. However, if the operation lasts beyond 2 to 3 hours or if there is any indication that satisfactory gas exchange is not being maintained, controlled ventilation should be instituted.

With regard to blood-gas measurements, the opinion is divided as to the relative merits of epidural analgesia in the postoperative period compared with narcotic analgesia. Some authors claim improved oxygenation after epidural analgesia compared with narcotic analgesia.[39] Clinically, respiratory status appears to be improved with postoperative epidural analgesia but review of the literature fails to prove this. A possible explanation is the difficulty of obtaining valid studies of respiratory variables in sick postoperative patients.[39]

As with high spinal anesthesia, the ability to cough is compromised because of intercostal and abdominal wall muscle paralysis. The airway obviously must be protected if there is any danger of aspiration of gastric contents.

Effects on Bladder Control

The effects of epidural anesthesia on bladder control are similar to those seen with spinal anesthesia: lumbar and sacral epidural anesthesia results in an atonic bladder with large volumes of residual urine, which needs to be drained by catheterization if the block continues for any length of time. However, if segmental thoracic epidural analgesia is induced to produce segmental blockade for, as an example, a cholecystectomy and continued postoperatively, then the lower parts of the spinal cord are left intact and bladder function should continue spontaneously.

Effects on Sodium and Water Retention

Bevan[55] has demonstrated that epidural anesthesia can prevent the usual postoperative retention of sodium, probably because this is mediated through spinal control rather than via vagal reflexes. Similarly, the hyperglycemia of the postoperative state can be reversed by epidural blockade but the hypersecretion of cortisol cannot.

ADDITION OF EPINEPHRINE TO EPIDURAL ANESTHETIC AGENTS

Epinephrine is usually added to epidural anesthetic agents in a concentration of 1:200,000. The local vasoconstrictive effect in the epidural space will reduce the uptake of anesthetic agent producing lower blood levels and therefore less potential systemic toxicity than plain solutions. Also a more profound and satisfactory block probably will result. With the shorter-acting agents, such as lidocaine and mepivacaine, the duration of block will be increased by approximately 50 percent. However, with the longer-acting agents, such as bupivacaine and etidocaine, the epinephrine effect dissipates before the local anesthetic effect and any increase in length of action is less significant. When drugs are administered via the lumbar epidural route, anesthesia of the lower lumbar and upper sacral roots are often imperfect and this is particularly so when plain solutions are used. The addition of epinephrine enhances the adequacy of the caudal spread of lumbar peridural block with lidocaine, bupivacaine, and etidocaine.[12]

There are some occasions when it is not desirable to add epinephrine to the solution. This includes anesthesia for those rare patients who are receiving monoamine oxidase inhibiting drugs, for those patients with a fixed cardiac output, and during those procedures, such as in ambulatory surgery facilities, where brevity of action and rapid restoration of function is a desirable characteristic.

Epinephrine is optimally added to the local anesthetic solution immediately prior to use because the lower pH of the commercially available epinephrine-containing solutions tends to increase the latency of onset by increasing the ionization of the local anesthetic solution.

From extensive studies on human volunteers, Ward[48] demonstrated significant cardiovascular differences between epidural blocks produced with plain as opposed to epinephrine-containing solutions, and these differences were attributed to the β-stimulating effects of the epinephrine. Tachycardia and increase in stroke volume and therefore cardiac output occur simultaneously with the decrease in peripheral resistance due to the vasodilation. The net result is usually a fall in mean arterial pressure. These β-stimulating systemic effects of the epinephrine reach a peak after about 15 minutes and last for 130 minutes (which in the case of lidocaine epidural anesthesia, lasts about as long as the block). For the longer acting agents—bupivacaine and etidocaine—the epinephrine effect is much shorter than the blockade. Compensatory vasoconstriction of the unblocked part of the body plays an important part in maintaining homeostasis during epidural blockade.

Phenylephrine has been considered as an alternative vasoconstrictor to epinephrine in epidural solution.[44] Epinephrine in a dose of 5 μg/ml is equipotent as a vasoconstrictor to 50 μg/ml of phenylephrine. In these concentrations, epinephrine is more effective in limiting vascular uptake of lidocaine from the peridural space. The β-stimulating effect of epinephrine (i.e., increased cardiac output, stroke volume, and cardiac rate and a decreased total peripheral resistance) is absent with the phenylephrine. Limb blood flow increases considerably more with the epinephrine than with the phenylephrine solution.

THE CARDIOVASCULAR RESPONSES TO EPIDURAL ANESTHESIA DURING BLOOD LOSS

The cardiovascular responses described above have been, for the most part, determined in studies done on healthy young volunteers and may not reflect the true state of affairs in the clinical situation. The hemodynamic responses of epidural anesthesia described above may not occur in individuals who are depleted of intravascular volume or suffering from hemorrhagic shock. The release of sympathetic tone that is produced by epidural anesthesia could, of course, produce catastrophic hypotension. Preliminary investigations by Bonica[56] showed in fact that high epidural block was poorly tolerated in individuals who had previously lost 15 percent of their blood volume and therefore these blocks probably are contraindicated in uncompensated hemorrhagic shock.

COMPLICATIONS OF EPIDURAL ANESTHESIA

Accidental Subarachnoid Puncture

After completion of placement of the epidural needle, clear fluid can sometimes be aspirated via the needle. In some cases the fluid frankly drips out from the needle when the syringe has been detached. This fluid may be CSF, the saline that was injected to obtain the loss of resistance, or the local anesthetic fluid if that had been injected.

To determine the nature of this fluid, drops should be permitted to fall onto the forearm of the anesthesiologist. Cerebrospinal fluid will feel warm but fluid that has just recently been injected will feel colder. If the drops of fluid are allowed to drip onto a fresh test strip for glucose, a color change will identify the presence of glucose as would be the case in CSF (45 to 65 mg percent glucose in CSF). Another interesting test for this fluid is described by Catterberg[57] in which a few drops of the fluid are dripped into some 2.5 percent thiopental. If the fluid is a local anesthetic, with a low pH, immediate precipitation occurs; whereas if it is CSF, with a higher pH (above 7.0), no precipitation occurs.

If a large dose of local anesthetic destined for the epidural space is administered into the subarachnoid compartment, then a high or total spinal anesthesia could result. The main problem here is the potential for immediate catastrophe due to profound hypotension with its subsequent respiratory paralysis. However, with vigilant monitoring, such an event should become readily evident. By treating the patient with head-down position, adequate intravascular volume replacement and, if need be, the addition of vasopressor agents (e.g., ephedrine in 10 to 50 mg quantities intravenously) the adverse effects of the high spinal anesthesia are well managed. If total spinal anesthesia occurs, endotracheal intubation and controlled ventilation may be required until the anesthesia recedes. Healthy patients tolerate such complications well if they are treated expeditiously. Should such a high or total spinal anesthesia result, it is quite feasible to proceed with the surgery once the physiological parameters have been stabilized (see comments regarding total spinal anesthesia in this chapter).

Intravascular Injection

Because of the highly vascular epidural space, the needle or the catheter occasionally may be placed within the lumen of one of these epidural vessels. If undetected, a large dose of local anesthetic could be injected into the intravascular compartment and produce systemic toxicity. In its more florid form, frank convulsions may result, and the dangers to the patient at this stage are that of hypoxia and/or cardiovascular collapse.

If the patient begins to show signs of systemic toxicity—that is, complains of tingling sensation around the mouth or lips, becomes tremulous, or starts shaking—the first priority is to administer 100 percent oxygen via a mask and then to titrate small doses of CNS depressants, usually diazepam in doses of 1 to 5 mg or thiopental 25 to 50 mg for a 70 kg adult. This approach will usually prevent the progress of the toxic reaction to convulsions. If frank convulsions should appear, however, positive pressure ventilation and even endotracheal intubation may be required. It is rare that muscle relaxants as such are needed to acquire control of the airway, but it is conceivable that succinylcholine might be used in the more refractory cases. This only prevents the skeletal muscle manifestations of the convulsions, but can enable the more expeditious control of the airway. If hypotension occurs, then intravascular fluid and/or ephedrine in IV doses of 10 to 50 mg should be administered to maintain blood pressure. Because of the possibility of such intravascular injections, test doses are mandatory whenever catheters are reinjected.

Postspinal Headache After Accidental Dural Puncture During Epidural Anesthesia

After an accidental puncture to the dura with a large 18 gauge needle, postpuncture headache occurs in about 70 percent of puncture cases.[40] This debilitating headache usually appears on the day following the procedure and can last a week or more. It is characteristically produced or exacerbated by assuming the upright position and relieved by lying flat. Treatment of a postspinal headache is described earlier in this chapter. An additional approach is to increase the CSF pressure by the injection of large quantities (60 ml) of epidural saline. By administering an epidural drip of 0.5 L of physiological saline, the incidence of postlumbar puncture headache can be reduced significantly from 73 to 21 percent.[40]

CAUDAL ANESTHESIA

First described by Cathelin in 1901[4] the caudal approach to the epidural space has been used intermittently over the intervening years. It became popular for regional anesthesia for the parturient in the 1940's.[58] It continues to be used for this latter indication as well as for surgery by practitioners of regional anesthesia.[24, 59] However, with the recent studies of the effects of large doses of local anesthetics administered to the mother on the fetus,[60, 61] caudal anesthesia has become less popular as a means of obstetric anesthesia. Many centers now use the lumbar approach as a preferred method. These objections to large doses of anesthetics administered via the caudal canal for anesthesia during the first stages of childbirth can be somewhat overcome by using a two-catheter technique;[62] in this technique, a catheter is placed in the lumbar epidural space for the early stages of labor and a caudally placed catheter is injected for the discomforts associated with delivery.

Caudal anesthesia lends itself well to surgical procedures on the lower extremities, perineum, and lower abdomen. However, it is less suitable than lumbar epidural anesthesia for upper abdominal procedures because it is difficult to predictably obtain sufficient cephalad spread; this lack of cephalad spread is probably due to anatomic impediments that exist in the adult, since spread in children appears to be sufficient for surgery.[63,64] For orthopedic procedures on the lower extremity, caudal anesthesia affords excellent predictable analgesia that may be continued into the postoperative phase if a catheter is left in situ. This has advantages over the lumbar epidural approach with the long-acting agents bupivacaine and etidocaine, because of the sacral sparing[12,43] that sometimes occurs when these agents are used in a higher lumbar epidural technique.

The main objections to caudal anesthesia are the difficulty in needle placement because of the often obscure landmarks in obese individuals. These landmarks are also variable because the sacral hiatus is not in a constant position in all patients and some talent and experience is needed to identify it. Considerable experience is needed with this technique before a high success rate can be obtained. Many practitioners abandon attempts to persevere with this technique after a few initial failures. There is less chance of accidentally producing a dural puncture with a caudal approach than there is with the conventional lumbar approaches. For this reason, it often offers advantages, particularly for those patients who have previously had lumbar surgical procedures and for any in whom the performance of a lumbar peridural approach poses considerable difficulties.

ANATOMY OF THE CAUDAL CANAL

The caudal canal is the caudal continuation of the spinal canal and is contained within the sacrum. It is bordered anteriorly by the ventral plate of the sacrum (analogous to the vertebral bodies of the other spinal vertebrae) and bordered posteriorly by the dorsal plate of the sacrum, which is analogous to the lamina and spines of the other vertebrae. It communicates above with the lumbar spinal canal, and via the anterior sacral foramina it communicates with the pelvis anteriorly. The sacral canal terminates at the sacral hiatus, which is marked by the caudal limit of the dorsal plate; a ligamentous band, the sacrococcygeal ligament, covers this hiatus. It is through this ligament and hiatus that drugs are introduced into the caudal canal for caudal peridural anesthesia (see Fig. 21-7).

The contents of the sacral canal are the cauda equina, and these are contained within the dura mater as far down as the level of the second sacral segment. This level is identified by a horizontal line 1 cm caudad to the posterior superior iliac spines. This lower dural level varies from S1 to S3 sacral levels in different individuals and is usually lower than this in children up to puberty. The distance from the sacral hiatus to the termination of the dura can vary considerably. Trotter[65] showed this to be anywhere from 16 to 75 mm.

The angle of the sacral canal with the dorsal surface of the patient varies in males and females. There is a greater angle in females (due to the different pelvic configuration) and a more acute angle in males.

The critical anatomic landmark for this procedure is the sacral hiatus and this varies considerably between individuals. This landmark is usually in the midline 5 cm from the tip of the coccyx; however, it can occupy a more rostral position in those patients with a defective dorsal sacral plate (as occurs in minor degrees of spina bifida.) Also it may be situated to one or the other side of the midline if there has been some asymmetry in the formation of the sacral dorsal plate. For these reasons, it is not a predictably localized anatomic landmark and must sometimes be searched for with an exploring needle to look for losses of resistance.

TECHNIQUE OF CAUDAL ANESTHESIA

The patient can be positioned in either the lateral or the prone position for caudal anesthesia. For nonpregnant women and for men, the prone position is probably the easiest for establishing landmarks and accomplishing the block. For pregnant women, the lateral position is optimal or even the knee-chest position is preferred by some.

In the prone position, the table is flexed and/or a pillow is positioned under the pelvis to produce flexion of the hip. The heels are turned outwards and the toes inverted. This maneuver relaxes the gluteal muscles and permits more ready palpation of the coccygeal area. In slim individuals, the sacral cornu can often be visualized. They are usually seen at a distance of approximately 5 cm from the tip of the coccyx. If they cannot be visualized, they are located by palpation. With a fingertip placed on the tip of the coccyx, the sacral hiatus will lie at the proximal interphalangeal crease of the palpating finger. Optimally the cornu are identified by examining with the palmar aspect of the examiner's left fingers, and pressure is exerted upon these digits by the examiner's right hand. If the left hand is moved at right angles to the spinal axis at or about the level of the expected position of the sacral cornu, these protuberances can often be located. When located, the palmar aspects of the index and middle fingers of the examiner's left hand are placed on each of the sacral cornu and a small skin wheal of local anesthetic inserted between them. It is advisable not to be too generous with infiltrations here as this can obscure the landmarks. An examining needle is then inserted at an angle of 45 degrees between these two cornu and advanced until a loss of resistance occurs when the needle first engages the sacrococcygeal ligament and then "pops" through into the sacral canal. With further advancement the needle will then strike the dorsal aspect of the ventral plate of the sacrum. This latter confirmatory sign is essential because the needle may have passed through the sacrococcygeal ligament and yielded a loss of resistance; but there will be no further bony landmarks beyond and the needle will pass into the pelvis—either into the rectum or even into the advancing fetal head in the parturient. For this reason caudal anesthesia is relatively contraindicated when the fetal head has descended to the perineum.

When the sacral hiatus has been located with the exploring 25 or 22 gauge needle, then a short bevel 18 gauge Tuohy 7 cm needle is inserted. A more evident loss of resistance will be appreciated with this blunt needle. When the needle then strikes the sacrum beyond the ligament, the angle of the needle is altered so that the needle almost becomes parallel to the skin with an angle of 5 degrees or less in the male and a somewhat steeper angle of 15 degrees in the female. The needle is now advanced into the sacral canal for a distance of about 2 cm. This distance is usually sufficient, and appropriate, to avoid the risk of dural puncture, the dural sac ending at the S2 level. Aspiration tests are necessary at this stage, since the caudal canal is a highly vascular area. If blood is aspirated, the needle is repositioned until no such aspiration occurs. Aspiration tests are also necessary to test for CSF in the rare event of a dural puncture having occurred, since the dural sac can extend lower than S2 in some individuals and frequently does so in children. With these tests completed, the operator can continue with injection in the case of a "single shot" technique or insert a peridural catheter with all the precautions as described above. A test dose is, of course, appropriate and 5 ml of 2 percent lidocaine is a frequently used dose for this purpose in the adult.

Approximately twice the dose of local anesthetic drug is needed for caudal compared to lumbar epidural anesthesia because of the relatively large sacral canal and the free leakage of solution out of the large sacral foramina. Three ml of drug is required per spinal segment (1.5 ml/segment for lumbar epidural).

USE OF CAUDAL ANESTHESIA IN PEDIATRIC SURGERY

Because of the good landmarks and predictable dose per segment (0.1 ml per year of age per segment), this technique lends itself well to pediatric practice.[63] With neonates and young toddlers, some premedication for sedation is helpful to ensure cooperation. Ketamine, 2 mg/kg IM, or 2 percent thiopental, 1 mg/kg IV, is helpful. Caudal anesthesia can also be used for postoperative pain relief.[66]

In contrast to the variable and often difficult to locate sacral hiatus in adults, this landmark is often surprisingly easy to palpate in children and caudal anesthesia can be used successfully in children from the neonate through to puberty. In this age group, there is often a predictable relationship between the dose injected and the resultant analgesia, which is not the case in adults. The main caveat to the use of caudal anesthesia in pediatric practice is the fact that the dural sac extends more caudad in children and therefore to avoid dural puncture and subarachnoid administration of the drug the needle should not be passed more than 1 cm or so into the sacral hiatus.

SUBARACHNOID AND EPIDURAL INJECTION OF NARCOTICS

This is a very new and exciting field of pain relief. It has been demonstrated in animals that morphine in small doses deposited around the spinal cord appears to react with enkephalin receptors and to produce significant selective spinal analgesia that does not appear to be due to any systemic uptake of the narcotic from the injection site. This phenomena has been demonstrated by several investigators in man.[7, 9, 10]

Behar[9] used 2 mg of morphine in 10 ml of normal saline and Cousins[10] used 100 mg of meperidine in a similar volume. This pro-duced effective analgesia without any sensory, motor, or sympathetic involvement. It seems to produce satisfactory analgesia for a period of 18 hours or more and its potential for use in the postoperative, obstetric, and terminal cancer[7] control of pain is considerable.

A significant characteristic of this procedure appears to be its long latency of onset of about 45 minutes. The patients are able to move and there is no associated muscle relaxation. The analgesia apparently is insufficient to permit its use alone for operative anesthesia, but because of the stability of the sympathetic and cardiovascular systems, it would appear to lend itself well to postoperative or maybe obstetric pain relief. In the field of postoperative pain relief, it may prove useful in posttrauma management in intensive care units, where its use may possibly reduce the need for intubation and ventilation in patients with broken ribs and chest trauma.

Other problems mentioned with its use appear to be a significant itch, which is very severe in some cases. There is some doubt as to whether this is due to contaminant preservatives in the morphine sulphate used because at this moment in time, there is not a preservative-free opiate readily available and it must be specially prepared. Wang[7] has suggested that if the pure morphine sulphate powder is used to mix the solutions, then itch should not occur. Retention of urine seems to be a problem in some patients and nausea has been reported when the morphine injection has been made in the region of the cervical cord. No mortality has been reported from this treatment as yet, but five cases of profound respiratory depression have been reported.[67] This author is aware of one death occurring 10 hours following the subarachnoid injection of the drug and one cardiac arrest has been reported in the recovery room following use of epidural morphine for operative and postoperative anesthesia. This technique seems to be less effective for visceral than for somatic pain.

The appropriate indications, techniques of

administration, benefits, and side effects of this therapy are still unclear and its widespread use needs to await better guidelines.

REFERENCES

1. Corning JL: Spinal anaesthesia and local medication of the cord. NY Med J 42:483, 1885
2. Bier A: from Dtsch Z Chir T 51:361, 1899 as translated in Surv Anesth 6:352, 1962
3. Siccard A: Les injestions médicamenteuses extradurales par voie sacro-coccygienne. Cr Soc Biol Paris 53:396, 1901
4. Cathelin MF: Une novelle voie d'injection rachidienne. Méthode des injections épidurales par le procédé du canal sacré applications l'homme. Cr Soc Biol (Paris) 53:452, 1901
5. Gelman S, Laws HL, Potzick J, et al: Thoracic epidural analgesia in morbid obesity. Anesthesiology (suppl.) 51:S234, 1979
6. Gelman S, Patel K: Clinical aspects of thoracic epidural analgesia in morbid obesity. Anesth Rev 7:12, 1980
7. Wang JK, Nauss LA, Thomas JE: Pain relief by an intrathecally applied morphine in man. Anesthesiology 50:149, 1979
8. Magora F, Olshwang D, Emeimerl D, et al: Observations on extradular morphine analgesia in various pain conditions. Br J Anaesth 52:247, 1980
9. Behar M, Magora F, Olshwang D, et al: Epidural morphine in the treatment of pain. Lancet 1:527, 1979
10. Cousins MJ, Mather LE, Glynn CJ, et al: Selective spinal analgesia. Lancet 1:1141, 1979
11. Last RJ: Anatomy, Regional and Applied. 6th edition. Edinbrugh, Churchill Livingstone, 1978, pp 37–47
12. Murphy TM, Mather LE, Stanton-Hicks Mdá, et al: The effects of adding adrenalin to etidocaine and lignocaine in extradural anaesthesia. 1: Block characteristics and cardiovascular effects. Br J Anaesth 48:893, 1976
13. Moore DC, Bridenbaugh PO, Bridenbaugh LD, et al: A double-blind study of bupivacaine and etidocaine for epidural (peridural) block. Anesth Analg 53:690, 1974
14. Taylor JA: Lumbosacral subarachnoid tap. J Urol 43:561, 1940
15. Dripps RD, Vandam LD: Long-term follow-up of patients who have received 10,098 spinal anesthetics. JAMA 156:1486, 1954
16. Lund PC: Principles and Practice of Spinal Anesthesia. Springfield, IL, Charles C Thomas, 1971
17. Nolte H: Current and future status of spinal anesthesia for surgery. Reg Anesth 4:10, 1979
18. Phillips OC, Ebner H, Nelson AT, et al: Neurologic complication following spinal anaesthesia with lidocaine. Anesthesiology 30:284, 1967
19. Greene NM: Present concepts of spinal anesthesia. Refresher Courses in Anesthesiology 7:131, 1979
20. Greene BA: Twenty-six gauge lumbar puncture needle. Its value in prophylaxis of headache following spinal analgesia for vaginal delivery. Anesthesiology 11:464, 1950
21. Frumin MJ: Spinal anesthesia using a 32-gauge needle. Anesthesiology 30:599, 1969
22. Neigh JL, Kane PB, Smith TC: Effects of speed and direction of injection on the level and duration of spinal anesthesia. Anesth Analg 49:912, 1970
23. Pflug EA, Aasheim GM, Beck HH: Spinal anesthesia bupivacaine vs tetracaine. Anesth Analg 55:489, 1976
24. Moore DC: Regional Block. 4th edition. Springfield, IL, Charles C Thomas, 1978
25. Swerdlow M: Intrathecal and extradural block in pain relief, Relief of Intractable Pain. Edited by Swerdlow M. Amsterdam, Excerpta Medica, 1974, p 148
26. Bonica JJ: Clinical application of diagnostic and therapeutic nerve blocks. Springfield, IL, Charles C Thomas, 1959
27. Wood KM: The use of phenol as a neurolytic agent: A review. Pain 5:205, 1978
28. Jonnesco T: General spinal anesthesia. Br Med J 1:1396, 1909
29. Greene NM: The area of differential block during spinal anesthesia with hyperbaric tetracaine. Anesthesiology 19:45, 1958
30. Hackel DB, Sancetta SM, Kleinerman J: Effect of hypotension due to spinal anesthesia on coronary blood flows and myocardial metabolism in man. Circulation 13:92, 1956
31. Freund FG, Bonica JJ, Ward RJ, et al: Ventilatory reserve and level of motor block during high spinal and epidural block. Anesthesiology 28:834, 1967
32. Kleinerman J, Sancetta SM, Hackle DB: Ef-

fects of high spinal anesthesia on cerebral circulation and metabolism in man. J Clin Invest 37:285, 1958

33. Ward RJ, Kennedy WF, Bonica JJ, et al: Experimental evaluation of atropine and vasopressor for the treatment of hypotension of high subarachnoid block. Anesth Analg 45:621, 1965

34. Claine WE, Hamilton WK: Central and peripheral venous oxygen saturations during spinal anesthesia. Anesthesiology 27:209, 1966

35. Abouleish E: Long-term follow-up of epidural blood patch. Anesth Analg 54:459, 1975

36. Abouleish E: Epidural blood patch for treatment of chronic postlumbar puncture cephalgia. Anesthesiology 49:291, 1978

37. Gormley JB: Treatment of postspinal headache. Anesthesiology 21:565, 1960

38. Moore DC: Complications of regional anesthesia, Bonica J.J., Clinical Anesthesia, Regional Anesthesia, Recent Advances, and Current Status. Edited by Bonica JJ. Philadelphia, FA Davis, 1967

39. Bromage PR: Epidural Anesthesia. Philadelphia, WB Saunders, 1978

40. Crawford JS: The prevention of headache consequent to dural puncture. Br J Anaesth 44:598, 1972

41. Batnitzky S, Keucher TR, Mealey J, et al: Iatrogenic intraspinal epidermoid tumor. JAMA 237:148, 1977

42. Dawkins CMJ: Thoracic extradural (epidural) block for upper abdominal surgery. Anaesthesia 26:41, 1971

43. Gallindo A, Hernandez J, Benevides O, et al: Quality of spinal and extradural anaesthesia: The influence of spinal nerve root diameter. Br J Anaesth 47:41, 1975

44. Stanton-Hicks Mdá, Berges PU, Bonica JJ: Circulatory effects of peridural block: Comparison of the effects of epinephrine and phenylephrine. Anesthesiology 39:308, 1973

45. Stanton-Hicks M, Murphy TM, Bonica JJ, et al: Effects of extradural block: Comparison of the properties, circulatory effects and pharmacokinetics of etidocaine and bupivacaine. Br J Anaesth 48:575, 1976

46. Cohen SE, Thurlow A: Comparison of a chlorprocaine-bupivacaine mixture with chlorprocaine and bupivacaine used individually for obstetric epidural anesthesia. Anesthesiology 51:288, 1979

46a. Covino BG, Marx GF, Finster M, et al: Prolonged sensory/motor deficits following inadvertent spinal anesthesia. Anesth Analg 59:399, 1980

47. Bozeman PM, Chandra P: Unilateral analgesia following epidural and subarachnoid block. Anesthesiology 52:356, 1980

48. Ward RJ, Bonica JJ, Freund FF: Epidural and subarachnoid anesthesia. JAMA 191:275, 1965

49. Defalque RJ: Compared effects of spinal and extradural anesthesia upon blood pressure. Anesthesiology 23:627, 1962

50. Bonica JJ, Berges PU, Morikawa K: Circulatory effects of peridural block. I: Influence of level of analgesia and dose of lidocaine. Anesthesiology 33:619, 1970

51. Otton PE, Wilson EJ: The cardiocirculatory effects of upper thoracic epidural analgesia. Can Anaesth Soc J 13:541, 1966

52. Stanton-Hicks Mdá: Cardiovascular effects of extradural anaesthesia. Br J Anaesth 47:253, 1975

53. Kennedy WF Jr, Sawyer TK, Gerbershagen HU, et al: Systemic cardiovascular and renal hemodyanmic alterations during peridural anesthesia in normal man. Anesthesiology 31:414, 1969

54. Kennedy WF Jr, Everett GM, Cobb LA, et al: Simultaneous systemic and hepatic hemodynamic measurements during high peridural anesthesia in normal man. Anaesth Analg 50:1069, 1971

55. Bevan DR: The sodium story: Effects of anesthesia and surgery on intrarenal mechanisms concerned with sodium homeostasis. Proc Roy Soc Med 66:1215, 1973

56. Bonica JJ, Kennedy WF, Akamatsu TJ, et al: Circulatory effects of peridural block. III: Effects of acute blood loss. Anesthesiology 36:219, 1972

57. Catterberg J: Local anesthetic vs spinal fluid. Anesthesiology 46:309, 1977

58. Hingson RA, Edwards WB: An analysis of the first ten thousand confinements managed with continuous caudal analgesia with a report of the authors' first one thousand cases. JAMA 123:538, 1943

59. Bonica JJ: Principles and Practice of Obstetric Analgesia and Anesthesia. Philadelphia, FA Davis, 1967

60. Scanlon JW, Brown WM, Weiss JB, et al.

Neurobehavioral responses of newborn infants after maternal epidural anesthesia. Anesthesiology 40:121, 1974

61. Sinclair JC, Fox HA, Lentz JF: Intoxication of the fetus by a local anesthetic. A newly recognized complication of maternal caudal anesthesia. N Engl J Med 273:1173, 1975

62. Cleland JGP: Continuous peridural and caudal analgesia in obstetrics. Anesth Analg 28:61, 1949

63. Schulte-Steinberg O, Rahlfs VW: Spread of extradural analgesia following caudal injection in children: A statistical study. Br J Anaesth 49:1027, 1977

64. Touloukian RJ, Wugmeister M, Pickett LK, et al: Caudal anesthesia for neonatal anoperineal and rectal operations. Anesth Analg 50:565, 1971

65. Trotter M: Variations of the sacral canal: Their significance in the administration of caudal analgesia. Anesth Analg 26:192, 1947

66. Kay B: Caudal block for postoperative pain relief in children. Anaesth 29:610, 1974

67. Davies GK, Tohurt-Cleaver CL: Respiratory depression following injection of intrathecal narcotics (abstr.). Am Soc Reg Anesth, Proc 5th Ann Meeting, 1980, p 25

68. Bromage PR: Exaggerated spread of epidural analgesia in arteriosclerotic patients: Dosage in relation to biological and chronological age. Br Med J 2:1634, 1962

69. Bromage PR: Aging and epidural dose requirements. Br J Anaesth 41:1061, 1969

70. Sharrock NE: Epidural anesthetic dose responses in patients 20–80 years old. Anesthesiology 49:425, 1978

Section II

Physiological Functions During Anesthesia

22

Respiratory Physiology and Respiratory Function During Anesthesia

Jonathan L. Benumof, M.D.

RESPIRATORY PHYSIOLOGY

INTRODUCTION

Understanding normal respiratory physiology is prerequisite to understanding disordered processes and mechanisms of gas exchange during anesthesia and surgery. Towards this end, the normal distribution of ventilation and perfusion, the major determinants of blood and air flow resistance, respiratory gas transport, and pulmonary structure and function are presented first. These processes and concepts are then discussed in regard to mechanisms of disordered pulmonary gas exchange during anesthesia and surgery.

DISTRIBUTION OF PULMONARY PERFUSION, VENTILATION, AND THE VENTILATION/PERFUSION RATIO

DISTRIBUTION OF PULMONARY PERFUSION

Contraction of the right ventricle imparts kinetic energy to the blood flow in the main pulmonary artery. As the kinetic energy in the main pulmonary artery is dissipated in climbing a vertical hydrostatic gradient, the absolute pressure in the pulmonary artery (Ppa) decreases 1 cm H_2O per cm of vertical distance up the lung (Fig. 22-1). At some height, Ppa becomes zero (atmospheric) and still higher in the lung Ppa becomes negative.[1] In this region PA then exceeds Ppa and pulmonary venous pressure (Ppv) (which is very negative at this vertical height). The pulmonary vessels in this region of the lung are collapsed and there is no blood flow (zone 1). Since no gas exchange is possible in this region, it constitutes an alveolar dead space or "wasted" ventilation. Little or no zone 1 exists in the lung under normal conditions, but this may be greatly increased if Ppa is reduced, as in oligemic shock, or if PA is increased, as in positive-pressure ventilation.

Further down the lung absolute Ppa becomes positive and blood flow will begin when Ppa exceeds PA (zone 2). At this vertical level in the lung, PA exceeds Ppv and blood flow is determined by the Ppa-PA difference rather than the more conventional (see below) Ppa−Ppv difference.[2] This phenomenon has various names, including the "Starling resistor," "waterfall," "Weir," and "sluice" effect. Since Ppa increases down this region of the lung but PA is constant, the driving pressure (Ppa−PA) increases and therefore blood flow increases.

Finally, near the bottom of the lung there is a vertical level where Ppv becomes positive

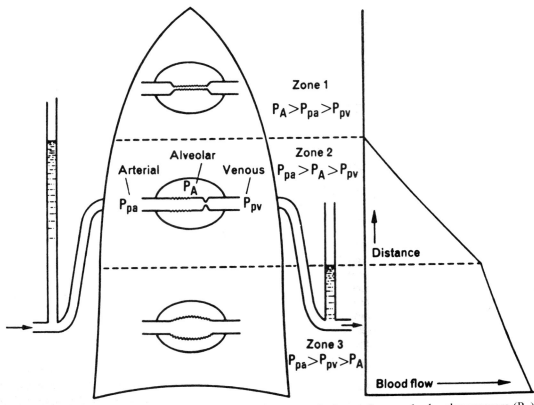

Fig. 22-1 The distribution of blood flow in the isolated lung is shown. In zone 1, alveolar pressure (P_A) exceeds pulmonary artery pressure (P_{pa}) and no flow occurs presumably because collapsible vessels are directly exposed to alveolar pressure. In zone 2, arterial pressure exceeds alveolar pressure, but alveolar pressure exceeds venous pressure (P_{pv}). Flow in zone 2 is determined by the arterial-alveolar pressure difference, which steadily increases down the zone. In zone 3, pulmonary venous pressure now exceeds alveolar pressure and flow is determined by the arterial-venous pressure difference ($P_{pa}-P_{pv}$), which is constant down the lung. However, the pressure across the walls of the vessels increases down zone 3 so that their caliber increases and so does flow. (Redrawn from West JB, Dollery CT, Naimark A: Distribution of blood flow in isolated lung: Relation to vascular and alveolar pressures. J Appl Physiol 19:713, 1964.)

and also exceeds PA. In this region blood flow is governed by the pulmonary arteriovenous pressure difference (Ppa−Ppv) (zone 3), for in this zone both of these vascular pressures exceed the PA and the capillary systems are thus permanently open and blood flow is continuous. Descending zone 3 gravity causes both absolute Ppa and Ppv to increase at the same rate so that the perfusion pressure (Ppa−Ppv) is unchanged. The pressure outside the vessels, namely pleural pressure (Ppl), increases less than Ppa and Ppv so that the transmural distending pressures (Ppa−Ppl and Ppv−Ppl) increase down zone 3, the radius of the vessels increase, vascular resistance decreases, and blood flow therefore increases further.

DISTRIBUTION OF VENTILATION

Gravity also causes Ppl differences, which in turn cause regional alveolar volume and compliance differences. The vertical gradient of Ppl can be best understood by imagining

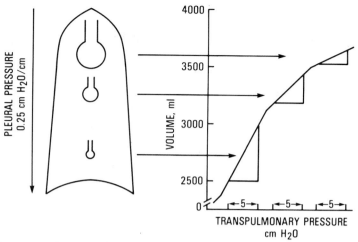

Fig. 22-2 Pleural pressure increases 0.25 cm H_2O every centimeter down the lung. The increase in pleural pressure causes a fourfold decrease in alveolar volume. The caliber of the air passages also decreases as lung volume decreases. When regional alveolar volume is translated over to a regional transpulmonary pressure–alveolar volume curve, small alveoli are on a steep (large slope) portion of the curve and large alveoli are on a flat (small slope) portion of the curve. The regional slope equals regional compliance. Over the normal tidal volume range (2500 to 3000 ml), the pressure-volume relationship is linear. Lung volume values in this diagram relate to the upright position.

the lung as a bag filled with semifluid contents and anchored by the hilium. The effect of gravity on the contents would cause the bag to bulge outwards at the bottom and inwards at the top. With the lung inside the chest, such gravitational forces create a greater subatmospheric pressure at the top of the pleural space than at the bottom. The magnitude of this pressure gradient is determined by the density of the lung. Since the lung is about one quarter of the density of water, the gradient of Ppl (in cm H_2O) will be about one quarter of the upright lung height (30 cm). Thus, Ppl increases positively by $30/4=7.5$ cm H_2O from the top to the bottom of the lung.[3] Since PA is the same throughout the lung, the Ppl gradient causes regional differences in transpulmonary distending pressures (PA−Ppl). Since Ppl is most positive (least negative) in the dependent basilar lung regions, alveoli in these regions are more compressed and therefore are considerably smaller than superior relatively noncompressed apical alveoli (approximately fourfold volume difference).[4] If the regional differences in alveolar volume are translated over to a pressure-volume curve for normal lung (Fig. 22-2), the dependent small alveoli are on the midportion and the nondependent large alveoli are on the upper portion of the S-shaped pressure-volume curve. Since the different regional slopes of the composite curve are equal to the different regional lung compliances, dependent alveoli are very compliant (steep slope) and nondependent alveoli are noncompliant (flat slope). Thus, the majority of the tidal volume is preferentially distributed to dependent alveoli, since they expand more per unit pressure change than nondependent alveoli.

DISTRIBUTION OF THE VENTILATION TO PERFUSION RATIO

Figure 22-3 shows both blood flow and ventilation (left-hand vertical axis) increase linearly with distance down the normal upright lung (horizontal axis from the top to the bottom of the lung).[5] Since blood flow in-

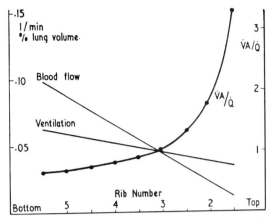

Fig. 22-3 Distribution of ventilation and blood flow (left-hand vertical axis) and the ventilation/perfusion ratio (right-hand vertical axis) in normal upright lung. Both blood flow and ventilation are expressed in L/min/percent alveolar volume and have been drawn as smoothed out linear functions of vertical height. The closed circles mark the ventilation/perfusion ratios of horizontal lung slices (three of which are shown in Fig. 22-4). A cardiac output of 6 L/min and a total minute ventilation of 5.1 L/min was assumed. (West JB: Ventilation/Blood Flow and Gas Exchange. 2nd edition. Oxford, Blackwell Scientific Publications, 1970.)

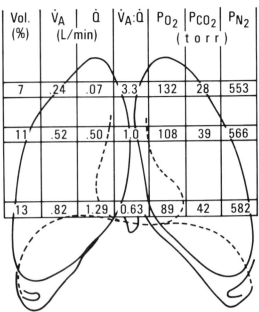

Vol. (%)	$\dot{V}_A$ (L/min)	$\dot{Q}$	$\dot{V}_A:\dot{Q}$	P_{O_2}	P_{CO_2} (torr)	P_{N_2}
7	.24	.07	3.3	132	28	553
11	.52	.50	1.0	108	39	566
13	.82	1.29	0.63	89	42	582

Fig. 22-4 The ventilation/perfusion ratio and the regional composition of alveolar gas. Values for the regional flow, ventilation, P_{O_2} and P_{CO_2} are derived from Figure 22-3. P_{N_2} has been obtained by what remains from the total gas pressure (including water vapor, equals 760 torr). The volumes of the three lung slices are also shown. Compared to the top of the lung, the bottom of the lung has a low ventilation/perfusion ratio and is relatively hypoxic and hypercarbic. (West JB: Regional differences in gas exchange in the lung of erect man. J Appl Physiol 17:893, 1962.)

creases more rapidly than ventilation with distance down the lung, the ventilation perfusion ($\dot{V}_A/\dot{Q}$) ratio (right-hand vertical axis) decreases rapidly at first, then more slowly. The degree of overperfusion or underventilation of alveoli is most conveniently expressed in terms of the ($\dot{V}_A/\dot{Q}$) ratio. Thus alveoli at the base of the lung are somewhat overperfused in relation to their ventilation ($\dot{V}_A/\dot{Q}<1$), whereas the alveoli at the apex are greatly underperfused in relation to their ventilation ($\dot{V}_A/\dot{Q}>1$).

Figure 22-4 shows the calculated ventilation ($\dot{V}_A$) and blood flow ($\dot{Q}$) in L/min, $\dot{V}_A/\dot{Q}$ ratio, and the alveolar P_{O_2} and P_{CO_2} in torr for horizontal slices of the top (7 percent of lung volume), middle (11 percent of lung volume) and bottom (13 percent of lung volume) of the lung.[6] It can be seen that the P_{O_2} in-

creases by over 40 torr from 89 torr at the base to 132 torr at the apex, while P_{CO_2} decreases by 14 torr from 42 torr at the bottom to 28 torr at the top. Thus, the bottom of the lung is relatively hypoxic and hypercarbic compared to the top of the lung.

Recently, Wagner and colleagues[7] have described a method of determining the continuous distribution of $\dot{V}_A/\dot{Q}$ ratios within the lung based on the pattern of elimination of a series of intravenously infused inert gases. Gases of differing solubility are dissolved in physiological saline solution and infused into a peripheral vein until a steady state is achieved (20 minutes). Towards the

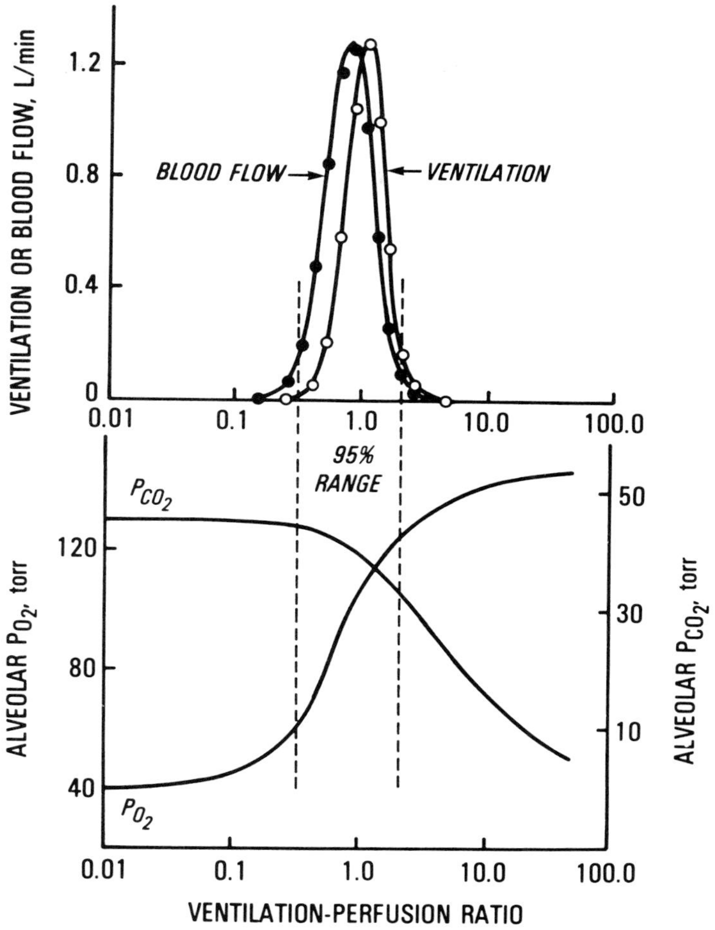

Fig. 22-5 The upper graph shows the average distribution of ventilation/perfusion ratios in young semirecumbent normal subjects. The 95 percent range covers ventilation/perfusion ratios from 0.3 to 2.1 (between dashed lines). The corresponding variations of PO_2 and PCO_2 in the alveolar gas can be seen in the lower panel. (West JB: Blood flow to the lung and gas exchange. Anesthesiology 41:124, 1974.)

end of the infusion period, samples of arterial and mixed venous blood and mixed expired gas are collected and total ventilation and cardiac output are measured. For each gas the ratio of arterial to mixed venous concentration (retention) and the ratio of expired to mixed venous concentration (excretion) are calculated and retention-solubility and excretion-solubility curves are drawn. This retention/excretion-solubility curve can be regarded as a "fingerprint" of the particular distribution of ventilation perfusion ratios that give rise to it.

Figure 22-5 (upper graph) shows the type of distributions found in young normal subjects breathing air in the semirecumbent po-

sition.[8] The distributions of both ventilation and blood flow are relatively narrow. The upper and lower 95 percent limits shown (vertical interrupted lines) correspond to $\dot{V}A/\dot{Q}$ ratios of 0.3 and 2.1 respectively. Notice that these young normal subjects had no blood flow perfusing areas with very low $\dot{V}A/\dot{Q}$ ratios nor did they have any blood flow to unventilated areas or shunt ($\dot{V}A/\dot{Q}=0$) or unperfused areas ($\dot{V}A/\dot{Q}=\infty$). Figure 22-5 also shows alveolar PO_2 and PCO_2 in respiratory units having different $\dot{V}A/\dot{Q}$ ratios. It can be seen that within the 95 percent range of $\dot{V}A/\dot{Q}$ ratios (0.3 to 2.1), the PO_2 ranges from 60 to 123 torr while the corresponding PCO_2 range is 44 to 33 torr.

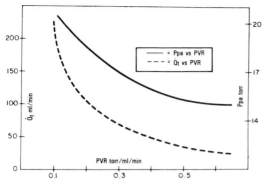

Fig. 22-6 Passive changes in pulmonary vascular resistance (PVR) as a function of pulmonary artery pressure (Ppa) and pulmonary blood flow ($\dot{Q}_t$) (PVR=Ppa/$\dot{Q}_t$). As flow increases pulmonary artery pressure also increases, but to a lesser extent, so that resistance decreases. As flow decreases, pulmonary artery pressure also decreases, but to a lesser extent. The net result is that resistance increases. (Fishman AP: Dynamics of the pulmonary circulation, Handbook of Physiology, Section 2: Circulation. Volume 2. Edited by Hamilton WF. © (1963) American Physiological Society, Bethesda, pp 1667–1743.)

CLINICALLY IMPORTANT DETERMINANTS OF PULMONARY VASCULAR RESISTANCE AND BLOOD FLOW DISTRIBUTION

CARDIAC OUTPUT

As cardiac output ($\dot{Q}_t$) increases, Ppa increases passively (Fig. 22-6).[9] Since the pulmonary vasculature is distensible, as Ppa increases, the radii of the vessels increase and pulmonary vascular resistance (PVR) decreases (PVR=Ppa/$\dot{Q}_t$). Conversely, a decrease in cardiac output passively causes a decrease in Ppa, which in turn causes the radii of the pulmonary vessels to decrease and pulmonary vascular resistance to then increase.

Understanding the relationship between pulmonary vascular resistance, Ppa, and cardiac output during passive events is prerequisite to recognition of active vasomotion in the pulmonary circulation. Active vasoconstriction occurs any time cardiac output decreases and Ppa remains either constant or increases. Active vasodilation occurs any time cardiac output increases and Ppa remains either constant or decreases.

ALVEOLAR HYPOXIA

Alveolar or environmental hypoxia of in vivo and in vitro whole lung, unilateral lung, lobe, or lobule of lung causes pulmonary vasoconstriction. This phenomenon is called hypoxic pulmonary vasoconstriction (HPV) and is due to either a direct action of alveolar hypoxia on pulmonary vasculature or an alveolar hypoxia-induced release of the vasoactive substance.[10]

There are three ways in which HPV operates in humans. First, life at high altitude or whole-lung respiration of a low inspired concentration of O_2 (FIO_2) greatly increases Ppa. The increased Ppa increases perfusion of the apices of the lung and results in gas exchange in a region of lung not normally utilized (i.e., zone 1). Thus, with a low FIO_2, the PaO_2 is greater and the alveolar-arterial O_2 tension difference and dead-space-to-tidal-volume ratio are less than would be expected or predicted on the basis of a normal (sea level) distribution of ventilation and blood flow. Second, hypoxic ventilation (FIO_2=0.1) or atelectasis of one lung generally causes a 30 to 40 percent diversion of blood flow away from hypoxic to nonhypoxic lung. This is of great importance in minimizing transpulmonary shunt during diseases of one lung, one-lung anesthesia, and inadvertant intubation of a mainstem bronchus. Third, in patients with chronic obstructive pulmonary disease, asthma, pneumonia, and mitral stenosis, who do not have bronchospasm, administration of pulmonary vasodilator drugs such as isoproterenol, sodium nitroprusside, nitroglycerin, or aminophylline causes a decrease in both PaO_2, and pulmonary vascular resistance and an increase in right-to-left transpulmonary shunt.[11] The mechanism for these changes is thought to be release of preexisting HPV.[11] In accordance with the latter two lines of evidence (one-lung hypoxia, vasodilator drug effects on whole-lung disease), HPV is thought to divert blood flow away from hypoxic regions of the lung and thereby serve as an autoregulatory mechanism that protects PaO_2 by favorably adjusting regional $\dot{V}_A/\dot{Q}$ ratios.

LUNG VOLUME

The functional residual capacity (FRC) is the lung volume that exists at the end of a normal exhalation after a normal tidal volume and when there is no muscle activity or pressure difference between alveoli and atmosphere. Total pulmonary vascular resistance is increased when lung volume is either increased or decreased from FRC (Fig. 22-7).[12-14] The increase in total pulmonary vascular resistance above FRC is due to alveolar compression of small intra-alveolar vessels, which results in an increase in small vessel pulmonary vascular resistance (i.e., creation of zone 1 or zone 2).[15] The increase in total pulmonary vascular resistance below FRC is due to either HPV or mechanical tortuosity of large extra-alveolar vessels, which results in an increase in large vessel pulmonary vascular resistance.[13, 16]

POTENTIAL PATHWAYS OF BLOOD FLOW THROUGH THE LUNG

There are both alveolar and nonalveolar pathways for blood to flow from the right side of the heart to the left side of the heart. The alveolar pathways are by (1) well-ventilated alveoli; (2) poorly-ventilated alveoli (low $\dot{V}_A/\dot{Q}$, when $FiO_2 < 30$ percent; low $\dot{V}_A/\dot{Q}$ lung units have a shunt effect); and (3) nonventilated alveoli ($\dot{V}_A/\dot{Q} = 0$, or a true shunt). Nonalveolar pathways consist of (1) the bronchial, pleural, and thebesian circulations,

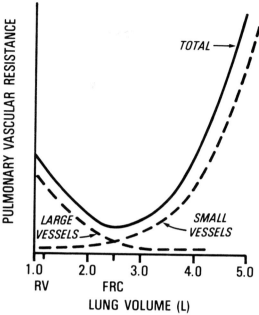

Fig. 22-7 An asymmetrical U-shaped curve relates total pulmonary vascular resistance to lung volume. The trough of the curve occurs when lung volume equals functional residual capacity (FRC). Total pulmonary resistance is the sum of resistance in small vessels (increased by increasing lung volume) and in large vessels (increased by decreasing lung volume). Curve represents a composite of data from references 12–14. RV=residual volume.

which empty into the left side of the heart without being oxygenated and constitute the 1 to 3 percent right-to-left shunt normally present (with chronic bronchitis the bronchial circulation may be as great as 10 percent of the cardiac output); (2) intrapulmonary arteriovenous anastomoses, which are considered normally closed but in the face of acute pulmonary artery hypertension (such as may be caused by a pulmonary embolus) they may open and cause a direct increase in shunt; and (3) esophageal to mediastinal to bronchial to pulmonary vein pathways, which may explain in part the hypoxemia associated with hepatic disease. With the exception of pathways by well-ventilated alveoli, all of the above pathways for blood flow represent right-to-left shunt pathways. The significance of shunt in terms of arterial oxygenation is discussed under oxygen transport.

CLINICALLY IMPORTANT DETERMINANTS OF COMPLIANCE, RESISTANCE, AND LUNG VOLUMES

PULMONARY COMPLIANCE

For air to flow into the lungs, a pressure gradient must be developed to overcome the elastic or static resistance of the lungs and chest wall to expansion. These structures are arranged concentrically, and their elastic resistances are therefore additive. The relationship between the pressure gradient (ΔP) and the resultant volume increase (ΔV) of the lungs and thorax is independent of time and is known as total compliance (C_T):

$$C_T(L/cm\ H_2O) = \Delta V(L)/\Delta P(cm\ H_2O) \quad (1)$$

Clinically the elasticity of lungs cannot be distinguished from that of the chest wall. Actually the anesthesiologist can assess C_T of the lung plus chest wall by estimating the pressure required to inflate the lung by manual compression of the reservoir bag on the anesthesia machine (dynamically, see below). It is important to realize that the C_T of lung plus chest wall is related to the individual compliances of lungs (C_L) and chest wall (C_{CW}) according to the following expression:

$$1/C_T = 1/C_L + 1/C_{CW}$$
$$[\text{or } C_T = (C_L)(C_{CW})/C_L + C_{CW}]$$

Normally, C_L and C_{CW} each equal 0.2 L/cm H_2O; thus C_T=0.1 L/cm H_2O. To determine C_L, ΔV and the transpulmonary pressure gradient (Palveolar−Ppleural) must be known; to determine C_{CW}, ΔV and the *transmural* pressure gradient (Ppleural−Pambient) must be known; to determine C_T, ΔV and the transthoracic pressure gradient (Palveolar−Pambient) must be known.

Dynamic compliance is the volume change divided by transthoracic pressure gradient change, at the point of zero air flow, but after the previous inflow of air has been sufficiently rapid for dynamic factors to influence its distribution throughout the lung. Static compliance is the volume change divided by the transthoracic pressure gradient, at the point of zero air flow, but after the preceding inflow of air has been sufficiently slow for distribution throughout the lung to be solely in accord with regional elasticity. The transthoracic pressure gradient usually decreases as gas redistributes into more compliant alveoli, and therefore static compliance is usually greater than dynamic compliance.

AIRWAY RESISTANCE

In order for air to flow into the lungs, a pressure gradient must also be developed to overcome the nonelastic or dynamic resistance of the lungs to air flow. The relationship between the pressure gradient (ΔP) and the rate of air flow ($\dot{V}$) is dependent on time and is known as airway resistance (R):

$$R(cm\ H_2O/L/sec) = \frac{\Delta P(cm\ H_2O)}{\dot{V}(L/sec)} \quad (2)$$

Resistance to tissue viscosity is small (20 to 30 percent of total) and constant.[17] Resistance to airflow normally accounts for 70 to 80 percent of the total nonelastic resistance of the lungs. It depends on the characteristics of the airway and the rate and pattern of airflow. There are three main patterns of airflow: laminar flow occurs when the gas passes down parallel-sided tubes at less than a certain critical velocity. With laminar flow, the pressure drop down the tube is proportional to the flow rate and may be calculated from the equation derived by Poiseuille: $P = \dot{V} \times 8\ L \times \mu/\pi r^4 \times 980$, where P=pressure drop (in cm H_2O); $\dot{V}$=volume flow rate (in ml/sec); L=length of tube (in cm); r=radius of tube (in cm); and μ=viscosity (in poises).

When flow exceeds the critical velocity, it becomes turbulent. The significant feature of turbulent flow is that the pressure drop along the airway is no longer directly proportional to flow rate but is proportional to the square of flow rate according to the equation $P = \dot{V}^2 \, fl / 4\pi^2 r^5$, where f is a friction factor that depends on the roughness of the tube wall.[18]

Orifice flow occurs at constrictions such as the larynx. In these situations the pressure drop is also proportional to the square of flow rate but density replaces viscosity as the important factor in the numerator. This explains why low-density gas such as helium diminishes the resistance to flow (by threefold compared to air) in severe obstruction of the upper airway.

Since the total cross-sectional area of the airways increases as branching occurs, the velocity of airflow decreases; laminar flow is therefore chiefly confined to the airways below the main bronchi. Orifice flow occurs at the larynx, and flow in the trachea is turbulent during most of the respiratory cycle. Viewing the above equations, one can see that many factors obviously may affect the pressure drop down the airways during respiration. However, variations in diameter of the smaller bronchi and bronchioles are particularly critical and the pressure drop along the airways is intimately related to flow rate.

DIFFERENT REGIONAL LUNG TIME CONSTANTS

So far, the static and dynamic properties of the chest have been discussed separately. In this analysis, I assume that the pressure at the mouth is suddenly increased to a fixed value (Fig. 22-8)[19] that overcomes both elastic and nonelastic resistance and is maintained at this value during inflation of the lungs. The pressure gradient required to overcome nonelastic (airflow) airway resistance is the difference between the fixed mouth pressure and the instantaneous height of the dashed line in Figure 22-8 and is proportional to the flow rate during most of the respiratory cycle. The pressure gradient required to overcome non-

elastic airway resistance will thus be maximal initially but will decline (Fig. 22-8, hatched lines) as the alveolus fills and the retractive force increases. The remainder of the pressure gradient overcomes the elastic resistance (the instantaneous height of the dashed line in Fig. 22-8) and is proportional to the change in lung volume. Alveolar filling will cease when the pressure resulting from the retractive force balances the applied (mouth) pressure (Fig. 22-8, dashed line). The rate of filling, therefore, declines in an approximately exponential manner. Thus, if only a finite time is available for alveolar filling, the degree of filling obviously must be affected by the duration of the inspiration.

An exponential curve can be described mathematically by utilizing its time constant (τ) (see Ch. 11). Tau (τ) is the time required to complete 63 percent of an exponentially changing function if the total time allowed for the function change is unlimited ($2\tau = 87$ percent, $3\tau = 95$ percent, $4\tau = 99$ percent). For lung inflation $\tau = C_T \times R$; normally, $C_T = 0.1$ L/cm H_2O, R = 2.0 cm H_2O/L/sec and $\tau = 0.2$ second and $3\tau = 0.6$ second.

Applying this equation to individual alveolar units, the time taken to fill such a unit clearly increases as airway resistance increases. The time to fill an alveolar unit also increases as compliance increases, since a greater volume of air will be transferred into a more compliant alveolus before the reactive force equals the applied pressure. The compliance of individual alveoli differs from top to bottom of the lung and the resistance of individual airways will vary widely depending on their length and caliber. Therefore a variety of time constants exist throughout the lung.

THE WORK OF BREATHING

Ventilatory work may be analyzed by plotting pressure against volume, since work is the product of pressure times volume. Conventionally:

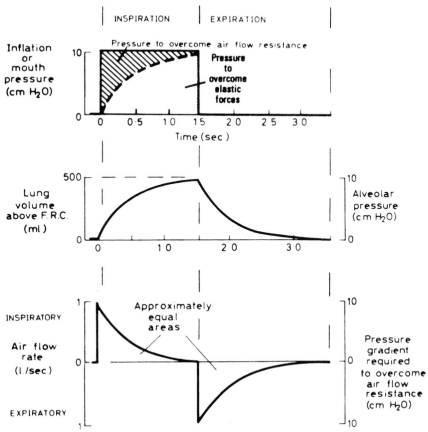

Fig. 22-8 Artificial ventilation by intermittent application of a constant pressure (square wave). Expiration is passive. Inspiratory and expiratory flow rates are both exponential. Assuming that airflow resistance (R) is constant, it follows that the flow rate ($\dot{V}$) and the pressure gradient ($\triangle P$) required to overcome resistance may be shown on the same graph ($R = \triangle P/\dot{V}$). Lung volume change ($\triangle V$) and alveolar pressure change ($\triangle P$) may be shown on the same graph if compliance (C_T) is constant ($C_T = \triangle V/\triangle P$). Values are typical for an anesthetized supine paralyzed patient: total dynamic compliance, 50 ml/cm H_2O; pulmonary resistance, 3 cm H_2O/L/sec; apparatus resistance, 7 cm H_2O/L/sec; total resistance, 10 cm H_2O/L/sec; time constant, 0.5 sec. (Reprinted by permission of the publisher, from Nunn JF: Applied Respiratory Physiology. 2nd edition. London: Butterworths (Publishers) Ltd. 1977.)

(1) Work   = Force × Distance
(2) Force   = Pressure × Area;
    Volume   = Area × Distance;
    Distance = Volume/Area
(3) Work   = (Pressure × Area)
               (Volume/Area)
             = Pressure × Volume

Two different pressure-volume diagrams are shown in Fig. 22-9. During normal inspiration (left graph) intrathoracic pressure increases from 0 to 5 cm H_2O while 500 ml of air is drawn into the lung. Potential energy is stored by the lung during inspiration and expended during expiration; as a consequence, the entire expiratory cycle is passive. The hatched area plus the triangular area ABC represents pressure multiplied by volume and is the work of breathing. Line AB is a section of the pressure-volume diagram of Figure

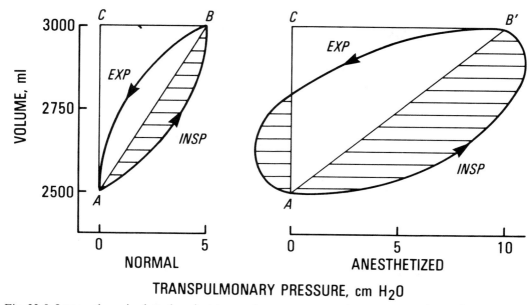

Fig. 22-9 Lung volume is plotted against transpulmonary pressure in a pressure volume diagram for an awake (normal) and an anesthetized patient. The lung compliance of the awake patient (slope of line AB=100 ml/cm H_2O) equals that shown for the small dependent alveoli in Figure 22-2. The lung compliance of the anesthetized patient (slope of line AB'= 50 ml/cm H_2O) equals that shown for the medium midlung alveoli in Figure 22-2 and for the anesthetized patient in Figure 22-8. The total area within the oval and triangles has the dimensions of pressure multiplied by volume and represents the total work of breathing. The hatched area to the right of lines AB and AB' represents active inspiratory work necessary to overcome resistance to airflow during inspiration (INSP). The hatched area to the left of the triangle AB'C represents active expiratory work necessary to overcome resistance to airflow during expiration (EXP). Expiration is passive in the normal subject because sufficient potential energy is stored during inspiration to produce expiratory airflow. The fraction of total inspiratory work necessary to overcome elastic resistance is shown by the triangles ABC and AB'C. The anesthetized patient has a decreased compliance and increased elastic resistance work (triangle AB'C) compared to the normal patient's compliance and elastic resistance work (triangle ABC). The anesthetized patient shown in this figure has an increased airway resistance to both inspiratory and expiratory work.

22-2. The triangular area ABC is the work required to overcome elastic forces (C_T), whereas the hatched area is the work required to overcome airflow or frictional resistances (R). The graph on the right shows an anesthetized patient with diffuse airway obstructive disease due to the accumulation of mucous secretions. There is a marked increase in both the elastic (triangle AB'C) and airway (hatched area) resistive components of respiratory work. During expiration, only 250 ml of air leave the lungs during the passive phase when intrathoracic pressure reaches the equilibrium value of 0 cm H_2O. Active effort-

producing work, is required to force out the remaining 250 ml of air, and intrathoracic pressure actually becomes positive.

For a constant minute volume, the work done against elastic resistance is increased when breathing is deep and slow. On the other hand, the work done against flow resistance is increased when breathing is rapid and shallow. If the two components are summated and the total work plotted against the respiratory frequency, there is an optimal respiratory frequency at which the total work of breathing is minimal (Fig. 22-10).[21] In patients with diseased lungs, when elastic resis-

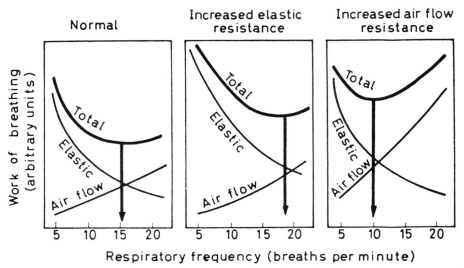

Fig. 22-10 The diagrams show the work done against elastic and airflow resistance separately and summated to indicate the total work of breathing at different respiratory frequencies. The total work of breathing has a minimum value at about 15 breaths per minute under normal circumstances. For the same minute volume, minimum work is performed at higher frequencies with stiff (less compliant) lungs and at lower frequencies when the airflow resistance is increased. (Reprinted by permission of the publisher, from Nunn JF: Applied Respiratory Physiology. 2nd edition. London: Butterworths (Publishers) Ltd. 1977.)

tance is high (pulmonary fibrosis, pulmonary edema, infants, etc.), the optimum frequency is increased and rapid shallow breaths are favored. When airway resistance is high (asthma, obstructive lung disease), the optimum frequency is decreased and slow deep breaths are favored.

THE FUNCTIONAL RESIDUAL CAPACITY AND THE CLOSING CAPACITY RELATIONSHIP

The Functional Residual Capacity

The functional residual capacity (FRC) is defined as the volume of gas in the lung that exists at the end of a normal expiration when there is no airflow and alveolar pressure equals the ambient pressure. Under these conditions, expansive chest wall elastic forces are exactly balanced by retractive lung tissue elastic forces (Fig. 22-11).[22]

The expiratory reserve volume is part of the FRC and is that additional gas beyond the end-tidal volume that can be consciously exhaled and results in the minimum volume of lung possible, known as the residual volume. Thus, the FRC equals the residual volume plus the expiratory reserve volume (Fig. 22-12). With regard to the other lung volumes shown in Figure 22-12, tidal volume, vital capacity, inspiratory capacity, inspiratory reserve volume, and expiratory reserve volume can all be measured by simple spirometry. Total lung volume, FRC, and residual volume all contain a fraction (the residual volume) that cannot be measured by simple spirometry. However, if one of these three volumes is measured, the others can be easily derived because the other lung volumes, which relate these three volumes to one another, can be measured by simple spirometry. FRC can be measured by one of three techniques. The first method is to wash the N_2 out of the lungs by several minutes of O_2 breath-

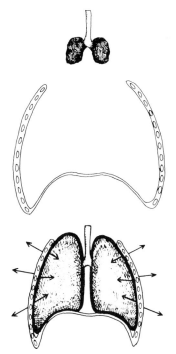

Fig. 22-11 (*Top*) the resting state of normal lungs when they are removed from the chest cavity; i.e., elastic recoil causes total collapse. (*Middle*) the resting state of a normal chest wall and diaphragm when the thoracic apex is open to the atmosphere and the thoracic contents are removed. (*Bottom*) the lung volume that exists at the end of expiration; the functional residual capacity. At functional residual capacity the elastic forces of lung and chest walls are equal and in opposite directions. The pleural surfaces link these two opposing forces. (Reproduced with permission from Shapiro BA, Harrison RA, Trout CA: Clinical Application of Respiratory Care. 2nd edition. Copyright © 1979 by Year Book Medical Publishers, Inc., Chicago.)

ing with measurement of the total quantity of N_2 eliminated. Thus, if 2 L of N_2 are eliminated and the initial alveolar N_2 concentration was 80 percent, it follows that the initial volume of the lung was 2.5 L. The second method uses the wash-in of a tracer gas such as helium. If 50 ml of helium is introduced into the lungs and the helium concentration is then found to be 1 percent, it follows that the volume of the lung is 5 L. The third method of measurement of FRC uses Boyle's law; namely, PV=K, where P=pressure, V=volume and K=a constant. The subject is confined within a gas-tight box (plethysmograph) so that changes in the volume of his body may be readily determined as a change in pressure within the box. Disparity between FRC as measured in the body plethysmograph and by the helium method is often used as a way of detecting large, nonventilating air-trapped blebs.[23] Clearly, there are difficulties in the application of the body plethysmograph to anesthetized patients.

Airway Closure and Closing Capacity

As discussed in the section on the distribution of ventilation, pleural pressure increases from the top to the bottom of the lung and determines regional alveolar size, compliance, and ventilation. Of even greater importance to the anesthesiologist is the recognition that these gradients in pleural pressure may lead to airway closure and collapse of alveoli.

Airway Closure in Patients with Normal Lungs. Figure 22-13*A* illustrates the normal resting end-expiratory (FRC) position of the lung–chest wall combination. The distending transpulmonary and the intrathoracic air passage transmural pressure gradients are 5 cm H_2O and the airways remain patent. During the middle of a normal inspiration (Fig. 22-13*B*), there is an increase in the transmural pressure gradient (6.8 cm H_2O), which encourages distending of intrathoracic air passages. During the middle of a normal expiration (Fig. 22-13*C*), expiration is passive; alveolar pressure is due only to the elastic recoil of the lung (2 cm H_2O) and there is a decrease (5.2 cm H_2O) but still a favorable (distending) intraluminal transmural pressure gradient. During the middle of a severe forced expiration (Fig. 22-13*D*), pleural pressure increases far above atmospheric pressure and is communicated to the alveoli, which have a pressure higher still due to the elastic recoil of the alveolar septa. At high gas

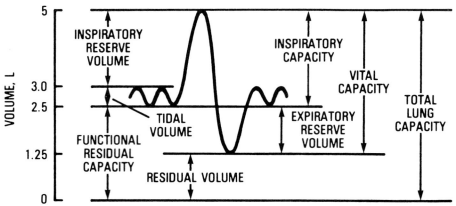

Fig. 22-12 The dynamic lung volumes that can be measured by simple spirometry are the tidal volume, inspiratory reserve volume, expiratory reserve volume, inspiratory capacity, and vital capacity. The static lung volumes are the residual volume, functional residual capacity, and total lung capacity. The static lung volumes cannot be measured by observation of a spirometer trace and require separate methods of measurement.

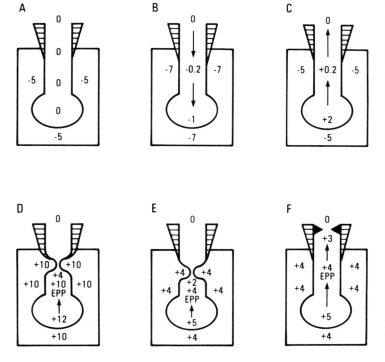

Fig. 22-13 Pressure gradients across the airways. The airways consist of a thin-walled intrathoracic portion (near the alveoli) and a more rigid (cartilagenous) intrathoracic and extrathoracic portion. During expiration the pressure due to elastic recoil is assumed to be $+2$ cm H_2O and the total pressure inside the alveolus is pleural pressure plus the elastic recoil. The arrows indicate direction of airflow. EPP=equal pressure point. (*A*) End expiration, normal lung; (*B*) middle of inpiration, normal lung; (*C*) middle of passive expiration, normal lung; (*D*) middle of forced expiration, normal lung; (*E*) mild forced expiration, emphysematous lung, and; (*F*) mild forced expiration in emphysematous lung against a partly closed larynx. See text for explanation.

flow rates, the pressure drop down the air passage is increased and there will be a point where intraluminal pressure equals pleural pressure. At that point, namely, the equal pressure point (EPP), the air passages are held open by either the elastic recoil of the lung parenchyma in the small air passages or by cartilage in the larger air passages. Downstream of the EPP, the transmural pressure gradient is reversed (-6 cm H_2O) and will result in airway closure. If lung volume were decreased and expiration were forced, the alveolar pressure due to elastic recoil and the caliber of the airways would be reduced causing the equal pressure point and point of collapse to move progressively from larger to smaller air passages.

Airway Closure in Patients with Abnormal Lungs. Airway closure occurs with milder active expiration and lower gas flow rates in patients with emphysema, bronchitis, and asthma. In all three conditions, airway resistance is increased, creating the potential for negative intrathoracic transmural pressure gradients and narrowed and collapsed airways. In emphysema, the elastic recoil of the lung is reduced, the point of airway resistance is close to the alveolus, and the air passages are poorly supported by the lung parenchyma. So during a *mild* forced expiration by a patient with emphysema, the equal pressure point and the point of collapse (where the transmural pressure gradient is sufficiently negative) are near the alveolus (Fig. 22-13*E*). Use of pursed lip or grunting expiration (the equivalents of partly closing the larynx during expiration), positive end-expiratory pressure, and a continuous positive airway pressure in an emphysematous patient restores a favorable (distending) intrathoracic air passage transmural gradient (Fig. 22-13*F*). In bronchitis the elastic recoil of the lung is nearly normal, and thus a mild forced expiration may still result in airway closure because structurally weakened airways may close when only a small negative transmural pressure gradient is present. Finally, in asthma, the middle-sized airways are narrowed by bronchospasm and if expiration is

forced they are further narrowed by a negative transmural pressure gradient.

The Measurement of Closing Capacity (CC) is a sensitive test of early small-airway disease and is performed by having the patient exhale to residual volume (Fig. 22-14).[24] A bolus of tracer gas (^{133}Xe, helium) is inhaled at residual volume and inhalation is continued to total lung capacity. During the initial part of this inhalation, the first gas to enter the alveolus is the dead space gas and the tracer bolus. This gas preferentially goes to the apices of the lung, presumably because the dependent alveoli are closed. As the inhalation continues, apical alveoli complete filling and basilar alveoli open and begin to fill.

A differential tracer gas concentration is thus established: the gas in the apices has a higher tracer concentration than that in the bases. As the subject exhales, and the diaphragm ascends, a point is reached where the small airways just above the diaphragm tend to close, limiting airflow from these areas. The airflow now comes from the upper lung fields, where the alveolar gas has a much higher tracer concentration, thus resulting in a sudden increase in the tracer gas concentration toward the end of exhalation (phase IV).

The absolute volume (in ml) above residual volume where this increase in N_2 concentration occurs is known as the closing volume (CV). The CV plus the residual volume is known as the closing capacity. Smoking, obesity, aging and the supine position increase the CC.[25] In healthy individuals at a mean age of 44 years, CC=FRC in the supine position and at a mean age of 66 years CC=FRC in the upright position.[26]

The Relationship Between the Functional Residual Capacity and the Closing Capacity

The relationship between FRC and CC is as follows: as lung volume decreases during expiration towards residual volume, small

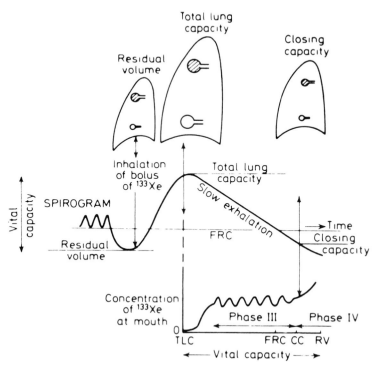

Fig. 22-14 Measurement of closing capacity by the use of a tracer gas such as xenon 133. The bolus of tracer gas is inhaled near residual volume and, due to airway closure, is distributed *only* to those alveoli whose air passages are still open (upper, nondependent alveoli shown shaded in diagram). During expiration, the concentration of the tracer gas becomes constant after the dead space is washed out. This plateau (phase III) gives way to a rising concentration of tracer gas (phase IV) when there is closure of airways leading to alveoli that did not receive the tracer gas. (Reprinted by permission of the publisher, from Nunn JF: Applied Respiratory Physiology. 2nd edition. London: Butterworths (Publishers) Ltd. 1977.)

airways (0.5 to 0.9 mm in diameter) show a progressive tendency to close, whereas larger airways remain patent.[27,28] Airway closure occurs first in the dependent lung regions, since the distending transpulmonary pressure is less and the volume change during expiration is greater. In the presence of lung disease, when the volume of lung at which some airways close is greater than the whole of the tidal volume, lung volume never increases enough during tidal inspiration to open any of these airways. Thus, these airways stay closed during all of the tidal respiration. Airways that are closed all of the time are equivalent to atelectasis (Fig. 22-15). If the closing volume of some airways lies within the tidal volume, then as lung volume increases during inspiration, some previously closed airways will open for a short period of time until lung volume recedes once again below the closing volume of these airways. Since these opening

and closing airways are only open for a shorter period of time than normal airways, they have less chance or time to participate in fresh gas exchange, which is a circumstance equivalent to a low ventilation to perfusion region. If the closing volume of the lung is below the whole of tidal respiration, then no airways are closed at any time during tidal respiration, and this is a normal circumstance.

The reason mechanical intermittent positive pressure breathing (IPPB) may be efficacious is that it can take a previously spontaneously breathing patient with a low ventilation to perfusion relationship (where the closing capacity is greater than FRC, as depicted on the left-hand side of Fig. 22-16) and increase the amount of time that some previously closed airways spend in fresh gas exchange and thereby increase the ventilation to perfusion relationship (middle panel of

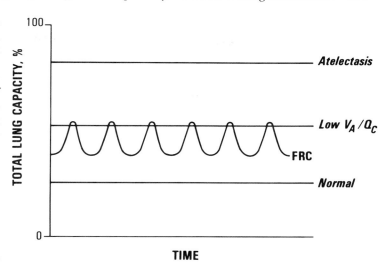

Fig. 22-15 The relationship between the functional residual capacity (which is the percent of total lung capacity [TLC] that exists at the end of exhalation), shown by the level of each trough of the sine wave tidal volume, and the closing capacity (CC) of the lung (three different closing capacities are indicated by the three different straight lines). See text for explanation of why the three different functional residual capacity to closing capacity relationships depicted result in normal, low ventilation to perfusion relationships ($\dot{V}_A/\dot{Q}$), or atelectasis. The abscissa is time.

Fig. 22-16). If positive end-expiratory pressure (PEEP) is added to the IPPB, the PEEP increases FRC above or to a lung volume greater than closing capacity and thereby restores a normal FRC to closing capacity relationship so that no airways are closed at any time during the tidal respiration depicted on the right-hand side of Figure 22-16 (IPPB+PEEP*)*.

OXYGEN AND CARBON DIOXIDE TRANSPORT

ALVEOLAR AND DEAD SPACE VENTILATION AND ALVEOLAR GAS TENSIONS

In patients with normal lungs, approximately two-thirds of each breath reaches perfused alveoli and thereby takes part in gas exchange. This constitutes the effective or alveolar ventilation. The remaining one-third of each breath takes no part in gas exchange and is therefore termed the total (or effective or physiological) dead space ventilation. This dead space ventilation may be divided into two components: a volume of gas that ventilates the conducting airways (the anatomical

dead space ventilation) and a volume of gas that may be thought of as not taking part in effective gas exchange at the alveolar level (the alveolar dead space ventilation). Figure 22-17 shows a two-compartment model of the lung in which the anatomic and alveolar dead

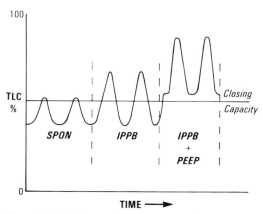

Fig. 22-16 The functional residual capacity to closing capacity relationship during spontaneous ventilation (SPON), intermittent positive pressure breathing (IPPB), and intermittent positive pressure breathing and positive end-expiratory pressure (IPPB + PEEP). See text for explanation of the effect of the two ventilatory maneuvers (IPPB and PEEP) on the functional residual capacity to closing capacity relationship.

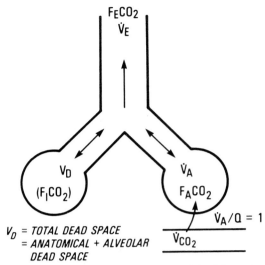

V_D = TOTAL DEAD SPACE
= ANATOMICAL + ALVEOLAR
DEAD SPACE

Fig. 22-17 Two compartment model of lung in which the anatomical and alveolar dead space compartments have been combined onto the total (physiological) dead space (V_D). $\dot{V}_A$, alveolar ventilation; $\dot{V}_E$, expired minute ventilation; $\dot{V}_{CO_2}$, carbon dioxide production; F_ICO_2, inspired carbon dioxide fraction; F_ACO_2, alveolar carbon dioxide fraction; F_ECO_2, mixed expired carbon dioxide fraction; and $\dot{V}_A/Q = 1$, equal ventilation and perfusion in L/min.

space compartments have been combined into the total (physiological) dead space compartment; the other compartment is the alveolar ventilation ($\dot{V}_A$) compartment, whose idealized ventilation/perfusion ratio is $\cong 1.0$.*

The anatomic dead space varies with lung size and is approximately 1 ml/lb body weight. In the normal patient lying supine, the anatomic and total (physiological) dead

---

* Figure 22-17 indicates that in a steady state the volume of CO_2 entering the alveoli ($\dot{V}CO_2$) must equal the volume of CO_2 eliminated in the expired gas ($\dot{V}_E$) (F_ECO_2). Hence: $\dot{V}CO_2 = (\dot{V}_E) (F_ECO_2)$. But the expired gas volume consists of alveolar gas ($\dot{V}_A$) (F_ACO_2) and dead space gas (V_D) (F_ICO_2). Hence: $\dot{V}CO_2 = (\dot{V}_A) (F_ACO_2) + (V_D) (F_ICO_2)$. Setting the first equation equal to the second equation and using the relationship $\dot{V}_E = \dot{V}_A + V_D$ and subsequent algebraic manipulation (e.g., $PAO_2 = PaO_2$) results in the physiological dead space equation:

$$V_D/V_T = PaCO_2 - P\bar{E}CO_2/PaCO_2 \qquad (3)$$

spaces are approximately equal (alveolar dead space is minimal). In the erect posture, when the uppermost alveoli are not perfused alveolar dead space may increase to 60 to 80 ml.

In severe lung disease, the physiological dead space to tidal volume ratio V_D/V_T provides a useful expression of the inefficiency of ventilation. In the normal patient, this ratio is usually less than 30 percent; i.e., ventilation is more than 70 percent efficient. In the patient with obstructive airway disease, V_D/V_T may increase to 60 to 70 percent. Under these conditions, ventilation is obviously grossly inefficient. Figure 22-18 shows the relation between minute ventilation ($\dot{V}_E$) and V_D/V_T for several $PaCO_2$ values. If $\dot{V}_E$ is constant and V_D/V_T increases, $PaCO_2$ increases. If V_D/V_T is constant and $\dot{V}_E$ increases, $PaCO_2$ decreases. If $PaCO_2$ is constant and V_D/V_T increases, then $\dot{V}_E$ must increase.*

The alveolar concentration of a gas is equal to the difference between the inspired concentration of a gas and the ratio of the output (or uptake) of the gas to the $\dot{V}_A$. Thus, for gas X, $PaX = (Pdry atm) (F_IX) \pm \dot{V}X$ (output or uptake)/$\dot{V}_A$, where PaX = alveolar partial pressure of gas X; F_IX = inspired concentration of gas X; $Pdry atm$ = dry atmospheric pressure = $Pwet atm - PH_2O = 760 - 47 = 713$ torr; $\dot{V}X$ = output or uptake of gas X; $\dot{V}_A$ = alveolar ventilation. For CO_2, $PaCO_2 = 713(F_ICO_2 + \dot{V}CO_2/\dot{V}_A)$. Since $F_ICO_2 = 0$ and using standard conversion factors,

$$PaCO_2 = \dot{V}CO_2 \text{ (ml/min STPD)}/\dot{V}_A$$
$$\text{(L/min/BTPS) (0.863)}. \qquad (4)$$

For O_2:
$$PaO_2 = 713(F_IO_2 - \dot{V}O_2/\dot{V}_A) \qquad (5)$$

For example, 100 torr = $713(0.21 - 225/3200)$ (ml/min÷ml/min). Figure 22-19 shows the hyperbolic relationships expressed in equations (4) and (5) between $PaCO_2$ and PaO_2 and $\dot{V}_A$ for different levels of $\dot{V}O_2$ and $\dot{V}CO_2$, respectively. Note that as $\dot{V}_A$ increases, the second term of the right-hand side of equations (4) and (5) approaches zero and the composition of the alveolar gas approaches that of the inspired gas.

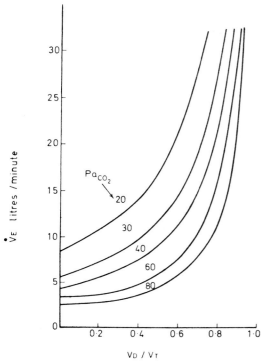

Fig. 22-18 The relationship between the total dead space to tidal volume ratio (VD/VT) and the minute ventilation (V̇E, L/min) required to maintain PaCO₂ levels of 20, 30, 40, 60, and 80 torr. These curves are hyperbolic and rise steeply at high VD/VT values. It is apparent from this graph that if a patient with a high VD/VT (for example, 0.65) accepts a PaCO₂ of 60 torr rather than works to maintain a PaCO₂ at 40 torr, the patient will save a great deal of V̇E work (5 L/min in this example).

Note that Figure 22-19 retains $P_{A}O_2$ from equation (5) and substitutes $PaCO_2$ for $P_{A}CO_2$ from equation (4). The reason for this difference is important and involves the differential effects of ventilation to perfusion inequalities upon CO_2 and O_2 exchange. This is due to the disparity between the venous-to-arterial O_2 and CO_2 tension differences (60 torr and 6 torr, respectively) and to the different characteristics of the O_2 and CO_2 dissociation curves. Blood passing through underventilated alveoli tends to retain its CO_2 and does not take up enough O_2; blood traversing

overventilated alveoli gives off an excessive amount of CO_2 but cannot take up a proportionately increased amount of O_2 owing to the flatness of the oxyhemoglobin dissociation curve in this region (see Fig. 22-20). Hence, a lung with uneven ventilation to perfusion relationships can eliminate CO_2 from the overventilated alveoli to compensate for the underventilated alveoli. Thus, with uneven ventilation to perfusion relationships, $P_{A}CO_2$

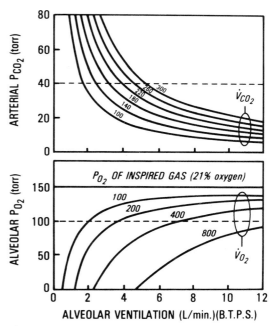

Fig. 22-19 The relationship between alveolar ventilation and alveolar PO₂ and arterial PCO₂ for a family of different O₂ consumption (V̇O₂) and CO₂ production (V̇CO₂) is derived from equations 4 and 5 in the text and is hyperbolic. Note that as alveolar ventilation increases the alveolar PO₂ and arterial PCO₂ approach inspired concentrations. Decreases in alveolar ventilation below 4 L/min are accompanied by precipitous decreases in alveolar PO₂ and increases in arterial PCO₂. If the inspired O₂ concentration is increased, then alveolar ventilation must decrease much more to produce hypoxemia. (Reprinted (with modification) by permission of the publisher, from Nunn JF: Applied Respiratory Physiology. 2nd edition. London: Butterworths (Publishers) Ltd. 1977.)

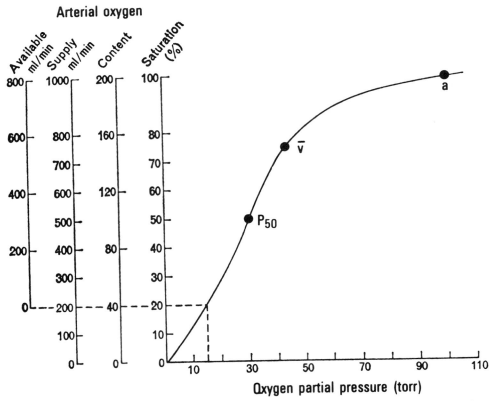

Arterial oxygen

Fig. 22-20 The oxygen-hemoglobin dissociation curve. Four different ordinates are shown as a function of oxygen partial pressure (the abscissa). In order of right to left, they are: saturation (%); O_2 content (ml O_2/L); O_2 supply to the peripheral tissues (ml/min); and O_2 available to the peripheral tissues (ml/min), which is O_2 supply minus approximately 200 ml/min which cannot be extracted below a partial pressure of 20 torr. Three points are shown on the curve; (a) normal arterial, ($\bar{v}$) normal mixed venous; and (P_{50}) the partial pressure (27 torr) at which hemoglobin is 50 percent saturated.

to $PaCO_2$ gradients are small and PaO_2 to PaO_2 gradients are usually large.

ALVEOLAR PERFUSION AND
RIGHT-TO-LEFT TRANSPULMONARY
SHUNT BLOOD FLOW

The Oxyhemoglobin Dissociation Curve

The oxyhemoglobin dissociation (oxy-Hb) curve normally relates the *saturation* (percent sat) of hemoglobin (y axis most right in Fig. 22-20) to the PaO_2. Hemoglobin (Hb) is fully saturated (100 percent) by a PO_2 of about 700 torr. The normal arterial point on the right side and flat part of the oxy-Hb curve in Figure 22-20 is 95 to 98 percent saturated by a PaO_2 of about 90 to 100 torr. When the PO_2 is less than 60 torr (90 percent sat), the saturation falls steeply so that the amount of Hb uncombined with O_2 increases greatly for a given decrease in PO_2. Mixed venous blood has a PO_2 ($P\bar{v}O_2$) of about 40 torr and is aproximately 75 percent saturated, and is indicated by the middle of the three points on the oxy-Hb curve in Figure 22-20.

The oxy-Hb curve can also relate the O_2 *content* (vol percent, ml O_2/0.1 L of blood; y axis second most right in Fig. 22-20) to the PO_2. Oxygen is carried in solution in the plasma, 0.003 ml O_2 per torr $PO_2/0.1$ L, and combined with Hb, 1.34 ml O_2 per gm Hb to the extent (percent) Hb is saturated. Thus:

$$C_{O_2} = (1.34) (Hb)(\% \, sat) + 0.003(PO_2) \quad (6)$$

For a patient with a Hb of 15 gm/0.1 L, PaO_2 of 100 torr, and $P\bar{v}O_2$ of 40 torr—$CaO_2 =$ (1.34) (15) (1) + (0.003) (100) = 20.1 + 0.3 = 20.4 ml $O_2/0.1$ L; $C\bar{v}O_2 = (1.34) (15) (0.75) +$ (0.003) (40) = 15.1 + 0.1 = 15.2 ml $O_2/0.1$ L. Thus, the normal arteriovenous O_2 content difference is approximately 5.2 ml/0.1 L.

The oxy-Hb curve can also relate the *O*$_2$ *transport* (L/min) to the peripheral tissues (y axis third most right in Fig. 22-20) to the PO_2. This is obtained by multiplying O_2 content by the cardiac output ($\dot{Q}_t$). If $\dot{Q}_t = 5$ L/min and $CaO_2 = 20.4$ ml $O_2/0.1$ L, then the arterial point corresponds to 1.02 L/min going to the periphery and the venous point corresponds to 0.76 L/min returning to the lungs for a $\dot{V}O_2 = 0.26$ L/min.

The oxy-Hb curve can also relate to the *O*$_2$ actually *available* to the tissues (y axis most left in Fig. 22-20) as a function of PO_2. Of the 1.0 L/min of O_2 normally going to the periphery, 0.2 L/min of O_2 cannot be extracted because it would lower the PO_2 below the level (dashed line in Fig. 22-20) at which such organs as the brain can survive: the O_2 available to the tissues is therefore 0.8 L/min. This is approximately three to four times the normal resting $\dot{V}O_2$. When $\dot{Q}_t = 5$ L/min and the arterial saturation is less than 40 percent, the total flow of O_2 to the periphery is reduced to 0.4 L/min so that the available O_2 is now 0.2 L/min. Supply then just equals demand. At an arterial saturation below 40 percent, tissue demand can only be met by an increase in cardiac output or, in the long term, by an increase in Hb concentration.

The *position* of the oxy-Hb curve is best described by the PO_2 at which Hb is 50 percent saturated (the P_{50}). The normal P_{50}, which is the point on the left side and steep portion of the oxy-Hb curve in Figure 22-20, is 26.7 torr.

The effect of a shift in the position of the oxy-Hb curve depends greatly on the PO_2. In the region of the normal PaO_2 (75 to 100 torr), the curve is relatively horizontal so that shifts of the curve have little effect on saturation. In the region of the mixed venous PO_2, where the curve is relatively steep, a shift of the curve leads to a much greater difference in saturation. A $P_{50}<27$ torr describes a left-shifted oxy-Hb curve, which means that at any given PO_2, Hb has a higher affinity for O_2 and is therefore more saturated than normal. This may require a higher tissue perfusion than normal to produce the normal amount of O_2 unloading. The causes of a left-shifted oxy-Hb curve are alkalosis (metabolic and respiratory), hypothermia, abnormal and fetal Hb, CO-Hb, methemoglobin, and decreased red blood cell 2,3-diphosphoglycerate (DPG) content (tranfusion of old stored blood) (see Ch. 28).

A $P_{50}>27$ torr describes a right-shifted oxy-Hb curve, which means that at any given PO_2, Hb has a low affinity for O_2 and is less saturated than normal. This may allow a lower tissue perfusion than normal to produce the normal amount of O_2 unloading. The causes of a right-shifted oxy-Hb curve are acidosis (metabolic and respiratory), hyperthermia, abnormal Hb, and increased red blood cell 2,3-DPG content.

The Effect of $\dot{Q}_s/\dot{Q}_t$ on the PaO_2

Figure 22-21[29] shows the relationship between FIO_2 and PaO_2 for a family of right-to-left transpulmonary shunts ($\dot{Q}_s/\dot{Q}_t$) with a constant cardiac output. With no $\dot{Q}_s/\dot{Q}_t$, a linear increase in FIO_2 results in a linear increase in PaO_2 (solid straight line). As shunt is increased, the lines become flat. With a shunt of 50 percent of the cardiac output, an increase in FIO_2 results in almost no increase in PaO_2. The solution to the problem of hypoxemia secondary to a large shunt is not increasing the FIO_2, but rather a reduction in shunt (fiberoptic bronchoscopy, PEEP, turning, antibiotics, suctioning, diuretic, etc.).

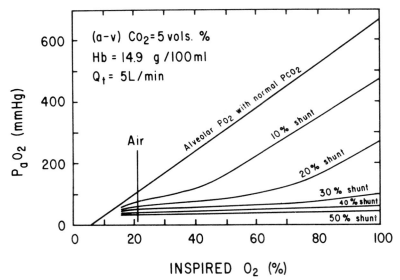

Fig. 22-21 Effect of changes in inspired oxygen concentration on arterial PO_2 for various right to left transpulmonary shunts. Cardiac output ($\dot{Q}_t$), hemoglobin (Hb), and oxygen consumption and arteriovenous oxygen content differences [(a−v)Co_2] were assumed to be normal. (Modified by Benumof[43] from Nunn JF: Applied Respiratory Physiology. 2nd edition. London: Butterworths (Publishers) Ltd. 1977. Reprinted by permission of the publisher, Butterworths.)

The Effect of $\dot{Q}_t$ and $\dot{V}O_2$ on CaO_2

In addition to an increased $\dot{Q}_s/\dot{Q}_t$, the CaO_2 is decreased by a decreased $\dot{Q}_t$ (for a constant $\dot{V}O_2$) and by an increased $\dot{V}O_2$ (for a constant $\dot{Q}_t$). In either case (decreased $\dot{Q}_t$ or increased $\dot{V}O_2$), and with a constant right-to-left shunt ($\dot{Q}_s/\dot{Q}_t$), the tissues must extract more O_2 from the blood per unit blood volume and, therefore, the O_2 content of mixed venous blood ($C\bar{v}O_2$) must decrease. When the blood with lower $C\bar{v}O_2$ passes through whatever shunt that exists in the lung (50 percent is the example in Fig. 22-22) and remains unchanged in its oxygen composition, it must inevitably mix with oxygenated end-pulmonary capillary blood (c′ flow) and decrease the CaO_2 (Fig. 22-22).* The larger the right-to-left $\dot{Q}_s/\dot{Q}_t$, the greater effect a low

---

* The amount of O_2 flowing through any given channel per minute in Figure 22-22 is a product of the

$C\bar{v}O_2$ will have on the CaO_2 (Figs. 22-21 and 22-22).[30] Thus, the $P(A-a)O_2$ is not only a function of the size of the $\dot{Q}_s/\dot{Q}_t$ but also what is flowing through the $\dot{Q}_s/\dot{Q}_t$ (namely $C\bar{v}O_2$), and that is a primary function of $\dot{Q}_t$ and $\dot{V}O_2$.

Use of the Fick Principle to Determine $\dot{V}O_2$

The Fick principle can be used to determine $\dot{V}O_2$ in two ways. First, the amount of O_2 consumed by the body ($\dot{V}O_2$) is equal to the amount of O_2 leaving the lungs

---

blood flow times the O_2 content. Hence, from Figure 22-22:

$$\dot{Q}_t C\bar{v}O_2 \begin{array}{c} \longrightarrow \dot{Q}c'Cc'O_2 \\ \\ \longrightarrow \dot{Q}_s C\bar{v}O_2 \end{array} \longrightarrow \dot{Q}_t CaO_2$$

$\dot{Q}_t CaO_2 = Qc'Cc'O_2 + \dot{Q}_s C\bar{v}O_2$. With $Qc = \dot{Q}_t - \dot{Q}_s$ and further algebraic manipulation:[31]

$$\dot{Q}_s/\dot{Q}_t = Cc'O_2 - CaO_2/Cc'O_2 - C\bar{v}O_2 \qquad (8)$$

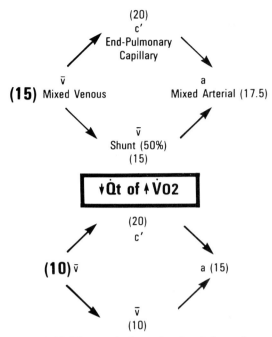

Fig. 22-22 The equivalent circuit of the pulmonary circulation. Oxygen content is in ml/100 ml blood (vol percent). In the example, 50 percent of the cardiac output flows through the right-to-left shunt. A decrease in cardiac output ($\dot{Q}t$) or an increase in O_2 consumption ($\dot{V}O_2$) can cause a decrease in mixed venous oxygen content (from 15 vol percent to 10 vol percent in this example), which in turn will cause a decrease in the arterial content of oxygen (from 17.5 vol percent to 15.0 vol percent). In this example the decrease in mixed venous oxygen content was twice the decrease in arterial oxygen content.

($\dot{Q}_t$) (CaO_2) minus the amount of O_2 returning to the lungs ($\dot{Q}_t$) ($C\bar{v}O_2$). Thus:

$$\dot{V}O_2 = (\dot{Q}_t)(CaO_2) - (\dot{Q}_t)(C\bar{v}O_2)$$
$$= \dot{Q}_t(CaO_2 - C\bar{v}O_2);$$

condensing the content symbols yields the usual expression of the Fick equation:

$$\dot{V}O_2 = (\dot{Q}_t)[C(a - v)O_2] \qquad (7)$$

which states that oxygen consumption is equal to the cardiac output times the arteriovenous O_2 content difference. Normally (5 L/min) (5.2 ml)/0.1 L=0.26 L/min. Additionally, the Fick equation is useful in un-

derstanding the impact of changes in $\dot{Q}_t$ on PaO_2 and $P\bar{v}O_2$. If $\dot{V}O_2$ remains constant (K) and $\dot{Q}_t$ decreases ($\downarrow$), then the arteriovenous O_2 content difference has to increase ($\uparrow$): $\dot{V}O_2$ = K = $\dot{Q}_t(\downarrow) \times C(a - \bar{v})O_2(\uparrow)$. The $C(a - \bar{v})O_2$ increases because a decrease in $\dot{Q}_t$ causes a much larger and primary decrease in $P\bar{v}O_2$ and $C\bar{v}O_2$ compared to a smaller and secondary decrease in PaO_2 and CaO_2 [($\uparrow$)C(a − $\bar{v}$)O₂ = C($\downarrow$a − $\downarrow\downarrow\bar{v}$)O₂].[30] Thus, the $P\bar{v}O_2$ and $C\bar{v}O_2$ are much more sensitive indicators of $\dot{Q}_t$, since they change more with the changes in $\dot{Q}_t$ than do PaO_2 and CaO_2.

Second, the amount of O_2 consumed by the body ($\dot{V}O_2$) is equal to the amount of O_2 brought into the lungs by ventilation ($\dot{V}I$) (FIO_2) minus the amount of O_2 leaving the lungs by ventilation ($\dot{V}E$) ($F\bar{E}O_2$). Thus, $\dot{V}O_2$ = ($\dot{V}I$) (FIO_2) − ($\dot{V}E$) ($F\bar{E}O_2$). Since the difference between $\dot{V}I$ and $\dot{V}E$ is due to the difference between $\dot{V}O_2$ (normally, 0.26 L/min) and $\dot{V}CO_2$ (normally, 0.20 L/min) and is only 0.06 L/min, $\dot{V}I$ essentially equals $\dot{V}E$:

$$\dot{V}O_2 = \dot{V}E(FIO_2) - \dot{V}E(F\bar{E}O_2)$$
$$= \dot{V}E(FIO_2 - F\bar{E}O_2)$$

For example and normally, $\dot{V}O_2$=5.0 L/min (0.21−0.16 ml)=0.25 L/min. In determining $\dot{V}O_2$ in this way, $\dot{V}E$ can be measured with a spirometer, FIO_2 can be measured with an O_2 analyzer or from known fresh gas flows, and $F\bar{E}O_2$ can be measured by collecting expired gas in a bag over the course of a few minutes. A sample of the mixed expired gas is used to measure $P\bar{E}O_2$. To convert $P\bar{E}O_2$ to $F\bar{E}O_2$, simply divide $P\bar{E}O_2$ by dry atmospheric pressure: $P\bar{E}O_2/713 = F\bar{E}O_2$.

PULMONARY STRUCTURE AND FUNCTION

PULMONARY MICROCIRCULATION AND PULMONARY EDEMA

A schematic of the ultrastructural appearance of an alveolar septum is shown in Figure 22-23.[32] Capillary blood is separated from al-

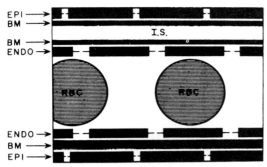

Fig. 22-23 Schematic of the anatomic ultrastructure of the pulmonary microcirculation. ENDO = capillary endothelium; BM = basement membrane; IS = interstitial space; EPI = alveolar epithelium; and RBC = red blood cells. (Modified from Fishman AP: Pulmonary edema: The water exchanging function of the lung. Circulation 46:390, 1972, by permission of the American Heart Association, Inc.)

veolar gas by a series of anatomic layers: capillary endothelium, endothelial basement membrane, interstitial space, epithelial basement membrane, and alveolar epithelium (type I pneumocyte).

On one side of the alveolar septum (the thick, upper, fluid- and gas-exchanging side), the epithelial and endothelial basement membranes are separated by a space of variable thickness containing connective tissue fibrils, elastic fibers, fibroblasts, and macrophages. This connective tissue is the "backbone" of the lung parenchyma and forms a continuum with the connective tissue sheaths around the conducting airways and blood vessels. Thus, the pericapillary perialveolar interstitial space is continuous with the interstitial tissue space that surrounds terminal bronchioles and vessels and is identical to the connective tissue space. There are no lymphatics in the interstitial space of the alveolar septum. Instead, lymphatic capillaries first appear in the interstitial space surrounding terminal bronchioles, small arteries, and veins.

The oppposite side of the alveolar septum (the thin, down, gas-exchanging side) contains only fused epithelial and endothelial basement membranes. The interstitial space is thus restricted due to fusion of the basement membranes: interstitial fluid cannot separate the endothelial and epithelial cells from one another, and as a result the barrier between alveolar and capillary compartments is minimal and in this part is composed only of the two cell barriers with their associated basement membranes.[33,34]

Between the individual endothelial and epithelial cells are holes (slits, or loose junctions) that provide a potential pathway for fluid to move from the intravascular space to the interstitial space and finally from the interstitial space to the alveolar space. Pulmonary capillary permeability (K) is therefore a direct function of and essentially equivalent to the size of the holes in the endothelial and epithelial linings. When flow of interstitial fluid through the endothelial holes is excessive and cannot be cleared adequately by lymphatics, it will accumulate in the interstitial connective tissue compartment around the large vessels and airways, forming peribronchial and periarteriolar edema fluid cuffs. There is now good evidence that indicates that one of the mechanisms of hypoxemia during pulmonary edema is as follows: the perialveolar interstitial edema compresses alveoli and acutely reduces functional residual capacity; the peribronchial edema fluid cuffs compress bronchi and acutely increase closing volume.[35,37] A decreased FRC and an increased CV must create areas of low $\dot{V}_A/\dot{Q}$ and/or atelectasis.

Following filling of the pulmonary interstitial compartment with edema fluid, fluid from the interstitial space, under an increased driving force, will cross the relatively impermeable epithelial wall holes and the alveolar space will fill. Intra-alveolar edema fluid will additionally cause alveolar collapse and atelectasis.

The forces governing net transcapillary fluid movement are as follows: the net transcapillary flow of fluid (F) out of pulmonary capillaries is equal to the difference between pulmonary capillary hydrostatic pressure

(Pinside) and the interstitial fluid hydrostatic pressure (Poutside) and to the difference between the capillary colloid osmotic pressure (πinside) and the interstitial colloid osmotic pressure (πoutside). These four forces will produce a steady state fluid flow (F) during a constant capillary permeability (K).

$$F = K(Pinside - Poutside) - (\pi inside - \pi outside) \quad (10)$$

K is a capillary filtration coefficient expressed in ml/min/mm Hg/100 g. The filtration coefficient is the product of the effective capillary surface area in a given mass of tissue and the permeability per unit surface area of the capillary wall to filter the fluid. Under normal circumstances, the intravascular colloid osmotic pressure (about 21 to 25 torr) acts to keep water in the capillary lumen, and working against this force, the pulmonary capillary pressure (about 9 torr) acts to force water across the loose endothelial junctions into the interstitial space. If these forces were the only ones operative, the interstitial space, and consequently the alveolar surfaces, would be constantly dry and there would be no lymph flow. In fact, alveolar surfaces are moist, and lymphatic flow from the interstitial compartment is constant (approximately 500 ml/day). This can be explained in part by the πoutside and in part by the studies that indicate that the interstitial Poutside is uniquely negative.[38] Subatmospheric interstitial space pressure would promote, by suction, a slow loss of fluid across the endothelial holes.[39] Any change in the size of the endothelial holes or in the forces acting across them results in leakage of water into pericapillary interstitial space.

ALVEOLAR SURFACTANT

The alveolar surfaces are moist and are lined with a layer of water. The alveolar water-lining layer appears to be a fluid continuum extending over the entire alveolar surface, finally extending toward the conducting airways, where it is continuous with the bronchiolar, and thus eventually with the

bronchial, surface-lining layer. The lining of a curved surface (sphere or cylinder, as are the alveoli, bronchioles, bronchi) with water creates a surface tension that tends to make the surface area exposed to the atmosphere as small as possible. Simply stated, water molecules crowd much closer together on the surface of a curved layer of water than elsewhere in the fluid.

The pressure in a bubble is above ambient pressure by an amount depending on the surface tension of the liquid and the radius of curvature of the bubble, according to the Laplace equation:

$$P=2T/R \quad (11)$$

where P is the distending pressure within the bubble (dyn/sq cm), T is surface tension of the liquid (dyn/cm), and R is radius of the bubble (cm).

Although surface tension probably contributes to the retractive forces of the lung, two difficulties must be resolved. The first problem is that the distending pressure for small bubbles is higher than for large bubbles, a conclusion that stems directly from the Laplace equation. From this reasoning, pressure in a small alveolus should be greater than in a large one and would result in a progressive discharge of each small alveolus into a larger one, until eventually only one gigantic alveolus would be left (Fig. 22-24*A*).

The second problem concerns the relationship between lung volume and the transmural pressure gradient. According to the Laplace equation, the retractive forces of the lung should increase as the lung volume decreased, a relationship which is certainly true of a bubble. If this were true of the lung, the lung should decrease in volume according to a vicious cycle, with the tendency to collapse increasing progressively as the lung volume diminished.

These two problems can be resolved by showing that surface tension of the fluid lining the alveoli is variable and decreases as its surface area is reduced. Surface tensions reach very low levels that are well below the normal range for body fluids such as water and plasma. When an alveolus decreases in

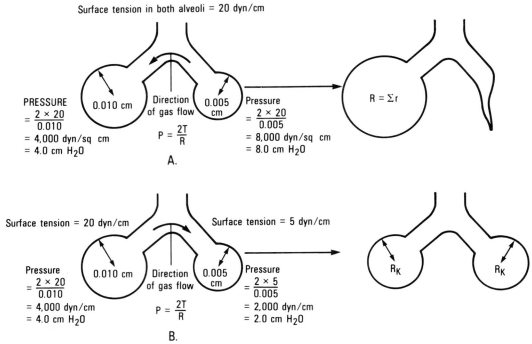

Fig. 22-24 Surface tension and alveolar transmural pressure. (*A*) The pressure relations in two alveoli of different size but with the same surface tension of their lining fluids. The direction of gas flow will be from the higher pressure, small alveolus to the lower pressure, large alveolus and the result is one large alveolus. (*B*) The pressure relations of two alveoli of different size when allowance is made for the expected changes in surface tension. The direction of gas flow is from the larger alveolus to the smaller alveolus until the two alveoli are of equal size and are volume stable (R_K).

size, the surface tension of the lining fluid falls to a greater extent than the corresponding reduction of radius so that the transmural pressure gradient ($=2T/R$) diminishes. This explains why small alveoli do not discharge their contents into large alveoli (Fig. 22-24*B*) and why the elastic recoil of small alveoli is less than that of large alveoli.

The substance responsible for the reduction (and variability) of alveolar surface tension is secreted by the intra-alveolar type II pneumocyte and is a lipoprotein called surfactant that floats as a 50 Å thick film on the surface of the alveolar-lining fluid. When the surface film is reduced in area and the concentration of surfactant at the surface is increased, there is an increased surface reducing pressure that counteracts the surface tension of the fluid lining the alveoli.

DEPENDENCY OF ALVEOLAR DUCTS, BRONCHIOLE, AND BRONCHIAL STRUCTURAL (AND FUNCTIONAL) INTEGRITY ON LUNG VOLUME

In the bronchial tree, the Clara cells are thought to secrete a surface tension-reducing material. Smokers have been demonstrated to have an increase in the number of goblet cells and a decrease in the number of Clara cells.[40] The hypothesis has been advanced[40] that the disappearance of Clara cells and their replacement by goblet cells may result in the bronchioles becoming lined by a film of mucus. Normally, bronchioles are lined by a material that is consistent in appearance with surfactant and they behave as though they were lined by surface-active material. Replacement of the surfactant layer by a film of mucus would render the bronchioles unstable and they would close unduly easily and open with great difficulty, leading to functional obstruction.

An important change occurs in the airways at about the eleventh generation, when the diameter is of the order of 1 mm. Cartilage disappears from the wall of the air passages (bronchi) at this level, and structural rigidity ceases to be the principal factor in maintaining patency. Fortunately, at this level the air passages (bronchioles) leave their fibrous sheath and become embedded directly in the lung parenchyma. Elastic recoil of the alveolar septa is then able to hold the air passages open like the guy ropes of a bell tent. Similarly, the patency of the alveolar duct is maintained by the retraction of the surrounding alveolar septa, which also act like the guy ropes of a tent. The destruction of alveolar septa in individuals with emphysema renders the alveolar ducts more liable to closure. The caliber of airways and alveolar ducts beyond the eleventh generation is, therefore, mainly influenced by lung volume, since the forces acting to hold their lumina open are stronger at high lung volume. The caliber of the bronchioles is, however, less influenced by intrathoracic pressure than is the case in the bronchi.

Down to the level of the smallest true bronchi, air passages lie with pulmonary vessels in a sheath that may be distended by edema fluid. They are not directly attached to the lung parenchyma and thus are not subjected to direct traction. They are, nevertheless, subject to intrathoracic pressure and if the extramural pressure is substantially above the intraluminal pressure, collapse will occur in spite of structural support from cartilagenous plates in the bronchial walls.

PATHWAYS OF COLLATERAL VENTILATION

There are four known pathways of collateral ventilation. First, *interalveolar* communications (pores of Kohn) exist in most species, and in the dog range 8 to 50 per alveolus and

may increase in humans with age and with the development of obstructive lung disease. Their precise role has not been defined. Second, *distal bronchiole to alveolar* communications exist (channels of Lambert) but their function in vivo is speculative. Third, there are connections between *respiratory bronchioles to terminal bronchioles* from adjacent lung segments (channels of Martin) in healthy dogs and in humans with lung disease. Fourth, the functional characteristics of interlobar collateral ventilation through *interlobar* connections have recently been described in dogs[41] and these interlobar connections have been observed in humans.[42]

RESPIRATORY FUNCTION DURING ANESTHESIA

INTRODUCTION

The effect of a given anesthetic on respiratory function will depend on the depth of anesthesia, the patient's preoperative respiratory condition, the presence of special intraoperative anesthetic and surgical conditions, and the proper functioning of anesthesia equipment. Irrespective of these first four modifying factors, anesthetics (and allied drugs) and the state of general anesthesia both have intrinsic mechanisms of producing poor gas exchange (hypoxemia and hypercarbia).

EFFECT OF ANESTHETIC DEPTH ON RESPIRATORY PATTERN AND FUNCTION

The respiratory pattern is altered by the induction and deepening of anesthesia.[43] When the depth of anesthesia is inadequate (less than MAC), respiratory pattern may vary from excessive hyperventilation and vocalization to breath-holding. As anesthetic depth approaches or equals MAC (light anesthesia), irregular respiration progresses to a more regular pattern, which is associated with

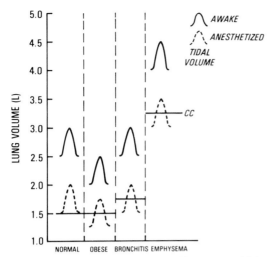

Fig. 22-25 The lung volume (ordinate) at which the tidal volume is breathed decreases (by ≅ 1 L) from the awake state to the anesthetized state. The functional residual capacity, which is the volume of lung existing at the end of the tidal volume, therefore also decreases (by ≅ 1 L) from the awake to the anesthetized state. In the normal, obese, bronchitis, and emphysema patients the awake functional residual capacity considerably exceeds the closing capacity (CC). In the obese, bronchitis, and emphysema patients the anesthetized state causes functional residual capacity to be less than closing capacity. In the normal patient anesthesia causes the functional residual capacity to equal the closing capacity.

a larger than normal tidal volume. However, during light, but deepening anesthesia, the approach to a more regular respiratory pattern may be interrupted by a pause at the end of inspiration (a sort of "hitch" in the inspiration), followed by a relatively prolonged and active expiration in which the patient seems to forcefully, rather than passively, exhale. As anesthesia deepens to moderate levels, respiration becomes faster, more regular, but more shallow. The respiratory pattern is a sine wave losing the inspiratory hitch and lengthened expiratory pause. There is little or no inspiratory or expiratory pause, and the inspiratory and expiratory periods are equivalent. Intercostal muscle activity is still present, and there is normal movement of the

thoracic cage with lifting of the chest during inspiration. The respiratory rate is generally slower and the tidal volume larger with nitrous oxide–narcotic anesthesia compared with anesthesia with halogenated drugs. During deep anesthesia with halogenated drugs, increasing depression of respiration is manifested by even more rapid, shallow breathing (panting). On the other hand, with deep nitrous oxide–narcotic anesthesia, respirations become slower but may remain deep. With very deep anesthesia with all drugs, respirations are jerky or gasping in character and irregular in pattern. This results from loss of active intercostal muscle contribution to inspiration. As a result, a "rocking boat" movement occurs in which there is an out-of-phase depression of the chest wall during inspiration and a flaring of the lower chest margins and a billowing of the abdomen. The reason for this type of movement is that inspiration is dependent solely on diaphragmatic effort. Independent of anesthetic depth, similar chest movements may be similated by upper and lower airway obstruction and by partial paralysis.

PREEXISTING RESPIRATORY DYSFUNCTION

Among the patients that anesthesiologists are frequently required to care for are (1) patients with acute chest disease (pulmonary infection, atelectasis) or systemic diseases (sepsis, cardiac and renal failure, or multiple trauma) that require emergency operations; (2) heavy smokers with subtle pathologic airway and parenchymal conditions and hyperreactive airways; (3) patients with classic emphysematous and bronchitic problems as well as patients with borderline congestive heart failure; (4) obese people prone to decreases in functional residual capacity during anesthesia;[44, 45] (5) patients with chest deformities; and (6) very old patients.

The nature and magnitude of these preexisting respiratory conditions will determine, in part, the effect of a given standard anesthetic on respiratory function. For example, in Figure 22-25 the FRC-CC relationship is depicted for normal, obese, bronchitic, and emphysematous patients. In the normal patient FRC exceeds CC by approximately 1 L. In the latter three respiratory conditions, CC is 0.5 to 0.75 L less than FRC. If anesthesia causes a 1 L decrease in FRC then the normal patient will have no change in the qualitative relationship between FRC and CC. In the patients with the special respiratory conditions, a 1 L decrease in FRC will cause CC to exceed FRC and change the previously marginally normal FRC-CC relationship to either a grossly low $\dot{V}A/\dot{Q}$ or an atelectatic FRC-CC relationship. Similarly, patients with chronic bronchitis, who have copious airway secretions, may suffer more from an anesthetic-induced decrease in mucous velocity flow than other patients. Finally, if an anesthetic drug inhibits HPV, the drug may increase shunting more in patients with preexisting HPV than in those without preexisting HPV. Thus, the effect of a standard anesthetic can be expected to produce varying degrees of respiratory change among patients who have different degrees of preexisting respiratory dysfunction.

SPECIAL INTRAOPERATIVE CONDITIONS

A mechanism of abnormal gas exchange is a final common pathway that is constructed from multiple specific intraoperative conditions and diseases. For example, a decreased cardiac output (a mechanism of hypoxemia) may have multiple specific causes (surgical exposure requirements causing compression of great veins, hemorrhage, arrhythmias). On the other hand, a single intraoperative condition may contribute to a number of different mechanisms of deranged gas exchange.

For example, unusual surgical positions and surgical exposure requirements may contribute to mechanisms of hypoxemia (decreased cardiac output, hypoventilation, and reduced functional residual capacity) and hypercarbia. The intrinsic deleterious respiratory effects of any anesthetic will be magnified by the type and severity of preexisting respiratory dysfunction as well as by the number and severity of special intraoperative conditions that can embarrass respiratory function.

MECHANISMS OF HYPOXEMIA DURING ANESTHESIA

MALFUNCTION OF EQUIPMENT

Mechanical Failure of Anesthesia Apparatus

Hypoxemia (decreased PaO_2) due to mechanical failure of the O_2 supply system or the anesthesia machine is a recognized hazard of anesthesia. Reported causes of O_2 failure during anesthesia include (1) empty or depleted O_2 cylinder, (2) substitution of a non-O_2 cylinder at the O_2 yoke because of absence or failure of the pin index, (3) an erroneously filled O_2 cylinder, (4) insufficient opening of the O_2 cylinder, which hinders a free flow of gas as pressure decreases, (5) failure of gas pressure in a piped O_2 system, (6) failure to open the valve of a piped O_2 system, (7) faulty locking of the piped O_2 system to the anesthesia machine, (8) inadvertent switching of the Schrader adapters on piped lines, (9) crossing of piped lines during construction, (10) failure of a reducing valve or gas manifold, (11) inadvertent disturbance of the setting of the O_2 flowmeter, (12) employment of the fine O_2 flowmeter instead of the coarse flowmeter, (13) fractured or sticking flowmeters, (14) transposition of rotameter tubes, (15) erroneous filling of a liquid O_2 reservoir with N_2, and (16) fresh gas line disconnect from airway.[46-50]

Mechanical Failure of Endotracheal Tube. Main Stem Bronchus Intubation

Virtually all mechanical problems (except disconnect) with endotracheal tubes (such as kinking, secretion blockage, and herniated or ruptured cuffs) cause an increase in airway resistance and may result in hypoventilation. However, intubation of a main stem bronchus results in the absence of ventilation of the contralateral lung. Although potentially minimized by HPV, some perfusion to the contralateral lung will always remain and shunting will increase and PaO_2 will decrease. A change in the position of the patient can cause the endotracheal tube to move. A tube previously well positioned in the trachea may enter a bronchus after the patient or the head is turned or moved into a new position.[51] Flexion of the head causes caudad movement and extention of the head causes cephalad movement of an endotracheal tube.[51] A high incidence of main stem bronchus intubation following institution of a 30 degree Trendelenburg position has been reported.[52] Cephalad shift of the carina during the Trendelenburg position caused the previously "fixed" endotracheal tube to locate in a main stem bronchus.

HYPOVENTILATION (DECREASED TIDAL VOLUME)

Patients under general anesthesia may have a reduced tidal volume for a number of reasons. First, rapid shallow breathing is a regular feature of moderate depths of anesthesia. Second, airway resistance is increased because of the presence of external apparatus, possible airway obstruction, and reduced lung volume. Third, lung compliance is reduced due to all of the factors that decrease FRC. Fourth, surgical posture may restrict or interfere with inferior-superior movement of the diaphragm, with upward and lateral movements of the ribs, and with the similar upward but forward movement of the ribs and sternum and cause a decrease in tidal volume.

There are two ways a decreased tidal volume may cause hypoxemia. First, if tidal volume is reduced and respiratory rate increases proportionately, minute ventilation will remain constant and breathing will be rapid and shallow. Second, if tidal volume is decreased and respiratory rate does *not* increase proportionately, minute ventilation will decrease, PaO_2 may decrease, and $PaCO_2$ may increase (Fig. 22-19). This is likely to occur during deeper levels of anesthesia, during which the chemical control of breathing is altered. Figure 22-26 shows that increasing halothane concentration displaces the PCO_2 ventilation response curve to the right, decreases the slope of the curve, and shifts the apneic threshold to a higher PCO_2 level[53] (see Ch. 13 for more details). Similar alterations are observed with other halogenated anesthetics and narcotics. Thus, with spontaneous ventilation, the changes in respiratory pattern and work of breathing and the alterations in the control of breathing may result in patients who hypoventilate because they have less *desire* to breathe and for whom it is *more difficult* to breathe. Since anesthesia is usually administered with an O_2 enriched gas mixture, hypercarbia is a more common result of hypoventilation than hypoxemia.

HYPERVENTILATION

Hypocapnic alkalosis (hyperventilation) may result in a decreased PaO_2 by causing (1) decreased cardiac output,[30,54] (2) increased oxygen consumption,[55,56] (3) a left-shifted oxy-Hb dissociation curve, (4) decreased HPV,[57] and/or (5) increased airway resistance and decreased compliance.[58]

DECREASE IN FRC

Induction of a general anesthesia is consistently accompanied by a significant (15 to 20 percent) decrease in FRC,[59] which usually causes a decrease in compliance.[60] The maximum decrease in FRC appears to occur

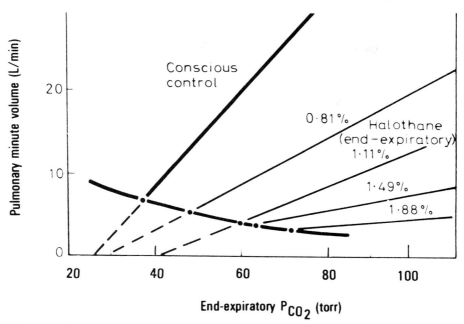

Fig. 22-26 In conscious controls (heavy solid line) increasing end-expiratory PCO_2 increases pulmonary minute volume. The dashed line is an extrapolation of the $CO_2 =$ response curve to zero ventilation and represents the apneic threshold. An increase in anesthetic (halothane) concentration (end-expiratory concentration) progressively diminishes the slope of the $CO_2 =$ response curve and shifts the apneic threshold to a higher PCO_2. The heavy line interrupted by dots shows the decrease in minute ventilation and the increase in PCO_2 that occurs with increasing depth of anesthesia. (Modified from Munson ES, Larson CP Jr, Babad AA, et al: The effects of halothane, fluroxene and cyclopropane on ventilation: A comparative study in man. Anesthesiology 27:716, 1966.)

within the first few minutes of anesthesia,[61-63] and in the absence of any other complicating factor, does not seem to decrease progressively during anesthesia. During anesthesia, the reduction in FRC is of the same order whether ventilation is spontaneous or controlled. Conversely in awake patients, FRC is only slightly reduced during controlled ventilation.[63] The reduction of FRC continues into the postoperative period.[64] For individual patients, the reduction in FRC correlates well with an increase in the alveolar-arterial PO_2 gradient during anesthesia with spontaneous breathing,[65] during anesthesia with artificial ventilation,[62] and in the postoperative period.[64] The reduced FRC may be restored to normal or above normal by the application of PEEP.[66] In the following discussion, some of the causes of the reduced FRC are discussed.

Supine Position

Anesthesia and surgery are usually performed with the patient in the supine position. In changing from the upright to the supine position, FRC decreases by 0.5 to 1.0 L[67] because of a 4 cm cephalad displacement of the diaphragm by the abdominal viscera. Pulmonary vascular congestion may also contribute to the decrease in FRC in the supine position, particularly in patients who preoperatively experienced orthopnea.

The FRC-CV relationship, however, is more important than FRC changes alone. The change in FRC-CV relationship and PaO_2 occurring in moving from the seated to the supine position has been shown to depend on the initial FRC-CV relationship in the seated position.[67] In this study,[67] subjects were divided into four groups. In group 1,

FRC exceeded CV in both supine and erect position. In group 2, FRC exceeded CV only in the seated position. In group 3, CV occurred within the tidal volume in the seated position and exceeded the tidal volume in the supine position. In group 4, CV occurred above the tidal volume in both positions.

Group 1 subjects, whose tidal breathing was above the level of the CV in both postures, showed improved gas exchange in the supine position. This was explained by the presumed improvement in overall uniformity of $\dot{V}_A/\dot{Q}$ and by the observed increase in cardiac output. With a constant systemic oxygen consumption, an increase in cardiac output causes an increased mixed venous O_2 tension, which, when shunted through the pulmonary circulation, produces less lowering of PaO_2 than it does a lower mixed venous O_2 tension (low $\dot{Q}_t$). In group 2 subjects, FRC was greater than CV in the erect position and less than CV in the supine position. The $P(A-a)O_2$ and shunt increased on making this posture change. In group 3 subjects, CV occurred within the tidal breathing range in the erect position, and the erect $P(A-a)O_2$ and shunt were similar to those of group 2 subjects when supine, while change to supine position resulted in a further increase in $P(A-a)O_2$ and shunt fraction. In group 4 subjects, CV exceeded the whole of tidal respiration in the upright position. Changing to the supine position caused no significant change in $P(A-a)O_2$, but a significant increase in shunt occurred. Presumably, the factors tending to improve gas exchange in the supine position (increase in cardiac output and more uniform perfusion) counteracted any further airway closure.

Induction of General Anesthesia—Change in Thoracic Cage Muscle Tone

At the end of a normal (awake) expiration, there is slight tension in the inspiratory muscles and no tension in the expiratory muscles.

Thus, at the end of a normal expiration, there is a force tending to maintain lung volume and no force decreasing lung volume. Following the induction of general anesthesia, there is a loss of the end-expiratory tone in the inspiratory muscles and an appearance of end-expiratory tone in the abdominal expiratory muscles. The end-expiratory tone in the abdominal expiratory muscles increases intra-abdominal pressure, forces the diaphragm cephalad, and decreases FRC.[61,68] Thus, following the induction of general anesthesia, there is loss of a force tending to maintain lung volume and gain of a force tending to decrease lung volume. Indeed, Innovar may increase tone in expiratory muscles to such an extent that the reduction in FRC with Innovar anesthesia alone is greater than that with Innovar plus paralysis induced by succinylcholine.[69]

With emphysema, expiration may be accompanied by pursing the lips or grunting (partially closed larynx). The emphysematous patient exhales in either of these ways because both these maneuvers cause an expiratory retard (but not active exhalation), which produces PEEP in the intrathoracic air passage and decreases the possibility of airway closure and a decrease in FRC (Fig. 22-13F). Endotracheal intubation bypasses the lips and glottis and may abolish normally present pursed-lip or grunting exhalation and in that way contribute to airway closure and a loss in FRC in select patients.

Paralysis

In the upright subject, the FRC and the position of the diaphragm are determined by the balance between the lung elastic recoil pulling it cephalad and the weight of the abdominal contents pulling it caudad.[70] There is no transdiaphragmatic pressure gradient.

The situation is more complex in the supine position. The diaphragm separates two compartments of markedly different hydrostatic gradients. On the thoracic side, pressure increases approximately 0.25 cm H_2O/cm lung height[3,4,71] and on the abdominal side, 1.0 cm H_2O/cm.[70] This means that in horizontal postures, progressively higher transdiaphragmatic pressures must be generated towards dependent parts of the diaphragm to keep the abdominal contents out of the thorax. This tension could be developed by passive stretch and shape changes of the diaphragm, or by active tension. With acute muscle paralysis, a shift of the diaphragm to a more cephalad position occurs.[72] The latter position must express the true balance of elastic forces in the system, unmodified by any muscle activity.

The cephalad shift in the FRC position of the diaphragm due to expiratory muscle tone during general anesthesia is equal to the shift observed during paralysis (awake *or* anesthetized patients).[61,72] The equal shift suggests that the pressure on the diaphragm caused by an increase in expiratory muscle tone during general anesthesia is equal to the pressure on the diaphragm caused by the weight of the abdominal contents during paralysis. It is quite probable that the magnitude of these changes in FRC is dependent on the anesthetic drugs used, as well as body habitus.

Light or Inadequate Anesthesia and Active Expiration

The induction of general anesthesia can result in increased expiratory muscle tone,[68] but the expiratory muscle tone does not contribute to the exhaled volume of gas. Spontaneous ventilation during light general anesthesia usually results in moderately forceful active exhalation. Excessively inadequate anesthesia (relative to a given stimulus) results in very forceful active exhalation, which may produce exhaled volumes of gas equal to an awake expiratory vital capacity.

As during an awake expiratory vital capacity maneuver, a forced expiration during anesthesia raises the intrathoracic and alveolar pressures considerably above atmospheric pressure (Fig. 22-13). This results in a rapid outflow of gas and, since part of the expiratory resistance lies in the smaller air passages, a pressure drop will occur between the alveoli and the main bronchi. Under these circumstances, the intrathoracic pressure rises considerably above the pressure within the main bronchi. Collapse will occur if this reversed pressure gradient is sufficiently high to overcome the structural rigidity of these tubes. Such collapse occurs in the normal subject during a maximal forced expiration and it is responsible for the associated wheeze both in awake and anesthetized patients.[73] This effect is particularly prominent in bronchi with a posterior membranous sheath that appears to invaginate into the lumen.[74]

The limitation of air flow rate by bronchial collapse is much more marked in emphysematous and asthmatic patients (Fig. 22-13). The resistance in the small bronchi of these patients is higher and, therefore, the pressure drop from the alveoli to the larger bronchi is greater. During a forced expiration, the adverse pressure gradient across the walls of the bronchi will thus tend to be greater. To make matters worse, the bronchi of the emphysematous patient lack the tethering effect of lung parenchyma elastic recoil and are much less able to withstand collapse than those of the normal patient. These factors combine to render the emphysematous patient particularly liable to bronchial collapse during a forced expiration. In the asthmatic patient the increased airway resistance is due to bronchiolar spasm and mucosal edema.

In the paralyzed anesthetized patient, the use of a subatmospheric expiratory pressure phase is analogous to a forced expiration in the conscious subject, and a "negative phase" may set up the same adverse pressure gradients and thus cause airway closure, gas trapping, and a decrease in FRC. An excessively rapidly descending bellows of a ventilator during expiration has caused a subatmospheric expiratory pressure and has resulted in wheezing.[75]

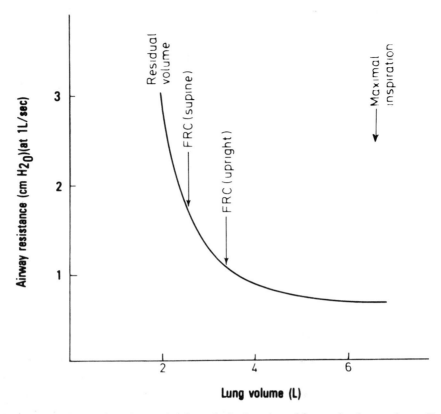

Fig. 22-27 Airway resistance is an increasing hyperbolic function of decreasing lung volume. Functional residual capacity (FRC) decreases in changing from the upright to supine position. (Reprinted (with modification) by permission of the publisher, from Nunn JF: Applied Respiratory Physiology. 2nd edition. London: Butterworths (Publishers) Ltd. 1977.)

Increased Airway Resistance

The overall reduction in all components of lung volume during anesthesia results in a reduced caliber of airway (Figs. 22-2 and 22-14), which increases airway resistance and any tendency towards airway collapse. The relationship between airway resistance and lung volume is well established (Fig. 22-27) and the observed reductions in FRC, firstly, on assuming the supine position (about 0.8 L) and secondly, following the induction of anesthesia (about 0.4 L), are often sufficient to explain the increased resistance seen in the healthy anesthetized patient.[76]

In addition to this expected increase in air-

way resistance in anesthetized patients, there are a number of additional special potential sites of increased airway resistance. These consist of the upper and lower airway passages and the external anesthesia apparatus. Pharyngeal obstruction, which can be considered to be a normal feature of unconsciousness, is most common. A minor degree of this type of obstruction occurs in snoring. Laryngospasm and obstructed endotracheal tubes (secretions, kinking, herniated cuffs) are not uncommon and may be life-threatening.

Respiratory apparatus often causes resistance that is considerably higher than the resistance in the normal human respiratory tract (Fig. 22-28).[77] When a number of resis-

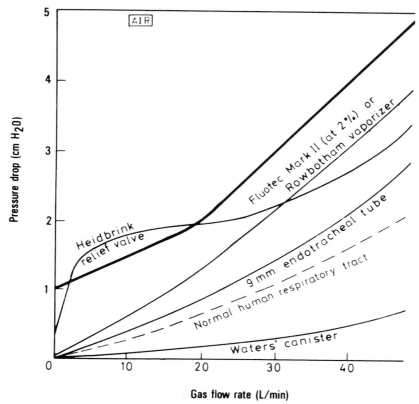

Fig. 22-28 The pressure drop across various pieces of anesthetic apparatus (solid lines) compared with the normal human respiratory tract (dashed line). If flow rate is constant then a pressure drop equals airway resistance. The heavy line is a suggested upper limit of acceptable resistance for an adult patient. (Reprinted (with modification) by permission of the publisher, from Nunn JF: Applied Respiratory Physiology. 2nd edition. London: Butterworths (Publishers) Ltd. 1977.)

tors such as those shown in Figure 22-28 are joined in a series to form an anesthetic gas circuit, they generally summate to produce a larger resistance (as with resistances in an electrical circuit). As a general guide, the heavy line in Figure 22-28 indicates a level of resistance (which is equal to the pressure drop—the ordinate—for any given flow rate) that may be considered excessive.

It is unusual to measure airway resistance in clinical practice, and the degree of resistance is commonly assessed in terms of the response of the patient. However, the ventilatory response of a patient is dependent on the duration of the obstruction for two reasons. First, patients may fatigue in time. Sec-

ond, increases in inspiratory resistance (e.g., kinked endotracheal tube) may cause the patient to generate extremely negative pleural pressure, which in turn will cause the pulmonary perivascular hydrostatic pressures to become extremely negative, and the latter has caused pulmonary edema.[78] Thus, a fixed degree of obstruction may appear to progress from causing a slight to moderate to severe airway resistance.

A moderate resistance is present when a considerable respiratory effort is required to avert a deterioration in blood gas levels. In some patients, with substantial airway resistance, an increased effort is well sustained and $PaCO_2$ does not rise appreciably. Some of these patients, who have chronic obstructive airway disease, have been referred to as "pink puffers," in contrast to patients who have chronic bronchitis who allow their ventilation to decrease in the face of a similar degree of resistance and have been referred to as "blue bloaters." In both of these types of patients, the corresponding decrease in PaO_2 is often additionally influenced by abnormalities of distribution as well as by hypoventilation. Inability to increase respiratory effort during anesthesia is conspicuous in these patients and is considered under hypoventilation.

The Supine Position, Immobility and Excessive Intravenous Fluid Administration

Patients undergoing anesthesia and surgery are often kept supine and immobile for long periods of time. Thus, a great deal of the lung may be continually dependent and below the left atrium, and therefore be in zone 3. Being in a dependent position, the lung is predisposed to fluid accumulation. Coupled with excessive fluid administration, conditions sufficient to promote transudation of fluid into the lung are present and will result in pulmonary edema and a decreased FRC. Figure 22-29 shows that when mongrel dogs are placed in a lateral decubitus position and are anesthetized for several hours (bottom horizontal axis), an extracellular fluid space expansion (top horizontal axis) will cause the PO_2 (left hand axis) of blood draining the down (dependent) lung (closed circles) to decrease precipitously to mixed venous levels (no O_2 uptake).[79] Blood draining the up (nondependent) lung maintained its PO_2 for a period of time but in the face of the extracellular fluid expansion also suffered a decline in its PO_2 after 5 hours. Transpulmonary shunt (right-hand axis) progressively increased. Thus during clinical anesthesia, excessive fluid administration may cause the dependent lung to become somewhat edema-

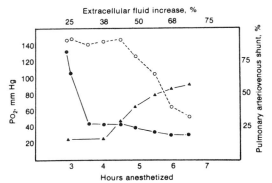

Fig. 22-29 Mongrel dogs anesthetized with pentobarbital (bottom axis), placed in a lateral decubitus position, and subjected to progressive extracellular fluid expansion (top axis) have a marked decrease in the PO_2 (left vertical axis) of blood draining the dependent lung (solid circles) and a smaller, much slower decrease in PO_2 of blood draining the nondependent lung (open circles). The pulmonary arteriovenous shunt (right vertical axis) rises progressively (triangles). (Modified from Ray JF, Yost L, Moallem S et al: Immobility, hypoxemia, and pulmonary arteriovenous shunting. Arch Surg 109:537, 1974. Copyright 1974, American Medical Association.)

tous. Again, pulmonary edema can cause FRC to decrease and CC to increase.

High Inspired Oxygen Concentration and Absorption Atelectasis

General anesthesia is very frequently administered with an increased inspired concentration of O_2 (FIO_2). When patients, with a significant amount of blood flow perfusing lung units with low $\dot{V}A/\dot{Q}$ ratios (large left-sided tail to blood flow distribution curve in Fig. 22-3), breathe 100 percent oxygen, these low $\dot{V}A/\dot{Q}$ units are virtually abolished and a moderately large right-to-left shunt results. [7, 8, 80] Thus, in these studies the effect of breathing O_2 was to convert units that had low $\dot{V}A/\dot{Q}$ ratios into shunt units. The increase in shunting was equal to the amount of blood flow previously perfusing low $\dot{V}A/\dot{Q}$ ratio areas during the breathing of air. Even an FIO_2 as low as 50 percent probably can produce large shunts provided low enough $\dot{V}A/\dot{Q}$ ratios exist in the lung.[80, 81]

The cause of the shunting during O_2 breathing is presumably the increase in O_2 uptake by lung units with low $\dot{V}A/\dot{Q}$ ratios.[80, 81] A unit that has a low $\dot{V}A/\dot{Q}$ ratio during breathing of air will have a low alveolar PO_2. When an enriched O_2 mixture is inspired, alveolar PO_2 will rise and, therefore, the rate at which O_2 moves from the alveolar gas to the capillary blood will greatly increase. Under some circumstances this O_2 flux may increase so much that the net flow of gas into the blood exceeds the inspired amount of gas, and under some conditions, the unit can then close. Collapse is most likely to occur if the FIO_2 is high and the content of O_2 in the mixed venous blood is low. This phenomenon is of considerable significance in the clinical situation for two reasons. First, enriched O_2 mixtures are often used therapeutically, and it is important to know whether this therapy is causing atelectasis. Second, the amount of shunt is often estimated during breathing of 100 percent O_2, and if this maneuver results in additional shunt, the measurement will clearly be in error.

Surgical Position (see Ch. 4)

The Supine Position. The diaphragm lies lower in the erect position than in the supine position, and thus in the latter the abdominal contents force the diaphragm cephalad and reduce FRC.[61, 67, 68, 72]

The Trendelenburg Position. Not surprisingly, a moderate decrease in FRC occurs in the Trendelenburg position. A steep Trendelenburg position allows the abdominal contents to push the diaphragm further cephalad so that the diaphragm then not only must ventilate the lungs but also must lift the abdominal contents out of the thorax. The result is a predisposition to decreased FRC and atelectasis.[82] Increased pulmonary blood volume and gravitational force on the mediastinal structures are additional factors that may decrease pulmonary compliance and FRC. Finally, in the steep Trendelenburg position, most of the lung may be below the left atrium and therefore in a zone 3 condition. As such, the lung may be prone to develop pulmonary interstitial edema. Thus, patients with elevated pulmonary artery pressure, such as those with mitral stenosis, do not tolerate the Trendelenburg position well.[83]

The Lateral Decubitus Position. In this position, after the induction of general anesthesia, the dependent lung experiences a moderate decrease in FRC and is predisposed to atelectasis.

The Kidney, Lithotomy, and Prone Positions. In anesthetized patients, these positions have either caused small clinically insignificant changes in lung volume or studies have not been reported.

Ventilatory History (Rapid Shallow Breathing)

Rapid shallow breathing is often a regular feature of anesthesia. Regular shallow breathing may promote atelectasis, which in turn may cause a decrease in FRC and compliance.[84, 85] Initially, these changes may cause hypoxemia (decreased FRC) with normocarbia and may be reversed by periodic large inspirations.

Decreased Removal of Secretions (Decreased Mucociliary Flow)

Tracheobronchial mucous glands and goblet cells produce mucus, which is swept by cilia up to the larynx where it is swallowed or expectorated. This process clears inhaled organisms and particles from the lungs. The secreted mucus consists of a surface gel layer, which lies on top of a more liquid sol layer in which the cilia beat. The tips of the cilia propel the gel layer towards the larynx (upward) during the forward stroke. As the mucus streams upward and the total cross-sectional area of the airways diminishes, absorption takes place from the sol layer so as to maintain a constant depth of 5 mm.[86]

Poor systemic hydration and low inspired humidity reduce mucociliary flow by increasing the viscosity of secretions and by slowing the ciliary beat.[87–89] Mucociliary flow varies directly with body or mucosal temperature (low inspired temperature) over a range of 32° to 42°C.[90,91] A high FIO_2 decreases mucociliary flow.[92] Inflation of an endotracheal tube cuff suppresses tracheal mucous velocity.[93] The depression in tracheal mucous velocity occurs within 1 hour, and apparently it does not matter whether a low- or high-compliance cuff is used. Passage of an uncuffed tube through the vocal cords and kept in situ for several hours does not affect tracheal mucous velocity.

The mechanism for endotracheal tube cuff suppression of mucociliary clearance is speculative. Measurements of mucous velocity were made in the distal trachea, whereas the cuff was inflated in the proximal portion. Thus, the phenomenon cannot be attributed solely to damming of mucus at the cuff site. One possibility is that the endotracheal tube cuff caused a critical increase in the thickness of the layer of mucus proceeding distally from the cuff. Another possibility is that mechanical distention of the trachea by the endotracheal tube cuff initiated a neurogenic reflex arc that altered mucous secretions or frequency of ciliary beating.

Other investigators have recently shown that when all of the above-mentioned factors are controlled, halothane reversibly and progressively decreases, but does not stop, mucous flow over an inspired concentration of 1 to 3 MAC.[94] The halothane-induced depression of mucociliary clearance was likely due to depression of the ciliary beat, an effect which caused slow clearance of mucus from the distal and peripheral airways. In support of this hypothesis is the fact that cilia are morphologically the same throughout the an-

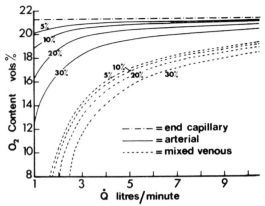

Fig. 22-30 Effects of changes in cardiac output ($\dot{Q}$) on the O_2 content of end-pulmonary capillary, arterial, and mixed venous blood for a family of different transpulmonary right-to-left shunts. Note that a decrease in $\dot{Q}$ results in a greater decrease in the arterial content of O_2, the larger the shunt. (Modified from Kelman GF, Nunn JF, Prys-Roberts C, et al: The influence of the cardiac output on arterial oxygenation: A theoretical study. Br J Anaesth 39:450, 1967.)

imal kingdom and in clinical dosages, inhaled anesthetics, including halothane, have been found to cause reversible depression of the ciliary beat of protozoa.[95]

DECREASED CARDIAC OUTPUT

A decrease in cardiac output ($\dot{Q}_t$), assuming a constant O_2 consumption ($\dot{V}O_2$), must result in lower mixed venous O_2 content ($C\bar{v}O_2$). The lowered $C\bar{v}O_2$ will then flow through whatever shunt pathways exist, mix with the oxygenated end-pulmonary capillary blood, and lower the O_2 content of the arterial blood (CaO_2) (Fig. 22-22). Figure 22-30 shows these relationships quantitatively for several different intrapulmonary shunts.[30,54] The larger the intrapulmonary shunt, the greater is the decrease in CaO_2 because more venous blood with lower $C\bar{v}O_2$ can admix with end-pulmonary capillary blood. Increased O_2 extraction ($\dot{V}O_2$) may also decrease $C\bar{v}O_2$ and may occur with excessive sympathetic nervous system stimulation, hyperthermia, or shivering and can further contribute to impaired oxygenation of arterial blood.[97]

INHIBITION OF HYPOXIC PULMONARY VASOCONSTRICTION (HPV)

Decreased regional alveolar PO_2 causes regional pulmonary vasoconstriction, which diverts blood flow and so minimizes venous admixture from underventilated or nonventilated lung units. Inhibition of regional HPV might impair arterial oxygenation by permitting increased venous admixture from hypoxic or atelectatic areas of the lung. Since the pulmonary circulation is poorly endowed with smooth muscle, any condition that increases the pressure against which the vessels must constrict (i.e., the Ppa) will decrease HPV. There are numerous clinical conditions that can increase Ppa and therefore decrease HPV. Mitral stenosis,[97] volume overload,[97] low (but above room air) F_{IO_2} in nondiseased lung,[99] progressively increasing the amount of lung that is diseased,[98] thromboembolism,[98] hypothermia,[99] and vasoactive drugs[100] can all increase Ppa. Direct vasodilating drugs such as aminophylline, isoproterenol, nitroglycerin, and nitroprusside,[11, 101] inhaled anesthetics[102, 103] and hypocapnia[57] can directly decrease HPV.

PARALYSIS

In the supine position, the weight of the abdominal contents against the diaphragm is greatest in the dependent or posterior part of the diaphragm and least in the nondependent or anterior part of the diaphragm. In the awake patient breathing spontaneously, the active tension in the diaphragm is able to overcome the weight of the abdominal contents and the diaphragm moves the most in the posterior portion and least in the anterior portion. This is a healthy circumstance because the greatest amount of ventilation is occurring where there is the most perfusion (posteriorly or dependent) and the least amount of ventilation is occurring where there is the least perfusion (anteriorly or nondependent). During paralysis and positive pressure breathing, the passive diaphragm is displaced preferentially in the anterior nondependent portion and is displaced minimally in the posterior dependent portion. This is an unhealthy circumstance because the greatest amount of ventilation is occurring where there is the least perfusion and the least amount of ventilation is occurring where there is the most perfusion.[72]

THE INVOLVEMENT OF MECHANISMS OF HYPOXEMIA IN SPECIFIC DISEASES

Pulmonary embolism (air, fat, thrombi) and the evolution of the adult respiratory distress syndrome are two examples of diseases that involve many of the mechanisms of hypoxemia listed above. A significant pulmonary embolus can cause severe increases in pulmonary artery pressure and these increases can cause right-to-left transpulmonary shunting through opened a-v anastomoses and the foramen ovale (possible in 20 percent of patients); pulmonary edema in nonembolized regions of the lung; and inhibition of HPV. The embolus may cause hypoventilation via increased dead space ventilation. If the embolus contains platelets, serotonin may be released and this release can cause hypoventilation via bronchoconstriction and pulmonary edema via increased pulmonary capillary permeability. Finally, the pulmonary embolus can increase pulmonary vascular resistance and decrease the cardiac output.

Following major hypotension, shock, or blood loss, respiratory failure often ensues and this syndrome has been called the adult respiratory distress syndrome (ARDS) (see Ch. 38, 42, and 43). This syndrome can evolve during and after anesthesia and has many etiologies. Following shock and trauma, increased plasma levels of serotonin, histamine, plasmakinins, lysozymes, and fatty acids occur. If pulmonary contusion occurs, these factors may individually or collectively increase pulmonary capillary permeability. Following shock, it has been shown that acidosis, increased circulating catecholamines and sympathetic nervous system activity, prostaglandin release, histamine release, microembolism (with serotonin release), increased intracranial pressure (with head injury), and alveolar hypoxia may occur and may individually or collectively, particularly postresuscitation, cause a moderate increase in pulmonary artery pressure. Following shock, the normal compensatory response is a protein-free interstitial fluid movement into the vascular space in order to restore vascular volume. The dilution of vascular proteins by protein-free interstitial fluid can cause a decreased capillary colloid osmotic pressure (see Ch. 38). Increased pulmonary capillary permeability and pulmonary artery pressure and decreased capillary colloid osmotic pressure will cause fluid transudation and pulmonary edema. Additionally a decreased cardiac output, inhibition of HPV, immobility, supine position, excessive fluid administration, and an excessively high F_IO_2 can contribute to the development of ARDS.

MECHANISMS OF HYPERCAPNIA AND HYPOCAPNIA DURING ANESTHESIA

HYPERCAPNIA

The following factors can all cause hypercapnia.

Hypoventilation

The causes of hypoventilation during anesthesia are numerous and include position, airway resistance, compliance changes, and the effects of drugs (e.g., opiates, volatile anesthetics, and neuromuscular blockers). Other factors such as direct trauma, various neural and motor endplate diseases, and biochemical changes on the component parts of the respiratory apparatus (the medullary respiratory center, upper and lower motorneurons, neuromuscular junction, respiratory muscles, airways, lung parenchyma, and chest wall) may contribute to hypoventilation. A specific listing of these possibilities is beyond the scope of this discussion.

Increased Dead Space Ventilation

A *decrease* in pulmonary artery pressure, as during deliberate hypotension,[104] may cause an increase in zone 1 and alveolar dead space ventilation.

An *increase* in *airway pressure* (as with PEEP) may cause an increase in zone 1 and alveolar dead space ventilation.

Pulmonary embolus, thrombosis and *vascular obliteration* (kinking, clamping, blocking of pulmonary artery during surgery) may increase the amount of lung that is ventilated but unperfused.

Rapid short inspirations may be distributed preferentially to noncompliant (short time constant for inflation) and badly perfused alveoli, while a slow inspiration allows time for distribution to more compliant (long time constant for inflation) and better perfused alveoli. Thus, rapid short inspirations may have a dead space ventilation effect.

Total dead space ventilation increases with *age* (V_D/V_T 33+age/3).

The *anesthesia apparatus* increases total dead space (V_D/V_T) (see Ch. 5). Inclusion of normal apparatus dead space increases the total V_D/V_T ratio to about 46 percent in intubated patients and to about 64 percent in patients breathing from a mask.[105] These values relate to the total dead space, which equals the combination of alveolar, anatomic, and apparatus dead space plus a rebreathing effect (see immediately below).

Anesthesia circuits cause *rebreathing* and the classification by Mapleson is widely accepted[106] (see Ch. 5). The order of increasing rebreathing (decreasing merit) with spontaneous ventilation with Mapleson circuits is A (Magill), D, C, and B. The order of increasing rebreathing (decreasing merit) with controlled ventilation is D, B, C, and A. System E (Ayre T-piece) will have no rebreathing if the fresh gas flow is greater than the peak inspiratory flow rate.

The effects of an increase in dead space can usually be counteracted by a corresponding increase in the respiratory minute volume. If, for example, the minute volume is 10 L/min and the V_D/V_T ratio 30 percent, the alveolar ventilation will be 7 L/min. If a pulmonary embolism occurred resulting in an increase of the V_D/V_T ratio to 50 percent, the minute volume would need to be increased to 14 L/min to maintain an alveolar ventilation of 7 L/min (14 L/min × 0.5).

Increased Carbon Dioxide Production

All of the causes of increased O_2 consumption will also increase CO_2 production—shivering, catecholamine release (light anesthesia), hypertension, thyroid storm. If minute ventilation, total dead space, and ventilation/perfusion relationships are constant, an increase in CO_2 production will result in hypercapnia.

Inadvertent Switching Off of a Carbon Dioxide Absorber

Many factors, such as patient ventilatory responsiveness to CO_2 accumulation, fresh gas flow, circle system design, and CO_2 production, determine whether hypercapnia will result from inadvertent switching off or using up of a circle CO_2 absorber. However, high fresh gas flows (> 5 L/min) minimize the

problem with almost all systems for almost all patients.

HYPOCAPNIA

The mechanisms of hypocapnia are the reverse of those that produce hypercapnia. Thus, with all other factors being equal, hyperventilation (spontaneous or controlled ventilation), decreased dead space ventilation (i.e., change from mask airway to endotracheal tube airway or increased pulmonary artery pressure), and decreased CO_2 production (hypothermia, deep anesthesia, hypotension) will lead to hypocapnia. By far the most common mechanism is passive hyperventilation by mechanical means.

PHYSIOLOGICAL EFFECTS OF ABNORMALITIES IN THE RESPIRATORY GASES

HYPOXIA

The essential feature of hypoxia is the cessation of oxidative phosphorylation when mitochondrial PO_2 falls below a critical level. Anaerobic pathways, which produce energy (ATP) inefficiently, are then utilized. The end-products of aerobic metabolism are carbon dioxide and water, both of which are easily diffusible and lost from the body. The main anaerobic metabolites are hydrogen and lactate ions, which escape into the circulation where they may be conveniently quantified in terms of the base deficit and the lactate/pyruvate ratio.

The degree of hypoxia will vary from one organ to another so that clinical diagnosis of hypoxia is usually related to the organ considered most vulnerable. This is usually the brain, but in special circumstances may be the heart (myocardial infarction), kidney (acute tubular necrosis), liver (hepatitis), or limb (claudication, gangrene).

Hypoxia presents a serious threat to the

body and vigorous compensatory mechanisms are activated. These mechanisms are usually robust and not easily impaired by drugs or disease. Where they conflict with other mechanisms acting in the opposite direction, the compensation for hypoxia is usually dominant. Thus, for example, hypoxia with concomitant hypocapnic hyperventilation results in an increase of cerebral blood flow in spite of the lowered PCO_2. Hyperventilation will be stimulated whatever the reason for the hypoxia ($PaO_2 < 50$ torr), although the effectiveness will depend to a large extent upon its actual cause. For example, hyperventilation will be largely ineffective in stagnant hypoxia because hyperventilation (while breathing air) can do little to increase the O_2 content of the arterial blood and usually nothing to increase perfusion. The interrelationship between hypoxia and other factors in the control of breathing is discussed in Chapter 2.

Cardiac output is increased by hypoxia together with the regional blood flow to almost every major organ, particularly the brain.[107] The immediate cardiac output response to hypoxia is reflex and is initiated by carotid body chemoreceptors; it occurs before there has been any measurable rise in circulating catecholamines. In addition, cerebral and probably the myocardial vascular resistance decreases and is also not dependent upon the autonomic innervation or upon circulating catecholamines. The effect appears to be due to a local response within the vessels themselves. Nevertheless, catecholamine levels are raised in due course.

Pulmonary distribution of blood flow is improved by hypoxia as a result of the increase in pulmonary artery pressure. Hemoglobin concentration is elevated by chronic (not acute) hypoxia such as that present with residence at altitude, chronic respiratory disease, etc. Chronic hypoxia may also cause the oxy-Hb dissociation curve to be displaced to the right by an increase in 2,3-diphosphoglycerate or as a result of acidosis. This tends to raise tissue PO_2.

Hyperoxia (Oxygen Toxicity)

The dangers associated with the inhalation of excessive O_2 are multiple. Exposure to a high O_2 tension clearly causes *pulmonary damage* in healthy individuals.[109] Since the lungs of normal human volunteers cannot be examined to determine the rate of onset and course of toxicity, indirect measures have been employed. Many have used the onset of symptom formation to describe tolerance curves.[109] The rate of the onset of the disease process is proportional both to the tension of O_2 and to the duration of exposure. The dominant symptom is substernal distress, which begins as a mild irritation in the area of the carina and may be accompanied by occasional coughing. As exposure continues, pain becomes more intense and the urge to cough and deep breathe also becomes intense. This progresses to severe dyspnea and paroxysmal coughing. The most sensitive pulmonary function test of lung damage under these circumstances has been a progressive decrease in vital capacity. As toxicity progresses, other pulmonary function studies such as compliance and blood gases deteriorate. Pathologically, the lesion progresses from a tracheobronchitis, to pulmonary interstitial edema, to pulmonary fibrosis.[110]

A dose-toxicity curve for humans is available from a number of studies.[108] Examination of the curve indicates that no measurable changes in pulmonary function or blood-gas exchange occur in man during exposures to less than 0.5 atm even for long periods. Despite wide variations in human susceptibility there is apparently no identifiable risk associated with the administration of pure O_2 at 1 atm for 12 hours.

Ventilatory depression may occur in those patients who, by reason of drugs or disease, have been ventilating in response to a hypoxic drive. By definition, ventilatory depression resulting from removal of a hypoxic drive by increasing the inspired O_2 concentration will cause a relative hypercapnia but does not produce hypoxia.

Absorption atelectasis has been previously discussed. *Retrolental fibroplasia* (see Chs. 35 and 36), an abnormal proliferation of the immature retinal vasculature of the prematurely born infant, can occur following exposure to hyperoxia. Very premature infants are most susceptible to retrolental fibroplasia (i.e., those of less than 1.0 kg birth weight and 28 weeks gestation). The risk of retrolental fibroplasia exists whenever an FiO_2 causes $PaO_2 > 80$ torr for more than 3 hours in an infant whose gestational age plus life age combined is less than 44 weeks. If the ductus arteriosus is patent, arterial blood samples must be drawn from the right radial artery.

The mode of action of toxicity of O_2 in tissues is complex but interference with metabolism seems to be widespread. Most importantly, there is inactivation of many enzymes, particularly those with sulphydryl groups. The most toxic enzyme effect of O_2 in man is a *convulsive effect* that occurs during exposure to pressures in excess of 2 atmospheres absolute.

High inspired O_2 concentrations can be of use therapeutically. Clearance of gas loculi in the body may be greatly accelerated by inhalation of 100 percent O_2. The principle of this form of therapy (denitrogenation) depends upon elimination of N_2 from the venous blood. This causes an N_2 gradient to exist from the gas space to the perfusing blood. As a result, N_2 leaves the gas space and the space diminishes in size. The use of O_2 to remove gas may be used to ease intestinal gas pressure in patients with intestinal obstruction, to hasten recovery from pneumoencephalography, to decrease the size of an air embolus, and to aid absorption of pneumoperitoneum and pneumothorax.

HYPERCAPNIA

Survival in severe hypercapnia is, to a large extent, dependent on the autonomic response because a great many of the effects of carbon dioxide on various organ systems are either due to or influenced by the autonomic response to carbon dioxide. An elevation of PCO_2 causes an increase in plasma levels of both epinephrine and norepinephrine. Plasma catecholamine levels of patients under halothane anesthesia increase in much the same way in response to increased CO_2 levels as in conscious subjects.

The maximal stimulant effect is attained by $PaCO_2$ of about 100 torr. With a higher $PaCO_2$, stimulation is reduced, and at very high levels respiration is depressed and later ceases altogether. The PCO_2/ventilation response curve is generally displaced to the right and its slope reduced by anesthetics and other depressant drugs[111] (see Chs. 13 and 15). With profound anesthesia the response curve may be flat, or even sloping downwards, and carbon dioxide then acts as a respiratory depressant. Quite apart from the effect of carbon dioxide upon ventilation, it exerts two other important effects that influence the *oxygenation of the blood*. Firstly, if the concentration of nitrogen (or other "inert" gas) remains constant, the concentration of CO_2 in the alveolar gas can only increase at the expense of O_2, which must be displaced. Secondly, hypercapnia shifts the oxy-Hb to the right.

The effects of carbon dioxide upon the *circulation* are complicated due to opposing actions on different components of the system. The depressant direct action of CO_2 on myocardial contractility and heart rate is usually overshadowed by the stimulant effect mediated through the sympathetic system. At very high levels of $PaCO_2$, cardiac output generally decreases.

Blood pressure is generally increased as $PaCO_2$ increases in both conscious and anesthetized patients. However, the response is variable and certainly cannot be relied upon as an infallible diagnostic sign of hypercapnia. At very high levels of $PaCO_2$, the blood pressure declines. Hypercapnia causes a rise in pulmonary arterial pressure and pulmonary vascular resistance and locally augments

HPV. Arrhythmias have been reported in unanesthetized humans during acute hypercapnia but have seldom been of serious import. A high $PaCO_2$ level is, however, more dangerous during general anesthesia. With halothane anesthesia, arrhythmias will frequently occur above a $PaCO_2$ arrhythmic threshold which is often constant for a particular patient.

In patients with ventilatory failure, carbon dioxide narcosis occurs when the $PaCO_2$ rises above 90 to 120 torr. Thirty percent carbon dioxide is sufficient for the production of anesthesia, and this concentration causes total but reversible flattening of the electroencephalogram.[112] However, at this level of CO_2 concentration, grand mal convulsions are frequent. Cerebral blood flow and intracranial pressure changes due to hypercapnia are discussed in Chapter 25.

Chronic hypercapnia results in increased resorption of bicarbonate by the kidneys, further raising the plasma bicarbonate level and constituting a secondary or compensatory "metabolic alkalosis." Chronic hypocapnia decreases renal bicarbonate resorption, resulting in further fall of plasma bicarbonate and producing a secondary or compensatory "metabolic acidosis." In each case arterial pH returns towards the normal value, but the bicarbonate ion concentration departs even further from normal.

Hypercapnia is accompanied by a leakage of potassium from the cells into the plasma. A good deal of the potassium comes from the liver, probably from glucose, the latter of which is mobilized in response to the rise in plasma catecholamine levels.[113] Since the plasma potassium level takes an appreciable time to return to normal, repeated bouts of hypercapnia at short intervals result in a stepwise rise in plasma potassium.

The influence of hypercapnia on pressure-flow relationships in the splanchnic and hepatic circulation varies considerably according to the anesthetic agent used. During thiopentone and nitrous oxide anesthesia, in which the sympathetic adrenergic mecha-

nisms are not unduly suppressed, hypercapnia is associated with splanchnic vasoconstriction and reduced hepatic blood flow, whereas during halothane anesthesia the balance is such that the direct vasodilator effect of carbon dioxide promotes splanchnic vasodilation and a marked increase in hepatic blood flow.[114] At high levels of PCO_2, there is constriction of the glomerular afferent arterioles, leading to oliguria.

The two major vascular circuits in the limbs are those to skin and skeletal muscle; in both circuits the response to hypercapnia is a balance between the direct vasodilator effects of CO_2 and the vasoconstrictor effects secondary to sympathetic adrenergic activity. During anesthesia, the response is predominantly vasodilative in the skin circuit and vasoconstrictive in the muscle.

Changes in PCO_2 may affect drug action as a result of a number of different mechanisms. First, the distribution of the drug may be influenced by changes in perfusion of organs. Second, the ionization of drugs may be altered by the change in blood pH. Third, the solubility of the drug in the body fluids and the degree of protein binding may be influenced.

There are no infallible diagnostic signs of hypercapnia. The skin is usually flushed and the pulse is generally full and bounding, with occasional extrasystoles and possibly other cardiac arrhythmias. Hypertension usually results but not always. However, hypercapnia should always be considered when there is an unexplained hypertension during anesthesia. Hyperventilation will obviously be absent if hypercapnia is caused by hypoventilation. Muscle twitchings and a characteristic flap of the hands may be seen when the $PaCO_2$ approaches the level at which coma occurs. Convulsions may occur at still higher levels. It must be stressed that coma and depressed breathing may be the only signs of a severe hypercapnia and the diagnosis may not be obvious. Analysis of arterial blood gases is required to make the diagnosis of hypercapnia with certainty.

HYPOCAPNIA

In this section, hypocapnia is considered to be produced by passive hyperventilation (by the anesthesiologist or ventilator).

Hypocapnia may cause a decrease in the cardiac output by three separate mechanisms. First, if present, an increase in intrathoracic pressure will decrease the cardiac output. Second, hypocapnia is associated with a withdrawal of sympathetic nervous system activity and this can decrease the ionotropic state of the heart. Third, hypocapnia can increase pH, which can in turn decrease ionized Ca^{++}, which may in turn decrease the ionotrophic state of the heart. Hypocapnia will also shift the oxy-Hb to the left, which results in an increased Hb affinity for O_2 at the tissue level. Thus, cardiac output or tissue perfusion has to increase at a time it may not be possible to do so. Since hypocapnia may cause a selective reduction in the cerebral blood flow and also left shifts of the oxy-Hb curve, this has led to the view that the cerebral effects of hypocapnia may be related to a state of cerebral hypoxia. Finally, hypocapnia at a $PaCO_2$ of 20 torr will increase O_2 consumption by 100 percent. Thus, hypocapnia may simultaneously increase tissue O_2 demand and decrease tissue O_2 supply.

Hypocapnia may cause $\dot{V}A/\dot{Q}$ abnormalities by inhibiting HPV or by causing bronchoconstriction and a decreased lung compliance. Finally, passive hypocapnia will produce apnea.

ACKNOWLEDGMENT

The author gratefully acknowledges the typing and editorial assistance of Donna J. Barnum.

REFERENCES

1. West JB, Dollery CT, Naimark A: Distribution of blood flow in isolated lung: Relation to vascular and alveolar pressures. J Appl Physiol 19:713, 1964

2. Permutt S, Bromberger-Barnea B, Bane HN: Alveolar pressure, pulmonary venous pressure and the vascular waterfall. Med Thorac 19:239, 1962

3. Hoppin FG Jr, Green ID, Mead J: Distribution of pleural surface pressure. J Apl Physiol 27:863, 1969

4. Milic-Emili J, Henderson JAM, Dolovich MB, et al: Regional distribution of inspired gas in the lung. J Appl Physiol 21:749, 1966

5. West JB: Ventilation/Blood Flow and Gas Exchange. 2nd edition. Oxford, Blackwell Scientific Publications, 1970

6. West JB: Regional differences in gas exchange in the lung of erect man. J Appl Physiol 17:893, 1962

7. Wagner PD, Saltzman HA, West JB: Measurement of continuous distributions of ventilation-perfusion ratios: Theory. J Appl Physiol 36:588:599, 1974

8. West JB: Blood flow to the lung and gas exchange. Anesthesiology 41:124, 1974

9. Fishman AP: Dynamics of the pulmonary circulation, Handbook of Physiology, Section 2: Circulation. Vol 2. Edited by Hamilton WF. Baltimore, Williams & Wilkins, 1963, pp 1667–1743

10. Benumof JL, Mathers JM, Wahrenbrock EA: The pulmonary interstitial compartment and the mediator of hypoxic pulmonary vasoconstriction. Microvasc Res 15:69, 1978

11. Benumof JL: Hypoxic pulmonary vasoconstriction and sodium nitroprusside perfusion. Anesthesiology 50:481, 1979

12. Simmons DH, Linde CM, Miller JH, et al: Relation of lung volume and pulmonary vascular resistance. Circ Res 9:465, 1961

13. Burton AC, Patel DJ: Effect on pulmonary vascular resistance of inflation of the rabbit lungs. J Appl Physiol 12:239, 1958

14. Wittenberger JL, McGregor M, Berglund E, et al: Influence of state of inflation of the lung on pulmonary vascular resistance. J Appl Physiol 15:878, 1960

15. Benumof JL, Rogers SN, Moyce PR, et al: Hypoxic pulmonary vasoconstriction and regional and whole lung PEEP in the dog. Anesthesiology 52:503, 1979

16. Benumof JL: Mechanism of decreased blood flow to atelectatic lung. J Appl Physiol 46:1047, 1978

17. Marshall R: The physical properties of the lungs in relation to the subdivisions of lung volume. Clin Sci 16:507, 1957

18. Sykes MK: The mechanics of ventilation, Scientific Foundations of Anesthesia. Edited by Scurr C, Feldman S. Philadelphia, FA Davis, 1970, pp 174–186

19. Nunn JF: Mechanisms of pulmonary ventilation, Applied Respiratory Physiology. 2nd edition. London, Butterworths, 1977, pp 139–177

20. Peters RM: Work of breathing following trauma. J Trauma 8:915, 1968

21. Nunn JF: The minute volume of pulmonary ventilation, Applied Respiratory Physiology. 2nd edition. London, Butterworths, 1977, pp 178–212

22. Shapiro BA, Harrison RA, Trout CA: The mechanics of ventilation, Clinical Application of Respiratory Care. 2nd edition Chicago, Year Book Medical Publishers, 1979, pp 57–89

23. Comroe JH, Forster RE, Dubois AB, et al: The Lung. 2nd edition. Chicago, Year Book Medical Publishers, 1962

24. Nunn JF: Resistance to gas flow, Aplied Respiratory Physiology. 2nd edition. London, Butterworths, 1977, pp 94–138

25. Rehder K, Marsh HM, Rodarte JR, et al: Airway Closure. Anesthesiology 47:40, 1977

26. Leblanc P, Ruff F, Milic-Emili J: Effects of age and body position on "airway closure" in man. J Appl Physiol 28:448, 1970

27. Craig DB, Wahba WM, Don HF, et al: "Closing volume" and its relationship to gas exchange in seated and supine positions. J Appl Physiol 31:717, 1971

28. Burger EJ Jr, Macklem P: Airway closure: Demonstration by breathing 100% O_2 at low lung volumes and by N_2 washout. J Appl Physiol 25:139, 1968

29. Nunn JF: Oxygen, Applied Respiratory Physiology. 2nd edition. London, Butterworths, 1977, pp 375–444

30. Kelman GF, Nunn JF, Prys-Roberts C, et al: The influence of the cardiac output on arterial oxygenation: A theoretical study. Br J Anaesth 39:450, 1967

31. Berggren SM: The oxygen deficit of arterial blood caused by non-ventilating parts of the lung. Acta Physiol Scand 4 (supp 11):1, 1942

32. Fishman AP: Pulmonary edema: The water exchanging function of the lung. Circulation 46:390, 1972

33. Low FN: Lung interstitium, development, morphology, fluid content, Lung Water and Solute Exchange. Edited by Staub NC. New York, Dekker, 1978, pp 17–48

34. Weibel ER: Morphological basis of alveolar-capillary gas exchange. Physiol Rev 53:419, 1973

35. Hales CA, Kazemi H: Small airways function in myocardial infarction. N Engl J Med 290:761, 1974

36. Harken AH, O'Conner NE: The influence of clinically undetectable edema on small airway closure in the dog. Ann Surg 184:183, 1976

37. Biddle TL, Yu PN, Hodges M, et al: Hypoxemia and lung water in acute myocardial infarction. Am Heart J 92:692, 1976

38. Guyton AC: A concept of negative interstitial pressure based on pressures in implanted perforated capsules. Circ Res 12:399, 1963

39. Smith-Erichsen N, Bo G: Airway closure and fluid filtration in the lung. Br J Anaesth 51:475, 1979

40. Ebert RV, Terracio MJ: The bronchiolar epithelium in cigarette smokers. Observations with the scanning electron microscope. Am Rev Resp Dis 111:4, 1975

41. Scanlon TS, Benumof JL: Demonstration of interlobar collateral ventilation. J Appl Physiol 46:658, 1979

42. Kent EM, Blades B: The surgical anatomy of the pulmonary lobes. J Thorac Surg 12:18, 1941

43. Benumof JL: Monitoring respiratory function during anesthesia, Monitoring in Anesthesia. Edited by Saidman LJ, Smith NT. New York, John Wiley and Sons, 1978, pp 31–51

44. Couture J, Picken J, Trop D, et al: Airway closure in normal, obese, and anesthetized supine subjects. Fed Proc 29:269, 1970

45. Don HF, Craig DB, Wahba WM, et al: The measurement of gas trapped in the lungs at functional residual capacity and the effects of posture. Anesthesiology 35:582, 1971

46. Ward CS: The prevention of accidents associated with anesthetic apparatus. Br J Anaesth 40:692, 1968

47. Mazze RI: Therapeutic misadventures with oxygen delivery systems: The need for continuous in-line oxygen monitors. Anesth Analg 51:787, 1972

48. Epstein RM, Rackow H, Lee ASJ, et al: Prevention of accidental breathing of anoxic gas

mixture during anesthesia. Anesthesiology 23:1, 1962

49. Sprague DH, Archer GW: Intraoperative hypoxia from an erroneously filled liquid oxygen reservoir. Anesthesiology 42:360, 1975

50. Eger EI II, Epstein RM: Hazards of anesthetic equipment. Anesthesiology 25:490, 1964

51. Martin JT: Positioning in Anesthesia and Surgery. Philadelphia, WB Saunders, 1978

52. Heinonen J, Takki S, Tammisto T: Effect of the Trendelenburg tilt and other procedures on the position of endotracheal tubes. Lancet 1:850, 1969

53. Munson ES, Larson CP Jr, Babad AA, et al: The effects of halothane, fluroxene and cyclopropane on ventilation: A comparative study in man. Anesthesiology 27:716, 1966

54. Philbin DM, Sullivan SF, Bowman FO, et al: Post-operative hypoxemia: Contribution of the cardiac output. Anesthesiology 32:136, 1970

55. Cain SM: Increased oxygen uptake with passive hyperventilation of dogs. J Appl Physiol 28:4, 1970

56. Karetzky MS, Cain SM: Effect of carbon dioxide on oxygen uptake during hyperventilation in normal man. J Appl Physiol 28:8, 1970

57. Benumof JL, Mathers JM, Wahrenbrock EA: Cyclic hypoxic pulmonary vasoconstriction induced by concomitant carbon dioxide changes. J Appl Physiol 41:466, 1976

58. Cutillo A, Omboni E, Perondi R, et al: Effect of hypocapnia on pulmonary mechanics in normal subjects and in patients with chronic obstructive lung disease. Am Rev Resp Dis 110:25, 1974

59. Don H: The mechanical properties of the respiratory system during anesthesia, International Anesthesiology Clinics, Vol 15: Anesthesia and Respiratory Function. Edited by Kafer ER. Boston, Little Brown, 1977, pp 113–136

60. Don HF, Robson JG: The mechanics of the respiratory system during anesthesia. Anesthesiology 26:168, 1965

61. Don HF, Wahba M, Cuadrado L, et al: The effects of anesthesia and 100 percent oxygen on the functional residual capacity of the lungs. Anesthesiology 32:521, 1970

62. Hewlett AM, Hulands GH, Nunn JF, et al: Functional residual capacity during anaesthesia. III: Artificial ventilation. Br J Anaesth 46:495, 1974

63. Westbrook PR, Stubbs SE, Sessler AD, et al: Effects of anesthesia and muscle paralysis on respiratory mechanics in normal man. J Appl Physiol 34:81, 1973

64. Alexander JI, Spence AA, Parikh RK, et al: The role of airway closure in postoperative hypoxemia. Br J Anaesth 45:34, 1973

65. Hickey RF, Visick W, Fairley HB, et al: Effects of halothane anesthesia on functional residual capacity and alveolar-arterial oxygen tension difference. Anesthesiology 38:20, 1973

66. Wyche MQ, Teichner RL, Kallos T, et al: Effects of continuous positive-pressure breathing on functional residual capacity and arterial oxygenation during intra-abdominal operations. Anesthesiology 38:68, 1973

67. Craig DB, Wahba WM, Don HF, et al: "Closing volume" and its relationship to gas exchange in seated and supine positions. J Appl Physiol 31:717, 1971

68. Freund F, Roos A, Dodd RB: Expiratory activity of the abdominal muscles in man during general anesthesia. J Appl Physiol 19:693, 1964

69. Kallos T, Wyche MQ, Garman JK: The effects of innovar on functional residual capacity and total chest compliance. Anesthesiology 39:558, 1973

70. Campbell EJM, Agostini E, David JN: The Respiratory Muscles: Mechanics and Neural Control. 2nd edition. Philadelphia, WB Saunders, 1970

71. Milic-Emili J, Mead J, Tanner JM: Topography of esophageal pressure as a function of posture in man. J Appl Physiol 19:212, 1964

72. Froese AB, Bryan CA: Effects of anesthesia and paralysis on diaphragmatic mechanics in man. Anesthesiology 41:242, 1974

73. Dekker E, Defares JG, Heemstra H: Direct measurement of intrabronchial pressure. Its application to the location of the check-value mechanism. J Appl Physiol 13:35, 1958

74. Macklem PT, Fraser RG, Bates DV: Bronchial pressures and dimensions in health and obstructive airway disease. J Appl Physiol 18:699, 1963

75. Ward CF, Gagnon RL, Benumof JL:

Wheezing after induction of general anesthesia: Negative expiratory pressure revisited. Anesth Analg 58:49, 1979

76. Mead J, Agostoni E: Dynamics of breathing, Handbook of Physiology, Section 3: Respiration. Vol 1. Edited by Fenn WO, Rahn H. Baltimore, Williams & Wilkins, 1964, pp 411–427

77. Nunn JF: Mechanisms of pulmonary ventilation, Applied Respiratory Physiology. 2nd edition. London, Butterworths, 1977, pp 94–138

78. Oswalt CE, Gates GA, Holmstrom FMG: Pulmonary edema as a complication of acute airway obstruction. Rev Surg 34:364, 1977

79. Ray JF, Yost L, Moallem S, et al: Immobility, hypoxemia, and pulmonary arteriovenous shunting. Arch Surg 109:537, 1974

80. Wagner PD, Laravuso RB, Uhl RR, et al: Continuous distributions of ventilation-perfusion ratios in normal subjects breathing air and 100% O_2. J Clin Invest 54:54, 1974

81. Briscoe WA, Cree EM, Filler, et al: Lung volume, alveolar ventilation and perfusion interrelationships in chronic pulmonary emphysema. J Appl Physiol 15:785, 1960

82. Slocum HC, Hoeflich EA, Allen CR: Circulatory and respiratory distress from extreme positions on the operating table. Surg Gynecol Obstet 84:1065, 1947

83. Laver MB, Hallowell P, Goldblatt A: Pulmonary dysfunction secondary to heart disease: Aspects relevant to anesthesia and surgery. Anesthesiology 33:161, 1970

84. Bendixen HH, Hedley-Whyte J, Chir B, et al: Impaired oxygenation in surgical patients during general anesthesia with controlled ventilation. N Engl J Med 269:991, 1963

85. Bendixen HH, Bullwinkel B, Hedley-Whyte J, et al: Atelectasis and shunting during spontaneous ventilation in anesthetized patients. Anesthesiology 25:297, 1964

86. Yeaker H: Tracheobronchial secretions. Am J Med 50:493, 1971

87. Forbes AR: Humidification and mucous flow in the intubated trachea. Br J Anaesth 45:874, 1973

88. Bang BG, Bang FB: Effect of water deprivation on nasal mucous flow. Proc Soc Exp Biol Med 106:516, 1961

89. Hirsch JA, Tokayer JL, Robinson MJ, et al: Effects of dry air and subsequent humidification on tracheal mucous velocity in dogs. J Appl Physiol 39:242, 1975

90. Dalhamn T: Mucous flow and ciliary activity in the tracheas of rats exposed to respiratory irritant gases. Acta Physiol Scand 36 (suppl 123):1, 1956

91. Hill L: The ciliary movement of the trachea studies *in vitro*. Lancet 2:802, 1928

92. Sackner MA, Landa J, Hirsch J, et al: Pulmonary effects of oxygen breathing. Ann Intern Med 82:40, 1975

93. Sackner MA, Hirsch J, Epstein S: Effect of cuffed endotracheal tubes of tracheal mucous velocity. Chest 68:774, 1975

94. Forbes AR: Halothane depresses mucociliary flow in the trachea. Anesthesiology 45:59, 1976

95. Nunn JF, Sturrock JE, Wills EJ, et al: The effect of inhalation anaesthetics on the swimming velocity of Tetrahymena pyriformis. J Cell Sci 15:537, 1974

96. Prys-Roberts C: The metabolic regulation of circulatory transport, Scientific Foundations of Anesthesia. Edited by Scurr C, Feldman S. Philadelphia, FA Davis, 1970, pp 87–96

97. Benumof JL, Wahrenbrock EA: Blunted hypoxic pulmonary vasoconstriction by increased lung vascular pressures. J Appl Physiol 38:846, 1975

98. Scanlon TS, Benumof JL, Wahrenbrock EA, et al: Hypoxic pulmonary vasoconstriction and the ratio of hypoxic lung to perfused normoxic lung. Anesthesiology 49:177, 1978

99. Benumof JL, Wahrenbrock EA: Dependency of hypoxic pulmonary vasoconstriction on temperature. J Appl Physiol 42:56, 1977

100. Ward CF, Benumof JL, Wahrenbrock EA: Inhibition of hypoxic pulmonary vasoconstriction by vasoactive drugs. Abstracts of Scientific Papers, 1976 ASA Meeting, p 333

101. Johansen I, Benumof JL: Reduction of hypoxia induced pulmonary artery hypertension by vasodilator drugs. Amer Rev Resp Dis 119:375, 1979

102. Benumof JL, Wahrenbrock EA: The local effect of anesthetics on regional hypoxic pulmonary vasoconstriction. Anesthesiology 43:525, 1975

103. Mathers JM, Benumof JL, Wahrenbrock EA: General anesthetics and regional hypoxic pulmonary vasoconstriction. Anesthesiology 46:111, 1977

104. Eckenhoff JE, Enderby GEH, Larson A, et al: Pulmonary gas exchange during deliberate hypotension. Br J Anaesth 35:750, 1963

105. Kain ML, Panday J, Nunn JF: The effect of intubation on the dead space during halothane anaesthesia. Br J Anaesth 41:94, 1969

106. Conway CM: Anesthetic circuits, Scientific Foundations of Anesthesia. 2nd edition. Edited by Scurr C, Feldman S. London, William Heinemann Medical Books, 1974, pp 509–515

107. Cohen PJ, Alexander SC, Smith TC, et al: Effects of hypoxia and normocarbia on cerebral blood flow and metabolism in conscious man. J Appl Physiol 23:183, 1967

108. Winter PM, Smith G: The toxicity of oxygen. Anesthesiology 37:210, 1972

109. Lambertsen CJ: Effects of oxygen at high partial pressure, Handbook of Physiology, Section 3: Respiration. Vol 2. Edited by Fenn WO, Rahn H. Baltimore, Williams & Wilkins, 1965, pp 1027–1046

110. Nash G, Blennerhasset JB, Pontoppidan H: Pulmonary lesions associated with oxygen therapy and artificial ventilation. N Engl J Med 276:368, 1967

111. Severinghaus JW, Larson CP: Respiration in anesthesia, Handbook of Physiology, Section 3: Respiration. Vol 2. Edited by Fenn WO, Rahn H. Baltimore, Williams & Wilkins, 1965, pp 1219–1264

112. Clowes GHA, Hopkins AL, Simeone FA: A comparison of the physiological effects of hypercapnia and hypoxia in the production of cardiac arrest. Ann Surg 142:446, 1955

113. Fenn WO, Asano T: Effects of carbon dioxide inhalation on potassium liberation from the liver. Am J Physiol 185:567, 1956

114. Alfery D, Benumof JL: Hepatic blood flow alterations during anesthesia. Contemp Anesth Prac Series 4:31, 1981

23

Cardiovascular Physiology*

Joel A. Kaplan, M.D.

In this chapter, cardiac physiology is emphasized. The physiology of the peripheral vasculature and regulation of blood flow to specific organs is discussed in other chapters (e.g. cerebral blood flow in Ch. 25 and renal blood flow in Ch. 24). Therefore, the purposes of this chapter are to:

1. Review concepts of cardiac physiology as they apply to anesthesia.

2. Clarify the language of cardiac physiology.

3. Indicate the techniques used to measure cardiac function.

4. Review these techniques as they apply to anesthetic agents.

Under normal conditions, the heart acts as a servant by varying the cardiac output in accordance with total tissue needs.[1] Tissue needs may change secondary to exercise, infection, heart disease, trauma, surgery, drugs, or anesthetic agents. Although the heart receives much of our emphasis, the needs of peripheral tissues are actually regulating circulatory requirements. The heart serves only as the limiting factor in many patients with severe cardiac disease. In this regard, there are three definitions that are often confused and should be clearly separated:[2]

Circulatory function—This is the function of the entire circulatory system, including the heart, blood vessels, and blood volume. Failure of any one of these can lead to significant circulatory dysfunction. For example, hypovolemia can lead to circulatory failure or shock in the presence of normal blood vessels and a normal heart.

Cardiac function—This includes the function of the myocardium, valves, conduction tissue, and supporting structures. Dysfunction of any of these can lead to cardiac and circulatory failure. The myocardium can be entirely normal, but with insufficient valves the heart can fail badly.

Myocardial function—This depends on the cardiac muscle itself and its blood supply. There can be myocardial failure based on actual muscle damage or based on myocardial ischemia and inadequate muscle function. Certainly myocardial dysfunction will then produce cardiac dysfunction and circulatory problems.

The primary function of the heart is to deliver sufficient oxygenated blood to meet the metabolic requirements of the peripheral tissues. One definition of heart failure is that the heart is unable to pump blood at a rate sufficient to meet these requirements. Therefore, the cardiac output is usually considered the key test of cardiac function. However, cardiac output and myocardial function or contractility cannot be related in a simple straight-forward manner. The contractile state of the myocardium is only one of several determinants of the heart's ability to eject an adequate cardiac output.[3]

---

* Parts of this chapter are reproduced with modification from Kaplan, JA (Editor): Cardiac Anesthesia. New York, Grune & Stratton, 1979, by permission of the publisher.

CARDIAC OUTPUT

The cardiac output is the amount of blood pumped to the peripheral circulation per minute. It is a measurement reflecting the status of the *entire circulatory system,* not only the heart and is governed by autoregulation in the tissues.[4] Although affected by a number of peripheral factors, cardiac output may not be able to change much in the presence of severe cardiac dysfunction. The cardiac output (CO) equals the stroke volume (SV) per beat times the heart rate (HR) per minute:

$$CO = SV \times HR$$

Normal average values are a cardiac output of 5 to 6 L/min in a 70 kg man, with a stroke volume of 60 to 90 ml/beat and a heart rate of 80 beats/min. To compare patients with different body sizes, cardiac output may be corrected in relation to body surface area and is called the cardiac index (CI), which equals the cardiac output divided by the body surface area (BSA):

$$CI = \frac{CO}{BSA}$$

The normal value for a 70 kg man is 2.5 to 3.5 L/min/m^2. A normal person has a tremendous reserve capacity to increase cardiac output to as much as 25 to 30 L/min. Factors controlling the cardiac output include venous return to the heart, peripheral vascular resistance, peripheral tissue oxygen needs, blood volume, body position, pattern and type of respiration, heart rate, and myocardial contractility.

The two main determinants of cardiac output are heart rate and stroke volume. Heart rate depends on the intrinsic rhythmicity of the sinoatrial node and is further affected by extrinsic neural or humoral factors.

The neural input to the cardiac conduction system is via both the sympathetic and parasympathetic nervous systems. These changes can lead to increases or decreases in the heart rate and therefore the cardiac output. The cardiac output can also be affected by changes in stroke volume caused by alterations in myocardial fiber shortening. The four factors affecting the stroke volume through this mechanism are: preload, afterload, contractility, and wall motion abnormalities. The resultant cardiac output is then distributed throughout the various vascular beds of the body including the central nervous system, myocardium, renal and splanchnic beds, skeletal muscle, and skin. The peripheral vasculature is affected by a number of intrinsic factors, such as metabolic demand, and extrinsic factors, such as neural and humoral stimuli, all of which produce the appropriate distribution of the cardiac output.[5]

The cardiac ouput may be *increased* by increases in heart rate; increases in left ventricular volume (preload) produced by an increased venous return; decreases in afterload such as that which occurs with peripheral vasodilatation, or in the presence of an arteriovenous fistula; or increases in myocardial function as occurs with increased endogenous or exogenous catecholamine stimulation.

Decreases in cardiac ouput can be produced by parasympathetic stimulation producing a decrease in heart rate; a decrease in preload; an increase in afterload; or intrinsic myocardial disease or drugs limiting myocardial contractility.

An example of the tremendous increase possible in cardiac output is seen in young patients during extreme exercise, as shown below:

	Heart Rate (Beats/min) $\times$	Stroke Volume (ml/beat) $=$	Cardiac Output (ml/min)
At rest	70	80	5,600
Moderate exercise	130	130	16,900
Extreme exercise	200	150	30,000

CONTROL OF HEART RATE

At a constant stroke volume, cardiac output has a linear relationship to heart rate. The heart rate is primarily determined by the rhythmicity of the sinoatrial (SA) node due to the spontaneous phase IV depolarization of its pacemaker cells. The intrinsic control of heart rate produced by the SA node is affected by extrinsic neural and humoral factors. The neural factors stimulating the heart via the autonomic nervous system are of great importance in altering the heart rate. Humoral factors such as circulating catecholamines are of less importance in most situations. Sympathetic stimulation of the heart increases heart rate by increasing the slope of phase IV depolarization, while parasympathetic stimulation decreases phase IV depolarization and produces a slowing of the heart rate. Sympathetic neural influences on the heart travel through the cervical (superior, middle, and inferior) ganglia and the thoracic cardiac accelerator nerves (T_1 to T_4) and affect the sinoatrial node, the atrioventricular node, and the ventricular muscle and conduction system. Parasympathetic neural influences on the heart travel via the vagus nerves to the sinoatrial and atrioventricular nodes with minimal influence on the ventricular conduction system. Vagal influences produce a decreased heart rate, decreased atrial force of contraction, and delayed atrioventricular conduction. Studies by Higgins et al. have shown the relative dominance of the parasympathetic nervous system in the control of normal heart rate.[6] They have found that the normal baroreceptor-induced slowing of heart rate is mediated largely by the parasympathetic system. In patients with heart disease, both a depletion of cardiac catecholamine stores and a markedly abnormal baroreceptor reflex mechanism produce gross alterations in autonomic control of cardiac rate.[7]

CONTROL OF STROKE VOLUME

The second basic variable in the control of cardiac output is the stroke volume. Stroke volume is a function of the extent of myocardial fiber shortening, which, in turn, is determined by the four factors previously mentioned.

PRELOAD

Starling's Law of the heart states that the force of ventricular contraction depends on the initial muscle fiber length.[8] In the isolated cat papillary muscle preparation, the preload is the weight exerted on the myocardial muscle fiber before contraction takes place. It determines the resting fiber length. As the resting fiber length is increased, the force of contraction of the isolated muscle is increased. In the intact heart, the preload is determined by the left ventricular end-diastolic *volume* (LVEDV) (Fig. 23-1). This is the initial stretch on the ventricular muscle. The left ventricular end-diastolic volume is very difficult to measure clinically and measurement is only beginning to be possible with techniques such as echocardiography, ventriculography, or radionucleotide scans, all of which can be used both in the operating room and in the intensive care unit. Left ventricular end-diastolic *pressure* (LVEDP) clinically is usually measured as an approximation of the left ventricular end-diastolic volume (preload) of the heart.[9] This assumes that left ventricular compliance is entirely normal, which is *not* a valid assumption in many patients with cardiac disease (Fig. 23-2). With ischemic heart disease or aortic stenosis, the left ventricular compliance curve is frequently shifted to the left where small increases in volume can produce large increases in left ventricular filling pressure (decreased compliance). With aortic insufficiency or immediately after cardiopulmonary bypass when myocardial cardioplegic solutions have been

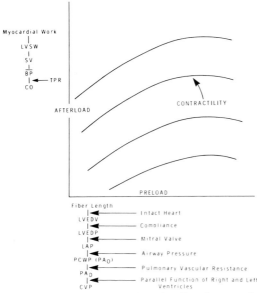

Fig. 23-1 The Frank-Starling family of curves is demonstrated. The horizontal axis represents the preload of the heart and the various factors used to estimate preload are shown. The vertical axis represents the myocardial work and the various factors used to represent this are shown. The vertical axis is also affected by the afterload of the heart. See the text for details. LVSW = left ventricular stroke work; SV = stroke volume: BP = mean blood pressure; TPR = total peripheral resistance; CO = cardiac output; LVEDV = left ventricular end-diastolic volume; LVEDP = left ventricular end-diastolic pressure; LAP = left atrial pressure; PCWP = pulmonary capillary wedge pressure; Pa_O = pulmonary artery occluded pressure; Pa_D = pulmonary artery diastolic pressure; CVP = central venous pressure. (Modified from Bonner J: Anesthesiology Review, July 1977, pp 26–29.)

used, compliance increases and large volumes can be placed in the left ventricle with minimal increases in pressure. Therefore, left ventricular end-diastolic pressure is *not always* a good reflection of left ventricular end-diastolic volume.[10] The left ventricular end-diastolic pressure can be measured with a catheter in the left ventricle, but this is usually done only at cardiac catheterization and not during surgery because there is a high incidence of ventricular dysrhythmias produced by this technique.

During cardiac surgery, the preload of the heart is frequently measured by inserting a catheter into the left atrium and measuring left atrial pressure (LAP), which gives a good approximation of the LVEDP as long as there is a normal mitral valve.[11] However the Swan-Ganz flow-directed pulmonary artery catheter is now being used clinically to ascertain the left ventricular filling pressure.[12] The pulmonary capillary wedge pressure (PCWP) or pulmonary artery occluded pressure (PAoP) is usually a good reflection of the left atrial pressure.[13] Marked alterations in airway pressure such as the use of high levels of positive end-expiratory pressure may, however, disturb the relationship between the PCWP and left atrial pressure.[14] Depending on the compliance of the pulmonary parenchyma, either part or all of the airway pressure may be transmitted to the pulmonary artery catheter. This must be considered when evaluating left ventricular filling pressure by the use of the Swan-Ganz catheter in patients receiving mechanical ventilation and positive end-expiratory pressure. Also, the location of the tip of the catheter in relation to the left atrium must be ascertained. If the catheter tip is in zone I of the

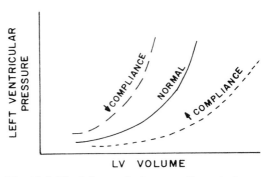

Fig. 23-2 The left ventricular compliance is the relationship between the left ventricular end-diastolic pressure and the left ventricular volume. An increase in compliance shifts the curve down and to the right, while a decrease in compliance shifts it up and to the left. (Thomas SJ, Lowenstein E: Anesthetic management of the patient with valvular heart disease. Int Anesthesiol Clin 17:67, 1979.)

lung (see Ch. 22), it will reflect airway pressure instead of left atrial pressure.[15] When the catheter cannot be placed in the wedge position, the pulmonary artery diastolic pressure (PAdP) may be used to estimate the left atrial pressure and is usually quite accurate.[13] However, if the pulmonary vascular resistance is markedly elevated, large disparity between the pulmonary artery diastolic pressure and the left atrial pressure will exist.

The central venous pressure (CVP) is the poorest approximation of left ventricular end-diastolic pressure, but may be used to estimate the left ventricular end-diastolic pressure in patients with good function of both the right and left ventricles. However, when cardiac disease is characterized by disparate right and left ventricular function, the central venous pressure may be misleading when quantitating left ventricular filling pressure.[16] An important concept to remember is that left ventricular and right ventricular preloads and function curves are not always equal or even parallel.[17] The CVP can be higher or lower than the LVEDP depending on the underlying pathology.

Factors affecting the preload of the heart include the total blood volume, body position, intrathoracic pressure, intrapericardial pressure, venous tone, pumping action of skeletal muscles, and the atrial contribution to ventricular filling.[18] There is probably a descending limb of the Starling curve in man which can be explained by Laplace's Law of P = T/R, where P equals the pressure developed by a particular level of wall tension (T) and R is the radius of the chamber. This formula states that if the diastolic volume is markedly increased, a greater myocardial tension is needed to develop a particular level of intraventricular pressure. In other words, overdistention of the ventricle produces a need for greater wall tension and work of the ventricle in order to eject blood at an adequate pressure.

The vertical or work axis on the Starling

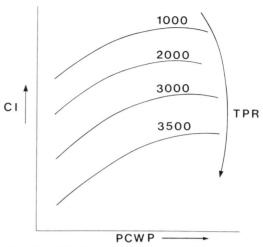

Fig. 23-3 The family of Frank-Starling curves is demonstrated with the cardiac index (CI) on the vertical axis and the pulmonary capillary wedge pressure (PCWP) on the horizontal axis. As total peripheral resistance (TPR) is increased from 1,000 toward 3,500 dynes-sec/cm^{-5} the curves are shifted down and to the right.

curve shown in Figure 23-1 would ideally reflect myocardial work that cannot be derived clinically. Variables often placed on this axis are either blood pressure, cardiac output (CO), stroke volume (SV), or left ventricular stroke work (LVSW) derived from the cardiac output, all of which can be derived clinically with hemodynamic monitors such as Swan-Ganz catheters and thermal dilution cardiac outputs. The afterload, as expressed by total peripheral resistance (TPR) is shown also to have an effect on this axis. Bolooki has modified the curve to include an axis for TPR (Fig. 23-3).[19]

According to Starling's Law, increases on the filling pressure axis should lead to increases in work. Sarnoff and Bergland described a series of curves that fit on this diagram (Figs. 23-1 and 23-4).[17] Curves moving up and toward the left show an increase in myocardial contractility when more work is done at a lower filling pressure. Curves moving down and to the right show decreased work at higher filling pressures.

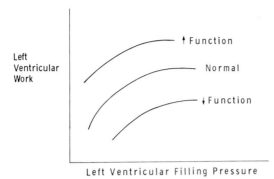

Fig. 23-4 The Frank-Starling family of curves is demonstrated with increasing left ventricular function moving the curve up and to the left and decreasing left ventricular function moving the curve down and to the right.

AFTERLOAD

Afterload is the wall stress faced by the myocardium during left ventricular ejection and, therefore, depends on a complicated relationship of left ventricular size, shape, pressure, and wall thickness. Afterload can be thought of, however, as the impedance to left ventricular ejection which, in the absence of aortic stenosis, depends on the distensibility of the large arteries and the systemic vascular resistance.[20] Clinically, mean arterial blood pressure is measured or, preferably the systemic vascular resistance (SVR) or total peripheral resistance (TPR), is calculated to assess the afterload of the heart.

Because blood pressure depends on both impedance to left ventricular ejection and the stroke volume and therefore is not a good measure of afterload, calculation of the systemic vascular resistence is preferred. For example, a patient with a low mean blood pressure might have a high afterload combined with a very low stroke volume, or a very low afterload combined with a normal stroke volume. However, a high arterial blood pressure clinically may be the only available indicator of increased impedance to left ventricular ejection.

Afterload reduction has become a major intervention in the modern therapy of left ventricular failure.[21] The failing left ventricle cannot pump against an increased peripheral resistance and, therefore, modern therapeutic interventions using vasodilators to reduce arterial afterload have become extremely useful. Figure 23-5 demonstrates how a normal ventricle maintains normal function or even increases output with an increased TPR (Anrep effect); however, a failing ventricle is severely compromised by an increased resistance.

CONTRACTILITY

When preload and afterload are held constant, stroke volume is a function of the contractile state of the myocardium. This is an intrinsic property of the myocardium and reflects its ability to do mechanical work at any given level of preload. A true measure of contractility, therefore, must be made with a constant preload, afterload, and heart rate,

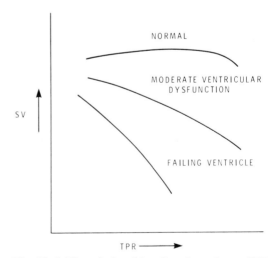

Fig. 23-5 The relationship of stroke volume (SV) to total peripheral resistance (TPR) is demonstrated in normal and failing ventricles. (Modified from Cohn JN, Francisosa JA: Vasodilator therapy of cardiac failure. Reprinted by permission of the New England Journal of Medicine, 297:27, 1977.)

since all of these factors affect the heart's function.[22] This, then, is a difficult parameter to measure clinically.

Factors affecting the contractile state of the myocardium are numerous. Factors *increasing* contractility include:

Sympathetic stimulation—direct increases of force of contraction, as well as indirect increases due to increased heart rate (rate-treppe effect or Bowditch phenomenon).

Parasympathetic inhibition producing increased heart rate.

Administration of positive inotropic drugs such as digitalis.

Factors *decreasing* contractility include:

Parasympathetic stimulation—decreased rate effect.

Sympathetic inhibition—via withdrawal of catecholamines or blockade of adrenergic receptors.

Administration of β-adrenergic blocking drugs.

Myocardial ischemia and infarction.

Intrinsic myocardial diseases such as cardiomyopathies.

Hypoxia or acidosis.

The relationship between myocardial activation and contraction is dependent on the presence of calcium.[23] Excitation of the cell membrane and depolarization are accompanied by a rapid entry of extracellular calcium into the cell, and the spread of electrical activity by way of the sarcoplasmic tubules causes the release of intracellular calcium and activation of contraction. For the cardiac muscle to relax, intracellular calcium must be recaptured by the sarcoplasmic reticulum or mitochondria. Myocardial contraction is initiated when the ionic calcium reaches the reactive sites on the myofilaments. The present concept of myocardial contraction is based on the fact that in diastole the troponin-tropomyosin complex inhibits the interaction between the two major contractile proteins, actin and myosin. The presence of ionic calcium released from the sarcoplasmic reticulum causes a confirmational change in the troponin-tropomyosin complex so that it no

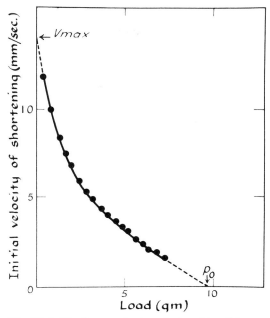

Fig. 23-6 The force-velocity relationship of the cat papillary muscle. Vmax is maximum possible contractility extrapolated from the curve, and P_O is the isometric load on the heart muscle.

longer inhibits the actin-myosin interaction, and myocardial contraction results.

To study mycardial contraction, the A. V. Hill model of the isolated cat papillary muscle is usually utilized.[24] The maximum velocity of shortening of the muscle depends on the load and the relationship between the tension (force) developed and the velocity of contractions expressed by the force velocity curve shown in Figure 23-6. The lower the load, the higher the velocity of shortening. The maximum velocity of shortening with zero load is called V max, which is not directly measured but extrapolated from the curve.Therapeutic interventions affect this curve in a number of ways as shown in Figure 23-7. It is shifted by drugs that affect preload and afterload as well as contractility. Increasing afterload (e.g., methoxamine) shifts the curve from point 1 to point 2, while decreasing afterload with a vasodilator (e.g., nitroprusside) shifts the curve from point 1 to point 3. Therapy with a positive inotropic drug (e.g., calcium chloride)

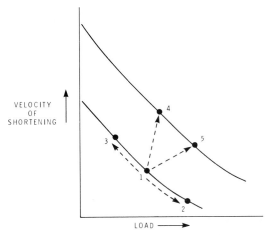

VELOCITY
OF
SHORTENING

LOAD ⟶

Fig. 23-7 The effects of altering load and/or contractility on the force-velocity relationship are demonstrated. See the text for details.

shifts the curve up from point 1 to point 4, and combined inotropic stimulation and vasoconstriction (e.g., epinephrine) shifts the curve up and to the right from point 1 to point 5.

The behavior of the left ventricle during *diastole* depends on properties of ventricular relaxation, affecting early diastolic filling, and ventricular stiffness, which mainly affects mid-diastolic and late-diastolic filling. Ventricular relaxation is an energy-dependent process that can be altered separately from contraction and is probably dependent on the rate of sequestration of calcium ion by the sarcoplasmic reticulum and mitochondria after systole.[25] Relaxation of the ventricle is

enhanced by β_1-adrenergic stimulation, and can be impaired by heart failure, myocardial ischemia, hypercalcemia, and tachycardia. In these conditions, therefore, early diastolic filling can be impaired.

LEFT VENTRICULAR WALL MOTION ABNORMALITIES

Left ventricular dyssynergy or wall motion abnormalities occur when localized areas of the left ventricle are hypokinetic, akinetic, or dyskinetic (bulging outward during systole) (Fig. 23-8). Thus, at any given level of preload, afterload, or contractility, stroke volume will be less if left ventricular dyssynergy exists.[26] This is not found in normal ventricles but is common in patients with coronary artery disease or mitral stenosis.

CARDIAC OUTPUT MEASUREMENTS

Cardiac output is increasingly being monitored during and after surgery. Serial measurements can be used to assess the general status of the circulation and to determine the appropriate hemodynamic therapy and estimate its efficacy. However, equally useful are the variables that may be determined once the cardiac output is known.[27] These variables include the peripheral and pulmonary vascular resistances, stroke volumes, and stroke work. Formulae for these parameters are shown below:

Formula	Normal Value
$SV = \dfrac{CO}{HR} \times 1000$	60–90 ml/beat
$SI = \dfrac{SV}{BSA}$	40–60 ml/beat/m^2
$LVSWI = 1.36 \times \dfrac{(\overline{MAP} - \overline{PCWP}) \times SI}{100}$	45–60 gm-meters/m^2/beats
$RVSWI = 1.36 \times \dfrac{(\overline{PAP} - \overline{CVP}) \times SI}{100}$	5–10 gm-meters/m^2/beats
$SVR = \dfrac{(\overline{MAP} - \overline{CVP}) \times 80}{CO}$	900–1,500 dynes-sec/cm^{-5}
$PVR = \dfrac{(\overline{PAP} - \overline{PCWP}) \times 80}{CO}$	50–150 dynes-sec/cm^{-5}

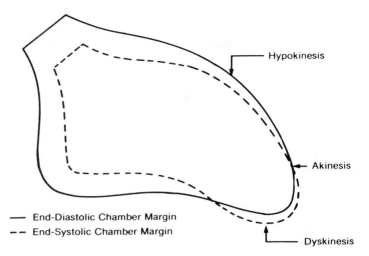

Fig. 23-8 Areas of hypokinesia, dyskinesia, and akinesia are demonstrated from a ventriculogram. (Alderman EL: Angiographic indicators of left ventricular function. JAMA 236:1055, 1976. Copyright 1976, American Medical Association.)

Hypokinesis

Akinesis

Dyskinesis

—— End-Diastolic Chamber Margin
-- End-Systolic Chamber Margin

where SV = stroke volume; CO = cardiac output; HR = heart rate; BSA = body surface area; LVSWI = left ventricular stroke work index; $\overline{MAP}$ = mean arterial pressure; $\overline{PCWP}$ = mean pulmonary capillary wedge pressure; RVSWI = right ventricular stroke work index; $\overline{PAP}$ = mean pulmonary artery pressure; $\overline{CVP}$ = mean central venous pressure; SVR = systemic vascular resistance; $\overline{PVR}$ = pulmonary vascular resistance, and SI = stroke index. All these parameters are rapidly derived in both the operating room and intensive care unit using programmable portable calculators available at the present time.

Cardiac output can be measured by several techniques. The thermodilution method, employing the Swan-Ganz catheter, is the clinical method of choice. With this technique, multiple outputs can be obtained at frequent intervals along with measures of both right and left ventricular filling pressure. Swan, Ganz, and Forrester introduced their catheter for thermodilution cardiac output measurements in 1970 and found that thermodilution-measured flow was accurate to within 2 percent of the known pump flow in vitro.[12] In 20 patients, they showed the standard deviation of triplicate measurements was 4.6 percent in the range of 2 to 8 L/min of cardiac output.[28] Other investigators have shown excellent correlation between dye and thermodilution cardiac outputs in patients after cardiac surgery.[29] The thermodilution method may be even more accurate than the dye dilution method at low cardiac outputs, since there is no recirculation of the indicator in the thermodilution technique.

To provide a high rate of reproducibility, the technique of thermodilution cardiac output measurements must be standardized. The injectate temperature and volume, as well as the speed of injection, should be carefully controlled and duplicated. The most reproducible results have been obtained using injections of 10 ml of cold (1 to 2 °C) 5 percent dextrose in water. All measurements should be made in duplicate or triplicate during expiration. Necessary equipment includes a sterile system for maintaining the cold syringes at 0 to 2 °C, a cardiac output computer, and precise temperature measurement of the injectate and the patient. Additional equipment that may be used are a mechanical injector for greater injection speed and reproducibility, and a recorder for observation and hand calculation of the curves.

The Swan-Ganz 7-French thermodilution cardiac output catheter contains two fine wires that extend the length of the catheter and terminate in a thermistor embedded in the catheter wall just proximal to the balloon. The principle of measurement is similar to the dye dilution method of cardiac outputs except that a cold solution acts as the indicator.[30] A known change in the temperature is induced at one point in the circulation, and the resulting change in temperature is detected at a point downstream. The baseline pulmonary artery body temperature is recorded in the computer, the cold solution is then injected via the proximal port into the right atrium, and the resulting temperature change is detected by the thermistor in the pulmonary artery. The newest thermodilution catheters automatically measure the body temperature and the injectate temperature. The thermistor acts as a variable resistor in a Wheatstone bridge with a linear relationship between temperature and electric resistance. The change in temperature alters the resistance and thus the output from the bridge, which is amplified and recorded, and the cardiac output is calculated by the computer.

The thermal dilution technique measures *right* sided cardiac outputs. This is very important in patients with intracardiac shunts and can lead to totally erroneous numbers. For example, a patient with a ventricular septal defect and a left-to-right shunt, will have a falsely elevated cardiac output measured by this technique.

Other methods to measure cardiac output include the standard Fick and dye dilution techniques, as well as direct flow meter techniques including Doppler and aortic pulse contour measurements.[31] The Fick technique is the standard for *steady state* measurements of cardiac output and is said to be accurate within ± 10 percent. The technique is complex and cumbersome, however, involving both the collection of expired gases and right heart catheterization to obtain mixed venous blood. Recently, Davis et al. has shown that cardiac output measurements by the Fick technique can also be employed using carbon dioxide in a rebreathing system versus the standard oxygen Fick method.[32]

The indicator dye dilution method using indocyanine green dye had been the most popular technique of cardiac output measurements prior to the thermodilution method. This technique consists of a rapid injection of a precise amount of dye into the venous circulation, where the indicator mixes with blood, passes rapidly through the heart and lungs into the arterial circulation, and is detected by sampling arterial blood and passing it through a densitometer. Complex mathematical formulae are necessary to calculate the cardiac output by this method, since there is a significant amount of recirculation which occurs. This technique is still useful when intracardiac shunts are present and, in fact, may be used to confirm their presence.

Another method of cardiac output measurement utilizing computers is the Warner aortic pulse contour analysis technique. This allows on-line measurement of stroke volume by placing a central aortic catheter. However, this technique makes assumptions concerning a constant compliance of the systemic vascular bed that are not valid with certain therapeutic interventions or anesthetic techniques. Therefore, this technique has been questioned by some and has not gained great popularity. Recently, English and colleagues have compared the pulse contour method to thermodilution cardiac output measurements.[33] The pulse contour method was found to be *inaccurate* in any situation where systemic vascular resistance changed by 30 percent or more. Patients with frequent marked changes in cardiovascular dynamics such as occur in the operating room and intensive care unit should not have cardiac outputs measured by this technique. Pharmacologic studies in which peripheral resistance may change, such as occurs in studies of anesthetic induction with narcotics or neuroleptanesthetic drugs, should also be performed with a more reliable technique of cardiac output measurement.

VENTRICULAR FUNCTION

Myocardial contractility is difficult to measure directly in the clinical situation. Therefore, two categories of measurement techniques are used to assess myocardial function in patients: ventricular function curves and contractility measurements.

VENTRICULAR FUNCTION CURVES

Multiple measurements of cardiac output and its derivatives, along with ventricular filling pressure, allow the construction of Starling ventricular function curves.[34] The Frank-Starling mechanism of the heart relates the filling volume of the heart (preload) to the stroke volume of the *corresponding* ventricle. A Starling diagram showing both right and left ventricular function curves is shown in Figure 23-9. Measurements of *left* ventricular function should have the pulmonary capillary wedge pressure or another measurement of left ventricular filling pressure on the horizontal axis and the left ventricular stroke work index on the vertical axis. In order to measure *right* ventricular function, these could be replaced by the central venous pressure on the horizontal axis and the right ventricular stroke work index on the vertical axis. It is not accurate, however, to mix one measurement from each side of the heart; e.g., central venous pressure and left ventricular stroke work index. Interventions that increase contractility shift the curves up and to the left. Disease states or drugs that depress the heart shift the curves down and to the right. These ventricular function curves can be used to:

1. Guide cardiovascular therapy during anesthesia or in the postoperative period.

2. Aid in the treatment of patients in heart failure with inotropes or vasodilators.

3. Guide therapeutic decisions when terminating cardiopulmonary bypass.

4. Guide therapy in patients requiring the intraaortic balloon.

A number of therapeutic interventions can be performed on the patient with a low output syndrome.[9] The proper choice depends on an understanding of the underlying cardiac

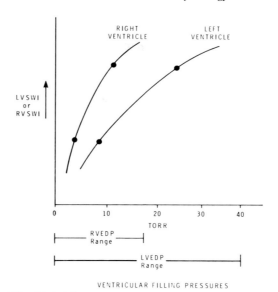

Fig. 23-9 The Frank-Starling diagram of both the right and left ventricles is demonstrated. Notice that the curves are not parallel and cover different ventricular filling pressure ranges.

physiology and the use of the Starling curve. The algorithm shown in Figure 30-8 (see Ch. 30) is useful in determining therapy. The first step in the treatment of a patient who is hypotensive with a low filling pressure and low cardiac output is to increase the patient's filling volume or preload by the administration of a volume infusion. This is done in an effort to move the patient up on the Starling curve to a maximum point of function with a pulmonary capillary wedge pressure of about 12 to 18 torr. The infusion is usually given in incremental doses of 100 to 200 ml while monitoring the filling pressure and the resultant change in blood pressure, stroke volume, or cardiac output. With hypovolemia alone, volume infusion should improve the hemodynamic variables and will probably be the only therapy necessary. With heart failure or low output syndromes, further therapeutic interventions will be necessary and these can be seen in Figure 23-10 where the patient starts with a high filling pressure and a low cardiac output at point 1. Further volume administration at this point would be fruitless and, in

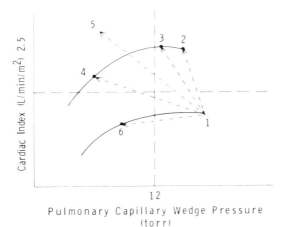

Fig. 23-10 The figure demonstrates a patient at point 1 on a hypofunctioning Starling curve. Five therapeutic interventions are made, and the results are demonstrated on the Starling curve showing increased function. These therapeutic interventions are labeled 2, 3, 4, 5, and 6. See the text for full explanation.

fact, possibly dangerous because it would take the patient over the hump of the Starling curve and overdistend the ventricle even further. A number of therapeutic interventions such as inotropes, vasodilators, diuretics, or the intraaortic balloon could be used in this patient and they would have different effects on the cardiovascular system. Most physicians would choose an inotropic drug such as dopamine in the patient with a low output syndrome and a low blood pressure. A dose of 5 μg/kg/min of dopamine might move the patient from point 1 on the curve to a higher Starling curve up and toward the left at point 2. Other inotropic drugs such as calcium chloride, digitalis, dobutamine, or epinephrine would have similar effects. A diuretic, such as furosemide, administered to the patient at point 1 may move the patient to point 6 by reducing his left ventricular filling pressure and not augment stroke volume, cardiac output, or blood pressure. It would serve only to reduce signs of congestive heart failure such as pulmonary edema. This would also be true of any other venodilator, such as morphine, given at this point.

The new therapeutic intervention of impedance reduction or afterload reduction can be used to move the patient from point 1 up to point 3.[21] An arteriolar dilator such as phentolamine, or a low dose of nitroprusside, would tend to reduce the impedance to ejection and allow the patient to move up and to the left on the Starling curve similar to what occurs with an inotropic agent (Figs. 23-3 and 23-10). The advantage of using a vasodilator instead of the inotrope is that there is no increase in myocardial oxygen demand required by the vasodilator. However, administering a vasodilator to a patient with heart failure is a tricky therapeutic undertaking. Excessive administration of the vasodilator can move the patient from point 1 to point 4 where extra volume infusions may be necessary to maintain the preload. In fact, often an attempt to maximally reduce the afterload is made by administering a large dose of arterial vasodilator and then augmenting the preload by additional volume infusions to bring the patient from point 1 to point 4 and then back to point 3. An approach of *minimizing* the afterload while *maximizing* the preload is a very good clinical tool.[35] Not all the vasodilators have similar hemodynamic effects. Figure 23-11 shows the difference between an arterial dilator such as phentolamine (A) and a venodilator such as nitroglycerin (V). An arterial dilator will reduce afterload and allow the patient to move up and to the left on the Starling curve from point 1 to point 3 on Figure 23-10. A venodilator such as a low dose of nitroglycerin will simply reduce preload, not overload, and move the patient from point 1 to point 6 on the Starling curve in Figure 23-10. A drug such as nitroprusside (A and V), which has effects on both preload and afterload, is probably the best in this situation because it will reduce afterload, allow an increased stroke volume and cardiac output, and, at the same time, reduce the symptoms of pulmonary congestion by its venodilating properties.[36] Combinations of inotropes, like dopamine, and mixed arterial and venous vasodilators, like nitroprusside, have become

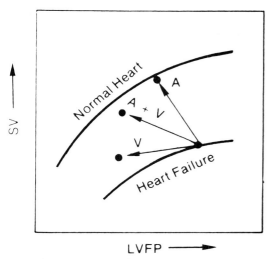

SV

LVFP ⟶

Fig. 23-11 Frank-Starling ventricular function curves of a normal heart and a heart in failure are demonstrated. The effects of three different types of vasodilators are demonstrated. An arteriolar dilator (A), a venodilator (V), and a mixed arterial and venodilator (A & V) are shown. See the text for details. (Mehta J: Vasodilators in the treatment of heart failure. JAMA 238:2534, 1977. Copyright 1977, American Medical Association.)

extremely popular and tend to give the largest increases in filling pressure, as shown on point 5 in Figure 23-10. Mechanical interventions such as the intraaortic balloon pump

(IABP) tend to reduce preload and afterload while augmenting coronary blood flow and increasing contractility and thus also shift the curve up and to the left, similar to combinations of inotropes and vasodilators at point 5. Figure 23-12 shows two groups of patients who received treatment with the IABP before and after cardiopulmonary bypass.[37]

By utilizing direct measurements of preload (such as the pulmonary capillary wedge pressure), indirect measurements of afterload (such as systemic vascular resistance), and ventricular function curves to assess myocardial contractility, the clinician can think about the cardiovascular system in specific terms and apply rational therapeutic interventions to clinical situations (Fig. 23-13). Alterations of preload, afterload, and contractility can then be specifically corrected. For example, if the preload is decreased, volume can be infused into the patient using either crystalloid, colloid, or whole blood, depending on the patient's hematocrit and possibly the colloid oncotic pressure (COP).[38] If necessary, while the preload is being augmented, systemic vascular resistance could be increased with a small dose of an α-adrenergic vasoconstrictor. This latter step would only be a very temporary measure while the preload was being augmented by volume infu-

Fig. 23-12 Left ventricular function diagram is shown with the normal range shaded dark. Intraaortic counterpulsation moved patients, both in the prebypass and postbypass groups, up and to the left on the curves. (Kaplan JA, Craver JM, Jones EL, et al: The role of the intraaortic balloon in cardiac anesthesia and surgery. Am Heart J 98:580, 1979.)

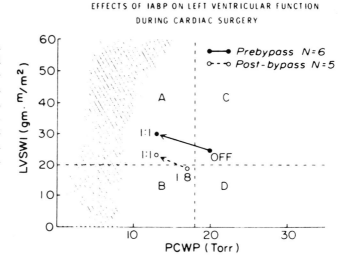

EFFECTS OF IABP ON LEFT VENTRICULAR FUNCTION DURING CARDIAC SURGERY

RATIONAL CV THERAPY

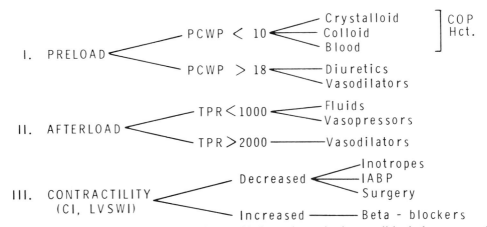

Fig. 23-13 Rational cardiovascular therapy for specific hemodynamic abnormalities is demonstrated. CI = cardiac index; LVSWI = left ventricular stroke work index; PCWP = pulmonary capillary wedge pressure; TPR = total peripheral resistance; IABP = intraaortic balloon pump; COP = colloid oncotic pressure; Hct = hematocrit.

sion and possibly by position change of the patient. If the problem is that the preload is too high—for example, a pulmonary capillary wedge pressure over 18 torr—then a diuretic, like furosemide, or the administration of a venodilator, like nitroglycerin, would correct the hemodynamic abnormality. If the wedge pressure is elevated due to heart failure, it may even be necessary to intervene with an inotropic agent. In some situations, it may be that the afterload is the abnormal hemodynamic parameter. If the systemic vascular resistance and mean arterial blood pressure are found to be very low, then fluids can be infused and, if necessary, α-adrenergic vasoconstrictors can be used. If the afterload is very high, and impedance to left ventricular ejection is altering left ventricular function, then an arterial vasodilator such as nitroprusside or phentolamine could be used to augment stroke volume and cardiac output, which probably would cause little change in blood pressure. If contractility is the primary abnormality, administration of inotropic drugs or the use of the intraaortic balloon may provide effective therapy. In the rare sit-

uation where contractility is markedly elevated, and this is the hemodynamic abnormality, direct myocardial depressants such as halogenated anesthetic agents or intravenous propranolol could be administered.

MEASUREMENTS OF MYOCARDIAL CONTRACTILITY

The contractile state is only one of several determinants of the heart's ability to eject blood. The cardiac output and the heart's contractile state cannot be related to one another in a simple manner. Measurements of cardiac output, alone, are of limited value in deducing myocardial contractility. It is important to realize the difference between cardiac output and myocardial contractility and not to equate the two.[3]

Considerable controversy exists over the definition and measurement techniques of myocardial contractility. Many techniques have been proposed to measure this elusive factor, and all have had their problems, since most of the techniques are also affected by changes in preload, afterload, and heart rate. Some of these techniques are highly invasive and others are totally noninvasive.[39]

Force Velocity Curve

This is the standard laboratory measurement based on Hill's model of contraction of an isolated muscle in which Vmax can be readily determined (Fig. 23-6). However, even Vmax has been questioned as to its validity as a pure measure of contractility.[40]

Walton-Brodie Strain Gauge Arch

Using this technique, a strain gauge can be sutured to the surface of the ventricle to directly measure contractile force. Morrow and Morrow used this technique to measure the effects of halothane on the intact heart of patients on cardiopulmonary bypass.[41] The strain gauge was sutured to the anterior surface of the right ventricle of six patients undergoing closure of an atrial septal defect while on total cardiopulmonary bypass. Two percent halothane was added to the oxygenator while the extracorporeal perfusion was kept constant at 2 L/min/m^2. Halothane depressed myocardial contractile force of the beating empty heart by 16 to 50 percent over 5 minutes. Partial recovery of ventricular function took 15 minutes.

Rate of Pressure Development (dP/dt)

The rate at which ventricular pressure rises (the first derivative of the ventricular pressure curve) is called dP/dt and is expressed in mm Hg/sec. Normal range is 800 to 1,700 mm Hg/sec. This number can now be obtained during cardiac surgery or catheterization using catheters with microtransducers at their tips which are inserted into the left ventricle and attached to an external differentiating circuit (Fig. 23-14). Many studies have shown that when contractility is augmented, the dP/dt increases. However, dP/dt is also affected by changes in preload, afterload, and heart rate.[42] Increases in any of these three factors also increase dP/dt. This problem has been partially solved by a series of correction factors such as $\dfrac{dP/dt}{CPIP}$ where CPIP is the common peak isovolemic pressure. This is the peak pressure common to both the control measurement and the therapeutic intervention. It corrects for any differences in afterload but not in preload or heart rate, which must still be held relatively constant. A series of other correction factors have been used to try to hold these other factors constant so as to measure only contractility, but none has been universally successful. The measurement of dP/dt has been primarily used during cardiology studies in cardiac catheterization laboratories. However, we have done some intraoperative studies using this parameter to assess myocardial function before and after cardiopulmonary bypass in situations where preload, afterload, and heart rate can be held relatively constant. In addition, recent studies in patients undergoing noncardiac surgery has shown a dose-related decrease in dP/dt with increasing concentrations of halothane.[43]

Catheter Tip Flow Meters

Tomlin et al. has found a good correlation between indices derived from velocity and flow of blood compared to dP/dt.[44] Noble has shown that the maximum acceleration of aortic blood flow is a good measure of contractility which is relatively independent of preload and afterload.[45] In fact, these measurements have been used to compare invasive and noninvasive measurements of contractility and to prove the validity of some noninvasive techniques.

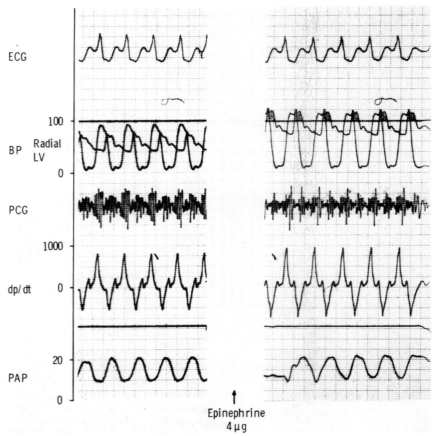

ECG

BP   Radial   100

LV   0

PCG

dp/dt   1000

0

PAP   20

0

Epinephrine
4 μg

Fig. 23-14 Hemodynamic responses of a patient during cardiac surgery are demonstrated. The panel on the left was before the administration of 4 μg epinephrine and the panel on the right was afterward. Note that the dP/dt changed from 800 to about 950. This was associated with an increase in the radial artery and left ventricular blood pressures to about 110 to 120 torr. Also shown are the electrocardiogram, phonocardiogram, and pulmonary artery pressure curves.

Angiography

Left ventriculography is an important part of a cardiac catheterization and can provide useful information about ventricular function. The ejection fraction (EF) is a measurement of overall systolic function and is the difference between the end-diastolic volume (EDV) and the end-systolic volume (ESV) $(EF = \dfrac{EDV - ESV}{EDV})$. Normal ventricles eject more than 55 percent of their volume and therefore have an ejection fraction equal to or greater than 0.55 (Fig. 23-15). In addition, abnormalities of the left ventricular wall motion can also be observed at catheterization. Potential reversibility of these abnormal wall segments is often tested with nitroglycerin or postextrasystolic potentiation tests. These measurements are found to be more sensitive measures of myocardial function than is the resting cardiac output; and they are, therefore, sometimes abnormal in patients with normal cardiac outputs (Fig. 23-16).[46] Some authors have used radiopaque markers placed on the ventricles at the time of surgery

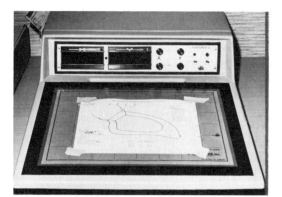

Fig. 23-15 The X-Y plotter is shown, which is used to calculate the ejection fraction from the end-systolic and end-diastolic outlines of the heart taken from the arteriogram.

and then myocardial function, fiber length, or ejection fraction can be calculated by postoperative radiologic studies.

NONINVASIVE TECHNIQUES

Systolic Time Intervals

These measure the phase of the left ventricular systole in man and are determined from simultaneous high-speed recordings of the electrocardiogram, phonocardiogram, and an arterial pressure tracing (Fig. 23-17). Total electromechanical systole (QS_2) is the interval from the onset of the QRS-complex on the ECG to the first major deflection of the second heart sound. The left ventricular ejection time (LVET) is the phase of systole when the ventricle ejects blood into the aorta and is measured from the beginning of the arterial upstroke to the dicrotic notch. The preejection period (PEP) is the interval from the onset of ventricular depolarization to the beginning of ejection and is derived by subtracting the LVET from the QS_2.[47] These intervals vary with heart rate, and, therefore, Weissler developed correction factors to adjust for this fact. An ECG lead showing a clear onset of the QRS complex is selected. A chest phonocardiogram is used over the upper precordium when possible; and during thoracic or cardiac surgical procedures an esophageal phonocardiogram is used similar to the one described by Tonnesen and colleagues.[48] We use a miniature hearing-aid microphone with a frequency response of 50 to 15,000 Hz and filter this to the 25 to 200 Hz range needed to detect the second heart sound, which has a frequency of 100 to 150 Hz. Central aortic, carotid, or subclavian arterial tracings are preferred, but more peripheral arterial tracings have been used.

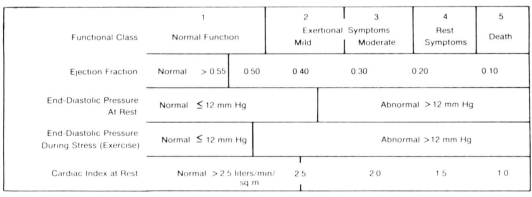

Functional Class	1 Normal Function		2 Exertional Symptoms Mild	3 Exertional Symptoms Moderate	4 Rest Symptoms	5 Death
Ejection Fraction	Normal > 0.55	0.50	0.40	0.30	0.20	0.10
End-Diastolic Pressure At Rest	Normal ≤ 12 mm Hg		Abnormal > 12 mm Hg			
End-Diastolic Pressure During Stress (Exercise)	Normal ≤ 12 mm Hg		Abnormal > 12 mm Hg			
Cardiac Index at Rest	Normal > 2.5 liters/min/ sq m	2.5	2.0	1.5	1.0	

Fig. 23-16 The relationship between functional class, ejection fraction, and cardiac index at rest is demonstrated. Many patients have normal cardiac indices of 2.5 L/min/m² with depressed ejection fractions under 0.50. (Alderman EL: Angiographic indicators of left ventricular function. JAMA 236:1055, 1976. Copyright 1976, American Medical Association.)

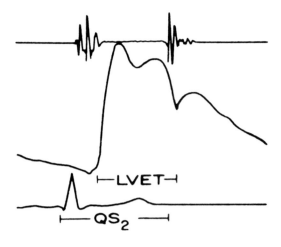

$$PEP = QS_2 - LVET$$

Derived Intervals

$$PEP/LVET$$

$$1/PEP^2$$

$$EF = 1.125 - 1.250 \ PEP/LVET$$

Fig. 23-17 High-speed recordings of the phono-cardiogram, arterial pressure tracing, and electro-cardiogram are demonstrated. Measurement of the QS_2 and LVET is shown. The PEP is derived by subtracting the LVET from the QS_2. Further derived intervals are shown at the bottom of the figure and discussed in the text.

The PEP has been found to be the best of the measured systolic time intervals as an estimate of contractility. It changes inversely to the dP/dt measurement, and there is a good direct correlation between the externally derived systolic time intervals and internal measures of left ventricular function. The PEP/LVET ratio shows an even better relationship to internal measurements of contractility.[49] Increases in contractility decrease the PEP, increase the LVET, and decrease the PEP/LVET ratio from its normal value of 0.35. With decreased left ventricular performance, the PEP increases, the LVET shortens, and PEP/LVET increases. These correlate closely with decreased stroke volume, cardiac output, and ejection fraction. The closest correlation was found between PEP/LVET and the ejection fraction. Figure 23-17 shows a formula that can even be used to noninvasively derive the ejection fraction from PEP/LVET.

A new indirect index of contractility using the PEP along with the PCWP has been described by Diamond et al.[50] The mean electromechanical $\Delta p/\Delta t$ is derived as follows:

$$\frac{\Delta p}{\Delta t} = \frac{DBP - PCWP}{PEP}$$

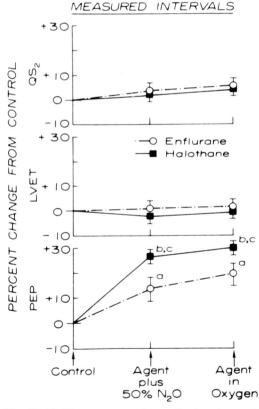

Fig. 23-18 Three measured systolic time intervals are shown as percent change from control values. All points represent mean values, ± 1 S.E., of six subjects. (Kaplan JA, Miller ED, Bailey DR: A comparative study of enflurane and halothane using systolic time intervals. Anesth Analg 55:263, 1976.)

where DBP = diastolic blood pressure, PCWP = pulmonary capillary wedge pressure, and PEP = preejection period. This index had a correlation of 0.96 with dP/dt in the Diamond et al. study of 18 cardiac patients.

Several studies have shown that the systolic time intervals, especially PEP, are influenced by changes in the preload and afterload.[51] The PEP is lengthened by increased afterload and shortened by increased preload. PEP/LVET is somewhat less affected by these changes, but is still altered. Reitan et al. proposed the use of $1/PEP^2$, which correlated well with peak ascending aortic blood flow; the latter measurement has previously been shown to be minimally affected by changes in loading conditions.[52] Therefore, $1/PEP^2$ may be the systolic time interval least affected by alterations in preload and afterload.

Systolic time intervals have been used to measure the effects of anesthetic agents on the heart. An early study my colleagues and I performed, compared halothane to enflurane (Fig. 23-18 and 23-19).[53] Recently, attempts have been made to use systolic time intervals as on-line monitors of ventricular function during anesthesia and surgery.[54] However, several problems have delayed routine use in the operating room:[55] difficulty in manually computing the systolic time intervals from the raw data; difficulty in obtaining satisfactorily the three necessary recordings; and nagging doubts as to whether the systolic time intervals represent pure ventricular function, without changes in preload and afterload.

Ballistocardiogram

The ballistocardiogram (BCG) is a complex apparatus designed to record body motion produced by cardiovascular phenomenae. A good correlation has been shown between the I-J wave of the BCG and dP/dt. The technique is technically very demanding, has been brought into question on a number

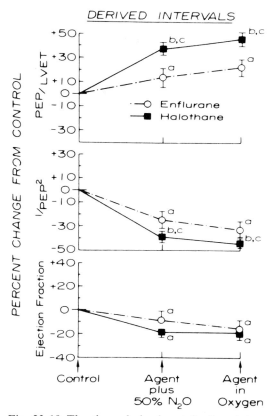

Fig. 23-19 The three derived systolic time intervals are shown as percent change from control values. (Kaplan JA, Miller ED, Bailery DR: A comparative study of enflurane and halothane using systolic time intervals. Anesth Analg 55:263, 1976.)

of points, and is therefore not used very often.[56]

Pneumocardiogram

This system is essentially a recording of movements of air into and out of the airway caused by cardiovascular events in the chest. It is an offspring of the ballistocardiogram and has considerable appeal to the anesthesiologist, who has access to the patient's airway. However, many technical problems remain to be solved before this becomes a useful clinical method.[57]

Impedance Cardiogram

Much attention has been recently devoted to the recording of changes in thoracic impedance. It has been claimed that many variables can be obtained from the impedance cardiogram. It may be used to give easier access to systolic time intervals as well as estimates of lung volume, cardiac output, and left ventricular function. However, placement of the electrodes and their maintenance during a surgical procedure are problems yet to be solved and, therefore, this technique has not yet been used practically.[58]

Electrocardiogram

The ECG for patients with coronary artery disease may prove useful as a simple, noninvasive guide to assessment of preoperative left ventricular function. Askenazi et al. correlated the sum of R waves in leads AVL, AVF, and V_1 to V_6 (summation of R) with the ejection fraction.[59] Among patients with a summation of R less than 4.0 mV, the PVC augmented ejection fraction was less than 0.45; while in patients with a summation of R of 4.0 mV or more, the augmented ejection fraction was greater than 0.45. This procedure needs more study to determine its true validity in the clinical situation. It has not been applied to studies of anesthetic agents as of the present time.

Echocardiography

Echocardiography is a relatively new technique that has become extremely popular in modern cardiology and is now beginning to be applied to anesthesiologic studies. It will probably prove to be very useful in studies of anesthetic agents and ventricular function, as has been demonstrated in some recent studies on the hemodynamic effects of halothane.[60] The echocardiogram is useful in measuring right or left ventricular function (ejection fraction or wall motion), analyzing valve function, and detecting pericardial effusions. Improvements in measurements and analysis have taken place at a startling rate, and will continue to do so in the foreseeable future. Two-dimensional techniques are currently being appraised, including a multiscan probe with an array of sectors and a sector scan that rotates through an arc. The echocardiogram probably yields more information than any other strictly noninvasive method. Among the variables that can help the anesthesiologist assess ventricular function are the systolic time intervals, ejection fraction, stroke volumes, left atrial dimensions, and mean velocity of circumferential shortening.[61] This is an amazing amount of information to be obtained from a noninvasive technique and, therefore, is of great appeal to anesthesiologists.

Nuclear Techniques

Measurements of ventricular function, including the ejection fraction, can be obtained using radiopharmaceuticals (such as labeled albumin) with scintillation counters and computers.[62] Nuclear cardiology is probably even further away from practical use in the operating room on a daily basis than is echocardiography. However, advances have been extremely rapid in this field and the information already available surpasses almost any other relatively noninvasive method. The image from the scintillation counter can be photographed for a permanent record or processed in a number of ways by computer. The computerized method can yield considerable information not available with other techniques, including volume versus time curves and rate of volume change versus volume loops. Many problems must be solved before these nuclear cardiology techniques can be used in the operating room. The cameras and ancillary equipment are large and barely mobile at present.

PHYSIOLOGY OF THE CORONARY CIRCULATION

The right and left coronary arteries which begin at the root of the aorta provide the entire blood supply to the myocardium. The right coronary artery principally supplies the right atrium and ventricle; while the left main coronary artery divides into the left anterior descending and circumflex arteries, which principally supply the left atrium and ventricle. There are many variations of the usual coronary anatomy and significant overlap exists between the different vessels and the areas of the heart they supply. In man, the right coronary artery supplies the sinus node in about 55 percent of individuals; while the left circumflex artery supplies the sinus node in the other 45 percent. Blood supply to the atrioventricular node is provided by the right coronary artery in 90 percent of individuals and by the circumflex branch of the left coronary artery in the remaining 10 percent. The papillary muscles of the left ventricle are of vital functional significance. The anterior papillary muscle is almost always supplied by branches of the left coronary artery, while the posterior muscle usually receives blood flow from both the left and right coronary artery branches. In both instances, the collateral supply is usually good.[63]

After passage of the blood through the coronary capillary beds, most of the venous return occurs via the coronary sinus into the right atrium. However, there are also vascular communications directly between the vessels and the cardiac chambers. These include arteriosinosoidal communications, arterioluminal communications, and the thebesian vessels. The thebesian vessels are small veins that connect the capillary beds directly with the cardiac chambers and also communicate with other cardiac veins and thebesian veins. Thus, intercommunication exists among all the minute vessels of the myocardium in the form of an extensive plexus of subendocardial vessels.

NORMAL CORONARY BLOOD FLOW

The resting coronary blood flow in the typical 70 kg man is approximately 225 ml/min, which is about 4 to 5 percent of the total cardiac output. When a normal person exercises vigorously there is a proportional increase in both the cardiac output and coronary blood flow. A number of factors affect the regulation of coronary blood flow as outlined below.[64]

Aortic Blood Pressure

Changes in aortic diastolic pressure generally evoke parallel changes in coronary blood flow. The normal coronary circulation demonstrates autoregulation of its blood flow in the intermediate coronary perfusion pressure range of 60 to 150 mm Hg.[65] However, under normal conditions, the blood pressure is kept within relatively narrow limits so that changes in coronary blood pressure are primarily caused by caliber changes in the coronary resistance vessels in response to metabolic demands of the heart.

Most coronary blood flow to the left ventricle occurs during diastole. The reason for this is that as the cardiac muscle contracts it compresses the myocardial vasculature and thereby impairs blood flow during systole. During diastole, the compression on the myocardial vasculature by ventricular muscle relaxes and coronary blood flow driven by the aortic diastolic blood pressure increases. The intramural systolic force is so great during early ventricular systole that blood flow, as measured in large coronary arteries supplying the left ventricle, is briefly reversed. The maximum left coronary inflow occurs in early diastole when the ventricles have relaxed and extravascular compression of the coronary vessels is absent. This flow pattern is seen in the phasic coronary blood flow curve for the left coronary artery seen in Figure 23-20.[64] After initial reversal in early systole, left coro-

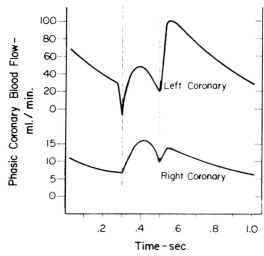

Fig. 23-20 Comparison of phasic coronary blood flow on the left and right coronary arteries. See text for details. (Berne RM, Levy MN: Cardiovascular Physiology. 4th edition. St. Louis, C. V. Mosby, 1981.)

nary blood flow follows aortic pressure until early diastole when it rises abruptly and then declines slowly as aortic pressure falls during the remainder of diastole. Blood flow in the right coronary artery shows a similar pattern; but because of the lower pressure developed during systole by the thin right ventricle, reversal of blood flow does not occur in early systole and systolic blood flow constitutes a much greater proportion of the coronary in-

flow than it does in the left coronary artery. In fact, in the right coronary artery, blood flow occurs relatively freely throughout both systole and diastole.

During systole there is a gradient of myocardial pressures that occurs with the greatest pressure development being in the subendocardium and the least pressure development being in the epicardium.[66] The importance of this pressure gradient is that the left ventricular muscle compresses the subendocardial vasculature much more than it does the epicardial vessels. Thus, reduced blood flow to the subendocardium of the left ventricle places this area of the myocardium at the greatest risk. It can be seen from Figure 23-21 that during systole the pressure in the subendocardium of the left ventricle approximates that in the left ventricular cavity. No blood will flow through the subendocardial region of the left ventricle during systole. In the midmyocardium of the left ventricle the pressure development during systole is less than in the subendocardium, and in the epicardium the pressure development is even smaller. However, under normal conditions this pressure gradient does not result in subendocardial ischemia, since the greater *diastolic* flow in the subendocardium compensates for the reduced systolic flow.[67] Radioactive microsphere studies have shown that blood flow to the epicardial and endocardial

RIGHT AND LEFT VENTRICULAR BLOOD SUPPLY

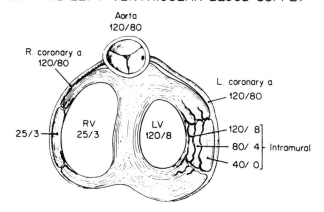

Fig. 23-21 Diagramatic cross-section of the heart to indicate intramyocardial compressive forces in different parts of the myocardium. (Hoffman JIE, Buckberg GD: Regional myocardial ischemia—causes, prediction, and prevention. Vasc Surg 8:115, 1974.)

CORONARY ARTERY DISEASE

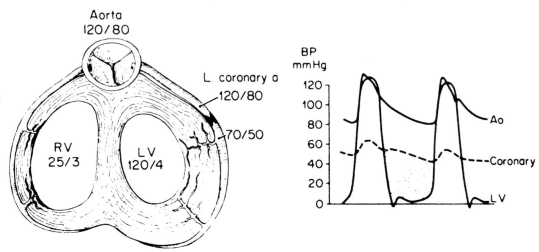

Fig. 23-22 Diagramatic cross-section of the heart to indicate coronary arterial pressure beyond a severe obstructive arterial lesion. On the left is shown the aortic, distal coronary, and left ventricular pressures. The stippled area indicates the diastolic pressure-time area for the region of the heart supplied by the partially obstructed coronary artery. (Hoffman JIE, Buckberg GD: Regional myocardial ischemia—causes, prediction, and prevention. Vasc Surg 8:115, 1974.)

halves of the left ventricle are approximately equal under normal circumstances.[68] This is probably due to the fact that the tone of the endocardial resistance vessels is less than that of the epicardial vessels. Under abnormal conditions, such as severe hypotension, the ratio of endocardial to epicardial blood flow falls below 1.0. This indicates that the blood flow through the endocardial region is more severely impaired than through the epicardial region of the ventricle during hypotension.[69]

LEFT VENTRICULAR END-DIASTOLIC PRESSURE

The coronary perfusion pressure (CPP) is usually defined as the aortic diastolic blood pressure minus the left ventricular end-diastolic pressure (LVEDP):

$$CPP = DBP - LVEDP$$

Elevation of the LVEDP will decrease the gradient of blood flow to the vulnerable subendocardial tissue during diastole as much as

will a decrease in the diastolic blood pressure.[70] This relationship can be seen below:

CPP	=	DBP	−	LVEDP
70	=	80	−	10
50	=	60	−	10
50	=	80	−	30

If coronary artery disease is present (Fig. 23-22), significant stenosis will decrease the coronary artery diastolic pressure well below the aortic diastolic pressure, and elevation of LVEDP can seriously jeopardize the subendocardium as seen below:[66]

Aortic Diastolic BP		Distal Coronary Diastolic BP	− LVEDP	= CPP
80	→	50	− 4	= 46
80	→	50	− 30	= 20

In fact, a vicious cycle of myocardial ischemia can be produced in patients with coronary artery disease by increases in left ven-

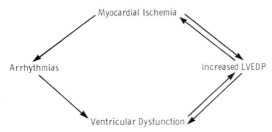

Fig. 23-23 The vicious cycle of myocardial ischemia which can be precipitated by elevations in the left ventricular filling pressure is demonstrated.

tricular end-diastolic pressure (Fig. 23-23). The left ventricular end-diastolic pressure elevation can produce subendocardial ischemia, which will then lead to both ventricular dysfunction and the production of ventricular arrhythmias. Also, however, it must be remembered that myocardial ischemia itself can produce left ventricular dysfunction and elevations in left ventricular end-diastolic pressure.[71]

Hoffman and Buckberg have described a relationship called the endocardial viability ratio (EVR), or diastolic pressure time index (DPTI) over tension time index (TTI), which describes the ratio of myocardial oxygen supply to the myocardial oxygen demand.[72] This ratio is used to estimate subendocardial blood flow. To assess the oxygen supply the DPTI is used; and for the oxygen demand the TTI is used. The formula described by them is:

$$EVR = \frac{DPTI}{TTI} = \frac{(DBP - \overline{LAP}) \times d_t}{\overline{SP} \times s_t} = \frac{oxygen\ supply}{oxygen\ demand}$$

where DBP = mean aortic diastolic pressure; LAP = mean left atrial pressure (or left ventricular end-diastolic pressure); SP = mean systemic arterial pressure; d_t = diastolic time; and s_t = systolic time.

A normal EVR is 1.0 or above when the DPTI equals or exceeds the TTI. When the EVR is less than 0.7, Hoffman and Buckberg found that the left ventricular endocardial blood flow fell in proportion to the epicardial flow (decreased endo/epi ratio), which indicates subendocardial ischemia. The endo/epi ratio fell whether the decreased EVR was secondary to decreased aortic diastolic pressure, increased left atrial pressure, or increased heart rate. Figure 23-24 shows the effect the intraaortic balloon has on increasing the EVR.[19]

ALTERATIONS IN HEART RATE

A change in the heart rate is accomplished chiefly by shortening or lengthening diastole. It has been estimated that approximately 70 percent of the coronary blood flow in man occurs during diastole.[73] With tachycardia, the proportion of time spent in diastole decreases and, therefore, the coronary blood flow is directly reduced. With a bradycardia the opposite is true and coronary blood flow increases. This relationship can be seen in the endocardial viability ratio formula above.

LOCAL METABOLIC FACTORS

There is a close relationship between the level of myocardial activity and the magnitude of the coronary blood flow. Blood flow through the coronary vasculature to the myocardium is regulated by the need of the cardiac muscle for oxygen. Thus, it is thought that hypoxia dilates the coronary arterial resistance vessels. The precise mechanism by which hypoxia dilates the coronary arterioles is not known, but it is postulated that either decreased oxygen tension directly causes relaxation of the coronary arterioles or hypoxia causes release of vasodilator substances (such as adenosine) which relax the resistance vessels within the myocardium. According to the adenosine hypothesis, a reduction in myocardial oxygen tension produced by either reduced coronary blood flow, hypoxemia, or increased metabolic activity of the heart leads

EFFECTS OF IABP ON MYOCARDIAL OXYGEN SUPPLY (DPTI) AND DEMAND (TTI)

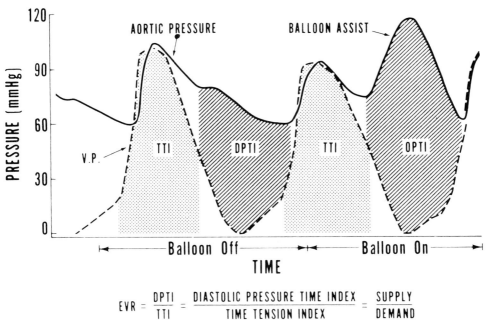

$$EVR = \frac{DPTI}{TTI} = \frac{DIASTOLIC\ PRESSURE\ TIME\ INDEX}{TIME\ TENSION\ INDEX} = \frac{SUPPLY}{DEMAND}$$

Fig. 23-24 The diastolic pressure-time index and tension-time index areas are shown on the figure. From these the endocardial viability ratio is calculated. The effect of the intraaortic balloon pump on the endocardial viability ratio is demonstrated. There is a marked increase in the DPTI as compared to the TTI. (Bolooki H: Clinical Applications of the Intraaortic Balloon Pump. New York, Futura, 1977.)

to the breakdown of adenonine nucleotides to adenosine, which diffuses out of the cardiac cells and induces dilatation of the coronary resistance vessels.[74] This dilatation results in an increase in coronary blood flow that enhances the washout of adenosine and reduces its formation by raising myocardial oxygen tension toward control levels. Under normal resting conditions only small amounts of adenosine are released by the heart and exert a minimal dilating effect.

NEURAL AND NEUROHUMORAL FACTORS

The autonomic nervous system affects coronary blood flow in two ways. There is a *direct* effect of released neurotransmitters on the coronary vessels themselves. Both α- and β-adrenergic receptors are known to exist in the coronary vasculature.[75] The epicardial coronary vessels have a preponderance of α-receptors and the intramuscular and subendocardial coronary arteries have a preponderance of β-receptors. The usual effect of sympathetic stimulation is a lowering of coronary vascular resistance, since most of the resistance to blood flow occurs in the intramuscular coronary arterioles which are stimulated by β-receptors. However, on occasion, it is believed that α-constriction of the epicardial arteries can predominate producing myocardial ischemia as is seen in Prinzmetal angina.[76] There appears also to be some parasympathetic nervous system innervation of the coronary vessels, and this may produce a slight vasodilatory effect.[77] The *indirect*

DETRIMENTAL CHANGES IN THE MYOCARDIAL

OXYGEN BALANCE

DECREASED MYOCARDIAL
OXYGEN SUPPLY

1. Decreased coronary blood flow
   a. Tachycardia
   b. Diastolic hypotension
   c. Increased preload
   d. Hypocapnia
   e. Coronary spasm
2. Decreased oxygen delivery
   a. Anemia
   b. Hypoxia
   c. Decreased 2,3 DPG

INCREASED MYOCARDIAL
OXYGEN DEMAND

1. Tachycardia
2. Increased wall tension
   a. Increased preload
   b. Increased afterload
3. Increased contractility

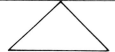

Fig. 23-25 Detrimental changes which can occur in the myocardial balance are demonstrated. Tachycardia and increased preload are marked to stand-out since they appear on both sides of the balance.

mechanism by which the autonomic nervous system exerts control over coronary blood flow is through myocardial stimulation due to released catecholamines.[73] For example, epinephrine produces an increase in heart rate and myocardial contractility that leads to a secondary increase in coronary blood flow to meet the increased oxygen demand. This indirect effect appears to be more important than the direct effect on the vessels themselves.

MYOCARDIAL OXYGEN BALANCE

The delicate balance between the myocardial oxygen supply and the myocardial oxygen demand is the overall controlling factor in the coronary circulation. In man, blood flow through the coronary circulation is regulated primarily in proportion to the demand by the myocardium for oxygen. The heart extracts approximately 65 percent of the oxygen from the arterial blood as the blood passes through it. This represents a near maximum extraction of oxygen, and the heart is able to remove little in the way of additional oxygen from blood as the demand for oxygen by the ventricles increase. Thus, the main reserve of the heart when it requires extra oxygen is to increase its coronary blood flow.

Figure 23-25 shows the detrimental changes that can occur in the myocardial oxygen balance. A decreased myocardial oxygen supply can be caused by a number of factors. Decreased coronary blood flow will be produced by tachycardia because this will limit the diastolic filling time to the left ventricle. The coronary perfusion pressure gradient can be decreased by either a decrease in the diastolic aortic blood pressure or an increase in left ventricular end-diastolic pressure. This is extremely important in patients with coronary artery disease and it is something that has not been realized in the past. The increase in the left ventricular end-diastolic pressure acts as a back pressure and tends to limit the subendocardial blood flow.[67] Subendocardial ischemia is easily produced by increases in left ventricular end-diastolic presure and is rapidly reversed by decreasing the left ventricular end-diastolic pressure with drugs such as nitroglycerin. Recent studies have been shown that hyperventilation to a $PaCO_2$ of 20 to 25 torr will decrease coronary blood flow, shift the oxygen hemoglobin-dissociation curve to the left, and decrease 2,3 DPG. These factors will interfere with the delivery of oxygen to the myocardium. Decreased oxygen delivery will also be present when severe anemia or hypoxemia exists.

Coronary artery spasm is becoming recognized as a more important cause of decreased myocardial blood flow than previously had been believed. Disease states such as Prinzmetal angina are primarily based on coronary spasm but there may be a degree of coronary spasm in many other patients with coronary artery disease. This may be due to autonomic innervation of the coronary vessels, since in some patients the administration of an α-adrenergic constricting drug can produce coronary spasm and reduce coronary blood flow to the epicardial vessels.

Since oxygen demand by the heart determines coronary blood flow, it is important to know the major hemodynamic alterations that will increase the myocardial oxygen demand. Increasing the heart rate will increase demand in direct proportion to the rise in rate. An increased heart rate is very detrimental in the presence of coronary artery disease since diastolic filling time (oxygen supply) is decreased as well as demand increased, and, therefore, perfusion of the myocardium suffers and ischemia frequently appears.[78]

Increases in left ventricular wall tension produced by an increased left ventricular end-diastolic pressure or an increase in blood pressure (afterload) will also increase myocardial oxygen demand. The pressure that the left ventricle develops during systole directly correlates with the demand for myocardial oxygen. This area under the systemic arterial blood pressure curve during systole was first called the tension time index by Sarnoff, and is one of the indirect indices of myocardial oxygen demand used by some authors.[79] Thus systolic hypertension is accompanied by a substantial increase in myocardial oxygen demand. The wall tension of the left ventricle is also proportional to the left ventricular end-diastolic pressure. A large dilated or distended left ventricle will have an increased oxygen demand. Thus, it can be seen that both a tachycardia and an increase in left ventricular filling pressure will decrease myocardial oxygen supply as well as increase myocardial oxygen demand.

The last factor that increases myocardial oxygen demand is increased myocardial contractility. The velocity of myocardial contraction is directly proportional to the myocardial oxygen demand. Braunwald has clearly shown that an increase in myocardial contractility results in a substantial increase in myocardial oxygen demand at any given level of developed tension.[73] A positive inotropic drug administered to an individual with a normal ventricle will produce an increase in contractility and myocardial oxygen demand. If, however, the positive inotropic agent is administered to a patient with an *overdistended failing* left ventricle, there may be a *net decrease* in myocardial oxygen demand as shown for digitalis administration (Fig. 23-26). Thus, there is a difference when a positive inotropic drug is administered to either a normal or a failing left ventricle in relation to myocardial oxygen demand. In fact, an inotrope may be beneficial if the ventricle is overdistended as long as it does not reduce diastolic blood pressure or increase heart rate too much.[26]

It is important to realize that changes in cardiac output alone do not increase myocardial oxygen demand. For example, if cardiac output is increased by decreasing total peripheral resistance, even though the heart

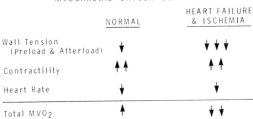

EFFECTS OF DIGITALIS ON
MYOCARDIAL OXYGEN DEMAND

	NORMAL	HEART FAILURE & ISCHEMIA
Wall Tension (Preload & Afterload)	↓	↓↓↓
Contractility	↑↑	↑↑
Heart Rate	↓	↓
Total MVO₂	↑	↓↓

Fig. 23-26 The effects of an inotropic drug such as digitalis on the myocardial oxygen demand of a normal and a failing ventricle are demonstrated. There is an overall increase in myocardial oxygen demand in the normal heart and a marked decrease in the failing, or ischemic, heart. (Mason D: Congestive Heart Failure. New York, Yorke Medical Books, Technical Publishing, a division of Dun-Donnelley Publishing Corporation, a Company of Dun & Bradstreet Corporation, 1976.)

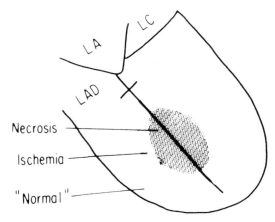

Fig. 23-27 Different zones of myocardial tissue following coronary artery occlusion are shown. These are the central necrotic dead zone, the surrounding periinfarction zone of ischemia with potentially viable tissue, and the zone of nonischemic normal tissue. (Mueller H, Ayres SM, Grace WJ: Principle defects which account for shock following acute myocardial infarction in man: Implications for treatment. Crit Care Med 1:27, 1973. © (1973) The Williams & Wilkins Co., Baltimore.)

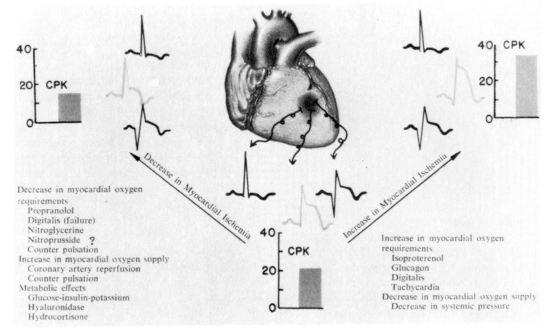

Decrease in myocardial oxygen requirements
  Propranolol
  Digitalis (failure)
  Nitroglycerine
  Nitroprusside ?
  Counter pulsation
Increase in myocardial oxygen supply
  Coronary artery reperfusion
  Counter pulsation
Metabolic effects
  Glucose-insulin-potassium
  Hyaluronidase
  Hydrocortisone

Increase in myocardial oxygen requirements
  Isoproterenol
  Glucagon
  Digitalis
  Tachycardia
Decrease in myocardial oxygen supply
  Decrease in systemic pressure

Fig. 23-28 Potential modifications of myocardial ischemia. (Parker JO: Myocardial infarction: Ways to reduce the damage. Resident & Staff Physician, May 1976, p. 63.)

will have an increased stroke volume and stroke work, there will be little change in myocardial oxygen demand. If, however, the cardiac output is increased by a significant increase in heart rate or if there is a significant increase in arterial blood pressure, then there will be an increase in myocardial oxygen demand. Thus, if the arterial pressure and heart rate are maintained constant, stroke volume can be increased with little accompanying increase in myocardial oxygen demand. This may be one of the significant beneficial effects of the use of vasodilators.

The myocardial oxygen balance represents a dynamic rather than a static process. In the case of severe ischemia or infarction, the damaged area is not totally defined at the time of the insult, but can be made better or worse by interventions or events.[80] Figure 23-27 shows an area of necrosis surrounded by the periinfarction zone of ischemia. This ischemic "twilight zone" can be salvaged or destroyed by appropriate or inappropriate interventions. Increases or decreases in the amount of ischemic tissue progressing to necrosis can be demonstrated by enzyme measurements and the electrocardiogram (Fig. 23-28). Myocardial ischemia will be decreased by reducing the myocardial oxygen demand (e.g., propranolol administration), increasing the myocardial oxygen supply (e.g., correcting hypoxemia), or possibly by improving the myocardial metabolic environment (e.g., glucose-insulin-potassium infusion). Myocardial ischemia may be worsened by increasing the oxygen demand (e.g., tachycardia) or decreasing the oxygen supply (e.g., severe hypotension).[71]

REFERENCES

1. Guyton AC: Regulation of cardiac output. N Eng J Med 277:805, 1967
2. Braunwald E: Determinates and assessment of cardiac function. N Eng J Med 296:86, 1977
3. Braunwald E: On the difference between the hearts output and its contractile state. Circulation 43:171, 1971
4. Guyton AC, Coleman TG, Granger HJ: Circulation: Overall regulation. Ann Rev of Phys 34:13, 1972
5. Braunwald E: Regulation of the circulation. N Eng J Med 290:1124, 1974
6. Higgins CB, Vatner SF, Braunwald E: Parasympathetic control of the heart. Pharmacol Rev 25:119, 1973
7. Chidsey CA, Braunwald E: Sympathetic activity and neurotransmitter depletion in congestive heart failure. Pharmacol Rev 18:685, 1966
8. Braunwald E, Ross J, Sonnenblick EH: Mechanisms of Contraction of the Normal and Failing Heart. 2nd edition. Boston, Little, Brown, 1976
9. Kaplan JA (ed.): Cardiac Anesthesia. New York, Grune and Stratton, 1979
10. Thomas SJ, Lowenstein E: Anesthetic management of the patient with valvular heart disease. Int Anesthesiol Clin 17:67, 1979
11. Humphrey CB, Oury JH, Virgill RW, et al: An Analysis of direct and indirect measurement of left atrial filling pressures. J Thor Cardiovas Surg 41:643, 1976
12. Swan HJC, Ganz W, Forrester JS, et al: Catheterization of the heart in man with the use of a flow directed balloon-tip catheter. N Eng J Med 283:447, 1970
13. Lappas D, Lell WA, Gabel JC, et al: Indirect measurement of left atrial pressure in surgical patients—pulmonary capillary wedge pressure and pulmonary artery diastolic pressure compared with left atrial pressure. Anesthesiology 38:384, 1973
14. Lorzman J, Powers, SR, Older T, et al: Correlation of pulmonary wedge and left atrial pressure: A study in the patient receiving positive end-expiratory pressure ventilation. Arch Surg 109:270, 1974
15. Pace NL: A critique of flow directed pulmonary artery catheterization. Anesthesiology 47:455, 1977
16. Civetta JM, Gabel JC, Laver MB: Disparate ventricular function in surgical patients. Surg Forum 22:136, 1971
17. Sarnoff SJ, Berglund E: Ventricular function. I. Starling's law of the heart studied by means of simultaneous right and left ventricular function curves in the dog. Circulation 9:706, 1954

18. Ross J, Sobel BE: Regulation of cardiac contraction. Ann Rev of Physiol 34:47, 1972
19. Bolooki H: Clinical application of the intra-aortic balloon pump. Mount Kisko, New York, Futura, 1977
20. Ross J, Braunwald E: The study of left ventricular function in man by increasing resistance to ventricular ejection with angiotensin. Circulation 29:739, 1964
21. Cohn JN, Franciosa JA: Vasodilator therapy of cardiac failure. N Eng J Med 297:27, 1977
22. Braunwald E: Myocardial function. Anesth Analg 51:489, 1972
23. Langer GA: The intrinsic control of myocardial contraction—ionic factors. N Eng J Med 285:1065, 1971
24. Sonnenblick EH, Strobeck JE: Derived indices of ventricular and myocardial function. N Eng J Med 296:978, 1977
25. Lewis BS, Gotsman MS: Current concepts of left ventricular relaxation and compliance. Amer Heart J 99:101, 1980
26. Mason DT: Regulation of cardiac performance in clinical heart disease, Congestive Heart Failure. Edited by Mason, DT. New York, Yorke Medical Books, 1976
27. Gorlin R: Practical cardiac hemodynamics. N Eng J Med 296:203, 1977
28. Ganz W, Donoso R, Marcus HS, et al: A new technique for measurement of cardiac output by thermodilution in man. Amer J Cardiol 27:392, 1971
29. Kohanna SH, Cunningham JN: Monitoring of cardiac output by thermodilution after open heart surgery. J Thor Cardiovasc Surg 73:451, 1977
30. Ganz W, Swan HJC: Measurement of blood flow by thermodilution. Amer J Cardiol 29:241, 1972
31. Guyton AC, Jones EC, Hallman TG: Circulatory Physiology: Cardiac Output and Its Regulation. 2nd edition. Philadelphia, WB Saunders, 1973
32. Davis CC, Jones NL, Sealey BJ: Measurements of cardiac output in seriously ill patients using a CO_2 rebreathing method. Chest 73:167, 1978
33. English JB, Hodges MR, Sentker C, et al: Comparison of aortic pulse-wave contour analysis and thermodilution methods of measuring cardiac output during anesthesia in the dog. Anesthesiology 52:56, 1980
34. Sarnoff SJ: Myocardial contractility as described by ventricular function curves: Observations on Starlings law of the heart. Physiol Rev 35:107, 1955
35. Ross J: Afterload mismatch and preload reserve: A conceptual framework for the analysis of ventricular function. Prog Cardiovasc Dis 18:255, 1976
36. Mehta J: Vasodilators in the treatment of heart failure. JAMA 238:2534, 1977
37. Kaplan JA, Craver JM, Jones EL, et al: The role of intra-aortic balloon in cardiac anesthesia and surgery. Amer Heart J 98:580, 1979
38. Raphael LD, Mantle JA, Moraski RE, et al: Quantitative assessment of ventricular performance in unstable ischemic heart disease by dextran function curves. Circulation 55:858, 1977
39. Weber KT, Janicki JS: The heart as a muscle-pump system and the concept of heart failure. Amer Heart J 98:371, 1979
40. Pollack GH: Maximum velocity as an index of contractility in cardiac muscle: A critical evaluation. Circ Res 26:11, 1970
41. Morrow DH, Morrow AG: The effects of halothane on myocardial contractile force and vascular resistance: Direct observations made in patients during cardiopulmonary bypass. Anesthesiology 22:537, 1961
42. Wallace AG, Skinner NS, Mitchell JH: Hemodynamic determinates of the maximal rate of rise of left ventricular pressure. Amer J Physiol 205:30 1963
43. Sonntag H, Donath U, Hillebrand W, et al: Left ventricular function in conscious man and during halothane anesthesia. Anesthesiology 48:320, 1978
44. Tomlin PJ, Duck S, McNulty M, et al: A comparison of methods of evaluating myocardial contractility. Can Anaes Soc J 22:436, 1975
45. Nobel M, Trenchard D, Guz A: Left ventricular ejection in conscious dogs: I. Measurement and significance of the maximum acceleration of blood from the left ventricle. Circulation Research 19:139, 1966
46. Alderman EL: Angiographic indicators of left ventricular function. JAMA 236:1055, 1976
47. Weissler AM: Systolic time intervals. N Eng J Med 296:321, 1977
48. Tonnesen AS, Gabel JC, Cooper JR, et al:

Intra-esophageal microphone for phonocardiographic recording. Anesthesiology 46:70, 1977

49. Martin CE, Shaver JS, Thompson ME: Direct correlation of external systolic time intervals with internal indicies of left ventricular function in man. Circulation 44:419, 1971

50. Diamond G, Forrester JS, Chatterjee K, et al: Mean elecromechanical $\triangle P/\triangle T$. Amer J Cardiol 30:338, 1972

51. Talley RL, Meyer JF, McNay JL: Evaluation of the pre-ejection period as an estimate of myocardial contractility in dogs. Amer J Cardiol 27:384, 1971

52. Reitan JA, Smith NT, Barrison BS, et al: Cardiac pre-ejection period. Anesthesiology 36:76, 1972

53. Kaplan JA, Miller ED, Bailey DR: A comparative study of enflurane and halothane using systolic time intervals. Anesth Analg 55:263, 1976

54. Dauchot PJ, Rasmussen JP, Nicholson DH, et al: On line systolic time intervals during anethesia in patients with and without heart disease. Anesthesiology 44:472, 1976

55. Lewis RP, Rittgess SE, Forrester WF, et al: A critical review of the systolic time intervals. Circulation 56:146, 1977

56. Eddleman EE, Harrison WK, Jackson WDH, et al: A critical appraisal of ballistocardiography. Amer J Cardiol 29:120, 1972

57. Wexler LF, Pohost GM: Hemodynamic monitoring: Non-invasive techniques. Anesthesiology 45:156, 1976

58. Harrison DC: Research related to non-invasive instrumentation. Circulation 60:1569, 1979

59. Askenazi J, Parisi AF, Cohn PF, et al: The value of the QRS complex in assessing left ventricular ejection fraction. Amer J Cardiol 41:494, 1978

60. Rathod R, Jacobs HK, Kramer NE, et al: Echocardiographic assessment of ventricular performance following induction with two anesthetics. Anesthesiology 49:86, 1978

61. Popp RL: Echocardiographic assessment of cardiac disease. Circulation 54:538, 1976

62. Pitt B, Strauss HW: Evaluation of ventricular function by radioisotopic techniques. N Eng J Med 296:1097, 1977

63. James TN: Anatomy of the coronary arteries and veins, The Heart. 4th Edition. Edited by Hurst JW. New York, McGraw-Hill, 1978, pp 32-47

64. Berne RM, Levy MN: Coronary circulation and cardiac metabolism, Cardiovascular Physiology. 4th edition. St. Louis, CV Mosby, 1981

65. Hoffman JIE: Determinates and prediction of transmural myocardial perfusion. Circulation 58:381, 1978

66. Hoffman JIE, Buckberg GD: Regional myocardial ischemia—causes, prediction and prevention, Vasc Surg 8:115, 1974

67. Klocke FJ, Ellis AK, Orlick AE: Sympathetic influences on coronary perfusion and evolving concepts of driving pressure, resistance, and transmural flow regulation. Anesthesiology 52:1, 1980

68. Schwartz PJ, Stone HL: Tonic influence of the sympathetic nervous system on myocardial reactive hyperemia and on coronary blood flow distribution in dogs. Circ Res 41:51, 1977

69. Hoffman JIE, Buckberg GD: Pathophysiology of subendocardial ischemia, Brit Med J 1:76, 1975

70. Gamble WJ, LaFarge CG, Fyler DC, et al: Regional coronary venous oxygen saturation and myocardial oxygen tension following abrupt changes in ventricular pressure in the isolated dog heart. Circ Res 34:672, 1974

71. Hillis LD, Braunwald E: Myocardial ischemia. N Eng J Med 296:971, 1034, 1093, 1977

72. Hoffman JIE, Buckberg GD: Transmural variations in myocardial perfusion, Progress in Cardiology. Edited by Yu PN and Goodwin JF. Philadelphia, Lea & Febiger, 1976, p 37

73. Braunwald E: Control of myocardial oxygen consumption: Physiologic and clinical considerations. Amer J Cardiol 27:416, 1971

74. Rubio R, Berne RM: Release of adenosine by the normal myocardium in dogs and its relationship to regulation of coronary resistance. Circ Res 25:407, 1969

75. Feigl EO: Sympathetic control of coronary circulation. Circ Res 20:262, 1967

76. Mudge GH, Grossman W, Mills RM, et al: Reflex increase in coronary vascular resistance in patients with ischemic heart disease. N Eng J Med 295:1333, 1976

77. Feigl EO: Parasympathetic control of coronary blood flow in dogs. Circ Res 25:509, 1969

78. Gobel FL, Nordstrom LA, Nelson RR, et al: The rate pressure product as an index of myocardial oxygen consumption during exercise in patients with angina pectoris. Circulation 57:549, 1978

79. Sarnoff SJ, Braunwald E, Welsh GH, et al: Hemodynamic determinates of oxygen con-sumption of the heart with special reference to the Tension-Time Index. Amer J Physiol 192:148, 1958

80. Kones RJ, Phillips JH: Reduction in myocardial infarct size: Prevention of heart cell death. S Med J 69:442, 1976

Index

Note: Page numbers in italics denote figures; those followed by t or f denote tables and footnotes, respectively.